Eleventh Edition

Rector's Community and Public Health Nursing

Promoting the Public's Health

Eleventh Edition

Rector's Community and Public Health Nursing

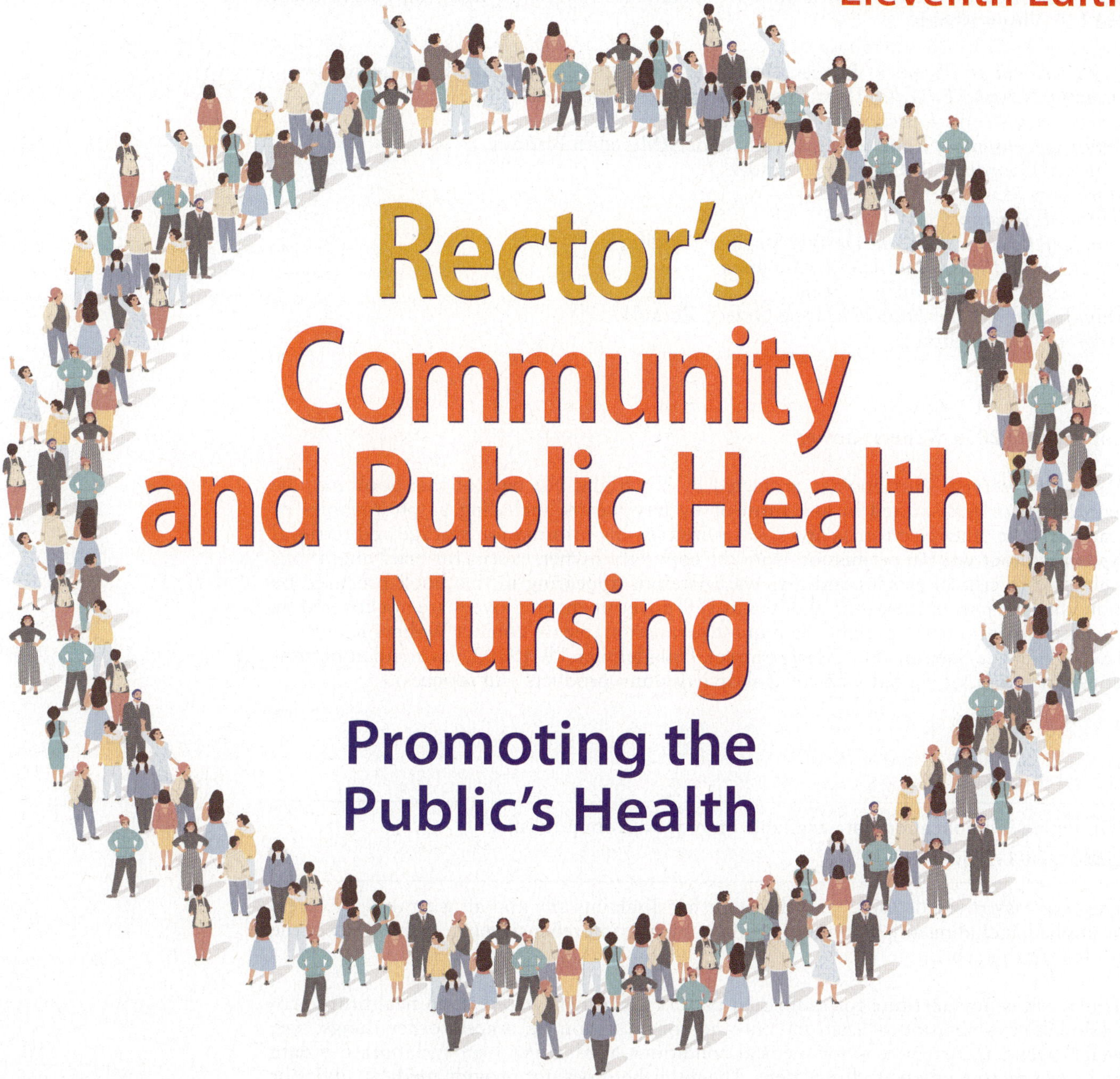

Promoting the Public's Health

Legacy Author

Cherie Rector, PhD, RN, PHN
Professor Emeritus
Department of Nursing
California State University, Bakersfield
Bakersfield, California

Authors

Mary Jo Stanley, PhD, RN, CNE
Professor
Department of Health Sciences
Colorado Mesa University
Grand Junction, Colorado
Professor Emeritus
School of Nursing
California State University, Stanislaus
Turlock, California

Charlene Niemi, PhD, MSN, RN, PHN
Associate Adjunct Professor
School of Nursing
University of California Los Angeles
Los Angeles, California
Emeritus Faculty
California State University, Channel Islands
Camarillo, California

Wolters Kluwer

Philadelphia • Baltimore • New York • London
Buenos Aires • Hong Kong • Sydney • Tokyo

Not authorised for sale in United States, Canada, Australia, New Zealand, Puerto Rico, and U.S. Virgin Islands.

Vice President and Segment Leader, Health Learning & Practice: Julie K. Stegman
Director, Nursing Education and Practice Content: Jamie Blum
Senior Acquisitions Editor: Jodi Rhomberg
Senior Development Editor: Jacquelyn Saunders/Meredith Brittain
Editorial Coordinator: Erin E. Hernandez
Marketing Manager: Wendy Mears
Editorial Assistant: Sara Thul
Manager, Graphic Arts and Design: Stephen Druding
Art Director, Illustration: Jennifer Clements
Production Project Manager: Frances M. Gunning
Manufacturing Coordinator: Margie Orzech-Zeranko
Prepress Vendor: Straive

Eleventh edition

9 8 7 6 5 4 3 2 1

Printed in Mexico

Cataloging in Publication data available on request from publisher
ISBN: 978-1-9752-3893-3

---

shop.lww.com

QUADM0125

To my family, with love.

—Mary Jo Stanley

To my students, a heartfelt thank you for trusting me with your stories to share in this textbook.

—Charlene Niemi

With love, to my husband, my children, and my grandchildren.

—Cherie Rector

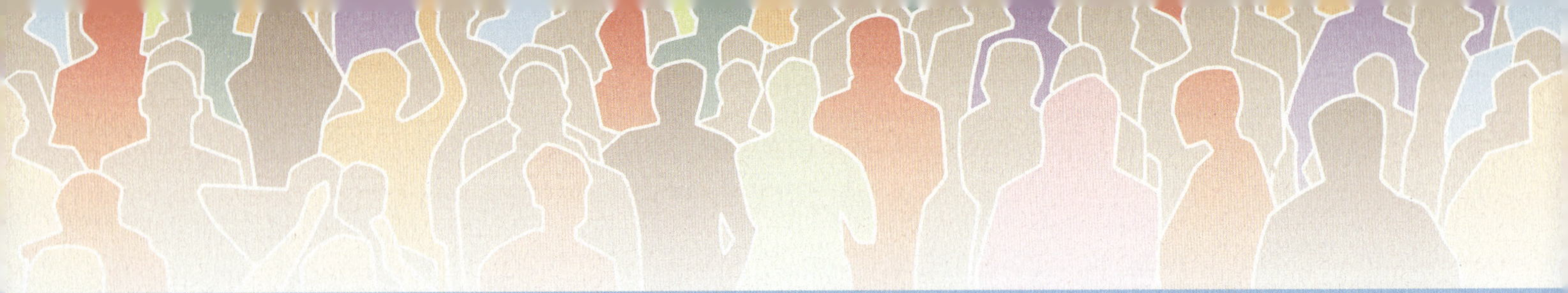

ABOUT THE AUTHORS

Dr. Mary Jo Stanley, PhD, RN, CNE, lives with her family in Colorado, where she gardens, raises alpacas, and enjoys Colorado's outdoor beauty. Dr. Stanley has been a nurse for over 38 years and in higher education for 16 years. Over Dr. Stanley's career, she has practiced in community, public, and school health settings, as well as in acute care ICU and PACU facilities. She earned a Bachelor of Science in Nursing, Master of Science in Nursing, Clinical Nurse Specialist, and School Nurse Credential from San Jose State University. Dr. Stanley completed her PhD in nursing with an emphasis in education from the University of Northern Colorado, where she was also on the faculty for many years. Dr. Stanley is a Certified Nurse Educator (CNE) with experience in curriculum creation and revision, and accreditation work. She is Professor Emeritus in the School of Nursing at California State University Stanislaus, where she served as the RN-BSN Program Director and the Director for the Nursing Department. Currently, she is a Professor at Colorado Mesa University.

Throughout her academic career, Dr. Stanley has taught classes to undergraduate and graduate students. Undergraduate teaching areas have included community/population theory and clinical, leadership and management theory and clinical, health assessment, foundations, health promotion, professional development, health education, capstone practicum, and professional roles. Graduate classes in nursing have included education theory and clinical, contemporary practices theory and clinical, nursing research, evidence-based practice, and graduate project Chair for Master of Science in Nursing students. Her research, publications, presentations, and grants have focused on educational development, strategies for teaching, and community health. Dr. Stanley has consulted for online instruction and is a certified online course reviewer. She is an active member of the Association of Community Health Nursing Educators and of Sigma Theta Tau International.

Dr. Charlene Niemi, PhD, MSN, RN, PHN, is a native Californian and has not ventured more than 30 miles from where she was born. Dr. Niemi enjoys spending time with her husband of 38 years, their two adult sons and their girlfriends, and the family dogs. She spends her free time people-watching while on walks, as well as having lengthy discussions on theology with friends. She has been in nursing and higher education for 34 years. Wanting to follow in her mother's footsteps, Dr. Niemi attended nursing school with the goal of becoming a trauma 1 emergency department RN. However, her last course in nursing school was community/public health nursing, which changed the course of her career.

Dr. Niemi has a Public Health Nurse (PHN) Certificate from the State of California and has vast experience in multiple public/community settings that include school health, correctional health, faith-based nursing, and public health nursing. At California State University, she developed the community health nursing curriculum and functioned as the lead for 12 years. In addition to community/public health, Dr. Niemi developed the psychiatric nursing curriculum and was lead at the same university.

Currently, Dr. Niemi is a faculty member at the University of California, Los Angeles, where she teaches public health nursing, psychiatric nursing, and geriatric nursing. Her research focuses on health literacy and social determinants of health; stigma in family members of those incarcerated; and childhood trauma. Dr. Niemi's education includes a BSN and an MSN (Nursing Education) from Mount Saint Mary's University and a school nurse credential from California State University, Fresno. Her PhD in Nursing is from Azusa Pacific University, with a dissertation on the role of forgiveness on the psychological well-being of men who had been abused by priests as children.

An important aspect of her life involves community outreach; she is the Director of Health Education and on the Board of Directors for Care Harbor, a mega clinical that provides free medical, dental, and vision care in a large metropolitan city. She is an active member of the American Public Health Association (PHN Section) and Sigma Theta Tau. Dr. Niemi is a recipient of the DAISY Faculty Award and an Emeritus faculty member at California State University Channel Islands.

Dr. Cherie Rector, PhD, RN, PHN, is a native Californian and an Emeritus Professor in the Department of Nursing at California State University, Bakersfield. While there, she served as lead faculty in community health nursing, Director of the School Nurse Credential Program and the RN to BSN Program, helping to develop and revise curriculum in those areas. She also developed an online curriculum for the RN to BSN program and taught in-person distance learning, and online courses in graduate and undergraduate programs. Prior to that, she served in an administrative position as Director of Allied Health and the Disabled Students Program at College of the Sequoias. She has also been the Coordinator of the School Nurse Credential Program and the RN to BSN Program at California State University, Fresno, overseeing curriculum development in those areas, for both online and in-person classes.

Undergraduate teaching areas have included community health nursing, foundations/health assessment, health teaching, leadership, and capstone classes. In addition, she has taught graduate courses in community health nursing, research, vulnerable populations, family theories, interprofessional development, and school nursing. She has served as a consultant to school districts and hospitals in the areas of child health, research, and evidence-based practice; has served on various state, local, and national boards and task forces; and has had leadership roles in professional nursing organizations.

Over the course of her career, Dr. Rector has practiced in community health and school nursing settings and in acute care neonatal nursing. Her grants, research, publications, and presentations have focused largely on child and adolescent health, school nursing, public health nursing, nursing education, and program development for underrepresented students.

Dr. Rector earned an associate degree in nursing from College of the Sequoias and a BSN from the Consortium of the California State Universities, Long Beach. She completed a master's degree in nursing (Clinical Nurse Specialist, Community Health) and a school nurse credential from California State University, Fresno. Her PhD in educational psychology is from the University of Southern California. She is an active member of the American Public Health Association (PHN Section), the Western Institute of Nursing, Sigma Theta Tau, and the Association of Community Health Nursing Educators.

CONTRIBUTORS

Anne Watson Bongiorno, PhD, APHN-BC, CNE
Professor
Department of Nursing
State University of New York at Plattsburgh
Plattsburgh, New York
Chapter 4, Research, Evidence-Based Practice, Quality Improvement, and Ethics

Yezenia Cadena-Malek, RN, BSN, MSHS
Army Public Health Nursing–Health Promotion Educator
Department of Public Health
Department of Preventive Medicine
Brooke Army Medical Center
San Antonio, Texas
Chapter 8, Communicable Disease

Denise Cummins, DNP, RN, WHNP-BC, CPHQ
Assistant Teaching Professor
College of Nursing
Brigham Young University
Provo, Utah
Chapter 12, Planning, Implementing, and Evaluating Community/Public Health Programs

Heide R. Cygan, DNP, RN, PHNA-BC
Associate Professor
Department of Community, Systems & Mental Health Nursing
Program Director, Advanced Public Health Nursing DNP
Program Director, Transformative Leadership: Population Health DNP
College of Nursing
Rush University
Chicago, Illinois
Chapter 13, Policy Making and Advocacy

Beverly A. Dandridge, MSN, FNP, MSAJS, CAPT
Commissioned Corps Liaison
Department of Homeland Security
Office of Health Security
Washington, District of Columbia
Chapter 17, Disasters and Their Impact

Lakisha Davis Flagg, DrPH, MPH, MS, RN, CPH, PHNA-BC, ACC
HRO Executive Leader Coach
Contractor Support to VHA Office of Quality & Patient Safety
Mandeville, Louisiana
Chapter 15, Community as Client

Carmen George, DNP, MSN, BSN, WHNP-C
Women's Health Nurse Practitioner
OB/GYN Clinic
Navy Medical Center
San Diego, California
Chapter 19, Maternal–Child Health
Chapter 28, Veterans Health

Kathleen Hall, PhD, APRN, GNP-BC, AGPCNP-BC
Associate Professor of Nursing
Department of Health Sciences
Colorado Mesa University
Grand Junction, Colorado
Chapter 4, Research, Evidence-Based Practice, Quality Improvement, and Ethics

Scott B. Harpin, PhD, MPH, RN
Professor
College of Nursing
University of Colorado Anschutz Medical Campus
Aurora, Colorado
Chapter 20, School-Age Children and Adolescents

Lenore Hernandez, PhD, MSN, RN, CNS, APRN, CDE
Clinical Nurse Specialist in Diabetes
Veterans Healthcare Administration Northern California
Martinez, California
Chapter 23, Working With Vulnerable People

Betty C. Jung, MPH, RN, MCHES
Director for Public Health Expertise Network of Mentors
Adjunct Lecturer
Department of Public Health
Southern Connecticut State University
New Haven, Connecticut
Chapter 7, Epidemiology in the Community

Mary Lashley, PhD, RN, PHNCS, BC, CNE
Professor
Public Health Nursing
Towson University
Townson, Maryland
Chapter 26, Unsheltered Populations

K. Bridget Marshall, DNP, APRN, CPNP-PC, PMHS
Associate Professor
Co-coordinator Graduate Nursing Programs
Department of Health Sciences
Colorado Mesa University
Grand Junction, Colorado
Chapter 4, Research, Evidence-Based Practice, Quality Improvement, and Ethics

Ruth McDermott-Levy, PhD, MPH, RN, FAAN
Professor
Co-director, Mid-Atlantic Center for Health and the Environment
M. Louise Fitzpatrick College of Nursing
Villanova University
Villanova, Pennsylvania
Chapter 9, Environmental Health and Safety

Charlene Niemi, PhD, MSN, RN, PHN
Associate Adjunct Professor
School of Nursing
University of California, Los Angeles
Los Angeles, California
Emeritus Faculty
Nursing Program
California State University, Channel Islands
Camarillo, California
Chapter 18, Violence and Abuse
Chapter 24, Clients With Disabilities
Chapter 25, Behavioral Health in the Community

Cherie Rector, PhD, RN, PHN
Professor Emeritus
Department of Nursing
California State University, Bakersfield
Bakersfield, California
Chapter 1, Introduction to Community/Public Health Nursing

Judith Martin Scott, PhD, RN
Associate Professor
Helen and Arthur E. Johnson Beth-El College of Nursing and Health Sciences
University of Colorado, Colorado Springs
Colorado Springs, Colorado
Chapter 22, Older Adults

Lisabeth M. Searing, PhD, RN
Assistant Professor
Villa Maria School of Nursing
Gannon University
Erie, Pennsylvania
Chapter 6, Structure and Economics of Community/Public Health Services

Jody Spiess, PhD, RN, GCPH
Associate Professor
RN-BSN Coordinator
Director of Keystone Seminars
Fellow, Institute for Human Rights & Humanitarian Studies
Webster University
Saint Louis, Missouri
Chapter 14, Family as Client

Mary Jo Stanley, PhD, RN, CNE
Professor
Department of Health Science
Colorado Mesa University
Grand Junction, Colorado
Professor Emeritus
School of Nursing
California State University, Stanislaus
Turlock, California
Chapter 5, Transcultural Nursing
Chapter 10, Communication, Collaboration, and Technology
Chapter 20, School-Age Children and Adolescents
Chapter 21, Adult Health

Rebecca E. Sutter, DNP, APRN, BC-FNP
Professor School of Nursing
College of Public Health
George Mason University
Fairfax, Virginia
Chapter 23, Working With Vulnerable People

Susan M. Swider, PhD, RN, PHNA-BC, FAAN
Professor, Community, Systems and Mental Health Nursing
Program Co-director, DNP in Advanced Public Health Nursing; Transformative Leadership: Population Health
College of Nursing
Rush University
Chicago, Illinois
Chapter 13, Policy Making and Advocacy

Ali R. Tayyeb, PhD, RN, NPD-BC, PHN, FAAN
Director, Nursing Academic Programs
AltaMed
Los Angeles, California
Chapter 28, Veterans Health

Dana Todd, PhD, APRN
Professor
BSN Program Director
School of Nursing & Health Professions
Murray State University
Murray, Kentucky
Chapter 2, Public Health Nursing in the Community
Chapter 11, Health Promotion Through Education
Chapter 19, Maternal–Child Health

Jeannine Uribe, PhD, RN
Associate Professor
Coordinator of the DNP Program
Accessions Director, Museum of Nursing History, Inc.
School of Nursing and Health Sciences
La Salle University
Philadelphia, Pennsylvania
Chapter 3, History and Evolution of Public Health Nursing

Katharine West, DNP, MPH, RN, PHN, CNS, NI-BC
Senior Adjunct Faculty
School of Nursing
Azusa Pacific University
Azusa, California
Chapter 16, Global Health Nursing

Robin M. White, PhD, MSN, RN
Director of BSN Program
Associate Professor
University of Tampa
Tampa, Florida
Chapter 27, Rural, Migrant, and Urban Communities

Lisa Ann Kirk Wiese, PhD, MSN, RN, GERO-BC, PHNA-BC, CNE, FGSA
Associate Professor
C.E. Lynn College of Nursing
Florida Atlantic University
Boca Raton, Florida
Chapter 21, Adult Health

REVIEWERS

Kathleen Adee, DNP, MSN, BSN
Professor
Salem State University
Salem, Massachusetts

Stacy Arriola, MS, RN, CNE
Visiting Clinical Instructor
Department of Population Health Nursing Science
University of Illinois Chicago
Chicago, Illinois

Gloria E. Barrera, MSN, RN, PEL-CSN
Visiting Clinical Associate
Department of Population Health Nursing Science
University of Illinois Chicago
Chicago, Illinois

Karen Bean, DNP, FNP-c, CNE
Assistant Professor
Oregon Health & Science University
La Grande, Oregon

Karen Britt, DNP, RN, MEDSURG-BC, CNE
Associate Professor
Massachusetts College of Pharmacy and Health Sciences
Manchester, New Hampshire

Adelita G. Cantu, PhD, RN, FAAN
Associate Professor
UT Health San Antonio
San Antonio, Texas

Donyale B. Childs, PhD, MSN, RN
Associate Professor
Albany State University
Albany, Georgia

Karin Ciance, DNP, MSN, RN
Associate Professor of Nursing
Anna Maria College
Paxton, Massachusetts

Georgina Colalillo, MS, RN
Professor
Queensborough Community College CUNY
Bayside, New York

Jennifer Delk, DNP, MSN, BSN
Associate Professor of Nursing
Chair for Undergraduate Programs
Union University
Jackson, Tennessee

Kathie DeMuth, MSN, BSN
Assistant Professor
Bellin College
Green Bay, Wisconsin

Florence Dood, DNP, MSN, BSN
Associate Professor
School of Nursing
Ferris State University
Big Rapids, Michigan

Charlene Douglas
Emerita Faculty
George Mason University
Fairfax, Virginia

Jami England, ARNP
Assistant Professor of Nursing
Lincoln Memorial University
Harrogate, Tennessee

Janelle Francis, MSN, RN
Assistant Professor
Bryan College of Health Sciences
Lincoln, Nebraska

Ann Garton, DNP, FPCC, RN, CNE
Associate Professor
St. Ambrose University
Davenport, Iowa

Dawn Goodolf, PhD, MSN, BSN
Associate Dean
Associate Professor
Moravian University
Bethlehem, Pennsylvania

Lucy Graham, PhD, MPH
Director
Department of Health Sciences
Colorado Mesa University
Grand Junction, Colorado

Lindsay Grainger, DNP, MSN, MPH
Adjunct Nursing Instructor
University of South Carolina Upstate
Greenville, South Carolina

Susan Gustafson, RN, MSN
Associate Professor of Nurse Education
Elmira College
Elmira, New York

Erika Huber, MS, RN
Nursing Instructor
South Dakota State University
Brookings, South Dakota

Monica Hughes, DNP, MSN
Clinical Assistant Professor
St. David's School of Nursing
Texas State University
Round Rock, Texas

Jennifer Hunter, DNP, RN
Associate Professor
Nurse Advocacy for the Underserved (NACU)
Northern Kentucky University
Highland Heights, Kentucky

Becky Johnson-Himes, DNP, RN
Associate Professor
RN to BSN Program Coordinator
School of Nursing
Ferris State University
Big Rapids, Michigan

Nicole Kreimer, MSN, RN, PHNA-BC
Assistant Professor
Research College of Nursing
Kansas City, Missouri

Kelly Krumwiede, PhD, RN, PHN
Assistant Professor
Minnesota State University Mankato
Mankato, Minnesota

Kimberly Lacey, DNSc, MSN, RN, CNE
Professor
Southern Connecticut State University
New Haven, Connecticut

Barbara Whitman Lancaster, DNP, MSN, ASN
Associate Professor
Middle Tennessee State University
Murfreesboro, Tennessee

Lisa LeBlanc, DNP, MSN, BSN
Assistant Professor
Wisconsin Lutheran College
Milwaukee, Wisconsin

Amy Luckowski, PhD, MSN, BSN
Associate Professor
Neumann University
Aston, Pennsylvania
Wilkes University
Wilkes Barre, Pennsylvania

Dana Martin, DNP, MSN, RN
Professor of Nursing
Pfeiffer University
Misenheimer, North Carolina

Julia Mattingly, DNP, RN, PHCNS-BC
Professor
Indiana University Southeast School of Nursing
New Albany, Indiana

Patti Moss, MSN, BSN
Assistant Professor
Lamar University
Beaumont, Texas

Amy Myers-Eisnaugle, DNP, MSN, APRN, RN
Assistant Professor of Nursing
Chair of the Nursing Department
Franciscan University of Steubenville
Steubenville, Ohio

Comfort Obi, DNP, MSN, MBA, BSN
Associate Professor
Clayton State University
Morrow, Georgia

Mary C. Owens, DNP, FNP-BC, MSN, CNE
Associate Professor of Nursing
Director of Nursing
Drake University
Des Moines, Iowa

Kimberly Paschall, MSN, BSN, RN
Instructor
Murray State University
Murray, Kentucky

Amanda Pitchford-Madrid, MSN
Assistant Professor of Nursing
Assistant Professor of Community/Public Health Nursing
California Baptist University
Riverside, California

Nanci Reiland, DNP, MSN, BSN
Associate Professor of Nursing
St Mary's University
San Antonio, Texas

Raquel Reynolds, PhD, MSN, BSN
Assistant Professor
Curry College
Milton, Massachusetts

Allison Sabin, DNP, RN, PHNA-BC, CNE
Associate Professor
Curriculum Coordinator
Chamberlain University College of Nursing
Chicago, Illinois

KathyAnn Sager, MS, BSN
Professor
Alfred State College of Technology
State University of New York
Alfred, New York

Joann Sands, DNP, RN, ANP-BC
Clinical Assistant Professor
SUNY–University at Buffalo
Buffalo, New York

Cheryl K. Schmidt, PhD, MSN, BSN
Clinical Professor
Edson College of Nursing and Health Innovation
Arizona State University
Phoenix, Arizona

Crystal Sherman, DNP, MSN, RN
Associate Professor
Shawnee State University
Portsmouth, Ohio

Diane Smith, DNP, MSN, RN
Assistant Professor
Bon Secours Memorial College of Nursing
Richmond, Virginia

Audrey Tolouian, EdD, MSN, RN, CNE
Instructor
American Canadian School of Medicine
Portsmouth, Dominica

Lisa Wallace, DNP, MSN, RNC-OB, NE-BC
Associate Professor
Morehead State University
Morehead, Kentucky

Susan G. Williams, PhD, MSN, BSN
Assistant Professor
University of South Alabama
Mobile, Alabama

Tammy Zamot, DNP, MSN, RN
Associate Professor
College of Central Florida
Ocala, Florida

PREFACE

The 11th edition of this book would not be possible without the contributions of previous authors. *Rector's Community and Public Health Nursing: Promoting the Public's Health* is the product of a legacy of nursing educators who bring their expertise, knowledge, and talents to each chapter. In recognition of Dr. Cherie Rector's numerous contributions to this textbook, we extend a heartfelt thank you for her many years of commitment to the writing and editing of this book. We pride ourselves on the accuracy of the textbook and rely on numerous subject matter experts from across the United States to peer review each chapter, providing the reader with a quality product.

The 11th edition provides foundational grounding in population-focused nursing with a heavy emphasis on the needs of aggregate and vulnerable groups. The textbook provides fundamentals of public health while gearing the presentation of the material to be classroom friendly. The text introduces students to key populations with whom they may engage while working in community settings. Through stories and features, it exposes students to commonly occurring situations in which they may find themselves as new nurses in the community and in other settings. Lastly, students will gain a solid understanding of how population-focused nursing occurs in the community.

We as authors recognize that students often deprioritize this course because the bulk of nursing education is focused on acute care, and most new graduates express interest in working in that setting. However, the COVID-19 pandemic reminded the world of the foundational need for public health nursing to protect and promote the public's health. In this textbook, we focus on showing the connection between community/public health population-focused nursing and the practice of acute care nursing, providing students with examples and information that will broaden their knowledge of their patients and enable them to provide more effective nursing care wherever they may choose to practice.

In this text, we also educate students that population-focused care does occur in acute care settings (e.g., infection control, programs to reduce length of stays, or readmission rates), and many hospital systems recognize the need for more community-based options. With more stringent Medicare reimbursement guidelines (e.g., nonpayment for medical errors and early readmissions), increased bundling, and a laser focus on value-based care, hospitals are striving to improve safety and quality and reduce readmission rates with more of a focus on transitional care and case management. Healthcare reform is changing the landscape for patients and providers, and care is becoming even more community based.

Population-focused tools and interventions are not only important in the community setting and within public health nursing; they are needed in acute care, as infection rates continue to rise, and nurse-sensitive outcome indicators are closely monitored. When a patient is discharged from the hospital, it is important for their nurse to understand their unique circumstances and how to best work with the patient and family to prevent further illness and promote better health. Transitional care is becoming more commonplace, and nonprofit hospitals must conduct community assessments, sometimes in conjunction with local public health departments or public health consultants.

Acute care settings and public health agencies are grappling with healthcare reform, a booming aging population, major natural disasters such as the pandemic and weather events, the opioid crisis and mental health, and the complex reality that the health of people, families, and communities extends beyond access to health services. In the United States, we are also seeing a renewed interest in the social determinants of health. It is now recognized that the largest factors influencing an individual's health status are behavior, genetics, adequate access to safe housing and healthy food, environment, and education status.

The United States is a melting pot of diverse people, religions, beliefs, and values. Despite our multiplicity, implicit biases and atrocities related to racism remain. Inclusivity and acknowledging one's positionality in partnership with diverse communities brings issues to the forefront in support of a more inclusive environment. We advocate to students that they will need to be ready to step up to contend with these issues, and this textbook will help them become prepared.

Over the years, we have carefully considered the feedback of community and public health instructors across the United States, and we have heard you that student engagement is a pressing issue. This textbook's features are designed to capture students' attention and encourage them to apply public health nursing principles to practice.

NEW TO THIS EDITION

The 11th edition concentrates on the most accurate, pertinent, and current information for students and nursing faculty with a focus on diverse, equitable, and inclusive practices, as well as the influence of social determinants of health (SDOH). All chapters are peer reviewed.

Expanded and new content in this 11th edition includes the following:

- **NEW!** In the following features, terminology and questions related to the Clinical Judgment Measurement Model (CJMM), developed by the National

Council of State Boards of Nursing (NCSBN), is used to support students' need to think critically and to use clinical judgment. (Terminology includes the following steps of the CJMM: Recognize Cues, Analyze Cues, Prioritize Hypotheses, Generate Solutions, Take Action, and Evaluate Outcomes; see https://www.ncsbn.org/public-files/NGN_Winter19.pdf for more information.)
  - **NEW! Case Studies** added at the end of some chapters focus on a contextual approach to understanding content, aligning with the 10 Essential Public Health Services. Case Studies examine situations and C/PHN roles based on chapter content within a real-world context, allowing students to use clinical judgment as they work through community and public health situations.
  - **Updated! C/PHN Use of the Nursing Process/Clinical Judgment** boxes quickly focus students' attention on key concepts and interventions related to public health nursing content and situations. This feature promotes student awareness of how the nursing process (something familiar to them) as well as the CJMM can be used in public health nursing.
- **Updated! Active Learning Exercises** at the end of each chapter challenge students, promote concept application and higher-level learning skills, as well as encourage active involvement in solving community health problems unique to specific areas. These may include internet-based exercises and can be assigned by instructors as learning activities or class assignments. A new feature in this edition is Bloom's taxonomy alignment of these activities to chapter competencies (chapter objectives), similar to the alignment of a course. One of the learning activities in each chapter focuses on the 10 Essential Public Health Services for student application and contextual understanding of content.
- **NEW! A chapter on veterans health** (Chapter 28) has been added in Unit 6, Vulnerable Populations.
- **NEW! Streamlining of content:** Unit 7 on settings has been removed; this information has been integrated into the chapters as appropriate to the C/PHN role to show context.
- **Special Boxes in This Book:** This section of this book's front matter, found immediately following the Table of Contents, makes it easier to find the features and stories that bring the theoretical content in the text to life. This section has been updated to include the new features.

Additional Key Features of the Text

In addition to the new and expanded features noted in the previous section, this edition includes the following key features from previous editions:

- **Evidence-Based Practice** boxes demonstrate how current research can be applied to public/community health nursing practice to achieve optimal client/aggregate outcomes.
- **Stories From the Field** boxes use storytelling to convey real-life situations and interventions accompanied by application-based questions. Storytelling has been shown to be very effective as a teaching/learning tool, especially in nursing education (Roddy et al., 2021; Yamashito, 2022). Through storytelling, students work to understand and apply the necessary art and skills for working with clients in a community setting.
- **Levels of Prevention Pyramid** boxes, unique to this text in their complexity and comprehensiveness, enhance understanding of the levels of prevention concepts that are basic to public/community health nursing. Each box addresses a chapter topic, describing nursing actions at each of the three levels of prevention. We place primary prevention (rather than tertiary prevention) at the pyramid's base to reflect its importance as a foundation for health.
- ***Healthy People 2030*** boxes highlight pertinent goals and objectives to promote health.
- **Perspectives** boxes share viewpoints from a variety of sources. The perspective may be from a nursing student, a novice or experienced public health nurse, a faculty member, a policy maker, or a client. These short features require students to think critically, reflect on commonly held misconceptions about C/PHN, and recognize the link between skills learned in this specialty practice and other practice settings, especially acute care hospitals.
- **Spotlight on Essential Nursing Competencies** (formerly QSEN: Focus on Quality) boxes focus on quality and safety in nursing education. These boxes help students understand that quality and safety are important not only in acute care but also in the public health setting.
- **What Do *You* Think?** boxes present thought-provoking current topics and common dilemmas found in C/PHN or ethical issues that may arise in healthcare settings. Students are asked to reflect and critically think about the issues presented to them.
- **Population Focus** boxes direct the student's attention to chapter concepts from a population-focused viewpoint.
- **Learning Objectives** and **Key Terms** sharpen the reader's focus and provide a quick guide for mastering the chapter content.
- The **Introduction** section presents the chapter topic, and the bulleted **Summary** section provides an overview of the material covered, serving as a concise and focused review.
- **Additional assessment tools** are provided throughout the chapters to enhance student assessment skills with people, families, or aggregates/populations.
- **References** for each chapter, found at the end of the book, provide current research and classic sources that offer a broad base of authoritative information for furthering knowledge on each chapter's subject matter.

Organization of This Book

For the 11th edition, the content has been streamlined into 6 units and 28 chapters.

Unit 1, "Foundations of Community/Public Health Nursing," covers fundamental principles and background about community/public health nursing.

- Chapter 1, "Introduction to Community/Public Health Nursing," discusses basic public health concepts of health, illness, wellness, community, aggregate, population, and levels of prevention. The chapter introduces leading health indicators, *Healthy People 2030* goals and objectives, and prevention as viewed through upstream/downstream approaches.
- Chapter 2, "Public Health Nursing in the Community," explains roles and settings for community/public health nursing, the core public health functions of public health, and the 10 Essential Public Health Services. Nursing standards of practice and community/public health nursing roles are presented.
- Chapter 3, "History and Evolution of Public Health Nursing," examines public health nursing's rich and meaningful history, its nursing leaders, the evolution of nursing education, and the social influences that have shaped our current practice. Features and pictures highlight historical landmarks and the C/PHN role during different time periods.
- Chapter 4, "Research, Evidence-Based Practice, Quality Improvement, and Ethics," considers values, ethical principles, and decision making unique to this nursing specialty. Evidence-based practice and research principles relating to community health nursing are also discussed, along with the nurse's role in utilizing current research, and addressing quality improvement in their practice.
- Chapter 5, "Transcultural Nursing," focuses on the concept of culture and the evolving demographics that constitute the changing population. A lens for diversity, equity, and inclusion and the influence of SDOH are discussed. The chapter presents the nurse's role in cultural awareness in providing care and relating to biases. The need for advocacy and social justice supports the C/PHN role.

Unit 2, "Community/Public Health Essentials," covers the structure of community/public health within the overall health system infrastructure and introduces the basic public health tools of epidemiology, communicable disease control, and environmental health.

- Chapter 6, "Structure and Economics of Community/Public Health Services," examines the economics of healthcare and compares U.S. health outcomes with those of other countries, while also discussing the impact of healthcare reform. The chapter also reviews official health agencies, some landmark public health legislation, and basic information on different types of health insurance.
- Chapter 7, "Epidemiology in the Community," highlights basic concepts of epidemiology and different methods of epidemiologic investigation and research, updates from the global pandemic, and what we learned for future events along with the C/PHN's role in epidemiology.
- Chapter 8, "Communicable Disease," presents a population focus on communicable disease control and immunization programs, highlighting vaccine hesitancy and effective approaches with clients along with updates from COVID-19 and lessons learned. The chapter discusses communicable disease investigations and common communicable diseases often seen in C/PHN practice.
- Chapter 9, "Environmental Health and Safety," covers concepts vital to environmental health along with the nurse's role in researching and intervening to promote a healthier environment for all.

Unit 3, "Community/Public Health Nursing Toolbox," includes tools used by the public health nurse to ensure practice effectiveness.

- Chapter 10, "Communication, Collaboration, and Technology," covers communication and collaboration, and collaborative communication with communities and cross-sectorial partners as well as clients. Also presented are health literacy and technology as they relate to community messaging, and the use of technology, especially in the wake of COVID-19. The chapter discusses the use of data and analytics, EHRs, mHealth, and GIS, among others, as examples of technology applications.
- Chapter 11, "Health Promotion Through Education," focuses on health literacy, with an emphasis on helping clients and aggregates achieve behavioral change through the application of educational and behavioral models.
- Chapter 12, "Planning, Implementing, and Evaluating Community/Public Health Programs," focuses on planning, implementing, and evaluating community health programs related to community/public health nursing practice. The chapter highlights use of SMART objectives and the implementation of programs.
- Chapter 13, "Policy Making and Advocacy," concludes this unit with an explanation of the public health nurse's role in political advocacy and policymaking, highlighting examples of successful political action campaigns and client empowerment strategies.

Unit 4, "The Health of Our Population," further expands the focus of the public health nurse, examining the family as client, the community as client, global health, emergency preparedness, and violence.

- Chapter 14, "Family as Client," applies family models to promoting family health and how C/PHNs work directly with families as clients. Conceptual frameworks and application of the nursing process to family health help promote healthy families. Home visiting protocols and safety are discussed.
- Chapter 15, "Community as Client," applies the nursing process to communities as clients and the foundations for community health promotion. Various community assessments are discussed, along with sources of data and community development.

- Chapter 16, "Global Health Nursing," highlights global health and international nursing using real-life case examples and perspectives on global health disparities.
- Chapter 17, "Disasters and Their Impact," examines preparedness with a closer look at disasters, terrorism, mass casualty events, and war. The Community/public health nurse's role in emergency preparedness, disaster management, preventive measures against terrorism, and *Healthy People 2030* objectives are also included in this chapter.
- Chapter 18, "Violence and Abuse," includes family- and community-level violence, with content on factors influencing violence, levels of prevention, and *Healthy People 2030* objectives related to this content.

Unit 5, "Aggregate Populations," covers maternal–child health, school-age children and adolescents, adults, and older adults, integrating the role of the nurse in various C/PHN settings.

- Chapter 19, "Maternal–Child Health," provides a PHN perspective in working with this aggregate. The Nurse–Family Partnership is highlighted, and material is updated and streamlined, with a focus on the C/PHN role.
- Chapter 20, "School-Age Children and Adolescents," examines the needs of this aggregate population and the C/PHN's roles and functions when working with this group.
- Chapter 21, "Adult Health," focuses on *Healthy People 2030* objectives and health promotion strategies for adults.
- Chapter 22, "Older Adults," includes updated content on memory care and dementia facilities, economic disparities, and health promotion strategies as they relate to healthy aging for these clients.

Unit 6, "Vulnerable Populations," covers basic concepts on vulnerability and social justice, and highlights vulnerable populations such as people who identify as LGBTQ+, veterans, refugees, people with disabilities, individuals with behavioral health issues, unsheltered populations, and rural, urban, and migrant populations.

- Chapter 23, "Working With Vulnerable People," introduces the foundations of vulnerable populations and groups commonly classified as vulnerable. It also covers social justice concepts and C/PHN strategies for working with vulnerable populations.
- Chapter 24, "Clients With Disabilities," covers civil rights legislation, the concept of universal design, support systems for this population, and risk for abuse of people in this group.
- Chapter 25, "Behavioral Health in the Community," addresses behavioral health issues (e.g., mental health, substance use) and the C/PHN's role in focusing on these problems using frameworks and screening tools. This chapter includes material on current mental health issues such as the opioid crisis and legislation that impacts public health practice.
- Chapter 26, "Unsheltered Populations," focuses on subpopulations of people experiencing homelessness across the United States and resources and services to help meet their needs. The chapter also examines the C/PHN role as an advocate and case manager.
- Chapter 27, "Rural, Migrant, and Urban Communities," encompasses the challenges and common problems facing these populations. It also explores issues of social justice, medically underserved populations, and frontier nursing.
- Chapter 28, "Veterans Health," provides an overview of veteran culture and health issues including interventions of the role of the C/PH nurse with this population.

A NOTE ABOUT LANGUAGE USED IN THIS BOOK

Wolters Kluwer recognizes that people have a diverse range of identities, and we are committed to using inclusive and nonbiased language in our content. In line with the principles of nursing, we strive not to define people by their diagnoses but to recognize their personhood first and foremost, using as much as possible the language diverse groups use to define themselves, and including only information that is relevant to nursing care.

We strive to better address the unique perspectives, complex challenges, and lived experiences of diverse populations traditionally underrepresented in health literature. When describing or referencing populations discussed in research studies, we will adhere to the identities presented in those studies to maintain fidelity to the evidence presented by the study investigators. We follow best practices of language set forth by the *Publication Manual of the American Psychological Association*, 7th Edition, but acknowledge that language evolves rapidly, and we will update the language used in future editions of this book as necessary.

A Comprehensive Package for Teaching and Learning

To further facilitate teaching and learning, a carefully designed ancillary package has been developed to assist faculty and students.

RESOURCES FOR INSTRUCTORS

Tools to assist with teaching this text are available upon its adoption at http://thePoint.lww.com/Rector11e.

- An **e-Book** gives you access to the book's full text and images online.
- The **Test Bank** lets you put together tests to help assess students' understanding of the material. Test questions are mapped to chapter learning objectives and page numbers.
- The following materials are provided for each book chapter:
  - **PowerPoint Presentations** provide an easy way for you to integrate the textbook with your students' classroom experience, either via slide shows or handouts. Multiple-choice and true/false questions are integrated into the presentations to promote class participation and allow you to use iClicker technology.

- An **Image Bank** lets you use the photographs and illustrations from this textbook in your PowerPoint slides or as you see fit in your course.
- Sample **Syllabi** provide guidance for structuring your community and public health nursing course.
- An **AACN Essentials Map** identifies content and special features in the book related to competencies identified by the American Association of Colleges of Nursing.

LIPPINCOTT® COURSEPOINT+

Lippincott® CoursePoint+ is an integrated, digital curriculum solution for nursing education that provides a completely interactive experience geared to help students understand, retain, and apply their course knowledge, and to be prepared for practice. The time-tested, easy-to-use and trusted solution includes engaging learning tools, evidence-based practice, case studies, and in-depth reporting to meet students where they are in their learning, combined with the most trusted nursing education content on the market to help prepare students for practice. This easy-to-use digital learning solution of Lippincott® CoursePoint+, combined with unmatched support, gives instructors and students everything they need for course and curriculum success!

Lippincott® CoursePoint+ includes the following:

- Leading content provides a variety of learning tools to engage students of all learning styles.
- A personalized learning approach gives students the content and tools they need at the moment they need them, giving students data for more focused remediation and helping to boost their confidence and competence.
- Powerful tools, including varying levels of case studies, interactive learning activities, and adaptive learning powered by PrepU, help students learn the critical thinking and clinical judgment skills to help them become practice-ready nurses.
- Preparation for Practice improves student competence, confidence, and success in transitioning to practice.
- Lippincott® Clinical Experiences: Community, Public, and Population Health Nursing offers clinical experiences that consistently expose students to diverse settings, situations, and populations in a safe, immersive, and engaging virtual environment, while actively developing their communication and intervention skills.
- Lippincott® Advisor for Education: With over 8500 entries covering the latest evidence-based content and drug information, Lippincott® Advisor for Education provides students with the most up-to-date information possible, while giving them valuable experience with the same point-of-care content they will encounter in practice.
- Unparalleled reporting provides in-depth dashboards with several data points to track student progress and help identify strengths and weaknesses.
- Unmatched support includes training coaches, product trainers, and nursing education consultants to help educators and students implement CoursePoint+ with ease.

ACKNOWLEDGMENTS

This textbook continues to evolve as it reflects our societal, historical, and community influences. Contributing authors are experts in various fields and specialty areas of community and public health nursing, providing a balanced and complete product. Most of our contributors have years of experience teaching community/public health nursing in the classroom and in community/public health settings. Contributors represent a cross section from across the United States, and the content reflects a broad spectrum of views and expertise. We have also carefully edited all chapters to make this a cohesive textbook with a common voice. We seek feedback from our readers and are proud to offer a peer-reviewed textbook.

The creation of a textbook takes a village. We have had the immense pleasure of working with an amazing team at Wolters Kluwer. A heartfelt thank you to Senior Acquisitions Editor Jodi Rhomberg, Senior Development Editors Meredith Brittain and Jacquelyn Saunders, and Editorial Coordinator Erin Hernandez for your hard work and attention to detail on the 11th edition of *Rector's Community and Public Health Nursing: Promoting the Public's Health*. We appreciate you!

CONTENTS

SPECIAL BOXES IN THIS BOOK

CASE STUDIES

C/PHN USE OF THE NURSING PROCESS/ CLINICAL JUDGMENT

EVIDENCE-BASED PRACTICE

HEALTHY PEOPLE 2030

LEVELS OF PREVENTION PYRAMID

PERSPECTIVES

POPULATION FOCUS

SPOTLIGHT ON ESSENTIAL NURSING COMPETENCIES

STORIES FROM THE FIELD

WHAT DO *YOU* THINK?

UNIT 1

Foundations of Community/ Public Health Nursing

CHAPTER 1

Introduction to Community/ Public Health Nursing

"For a community to be whole and healthy, it must be based on people's love and concern for each other."

—Millard Fuller (1935–2009), Founder, Habitat for Humanity

KEY TERMS

Aggregate
Community
Community health
Community health nursing
Geographic community
Health
Health continuum
Health promotion
Illness
Levels of prevention (primary, secondary, tertiary)
Population
Population focused
Public health
Public health nursing
Social determinants of health (SDOH)
Upstream focus
Wellness

LEARNING OBJECTIVES

Upon mastery of this chapter, you should be able to:

1. List examples of communicable diseases that have affected population health across different countries and regions of the world.
2. Research a problem in your community and list examples of nursing interventions that represent the three levels of prevention in your community.
3. Identify potential partners (e.g., people, governmental, and public health professionals) with whom you could collaborate on an identified community/public health problem.
4. Determine potential upstream factors and midstream effects that may have influenced health outcomes in your community.
5. Describe documented evidence-based examples of negative health outcomes for populations that have experienced health disparities and environmental or social justice inequities.

INTRODUCTION

By this point in your nursing education, you have cared for a variety of patients in acute care settings, and you may feel comfortable there. You have collaborated with other professionals when needed. Now you are entering a unique and exciting area of nursing that may seem very foreign to you—community/public health. As one of the oldest specialty nursing practices, public health nursing offers unique challenges and opportunities. Public health nursing is community based and population focused. As *The Future of Nursing 2020–2030: Charting a Path to Achieve Healthy Equity* recommends, nursing education and training must provide more student experiences "outside of acute care settings" to "build a culture of health and health equity" (p. 25) needed by "individuals, families, and communities that address social determinants of health and provide effective … accessible care for all across the care continuum" (National Academies Press, 2021, p. 24).

As you become familiar with community/public health, you will learn about:

- Expanding nursing's focus from the person and family to communities and populations
- Determining the needs of at-risk populations with health disparities and designing interventions to specifically address them
- Navigating the complexities of a constantly changing healthcare system and working toward a culture of health to improve the well-being and health status of all people in the United States (Robert Wood Johnson Foundation [RWJF], n.d.)

You will be asked to leave that familiar acute care setting and go out into the community—into homes, schools, correctional facilities, work settings, parishes, and even street corners that are commonplace to your clients and unfamiliar to you. Here, in the community, you will:

- Find few or no monitoring devices or charts full of laboratory data
- Have few professional and allied health workers at your side for assistance and consultation
- Use the skills of listening, assessing, planning, teaching, coordinating, evaluating, and referral
- Draw on the nursing skills you have learned throughout your experiences in the acute care setting (e.g., behavioral health and maternal, children's, and adult health nursing) and begin to "think on your feet" in new and compelling circumstances

Often, your practice will be solo, and you will need to combine creativity, ingenuity, intuition, and resourcefulness along with these skills. Talk about boundless opportunities and challenges! See Box 1-1.

You may sometimes feel that this new setting is difficult and have concerns about how you will perform in it. But perhaps, just perhaps, you will find that it is rewarding, that it constantly challenges you, interests you, and allows you to work holistically with clients of all ages, at all stages of illness and wellness, and that it absolutely demands the use of your critical thinking skills. Some of you may decide, when you finish your community/public health nursing course, that you have found your career choice. However, even if you are not drawn away from acute care nursing, your community/public health nursing experience can provide you with important new skills to make you a better nurse as you gain:

- A deeper understanding of the people for whom you provide care—where and how they live, the family and cultural dynamics at play, and the problems they are likely to face when discharged from your care
- A realization that clients are not only people or families but also may be aggregates, communities, and populations, giving you a broader view of nursing
- Greater knowledge of myriad community agencies and resources to better assist you in providing a continuum of care for members of your community

This chapter provides an overview of basic concepts related to community and health, the components of public health practice, and the salient characteristics of contemporary community/public health nursing practice. We begin by discussing community and public health and how it provides the context for community/public health nursing practice.

COMMUNITY AND PUBLIC HEALTH

Human beings are social creatures. We generally live out our lives in the company of other people. Indigenous tribes may be part of a small, tightly knit community of close relatives; a rural migrant worker may live in a small agricultural community with only a few hundred people. In contrast, someone from New York City might be a member of many overlapping communities, such as professional societies, a political party, a religious group, a cultural society, a neighborhood, and the city itself. Even those who try to escape community membership always begin their lives in some type of group, and they usually continue to depend on groups for material and emotional support.

We can draw two important conclusions from this fact:

- Communities are an essential and permanent feature of the human experience.
- A community that achieves a high level of wellness is composed of healthy citizens, functioning in an environment that protects and promotes health.

An example of one county's journey toward that goal is San Mateo County, California. In 2004, a coalition of county health system workers, hospitals, school districts, nongovernmental agencies, and city/county leaders developed an initial plan to eliminate health disparities and address the problem of childhood obesity. This eventually grew into a broader plan to build a healthier community through community engagement and policy changes that address the social determinants of health (SDOH), discussed in more detail later in this chapter and in Chapter 23. The goal is that "all residents, regardless

BOX 1-1 PERSPECTIVES

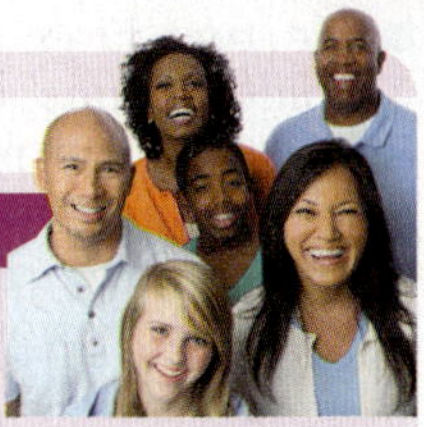

A Nursing Student Viewpoint on Community/Public Health Nursing

I was really terrified when I got to my community/public health rotation and found that I had to go knock on people's doors! I was close to graduating and felt comfortable in the hospital (the routines and machines). I was assigned a 16-year-old mother with a 4-month-old baby. I don't even have children! What can I tell her? She is a teenager who "knows it all." My clinical instructor told me to "build a relationship with her" and to "gain trust and rapport," difficult to do when you are scared to death. But I needed this class to finish nursing school, so I drove over there and knocked on her door.

The apartment building was disheveled. When she answered the door, she seemed uninterested—or maybe a little defensive. I told her who I was and why I was there, and she motioned me inside pointing toward the baby, propped up on the tattered couch. I spent the next 15 weeks visiting Anna and her baby every Thursday—weighing and measuring the baby, doing *Ages & Stages Questionnaires* and sharing the results with Anna about developmental milestones, getting her appointments for immunizations, listening to her story of abuse and abandonment, and I began to realize that what I was doing was actually interesting and rewarding. By the end of my rotation, I was going to miss Anna and little José! I had provided education on baby proofing her apartment, finding resources for food and clothing, and birth control. We even talked about how she could finish high school.

After graduation, I took a job in the emergency department (ED) and thought of Anna and José when young parents would bring in their sick babies. I used C/PHN skills in "connecting" with a teen mom to ensure follow through with antibiotics and antipyretics we were prescribing for her baby's high fever and serious infection. One day, I glanced up from my paperwork to see Anna and José. She looked so relieved to see me! She was frantic with worry about the serious burn José had on his right hand. The other nurses were mumbling about "child abuse" and how "irresponsible teen parents always were." Anna had left José with a neighbor while she went to an appointment about getting her GED. The neighbor was not used to dealing with a busy toddler, and José was able to reach the handle of a pan of refried beans. The team treated José's burn, and I gave Anna instructions for follow-up care. The bond we had developed was still there. She trusted me, and I knew that she would follow through with the instructions. The other nurses who were making comments about Anna did not know her circumstances. I feel that I am a more effective ED nurse because of the things I learned during my C/PHN rotation. Someday, when I get tired of the hospital, I may work as a public health nurse. You never know!

Madison, age 24

of income, race/ethnicity, age, ability, immigration status, sexual orientation, or gender have the opportunity to reach their full potential" (Get Healthy San Mateo County, n.d., p. 6). The building blocks include the following:

- "Healthy, stable, and affordable housing"
- "Complete neighborhoods and communities" (not just housing, but schools, stores, employment opportunities, recreational areas, and public transit)
- "High-quality education system"
- "Thriving and inclusive economy"
- Access to sufficient, healthy food (including school and neighborhood gardens and fresh, local produce)
- Public transit choices (easy to access, including biking and walking options)
- "Safe and diverse public places, parks, and open space"
- "Sense of community where everyone feels" safe and feels a sense of belonging
- "Clean environment"
- "Community-based public services and infrastructure for all people" (pp. 10–11).

Did any of the above building blocks mention hospitals, primary providers, nurses, or healthcare? Why is community health so important? The communities in which people reside and work have a profound influence on our collective health and well-being. In fact, only 20% of variation in county-level health outcomes can be ascribed to clinical care. However, SDOH (like the building blocks listed above) have been shown to affect up to 50% of the county-level variation in health outcomes as evidenced by scores of large studies conducted over many years (Scott et al., 2018; Sylvers et al., 2022; Whitman et al., 2022).

For example, do you suppose that green space in a city can influence one's health? Or that higher levels of social and physical disorder in your community may negatively affect your mental or cognitive health? Research has confirmed this:

- In a population-based study of 1680 urban adults in the United Kingdom living in an area with few green spaces, the overall prevalence of psychological distress was 22.7%. However, for those living near adequate green spaces, there was a 54% reduction in risk of psychological distress (Pope et al., 2018).
- Another UK study of 171 adults with a mean age of 84 who had a home garden during the start of the COVID-19 pandemic reported more frequent garden activities while in lockdown. An association was found between garden activities and better self-rated emotional, mental, and physical health, as well as quality of sleep (Corley et al., 2021).

- In two large-scale studies, researchers found that older adults had higher levels of depression and anxiety and poorer performance on cognitive tests when their neighborhoods were described as poorly maintained or they felt a lowered perception of social cohesion (Munoz et al., 2020; Sharifian et al., 2020).
- Other researchers, in a study of over 1.6 million U.S. veterans followed for over a decade, found that dementia risk was increased for those who lived in the "most disadvantaged neighborhood(s)" (Dintica et al., 2023, para 2).

Healthier communities can be created, and in many areas of this (and many other countries), it is an active goal.

It is helpful to distinguish between the concepts of community health and public health. Although both are organized community efforts aimed at the promotion, protection, and preservation of the public's health, **community health** has been defined as:

- The identification of needs, along with protection and improvement of collective health, within a geographically defined area
- The health status of a defined group of people and the actions and conditions to promote, protect, and preserve their health (Seabert et al., 2022)

The American Hospital Association, Center for Health Innovation (2023) states:

> "Community health refers to non-clinical approaches for improving health, preventing disease and reducing health disparities through addressing social, behavioral, environmental, economic, and medical determinants of health in a geographically defined population" (para. 1).

Public health is a broader concept and often goes beyond community boundaries, dealing with populations around the world. **Public health**, as a specialty of nursing practice, seeks to provide organizational structure, a broad set of resources, and the collaborative activities needed to accomplish the goal of an optimally healthy population or community. Public health:

- Views the community (small or large) as the recipient of service and health as the product
- Provides protection and improvement of individual, family, community, and population health in local areas and around the world
- Studies the interchange between population groups and their total environment and with the impact of that interchange on the total population's collective health

Though public health was historically associated with local, state, and national health departments and government agencies, it now has a broader meaning focusing on populations around the world (ANA, 2022). It was defined in the preface of a report on *The Future of the Public's Health in the 21st Century* by a committee of the Institute of Medicine (2003) as "what we as a society do (collectively) to assure the conditions in which people can be healthy" (p. 20). See Box 1-2.

- Winslow's classic 1920 definition of public health, adopted by the Centers for Disease Control and Prevention (CDC), still holds true and forms the basis for our understanding of public health in this text: public health is "the science and art of preventing disease, prolonging life, and promoting health through the organized efforts and informed choices of society, organizations, public and private communities, and individuals" (CDC, 2021a, para 1).

BOX 1-2 PERSPECTIVES

A Public Health Nursing Instructor Viewpoint

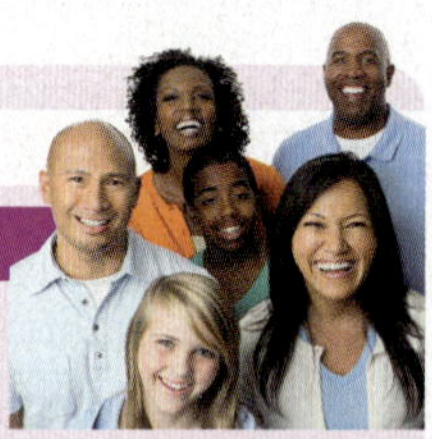

When I first introduce the topic of public health, many students don't understand why they need this "different" class; they are accustomed to acute care settings, and public health nursing seems so "odd." So, I ask students "Why do people end up being hospitalized?" Typical answers include "They needed surgery," "They had an accident," and the like.

Then, I tell them the story of 4-year-old Jackson:

"Why is Jackson in the hospital? (Because he has asthma and pneumonia.)

What caused the asthma and pneumonia? (He got a cold and it got worse, resulting in pneumonia, exacerbated by his asthma.)

Why did it get worse? (Because he lives in a low-income neighborhood.)

How does that cause more problems? (Because he is exposed to more asthma triggers [such as air pollution, mold, dust mites/cockroach allergens, and cigarette smoke] which exacerbate his asthma when he gets an upper respiratory infection—often leading to pneumonia.)

Why is he living there? (Because his family has limited resources and can only afford an apartment in a crowded building located in an area of town near factories and highways. The building is poorly maintained.)

Why can't his parents work harder so they can move to a better place? (Because he lives in a single-parent household with three siblings, and the single parent works two jobs. That income only covers rent, food, and a few bills.)

Why can't his parent get a better job? (Because they doesn't have the skills and education needed to get a higher paying job.) But why...?"

And then they become more aware of why this class is important and begin to comprehend how social and economic issues affect health.

Adapted from Federal, Provincial and Territorial Advisory Committee on Population Health (ACPH) (1999).

Other definitions of public health include:

- "Public health promotes and protects the health of people and the communities where they live, learn, work and play" (American Public Health Association [APHA], 2023, para. 1).
- "Public health aims to provide groups of people with the right to be healthy and live in conditions that support health" (CDC, Division of Scientific Education and Professional Development, 2021b, para. 1).

The core public health functions have been delineated as assessment, policy development, and assurance. These are discussed in more detail in Chapter 2. One of the challenges public health practice faces is to remain responsive to the community's changing health needs. As a result, its structure is complex; numerous health services and programs are currently available and more will be developed. Examples include health education, family planning, injury prevention, communicable disease control, environmental protection, immunization, nutrition, early periodic screening and developmental testing, school programs, mental health services, occupational health programs, and the care of vulnerable populations. The Department of Homeland Security, for example, is a community health and safety agency established in the aftermath of the terrorist attacks on New York City and Washington, District of Columbia, on September 11, 2001.

In response to the recent COVID-19 pandemic, chronically underfunded and understaffed public health departments received supplementary funding to help prevent the spread of the virus. However, they still had to choose between suspension or diversion of resources and personnel from primary and secondary services unrelated to COVID-19 services (e.g., high-risk pregnancies/infant–maternal mortalities, regular inspections of restaurants, tobacco prevention programs, mental health/substance use disorders) to address the overwhelming workload (Edmonds et al., 2020). See Chapters 6, 7, and 8.

THE CONCEPT OF COMMUNITY

The concepts of community and health together provide the foundation for understanding community health. Broadly defined, a **community** is a collection of people who share some important features of their lives (Fig. 1-1). In this text, the term community refers to a collection of people who interact with one another and whose common interests or characteristics form the basis for a sense of unity or belonging.

- A community can be a society of people holding common rights and privileges (e.g., citizens of a town), sharing common interests (e.g., a community of farmers), or living under the same laws and regulations (e.g., a prison community).
- The function of any community includes its members' collective sense of belonging and their shared identity, values, norms, communication, geography, and common interests and concerns (Anderson & McFarlane, 2019).

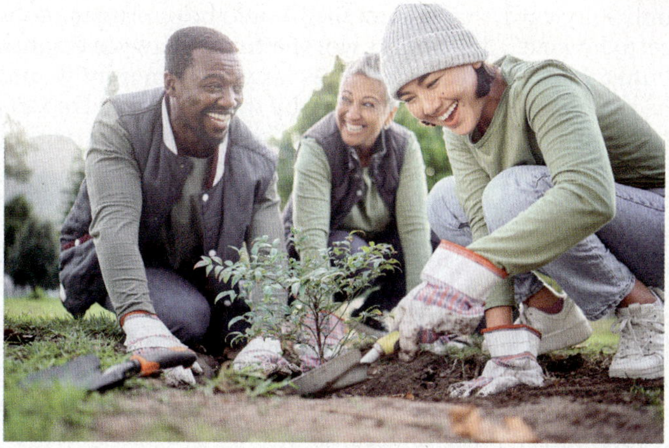

FIGURE 1-1 There are many different types of communities.

Some communities—for example, a small town in Appalachia—are composed of people who share almost everything. They live in the same location, work at a limited type and number of jobs, attend the same churches, and make use of the sole health clinic with its visiting nurse practitioner. Other communities, such as members of Mothers Against Drunk Driving, are large, scattered, and composed of people who share only a common interest and involvement in a certain goal (Horntvedt, 2023). Although most communities of people share many aspects of their experience, it is useful to identify three types of communities that have relevance to community health practice: geographic, common interest, and health problem or solution. Unit 4 contains more in-depth information about the community as a client.

Geographic Community

A community that is defined by its geographic boundaries is called a **geographic community**. A city, town, or neighborhood is a geographic community.

Consider the community of Hayward, Wisconsin. Located in northwestern Wisconsin, it is set in a wooded environment, far removed from any urban cities, and known for extremely harsh winters. With a population of approximately 2533, it is considered a rural community. The population fluctuates with the seasons: summers bring hundreds of tourists and seasonal residents. Hayward is a social system as well as a geographic location. The families, schools, hospital, churches, stores, and government institutions are linked in a complex network. This community, like others, has an informal power structure. It has a communication system that includes neighbors' casual conversations, the newspaper, the "co-op" store bulletin board, radio, television, internet sources, and social media. In one sense, then, a community consists of a collection of people located in a specific place and is made up of institutions organized into a social system.

A few miles south are other communities, including Northwoods Beach and Round Lake; these, along with Hayward and other towns and isolated farms, form a larger community called Sawyer County (population 18,559). If a nurse worked for a health agency serving only Hayward, that community would be of primary concern; however, if the nurse worked for the Sawyer County Public Health Department, this larger community would be the focus. A PHN employed by the Wisconsin Department of Health Services in Madison, Wisconsin, would have an interest in Sawyer County and Hayward, but only as part of the larger community of Wisconsin (state population 5.89 million).

Frequently, a single part of a city can be treated as a community. Cities are often broken down into census tracts or neighborhoods. In New York City, the neighborhood called Harlem is a community, as is the Haight-Ashbury district of San Francisco.

In community health, identifying a geographic area as a community is useful because it:

- Provides a clear target for the analysis of health needs
- Makes available data (e.g., morbidity and mortality figures) that can augment assessment studies to form the basis for planning health programs
- Facilitates mobilizing community members for action and forming groups to carry out intervention and prevention efforts that address needs specific to that community, such as shelters for people experiencing intimate partner violence, work site safety programs in local hazardous industries, or improved sexual health education in the schools
- Helps in gaining the support of politically powerful people and resources present in a geographic community

On a larger scale, the world can be considered as a global community. Indeed, it is very important to view the world this way. Borders of countries change with political upheaval, but communicable diseases are no respecter of arbitrary political boundaries. A person can travel around the world in less than 24 hours, and so can diseases, such as Zika virus, Ebola, or COVID-19. The recent pandemic is evidence of this. Global pandemics require cooperation and information sharing among affected nations. The world is one large, interconnected, diverse community that must work together to ensure a healthy today and a healthier and safer future.

Globalization and health were discussed at a landmark meeting of the World Health Organization (WHO) in 2008, predicting dire global consequences for health. Diseases, food and water shortages, climate change, and extreme weather are recognized as global, as well as local, problems. Globalization raises an expectation of health for all, for if good health is possible in one part of the world, the forces of globalization should allow it elsewhere and everyone then enjoys the benefits (WHO, 2023b; Youde, 2019). We will learn more about global health in Chapter 16.

Common-Interest Community

A community also can be defined by a common interest or goal. A collection of people, even if they are widely scattered geographically, can have an interest or goal that binds the members together. This is known as a *common-interest community.*

The members of a church in a large metropolitan area and families who have lost members to suicide are both examples of common-interest communities. People with disabilities who are scattered throughout a large city may emerge as a community through a common interest in promoting adherence to federal guidelines for wheelchair access, parking spaces, elevators, or other services for those with disabilities. The residents of an industrial community may develop a common interest in air or water pollution issues, whereas others who work but do not live in the area may not equally share that interest.

- Communities form to protect the rights of children, stop intimate partner violence, promote sensible gun laws, clean up the environment, or provide support for social and structural change (e.g., Black Lives Matter, National Right to Life). The kinds of shared interests that lead to the formation of communities vary widely.
- Common-interest communities whose focus is a health-related issue may join with community health agencies to promote their agendas. The single-minded commitment that characterizes such communities can be a mobilizing force for action. Many successful prevention and health promotion efforts, including improved services and increased community awareness of specific problems, have resulted from the work of common-interest communities.

Current examples of common-interest communities are groups such as Everytown for Gun Safety, Moms Demand Action, and Students Demand Action. Their common interest involves concerns over rising gun deaths and mass shootings in the United States. Current statistics on gun deaths include the following:

- In 2021, 48,830 Americans died from gun-related deaths (a 45% increase between 2019 and 2021). Over half of these deaths were due to suicide; 81% of murders involved firearms.
- During the same time period, gun deaths in children and teens increased by 50%.
- A definition of mass shooting incidents includes four or more people shot (even if no deaths occur), and there were 706 deaths from U.S. mass shooting incidents in 2021.
- Per 2019 data, the United States has higher gun death rates (10.6 per 100,000) than France (2.7), Canada (2.1), Australia (1.0), Germany (0.9), and Spain (0.6) (Gramlich, 2023).

Moms Demand Action began in response to the Sandy Hook school shooting in 2012, when Shannon Watts, a mother of five children, looked for an organization like Mothers Against Drunk Drivers that addressed the gun violence problem in America and the lack of regulations around gun sales in many states (see more on violence and abuse in Chapter 18). She could not find one, so she started a Facebook page that got instant and overwhelming responses from parents across the country. She had previously worked for 15 years as a communications executive, and even though she was now a stay-at-home mom, she felt passionately about the need to bring a new narrative to the public debate on guns. She organized a grassroots network to promote gun violence prevention and work together with other groups to enact common sense gun legislation at the local, state, and national levels. While supporting the second amendment, Moms Demand Action seeks to counter the powerful influence of the gun lobby and fight the public health crisis of gun violence. It has chapters with volunteers in every state and the District of Columbia (Moms Demand Action, 2023).

After the Parkland, Florida, high school shooting, a related organization, Students Demand Action, was organized and now has over 700 local groups nationwide. These young people call themselves "the school shooting generation," and they are endeavoring to register new voters and continue to raise awareness about gun violence. They are also working to enact more commonsense gun safety laws at national, state, and local levels (Students Demand Action, 2023, para. 2).

Both groups have joined with Everytown for Gun Safety that represents "nearly 10 million people who have joined the movement" (Everytown for Gun Safety, 2023, para. 10). They represent a community with a common interest and are very active in working toward their common goals.

Community of Solution

A type of community encountered frequently in community/public health practice is a group of people who come together to solve a problem that affects all of them. This type of community is known as a *community of solution*. The shape of this type of community varies with the nature of the problem, the size of the geographic area affected, and the number of resources needed to address the problem.

For example, a water pollution problem may involve several counties whose agencies and personnel must work together to control upstream water supply, industrial waste disposal, and city water treatment. This group of counties forms a community of solutions focusing on a health problem. Figure 1-2 depicts some communities of solution related to a single city.

In recent years, communities of solution have formed in many cities to address the spread of diseases, solve problems of homelessness, and have worked with community members to assess a variety of needs and create plans to make their community a safer and healthier place in which to live.

- In 2014, Flint, Michigan, was faced with a growing water crisis involving high levels of lead and an eventual outbreak of Legionnaires disease. Public health agencies, social service groups, schools, citizens, and media personnel banded together to create public awareness of the dangers and to promote preventive behaviors. However, it took more than 5 years to regain clean water in Flint's home faucets, and some community members remain skeptical due to the lack of health equity as this crisis largely affected Black and low-income neighborhoods (Robertson, 2020). See Chapter 9.

Across the country, the community of Blaine, Idaho, recognized a need and came together to develop a solution. An earlier community assessment had found that 35% of residents experienced food insecurity, but many people were hesitant to seek food assistance at local food pantries due to perceived stigma. The Hunger Coalition was formed with a local nonprofit food pantry and participation from local community members. Community gardens were created to grow fresh fruits and vegetables. A truck was purchased to bring this food to local neighborhoods in need. Much like an ice cream truck, the colorful vehicle delivered healthy sack lunches to children for free, along with books from the Bookmobile that was now combined with the produce truck. Throughout the summer, the colorful food truck/mobile library traveled throughout the county, serving children free lunches (and adult lunches for $1).

The project was so successful, that the community gardens produced over 7000 pounds of fresh produce in 2022, and the Hunger Coalition started operating pop-up fruit/vegetable stands in various neighborhoods from summer through the fall. Interns from the high school run the stands that also sell discounted meals along with produce. In 2023, they picked two locations for more permanent outdoor produce markets that accept Electronic Benefits Transfer from the Supplemental Nutrition Assistance Program. They also accept credit cards, cash, or checks, making it easy for families in need to access fresh fruits and vegetables. In June 2023, the food truck/mobile library served 250 children and 50 adults a total of 1599 meals in this one rural county of about 24,000 people. Other rural counties could adopt this successful program (Rural Health Information Hub, 2023).

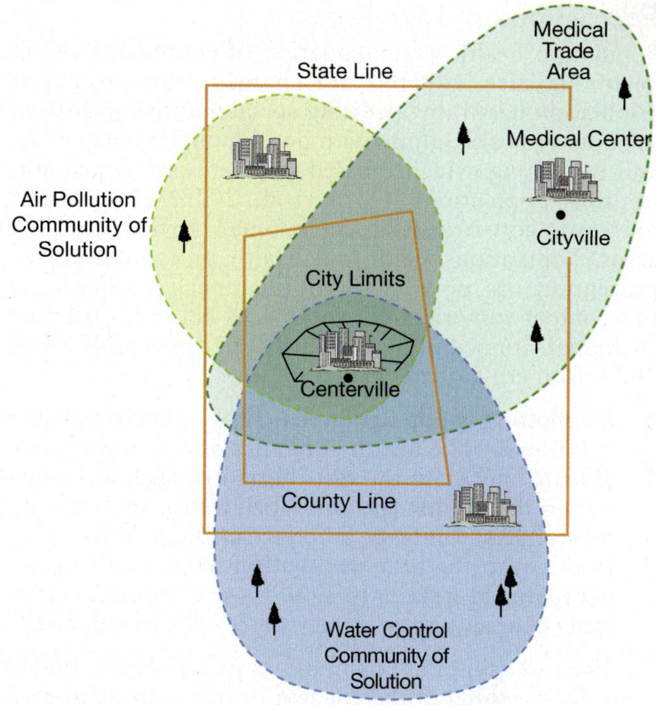

FIGURE 1-2 A city's communities of solution. State, county, and city boundaries (*solid lines*) may have little or no bearing on health solution boundaries (*dashed lines*).

As you can see, a community of solution is an important conduit for change in community/public health. Do you know of any communities of solution in your area?

Populations and Aggregates

Population health is a foundation of community/public health practice, C/PHNs are charged with promoting population health by assessing social and medical determinants of health, along with developing, implementing, and evaluating evidence-based interventions to promote healthier populations (Gwon et al., 2023). However, all nurses are now required to have some knowledge in these areas. Population health and health promotion/disease prevention are now included in nursing curricula, as this content comprises 6% to 12% of NCLEX questions (National Council of State Boards of Nursing [NCSBN], 2023; Romero-Collado et al., 2020).

- A definition of population that also applies to statistics is follows: "The health outcomes of a group of individuals, including the distribution of such outcomes within the group" (Institute for Healthcare Improvement, 2023; Kindig & Stoddart, 2003, p. 380).
- In this text, the term **population** refers to all people occupying an area or to all of those who share one or more characteristics (Anderson & McFarlane, 2019).

The three types of communities just discussed underscore the meaning of the concept of community: in each instance, a collection of people chose to interact with one another because of common interests, characteristics, or goals. The concept of population has a different meaning.

- In contrast to a community, a population is made up of people who do not necessarily interact with one another but share a sense of belonging to that group.
- A population may be defined geographically, such as the population of the United States or a city's population.
- This designation of a population is useful in community/public health for epidemiologic study and for collecting demographic data for purposes such as health planning.
- A population also may be defined by common qualities or characteristics, such as the older adult population, people who are homeless, or a particular racial or ethnic group.
- In community/public health, this meaning becomes useful when a specific group of people (e.g., people experiencing homelessness) is targeted for intervention; the population's common characteristics (e.g., health-related problems of homelessness) become a major focus of the intervention.

In this text, the term **aggregate** refers to a mass or grouping of distinct people who are considered as a whole and who are loosely associated with one another. It is a broader term that encompasses many different-sized groups. Both communities and populations contain subgroups of aggregates. Unit 5 discusses community/public health nursing with aggregates, and Unit 6 discusses vulnerable populations. The different settings for community/public health nursing can be found throughout the book.

The aggregate focus, or a concern for groupings of people in contrast to individual healthcare, is common in community/public health practice. C/PHNs may work with aggregates such as pregnant and parenting teens, older adults with diabetes, or families with toddlers who need information on how to child-proof their homes.

Because of community/public health nursing's focus on communities, aggregates, and families, new nursing and healthcare delivery systems may develop that are more cost-effective and beneficial in preventing health problems and expensive emergency room visits or hospitalizations. Community/public health workers, including C/PHNs, must clearly define the community targeted for study and intervention and understand its complexity before assessing its needs and designing interventions to address them. To help define the community, the C/PHN should answer the following questions:

- Who makes up the community?
- Where are they located, and what are their characteristics?
- What are the characteristics of the people in terms of age, gender, race, socioeconomic level, and health status?
- How does the community interact with other communities?
- What is its history? What are its resources?
- Is the community undergoing rapid change, and, if so, what are the changes?

These questions, as well as the tools needed to assess a community for health purposes, are discussed in detail in Chapter 15.

THE CONCEPT OF HEALTH

Health, in the abstract, refers to a person's physical, mental, and spiritual state; it can be positive (as being in good health) or negative (as being in poor health).

- The WHO offers a positive explanation of health as "a state of complete physical, mental, and social well-being and not merely the absence of disease or infirmity" (WHO, 2023a, para. 1).
- Building on this classic definition, our definition of health in this text is as follows: a holistic state of well-being, which includes soundness of mind, body, and spirit.

Health is determined by more than just medical care. It is influenced by various factors—location of residence, education, income, diet, exercise, accessibility of healthcare, and health behaviors (County Health Rankings, 2023). See Figure 1-3 for the County Health Rankings Model. Likewise, the WHO (2023a) has outlined the prerequisites for health as "peace, shelter, education, food, income, a stable eco-system, sustainable resources, social justice, and equity" (para. 5).

- Community health practitioners place a strong emphasis on **wellness**, which includes this definition of health but also incorporates the capacity to develop a person's potential to lead a fulfilling and productive life—one that can be measured in terms of quality of life.
- Today, our health is greatly affected by our lifestyles, preventive measures we take, and risk behaviors in which we engage (Whitman et al., 2022).
- Although this concept is not new, we are increasingly aware of the strong relationship of health to environment (Box 1-3; Dos Santos et al., 2023).

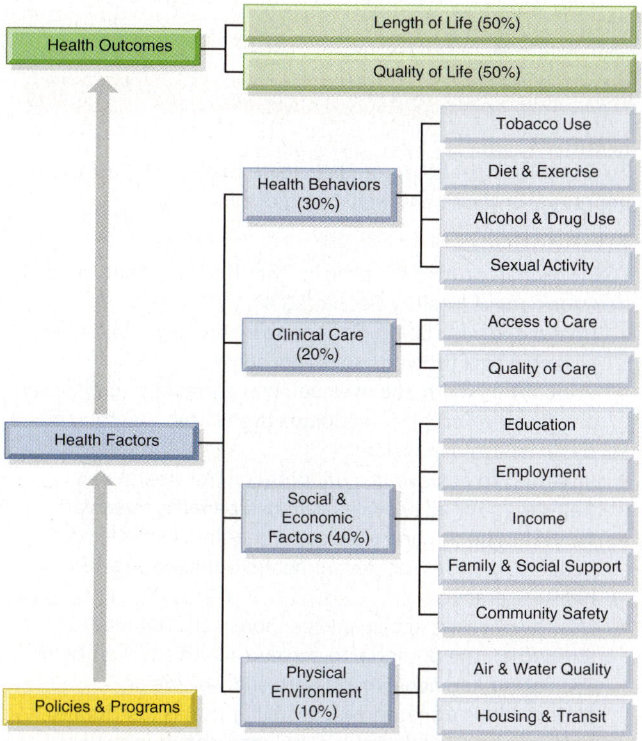

FIGURE 1-3 County Health Rankings Model demonstrates how many factors impact health outcomes. (Used with permission of The University of Wisconsin Population Health Institute. County Health Rankings & Roadmaps, 2024. www.countyhealthrankings.org.)

Over 160 years ago, Florence Nightingale explored the relationship between health/illness and the environment. She believed that a person's health was greatly influenced by ventilation, noise, light, cleanliness, diet, and a restful bed (Nightingale, 1859/1992). As is well documented, the built environment, or man-made structures and surroundings in a community (e.g., highways and bike paths, parks and open spaces, public buildings, and housing developments), significantly affects the health of people, aggregates, and populations (Castner et al., 2019; CDC, NCCDPHP, 2022; Whitman et al., 2022). Nightingale's model is explained in Chapters 3 and 7, and the environment's relationship to health is discussed in more detail in Chapter 9.

Culture also shapes our view of health. Some cultures see health as the freedom from and absence of evil and illness as punishment for being bad or doing evil or a result of witchcraft (Subu et al., 2022). Many people come from families in which beliefs regarding health and illness are heavily influenced by religion, superstition, folk beliefs, or "old wives' tales." C/PHNs commonly encounter such beliefs when working with various groups in the community. Chapter 5 explores these beliefs more thoroughly.

BOX 1-3 WHAT DO *YOU* THINK?

Dramatic Drop in U.S. Life Expectancy

We like to consider ourselves as a wealthy and healthy nation. However, there has been some incremental deterioration of life expectancy in the United States since 1983. But it significantly dropped from 78.7 to 76.1 years for a child born between 2020 and 2022, representing the largest 2-year drop since 1921–1923 (CDC, National Center for Health Statistics, 2022; Woolf, 2023). Strong factors in the dramatic decrease include the U.S. per capita deaths from COVID-19 (one of the largest rates) and higher rates of midlife deaths due to "drug overdose, alcohol-related causes, suicide, and cardiometabolic diseases" (Woolf, 2023, p. 977). Between 1933 and 2021, 56 countries reported a longer life expectancy than the United States (Woolf, 2023). Some of the reason for this rests with our policies, as many of those countries "offer more generous social welfare and income support programs and enforce stronger regulations to protect public health and safety" (Woolf, 2023, p. 975).

What things could we do to improve U.S. life expectancy? What policies and practices would need to be instituted?

The Health Continuum: Wellness—Illness

Western societies often exhibit a polarized or "either/or" way of thinking about health: either people are healthy and well or they are ill. Yet, wellness is a relative concept, not an absolute, and has been defined as the "quality or state of being in good health as an actively sought goal" (Merriam-Webster, 2023, para. 1). Conversely, **illness** is a state of being *relatively* unhealthy physically or mentally. The study of factors affecting health and illness is known as epidemiology and is discussed in Chapter 7. There are many levels and degrees of wellness and illness, from a robust 75-year-old who is fully active and functioning at an optimal level of wellness to a 45-year-old with diabetes and end-stage renal disease whose health is characterized as frail. Someone recovering from pneumonia may be mildly ill, whereas another person with functional limitations because of episodic depression may be described as mildly well. The **health continuum**, however, can change.

- Because healthiness involves a range of degrees from optimal health at one end to total disability or death at the other end, it is often described as a health continuum. This health continuum applies not only to people but also to families and communities.
- A nurse might speak of a "family in crisis," meaning one that is experiencing a relative degree of illness or altered functioning, or of a healthy family, meaning one that exhibits many wellness characteristics, such as effective communication and conflict resolution, as well as the ability to effectively work together and use resources appropriately.
- Likewise, a community, as a collection of people, may be described in terms of degrees of wellness or illness. The health of a person, family, group, or community moves back and forth along this continuum throughout the lifespan. Healthy people make healthy communities and a healthy society.

More information on working with families and communities is included in Chapters 14 and 15.

The Declaration of Alma Ata, which took place in 1978, noted that health is a "fundamental human right" of all people around the world and that "people have a right and duty to participate individually and collectively in the planning and implementation of their health care" (WHO, 2023e, para. 2). A common concern among the 134 participating countries included the "gross inequality of the health status of people" around the world and concluded that the level of health must be raised in all countries for any society to improve their health (WHO, 2023e, para. 2).

In the past, healthcare generally focused on treatment of acute and chronic conditions at the illness end of the continuum. However, the emphasis has been shifting to focus on the wellness end of the continuum, as outlined in the government document, *Healthy People 2030* (U.S. Department of Health and Human Services [USDHHS], Office of Disease Prevention and Health Promotion [ODPHP], 2023a).

- The vision for *Healthy People 2030* is for everyone to "achieve their full potential for health and well-being across the lifespan" (para. 4).
- This effort aims to improve the health of American citizens by establishing objectives and benchmarks that can be monitored over time. There have been Healthy People objectives for each decade beginning in 2000 (evaluated at that time but first published in 1990). New objectives were developed for evaluation in 2010, 2020, and now for 2030.
- A main foundational principle is that a population's health and well-being are a prerequisite to securing a flourishing and equitable society. The mission, foundational principles, and action plan of *Healthy People 2030* were used to guide the development of the current objectives (USDHHS/ODPHP, 2023c).

The goals overarch topics and objectives (Box 1-4). The objectives are stated in measurable terms that specify targeted incidence and prevalence changes and address age, gender, and culturally vulnerable groups along with improvement in public health systems. *Healthy People 2030* boxes can be found in selected chapters. There are three types of objectives:

- *Core objectives* that rely on health statistics data from established sources (e.g., U.S. Census, surveys, data sets) for accurate assessment of progress meeting targets.
- *Developmental objectives* are selected from "public health issues with evidence-based interventions but lacking reliable data" (ODPHP, 2023, para. 6).
- *Research objectives* are areas for potential studies without consistent evidence-based interventions.

Healthy People 2030 emphasizes that the health of a person is linked to the health of the larger community and that this larger community's health is related to the health of the corresponding state and ultimately our nation (Hinton, 2023; USDHHS, 2023a; Whitman et al., 2022). See Figure 1-4.

- Recognizing the important influence of SDOH, federal and state funded programs (e.g., Medicaid managed care) have now been given limited permission to use some funding in proactive, health promoting ways to address conditions like homelessness or inadequate nutrition and prevent poor health outcomes (Hinton, 2023).
- The recommended leading health indicators (LHIs) for *Healthy People 2030* are outcomes metric for measuring progress toward national public health goals. They are core objectives that extend across the lifespan and cover issues of utmost priority and importance. They often concern upstream behaviors and risk factors such as health equity and disparities, along with SDOH, and may be modified based on new data and evidence of effective interventions (ODP&HP, 2023).

BOX 1-4 HEALTHY PEOPLE 2030

Issues in Community/Public Health Nursing

Mission

To promote, strengthen, and evaluate the Nation's efforts to improve the health and well-being of all people

Foundational Principles

Foundational principles explain the thinking that guides decisions about Healthy People 2030.

- Health and well-being of all people and communities are essential to a thriving, equitable society.
- Promoting health and well-being and preventing disease are linked efforts that encompass physical, mental, and social health dimensions.
- Investing to achieve the full potential for health and well-being for all provides valuable benefits to society.
- Achieving health and well-being requires eliminating health disparities, achieving health equity, and attaining health literacy.
- Healthy physical, social, and economic environments strengthen the potential to achieve health and well-being.
- Promoting and achieving health and well-being nationwide is a shared responsibility that is distributed across the national, state, tribal, and community levels, including the public, private, and not-for-profit sectors.
- Working to attain the full potential for health and well-being of the population is a component of decision-making and policy formulation across all sectors.

Healthy People 2030 Overarching Goals

- Attain healthy, thriving lives and well-being, free of preventable disease, disability, injury, and premature death.
- Eliminate health disparities, achieve health equity, and attain health literacy to improve the health and well-being of all.
- Create social, physical, and economic environments that promote attaining full potential for health and well-being for all.
- Promote healthy development, healthy behaviors, and well-being across all life stages.
- Engage leadership, key constituents, and the public across multiple sectors to act and design policies that improve the health and well-being of all.

Reprinted from U.S. Department of Health and Human Services (USDHHS), Office of Disease Prevention & Health Promotion. (n.d.). *Healthy People 2030: Framework.* Retrieved September 4, 2023, from https://health.gov/healthypeople/about/healthy-people-2030-framework

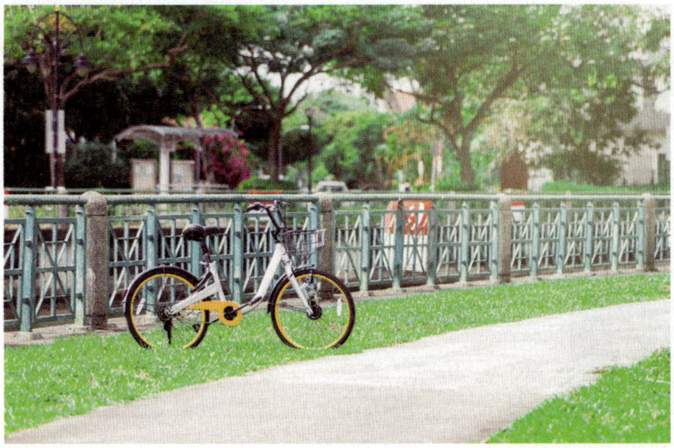

FIGURE 1-4 Healthy communities promote the health of their inhabitants.

BOX 1-6 WHO Social Determinants of Health

- Income and social protection
- Education
- Unemployment and job insecurity
- Working life conditions
- Food insecurity
- Housing, basic amenities, and the environment
- Early childhood development
- Social inclusion and nondiscrimination
- Structural conflict
- Access to affordable health services of decent quality

WHO. (2023). *Social determinants of health*. https://www.who.int/health-topics/social-determinants-of-health#tab=tab_1

The main topic areas under which the LHIs are outlined may be found in Box 1-4.

Probably the most frequently recognized metric for the health of a nation is the life expectancy of its citizens. According to the CDC (2011), life expectancy in the United States has increased from 47.3 years in 1900 to 76.8 years in 2000, and it is estimated that about 25 years of this growth can be attributed to public health advances (e.g., infectious disease control/prevention, sanitation). The remainder of the gain is the result of improvements in prevention and therapeutic interventions (e.g., lifestyle behaviors, medical advances). How has our life expectancy changed recently? Would you predict an even longer life expectancy? See Box 1-5.

Community characteristics of health have been described by the CDC as health-related quality of life indicators. A helpful source of community-level health indicators is the County Health Rankings and Roadmaps website (County Health Rankings, 2023).

- Compare your county's ratings with those of others in your state at https://www.countyhealthrankings.org/explore-health-rankings

BOX 1-5 *HEALTHY PEOPLE 2030*

Proposed Leading Health Indicators

The 23 LHIs are used to measure the health of the nation and will "drive action toward improving health and well-being" and reducing "major causes of death and disease" (para. 1). As a group, they are "core objectives" that "focus on upstream measures" (e.g., behaviors, risk factors) "of national importance" instead of just "disease outcomes" (para. 1). They "address high-priority public health issues" (e.g., health equity, health disparities, and SDOH) that may respond to "evidence-based interventions and strategies," as new data are periodically available (para. 7).

Reprinted from U.S. Department of Health and Human Services (USDHHS), Office of Disease Prevention & Health Promotion. (n.d.). *Leading health indicators (LHI)*. Retrieved September 4, 2023, from https://health.gov/healthypeople/objectives-and-data/leading-health-indicators

- The complete interactive County Health Rankings Model is available at https://www.countyhealthrankings.org/explore-health-rankings/county-health-rankings-model
- You can find information on the 2023 measures at https://www.countyhealthrankings.org/explore-health-rankings/county-health-rankings-measures

Many indicators of community health have been used over the years, such as income distribution, unemployment rates, number of health professionals, and lifestyle choices. The County Health Rankings examines health behaviors; clinical care, along with social/economic factors; and physical environment that influence health factors leading to health outcomes. See Figure 1-3 for the abbreviated County Health Rankings Model. You will learn more about community assessment in Chapter 15.

WHO defines SDOH as "the non-medical factors that influence health outcomes" (para. 1), and states that "addressing (them) … is fundamental for improving health and reducing longstanding inequities in health" found across all countries, rich and poor (WHO, 2023e, para. 6). A list of SDOH examples from WHO is found in Box 1-6. How wide is the disparity for many of these SDOH in your city or community? Are you surprised that only one of these elements contains the word "health"?

Health as a State of Being

Health refers to a state of being, including many different qualities and characteristics.

- A person might be described as energetic, outgoing, enthusiastic, beautiful, caring, loving, and intense. Together, these qualities become the essence of a person's existence; they describe a state of being.
- A geographic community, such as a neighborhood, might be characterized as congested, deteriorating, unattractive, dirty, and disorganized, all of which suggest diminishing degrees of vitality.
- A population, such as workers involved in a massive layoff, might be characterized as banding together to provide support and share resources to effectively seek new employment. Such a community shows signs of healthy adaptation and positive coping.

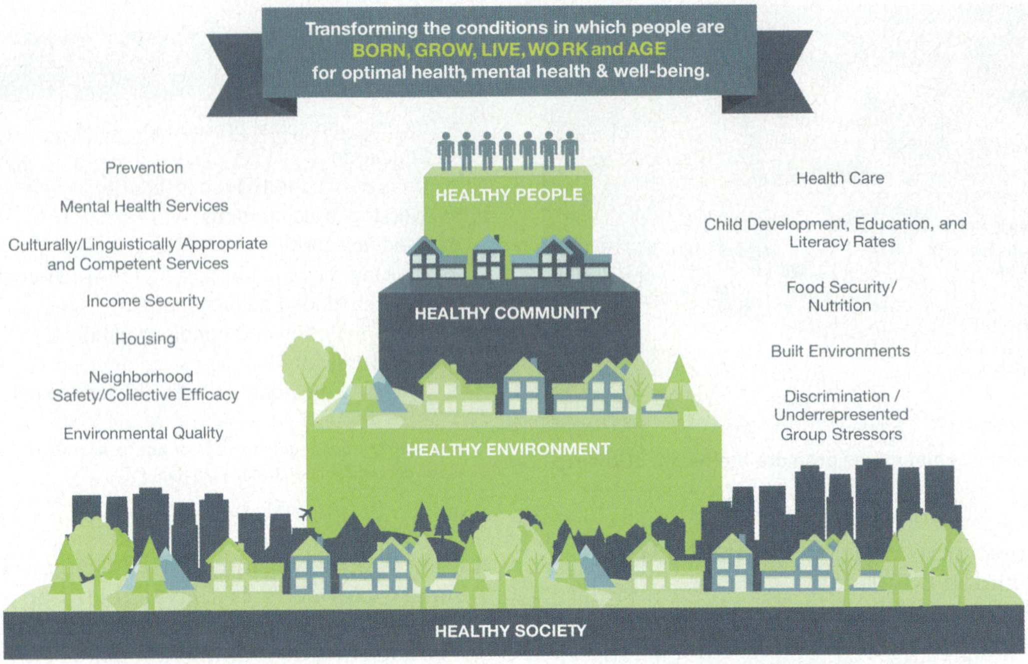

FIGURE 1-5 The health of the person is related to community, state, and national health. (Adapted from California Department of Public Health (CDPH). (2015, August). *Portrait of promise: The California statewide plan to promote health and mental health equity*. Report to the legislature and the people of California by the Office of Health Equity, CDPH. (p. 18). https://www.cdph.ca.gov/Programs/OHE/CDPH%20Document%20Library/ADA%20Approved%20POP%20Report.pdf#search=social%20determinants%20of%20health%20graphic)

Health involves the total person, aggregate, or community. All dimensions of life affecting everyday functioning determine a person's or a community's health, including physical, psychological, spiritual, economic, and sociocultural experiences. The approach should be holistic, including not only physical and emotional status but also the status of home, family, and work. For intervention purposes, it is important to consider the "health of a community" (Fig. 1-5).

Disasters occur around the world, affecting the health of countless people every year. In the summer of 2023, more than 885 wildfires burned in Canada, destroying over 27 million acres and causing smoke to cover large parts of Canada and the Northeastern United States. Unhealthy air quality even spread as far away as the Great Lakes area and reached Kentucky and Missouri (Czachor, 2023a; McDermott & Kelleher, 2023).

On August 9, 2023, other fires, whipped by high winds from a hurricane "hundreds of miles south" of the island and fueled by dry foliage and grasses, devastated the Hawaiian island of Maui (Czachor, 2023b, para. 3). The wildfires led to 101 fatalities (U.S. Fire Administration, 2024a), destroying over 2,200 structures totaling $5.5 billion in damages, significantly impacting the Lahaina historic district of Maui (U.S. Fire Administration, 2024b). As of August 2024, the Federal Emergency Management Agency (FEMA) continues to work in partnership with local and state partners as well as the US Army Corps of Engineers for cleanup and recovery. To date, clearing commercial and residential debris, school construction, infrastructure repair, and long-term housing has been ongoing. Investment in infrastructure for drinking water and waste continues to be part of the recovery process (FEMA, 2024a). With nearly three billion in federal support, FEMA-funded services continue to support survivors, offering crisis counseling, unemployment assistance, and disaster legal services (FEMA, 2024b). Fallen power lines appeared to spark the initial blaze (McDermott & Kelleher, 2023). See Figure 1-6.

Many dimensions of health (physical and SDOH) were significantly affected by these crises. We examine disaster and bioterrorism in Chapter 17.

Subjective and Objective Dimensions of Health

Health involves both *subjective* and *objective* dimensions; that is, it involves both how people feel (subjective) and how well they can function in their environment

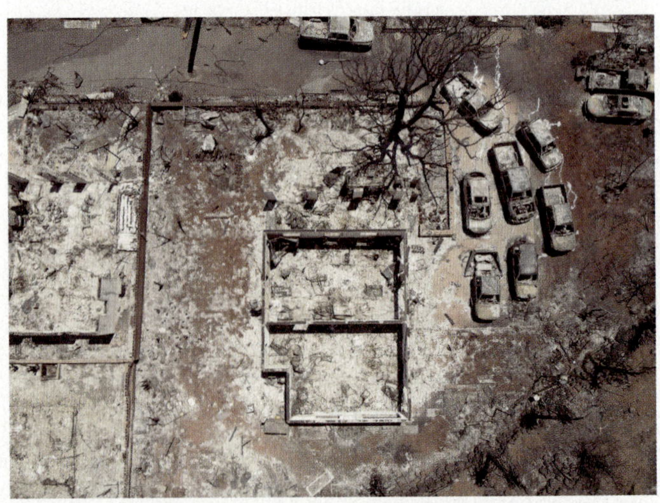

FIGURE 1-6 Home and cars burned in Lahaina, Maui wildfires, August 2023.

(objective). How they feel overall is a strong indicator of their overall state of health.

- Subjectively, a healthy person is one who feels well and who experiences the sensation of a vital, positive state.
- Health also involves the objective dimension of ability to function. A healthy person or community carries out necessary activities and achieves enriching goals. Unhealthy people not only feel unwell but they are limited, to some degree, in their ability to carry out daily activities.

Indeed, levels of illness or wellness are measured largely in terms of ability to function (Wei et al., 2023).

- A person confined to bed is often labeled sicker than an ill person managing self-care.
- A family that meets its members' needs is healthier than one that has poor communication patterns and is unable to provide adequate physical and emotional resources.
- A community actively engaged in affordable housing programs and services for people who are homeless or in policing of industrial wastes shows signs of healthy functioning.

The degree of functioning is directly related to the state of health.

The actions of a person, family, or community are motivated by their values. Some activities, such as daily walks and taking care of personal needs, are functions valued by most people. In assessing the health of people and communities, the C/PHN can observe people's ability to function but also must know their values, which may contrast with those of the nurse. The influence of values on health is examined more closely in Chapter 5.

Continuous and Episodic Healthcare Needs

Community/public health practice encompasses care for populations in all age groups with birth-to-death developmental healthcare needs.

- These *continuous needs* may include, for example, assistance with providing a toddler-proof home and meeting developmental milestones, help in effectively dealing with the progressive emancipation of preteens and teenagers, anticipatory guidance for reducing and managing the stress associated with retirement, or help coping with the death of an older parent. These are developmental events experienced by most people, and they represent typical life occurrences. The C/PHN has the skills to work at the individual, family, and group level to meet these needs.
- In addition, people, families, and populations may have a one-time, specific, negative health event, such as an illness or injury that is not an expected part of life. These *episodic needs* might derive from child abuse injuries for a teen placed in an emergency shelter or community outbreak of tuberculosis or other communicable disease. Disasters (e.g., hurricanes, wildfires, earthquakes) can affect large populations.

On any given day, the C/PHN may interact with clients having either continuous or episodic healthcare needs or both. For example, how do middle-aged adults, planning their retirement and preparing for the death of an older parent, deal with their adult child's HIV diagnosis? Or how do parents of a teenager confront their child's drug dependence? Complex situations such as these may be positively influenced by the interaction with and services of the C/PHN.

Public health departments must be ready to face new challenges, such as new COVID-19 variants or other emerging communicable diseases. They may also find new outbreaks of rare diseases such as leprosy:

- In 2022, the state of Florida reported increased cases of leprosy (Hansen disease) being reported, especially in central Florida, although it is generally uncommon in the United States. However, 159 new U.S. cases were reported in 2020, with Florida being one of the states with the most cases. Zoonotic transmission from armadillos was suspected for some infected people, as they had exposure and shared a distinctive strain of *Mycobacterium leprae*. But, for many others, the specific cause remained unknown despite contact tracing. This provided evidence of an endemic origin (Bhukhan et al., 2023).

Find more information on communicable diseases in Chapter 8, on epidemiology in Chapter 7, and on the public health system in Chapter 6.

Upstream Focus

PHNs incorporate an "upstream" focus into their work with populations. This approach emerged from the seminal publication by John McKinley in 1979, *A Case for Focusing Upstream*, which identified root causes of disease and the multiple factors that led to illness. The PHNs approach to prevention and health promotion relies on an **upstream focus** to address the root causes at the institutional and system level that influence health rather than looking solely at healthy lifestyle behaviors: in other words, PHNs address "upstream" factors in addition to the identified problem or issue (Butterfield, 2017; Ray et al., 2023).

- For example, a PHN is taking an upstream approach to asthma prevention by working with legislators to strengthen ambient air quality policies. Thus, the nurse is moving up along the system to address a leading factor (outdoor air pollution) that causes asthma.
- Two related concepts for public health nursing are health disparities and the SDOH. This "midstream" focus for public health was introduced in a classic article by Butterfield (1990) who reminds the nursing profession that nurses, particularly PHNs, serve to reduce risks. PHNs are often the "sentinels of surveillance" who detect unusual illness patterns and respond to environmental emergencies in work and community settings (Butterfield, 2002, p. 33). By using an upstream approach, PHNs can impact the prevalence of disease within a population by intervening where the root causes exist (Butterfield, 2017; McMahon, 2021).
- With emphasis upon data estimates that as much as 80% of disease and "25%–30% of the total disease burden" is attributable to environmental risk factors, the environment is an important part of a C/PHN's assessment (Dos Santos et al., 2023, p. 2; van Daalen et al., 2022).

- The increase of environmentally linked health problems such as allergies, asthma, chronic kidney disease, neurologic problems, certain cancers, heart disease, and chronic obstructive pulmonary disease makes the case for nurses to use an upstream framework to assess, monitor, educate, advocate, and create policies to reduce environmental health risks (Dos Santos et al., 2023; van Daalen et al., 2022).

More on environmental health can be found in Chapter 9, and disasters in Chapter 17.

Social Determinants of Health

According to the WHO, **social determinants of health (SDOH)** are defined as "the conditions in which people are born, grow, live, work, and age. These circumstances are shaped by the distribution of money, power, and resources at global, national, and local levels" (2023e, para. 1).

- SDOH include social factors that affect families and communities such as education, housing conditions, options for safe and active transportation, access to healthcare services, access to healthy food, employment and income, neighborhood environment and safety, and the quality of the built environment such as parks, buildings, and green spaces.
- These social factors and community-level stressors contribute to the inequities in health outcomes, burden of disease, and quality of life (Hinton, 2023).

Health Disparities

Health disparities are a serious concern for overall health in the United States and globally. As noted in the discussion of upstream approaches to health, environmental factors are basic determinants of health and well-being. However, great inequities occur between the environments of people with higher incomes and those of low-income communities, people of color, and tribal and Indigenous populations. There are complex relationships between genes and environment that are related to SDOH (National Institute of Environmental Health Sciences [NIEHS], 2023a, 2023b).

- Disparities that are directly correlated with environmental exposures include rates of asthma among children, elevated blood lead levels, cancers that are linked to environmental exposures, and lung diseases among adults.
- Social and economic factors have created disproportionate exposures to pesticides, toxic chemicals in the workplace, poor indoor air quality in schools, and lead in housing (Castner et al., 2019; Zota & Shamasunder, 2021).

Environmental Justice

Closely related to SDOH is the issue of environmental justice (EJ). The Environmental Protection Agency (EPA) defines EJ as "the fair treatment and meaningful involvement of all people regardless of race, color, national origin, or income with respect to the development, implementation, and enforcement of environmental laws, regulations, and policies" (EPA, 2023, para. 1).

- The key difference between social determinants and EJ is that the former addresses social factors that contribute to health disparities, whereas EJ is responsive to the inequities in the distribution of environmental hazards and exposure risks.
- In communities across the United States, people of color and underrepresented ethnic groups, low-resource communities, and tribal communities bear a higher burden of exposure to environmental risks where they live (Chan et al., 2023; EPA, 2023; Servadio et al., 2019).
- Health equity is also involved, as working-age White, Black, and Hispanic people in a recent large-scale study examining death data from 2000 to 2019 were shown to have higher rates of "deaths of despair" (e.g., deaths due to drug overdose, suicide, and alcohol-associated liver disease) related to their increased income inequality and decreased social mobility (Kuo & Kawachi, 2023, p. 1).
- Since 1999, median maternal mortality rates have increased among all ethnic and racial groups in the United States; however, Alaska Native, American Indian, and especially Black maternal deaths increased at substantially higher rates (Fleszar et al., 2023).

For more about environmental health and safety, see Chapter 9. Additional information on vulnerable populations is the focus of Chapter 23 and the remaining chapters in Unit 6.

COMPONENTS OF COMMUNITY/PUBLIC HEALTH PRACTICE

Community/public health practice can best be understood by examining two basic components—promotion of health and prevention of health problems. The levels of prevention are a key to community/public health practice.

Promotion of Health

Promotion of health is recognized as one of the most important components of community/public health practice. **Health promotion** includes all efforts that seek to move people closer to optimal well-being. Specifically, nursing has a social mandate for engaging in wellness and health promotion (Melariri et al., 2022).

- Health promotion programs and activities include many forms of health education—for example, teaching the dangers of drug use, demonstrating healthful practices such as regular exercise, and providing more health-promoting options such as heart-healthy menu selections. C/PHNs, working with a variety of populations, utilize health promotion regularly to improve the health of their clients and the communities they serve (Murdaugh et al., 2019).

Community/public health promotion encompasses the development and management of wellness promotion and preventive healthcare services that are responsive to community health needs. Wellness programs in schools and industry are examples. In addition, groups and health agencies that support a smoke-free environment, encourage physical fitness programs for all ages, or demand that food products be properly labeled underscore the importance of these practices and create public awareness. The main goal of health promotion is to raise levels of wellness for people, families, populations, and communities (WHO, 2023e).

- The Institute of Medicine's 2003 hallmark report, *The Future of the Public's Health in the 21st Century*, noted at that time the majority of healthcare spending, "as much as 95%," focused on "medical care and biomedical research," whereas evidence suggests that "behavior and environment are responsible for over 70% of avoidable mortality" and that healthcare is only one of many "determinants of health" (p. 2).

The implications of this national agenda for health have far-reaching consequences for people engaged in healthcare. For centuries, healthcare and its payment structure has focused on the illness end of the health continuum, but that is beginning to change, and health professionals can no longer justify concentrating most of their efforts exclusively on treating the sick and injured (Galea & van Schalkwyk, 2023; Lantz, 2020; McKillop & Lieberman, 2022). We now live in an age when it is not only possible to promote health and prevent disease and disability, but it is our mandate and responsibility to do so. For more on health promotion, see Chapter 11.

Prevention of Health Problems

Prevention of health problems constitutes a major part of community/public health practice. Prevention means anticipating and averting problems or discovering them as early as possible to minimize potential disability and impairment.

It is practiced on three **levels of prevention** in community/public health: primary, secondary, and tertiary prevention (AbdulRaheem, 2023; Lenartowicz, 2023; WHO Regional Office of the Eastern Mediterranean, 2023). These concepts recur throughout the chapters of this text, in narrative format and in the Levels of Prevention Pyramids, because they are basic to community/public health nursing (Box 1-7). It is our view that early intervention is where most of the emphasis should be placed in the healthcare system; therefore, we use it as the base of our pyramid, instead of the usual placement of tertiary prevention as the base (originally envisioned by Leavell and Clark (1953).

Primary prevention precludes the occurrence of a health problem; it includes measures taken to keep illness or injuries from occurring. It is applied to a generally healthy population and precedes disease or dysfunction. Primary prevention involves anticipatory planning and action on the part of community/public health professionals, who must envision potential needs and problems, and then design programs to counteract them so that they never occur. The concepts of primary prevention and proactive planning for the future are unfamiliar to many social groups, who may resist due to their differing values (AbdulRaheem, 2023; Iriarte-Roteta et al., 2020).

Examples of primary prevention activities by a C/PHN include the following:

- Providing childhood vaccinations and yearly flu shots
- Encouraging older people to install and use safety devices (e.g., grab bars by bathtubs, handrails on steps) to prevent injuries from falls
- Teaching young adults healthy lifestyle behaviors, so that they can make them habitual behaviors for themselves and their children
- Working through a local health department in consultation with a school district to help control and prevent communicable diseases such as measles, pertussis, or varicella by providing regular immunization programs and vaccine oversight
- Instructing a group of people with excess weight on how to follow a well-balanced diet while losing weight to prevent nutritional deficiency (Box 1-7)
- Teaching adolescents safe sex practices or the dangers of smoking/vaping and substance use
- Serving on a fact-finding committee exploring the effects of a proposed toxic waste dump on the outskirts of town

Vaccination is one method of preventing health problems. During the COVID-19 pandemic, when the new vaccines became available, some communities were hesitant to participate in vaccination. The pandemic "exacerbated disparities in existing social determinants of health." In some areas of Philadelphia, where historically tenuous relationships existed with government and medical professionals, trusted messages and messengers from community-based organizations were needed to build trust and provide facts to counter distrust and misinformation (Shen et al., 2023, para. 3). Another example is the "Vaccine Brigade" that organized in Chicago and Cook County. This group of mostly retired PHNs organized to help with administration of vaccines in "communities of color and other underserved communities" (Blacksin, 2022, p. 1).

Secondary prevention involves efforts to detect and treat existing health problems at the earliest possible stage—when intervention is most likely to be effective in controlling or eradicating it. This is the goal behind testing of water and soil samples for contaminants and hazardous chemicals in the field of community environmental health (AbdulRaheem, 2023; WHO Regional Office of the Eastern Mediterranean, 2023).

Examples of secondary prevention activities by a C/PHN include the following:

- Conducting community hypertension and cholesterol screening programs to help identify high-risk people and encourage early treatment to prevent heart attacks or strokes
- Encouraging breast self-examination, regular mammograms, and Pap smears for early detection of cancers and providing skin testing for tuberculosis
- Assessing for early signs of child abuse in a family, emotional disturbances among those grieving the loss of their spouse, or alcohol and drug use among adolescents and providing information about available resources and services

BOX 1-7 LEVELS OF PREVENTION PYRAMID

Link Between Poor Diet, Inactivity, and Obesity

SITUATION: Poor nutritional habits and inactivity are leading to obesity and a greater incidence of type 2 diabetes among children and adults.

GOAL: Using the three levels of prevention, avoid or promptly diagnose and treat negative health conditions, and improve population health.

Tertiary Prevention

Rehabilitation

- In person with diabetes, encourage weight, blood pressure, and cholesterol maintenance, along with good glucose control to prevent complications of diabetes.
- Reassess data to determine effectiveness of interventions.

Prevention

Health Promotion and Education

- Teach children and families the importance of maintaining a healthy weight through proper diet and exercise. Promote awareness of dangers of obesity and diabetes through use of public service announcements and billboards.

Health Protection

- Provide weight loss support.
- Provide access to periodic healthcare to check A1C levels and foot and eye examinations.

Secondary Prevention

Early Diagnosis

- Encourage weight loss in populations with obesity to prevent development of type 2 diabetes. Provide screening programs for high-risk groups.
- Refer clients with high glucose or other problems (e.g., hypertension, high cholesterol) to primary care provider or diabetes clinics.

Prompt Treatment

- Initiate educational and incentive programs to improve dietary practices.
- Teach clients (people or families) on a one-to-one basis to modify dietary practices and activity levels.

Primary Prevention

Health Promotion and Education

- Provide nutrition education programs to promote awareness at schools, work sites, etc.
- Encourage restaurants and schools to offer healthy menu items.
- Recommend nutrition classes offered at neighborhood centers or healthcare facilities

Health Protection

- Promote physical fitness, proper nutrition, and wellness activities.
- Work with local entities to provide easier access to fresh fruits and vegetables, as well as provide bike paths and walking clubs, and to reduce easy access to sodas, tax high-calorie foods.

Tertiary prevention attempts to reduce the extent and severity of a health problem to its lowest possible level to minimize disability and restore or preserve function. The people involved have an existing illness or disability whose impact on their lives is lessened through tertiary prevention (AbdulRaheem, 2023; Iriarte-Roteta et al., 2020; Krishna, 2022). See more on clients living with disabilities in Chapter 24.

Examples include the following:

- Treatment and rehabilitation of people after a stroke to reduce impairment
- Postmastectomy exercise programs to restore functioning
- Early treatment and management of diabetes to reduce complications or slow their progression

In community/public health, the need to reduce disability and restore function applies equally to families, groups, communities, and people. Many groups form for rehabilitation and offer support and guidance for those recuperating from a physical or mental illness. Examples include the following:

- Support group for people recovering from alcohol use disorder
- Halfway houses for patients with mental health problems discharged from acute care settings
- Drug rehabilitation programs
- Political action committees to develop public policies that promote health and prevent disease

In broader community health practice, tertiary prevention is used to minimize the effects of an existing unhealthy community condition. Examples of such prevention are as follows:

- Insisting that businesses provide wheelchair access
- Warning community residents about the dangers of a chemical spill
- Recalling a contaminated food or drug product
- Preventing injuries among survivors and volunteers during rescue in an earthquake, fire, hurricane, mass casualty incident due to gun violence, or a terrorist attack

Health assessment of people, families, and communities is an important part of all three levels of preventive practice. C/PHNs working with a group of young parents who themselves have been victims of child abuse can institute early treatment for the parents to prevent abuse and foster healthy parenting of their children.

Health problems are most effectively prevented by maintenance of healthy lifestyles and healthy environments. School-based education to promote healthy lifelong habits and socioeconomic improvement to address SDOH are effective preventive measures. To these ends, community/public health practice directs many of its efforts to providing safe and satisfying living and working conditions, nutritious food, and clean air and water (AbdulRaheem, 2023; Iriarte-Roteta et al., 2020; Rudner, 2021).

COMMUNITY/PUBLIC HEALTH NURSING PRACTICE

During the first 70 years of the 20th century, community health nursing was known as **public health nursing**. The PHN section of the American Public Health Association's (APHA, 2024) definition of public health nursing (PHN) follows:

> Public health nursing is a specialty practice within nursing and public health. It focuses on improving population health by emphasizing prevention and attending to multiple determinants of health. Often used interchangeably with community health nursing, this nursing practice includes advocacy, policy development, and planning, which addresses issues of social justice (para. 3).

ANA adapted this definition for their third edition of *Scope and Standards of Practice for Public Health Nursing* (2022). The C/PHN practice continues to evolve, as society's needs evolve. Public health nursing and primary care providers both have a shared interest in prevention, health promotion, population health, and collaboration to coordinate care that provides better health outcomes (APHA, 2024).

The PHN is prepared at the baccalaureate level and is trained to make systematic and comprehensive assessments of population health and the many SDOH affecting "the application of interventions at all levels—people, families, communities, and the systems that impact their health" (APHA, para. 4). The later title of community health nursing was adopted to better describe where the nurse practices. For the purposes of this text, the term used for community health nurse and public health nurse is combined as community/public health nurse (C/PHN).

BOX 1-8 Key Principles of Public Health Nursing

1. The main PHN goal is "systematic and comprehensive population-focused assessment, policy development, and assurance" (p. 19).
2. "Equity is both a core public health value and a goal" (p. 19). Primary prevention takes precedence, prioritizing health promotion and disease prevention.
3. There is a focus on creating "healthy social, environmental, and economic conditions" for populations to flourish (p. 20).
4. Clients (including communities and populations) are equal collaborative partners in prioritizing, planning, policymaking, and developing strategies and programs.
5. Collaboration with a variety of "professions, organizations, and stakeholder groups," along with the population served, is the best way to ensure health protection and community well-being (p. 20).
6. PHNs have an obligation to "actively identify and reach out to all" who could benefit from services, especially vulnerable populations (p. 20).
7. The "optimal use of ... resources and creation of new evidence-based ... strategies" is vital to improving population health (p. 20).

ANA (2022); Adapted from Quad Council (1997), now Council of Public Health Nursing Organizations (CPHNO).

The key principles of public health nursing in Box 1-8 are particularly salient to the practice of this specialty.

Many types of professionals are involved in public health, forming a complex team, such as:

- A city planner designing an urban renewal project
- A social worker providing counseling about child abuse or working with adolescent with substance use disorder
- A primary provider treating clients affected by a sudden outbreak of hepatitis and assisting public health epidemiologists and public health nurses (PHNs) to determine the source
- Those working in prenatal clinics, programs providing meals for older adults, genetic counseling centers, and educational programs for early detection of cancer

The professional nurse is an integral member of this team, a linchpin and a liaison between primary providers, social workers, government officials, and law enforcement officers. Community/public health nurses (C/PHNs) work in every conceivable kind of community agency, from a state public health department to a community-based advocacy group. Their duties vary:

- Examining infants in a well-baby clinic to teaching older adult stroke victims in their homes
- Planning community and population-focused interventions (e.g., marketing campaigns to reduce tobacco use)
- Conducting epidemiologic research, health policy analysis, and decision making

Despite its breadth, public health nursing is a specialized practice, generally requiring a bachelor's degree, and additional certification is needed in some states (ANA, 2022).

Historically, as a practice specialty, public health has been associated primarily with the efforts of official or government entities—for example, federal, state, or local tax-supported health agencies that target a wide range of health issues. In contrast, private health efforts or nongovernmental organizations, such as those of the American Lung Association or the American Cancer Society, often work toward solving selected health problems. The latter augments the former. Currently, community/public health practice encompasses both approaches and works collaboratively with all health agencies and efforts, public or private, concerned with the public's health. In this text, community health practice refers to a focus on specific, designated communities. It is a part of the larger public health effort and recognizes the fundamental concepts and principles of public health as its birthright and foundation for practice.

As a specialty field of nursing, community/public health nursing adds public health knowledge and skills that address the needs and problems of communities and aggregates and focuses care on communities and vulnerable populations. Recognition of this specialty field continues with a greater awareness of the important contributions made by community/public health nursing to improve the health of the public.

- Community/public health nursing is grounded in both public health science and nursing science, which makes its philosophical orientation and the nature of its practice unique. It has been recognized as a subspecialty of both fields (ANA, 2022).

Knowledge of the following elements of public health is essential to community/public health nursing (ANA, 2022; Campbell et al., 2020; Quad Council—now Council of Public Health Nursing Organizations [CPHNO], 2018):

- Priority of preventive, protective, and health-promoting strategies over curative strategies (see Chapters 11 and 12)
- Means for measurement and analysis of community health problems, including epidemiologic concepts and biostatistics (see Chapter 7)
- Influence of environmental factors on aggregate health, including emergency preparedness and recovery from disasters (see Chapters 9 and 17)
- Principles underlying management and organization for community health, because the goal of public health is accomplished through organized community engagement and cross-sector collaboration (see Chapters 6, 10, 12, and 15)
- Public policy analysis and development, along with health advocacy and an understanding of the political process (see Chapters 6 and 13)
- Research, evidence-based practice, and ethical decision-making, along with promotion of social and EJ (see Chapters 4 and 16, and Unit 6).

Confusion over the meaning of "community health nursing" arises when it is defined only in terms of where it is practiced. Because healthcare services have shifted from the hospital to the community, many nurses in other specialties now practice in the community. Examples of these practices include home healthcare, community mental health, geriatric nursing, long-term care, and occupational health. Although C/PHNs today practice in the same or similar settings, the difference often lies in applying the public health principles (health promotion and prevention) to large groups and communities of people—or having a population focus within the community one serves (Fig. 1-7).

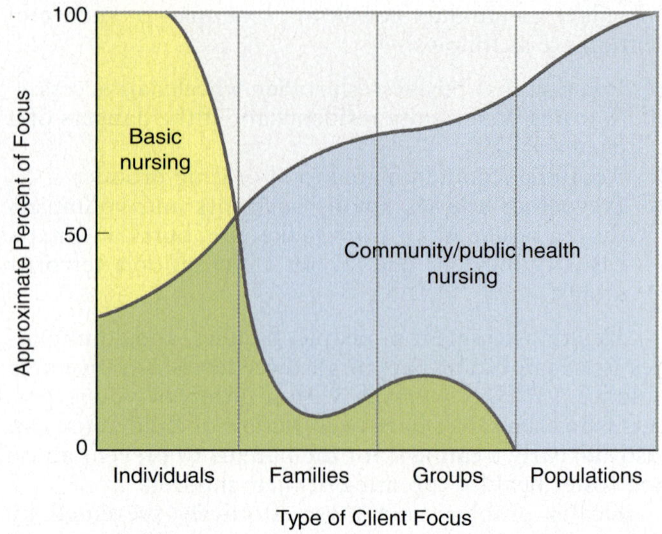

FIGURE 1-7 Difference in client focus between basic nursing and community/public health nursing.

For nurses moving into this nursing specialty, it requires a shift in focus—from people to a broader focus on aggregates and populations. Nursing and other theories undergird its practice, and the nursing process is one of its basic tools. See Chapters 14 and 15 for more details.

Community/public health nursing, then, as a specialty of nursing, combines nursing science with public health science to formulate a community-based and population-focused practice (Anderson & McFarlane, 2019).

Examples of community/public health nursing include:

- Developing a program for providing food and shelter for people who are homeless and sleeping in parks or vacant lots
- Collaborating to institute an educational program in the local school system on the dangers of vaping
- Assessing the needs of older people in retirement homes to ensure necessary services and provide health instruction and support

C/PHNs use primary, secondary, and tertiary levels of prevention that are evidence-based to develop programs, interventions, and services that help achieve health for all.

Population Focused

The central mission of public health practice is to improve the health of population groups. Community/public health nursing shares this essential feature with public health practice: it is **population focused**, meaning that it is concerned for the health status of population groups and their environment and prevention of disease (ANA, 2022; APHA Public Health Nursing Section, 2013).

A population may consist of older adults living throughout the community or of Syrian refugees clustered in one section of a city. It may be a scattered group with common characteristics, such as people at high risk of developing diabetes or people experiencing intimate partner violence living throughout a county. It may include all people living in a neighborhood, district, census tract, city, state, or province.

- A population-oriented focus requires the assessment of relationships. When working with groups and communities, the nurse does not consider people separately but rather in context—that is, in relationship to the rest of the community.
- When an outbreak of hepatitis occurs, the C/PHN does more than just work with others to treat it. The nurse tries to stop the spread of the infection, locate possible sources, and prevent its recurrence in the community.
- As a result of their population-oriented focus, C/PHNs seek to discover possible groups with a common health need, such as expectant parents, or groups at high risk for development of a common health problem (e.g., children at risk for type 2 diabetes due to obesity, victims of child abuse).
- C/PHNs continually look for problems in the environment that influence community health and seek ways to increase environmental quality. They work to prevent health problems and promote healthier lifestyles, such as promoting school-based education about nutrition and physical activity or exercise programs for older adults (Fig. 1-8).

The Greatest Good for the Greatest Number of People

A population-oriented focus involves a new outlook and set of attitudes. Individualized care is important, but prevention of aggregate problems in community/public health nursing practice reflects more accurately its philosophy, and it benefits more people. The ethical theory of utilitarianism promotes the greatest good for the greatest number (Savulescu et al., 2020). Further discussion of ethical principles in community/public health nursing can be found in Chapter 4.

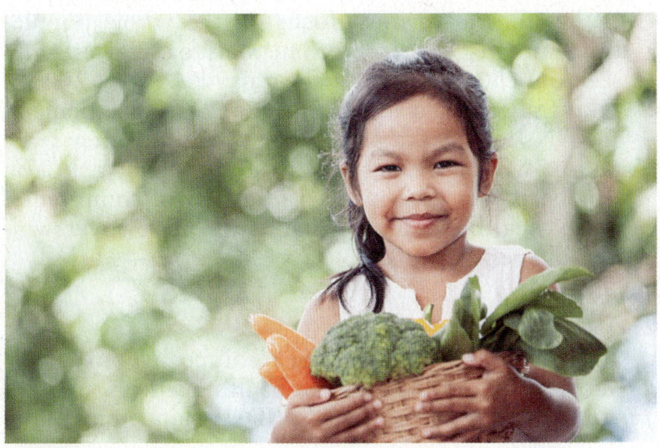

FIGURE 1-8 Healthy eating habits can begin in childhood.

Clients as Equal Partners

The goal of public health, increasing both the years and quality of healthy life and eliminating health disparities for populations, requires a partnership effort. Just as learning cannot take place in schools without student participation, the goals of public health cannot be realized without consumer participation. Community/public health nursing's efforts toward health improvement only go so far.

Clients' health status and health behavior will not change unless people accept and apply the proposals (developed in collaboration with clients) presented by the C/PHN. C/PHNs can encourage people's participation by promoting their autonomy rather than permitting dependency. For example, older people attending a series of nutrition or fitness classes can be encouraged to take the initiative and develop health or social programs on their own. Independence and feelings of self-worth are closely related. By treating people as independent adults, with trust and respect, C/PHNs promote self-reliance and the ability to function independently. Autonomy is an important objective of public health, as is equality (Rudner, 2021; Savulescu et al., 2020). These are discussed in more detail in Chapter 5.

When people believe that their health, and that of the community, is their own responsibility, not just that of health professionals, they will take a more active interest in promoting it. The process of taking responsibility for developing one's own health potential is called self-care (Ware et al., 2022).

- To this end, C/PHNs foster their clients' sense of responsibility by treating them as adults capable of managing their own affairs. Nurses can encourage people to negotiate healthcare goals and practices, identify and implement lifestyle changes that promote wellness, and learn how to monitor their own health. See Chapters 10 and 11.
- When planning for the health of communities, partnerships must be established and the values and priorities of the community incorporated into program planning and policymaking. Information and examples of program planning are found in Chapters 12 and 13.

Self-care includes meaningfully communicating with healthcare providers in a way that promotes understanding and then incorporating feedback to improve one's health. An important component of that involves health literacy. Health consumers may feel intimidated by health professionals and are unfamiliar with healthcare communication. They do not know what information to seek and are hesitant to act assertively. Obviously, the quality of care is affected when the consumer does not understand and cannot participate in the healthcare process. This is why health literacy is so important.

- Health literacy on an individual level is "the degree to which individuals have the ability to find, understand, and use information and services to inform health-related decisions and actions for themselves and others" (CDC, 2023, para. 1).

Health literacy is a two-way street. Organizational health literacy concerns the equitable enablement of clients to access, comprehend, and utilize services and information (CDC, 2023). Health literacy is discussed more fully in Chapter 10.

Prioritizing Primary Prevention

In community/public health nursing, the promotion of health and prevention of illness are a first-order priority. Less emphasis is placed on curative care.

Some corrective actions always are needed, such as cleanup of a toxic waste dump site, or stricter enforcement of day care standards, but community health best serves its constituents through preventive and health-promoting actions (AbdulRaheem, 2023; Ali & Katz, 2018; Anderson & McFarlane, 2019; Irriarte-Roteta et al., 2020). These include services to birthing parents and infants, prevention of environmental pollution, school health programs, fitness classes for older adults, and "workers' right-to-know" legislation that warns against hazards in the workplace.

Another distinguishing characteristic of community/public health nursing is its emphasis on positive health or wellness (Anderson & McFarlane, 2019). In contrast to acute care, community/public health nursing always has had a primary charge to prevent health problems from occurring and promote a higher level of health. C/PHNs concentrate on the wellness end of the health continuum in a variety of ways. Their goal is to help the community reach its optimal level of wellness. In clinical nursing and medicine, individual patients seek out professional assistance because they have health problems. They present their problems to the healthcare practitioner for diagnosis and treatment. C/PHNs, in contrast, seek out potential health problems in the community. They identify high-risk groups and institute preventive programs. C/PHNs visit clients in their homes and other settings (Fig. 1-9).

- For example, they watch for early signs of child neglect or abuse or domestic violence and intervene when any occur, often long before a request for help is made. See Chapter 18.
- They are watching for signs of potential mental health problems or substance misuse, insufficient nutrition or support, or other early warning signs that may resolve with early intervention. See Chapter 25.

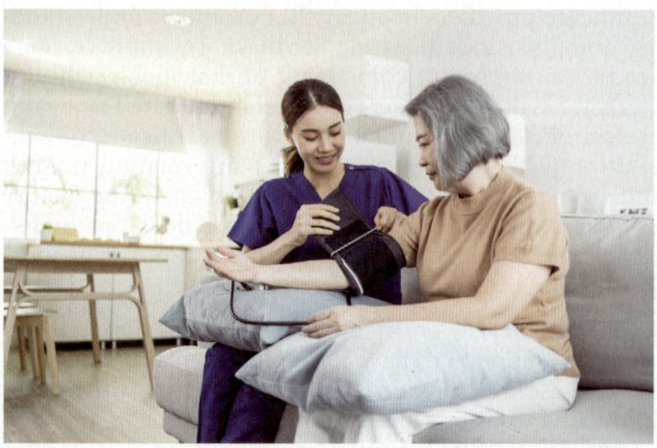

FIGURE 1-9 A C/PHN visits a client's home.

- They look for possible environmental hazards in the community, such as lead-based paint in older housing units, and work with appropriate authorities to correct them. See Chapters 9 and 13.

A wellness emphasis requires taking initiative and making sound judgments, which are characteristics of effective community/public health nursing (Iriarte-Roteta et al., 2020).

Selecting Interventions That Create Healthy Conditions in Which Populations May Thrive

With our population focus, it is prudent for C/PHNs to design interventions for the whole community, not limiting it only to those people seeking service or the poor and the most vulnerable. It is important to promote the health of entire populations and work to prevent injury, disease, and premature mortality.

- A recent study of 5705 PHNs from a national survey in 2377 counties found that where PHNs had higher levels of education and years of employment, there was a statistically significant association with lower rates of decreased physical inactivity and "reduced premature age-adjusted mortality rates" in those counties (Gwon et al., 2020, p. 829). An investment in C/PHNs pays health benefits.

Advocacy for our clients (people, families, aggregates, communities, or populations) is an essential function of community/public health nursing. We want to create healthy environments for our clients, and we do this by having a proactive stance with policy and legislative activities that promote health and prevent disease (ANA, 2022; Harris et al., 2022). More information about health advocacy and policymaking is provided in Chapter 13.

Actively Reaching Out

We know that some clients are more prone to develop disability or disease because of their vulnerable status (e.g., poverty, no access to healthcare, homelessness). Outreach efforts are needed to promote the health of these clients and to prevent disease.

- In acute care and primary healthcare settings, like emergency rooms or primary provider offices, clients come to you for service. However, in community/public health, nurses must focus on the whole population—not just those who come to us for services—and seek out clients wherever they may be (ANA, 2022).
- Like Lillian Wald and her Henry Street Settlement, C/PHNs must learn about the populations they serve and be willing to search out those most at risk. You can learn more about the rich history of community/public health nursing in Chapter 3. Unit 6 covers vulnerable populations.

Optimal Use of Available Resources

It is our duty to wisely use the resources we are given. For most state and local public health agencies, budgets are critically stressed, as the COVID-19 pandemic clearly revealed the many years of underfunding at all levels (Edmonds et al., 2020; Gaffney et al., 2020). For many decades, tertiary healthcare has gotten the largest percentage of our healthcare dollar, leaving decreased funds for primary and secondary services that are more cost-effective and pay dividends in better population health (as demonstrated by the above-mentioned study). The lack of regular sources of healthcare sends many people to expensive emergency departments for treatment, which could be averted with C/PHN intervention (Weiss & Jiang, 2021). The use of documented evidence as a basis for community/public health nursing practice promotes more efficient and cost-effective strategies in health promotion (American Nurses Association, 2022; Quad Council—now CPHNO, 2018).

Using personnel and resources effectively and prudently will pay off in the long run. It is vital that C/PHNs ground their practice in research and evidence (see Chapter 4) and use that information to educate policy makers about best practices (see Chapter 13).

Interprofessional Collaboration

C/PHNs must work in cooperation with other team members, coordinating services and addressing the needs of population groups. This interprofessional collaboration among healthcare workers, other professionals and organizations, and clients is essential for establishing effective services and programs.

Individualized efforts and specialized programs, when planned in isolation, can lead to fragmentation and gaps in health services. Interprofessional collaboration is an even greater necessity when working with population groups, especially those from vulnerable or at-risk segments. Collaboration improves client outcomes, staff communication, and the quality of care (Granrud et al., 2019; Moen & Jacobsen, 2022).

Collaboration involves working with members of other professions on community advisory boards and health planning committees to develop needs assessment surveys and to contribute toward policy development efforts. In addition to partnering with the population, other groups the C/PHN collaborates with include the following:

- Universities and researchers
- Local companies and trades/industries
- Advocacy groups and community action coalitions (e.g., food banks, childcare centers, homeless shelters) and community services (e.g., public schools, law enforcement, city planning, transportation, recreation, and emergency management services)
- Local churches and service groups
- City councils and other area or state policymakers
- Healthcare providers, hospitals/clinics, and public health agencies at the local, state, and federal levels
- Other public health professionals (e.g., environmental health specialists, health educators, social workers, epidemiologists, and nutritionists) (ANA, 2022).

Interprofessional collaboration requires clarification of each team member's role. When planning a citywide immunization program with a community group, for example, nurses need to explain the ways in which they might contribute to the program's objectives. They can share their knowledge of the public's preference about times and locations for the program, meet with various local agencies and organizations (e.g., health insurance companies, local hospitals) to gain financial support, help to organize and give immunizations, and influence planning for follow-up programs. Collaboration is discussed further in Chapter 10.

Another component includes development of policies to promote and protect the health of clients. Meeting with local legislators and providing testimony to local, state, and national bodies are common methods of ensuring enactment of effective health policies. See Chapter 13.

Client participation is promoted when people serve as partners on the healthcare team. An aim of community/public health nursing is to collaborate *with* people rather than do things *for* them. Community-based participatory research provides effective interventions to problems or issues identified by members of the community in partnership with academic researchers and C/PHNs (ANA, 2022; Zierold et al., 2020). See Chapter 4.

As consumers of health services are treated with respect and trust, their confidence and skill in self-care grows. C/PHNs encourage the involvement of healthcare consumers by soliciting their ideas and opinions, by inviting them to participate on health boards and committees, and by finding ways to promote their participation in decisions affecting their collective health. By assessing the needs of community, with input from members of the population, the C/PHN can discover the most pressing health needs and work toward more effective interventions. Community assessment and intervention are explored in depth in Chapters 12 and 15.

SUMMARY

- Community health is defined as the identification of needs and the protection and improvement of collective health within a geographically defined area.
- Public health is "the science of protecting and improving the health of people and … communities" (CDC Foundation, 2023, para. 1).
- A community is a collection of people who share some common interest or goal. Three types of communities were discussed: geographic, common-interest, and health problem-solving communities.
- A population refers to all people occupying an area or to all of those who share one or more characteristics but may or may not interact with each other.
- An aggregate refers to a grouping of distinct people who are considered as a whole and who are loosely associated with one another (e.g., older adults needing cholesterol and BP screenings).
- Health is an abstract concept that includes the many characteristics of a person, family, or community, whether physical, psychological, social, or spiritual.

- People have levels of illness or wellness known as the *health continuum*, and health has both subjective (how well people feel) and objective dimensions (how well they function).
- Healthcare needs may be continuing (developmental concerns that occur over a person's lifetime) or episodic (occurring unexpectedly over a lifetime).
- An upstream focus points to root causes for identified problems or conditions (e.g., air pollution that causes or aggravates asthma).
- SDOH are social conditions (e.g., education, employment/income, housing, safe neighborhoods, access to transportation, healthcare, healthy food) that contribute to the inequities in health outcomes, burden of disease, and quality of life.
- Health disparities are inequities that occur between the environments of people with higher incomes and those of low-income communities, people of color, and tribal and Indigenous populations.
- Environmental justice refers to all people (despite income, race/ethnicity) having equal protection from health/environmental hazards and equal participation in decisions about their environment.
- Levels of prevention refer to interventions at three levels: (primary) to prevent health problems, (secondary) to detect and treat the early stages of illness, or (tertiary) to preserve or restore function after an existing illness/disability.
- Eight important characteristics of community/public health nursing practice follow: the primary client is the population; achieving the greatest good for the greatest number of people; working with clients as equal partners (equity is both a value and goal); prioritizing primary prevention; focusing on strategies that create healthy environmental, social, and economic conditions; actively identifying and reaching out to all who might benefit; making "optimal use of available resources" and creating "new evidence-based ... strategies"; and collaborating with a variety of professions, populations, organizations, and other stakeholders to "promote and protect the health" of populations (Quad Council, 1997; cited in ANA, 2022, pp. 20–21).

ACTIVE LEARNING EXERCISES

1. Check local and state public health department websites for common (e.g., flu) and emerging or rare (e.g., communicable) diseases affecting population health. Search journals for articles on the origins of the infectious agent. How far did it travel? (Objective 1)
2. Research the County Health Rankings for your county. How did your county rank on health outcomes and health factors? How does it compare to your state and U.S. data for premature death rates, the percentage of adults over 18 reporting no physical exercise outside of work, rate of adult obesity, rate of sexually transmitted infections, and percentage of alcohol-impaired driving deaths? Describe one primary preventive C/PHN intervention, one secondary preventive intervention, and one tertiary preventive intervention for the most common health condition or risk behavior. Refer to the Levels of Prevention Pyramid and chapter content for examples. (Objective 2)
3. Find county, regional, or state websites for statistics on health outcomes in your county (e.g., chronic diseases like asthma, chronic obstructive pulmonary disease, heart disease; intentional [e.g., suicide] and unintentional injury [e.g., traffic/other injuries, poisoning, falls, fire, drowning]; life expectancy; infant mortality). Check county, regional, and other websites (e.g., U.S. News Healthiest Communities) for data on SDOH (e.g., demographics, equity, education, housing, environment) that may be upstream factors and midstream effects in the development of downstream conditions. (Objective 4)
4. Search scientific journals for research demonstrating negative health outcomes for populations reflecting similar demographics to your county or state. What interventions or actions are recommended? Talk to PHNs in your county about policies or programs developed to address specific inequities or poor health outcomes and their impact and community partners involved. With whom should you collaborate to assure effective interventions? (Objectives 3 and 5)

In Chapter 2, you will be introduced to the 10 Essential Public Health Services. For each case study/learning activity in the remaining chapters, you will need to identify the matching Essential(s).

CHAPTER 2

Public Health Nursing in the Community

"Healthcare is vital to all of us some of the time, but public health is vital to all of us all of the time."

C. Everett Koop

KEY TERMS

Advocate	Case management	Educator	Policy development
Assessment	Clinician	Leader	Researcher
Assurance	Collaborator	Manager	Transitional care

LEARNING OBJECTIVES

Upon mastery of this chapter, you should be able to:

1. Analyze the 10 Essential Public Health Services and their importance to the public health system.
2. Compare the core public health functions to the nursing process.
3. Examine the standards of practice for community/public health nursing.
4. Differentiate among the different roles of the community/public health nurse.
5. Explain the importance of each role in influencing people's health.
6. Analyze settings in which a community/public health nurse might practice.

INTRODUCTION

Historically, community and public health nurses (C/PHNs) have engaged in many professional roles. Nurses in this professional specialty have provided care to the sick, taught positive health habits and self-care, advocated on behalf of needy populations, developed and managed health programs, provided leadership, and collaborated with other professionals and consumers to implement changes in health services. Although the practice settings may have differed, the essential goal of the C/PHN has always been a healthier community. The home certainly has been one site for practice, but so too have public health clinics, schools, factories, and other community-based locations. Today, the roles and settings of C/PHN practice have expanded even further, offering a wide range of professional opportunities.

This chapter examines how the conceptual foundations, essential services, and core functions of community/public health practice are integrated into the various roles and settings of C/PHN. It provides an opportunity to gain greater understanding of how and where this nursing specialty is practiced. Moreover, it will expand awareness of the many existing and future possibilities for C/PHNs to improve the public's health. As you read through this chapter, think about client populations that you may have encountered in the acute care setting and consider your role with these same populations in a community setting. You may just discover a C/PHN specialty area that you have never considered.

ESSENTIAL PUBLIC HEALTH SERVICES

The Public Health Functions Steering Committee developed a list of 10 Essential Public Health Services in 1994 (Centers for Disease Control and Prevention [CDC], 2023). This initial effort was to define the service components essential to public health as these services apply to the core functions of public health. In March 2020, proposed revisions to the 10 Essential Public Health Services were distributed for comment; the final version was launched in September 2020 (CDC, 2023). As illustrated in Boxes 2-1 and 2-2, this framework and model shows the types of services necessary to achieve the core public health functions of assessment, policy development, and assurance. It also emphasizes the circular or ongoing nature of the process. The placement of equity in the center of the model represents the need to address health inequities, barriers, and discrimination in all public health services (Public Health National Center for Innovations, 2020). This implementation of the

BOX 2-1 *HEALTHY PEOPLE 2030*

Selected Public Health Infrastructure Objectives

Core and Developmental Objectives	
PHI-01, 02, 03, D07	Increase the proportion of state, tribal, and territorial public health agencies that are accredited.
PHI-04, 05, 06, D01, D02	Increase the proportion of state, local, tribal, and territorial public health agencies that use Core Competencies for Public Health Professionals in continuing education for personnel.
PHI-04, 05, D06	Increase the proportion of state, local, tribal and territorial jurisdictions that have a health improvement plan.
Research Objectives	
PHI-R04	Monitor and understand the public health workforce—composition, enumeration, gaps, and needs.
PHI-R05	Monitor the education of the public health workforce—degrees conferred, schools and programs of public health, and related disciplines and curricula.
PHI-R06	Enhance the use and capabilities of informatics in public health.
PHI-R08	Explore financing of the public health infrastructure.
PHI-R09	Explore the impact of community health assessment and improvement planning efforts.
PHI-R10	Explore the impact of accreditation and national standards.

PHI, public health infrastructure.

Reprinted from U.S. Department of Health and Human Services. (2020). *Public health infrastructure*. Retrieved from https://health.gov/healthypeople/objectives-and-data/browse-objectives/public-health-infrastructure

essential services for public health, combined with the core public health functions, is fundamental for successful population health outcomes.

CORE PUBLIC HEALTH FUNCTIONS

The various roles and settings for practice hinge on the three primary core functions of public health—assessment, policy development, and assurance—and are applied at three levels of service—person, family, and community (CDC, 2023; Institute of Medicine, 1988, 2002). Essential services that are linked to these core functions are found in Box 2-2.

Assessment

An essential first function in public health, assessment means that the C/PHN must first gather and analyze information that will affect the health of the people to be served. **Assessment** is the systematic collection, assembly, analysis, and dissemination of information about the health of a community. Health needs, environmental conditions, political agendas, financial, and other resources need to be assessed (Schneider, 2021). Data may be gathered in many ways (e.g., interviewing people in the community, conducting surveys, gathering information from public records, applying research).

At the community level, nurses perform assessment both formally and informally as they identify and interact with key community leaders. With families, the nurse can evaluate family strengths and areas of concern in the immediate living environment and in the neighborhood. At the individual level, the nurse identifies people within the family in need of services and evaluates their functional capacity using specific assessment measures and a variety of tools. Assessment of communities and families as the initial step in the nursing process is discussed more fully in Chapters 14 and 15.

Policy Development

Policy development is enhanced by the synthesis and analysis of information obtained during assessment to create comprehensive public health policy (Schneider, 2021). At the community level, the nurse provides leadership in convening and facilitating community groups to evaluate health concerns and develop a plan to address those concerns. Often, the nurse recommends specific training and programs to meet identified health needs of target populations (see Chapter 12) and raises the awareness of key policymakers about factors such as health regulations and budget decisions that negatively affect the health of the community (see Chapter 13).

With families, the nurse recommends new programs or increased services based on identified needs. Additional data may be needed to detect trends in groups or clusters of families, so that effective intervention strategies can be employed with these families.

At the individual level, the nurse assists in the development of standards for individual client care, recommends or adopts risk classification systems to assist with prioritizing individual client care, and participates in establishing criteria for opening, closing, or referring individual cases.

Assurance

Assurance is the pledge to our constituents that services necessary to achieve agreed-upon goals are provided by

BOX 2-2 10 Essential Public Health Services

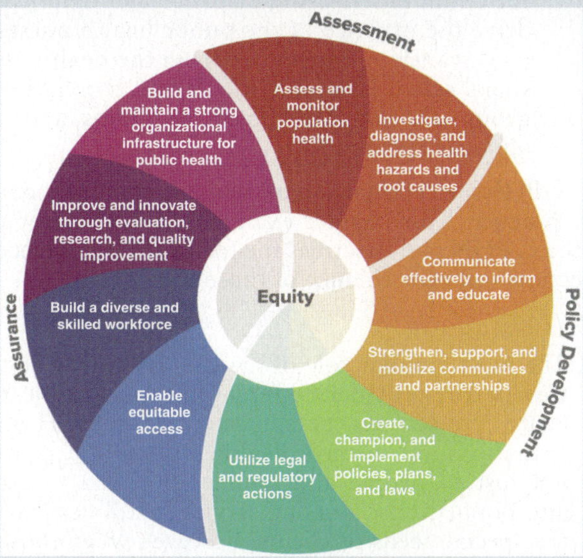

1. Assess and monitor population health status, factors that influence health, and community needs and assets.
2. Investigate, diagnose, and address health problems and hazards affecting the population.
3. Communicate effectively to inform and educate people about health, factors that influence it, and how to improve it.
4. Strengthen, support, and mobilize communities and partnerships to improve health.
5. Create, champion, and implement policies, plans, and laws that impact health.
6. Utilize legal and regulatory actions designed to improve and protect the public's health.
7. Assure an effective system that enables equitable access to the individual services and care needed to be healthy.
8. Build and support a diverse and skilled public health workforce.
9. Improve and innovate public health functions through ongoing evaluation, research, and continuous quality improvement.
10. Build and maintain a strong organizational infrastructure for public health.

Reprinted from CDC. (2023). *10 Essential Public Health Services* (revised, 2020). Retrieved from www.cdc.gov/public-health-gateway/php/about/

encouraging the actions of others (public or private) or requiring action through regulation or provision of direct services (Schneider, 2021). These activities often consume most of the C/PHN's time. Nurses perform the assurance function at the community level when they provide services to target populations, improve quality assurance activities, maintain safe levels of communicable disease surveillance and outbreak control, and collaborate with community leaders in the preparation of a community emergency preparedness plan. In addition, they participate in outcomes research, provide expert consultation, promote evidence-based practice, ensure competence and currency, and provide services within the community based on standards of care.

As you review these essential public health services and the core public health functions, think about what types of services might be provided. It is not necessary for the C/PHN to personally provide all of the listed services. Working in collaboration with an interdisciplinary team, the nurse can support the efforts of others to achieve improved health in the community. What is important is that the team members all recognize their respective roles and work toward the same goal.

STANDARDS OF PRACTICE

Since 1986, *The Essentials* series has been published and revised by the American Association of Colleges of Nursing (AACN) and serves as the educational foundation for baccalaureate and graduate nurses. The most recent published revision, *The Essentials: Core Competencies for Professional Nursing Education,* provides domains and competencies based on the ideal of nursing as a discipline with liberal education as a foundation utilizing competency-based education principles (AACN, 2021). This document provides ten domains with competencies for entry-level and advanced-level nursing education outcomes. The changes in *The Essentials* include a population health domain with associated competencies and a wellness, disease prevention sphere of care. These changes reflect and articulate the importance of preparing nurses to assume roles in the community setting and provide population healthcare (AACN, 2021).

C/PHN practice is further defined by specific standards developed under the auspices of the American Nurses Association (ANA) in collaboration with the Council of Public Health Nursing Organizations (CPHNO) formerly known as the Quad Council of Public Health Nursing Organizations (ANA, 2022). The CPHNO is composed of representatives from the Alliance of Nurses for Healthy Environments; the American Public Health Association, Public Health Nursing Section (APHA-PHN); the Association of Community Health Nursing Educators; and the Association of Public Health Nurses. These four organizations represent academics and professional practitioners, providing a broad spectrum of views regarding professional practice in C/PHN.

The CPHNO provides guidance on what constitutes public health nursing and how it can be differentiated from other nursing specialties. The standards of care it outlines are consistent with the nursing process and include assessment, population diagnosis and priorities, outcomes identification, planning, implementation, and evaluation. This document is an important reference for all those practicing in the community. It provides the basis for evaluating a person's performance in this field and is used by many employers to assess job performance.

The C/PHN also provides nursing services based on other standards developed by the ANA:

- Code of Ethics for Nurses with Interpretive Statements (2015)
- Nursing's Social Policy Statement (2010)
- Nursing: Scope and Standards of Practice (2021)

Each of these documents provides essential information regarding sound general nursing practice. When combined with *Public Health Nursing: Scope and Standards of Practice* (ANA, 2022), they provide the C/PHN with a clear understanding of accepted practice in this nursing specialty. Finally, Healthy People 2030 (USDHHS, 2020) emphasizes creating and supporting a competent public and personal healthcare workforce, and it includes competencies required for sound practice (see Box 2-1).

The Council of Public Health Nursing Organizations (CPHNO), formerly known as the Quad Council of Public Health Nursing Organizations, updated the Core Competencies for Public Health Professionals (see https://www.phf.org/resourcestools/Documents/Core_Competencies_for_Public_Health_Professionals_2021October.pdf). The competencies include eight domains:

1. Data Analytics and Assessment Skills
2. Policy Development and Program Planning Skills
3. Communication Skills
4. Health Equity Skills
5. Community Partnership Skills
6. Public Health Sciences Skills
7. Management and Finance Skills
8. Leadership and Systems Thinking Skills

The competencies consist of three tiers of practice, beginning with the front line and program support responsibilities in tier one, followed by the program manager and supervisory responsibilities in tier two, and ending with the senior management and executive leadership responsbilities in tier three.

With specific standards of practice and clear competencies to achieve, the C/PHN can integrate the core functions of assessment, policy development, and assurance, as well as the 10 essential services, throughout all of the various roles and community settings of practice.

ROLES OF C/PHNS

Just as the healthcare system is continually evolving, C/PHN practice evolves to remain effective with the clients it serves. Over time, the role of the C/PHN has broadened. This breadth is reflected in the description of public health nursing from the American Public Health Association Public Health Nursing (APHA-PHN, 2022):

> "Public health nursing is the practice of promoting and protecting the health of populations using knowledge from nursing and social and public health sciences" (para. 1).
> "Public health nurses interpret and articulate the health and illness experiences of diverse and often vulnerable residents to health planners and policymakers as well as assist members of the community. Using evidence and data [to] drive the practice of the public health nurses, who translate knowledge from the health and social sciences to individuals and population groups through direct care, programs, and advocacy" (para. 3).

C/PHNs wear many hats while conducting day-to-day practice. This chapter examines several major roles of the C/PHN and describes the factors that influence the selection and performance of those roles.

Clinician Role

- The most familiar role of the C/PHN is that of **clinician** or care provider. Different from such a role in the acute care setting, the clinician role in C/PH means that the nurse ensures health services are provided not just to people and families but also to groups and populations. Nursing service is still designed for the special needs of clients; however, when those clients compose a group or population, clinical practice takes different forms. It requires different skills to assess collective needs and tailor service accordingly. For instance, one C/PHN might visit residents in an apartment building for older adults. Another might serve as the clinic nurse in a rural prenatal clinic that serves migrant farm workers. These are opportunities to assess the needs of aggregates and design appropriate services.
- For C/PHNs, the clinician role involves certain emphases that are different from those of basic nursing. Three clinician emphases, in particular, are useful to consider here: holism, health promotion, and skill expansion.

Holistic Practice

- Most clinical nursing seeks to be broad and holistic. It is essential that community health nurses incorporate this holistic approach. The holistic approach considers a broad range of needs—physical, emotional, social, spiritual, and economic—that affect the collective health of the population, family, and person. The healthcare delivery system is complex; it is important that C/PHN provide a holistic approach that includes advocacy, coordination of services, and policy development while providing care to the client (Thorton, 2019).
- In C/PH, the client is a composite of people whose relationships and interactions with each other must be considered in totality. Holistic practice must emerge from this system's perspective (Fig. 2-1).

For example, when working with a group of pregnant teenagers living in a juvenile detention center, the nurse would consider the teens' relationships with one another, their parents, the fathers of their unborn children, and the detention center staff. The nurse would evaluate their ages, developmental needs, and

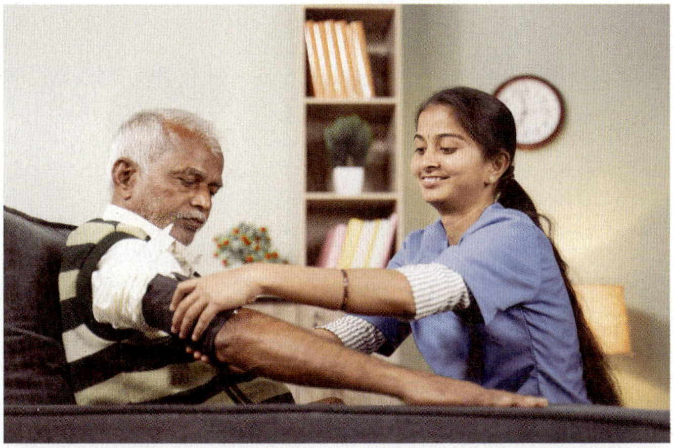

FIGURE 2-1 Community and public health nurse student making an in-home visit to an older client.

peer influences, as well as their knowledge of pregnancy, delivery, and issues related to the choice of keeping or giving up their babies. The teens' reentry into the community and their future plans for school or employment would also be considered. Holistic service would go far beyond the physical condition of pregnancy and childbirth. It would incorporate consideration of pregnant adolescents in this community as a population at risk. What factors contributed to these teens' situations, and what preventive efforts could be instituted to protect these or other teens from future pregnancies? The clinician role of the C/PHN involves holistic practice from an aggregate perspective.

Focus on Wellness

- The clinician role in C/PH also is characterized by its focus on promoting wellness. As discussed in Chapter 1, the C/PHN provides service along the entire range of the health continuum, especially emphasizing the promotion of health and prevention of illness.
- The C/PHN may provide education to healthy aggregate populations (e.g., schoolchildren, pregnant people). Effective services also include seeking out clients who are at risk for poor health and offering preventive and health-promoting services, rather than waiting for them to come for help after problems arise.

Nurses identify groups and populations who are vulnerable to certain health threats, and they design preventive and health-promoting programs to address these threats in collaboration with the community (Murdaugh et al., 2019). Examples include immunization of preschoolers, family planning programs, blood pressure screening, and prevention of behavioral problems in adolescents. Protecting and promoting the health of vulnerable populations is an important component of the clinician role and is addressed extensively in the chapters in Unit 6, which cover vulnerable aggregates.

Expanded Skills

Nursing requires multiple skills, including observation, listening, communication and counseling, and integrates psychological and sociocultural factors into practice.

- Additionally, environmental and community-wide considerations—such as problems caused by pollution, violence and crime, drug misuse, unemployment, poverty, homelessness, and limited funding for health programs—have created a need for stronger skills in assessing the needs of groups and populations and intervening at the community level (CDC, 2019).
- The clinician role in population-based nursing also requires skills in collaboration with consumers and other professionals, community organization and development, research, program evaluation, administration, leadership, and skill in epidemiology and biostatistics, as well as an ability to effect change (ANA, 2022). These skills are addressed in greater detail in later chapters.

Educator Role

A second important role of the C/PHN is that of **educator** or health teacher. Health teaching, a widely recognized part of nursing practice, is legislated through nurse practice acts and is one of the major functions of the C/PHN (ANA, 2022).

The educator role is especially useful in promoting the public's health for at least two reasons:

1. Community clients are usually not acutely ill and can absorb and act on health information. For example, a class of expectant parents, unhampered by significant health problems, can grasp the relationship of diet to fetal development. They understand the value of specific exercises to the childbirth process, are motivated to learn, and are more likely to perform those exercises. Thus, the educator role has the potential for finding greater receptivity and providing higher-yield results.
2. A wider audience can be reached. With an emphasis on populations and aggregates, the educational efforts of C/PHN are appropriately targeted to reach many people. Instead of limiting teaching to one-on-one or small groups, the nurse has the opportunity and mandate to develop educational programs based on community needs that seek a community-wide impact.

Whereas nurses in acute care often teach patients one-on-one, focusing on issues related to their illness and hospitalization, C/PHNs go beyond these topics to educate people in a variety of areas. Community-living clients need and want to know about issues such as family planning, weight control, smoking cessation, and stress reduction. Aggregate-level concerns also include such topics as environmental safety, sexual discrimination and harassment at school or work, violence, and drugs. C/PHN teaching addresses questions such as: What foods and additives are safe to eat? How can people organize the community to work for reduction of gun violence? What are health consumers' rights? Topics C/PHNs teach extend from personal and family health to environmental health and community organization. Since the COVID-19 pandemic, telehealth (which is discussed in Chapter 10) has become an integral part of healthcare and is useful when needing to reach distant clients or groups. However, research has shown disparities among certain population groups regarding the utilization of telehealth services (Karimi et al., 2022). Thus, emphasizing the importance of the next role, advocacy. Health teaching as a tool for C/PHN practice is discussed in detail in Chapter 11.

Advocate Role

The issue of clients' rights is important in healthcare. Every patient or client has the right to receive just, equal, and humane treatment.

The role of the nurse includes client *advocacy*, which is highlighted in the ANA *Code of Ethics for Nurses with Interpretive Statements* (2015), *Nursing's Social Policy Statement* (2010), and *Nursing's Social Policy Statement: Understanding the Profession from Social Contract to Social Covenant* (Fowler, 2016). The current healthcare system is often characterized by fragmented and depersonalized services, and many clients—especially people with low or no income, those in disadvantaged groups, those without health insurance, and people with language barriers—frequently are denied their rights. They become frustrated, confused, discouraged, and unable to cope with the system on their own. The C/PHN often acts as an **advocate** for clients, pleading their cause or acting on their behalf. Clients may need someone to explain which services to expect and which services they ought to receive, to make referrals as needed, or to guide them through the complexities of the system and ensure the satisfaction of their needs. This is particularly true for underrepresented and disadvantaged groups (Fig. 2-2; Kalaitzidis & Jewell, 2020; Nsiah et al., 2019).

Environmental health advocacy is an important advocacy role of the C/PHN. Now more than ever, environmental issues are detrimentally influencing the health of populations. Air and water pollution, chemical and biologic contamination, and climate change have long been associated with negative health effects. It is imperative that C/PHNs advocate for environmental health policies and educate others regarding the environmental impact on health (Yakusheva et al., 2022).

Advocacy Goals

Client advocacy has two underlying goals:

1. Help clients gain greater independence or self-determination. Until clients can research the needed information and access health and social services for themselves, the C/PHN acts as an advocate for them by showing them what services are available, those to which they are entitled, and how to obtain them.

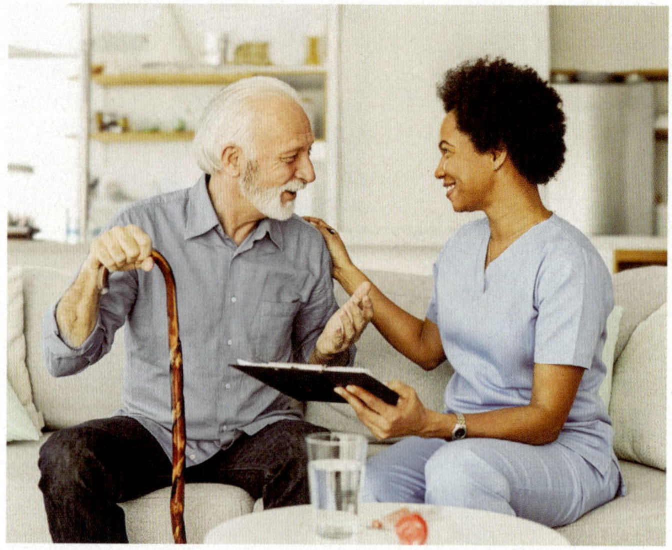

FIGURE 2-2 Like nurses working in every type of setting, community and public health nurses are advocates for their clients.

2. Make the system more responsive and relevant to the needs of clients (Nsiah et al., 2019). By calling attention to inadequate, inaccessible, or unjust care, C/PHNs can facilitate change can facilitate change through policy (see Chapter 13).

Advocacy Actions

The advocate role incorporates four characteristic actions: being assertive, taking risks, communicating and negotiating well, and identifying resources and obtaining results. Let's consider how a C/PHN might have taken each of these actions in the case of the Merrill family.

1. *Advocates must be assertive.* Fortunately, in the Merrill's dilemma, the clinic had a working relationship with the City Health Department and contacted Tracy Lee, a C/PHN liaison with the clinic, when Sarah broke down and cried. Tracy took the initiative to identify the Merrill's needs and find appropriate solutions. She contacted the Department of Social Services and helped the Merrill family to establish eligibility for coverage of surgery and hospitalization costs. She helped Sarah arrange for the baby's hospitalization and care for the other children.
2. *Advocates must take risks—go "out on a limb" if need be—for the client.* Tracy was outraged by the kind of treatment received by the Merrill family: the delays in service, the impersonal care, and the surgery that could have been planned as elective rather than as an emergency. She wrote a letter describing the details of the Merrill's experience to the clinic director, the chairman of the clinic board, and the nursing director. This action resulted in better care for the Merrill family and a series of meetings aimed at changing clinic procedures and providing better telephone screening.
3. *Advocates must communicate and negotiate well by bargaining thoroughly and convincingly.* Tracy stated the problem clearly and politely, yet firmly argued for its solution.

4. *Advocates must identify and obtain resources for the client's benefit.* By contacting the most influential people in the clinic and appealing to their desire for quality service, Tracy was able to facilitate change and hopefully improve service for other patients.

Advocacy at the population level incorporates the same goals and actions. Whether the population is people who are homeless, people experiencing intimate partner violence, or migrant children, the C/PHN in the advocate role speaks and acts on their behalf. The goals remain the same: to promote clients' self-determination and to shape a more responsive system through policy creation or policy change (Association of Public Health Nurses, 2021; see Chapter 13).

Manager Role

C/PHNs, like all nurses, engage in the role of a manager. The management process, like the nursing process, incorporates a series of problem-solving activities or functions: planning, organizing, leading, controlling, and evaluating (Bayot & Varacallo, 2022).

- As a **manager**, the nurse helps achieve clients' goals by assessing their needs, planning and organizing to meet those needs, directing and leading to achieve results, and controlling and evaluating the progress to ensure that goals are met.
- The nurse serves as a manager when overseeing client care as a case manager, supervising ancillary staff, managing caseloads, running clinics, or conducting community health needs assessment projects.

Nurse as Planner

The first function in the management process is planning. A planner sets the goals and direction for the organization or project and determines the means to achieve them.

- Planning includes defining goals and objectives. A good plan incorporates "SMART (specific, measurable, attainable, realistic, and time-bound) objectives (Bayot & Varacallo, 2022, para 2).
- Planning may be strategic. An example of *strategic planning* is setting 2-year agency goals to reduce opioid misuse in the county by 10%.
- Planning may be operational, focusing more on short-term planning needs. An example of *operational planning* is setting 6-month objectives to implement a new computer system for client recordkeeping.

The concepts of planning with people, families, and communities are discussed further in Chapters 12, 14, and 15.

Nurse as Organizer

The second function of the manager role is that of organizer. This involves designing a structure within which people and tasks function to reach the desired objectives. A manager must arrange matters so that the job can be done. People, activities, and relationships have to be assembled to put the plan into effect. In the process of organizing, the nurse manager provides a framework for the various aspects of service, so that each runs smoothly and accomplishes its purpose. The COVID-19 pandemic has solidified the fact that effective organizational skills are essential for adaptation to the constant changes in healthcare (Vázquez-Calatayud et al., 2022).

Nurse as Leader

In the manager role, the C/PHN also must act as a leader. As a **leader**, the nurse directs, influences, or persuades others to effect change that will positively impact people's health and move them toward a goal (Orukwowu, 2022).

- The leading function includes persuading and motivating people, directing activities, ensuring effective two-way communication, resolving conflicts, and coordinating the plan.
- Coordination means bringing people and activities together, so that they function in harmony while pursuing desired objectives.

An effective nurse leader is flexible and adaptive to change and incorporates the principles of nursing and leadership theories into practice. Effective leadership qualities range from effective communication and collaboration to ethical integrity and compassion. Leaders in nursing are needed to influence the change that is needed in healthcare (American Nurses Association, n.d.).

Nurse as Controller and Evaluator

The final manager functions are to control and evaluate projects or programs. A controller monitors the plan and ensures that it stays on course. In this function, the C/PHN must realize that plans may not proceed as intended and may need adjustments or corrections to reach the desired results or goals and must judge outcomes against original goals and objectives (Ballard et al., 2020).

An example of the controlling and evaluating function is evident in a program started in several preschool day care centers. The goal of the project is to reduce the incidence of illness among the children through intensive health education on prevention that addresses both the physical health and emotional health of the children with staff, parents, and children. At first, staff closely monitored the application of the prevention principles in day-to-day care, and the two C/PHNs managing the project were pleased with the progress of the classes. After several weeks, however, staff became busy and did not follow some plans carefully. Preventive activities, such as children coughing into a shirtsleeve and washing their hands after using the bathroom and before eating, were not being closely monitored. Several children who were clearly sick had not been kept at home. Staff often overlooked quiet or reserved children and did not include them in activities. To address these problems and get the project back on course, the nurses worked with staff and parents to motivate them. They held monthly meetings with the staff, observed the classes periodically, and offered one-on-one instruction to staff, parents, and children. One activity was to establish competition between the centers for the best health record, with the promise of a photograph of the winning center's children and an article in the local newspaper. Their efforts were successful.

Management Behaviors

As managers, C/PHNs engage in many different types of behaviors. First described in a classic book by Mintzberg (1973), the management roles were grouped into three sets of behaviors: decision making, transferring of information, and engaging in interpersonal relationships (Management at Work, 2019).

Decision-Making Behaviors. Mintzberg identified four types of decisional roles or behaviors: entrepreneur, disturbance handler, resource allocator, and negotiator.

- A manager serves in the *entrepreneur* role when initiating new projects. Until recently, nurse entrepreneurs were associated with advanced practice nurses. Starting a nurse-managed center to serve a population that is homeless is an example. However, nurse entrepreneurs have expanded to include a variety of areas. Nurse entrepreneurs are serving in a variety of areas including maternal–child, wellness, and education. Examples of these include the following: childbirth educator, doula, lactation consultant, health/mindfulness coach, aesthetician, spa owner, and online course developer/test question writer. The opportunities are endless for nurses to establish themselves as entrepreneurs (Carlson, 2023).
- C/PHNs play the *disturbance handler* role when they manage disturbances and crises—particularly interpersonal conflicts among staff, between staff and clients, or among clients (especially when being served in an agency).
- The *resource allocator* role is demonstrated by determining the distribution and use of human, physical, and financial resources.
- Nurses play the *negotiator* role when bargaining, perhaps with higher levels of administration or a funding agency, for new health policy or budget increases to support expanded services for clients (Management at Work, 2019).

Transfer of Information Behaviors. Three informational roles or behaviors include monitor, information disseminator, and spokesperson.

- The *monitor* role requires collecting and processing information, such as gathering ongoing evaluation data to determine whether a program is meeting its goals.
- In the *disseminator* role, nurses transmit the collected information to people involved in the project or organization.
- In the *spokesperson* role, nurses share information on behalf of the project or agency with outsiders (Management at Work, 2019). See Chapter 10 for more on communication.

Interpersonal Behaviors. While engaging in various interpersonal roles, the C/PHN may function as a figurehead, a leader, and a liaison.

- In the *figurehead* role, the nurse acts in a ceremonial or symbolic capacity, such as participating in a ribbon-cutting ceremony to mark the opening of a new clinic or representing the project or agency for news media coverage.
- In the *leader role*, the nurse motivates and directs people involved in the project.
- In the *liaison* role, a network is maintained with people outside the organization or project for information exchange and project enhancement (MindTools, n.d.).

Management Skills

Three basic management skills are needed for successful achievement of goals: human, conceptual, and technical.

- *Human skills* refer to the ability to understand, communicate, motivate, delegate, and work well with people (Cherry & Jacob, 2020). An example is a nursing supervisor's or team leader's ability to gain the trust and respect of staff and promote a productive and satisfying work environment. A manager can accomplish goals only with the cooperation of others. Therefore, human skills are essential to successful performance of the manager role.
- *Conceptual skills* refer to the mental ability to analyze and interpret abstract ideas for the purpose of understanding and diagnosing situations and formulating solutions (Liou et al., 2021). Examples are analyzing demographic data for program planning and developing a conceptual model to describe and improve organizational function.
- *Technical skills* refer to the ability to apply special management-related knowledge and expertise to a particular situation or problem. Such skills performed by a C/PHN might include implementing a staff development program or developing a computerized management information system (Liou et al., 2021). See Chapter 10 on technology in C/PHN.

Case Management

Case management has become the standard method of managing healthcare in the delivery systems in the United States, and managed care organizations have become an integral part of community-oriented care. **Case management** is a systematic process by which a nurse assesses clients' needs, plans for and coordinates services, refers to other appropriate providers, and monitors and evaluates progress to ensure that clients' multiple service needs are met in a cost-effective manner. Case management is integral to and encompasses other healthcare processes such as care management, disease management, and care coordination. Care management focuses on the holistic services, benefits, and programs that are available to clients and families. Examples include wellness programs, physical fitness/recreational activities, and social enrichment programs. Disease management focuses specifically on a disease process while incorporating case management to a disease process. Care coordination incorporates case management principles with a broader focus on population health. Patient care activities and healthcare services are communicated between multiple healthcare providers with patients and their families. For example, the C/PHN may work with people experiencing intimate partner violence who come to a shelter. First, the nurse must ensure that their immediate needs for safety, security, food, finances, and childcare are met. Then, the nurse must work with other professionals to provide more permanent housing, employment, ongoing counseling, and financial and legal resources for this group of people. Whether applied to families or aggregates, case management, like other applications of the manager role, uses the three sets of management behaviors and engages the C/PHN as planner, organizer, leader, controller, and evaluator (see Unit 6).

As clients leave hospitals earlier, as families struggle with multiple and complex health problems with meager resources, as more older people need alternatives to nursing home care, as competition and scarce resources contribute to fragmentation of services, and as the cost of healthcare continues to increase, there is a growing need for someone to oversee and coordinate all facets of needed service. The importance of case management is emphasized as a means to improve healthcare communication, control costs, and improve patient outcomes. (Giardino & De Jesus, 2023). Through case management, the nurse addresses this need in the community (Fig. 2-3).

Transitional Care

Case management is frequently associated with and used within transitional care. **Transitional care** involves managing the care of a client as they move within settings (i.e., Cardiac Care Unit to a medical-surgical floor), between healthcare settings (i.e., hospital to long-term care facility), across health continuums (i.e., home to assisted living), or between providers (i.e., primary care provider to oncologist) (National Association of Clinical Nurse Specialists, 2023). There are several models of transitional care (Ortiz, 2019):

- Colman's Care Transitions Intervention Model
- Naylor's Transitional Care Model
- Better Outcomes for Older Adults through Safe Transitions
- The New York State Department of Health (NYSDH) Transitional Care Model

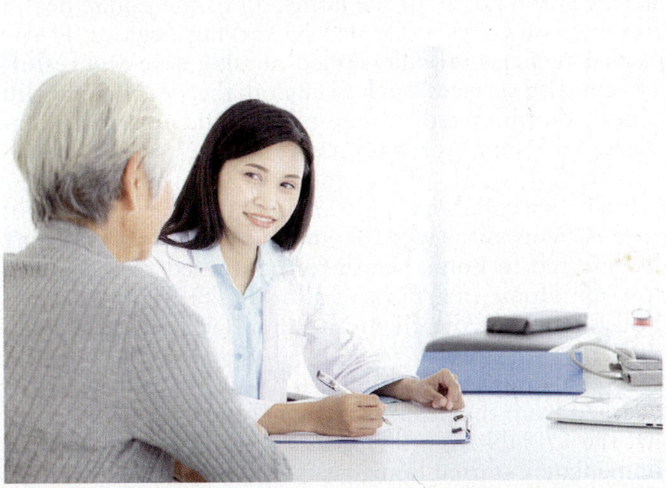

FIGURE 2-3 Community and public health nurses may serve as case managers for people experiencing intimate partner violence and other aggregates.

The NYSDH model is founded on five elements (Ortiz, 2019):

1. Determining the patient's strengths (e.g., emotional/cognitive, physical, medical, economic, abilities, support system)
2. Assessing the patient's functioning before admission to help determine potential resources needed on discharge
3. Informing decision making through ongoing collaboration among the patient, family, and interdisciplinary transition team
4. Providing both verbal and written information on available options and the range of community services
5. Allowing the patient and family to select preferred providers when possible

Transitional care is essential to ensure the continuity and coordination of healthcare services. It is essential for the C/PHN to collaborate with other healthcare providers to develop a plan of care that meets the client's healthcare goals (National Association of Clinical Nurse Specialists, 2023).

Collaborator Role

C/PHNs seldom practice in isolation. They work with many people, including clients, other nurses, primary providers, teachers, health educators, social workers, physical therapists, nutritionists, occupational therapists, psychologists, epidemiologists, biostatisticians, attorneys, secretaries, environmentalists, city planners, and legislators.

As members of the health team, C/PHNs assume the role of **collaborator**, which means working jointly with others in a common endeavor and cooperating as partners. When examining the success of collaboration in public health, the findings are mixed. However, these findings are related to the difficulty of measuring the variables of effective collaboration (i.e., leadership, allocation of resources, etc.). What is known is that when public health has collaborated, there have been successful C/PH outcomes (i.e., fluorinated water and seat belt laws) (Stabler, 2023).

The following examples show a C/PHN, employed by the local Area Agency on Aging, functioning as collaborator. Three families needed to find good nursing homes for their grandparents. The nurse met with the families, including the older adult members; made a list of desired features, such as a shower and access to walking trails; and then worked with a social worker to locate and visit several homes. The grandparents' respective primary providers were contacted for medical consultation, and, in each case, the older adult member made the final selection. In another situation, the C/PHN collaborated with the city council, police department, neighborhood residents, and manager of an older adults' high-rise apartment building to help a group of older people organize and lobby for safer streets.

Leadership Role

C/PHNs are becoming increasingly active in the leadership role, separate from leading within the manager role mentioned earlier. The leadership role focuses on effecting change; thus, the nurse becomes an agent of change. A broader attribute of the leadership role is that of visionary. A leader with *vision* sees what can be and leads people on a path toward that goal (Orukwowu, 2022).

As leaders, C/PHNs seek to initiate changes that positively affect people's health. They also seek to influence people to think and behave differently about their health and the factors contributing to it. The role of social determinants of health, such as the availability of health services and how the physical environment affects population health, is discussed in Chapter 11 in relation to health promotion of people and communities.

- At the community level, the leadership role includes health planning and may involve working with a team of professionals to direct and coordinate projects, such as a campaign to restrict marketing of e-cigarettes to adolescents or to lobby legislators for improved child day care facilities.
- When nurses guide C/PH decision making, stimulate an industry's interest in health promotion, initiate group therapy, direct a preventive program, or influence health policy, they assume the leadership role.

In one instance, it began as articulating the need for stronger C/PHN services to an underserved population in a neighborhood served by a C/PHN. In this densely populated, tenant-occupied neighborhood, drugs, crime, and violence were commonplace. One summer, an 8-year-old boy was shot and killed. The enraged immigrant families in the neighborhood felt helpless and hopeless. The nurse visited several families, and they shared their concerns with him. The nurse felt strongly about this community and offered to work with them to effect change. He gathered volunteers from neighborhood churches, and, together, they began to discuss the community's concerns. They prioritized their needs and began planning to make their community healthier. The nurse organized his workweek such that he could provide health screening and education to families in the basement of a church one morning each week. Initially, only a few families accessed this new service. In a matter of months, however, it became recognized as a valuable community service and was expanded to a full day; the increasing volunteer group soon outgrew the space. The C/PHN worked closely with influential community members and the families being served. They determined that many more services were needed in this neighborhood, and they began to broaden their outreach and think of ways to provide the needed services.

Within a year, the group had written several grants to the city and to a private corporation in an effort to expand the voluntary services. The funding that they obtained allowed them to rent vacant storefront space, hire a part-time nurse practitioner, contract with the health department for additional C/PHN services, and negotiate with the local university to have medical, nursing, and social work students placed there on a regular basis. The group, under the visionary leadership of the C/PHN, planned to add a one-on-one reading program for children, a class in English as a second language for immigrant families, a mentoring program for teenagers, and dental services. Even the police department had opened a substation in the neighborhood, making their presence more visible. This C/PHN's vision filled an immediate, critical need in the short term that developed into a comprehensive community center in the long term. Violence and crime diminished, and the neighborhood became a safer place where children could play.

Researcher Role

- In the **researcher** role, C/PHNs engage in the systematic investigation, collection, and analysis of data for solving problems and enhancing C/PH practice. Research is an investigative process in which all C/PHNs can become involved by asking questions and generating new knowledge (Ives Erickson & Pappas, 2020).
- The researcher role also includes evidence-based practice (EBP). It is important for C/PHNs to search the literature for evidence-based solutions and then implement those solutions into practice. The U.S. Department of Health and Human Services (USDHHS) incorporates resources utilizing EBP resources to evaluate *Health People 2030* objectives (USDHHS, n.d.). Chapter 4 will explain research in greater detail.

SETTINGS FOR COMMUNITY AND PUBLIC HEALTH NURSING PRACTICE

The previous section examined major C/PHN roles, which can now be placed in context by viewing the settings in which they are practiced. The sites are increasingly varied and include a growing number of nontraditional settings and partnerships with nonhealth groups. Employers of C/PHNs range from state and local health departments and home health agencies to managed care organizations, businesses and industries, and nonprofit organizations. This section provides a brief overview of the various settings.

Homes

Since Lillian Wald and the nurses at the Henry Street Settlement first started their practice in 1893 (see Chapter 3), the most frequently used setting for C/PHN practice has been the home. In the home, all of the public health nursing roles are performed to varying degrees. Home health agencies provide skilled nursing care and restorative health services, such as custodial care (home health aides), durable medical equipment, and pharmacy services. Additionally, rehabilitative services such as physical therapy, occupational therapy, and speech therapy services are collaborators to many home health plans of care. Clients discharged from acute care facilities may be referred to home health for continued care and follow-up. Home care nursing allows C/PHNs to obtain a holistic view of the client and family (Fig. 2-4; Maxell, 2022).

For example, Mr. White, 67 years of age, was discharged from the hospital with a colostomy. Jessica Levitz, the C/PHN from the county visiting nursing agency, immediately started home visits. She met with Mr. White and his wife to discuss their needs as a family and to plan for Mr. White's care and adjustment to living with a colostomy. Practicing the clinician and educator roles,

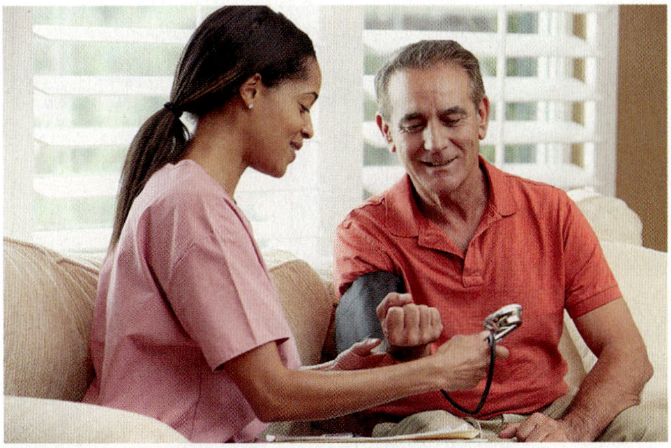

FIGURE 2-4 Community and public health nurses make home visits to assess and follow up with clients.

she reinforced and expanded on the teaching started in the hospital for colostomy care, including bowel training, diet, exercise, and proper use of equipment. As part of a total family care plan, Jessica provided some forms of physical care for Mr. White as well as counseling, teaching, and emotional support for both Mr. White and his wife. In addition to consulting with the primary provider and social service worker, she arranged and supervised visits from the home health aide, who gave personal care and homemaker services. She thus performed the manager, leader, and collaborator roles.

The home is also a setting for health promotion. Many C/PHN visits focus on assisting families to understand and practice healthier living behaviors. Nurses may, for example, instruct clients on parenting, infant care, child growth and development, diet, exercise, coping with stress, or managing grief and loss.

The character of the home setting is as varied as the clients served by the C/PHN. In one day, the nurse may visit a well-to-do widow in her spacious home, a middle-income family in their modest bungalow, an older transient man in his one-room fifth-story walk-up apartment, and a pregnant teenager and their infant living in a group foster home. In each situation, the nurse can view the clients in perspective and, therefore, better understand their constraints, capitalize on their resources, and tailor health services to meet their needs.

In the home, unlike in most other healthcare settings, clients are on their own "turf." They feel comfortable and secure in familiar surroundings and often are better able to understand and apply health information. A client's self-respect can be promoted, because the client is host and the nurse is a guest.

Sometimes, the thought of visiting clients' homes can cause anxiety. This may be your first experience outside the acute care, long-term care, or clinic setting. Visiting clients in their own environment may make you feel uncomfortable. You may be asked to visit families in unfamiliar neighborhoods and have to walk through those neighborhoods to locate the clients' homes. Frequently, fear of the unknown is the real fear—a fear that often has been enhanced by stories from previous nursing students. This may be the same feeling as that experienced when caring for your first client, first entering the operating room, or first having a client in the intensive care unit. However, in the community, more variables exist, and the nurse should follow the specific instructions given during the clinical experience and everyday commonsense safety precautions. General guidelines for safety and making home visits are covered in detail in Chapter 14.

Changes in the healthcare delivery system, along with shifting health economics and service delivery (discussed in Chapter 6), are moving the primary setting for C/PHN practice away from the home. Many local public health departments are finding it increasingly difficult to provide widespread home visits by their public health nurses.

Instead, many agencies are targeting populations that are most in need of direct intervention. Examples include families with low-birth-weight babies, clients requiring directly observed administration of tuberculosis medications, and families requiring ongoing monitoring because of identified child abuse or neglect. With limited staff and financial resources, the highest-priority clients or groups are targeted. Additional challenges to providing home care were created by the COVID-19 pandemic. Home health agencies responded by incorporating telehealth into practice. Telehealth or telemedicine refers to the communication of healthcare provider and client over the phone or internet (i.e., video chat). Telehealth allows for C/PHNs to monitor clients at home and may incorporate equipment to assess vital signs and other objective health data (USDHHS, 2023). With skills in population-based practice, C/PHNs serve the public's health best by focusing on sites where they can have the greatest impact. At the same time, they can collaborate with various types of home care providers, including hospitals, other nurses, primary providers, rehabilitation therapists, community aides, and durable medical equipment companies, to ensure continuous and holistic service. The nurse continues to supervise home care services and engage in case management. The increased demand for highly technical acute care in the home requires specialized skills that are best delivered by nurses with this expertise.

Ambulatory Service Settings

Ambulatory service settings include a variety of venues for C/PHN practice in which clients require day or evening services that do not include overnight stays. Examples include the following:

- A local public health department
- A clinic offering comprehensive services in an outpatient department of a hospital or medical center
- A comprehensive community or neighborhood health center
- A specialized clinic, such as a family planning clinic or a well-child clinic, in a community location convenient for clients, such as in a church basement or a pharmacy
- A day care center, such as for those with physical disabilities or behavioral health issues

- A nurse-managed health center, often provided as a community service component of a school of nursing, with the mission of enhancing student clinical experiences while meeting identified community needs in the areas of primary healthcare and health promotion
- A medical practice office, such as associated with a health maintenance organization and involving screening, referrals, case management services, counseling, health education, and group work
- An independent nursing practice in a community nursing center that also may include home visits
- A setting associated with a selected client group, such as a migrant camp, tribal land, correctional facility, children's day care center, faith community, coal-mining community, or remote frontier area

In each ambulatory setting, all of the C/PHN roles are used to varying degrees (Box 2-3).

Schools

- Schools of all levels make up a major group of settings for C/PHN practice. Nurses from C/PHN agencies frequently serve private schools at elementary and intermediate levels. Public schools are served by the same agencies or by C/PHNs who are hired directly by the school system.
- The C/PHN may work with groups of students in preschool settings, such as Montessori schools or Head Start centers, as well as in vocational or technical schools, junior colleges, and college and university settings. Specialized schools, such as those for students with developmental disabilities, are another setting for C/PHN practice (Fig. 2-5; ANA, 2017).

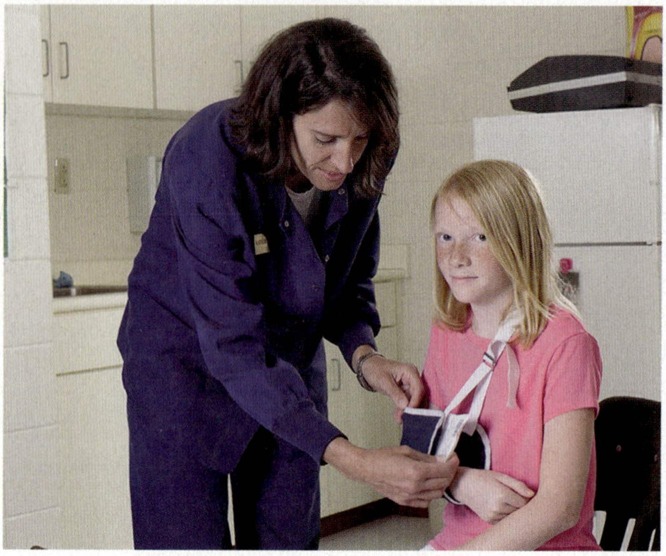
FIGURE 2-5 School nursing is another C/PHN role.

C/PHNs' roles in school settings are changing. School nurses, whose primary role initially was that of clinician (for person, family, and population health), are widening their practice to include more health education, interprofessional collaboration, and client advocacy. For example, one school had been accustomed to using the nurse as a first-aid provider and record keeper. Her duties were handling minor problems, such as headaches and cuts, and keeping track of such events as immunizations and medication administration at a local high school. This nurse sought to expand her practice and, after consultation and preparation, collaborated with a health educator and some of the teachers to offer a series of classes on personal hygiene, diet, and sexuality. She started a drop-in center for health counseling at the school and established a network of professional contacts for consultation and referral.

Nurses in school settings also assume managerial and leadership roles and recognize that the researcher role should be an integral part of their practice. The nurse's role with school-age and adolescent populations is discussed in detail in Chapter 20.

Occupational Health Settings

Occupational health settings range from industries and factories, such as an automobile assembly plant, to business corporations and even large retail sales systems. The field of occupational health offers a challenging opportunity, particularly in smaller businesses, where nursing coverage usually is not provided.

BOX 2-3 PERSPECTIVES

A Nurse Educator's Viewpoint on Public Health Accreditation

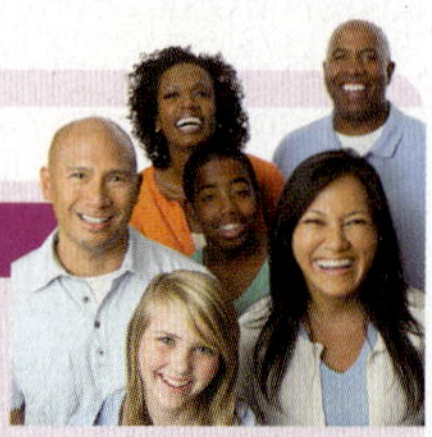

As a nurse educator with experience working in a rural, public health department, I have witnessed the evolution of public health accreditation from nonexistent to a standard of quality public health service. During the early 2000s, several healthcare and government stakeholders developed committees to examine the impact of national accreditation guidelines on public health departments. Findings from these organizations conceded that nationally developed accreditation standards were indicated. The Public Health Accreditation Board was later formed with the first public health accreditation standards approved. *Healthy People 2030* recognizes that public health accreditation strengthens the public health infrastructure and has several objectives focusing on public health accreditation. To date, accreditation is voluntary; however, hundreds of public health departments across the United States have received accreditation. I anticipate that in the next decade, public health accreditation will become a standard process.

Dana

Business and industry provide another group of settings for C/PHN practice. Employee health has long been recognized as making a vital contribution to individual lives, the productivity of business, and the well-being of the entire nation. Organizations are expected to provide a safe and healthy work environment, in addition to offering insurance for healthcare.

More companies, recognizing the value of healthy employees, are going beyond offering traditional health benefits to supporting health promotional efforts. Some businesses, for example, offer healthy snacks such as fruit at breaks and promote walking or jogging during the noon hour. A few larger corporations build exercise facilities for their employees, provide health education and wellness programs, and offer financial incentives for losing weight or staying well.

Residential Institutions

The most common residential institutions include assisted living and long-term care facilities. However, any facility where clients reside can be a setting in which C/PH nursing is practiced. Residential institutions also include transitional housing, in which clients live temporarily while recovering from substance use disorder. Additionally, there are community facilities for inpatient hospice programs, in which terminally ill clients live.

A continuing care center is another example of a residential site providing healthcare that may use C/PHN services. In this setting, residents are usually older adults; some live quite independently, whereas others become increasingly dependent and have many chronic health problems.

The nurse functions as an advocate and a collaborator to improve services. The nurse may, for example, coordinate available resources to meet the needs of residents and their families and help safeguard the maintenance of quality operating standards. Chapter 22 discusses the C/PHN's role with older adults. Sheltered workshops and group homes for children or adults with mental illness or developmental disability are other examples of residential institutions that serve clients who share specific needs.

C/PHNs also practice in settings where residents are gathered for purposes other than receiving care, where healthcare is offered as an adjunct to the primary goals of the institution. For example, many nurses work with camping programs for healthy children and adults offered by religious organizations and other community agencies, such as Scouting America and YMCA.

Other camp nurses work with children and adults who have chronic or terminal illnesses, through disease-related community agencies such as the American Lung Association, American Diabetes Association, and American Cancer Society. Camp nurses practice all available roles, often under interesting and challenging conditions and around the clock.

Another often overlooked practice setting is the correctional institution. People who are incarcerated, whether for the short or long term, have the same healthcare needs as the general public. The challenge to the nurse in this setting is to provide healthcare in an unbiased and nonjudgmental manner within the realities of the setting.

Because of the unique nature of this population, there are typically additional health and social service needs, often stemming from the reason for the incarceration in the first place (e.g., substance misuse) and placing them at increased risk for select health problems (e.g., AIDS, tuberculosis, poor nutrition). Residential institutions provide unique settings for the C/PHN to practice health promotion. Clients are more accessible, their needs can be readily assessed, and their interests can be stimulated. These settings offer the opportunity to generate an environment of caring and optimal quality healthcare provided by C/PHN services.

Faith Communities

Faith community nursing finds its beginnings in an ancient tradition. The beginnings of C/PHN can be traced to religious orders (see Chapter 3), and for centuries, religious and spiritual communities were important sources of healthcare.

In faith community nursing today, the practice focal point remains the faith community and the religious belief system provided by the philosophical framework. This nursing specialty may take different names, such as church-based health promotion, parish nursing, or faith community nursing practice. Whatever the service is called, it involves a large-scale effort by the church community to improve the health of its members through education, screening, referral, treatment, and group support.

The ANA, in collaboration with the Health Ministries Association, has published standards of care for faith community nursing practice in collaboration with the Health Ministries Association, Inc. (ANA, 2017). The standards act as guidelines for faith communities that plan to offer or are offering faith community nursing services. This specialty area of practice is guided by a variety of standards set up by several groups. Together, these standards provide guidance and direction for caregiving within the faith community. When C/PHNs work as faith community nurses, they enhance accessibility to available health services in the community while meeting the unique needs of the members of that religious community, practicing within the framework of the tenets of that religion.

Hospice Setting

Providing palliative and end of life care has long been associated with C/PHNs. Hospice involves palliative care at the end of life and may be provided in a variety of settings including an in-patient or home setting. The C/PHN serves as the case manager clients receiving hospice/palliative care. The focus of the plan of care is on comfort and the client's desires through a holistic lens. The ANA and the Hospice and Palliative Nurses Association (Dahlin, 2021) have established scope and standards of practice for palliative care.

Community at Large

When working with groups, populations, or the total community, the nurse may practice in many different places. For example, a C/PHN, as clinician and health educator, may work with a parenting group in a church or town hall. Another nurse, as client advocate, leader, and researcher, may study the health needs of a neighborhood's older adult population by collecting data throughout the area and meeting with university researchers or resource professionals in many places. Also, a nurse may work with community-based organizations such as an LGBTQ+ advocacy organization or a support group for parents experiencing the violent death of a child. Again, the community at large becomes the setting for practice for a nurse who serves on health-care planning committees, lobbies for health legislation at the state capital, runs for a school board position, or assists with flood relief in another state or another country (Fig. 2-6; see Box 2-4).

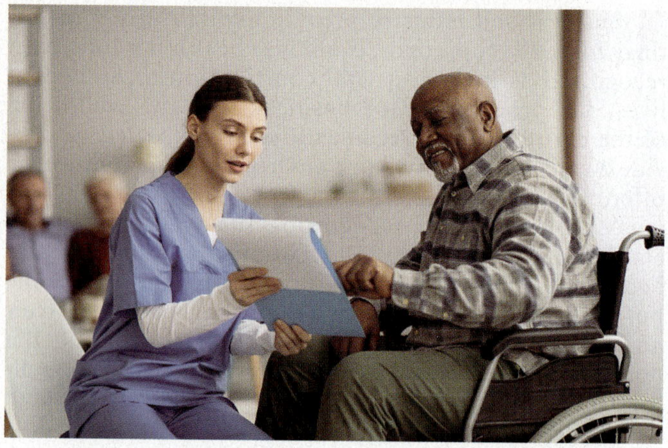

FIGURE 2-6 The community and public health nurse works with many different groups, including older adults.

Although the term "setting" implies a place, remember that C/PHN practice is not limited to a specific site but is a specialty of nursing that is defined by the nature of its practice, not its location, and it can be practiced anywhere. As you read through this chapter, perhaps an area of practice or a particular population captured your attention. If you are interested in tribal health, you might consider working as a U.S. Public Health Service nurse, or if you find that you are more interested in providing comprehensive health promotion programs to rural people, a nurse-managed health center may be of interest. Opportunities for C/PHN run the gamut from the American Red Cross, state and local health departments, the Peace Corps, to various international aid groups. Both private and public health agencies are actively seeking nurses with an interest in improving the health of their communities.

BOX 2-4 Innovative Community/Public Health Nursing Practice

In some C/PHN courses, students do not have access to an established agency such as a health department or community center from which to establish a client base. Student nurses and practicing C/PHNs can provide outreach services and do case finding in innovative settings such as these:

Settings	Clients	Roles of the Community Health Nurse
1. Centers for older adults when giving flu shots or when commodities are distributed	Older adults	Educator, clinician, advocate
2. Outside of grocery stores, department stores, movie theaters, large pharmacies (blood pressure checks and teaching/referrals; conducting surveys)	People of all ages and families	Educator, clinician, advocate, researcher
3. At parent–teacher association meetings, sporting events, dances, and school registration (in collaboration with school nurses; answer questions, provide health information and first aid, set up immunization clinics on site; check immunization records)	Young adults, children, and teenagers	Educator, clinician, advocate, collaborator, manager
4. Outside of concerts, plays, farmer's markets, etc. (answer questions, provide information, screenings, and referrals)	People of all ages	Educator, clinician, advocate
5. Conferences or seminars (present research, provide information)	Adults	Leader, educator, clinician, researcher
6. "On the street" (engaging with clients, making referrals)	People who are homeless, passersby, urban dwellers with low income	Educator, clinician, advocate

BOX 2-4 Innovative Community/Public Health Nursing Practice (*Continued*)

Settings	Clients	Roles of the Community Health Nurse
7. Truck stops (screenings, education, referrals)	Predominantly employed adults	Educator, clinician, advocate
8. Mobile clinics (seeing clients, making referrals)	People of all ages	Educator, clinician, advocate

Leader's role—initiate, plan, strategize, collaborate, and cooperate with community groups to present programs that are focused on specific populations' needs.

Educator's role—teach nutrition, stress management, safety, exercise, prevention of sexually transmitted diseases, and other adult health issues, child home/school/play and stranger safety, and child growth and development, and provide anticipatory guidance. Have pamphlets available to support verbal information on health and safety topics, specific diseases, social security, Medicare, and Medicaid.

Clinician's role—perform blood pressure screening, height, weight, blood testing for diabetes and cholesterol, occult blood test, hearing and vision tests, scoliosis measurements, and administration of immunizations.

Advocate's role—provide information regarding community resources as needed, cut "red tape" for those who need it, answer questions, and guide people to additional resources, such as websites and "800" phone numbers.

Collaborator's role—join with other social service and health professionals as team members to address the needs of clients (families, aggregates, communities).

Researcher's role—investigate an issue or problem, talk with community members, collect data, analyze results, and share outcomes (disseminate).

CASE STUDY 10 ESSENTIAL PUBLIC HEALTH SERVICES

Client Advocacy in the Home

Consider the experience of the Merrill family. Sarah Merrill has three small children. Early one Tuesday morning, the baby, Samuel, suddenly started to cry. Nothing would comfort him. Sarah went to a neighbor's apartment, called the local clinic, and was told to come in the next day. When she arrived, she was told that the clinic did not take appointments and was too busy to see any more patients that day. Sarah's neighbor reassured her that "sometimes babies just cry." For the rest of the day and night, Samuel cried incessantly. On Wednesday, Sarah and her children made the 45-minute bus ride to the clinic and waited 3 hours in the crowded reception room; the wait was punctuated by interrogations from clinic workers. Sarah's other children were restless, and the baby was crying. Finally, they saw the primary provider. Samuel had an inguinal hernia that could have strangulated and become gangrenous. The doctor admonished Sarah for waiting so long to bring the baby in. Immediate surgery was necessary. Someone at the clinic told Sarah that Medicaid would pay for it. Someone else told her that she was ineligible. At this point, all of her children were crying. Sarah had been up most of the night. She was frantic and confused and felt that no one cared. This family needed an advocate.

1. ***Recognize Cues:*** *Which findings require immediate follow-up, are unexpected, or are most concerning?*
2. ***Analyze Cues:*** *What information is noted or needed for interpreting findings?*
3. ***Prioritize Hypotheses:*** *Based on the information that you have, what is happening?*
4. ***Generate Solutions:*** *What intervention(s) will achieve the desired outcome?*
5. ***Take Action:*** *What actions should you take or do first?*
6. ***Evaluate Outcomes:*** *Were outcomes achieved? Why or why not?*
7. *Which Essential Public Health Services influence this situation? (See Box 2-2.)*

SUMMARY

- The various roles and settings for practice hinge on the 10 Essential Public Health Services, the three primary functions of public health—assessment, policy development, assurance, and equity—and are applied at three levels of service—person, family, and community.
- Assessment is the systematic collection, assembly, analysis, and dissemination of information about the health of a community.
- Policy development involves convening and facilitating community groups to evaluate health concerns and develop a plan to address those concerns, recommending new programs or increased services based on identified needs to address the needs of families, and developing standards for individual client care.
- Assurance is the pledge to provide services to clients that are necessary to achieve agreed-upon goals by encouraging the actions of others (public or private) or requiring action through regulation or provision of direct services.

- C/PHN practice is defined by specific standards of practice developed by organizations such as AACN, ANA, and the CPHNO in publications related to ethics, scope of practice, and core competencies.
- C/PHNs play many roles, including that of clinician, educator, advocate, manager, collaborator, leader, and researcher.
- There are many types of settings in which the C/PHN may practice. These settings can include homes, ambulatory service settings, schools, occupational health settings, residential institutions, hospice settings, faith communities, and the community at large.
- C/PHN practice is not limited to a specific site but is a specialty of nursing that is defined by the nature of its practice (i.e., population health), not solely its location.

ACTIVE LEARNING EXERCISES

1. Develop a plan of care using at least 3 of the 10 Essential Public Health Services (see Box 2-2) and the core public health functions when addressing a health risk in your community (e.g., opioid epidemic, low immunization rates, adolescent vaping, environmental hazards). (Objective 1)
2. Using the plan of care developed in Objective 1, compare this plan of care to the nursing process. (Objective 2)
3. Choose one of the C/PHN roles, discuss the similarities and differences between the C/PHN standards of practice compared to the ANA standards of practice. (Objective 3)
4. Think of a recent problem in your community and choose 3 roles outlined in this chapter that you, as a C/PHN, would use to help intervene in dealing with the problem. (Objective 4)
5. Compare the settings discussed in this chapter. What are the strengths and weaknesses of each setting? (Objective 6)
6. Discuss ways in which a C/PHN can make service holistic and focused on wellness with these groups:
   a. Preschool age children in a day care setting
   b. A group of adolescents who have a chemical dependence
   c. A group of older adults living in an older adults' high-rise building (Objective 5)

CHAPTER 3

History and Evolution of Public Health Nursing

"Our basic idea was that the nurse's peculiar introduction to the patient and her organic relationship with the neighborhood should constitute the starting point for a universal service to the region. We considered ourselves best described by the term 'public health nurses'."

—Lillian Wald (1867–1940), Pioneer of Public Health Nursing

KEY TERMS

American Nurses Association (ANA)
District nursing
Frontier Nursing Service
Henry Street Settlement
Industrial nursing
National League for Nursing (NLN)
National Organization for Public Health Nursing (NOPHN)
Population health
Rural nursing
Visiting nurse associations (VNAs)

LEARNING OBJECTIVES

Upon mastery of this chapter, you should be able to:

1. Describe community/public health nursing's professional development.
2. Compare the beginning of systems-based practice of selected past nursing leaders to current practice used by community/public health nursing.
3. Discuss the academic and advanced professional preparation of community/public health nurses.
4. Compare and contrast community health nursing with public health nursing.
5. Synthesize nursing's historical roots and the transformation of current community/public health nursing practice.
6. Identify the beginning of population-focused health and health promotion actions by public health nurses.

INTRODUCTION

You just left the home of a client who is concerned about a new family that just moved into the building where she lives. This family of six lives in an apartment with barely enough room for two. After years in this neighborhood, you are aware of the high rents charged for apartments with peeling paint, rodents, and garbage all around the buildings. Your client is concerned that the young mother looks "worn out" and coughs all the time. She said she tried to help, but the family doesn't speak much English. She describes four young children all under the age of about 5. She's never seen the husband, but you know that most of the men in this neighborhood leave early in the morning to try to get some day work, so you are not surprised. You thank her for the information and assure your client that you will do what you can to help her new neighbors. You start thinking about how you will prepare for the visit to the family who doesn't even expect you. At the top of your planning list is trying to find someone who speaks their language; you only know a few words. You suspect without even seeing the mother what the cough means, although you hope you are wrong. Then you think about the four young children living so close together and a mother who isn't well. The husband may want to help his wife more, but if he doesn't work, they don't have money to pay rent and buy food. You wonder if he has the cough too.

As you read this scenario, what picture comes to mind? What language is spoken in the home? What health concerns do you have for the family? Now, think about when this event might have occurred. If you thought this was a current scenario, it certainly could be, but this scenario was actually set in the early 1900s. This family emigrated and had not yet mastered the English language. The mother exhibits signs of consumption (the common name for tuberculosis at that time). Birth control information was not available to her. The typical tenement housing was small, crowded, and poorly lit. The husband found work as a laborer where he could. Few social services were available—if there was no work, then there was no food for the family, and no money to pay the rent. The family came to America with the hope of a new start, but they found harsh, urban living conditions. Social and charitable programs were available but fear of removal of the children from the home came with asking for assistance. Community/public health nurses (C/PHNs) in the early 20th century had to deal with many of the same issues we face today.

- Poverty, communicable diseases, poor housing, underfunded schools, lack of social services, and limited access to family planning and health information remain as challenges to improving the health of our population (see Fig. 3-1).

As a C/PHN, you will be facing similar challenges to those faced by nurses of the past. History is exciting because we get to hear the "voices" of nurses who have gone before us and to see what they endured and the extent of their dedication and service while establishing the profession. History is essential, for without it, we often fail to see patterns and learn from past actions.

- This chapter traces community/public health nursing's rich historical development, highlighting the contributions of several nursing leaders and examining the global and societal influences that shaped early and evolving community/public health nursing practice.
- The final section of the chapter describes the academic and advanced professional preparation required of C/PHNs today. Nursing's past influences its present, and both guide its future in the 21st century.

HISTORICAL DEVELOPMENT OF COMMUNITY/PUBLIC HEALTH NURSING

The history of community/public health nursing encompasses continuing change and adaptation (Donahue, 2011; Keeling et al., 2018). The historical record reveals a professional nursing specialty that has been on the cutting edge of innovations in public health practice and has provided leadership to public health efforts. (See Table 3-1 for information about the four general stages that mark the development of C/PHN.)

See Chapter 1 for a more complete discussion of the terms *public health nurse* and *community health nurse* and Chapter 2 for descriptions and discussion of the development of public health and community health.

In the historical evolution of this specialty, a shift in thinking about the focus of practice resulted in the broader use of the term *community health nurse* to refer to the generalist practice in this specialty. The title *public health nurse* now refers not just to those working in public health agencies but also to those working in many diverse community settings where population-focused nursing occurs (Edmonds et al., 2017; Kulbok et al., 2012). It is important to recognize that the work

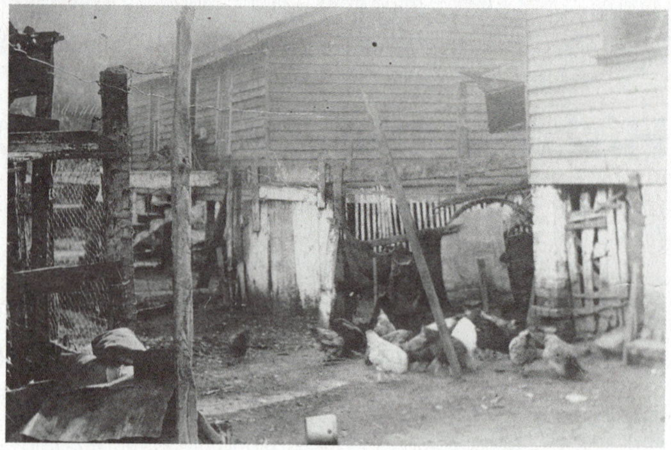

FIGURE 3-1 Public health nursing: where inspection begins. (From the American Red Cross and U.S. Medical Department of Sanitary Service (1917–1918). Retrieved from https://commons.wikimedia.org/wiki/File:Medical_Department_-_Sanitary_Service_-_Sanitation_-_Public_health_nursing._Where_inspection_begins_-_NARA_-_45499047.jpg)

TABLE 3-1 Development of Community Health Nursing

Period	Focus	Nursing Orientation	Service Emphasis	Institutional Base (Agencies)
Early home care (before mid-1800s)	Sick poor	Individuals	Curative	Lay and religious orders
District nursing (1860–1900)	Sick poor	Individuals; preventive	Curative; beginning of organized home visiting	Voluntary; some government
Public health nursing (1900–1970)	Destitute public	Families	Curative; preventive	Government; some voluntary
Emergence of community health nursing (1970–present)	Total community	Populations; illness prevention	Health promotion; practice	Variety; some independent

of the nurse is, as it always has been, to improve the health of the whole community, however, that community is defined. The term community/public health nurse (C/PHN) will be used throughout this text.

Early Home Care Nursing (Before Mid-1800s)

The Origins of Early Nursing

The early roots of home care nursing began with religious and charitable groups and the development of institutions devoted to the sick (Table 3-2; Pugh, 2001; Theofanidis & Sapountzi-Krepia, 2015):

- Deaconesses: Women in ancient Rome who cared for needy patients
- Knights Hospitaller: Warrior monks in Western Europe who protected and cared for pilgrims on their way to Jerusalem, founded in the early 11th century
- The Misericordia: A group of monks in Florence, Italy, who provided first aid care for injured victims on a 24-hour basis around the year 1244

During the 17th century, nursing care for low-income populations expanded in Europe and the New World:

- The colonial Spanish court sponsored the nursing brothers of the Order of San Juan de Dios (Saint John of God) to build a hospital in the capital city of Santiago, Chile, in 1617 to provide nursing care to people with no or low income (Huaiquián-Silva et al., 2013).
- In England, the Elizabethan Poor Law, written in 1601, provided medical and nursing care to people who lived in poverty or who were disabled.
- In France, St. Frances de Sales organized the Friendly Visitor Volunteers in the early 1600s (Dolan, 1978).
- In 1617, St. Vincent de Paul started the Sisters of Charity in Paris, France, an organization composed of nuns and laywomen dedicated to serving people who lived in poverty (Bullough & Bullough, 1978).

The Industrial Revolution (about 1760–1840) led to increased migration to cities from rural areas and from other countries. Small hospitals were built in large cities, and dispensaries provided greater access to medical treatments and medications from primary providers; however, medical education had no standardized curriculum until 1904 (Schwartz et al., 2018). Almshouses cared for people who could not care for themselves. Public health challenges included the following:

- Ships sailing into colonial American ports, such as Philadelphia, brought the threat of communicable diseases. The board of health required ships with ill crew members to wait outside of the port often spoiling merchandise onboard. To reduce loss, Philadelphia developed a quarantine site called the Lazaretto, which required all ships to stop and disembark anyone who was ill. The ship could then continue to Philadelphia ports, and on return, pick up crew members who had now recovered at the Lazaretto (Morman, 1984).
- Rural areas lacked primary providers and suffered injuries and illness.
- In urban Europe and America, overcrowding and poverty led to epidemics, high infant mortality, occupational diseases and injuries, and increasing mental illness.

TABLE 3-2 Landmarks in Nursing History: Pre-1800s

Time Frame	Landmark
Pre—middle ages	• Religious and charitable groups provided early care in the home. • Indigenous peoples used "shamans" or medicine men and women to provide care. • Little was known about disease origins.
500—1000	• The "Lady of the Manor" gave care. • Hildegard of Bingen, among other religious caregivers, provided nursing care.
650	• Hotel Dieu ("House of God") Hospital was established in Paris.
1000—1500	• Military orders, such as Knights Hospitaller of Jerusalem, cared for those returning from the Crusades. Men provided care. • St. Francis of Assisi (1182—1226) and St. Clare of Assisi (1194—1253) ministered to the sick. • The Maltese cross (shown below) was adopted as the insignia of the sick (later used on military nursing uniforms). 
1500—1800	• Religious nursing orders (e.g., Sisters of Charity) were founded and extended to America, Ireland, and Britain.

Source: Donahue (2011); Nutting and Dock (1907).

- Disease was rampant; mortality rates were high; and institutional conditions, especially in prisons, hospitals, and "asylums" for the insane, were deplorable.
- The sick and afflicted were kept in filthy rooms without adequate food, water, cover, or care for their physical and emotional needs (Bullough & Bullough, 1978; Duffy, 1992).

Dorothea Dix (1802–1887) fought for social justice for people who had mental illness and those who were abused and neglected in U.S. jails and almshouses. Her accomplishments included the following:

- In one of the first social research efforts in the United States, Dix toured places caring for those with mental illnesses and in the 1840s presented her firsthand accounts of the terrible living conditions to the legislatures of Massachusetts, New York, New Jersey, and Pennsylvania asking for government support to care for them (Dix, 2006; Reddi, 2005).
- Care for people who had mental illness improved as the number of institutions increased.

Florence Nightingale's Influence on Public Health

> "*Health is not only to be well but to use well the powers we have.*"
>
> —Florence Nightingale (1820–1910).

In England, Florence Nightingale came from a wealthy family and was educated. She desired a vocation for women outside of religious life. She trained at a nursing school in Germany and set out to provide nursing care (Fig. 3-2; Table 3-3).

Reading accounts of the war between Britain, Russia, France, and Turkey, Nightingale noted the high military mortality rates and wrote the Secretary of War to get involved. Taking 38 women with her to Scutari (1854–1856), Nightingale observed the deplorable conditions in the military hospitals, including thousands of sick and wounded men crowded together, lying in filth, without beds, food, water, or laundry facilities (Florence Nightingale Museum Trust, 1997; Goodnow, 1930, Chapter 2; Lee et al., 2013; Woodham-Smith, 1951). In response, she organized competent nursing care and sanitation, resulting in hundreds of lives saved. At the same time, Mary Seacole, of Jamaican Creole and Scottish parents, went to Scutari and nursed soldiers back to health using nursing and medical treatments she learned as a child from doctors (Staring-Derks et al., 2014). Both Nightingale and Seacole demonstrated that capable, holistic nursing intervention could prevent illness and improve the health of a population at risk—precursors to modern community/public health nursing practice (Hogan, 2015; Staring-Derks et al., 2014).

Nightingale's work with the military system was supported by the implementation of another public health

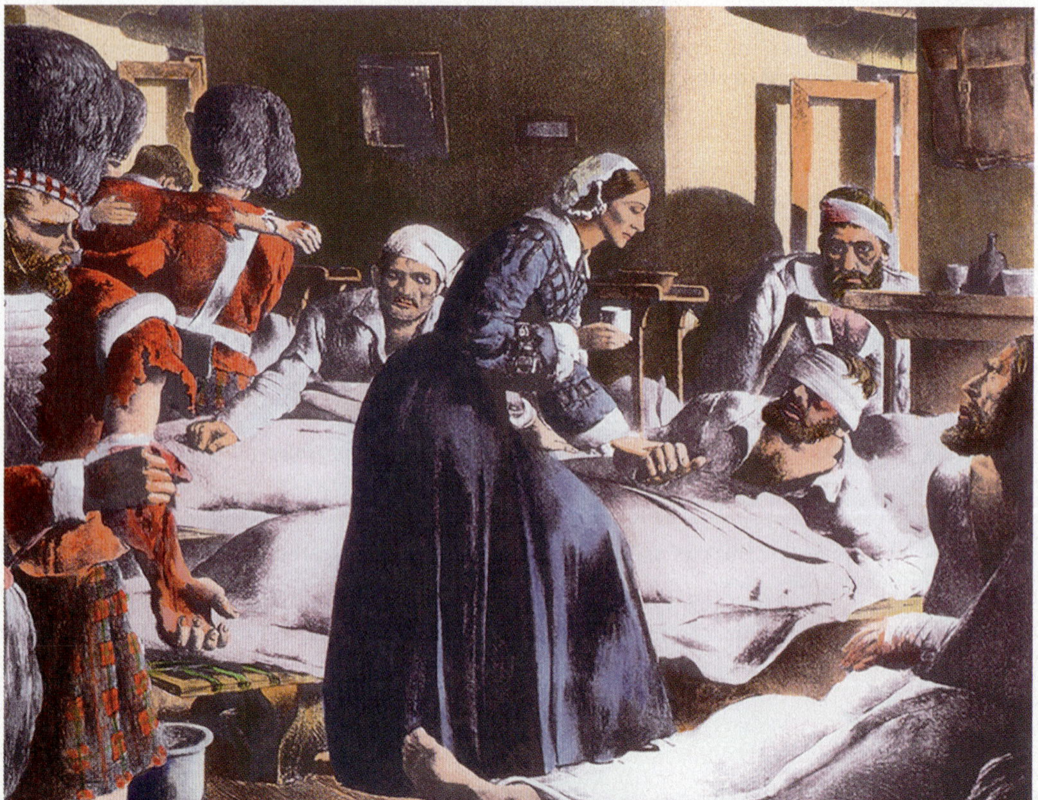

FIGURE 3-2 Florence Nightingale's concern for populations at risk, as well as her vision and successful efforts at health reform, provided a model for community health nursing today.

TABLE 3-3 Contributions of Florence Nightingale

Role	Result
Lobbyist	• Increased health standards and practice • Reformed military healthcare
Feminist	• Changed perceptions of women as nurses
Educator	• Developed standards of education for nursing practice • School at St. Thomas' Hospital, London, opened using Nightingale model
Military nurse	• Served in the Crimean War as nurse and administrator
Public health nurse	• Advocated holistic, population-focused care • Incorporated health promotion and disease prevention into practice model • Promoted five essential components to optimal health and healing: 1. Pure air 2. Pure water 3. Efficient drainage 4. Cleanliness 5. Adequate lighting
Author	• Wrote influential *Notes on Nursing* and *Notes on Hospitals*, among many other publications
Statistician	• Pioneered the use of statistics to change practice. • Harriet Martineau's *England and Her Soldiers* and Nightingale's *Sanitary Statistics of Native Colonial Schools and Hospitals* both incorporated her statistics and EBP to change medical and nursing care (Donahue, 2011; Rooney, 2016).
Architect	• After publication of *Notes on Hospitals*, her work became associated with long pavilion-style hospital wings, emphasizing light and ventilation (one is still visible today at St. Thomas' Hospital, London) (Richardson, 2010)
Social advocate/ reformer	• Advocated for people who were impoverished and disenfranchised, especially those in the military • Authored *On Trained Nursing for the Sick Poor*

Source: Donahue (2011); Florence Nightingale Museum Trust (1997); Lee et al. (2013); Nightingale (1969); Richardson (2010); Rooney (2016); Woodham-Smith (1951).

strategy: the use of biostatistics. Through meticulously gathered data and statistical comparisons, Nightingale demonstrated that military mortality rates, even in peacetime, were double those of the civilian population because of the terrible living conditions in the barracks—what we describe today as evidence-based practice (EBP) (Rooney, 2016). This work led to important military reforms and prioritization of hygiene (Lee et al., 2013). Florence Nightingale had the public's support for her work and became a skillful lobbyist for healthcare reform. Her exemplary influence on English politics and policy improved the quality of existing healthcare and set standards for future practice. Furthermore, she demonstrated how population-focused nursing works (Lee et al., 2013).

District Nursing (Mid-1800s–1900)

Nightingale's Influence on District Nursing

Nightingale's nursing knowledge influenced district nursing as well. In 1859, William Rathbone, an English philanthropist, became convinced of the value of home nursing as a result of private care given to his wife. In 1861, with Florence Nightingale's help and advice, Rathbone opened a training school for nurses connected with the Royal Liverpool Infirmary and established a visiting nurse service for the sick who lived in poverty in Liverpool. Her influence extended to rural **district nursing** programs, where nurses strengthened charity work with nursing actions (Howse, 2008; see Fig. 3-3).

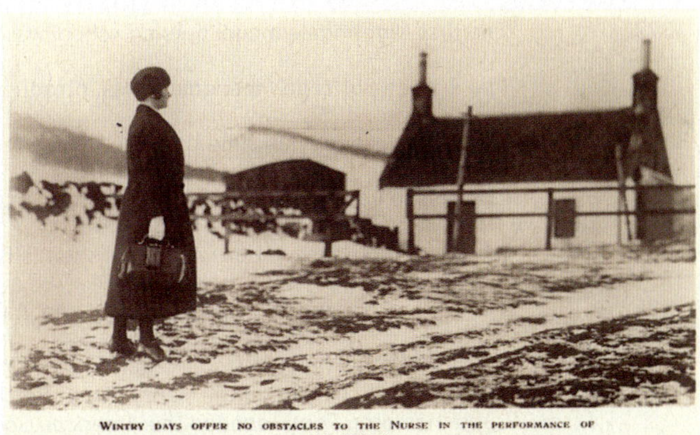
Wintry days offer no obstacles to the Nurse in the performance of her duties.

FIGURE 3-3 A Queen's District Nurse making a call in Scotland, 1927. (Retrieved from https://www.nlm.nih.gov/exhibition/picturesofnursing/exhibition2.html)

Florence Nightingale documented the need for community/public health nursing in her writings and recorded conversations:

- "Hospitals are but an intermediate stage of civilization. At present, hospitals are the only place where the sick poor can be nursed, or, indeed often the sick rich. But the ultimate object is to nurse all sick at home" (Nightingale, 1876, para. 8).
- "The aim of the district nurse is to give first-rate nursing to the sick poor at home" (Nightingale, 1876; also cited in Mowbray (1997, p. 24)).
- "The health visitor must create a new profession for women" (conversation with Frederick Verney, 1891; cited in Mowbray (1997, p. 25)).

Founding of the American Red Cross and Evolution of Disaster Nursing

In May 1881, Clara Barton and others founded the American Red Cross, modeling it after the International Red Cross, which was founded in 1863 and is responsible for global outreach and response in its humanitarian efforts (Table 3-4). Below are some milestones in the history of the American Red Cross:

- August 1881: A chapter was founded in Dansville, New York.
- September 1881: A devastating forest fire in Michigan claimed 800 victims; this was the newly formed organization's first disaster response, setting the stage for future fire response (Hanes, 2016).

TABLE 3-4 Landmarks in Nursing History: 1800–1900

Year	Landmark
1760–1840	The Industrial Revolution led to increased migration to cities, resulting in poverty, overcrowding, disease, mental illness, and increased mortality.
1845	Dorothea Dix addressed the New Jersey and Pennsylvania legislatures regarding abuse and neglect of people who had mental illness.
1848	The first women's rights convention in the United States was held in Seneca Falls, New York.
1849	Harriet Tubman escaped from slavery; she went on to lead many slaves to freedom through the Underground Railroad.
1853	John Snow linked a contaminated water pump to cholera epidemic in London.
1854	Florence Nightingale cared for the injured in the Crimean War.
1855	Mary Seacole established a boarding house and cared for sick and injured soldiers in the Crimean War.
1860	Florence Nightingale's *Notes on Nursing: What It Is, and What It Is Not* was published.
1861	The Civil War embroiled the United States until 1865. Harriet Tubman served as an unpaid nurse to wounded civilians and soldiers. Dorothea Dix was placed in charge of all women nurses in Union military hospitals.
1862	Louis Pasteur proposed the germ theory, which eventually led to the rejection of the "miasma" (bad air) theory of the origin of disease.
1865	Sojourner Truth served as a nurse for the Freedman's Relief Association during Reconstruction in Washington, DC.
1873	The first Nightingale model nursing school was established in the United States at Bellevue Hospital.
1878	The Woman Suffrage Amendment was introduced in the U.S. Congress.
1879	Mary Eliza Mahoney became the first African American to graduate from an American nursing school.
1881	Clara Barton and associates established the American Red Cross, and she became its first president.
1885	A visiting nurse association was established in Buffalo, New York.
1886	Visiting nurse associations were established in Philadelphia and Boston.
1893	Lillian Wald and Mary Brewster organized a visiting nurses service for people who lived in poverty in New York, which would be named the Henry Street Settlement in 1906. Isabel Hampton Robb founded the *American Society of Superintendents of Training Schools for Nursing* (later renamed the National League for Nursing).

Source: Bowery Boys (2018); D'Antonio (2017); Donahue (2011); Keeling et al. (2018); Lewinson et al. (2017).

- 1898: Clara Barton went to Havana, Cuba, during the Spanish–American War with supplies for victims, the first record of Red Cross military collaboration.
- 1905: Congress chartered the American Red Cross to provide relief during disasters and emergencies, support the military, help communities become more resilient, and conduct other well-known activities, such as blood collection.

Today the American Red Cross and the Medical Reserve Corps continue working toward the health and betterment of our local communities and our nation by giving assistance to those in need during both small and catastrophic crises (American Red Cross, 2020; Ye et al., 2014).

Home Visiting Takes Root

Although district nurses primarily cared for sick individuals, they also taught cleanliness and wholesome living to their patients, even during that early period (Kalisch & Kalisch, 2004). The problems of early home care patients in the United States were numerous and complex. Thousands of European and eastern European immigrants as well as African Americans migrating north from the South filled tenement housing in the poorest and most crowded areas of large eastern coastal cities during the late 1800s. Inadequate sanitation, infectious disease, unsafe and unhealthy working conditions, prejudices, and language and cultural barriers created inequalities between social classes (Table 3-5; Box 3-1).

Visiting nurses worked in Boston, Philadelphia, and Baltimore in the late 1800s often times connected to dispensaries and supported by philanthropic women. Isabel Hampton, superintendent of the Johns Hopkins Hospital Training School, worked to develop visiting nursing in Baltimore and publicized her ideas at the World's Fair in 1893. She fostered the need for further education for visiting nurses outside of their hospital diploma training and changed their jobs to include health promotion education alongside of providing sick care (Buhler-Wilkerson et al., 2021).

Public Health Nursing (1900–1970)

By the beginning of the 20th century, in the United States, advances in public health knowledge, laboratory sciences, and pharmacology increased the understanding of germs, communicability, and vaccination. These advances broadened district nursing to include the health and welfare of the general public, not just

TABLE 3-5 Some Public Health Issues of the 18th to the 20th Centuries

Communicable Diseases	Health Issues
Tuberculosis/consumption	Lack of sanitation/hygiene
Influenza	Contaminated/lack of clean water
Measles	Infections
Mumps	Nutrition/nutritional disorders/diseases
Rubella	Food preparation, harmful additives, and storage (spoiled food)
Typhoid	Temperature: heat and cold
Diphtheria	Vermin
Cholera	Cultural, religious, and superstitious beliefs
Smallpox	Respiratory diseases
Pneumonia	Chronic illness management
Pertussis, "whooping cough"	Maternity and postpartum care
Rheumatic fever	Well baby care
Scarlet fever	Alcohol use disorder
Meningitis	Domestic abuse
Tetanus	Medication administration
Yellow fever	Drug dependency (i.e., opiates in early medicines)
Polio	Surgical dressings/bandages (e.g., how to apply/change)
Malaria	Postoperative care (including illegal, as with abortions)
Conjunctivitis "pinkeye"	Household economy
Scabies, ringworm	Mental illness
Lice/typhus	Disasters
Fleas/plague	Poisoning (use of heavy metals in utensils and medicines common)
Epidemics/pandemics	Family planning/birth control
Isolation and quarantine	Trust

Source: Rosenberg (2008).

BOX 3-1 WHAT DO *YOU* THINK?

Communicable Diseases: Now Versus Then

What diseases can we treat today? Which have been eradicated worldwide? Discuss some recent outbreaks of historic diseases, including where, when, and why they occurred. Describe some new diseases that were not identified or did not occur in this time period. What are the roles of the C/PHN in health promotion and disease prevention?

people living in poverty (Duffy, 1992, Chapter 13). This new emphasis was part of a broader consciousness about public health. As demand rose, the number of private health agencies increased. These agencies supplemented the often-limited work of government health departments.

- In 1900, there were an estimated 200 public health nurses (PHNs); by 1912, that number had grown to 3000 (Gardner, 1936). This was an important development: "it brought healthcare and health teaching to the public, gave nurses an opportunity for more independent work, and helped to improve nursing education" (Bullough & Bullough, 1978, p. 143).
- Due to prejudice in hospital hiring in New York City, Jessie Sleet accepted a temporary nursing job with the Charity Organization Society's tuberculosis committee. Her nursing work was so effective at decreasing the TB morbidity and mortality rates in the African American population that she stayed in her position for 9 years and was replaced with two nurses when she left (Staupers, 1961). Credited as the first Black public health nurse, Jessie Sleet was a pioneer in early public health nursing practice (Table 3-6).
- By 1910, new federal laws made states and communities accountable for the health of their citizens. Catholic sisters and Lutheran deaconesses, as trained nurses operating out of motherhouses in various cities in the United States, provided care for local communities, sometimes working with other agencies such as the Red Cross (Keeling et al., 2018).

Nurses Making a Difference

Lillian D. Wald (1867–1940), a leading figure in the expansion of visiting nursing, first used the term *public health*

TABLE 3-6 Landmarks in Nursing History: 1900–1970

Year	Landmark
1900	Jessie Sleet Scales became the first African American public health nurse in the United States.
1900	Clara Barton led her final disaster relief effort with the American Red Cross, responding to a devastating Galveston, TX, hurricane.
1901	Clara Maass died after volunteering to test for yellow fever.
1902	The New York City Board of Education hired Lina Rogers Struthers as a school nurse and began the first public school nurse program in the country.
1902	The Pan American Sanitary Bureau, later the Pan American Health Organization is started with 11 countries of the Americas to collect data and exchange ideas to prevent epidemics.
1905	The American Red Cross received a congressional charter.
1906	The Pure Food and Drug Act was passed, prohibiting misbranding and adulteration of drugs and food.
1909	The Metropolitan Life Insurance Company provided the first insurance reimbursement for visiting nursing care.
1910	A public health nursing program was instituted at Teachers College, Columbia University.
1912	The National Organization for Public Health Nursing was formed, with Lillian Wald as the first president.
1914	Margaret Sanger published the monthly newsletter *The Woman Rebel* to promote contraception and was charged with distributing illegal "birth control" information.
1914	International Health Division of the Rockefeller Foundation spreads public health programs to Central and South America.
1917	The United States entered into World War I. Congress passed the 18th Amendment, ushering in Prohibition.

TABLE 3-6 Landmarks in Nursing History: 1900–1970 *(Continued)*

Year	Landmark
1918	The U.S. Public Health Service established the Division of Public Health Nursing to aid the war effort. World War I armistice occurred. Public health nurses went to Europe to help with recovery. Worldwide influenza pandemic began. Frances Reed Elliott became the first African American nurse accepted into the American Red Cross Nursing Service.
1919	The 19th Amendment was passed by Congress, giving women the right to vote.
1920	Women voted for the first time in a presidential election.
1921	Margaret Sanger founded the American Birth Control League to distribute contraception information. Sheppard-Towner Act legislation to decrease infant mortality using public health nurses.
1925	Mary Breckinridge established the Frontier Nursing Service.
1929	The U.S. stock market crashed (beginning of the Great Depression).
1930	The Tuskegee syphilis study began in Alabama (see Chapter 4).
1933	The 18th Amendment was repealed (Prohibition ends).
1935	The Social Security Act was signed into law.
1937	Birth control information was now legal in all but two states (Massachusetts and Connecticut).
1941	Elizabeth Brackett brings public health nursing to Chile and other countries under the Rockefeller Foundation's International Health Division.
1941	The United States entered into World War II and nurses were called to enlist.
1943	The Cadet Nurse Corps Program was established, providing federal funding for academic nursing education in exchange for work in "essential nursing services."
1944	The Public Health Service Act authorized qualified nurses to be commissioned in the U.S. Public Health Service.
1945	World War II ended. The United Nations voted to establish the World Health Organization.
1946	The Hill-Burton Act was approved, contributing to a shift to hospital-based care with federal funding of hospitals and medical centers. The Communicable Disease Center was established (a forerunner of the Centers for Disease Control and Prevention).
1949	Lucile Petry Leone became the Chief Nurse Officer of the Public Health Service, the first nurse and first woman to achieve a flag rank in the Public Health Service or military.
1950	The United States became involved in the Korean Conflict (which ended in 1953).
1954	In the case of Brown vs. Board of Education, a landmark Supreme Court decision prohibited racial segregation in public schools.
1955	The Salk polio vaccine was introduced (the first polio epidemic in the United States began in 1894, with a surge of cases noted in 1952).
1956	The Health Amendments Act provided funds to support public health nurse advanced training.
1960s	The Tuskegee syphilis study in Alabama ended.
1961	The Peace Corps was founded sending nurses to foreign countries. The United States entered into the Vietnam War and nurses were again needed for wartime nursing.
1965	Medicare and Medicaid were established.
1969	The National Environmental Policy Act provided first coordinated oversight effort. Based on the 1964 Surgeon General's report, passed national legislation requiring health warnings on cigarette packaging and ceasing broadcast media advertising.

Source: Donahue (2011); Keeling et al. (2008); The College of Physicians of Philadelphia (2020); Cueto and Palmer (2015); Uribe (2008).

nursing to describe this specialty (Ruel, 2014; Table 3-7). Visiting nurses, while caring for the sick, had pioneered in health teaching, disease prevention, and promotion of good health practices. Nurses working outside of the hospital increased their knowledge and skills in specialized areas such as tuberculosis, maternal and child health, school health, and mental disorders.

Lillian Wald's contributions to public health nursing were enormous:

- Appalled by the conditions of an immigrant neighborhood in New York's Lower East Side, she and a nurse friend, Mary Brewster, started the **Henry Street Settlement** in 1893 to provide nursing and social services.
- The Lower East Side was home to many European and Asian immigrants who lived in poverty, and the Henry Street Visiting Nurse Service visited sick children and families in their homes (Bowery Boys, 2018; Fig. 3-4).
- During one of the worst periods of economic depression, nurses from this organization supplied individuals and families with ice for keeping food fresh, meals, medicine, and sterilized milk; made referrals to hospitals and clinics, as needed; and "emphasized the human dignity of even the poorest" tenement families (Fee & Bu, 2010, p. 1206).

Wald's books, *The House on Henry Street* (1915) and *Windows on Henry Street* (1934), depict her work and convey her love of public health nursing (Fig. 3-5). The following website provides moving videos and photos of the neighborhood, Wald's *Baptism of Fire* and *The House on Henry Street*: https://www.henrystreet.org/about/our-history/exhibit-the-house-on-henry-street.

Wald's Growing Influence

Wald used her success at the Henry Street Settlement in reducing employee absenteeism as evidence to address the issue of childhood illness and school absenteeism (Bullough & Bullough, 1978; Hawkins & Watson, 2010). In the early 1900s, medical inspectors sent home about 15 to 20 children per day from each school in New York City for health-related reasons, but no one followed up with them to make sure that they were properly treated and returned to school. Wald suggested that placing

TABLE 3-7 Lillian Wald, Public Health Nurse and Social Activist

Year	Contribution
1893	Started Henry Street Settlement to serve low-income populations in NYC Lower East Side; first to use the term Public Health Nurse; expanded roles of nurses; used trained nurses instead of lay people to provide care (Ruel, 2014).
1900s	Developed project to address childhood illness, reducing school absenteeism; began first school nursing program (Bullough & Bullough, 1978; Hawkins & Watson, 2010; Kalisch & Kalisch, 2004; Vessey & McGowen, 2006).
1906	Hired Mrs. Elizabeth Tyler (Barringer), Miss Edith Carter, and Mrs. Emma Wilson as the first Black public health nurses to serve African American community leading to a satellite office at Stillman House (Fee & Bu, 2010).
1908	Worked to establish NYC Board of Child Hygiene (Ruel, 2014).
1909	Worked with Metropolitan Life Insurance Co. to reduce death rates by using visiting nurses to provide services to policyholders (Ruel, 2014).
1910–1912	Developed plan for national rural nursing service, which was developed with the American Red Cross to form American Red Cross Rural Nursing Service, later Town and Country Nursing Service (1913–1918), then the Bureau of Public Health Nursing. Program ended in 1947 (Ruel, 2014).
1912	Worked to establish Federal Children's Bureau; founder and first president of National Organization for Public Health Nursing; merged with the National League for Nursing (NLN) in 1952 (Christy, 1970; Feld, 2008; Lindenmeyer, n.d.).
1915	Wrote *The House on Henry Street* to highlight the achievements of the Henry Street Settlement (Wald, 1915).
1934	Published *Windows on Henry Street* describing work and views on public health nursing (Wald, 1934). Influenced social reforms: to establish health and social policies, improvements were made in child labor and pure food laws, tenement housing, parks, city recreation centers, treatment of immigrants, and teaching of children with cognitive disabilities (Kalisch & Kalisch, 2004; Ruel, 2014). Emphasized illness prevention and health promotion through health teaching and nursing intervention, as well as epidemiologic methodology as early EBP (Vessey & McGowen, 2006). Encouraged improved coursework at the Teachers College of Columbia University (New York) to prepare public health nurses for practice; modeled how nursing leadership, involvement in policy formation, and use of epidemiology led to improved health for the public (Ruel, 2014). Henry Street Settlement still in operation today: https://www.henrystreet.org/

Source: Bullough and Bullough (1978); Christy (1970); Donahue (2011); Fee and Bu (2010); Feld (2008); Hawkins and Watson (2003); Kalisch and Kalisch (2004); Ruel (2014); Wald (1915, 1934); Vessey and McGowen (2006); Staupers (1961).

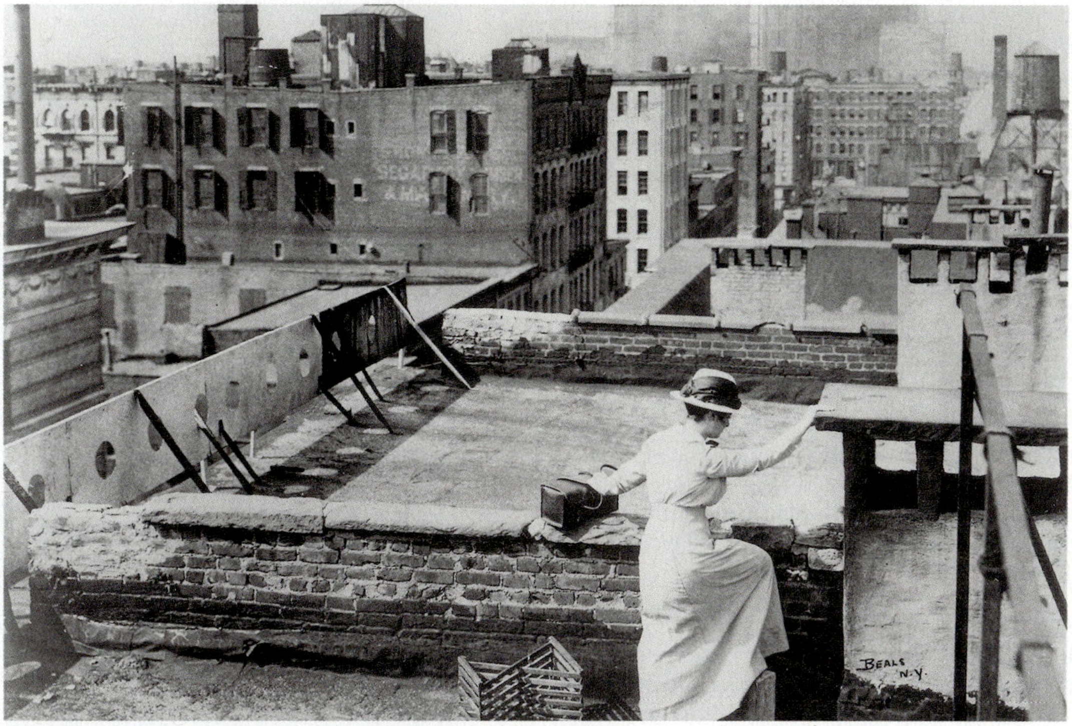

FIGURE 3-4 Iconic image of nurse crossing rooftops in New York City, 1908.

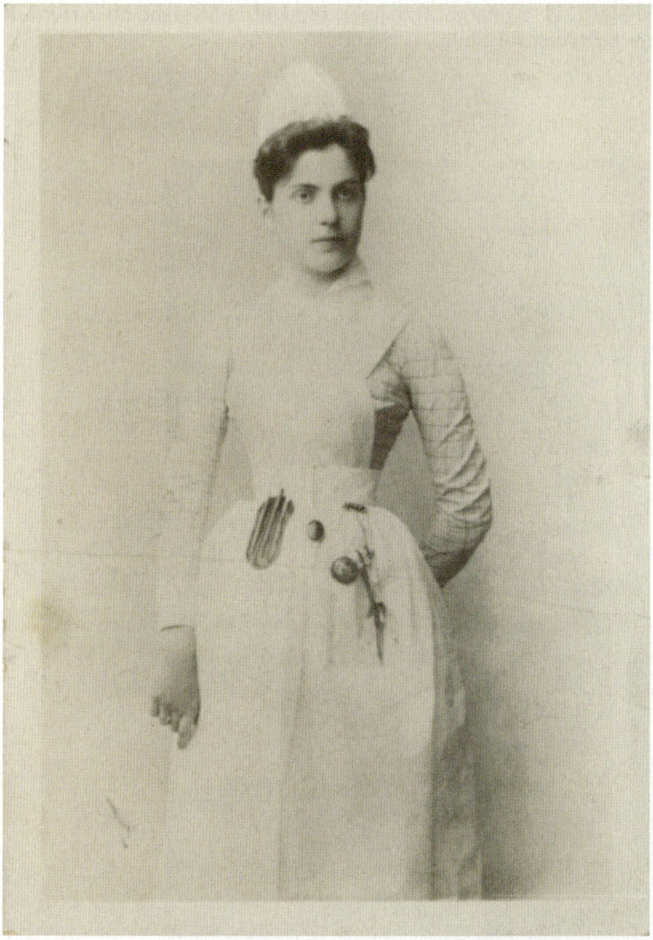

FIGURE 3-5 Lillian Wald as a student at New York Hospital Training School for Nurses, 1891.

nurses in the schools would allow for follow-up on recurring cases and home visits during the periods of exclusion. She argued that the nurses could supplement the work done by local primary providers, who occasionally examined the children. Offering the services of one nurse for 1 month, Wald hoped to demonstrate how effective a school nurse could be. Lina Rogers Struthers was the first school nurse appointed in this experiment (Kalisch & Kalisch, 2004). Within 1 year, the number of children sent home from school dropped dramatically, another example of EBP. By 1905, 44 nurses covered 181 public schools (Hawkins & Watson, 2010; Vessey & McGowen, 2006).

In 1909, Wald embarked on another visionary path. Using statistics from cases from Henry Street Settlement, she convinced the Metropolitan Life Insurance Company administrators that home visiting nurse intervention could reduce death rates (Buhler-Wilkerson, 2001; Hawkins & Watson, 2010; Hamilton, 2007). In collaboration with the Henry Street Settlement, the company organized the Visiting Nurse Department and provided services to policyholders in a section of Manhattan, beginning a program of **industrial nursing**. The success of this program resulted in expansion to other parts of the city and to 12 other eastern cities within a year. By 1912, the company had 589 Metropolitan nursing centers (Kalisch & Kalisch, 2004; Ruel, 2014). Industrial nurses proliferated after Wald's work with the Metropolitan Life Insurance Company in 1909 (Toering, 1919).

A Public Health Nursing Controversy

As Lillian Wald worked to alleviate suffering caused by disease and poverty, Margaret Sanger began a different battle to help women and children. Born in 1879, she saw her own mother die at age 49, after 18 pregnancies and a long battle with tuberculosis. She attended nursing school and began working as a visiting nurse (Ruffing-Rahal, 1986).

The Comstock Act of 1873 prevented her from providing her women clients any information on contraception to space their children, despite the fact that affluent and educated Americans had reliable contraception. Even discussing contraception was prohibited (Baker, 2011). In 1912, she watched helplessly as a 28-year-old mother of three died from abortion-induced septicemia—a woman who had earlier begged her for information on preventing future pregnancies (Ruffing-Rahal, 1986). Margaret Sanger opened her first birth control clinic in Brooklyn, but 10 days later, it was closed, and she was arrested (Fig. 3-6). She persisted and other clinics succeeded, resulting in the eventual formation of the International Planned Parenthood Federation (Baker, 2011).

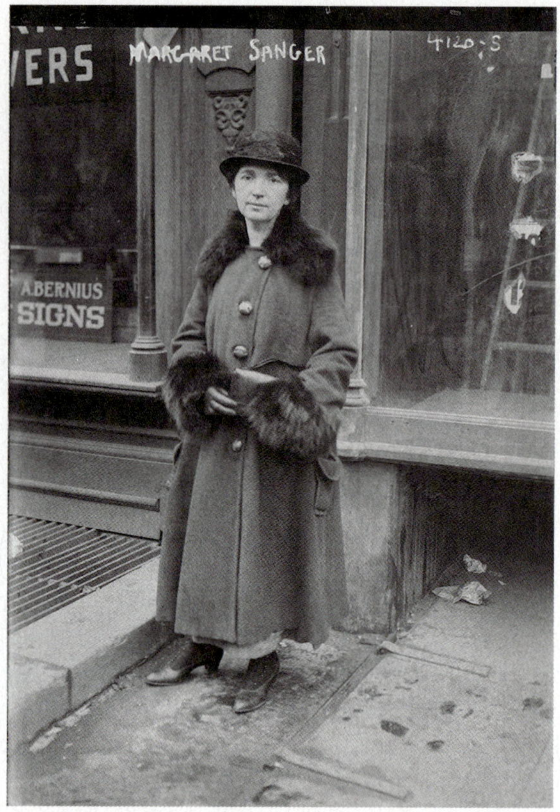

FIGURE 3-6 Margaret Sanger, thought to be standing in front of her birth control clinic.

Public Health Nursing Advances

PHNs gradually gained more cases in such areas as home care and instruction of good health practices to families and community groups (Figs. 3-7 and 3-8). One account relates a single PHN's experience providing care to those living in an isolated outpost on Kodiak Island, Alaska, during an outbreak of tuberculosis-related pneumonia (Carter, 2001; Curtis, 2008; Keeling et al., 2018). Industrial nursing also expanded, with 66 U.S. firms employing

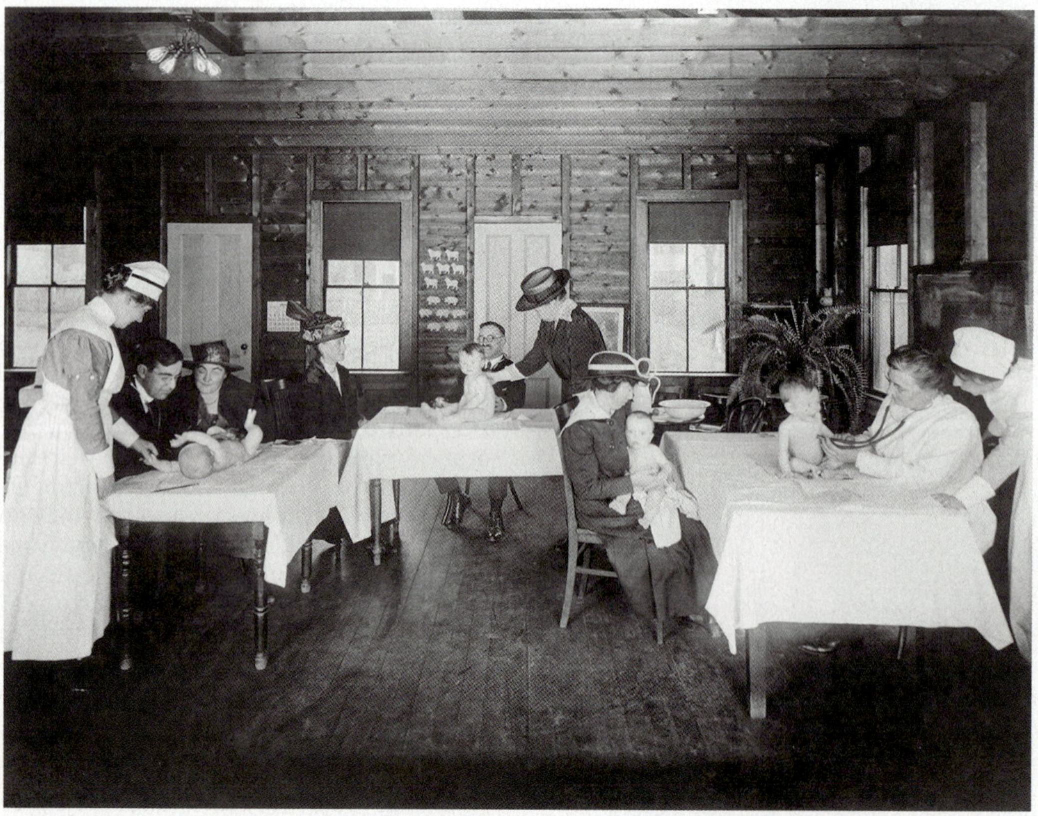

FIGURE 3-7 Well baby clinic in Framingham, Massachusetts (1920).

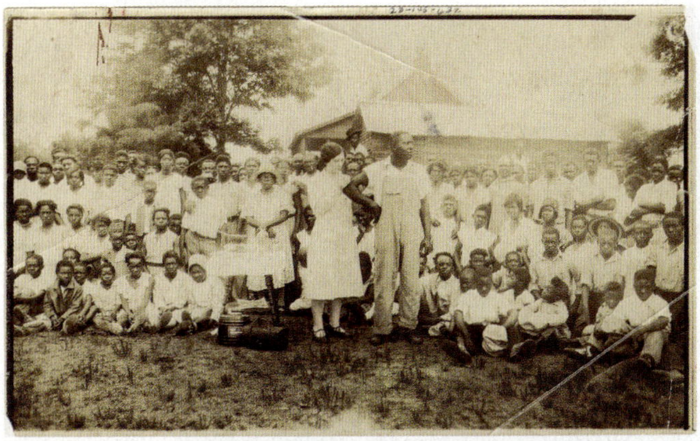

FIGURE 3-8 "Nurse Immunizing Man in Overalls in Front of a Large Group," Mississippi, ca. 1920s. (Retrieved from https://commons.wikimedia.org/wiki/File:Nurse_immunizing_man_in_overalls,_in_center_of_large_group_(16429738357).jpg)

nurses by 1910 (Bullough & Bullough, 1978). Out of necessity, PHNs began keeping better records of their services and continued home visiting for those in need. They also responded to **population health** needs, as more individual care was now available at hospitals and health centers (see Box 3-2). They worked with children and families affected by polio and administered the polio vaccine, once developed, at mass immunization clinics.

During the 20th century, the institutional base for much of public health nursing shifted to the government.

- By 1955, 72% of the counties in the continental United States had local health departments, staffed primarily by PHNs, who emphasized health promotion and provided care for the ill at home (Erwin & Brownson, 2017).
- Some of the district nursing services, known as **visiting nurse associations (VNAs)**, remained privately funded and administered, offering their own home nursing care. In some places, city or county health departments joined administratively and financially with VNAs to provide a combination of services, such as home care of the sick and health promotion to families (Fig. 3-9).
- The American Red Cross offered public health nursing services from 1912 to 1951: first via the Rural Nursing Services headed by Fannie Clement; second via the Town and Country Nursing Service, which served both rural areas and cities; and third via the Red Cross Public Health Nursing Service. The Red

BOX 3-2 STORIES FROM THE FIELD

New York City Public Health Nurses and the 1918 Influenza Pandemic

The 1918 influenza pandemic caused over 40 million deaths worldwide and 675,000 U.S. deaths. The country was at war (World War I), and the American Red Cross, the U.S. Public Health Service, and healthcare workers were stretched thin. The epidemic began in New York City with three cases during mid-September of 1918. It spread quickly and crossed social class and income boundaries; within a few days, there were 31 new cases reported (Keeling, 2009; Keeling & Wall, 2015).

Cities across the Eastern seaboard requested assistance, and a coordinated plan for a decentralized response was set in place. Lillian Wald, who directed the Henry Street visiting nurses, had weathered epidemics on the Lower East Side of New York City before and quickly responded to this new, even more virulent threat. When making home visits, nurses found "whole families were ill ... without anyone to give them the simplest nursing care" (Keeling, 2009, p. 2735). One person described, "People, desperate in their need watched from windows and doorways for the nurse. They surrounded her on the street, imploring her to go in six directions at once" (Geister, 1957, pp. 583–584).

Wald noted about 500 calls for nursing services to patients with influenza and pneumonia in the "first four days of October" and that nurses were instructed to wear masks but "31 out of ... 170 had succumbed to influenza" (Keeling, 2009, p. 2736). The Nurses' Emergency Council was organized for a citywide response, led by Lillian Wald, who requested that all who employed nurses allow them to work in caring for those afflicted by the epidemic. With this central structure, duplication of services was avoided, and services could be provided more quickly.

Wald requested automobiles for the visiting nurses to help them travel more quickly and carry "linens, pneumonia jackets, and quarts of soup"; the nurses started work early every morning and went out again at 4 PM to check on cases reported later each day (Keeling, 2009, p. 2737). They finished rounds around midnight, only to start again early the next morning. In Harlem, a nurse reported on a family of seven—"the mother has influenza, the father has lobar pneumonia, two children have measles and bronchopneumonia, and one child is only four weeks old," noting that they had no care until their case was reported to the visiting nurse association. This was a common situation across the city.

As the epidemic began to subside, the Nurses' Emergency Council discontinued central services on the 6th of November, and the Henry Street nurses opened postinfluenza clinics to address the follow-up needs of families. There were about 11,000 deaths from influenza and about 10,000 deaths from pneumonia reported in New York City over the 2-month period of the epidemic. All that the nurses could provide was comfort care—clean linens, bed baths, fluids, and monitoring. There was little help from the federal level of government; private, philanthropic, and religious organizations worked together with local government and nursing agencies to combat the deadly epidemic.

1. *How has your city or country responded to the novel coronavirus (COVID-19) pandemic? In what ways is this similar to the 1918 flu pandemic?*
2. *What disease threats are most likely to affect your community?*
3. *What resources are available?*
4. *How would public health nurses be involved?*

Source: Geister (1957); Keeling (2009); Keeling and Wall (2015).

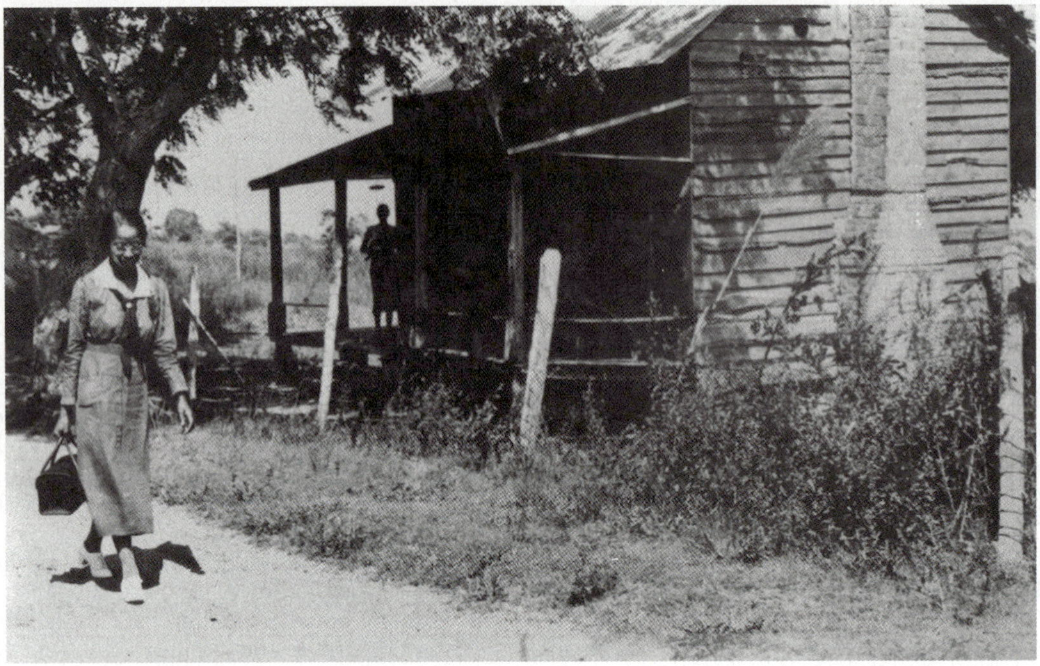

FIGURE 3-9 A public health nurse walks past a rural wooden house.

Cross also provided public health nursing services to families of soldiers during both World Wars (Ramsay, 2012; Sarnecky, 2018).

An innovative example of **rural nursing** was the **Frontier Nursing Service**, which was started by Mary Breckinridge (1881–1965) in 1925, who was influenced by English midwifery. From six mountain outposts in Kentucky, nurses on horseback (see Fig. 3-10) visited remote families to provide prenatal care, deliver babies, and provide food and nursing services. The work was hard, but rewarding; it combined general public health nursing and midwifery (January, 2009). From the beginning, Breckinridge insisted on accurate record keeping; this was used to assess patient risks and treatments.

Over the years, the service has expanded to provide medical, dental, and nursing care. The Frontier Nursing Service continues today, with its remarkable accomplishments of reducing mortality rates and promoting health among this disadvantaged population, as the parent holding company for the Frontier Nursing University. It is the largest nurse–midwifery program in the United States. In addition, Mary Breckinridge Healthcare, Inc. consists of multiple rural healthcare agencies (Carter, 2018; Dawley, 2003; see Box 3-3).

This period of public health nursing was characterized by service to the public, with the family targeted as a primary unit of care (Fig. 3-11). Official health agencies, which placed greater emphasis on disease prevention and health promotion, provided the chief institutional base.

- For instance, from 1928 to 1941, the East Harlem Nursing and Health Service offered "integrated family service(s)" by interdisciplinary independent PHNs to those living within an 87-city block area populated by mostly Italian immigrant and Italian American factory workers and laborers and their families (D'Antonio, 2013, p. 992).

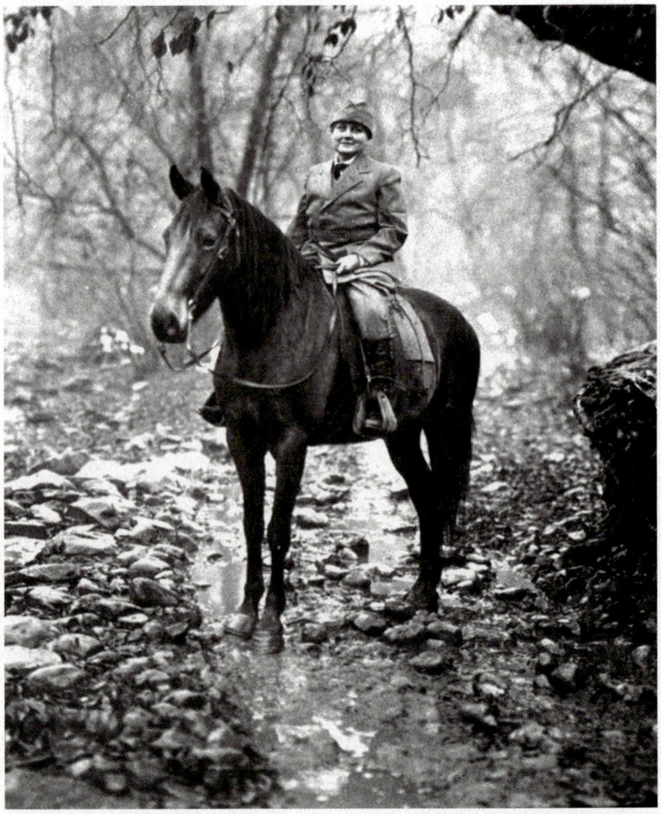

FIGURE 3-10 Mary Breckinridge on horseback. (Photo Courtesy of Frontier Nursing University Archives. Used with permission.)

BOX **3-3** PERSPECTIVES

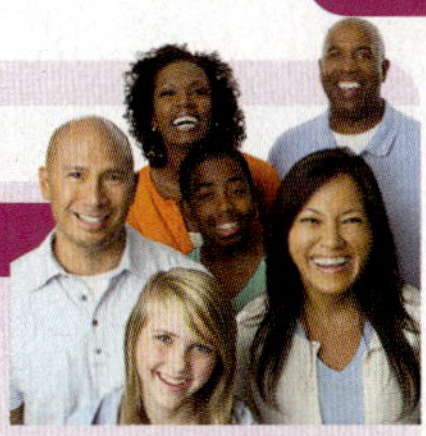

Roaming Through the Hills With the Public Health Nurse (1920)

As a state nursing supervisor, I visit PHNs during a typical week providing services in rural Virginia. The first PHN's territory consisted of a mountainous area, with winding, often muddy roads. Our first visit was made on horseback: "The road straight up the mountain was winding and lovely and way below in a gorge ran a stream" on our way to Star-Chapel School. After traveling by horseback all day, we crossed a final stream to reach a house that backed up to the mountain; "the stream dashing over the rocks at the front door" where we were invited to spend the night (Webb, 2011, pp. 291–292). The family was eager to help the nurse who had cared for others during the 1918 flu epidemic.

At the school, we checked the children, and the PHN talked to them about how to prevent disease and the importance of personal hygiene. We visited two more schools on the way back home. In the southwest corner of the state, I visited another PHN, and we traveled 30 miles by logging train, which seemed to be "balanced on the peak of a mountain top" to visit a small, isolated town that desperately wants a nurse to visit schoolchildren and families (Webb, 2011, p. 292).

In another county, the PHN visits with a girl who is recovering from meningitis, and her mother brags that she wants a clean glass and washes her hands now before she eats every meal. We then travel to a log cabin where mothers and children meet every week, and the PHN weighs babies and provides health pamphlets and talks about "babies, screening houses, homemade ice boxes," and other topics of interest (Webb, 2011, p. 293). At an old stone fireplace, the women cook gingerbread and make hot cocoa. We later visited a rundown camp and found women there each having between three and eight children, along with a 14-year-old who had stopped dipping snuff, as the nurse advised. The nurse had promised her a prize, and she proudly claimed it. The PHN talked with a 12-year-old girl who refused to go to school and found that the reason was that she couldn't see, and her eyes were hurting. The mother agreed that she needed to see a specialist, but the girl would not agree to this unless her father made her go.

The PHN was disappointed to see a 4-year-old, who had agreed to stop chewing tobacco, come by to visit her with a cigarette in his mouth! Our state needs many more PHNs, and we are budgeting the money for services, but we don't have enough nurses who are willing to do this type of rural pioneer nursing. It can be very rewarding (Webb, 2011).

A silent film showing these nurses making visits on horseback during difficult conditions (begin at about the 10-minute mark) can be found at this site: https://collections.nlm.nih.gov/catalog/nlm:nlmuid-8600028A-vid

1. *Where are rural nurses practicing today?*
2. *How has it changed from the 1920s?*
3. *What problems continue in this population? How can current resources (e.g., technologic, pharmacologic, social, political) be effectively used by PHNs?*

Adapted from a 1920 article found in Webb (2011).

- In New York City, 87% of babies were delivered at home, often by PHNs, and their services were in demand during the Great Depression as they worked to sustain families and address the social determinants of health that devastated them (D'Antonio, 2013).

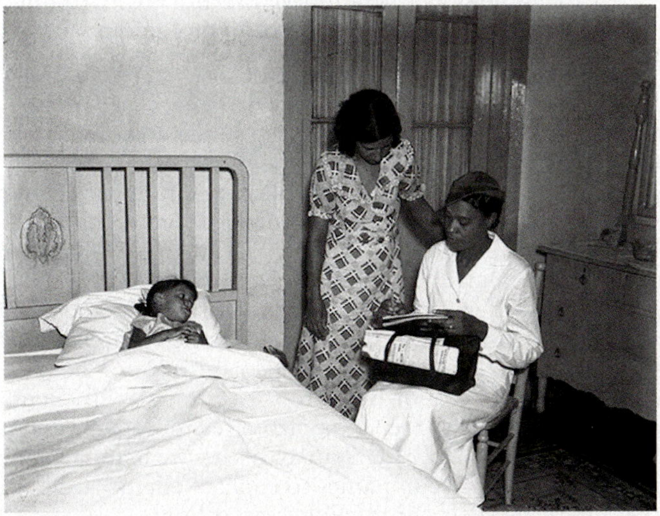

FIGURE 3-11 This Works Progress Administration photograph shows a New Orleans public health nurse making a house call during the Great Depression, 1936. (Retrieved from https://commons.wikimedia.org/wiki/File:NurseHousecall1936.jpg)

Nurses in Military Service

Since Florence Nightingale's service to the British soldiers during the Crimean War, nurses have continued to provide service during wartime.

- Women served in many capacities (nurses, cooks, seamstresses) during the Revolutionary War.
- Clara Barton, a founder of the American Red Cross, volunteered her services during the Civil War, as did about 20,000 women of different races and classes (D'Antonio, 2010, 2013).
- In 1901, an Act of Congress established the Army Nurse Corps, and in 1908, the Navy Nurse Corps was added (Lineberry, 2013; McIsaac, 1912).
- During World War I, many new graduates responded to the pleas of the American Red Cross for nurses to care for the sick and wounded and entered the Army Nurse Corps to serve the military locally or abroad. U.S. nurses would continue to serve in public health work and hospitals in the postwar recovery in Europe (Jamme, 1918).
- The Army Nurse Corps served the wounded and dying at Pearl Harbor when the island was bombed in 1941, and nurses continued to serve in the theaters of war until the end in 1945 (Liehr et al., 2016). Professional nurses volunteered for war service and 103,869 qualified for military service and by 1945, 65,216 were on duty as the war ended (see Fig. 3-12).

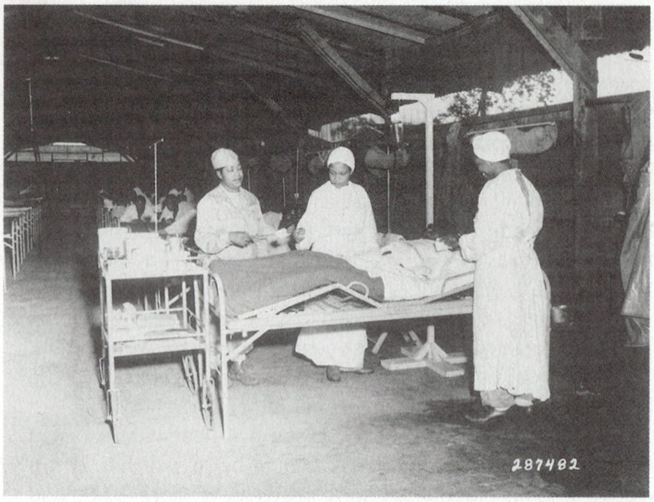

FIGURE 3-12 WW II, 1944. Surgical ward treatment at the 268th Station Hospital, Base A, Milne Bay, New Guinea. (Retrieved from https://commons.wikimedia.org/wiki/File:Surgical_ward_treatment_at_the_268th_Station_Hospital..._(5546316741).jpg)

- The Cadet Nurse Corps was created in 1943 under the Surgeon General's Office of the U.S. Public Health Service to educate nurses needed for war and civilian hospitals. Approximately 1100 hospitals allowed students applicants to study for 30 months then complete a 6-month internship either in their local hospital or in hospitals of the federal health system (Petry, 1945). This program helped to bring attention to the importance of nurses in society (Petry, 1945). Military nurses didn't receive permanent commissioned officer status until 1947 (Robinson, 2009).
- Knowledge of the value of Black nurses was discussed in the War Council, and the National Association of Colored Graduate Nurses leaders fought for equality to serve. Staupers (1961) documents several assignments gained for Black nurses in military and civilian hospitals but even when caring for prisoners of war, they experienced prejudice in the areas where they were assigned to provide care. In 1945, President Franklin D. Roosevelt "desegregated nursing in the U.S. Armed Forces" (D'Antonio, 2010; Staupers, 1961).

The Profession Evolves

The formation of national nursing organizations contributed to nursing's professional growth.

- The American Society of Superintendents of Training Schools for Nurses in the United States and Canada:
  - Founded in 1893 by Isabel Hampton Robb
  - Purpose: to establish educational standards for nursing
  - Became the National League of Nursing Education (NLNE) in 1912, the forerunner of the current **National League for Nursing (NLN)**, established in 1952 (Ellis & Hartley, 2012; Stegen & Sowerby, 2019)
- National Association of Colored Graduate of Nurses
  - Founded in 1909 by Martha Franklin
  - Purpose: "advance the standards and best interests of trained nurses; to breakdown discrimination in the nursing profession; and to develop leadership within the ranks of Black nurses" (Staupers, 1961, p. 17).
  - Merged with American Nurses Association in 1952 (Staupers, 1961).
- The **American Nurses Association (ANA)**:
  - Developed from a meeting of nursing leaders who initiated an alumnae organization of 10 schools of nursing to form the National Associated Alumnae of the United States and Canada in 1896
  - Purpose: to promote nursing education and practice standards
  - In 1899, renamed the Nurses' Associated Alumnae of the United States and Canada, became the ANA in 1911; Canadian nurses formed a separate nursing organization (Ellis & Hartley, 2012)
- The **National Organization for Public Health Nursing (NOPHN)**:
  - Founded by Lillian Wald and Mary Gardner in 1912
  - Purpose: setting standards for PHNs (Christy, 1970; Feld, 2008; NOPHN, 1939)
  - In 1931, developed "general and specialized objectives" regarding work with individuals, families, and communities
  - In 1940, added 12 functions of PHNs (Abrams, 2004, p. 507); began using community health nurse as a more inclusive gesture
  - In 1952, they merged with the NLNE and the ACSN to form the National League for Nursing (The 1952 Biennial, 1952). These organizations, in particular, strengthened ties between nursing groups and improved nursing education and practice. The accomplishments of Wald and many other nurse leaders reflect their concern for populations at risk and demonstrate how leadership, involvement in policy formation, and use of epidemiology led to improved health for the public (see Table 3-8 for information on famous PHNs).

The multiple problems faced by many families impelled a trend toward nursing care generalized enough to meet diverse needs and provide holistic services, but there was also a call for specialization in some densely populated areas, where tuberculosis, infant care, and school children were a primary concern (Brainard, 2012; King, 2011; Ruel, 2014; see Figs. 3-13 and 3-14). Another area of specialization included the home. Medicare legislation passed in 1965 and visiting nurses adapted their agencies to provide individualized skilled nursing visits posthospitalization. Nurses also pushed for hospice care to provide end-of-life care for terminally ill clients allowing patients to step away from technology to die in their homes (Buck, 2011). Nurses used case management through insurance companies to educate clients and help them manage their chronic illnesses at home.

As nursing education became increasingly rigorous, collegiate programs included public health as essential content in basic nursing curricula.

TABLE 3-8 A Partial List of Famous Nurses in the Development of U.S. Public Health Nursing 1800–1950

Name	Years	Why This Person Is Famous
Florence Nightingale	1820–1910	Often recognized as the "mother of modern nursing"; she was a social and health reformer who changed perceptions and practice of nursing (Keeling et al., 2018).
Mary Seacole	1805–1881	Jamaican nurse and entrepreneur led 39 other women to nurse and care for soldiers and families during the Crimean War (Staring-Derks et al., 2014).
Clara Barton	1821–1912	"Angel of the Battlefield" during U.S. Civil War; ran the Office of Missing Soldiers for family reunification. Founder of American Red Cross, 1871 (American Red Cross, 2020).
Mary Ann "Mother" Bickerdyke	1817–1901	U.S. Civil War nurse called "Cyclone in Calico"; changed conditions in military camps. Named by Gen. W.T. Sherman as matron of military hospital in Cairo, IL; set up 300 field hospitals on 19 battlefields. Campaigned for pensions on behalf of soldiers and nurses (Keeling et al., 2018; Nursingtheory.org, 2016).
Lillian Wald	1867–1940	Started Henry Street Settlement in NYC; used EBP to revolutionize public health nursing; health and social activist (Keeling et al., 2018).
Isabel Hampton Robb	1859–1910	Set standards for nursing practice, education, and ethics. First president of the Nurses' Associated Alumnae of the United States and Canada (now ANA), 1897. One of the founders of the American Journal of Nursing Company. President of Association of Superintendents of Training Schools (now NLN), 1908 (AAHN, 2018).
Adelaide Nutting	1858–1948	WWI: Chairman of the Committee of Nursing of the General Medical Board of the Council of National Defense, coordinating nursing services and recruiting nurses Many other accomplishments in nursing (Spring, 2017).
Jane Delano	1862–1919	President of the Associated Alumnae and president of the Board of Directors of the American Journal of Nursing, 1908. Chairman, American Red Cross Nursing Service and second superintendent of the Army Nurse Corps, 1909. Credited for recruiting the majority of the 21,480 army nurses who served during World War I (Sarnecky, 2018).
Mary Breckinridge	1881–1965	Founder of Frontier Nursing Service, nurse midwife Used EBP and data to change rural nursing Organizations still operating today including Frontier Nursing University (Carter, 2018).

Source: AAHN (2018); Carter (2018); Dickens (1907); Keeling et al. (2018); National Geographic (2008); Nursingtheory.org (2016); American Red Cross (2020); Sarnecky (2018); Spring (2017); Staring-Derks et al. (2014).

- A group of agencies met in 1946 to establish guidelines for public health nursing, and by 1963, public health content was required for NLN accreditation in all baccalaureate degree–level nursing programs (Kulbok & Glick, 2014; Spring, 2017).
- The nurse practitioner (NP) movement, starting in 1965 at the University of Colorado, was initially a part of public health nursing and emphasized primary healthcare to rural and underserved populations (Hawkins & Watson, 2010).

Community Health Nursing (1970 to the present)

The emergence of the term community health nursing heralded a new era (Table 3-9). By the late 1960s and early 1970s, while PHNs continued their work, many other nurses who practiced primary care and individualized care were based in the community. Medicare paid for posthospitalization home care visits allowing nurses to visit individuals over 65 years of age in their homes to assess them and educate them to return to their highest level of functioning at home. Other practice settings included community-based clinics, doctors' offices, worksites, and schools (Fig. 3-15). To provide a label that encompassed all nurses in the community, the ANA and others called them community health nurses. This term was not universally accepted, however, and many people—including nurses and the public—had difficulty distinguishing community health nursing from public health nursing and determining whether community health nursing was a generalized or a specialized practice.

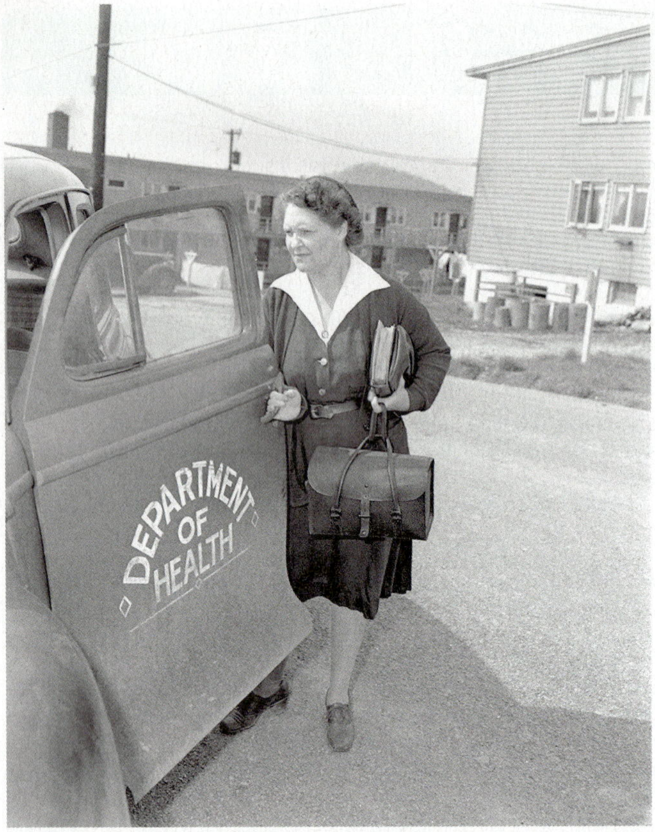

FIGURE 3-13 A public health nurse carrying the classic public health nursing bag in Oakridge, Tennessee, 1947. Note dark uniform, hat, and sensible shoes. (Retrieved from https://commons.wikimedia.org/wiki/File:Public_Health_Nursing_Oak_Ridge_1947_(12000263256).jpg)

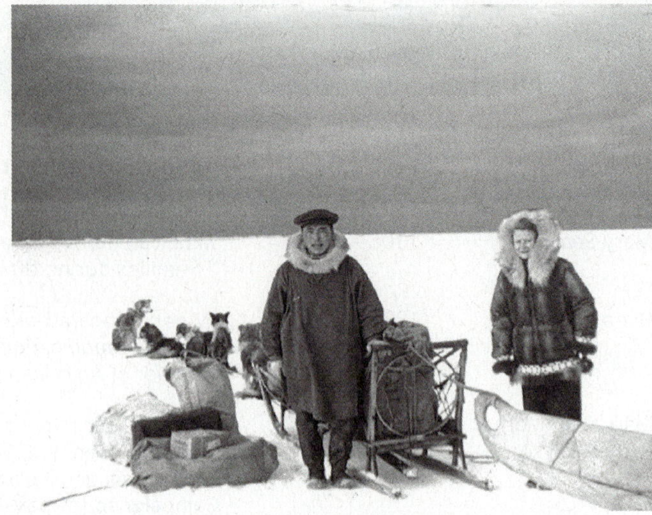

FIGURE 3-14 In Alaska in 1954, a public health nurse makes a home visit to clients, aided by an Inuit man and his dog team. (Retrieved from https://commons.wikimedia.org/wiki/File:1956_Alaska_-_Eskimo_and_dog_team.jpg)

To help resolve this confusion, the following actions were taken:

- The ANA's Division of Community Health Nursing:
  - Developed a Conceptual Model of Community Health Nursing in 1980 to distinguish generalized preparation at the baccalaureate level from advanced preparation at the master's or postgraduate level.

TABLE 3-9 Landmarks in Nursing History: 1970 and Beyond

Year	Landmark
1972	The Social Security Administration allowed Medicare coverage for those <65 years with long-term chronic disease and end-stage renal disease.
1973	U.S. military troops left South Vietnam. In the case of Roe vs. Wade, a landmark Supreme Court decision legalized abortion.
1977	Global smallpox eradication was achieved.
1978	Drug-resistant tuberculosis was reported in Mississippi.
1979	Healthy People: The Surgeon General's Report on Health Promotion and Disease Prevention was released.
1980s	A focus on in-patient care led to decreased funding for public health services.
1980	The American Nurses Association (ANA) published *Nursing: A Social Policy Statement.*
1985	American Red Cross Blood Services began testing for the HIV antibody.
1986	The ANA published *Standards of Community Health Nursing Practice.* The National Center for Nursing Research was created at the National Institutes of Health to support nursing research.
1988	The U.S. Department of Health and Human Services formed the Secretary's Commission to respond to a nursing shortage. IOM published *The Future of Public Health.*

TABLE 3-9 Landmarks in Nursing History: 1970 and Beyond *(Continued)*

Year	Landmark
1990s	Aging "Baby Boomers" created the need for improved geriatric care.
1990	The Persian Gulf War began.
1990	*Healthy People 2000:* National Health Promotion and Disease Prevention Objectives.
1993	National Center for Nursing Research became the National Institute of Nursing Research under the National Institutes of Health.
1996	The Health Insurance Portability and Accountability Act was signed into law. The U.S. Food and Drug Administration issued restrictive regulations for cigarettes and smokeless tobacco.
1997	Oregon legalized Death with Dignity, allowing terminally ill patients to end their lives with self-administered lethal injection.
1997	President Bill Clinton apologized for U.S. government sanctions of the "Tuskegee Study of Untreated Syphilis in the Negro Male," resulting in new federal guidelines on ethical treatment of human subjects.
1999	*The Scope and Standards of Public Health Nursing Practice* published by the ANA. Targeted drug therapies for some cancers introduced (Herceptin, TyKerb).
2000s	Nurse-run clinics unable to meet Medicaid/Medicare requirements to hire primary providers; many closed.
2000	*Healthy People 2000* results published; no nurses on the committee. *Healthy People 2010:* Understanding and Improving Health. Draft sequencing of human genome completed and released to public.
2001	September 11 terrorists attacks resulted in over 3000 deaths in New York City, Washington, and Pennsylvania. The Iraq War began.
2002	President George W. Bush signed Nurse Reinvestment Act. The U.S. government created the Department of Homeland Security as a cabinet-level department to protect national security.
2003	Worldwide epidemic of severe acute respiratory syndrome.
2005	Hurricane Katrina became the most expensive disaster in U.S. history.
2006	Medicare Part D Prescription Drug benefit implemented. *Public Health Nursing: Scope and Standards of Practice* published by the ANA. HIV cocktail drug, Atripla, and HPV vaccine, Gardasil, approved by the FDA.
2008	Barack Obama elected President, being the first African American to hold this position.
2009	*Essentials of Baccalaureate Nursing Education for Entry-Level Community/Public Health Nursing* published by the Association of Community Health Nursing Educators, Education Committee. H1N1 influenza "swine flu" outbreak declared a national emergency with over 22 million Americans contracting the disease and 4000 deaths.
2010	The Patient Protection and Affordable Care Act signed and included federal funding for nurse—family home visitation programs such as the Nurse Family Partnership to improve maternal/child health. Grant funding approved for existing school-based clinics as well as new construction. Institute of Medicine published *The Future of Nursing: Leading Change, Advancing Health.* Haiti earthquake triggered large nursing response.
2011	*The Future of Nursing: Leading Change, Advancing Health,* an Institute of Medicine report was released. Medicare reimbursement to Certified Nurse—Midwives increased from 65% to 100% of the Physician Fee Schedule. National Health Service Corps hired over 10,000 additional nurses and other healthcare professionals.
2012	*Patient-Centered Outcomes Research Institute* established, with two recognized nurse leaders/researchers serving on the Board of Governors and Methodology Committee. Institute of Medicine published *For the Public's Health: Investing in a Healthier Future.*

(Continued)

TABLE 3-9 Landmarks in Nursing History: 1970 and Beyond *(Continued)*

Year	Landmark
2013	Under the Affordable Care Act, grants and scholarships expanded for nursing and other health professionals. The ANA published second edition of *Public Health Nursing: Scope and Standards of Practice.*
2014	The *Advanced Nursing Education Grant* program funded to expand the number of nurses in advanced nursing education and practice. The *Nursing Education and Loan Repayment Program* expanded to include up to 85% of loan forgiveness for registered nurses, advanced practice nurses, and faculty members working a minimum of 2 years in either critical shortage areas or accredited schools of nursing. Flint water crisis; school nurses and volunteers responded. Ebola outbreak in West Africa. CDC incorporates pre-exposure prophylaxis into HIV clinical guidelines.
2015	Right-to-Die legislation for terminally ill patients enacted in California.
2017	*Healthy People 2020* midcourse review corrected and published; no nurse on committee.
2016	*Healthy People 2030*: Nurse Therese Richmond appointed to committee.

Source: Donahue (2011); Keeling et al. (2018); USDHHS (n.d.); American Nurses Association (n.d.); Baker (2019); Mason and McGinnis (1990); Cantelon (2010).

  - Defined the generalist as one who provides nursing service to individuals and groups of clients while keeping "the community perspective in mind" (American Nurses Association, Community Health Nursing Division, 1980, p. 9).
- In 1984, the U.S. Department of Health and Human Services, Bureau of Health Professions, Division of Nursing:
  - Convened a Consensus Conference on the Essentials of Public Health Nursing Practice and Education in Washington, District of Columbia (U.S. Department of Health and Human Services [USDHHS], Division of Nursing, 1984)
  - Identified community health nursing as the broader term, referring to all nurses practicing in the community, regardless of their educational preparation
  - Identified public health nursing as a part of community health nursing involving a generalist practice for nurses prepared with basic public health content at the baccalaureate level and a specialized practice for nurses prepared in public health at the master's level or beyond (Table 3-10)
- Nursing is currently adopting a competency-based curriculum to educate nurses. The *Essentials* promotes awareness of population-focused care as a competency for all nurses at all educational levels, which will benefit health outcomes.

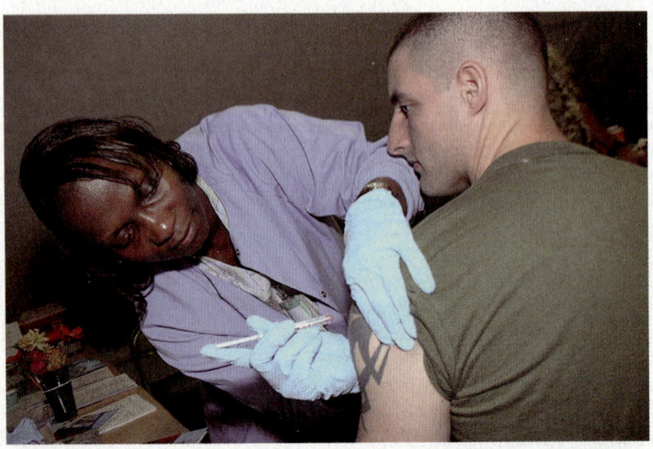

FIGURE 3-15 Germany, 2008. A nurse vaccinates a U.S. marine at Stuttgart Army Health Clinic. (Retrieved from https://commons.wikimedia.org/wiki/File:USMC-080918-M-0884D-002.jpg)

In this text, the terms public health nursing and community health nursing are combined (C/PHN), but whichever term is used to describe this nursing specialty, the fundamental issues and defining criteria remain the same:

- Are populations or communities the target of practice?
- Are the nurses prepared in public health and engaging in public health practice?

Finally, confusion also arose regarding the changing roles and functions of C/PHNs. Accelerated changes in healthcare organization and financing, technology, and social issues made increasing demands on C/PHNs to adapt to new patterns of practice. Many new kinds of community/public health services appeared with the passing of Medicare Act. Hospital-based home care visiting programs reached into the community. Private home care agencies proliferated, offering in-home visits and other community-based services.

Public health nursing continues to mean the synthesis of nursing and the public health sciences applied to promoting and protecting the health of populations. Community health nursing refers more broadly to nursing in the community. Community health nurses are carving out new roles for themselves in primary healthcare.

TABLE 3-10 Community/Public Health Nursing

Area of Practice	Sample Activities
Public health	Primary prevention activities, epidemiology; screenings, program planning
Disaster nursing	Nurses' roles in prevention/preparedness, response, recovery, and mitigation for/of disasters
Environmental health	Analysis of environmental hazards
Health education	Community education activities/academic education
Home health	Primary healthcare in residences
Hospice	End-of-life care
Midwifery	Ante- through postpartum care; women's health
Military nursing	International health relief projects
Missionary nursing	Operating clinics in underserved areas
Occupational/industrial health	Health education, safety evaluation for companies
Ombudsman/community advocate	Work with individuals and communities to educate and advocate for proper, reasonable, and timely healthcare
Policy formation/social justice/political activism	Serve on local boards and committees; join professional organizations
Population health	Health promotion activities for populations such as diabetes education or weight loss programs
Research	Study and disseminate information on issues relevant to PHN/CHN
Rural nursing	Home visits, immunization clinics
School nursing	Health promotion/disease tracking and prevention in schools
Visiting nurses	Provide short- or long-term care in the home
Volunteerism	Flu clinics, Disaster Management Assistance Teams

Collaboration and interdisciplinary teamwork are recognized as crucial to effective community nursing.

Community/public health nurses:

- Work through many kinds of agencies and institutions, such as centers for older adults, ambulatory services, mental health clinics, and family planning programs to engage people to live healthy lives and remain in their homes and communities.
- Conduct community needs assessment to plan programs and actions, document nursing outcomes, engage in program evaluation, advocate for clients, and work on quality improvement, assist in formulating public policy, and conduct community nursing research.
- Seek to promote health and prevent disease, by applying current research evidence; promoting healthier lifestyle practices such as eating healthy diets, exercising, and maintaining social support systems; promoting healthy conditions in schools and work sites; and designing meaningful activities for children, adolescents, adults, and older adults (Kulbok et al., 2012; Milbrath & DeGuzman, 2015).
- Seek to provide holistic care by collaborating with other healthcare professionals to offer coordinated, comprehensive, and personalized services—a case management approach.

History has demonstrated that nursing's most effective contributions to the overall health of our nation are based in the community. Nurses comprise the largest group of professionals in the public health workforce—about 16% or 47,000 employees in local, state, and federal agencies (Beck et al., 2014). A study conducted 2 years later estimated the total number of full-time equivalent nurses working at state and local health departments at 40,791 (Beck & Boulton, 2016). As funding is limited in community and public health, it is important for C/PHNs to continue to demonstrate their worth. According to the U.S. Bureau of Labor Statistics (2020), job growth for registered nurses continues to be robust (with employment of registered nurses projected to grow 12% from 2018 to 2028); a significant driver of growth is the continuing recognition of the importance of preventive healthcare (Box 3-4).

BOX 3-4 LEVELS OF PREVENTION PYRAMID

Promoting Community/Public Health Nursing

SITUATION: The general population is aware of nurses working in acute care settings or clinics, but fewer people interact regularly with population-focused, community-based nurses. As budgets are tightened, C/PHNs need to market their unique skill set and influence on health promotion and disease prevention in order to nurture this important nursing specialty.
GOAL: To clarify and enhance the community/public health nurse's role to promote greater impact of services.

Tertiary Prevention

- Promote increasing influence of the nurse through an expanded role in service delivery.
- Minimize the impact of community misunderstandings of the nurse's role through education.

Secondary Prevention

- Promote aggregate-level interventions.
- Foster nurse involvement on community boards and other political groups.

Primary Prevention

- Participate in policy formation.
- Be politically active.
- Assist in acquiring funding for community health programs.
- Conduct research on health and nursing outcomes to enhance EBP.
- Collaborate with the news media to publicize current public health issues.

SUMMARY

- Nursing leaders contributed to development of community/public health nursing, most notably:
  - Florence Nightingale, who outlined public health nursing
  - Clara Barton, a Civil War nurse who founded the American Red Cross and shaped disaster nursing
  - Lillian Wald, who developed public health nursing, influenced legislation and policy, and instituted school and industrial nursing as new areas of public health
- Community/public health nursing encompasses many areas dealing with individuals, families, communities, and populations. Some examples include public health, disaster nursing, environmental health, health education, home health, hospice, midwifery, military nursing, missionary nursing, occupational/industrial health, ombudsman/community advocate, policy formation/social justice/political activism, population health, research, rural nursing, school nursing, visiting nurses, and volunteerism.
- Academic preparation for community/public health nursing *begins* at the baccalaureate level. The need for advanced preparation was recognized in the early 20th century, as college-level coursework was provided for this specialty.
- C/PHNs work in interdisciplinary teams in a variety of agencies with various populations to promote health.

ACTIVE LEARNING EXERCISES

1. Select one societal influence on the development of community/public health nursing and explore its continuing impact. What other events are occurring today that shape community/public health nursing practice? Using current, credible resources, support your arguments with documentation. (Objective 1)
2. Research the life and works of a historical public health nursing leader. Using this information, determine how this practitioner dealt with a population-based issue current to her time. Is the problem similar to a current problem? Explain your thinking. (Objective 2)
3. Read a historical article about early public health nursing experiences. Compare these experiences with your public health clinical experiences today. What are the most striking similarities and differences? (Objective 3)
4. Choose two areas of community/public health nursing where you might like to practice (Table 3-10). Compare and contrast those two areas describing geographic locations (e.g., international, rural), type of employment (e.g., public, private, grant funded), and job description, duties, activities areas of focus, and nursing orientation (e.g., individual, families,

communities, populations). Compare your information with a classmate's selections. (Objective 4)

5. Review the 10 Essential Public Health Services (see Box 2-2) and give 4 additional examples of how the 3 core competencies and 10 Essential Public Health Services were implemented in historical community/public health settings. Include which key nurse leaders implemented them, what they did, where it occurred, and when. Give an example related to today's community/public health nursing practice. (Objectives 5 and 6)

CHAPTER 4

Research, Evidence-Based Practice, Quality Improvement, and Ethics

"I have often thought how wise a piece of education ... that the habit of ready and correct observation will by itself make us useful nurses, but that without it we shall be useless with all our devotion."

—Florence Nightingale (1898, in *Notes on Nursing*)

"Avoid basing decisions on untested but strongly held beliefs, what you have done in the past, or on uncritical 'benchmarking' of what winners do."

—J. Pfeffer, Top 5 EB Mgt. Tips

KEY TERMS

Auditability
Belmont Report
Common Rule
Confirmability
Creditability
Declaration of Helsinki
Ethics
Evidence-based practice
Fittingness
Institutional Review Boards
Levels of evidence
Mixed methods
Quality improvement
Reliability
Research
Transferable
Validity

LEARNING OBJECTIVES

Upon mastery of this chapter, you should be able to:

1. Differentiate research, evidence-based practice (EBP), and quality improvement (QI), including their purposes and methodologies.
2. Summarize the ethical standards governing research, EBP, and QI.
3. Identify the community/public health nurse's roles in research, EBP, and QI to improve nursing practice.
4. Employ research, EBP, and QI models to solve real or potential public health problems.

INTRODUCTION

As a new student in community/public health nursing, you may ask, "Can I really do something to make a difference in the lives of my clients?" You may feel shocked and discouraged by the prevalence of social problems and have a sense of helplessness about your ability to solve them. For the first time in your life, you may truly confront the inequalities and injustices of our health-care system. You will face many ethical dilemmas in community/public health nursing. You may ask, "Why should I bother to make home visits to teens who are pregnant? Why should I offer smoking cessation classes for people living in transitional housing? Will it really matter?" Hopefully, by the end of this chapter, you will see specific ways you can help improve the health and well-being of the public you serve as a nurse.

The purposes of this chapter are to elucidate the differences between research, evidence-based practice (EBP), and quality improvement (QI), summarize the ethical standards for each, and describe exemplar roles that use research, EBP, and QI. While all three use systematic processes, their applications vary based on their purposes and methodologies. Nurses are expected to be proficient in all three methodologies, as all three are included among the core competencies

TABLE 4-1 Comparison Among Research, Evidence-Based Practice, and Quality Improvement

	Research	EBP	QI
Purpose	Generation of new knowledge	Improvements in clinical practice	Evaluation and achievement of improved outcomes
Structure	Person, group, or team	Person or interdisciplinary team	Interdisciplinary group or team
Process	Disciplined research methods	Evidence-based methods	Process improvement methods
Outcome	Generalizable new knowledge	Potentially transferrable change in care	Potentially transferrable change in systems' change

Note. EBP, evidence-based practice; QI, quality improvement.
Adapted from Fain, J. A. (2021). *Reading, understanding, and applying nursing research* (6th ed., Tables 2-5 and 2-6, p. 27). F. A. Davis.

for nursing (American Association of Colleges of Nursing [AACN], 2021). Some of the differences between research, EBP, and QI are summarized in Table 4-1.

RESEARCH THAT MAKES A DIFFERENCE: THE NURSE–FAMILY PARTNERSHIP (NFP)

Recent public health nursing research validates that nursing care *does* matter and that you really *can* make a difference in the lives of your clients. For example, the Nurse–Family Partnership (NFP), a home visiting program based on the work of Olds and colleagues, is an intensive home visit program for first-time birthing parents facing socioeconomic disparities. The NFP has a significant history and continues to influence the health of families. The NFP model is based on theory and decades of research and is a testament to the power of research to influence practice (Nurse-Family Partnership, 2024). See Figure 4-1 for NFP Trial Outcomes.

- In a recent randomized controlled trial in Canada, improved behaviors were seen in 2-year-olds as a result of the NFP program (Nicole et al., 2023). Old's initial studies of similar populations in the United States found similar, statistically significant results of reduced reports of child abuse and improved parental life course through planned pregnancies (Olds et al., 1997).
- A recent qualitative study examined how an NFP program in Australia impacted self-efficacy in First Nations women (Massi et al., 2023). The main themes derived from a reflexive thematic analysis were personal growth/empowerment, making connections/building relationships, and self-efficacy. This study was quite important as self-efficacy in a First Nations cultural context includes a community sense of self that is derived from their collectivist societal norms.

These and other studies are powerful evidence noting the effectiveness of a program of regular C/PHN visits (Eckenrode et al., 2010; Karoly, 2017; Kitzman et al., 2010a, 2010b; Olds et al., 2014a, 2014b; Sierau et al., 2016). A classic study by the Olds research team examining pregnancy outcomes, childhood injuries, and repeated childbearing (Kitzman et al., 1997) was recognized by the National Institute of Nursing Research (NINR) (National Institutes of Health [NIH], n.d.) as one of 10 landmark nursing research studies. Olds and his colleagues have encouraged replication, using the established framework undergirding their results. The value of this program, which provides C/PHN visits to at-risk birthing parents and children in their homes, has been validated. C/PHNs really *do* make a difference! See Box 4-1.

RESEARCH

Nurses may not see themselves as nurse researchers. However, all nurses need to be prepared to read and understand research so they can integrate research evidence into their practice. In fact, AACN (2021) states in Domain 1: Knowledge for Nursing Practice that entry-level nurses are expected to "apply theory and research-based knowledge from nursing, the arts, humanities, and other sciences" (Key Element 1.2, p. 27).

Nursing research began with Florence Nightingale, who provided care for soldiers in the Crimean War (1854–1856). Through her knowledge of statistics, she tracked mortality rates as healthcare delivery changes were made. Based on her ability to quantify improvements in health outcomes, the data-driven discipline of nursing was born. In her *Notes on Nursing* (1898), Nightingale stated that "symptoms or sufferings generally considered to be inevitable and incident to the disease are very often not symptoms of the disease at all, but of something quite different—of the want of fresh air, or of light, or of warmth, or of quiet, or of cleanliness, or of punctuality and care in the administration of diet, of each or of all of these" (p. 2). One can argue that professional nursing practice is the inclusion of empirical science, along with aesthetics, ethics, and praxis, in the process of care delivery (Carper, 1978). Prior to Nightingale's work, the empirical science part was left to others. Now, it is core to nursing practice.

Nursing research has grown in its scope and complexity since Nightingale's original work. In fact, nursing now has its own division of the NIH called the NINR. The mission of NINR (n.d.) is to lead "nursing

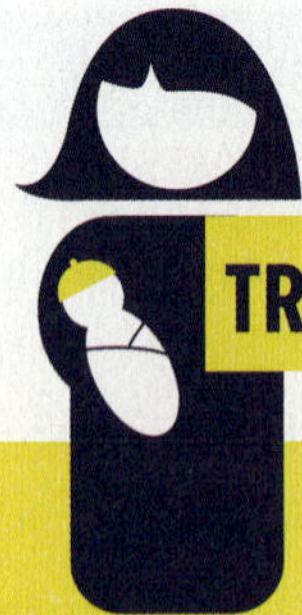

TRIAL OUTCOMES

Trial outcomes demonstrate that Nurse-Family Partnership delivers against its three primary goals of better pregnancy outcomes, improved child health and development, and increased economic self-sufficiency—making a measurable impact on the lives of children, families and the communities in which they live.

For example, the following outcomes have been observed among participants in at least one of the trials of the program.

48% reduction in child abuse and neglect

56% reduction in ER visits for accidents and poisonings

50% reduction in language delays of child age 21 months

67% less behavioral/intellectual problems at age 6

79% reduction in preterm delivery for patients who smoke

32% fewer subsequent pregnancies

82% increase in months employed

61% fewer arrests of the birthing parent

59% reduction in child arrests at age 15

FIGURE 4-1 Nurse–family partnership trial outcomes. (Adapted with permission from Nurse-Family Partnership. (2022). *Research Trials and Outcomes Fact Sheet.* https://www.nursefamilypartnership.org/wp-content/uploads/2020/06/NFP-Research-Trials-and-Outcomes-1.pdf)

BOX **4-1** PERSPECTIVES

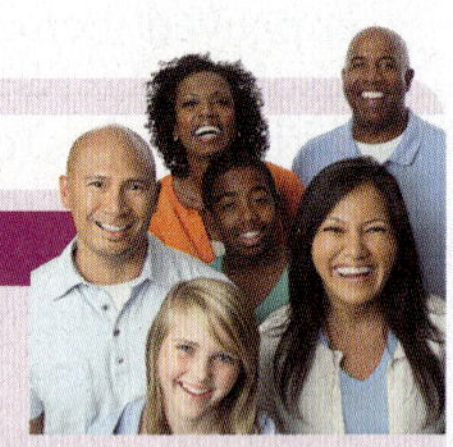

An NFP Nurse Viewpoint on Public Health Nursing

I walked into the high school not sure what to expect; after all, I was used to visiting my clients in their homes. A very young girl walked in, noticeably pregnant and extremely shy. I tried to meet her eyes, but she kept looking down as we walked to a room. We met there every week for 6 weeks.

Several months later, when my client called to tell me that her mom had physically abused her and that her brother had threatened her with a gun, I felt helpless. I listened to her and hooked her up with resources for a safe place to go. If she couldn't count on her own mom, how would she ever succeed, I wondered.

She called me a lot after that day, many times just to talk. She wanted desperately to go to school, but since leaving her mom's home, she lived too far away to walk. I gave her as many bus passes as I could to get her to school and back. I thought that would be enough until I could speak to school officials and find her some permanent transportation. Little did I know, but I was the ONLY one who cared if this child got to school or not. I tried tirelessly to get through to caseworkers, school officials, and social workers. I never thought that I would have this problem: a pregnant girl who wanted to go to school and adults who didn't care. How could this girl win?

My client gave birth to her baby and continued to faithfully keep our scheduled visits. We would laugh and have fun while covering the program curriculum. She was doing a great job of parenting her baby, and growth and development were on target. The baby was thriving. She was living somewhere new and again insisted that she wanted to go to school. We found out what district she was in, and they needed her to get a physical examination and records from her old school. I encouraged her but was not too sure if she could get it all done. Those types of errands are easy for most people, but for someone who has no means of transportation and little support, they are a huge ordeal.

BOX **4-1** PERSPECTIVES

An NFP Nurse Viewpoint on Public Health Nursing (*Continued*)

A week later I got a phone call, it was my client. I had to ask who it was because this young lady sounded so sure of herself and assertive. I couldn't believe that it was her! When had she started to speak up and articulate like this? She was calling to tell me that she had gotten her physical and her school records, and she was just waiting to hear from the school. I told her how proud I was of her for being so responsible.

The next time I saw my client, she rushed to the door and pulled me inside. She wanted to show me something and led me to her room. There, laid out on the bed, was her ROTC uniform, complete with shiny black shoes. Her grandmother was willing to help with the baby so that she could participate. She looked me right in the eyes and said in a powerful voice... "What do you think?" I told her that I had no doubt in my mind that she would do great things in life and that I was so proud of her. She said, "Ms. Shelly, I don't know why you are so proud; you are the one who taught me to be this way." Amazing! I have had so many success stories and seen so many healthy moms and babies. I love working with this program. What I do can make a big difference.

—*Shelly, RN, PHN, NFP Nurse*

research to solve pressing health challenges and inform practice and policy—optimizing health and advancing health equity into the future." In NINR's Strategic Plan 2022–2026, they list the following priority foci: health equity, social determinants of health, population and community health, prevention and health promotion, and systems and models of care (https://www.ninr.nih.gov/sites/default/files/docs/NINR_One-Pager_508c.pdf). Those working in C/PHN can expect to see professional opportunities expand within those foci.

Research is defined as the systematic collection and analysis of data related to a particular phenomenon. The purpose of research is to produce *generalizable* new knowledge to add to what is currently known about a phenomenon of interest (Fain, 2021). Note that research is not using interventions that depart from accepted clinical practice to "see what happens." Instead, it follows a formal protocol and set of procedures to draw *generalizable* conclusions about the study's stated purpose (USDHHS, 1979, p. 2). Research can be classified in many ways:

- Research in public health is usually nonexperimental, meaning it is descriptive, exploratory, or correlational in nature (Fain, 2021). In C/PHN, these are referred to as observational analytic studies.
- Observational study designs are classified as having no assigned exposure as it would be unethical (see the Tuskegee Syphilis Study) to expose a subpopulation to a specific disease that could cause harm.
- Although population studies do not assign exposure, they still follow a systematic process. If there is no assigned exposure, the distinguishing characteristics determining the study design are the element of time and the comparison group.
- A comparison group should not be confused with a control group, where the exposure and control group are determined prior to the study commencement. Comparison groups are those groups within the observational design that are monitored because of their exposure or treatment. For example, people who choose to vape may be compared to people who choose not to vape. The group that chooses to vape is not assigned to vape; rather, they already partake of this exposure. The comparison group (e.g., those who choose not to vape) would need to include the same demographics as the people in the vaping group.
- If the comparison groups start in the present and progress backward, it is a retrospective study design. If the exposure occurs and the time goes into the future, it is a longitudinal cohort study.
- A cross-sectional study is when the exposure and outcome comparison group are assessed at the same point in time. If there is no comparison group, then the study design is descriptive. See Figure 4-2.

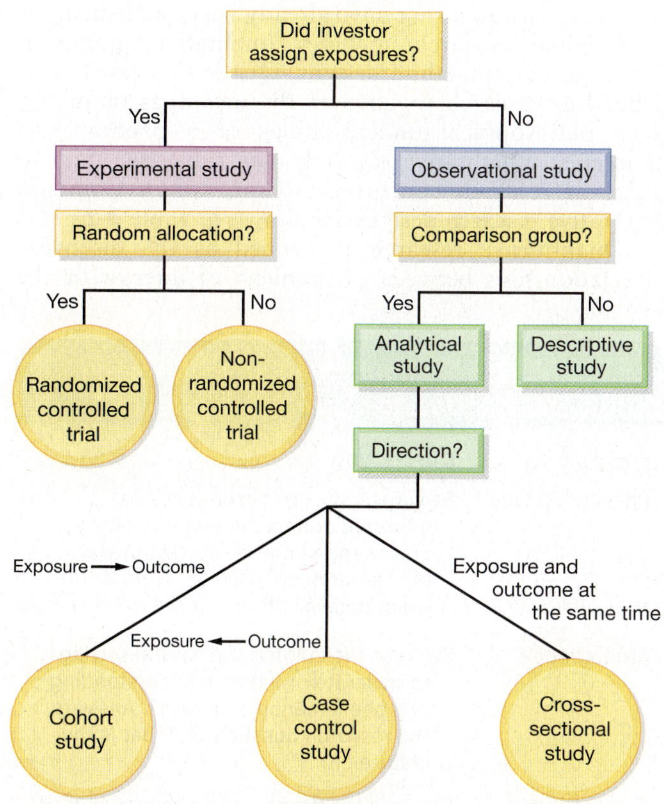

FIGURE 4-2 Study designs. (Reprinted with permission from Grimes, D. A., & Schultz, K. F. (2002). An overview of clinical research: The lay of the land. *Epidemiology, 39*, 57–61. https://www.thelancet.com/journals/lancet/article/PIIS0140-6736(02)07283-5/fulltext)

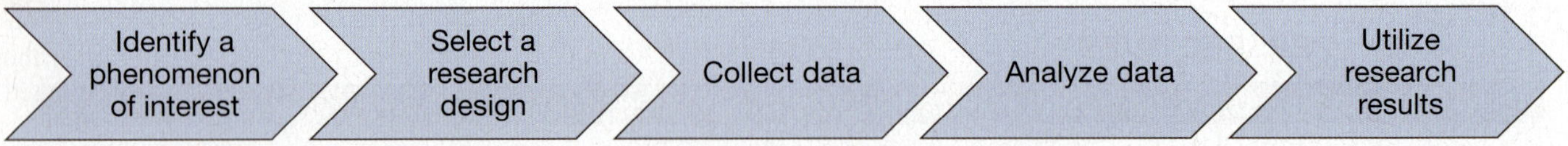
Identify a phenomenon of interest
Select a research design
Collect data
Analyze data
Utilize research results

FIGURE 4-3 Basic steps of research. (Adapted from Fain, J. A. (2021). *Reading, understanding, and applying nursing research* (6th ed., Fig. 3-1). F. A. Davis.)

Research Methods

Research, no matter the design, follows the scientific method, first described by Francis Bacon (1621/2013). The scientific method involves testing ideas using predefined systematic methods. Without systematic methods, one could not generalize the research conclusions drawn from the study (Fain, 2021). The basic steps of the research process, adapted from Fain (2021), are shown in Figure 4-3.

Step one is identifying a phenomenon of interest. This is largely based on the interests of the researcher and the most concerning problems the researcher experiences. Step two is selecting a research design (Fain, 2021). Research designs are selected based on what is known about the phenomenon of interest. If little is known about a phenomenon of interest, qualitative designs may be preferred. If much is known about a phenomenon of interest, quantitative designs may be preferred. Some research designs utilize original research, that is, research that does not yet exist. Other research designs synthesize reviews of research that have already been published.

Original research includes qualitative, quantitative, and mixed-method designs. Qualitative research is defined as research to uncover the meanings or underlying philosophical underpinnings of a phenomenon of interest. Qualitative research uses subjective data to arrive at research conclusions (Fain, 2021). Common qualitative research designs are shown in Table 4-2.

Quantitative research is defined as the discovery of relationships between phenomena of interest or the establishment of cause and effect based on the scientific method. Quantitative research uses objective data to arrive at research conclusions (Fain, 2021). Common quantitative research designs are shown in Table 4-3. **Mixed methods**, also called triangulation, use a combination of qualitative and quantitative designs (Fain, 2021).

Research designs that synthesize research previously published include systematic literature reviews, meta-analyses, scoping literature reviews, and integrative literature reviews (Fain, 2021). Table 4-4 outlines each of these. Collections of systematic literature reviews can be accessed through the Cochrane Library, available at

TABLE 4-2 Common Qualitative Research Designs

Design	Description
Phenomenology	Explores one's lived experience to generate or improve understanding of a phenomenon of interest. Answers the research question of "What is the experience of...?"
Ethnography	Explores the culture of a natural setting to generate or improve understanding of a phenomenon of interest. Answers the research question of "What is the culture of ...?"
Grounded theory	Explores the process of a phenomenon of interest. Answers the research question of "What is the process of ...?"

Adapted from Fain, J. A. (2021). *Reading, understanding, and applying nursing research* (6th ed., Table 10-1, p. 187). F. A. Davis.

TABLE 4-3 Common Quantitative Research Designs

Design	Description
Analytic epidemiological	Tests hypotheses to determine if specific exposures are related to specific diseases.
Descriptive correlational	Describes and explains the nature and magnitude of relationships between variables.
Descriptive epidemiological	Studies patterns and distributions of diseases or disabilities within a population.
Descriptive	Describes variables associated with a phenomenon of interest.
Experimental	Requires the researcher to manipulate one or more variable to observe the effect of that manipulation on other variables; requires random assignment and control and experimental groups.
Quasi-experimental	Requires the researcher to manipulate one or more variables to observe the effect of that manipulation on other variables; random assignment and control groups are absent.
Randomized controlled trial (RCT)	Studies the effectiveness of an intervention with a large sample of research subjects; assignment of subjects to either an experimental or control group.

Adapted from Fain, J. A. (2021). *Reading, understanding, and applying nursing research* (6th ed., Chapter 9). F. A. Davis.

TABLE 4-4 Research Designs Synthesizing Published Research

Design	Description
Systematic literature review	Uses systematic and well-defined methods to identify, appraise, and analyze quantitative literature; generally includes RCTs.
Meta-analyses	Uses studies with similar methods to increase the sample size and therefore, the statistical power of the findings.
Scoping literature review	Maps a body of literature on a specific phenomenon of interest and identifies relevant concepts and research gaps, regardless of research design.
Integrative literature review	Summarizes past literature, regardless of study design, to provide a comprehensive understanding of a phenomenon of interest.

Note: RCTs, randomized controlled trials.
Adapted from Johns Hopkins University Welch Medical Library. (2020). *Expert methodologies & review types.* https://browse.welch.jhmi.edu/searching/other-review-types

https://www.cochranelibrary.com/. Researchers wishing to use any of these three designs are referred to the Preferred Reporting Items for Systematic Reviews and Meta-Analyses (PRISMA), available at http://www.prisma-statement.org/, and PRISMA for scoping reviews (PRISMA-ScR), available at http://www.prisma-statement.org/Extensions/ScopingReviews.

Step three is collecting data. This requires the researcher to follow the steps described in their research design (Fain, 2021). Step four is analyzing data. This requires the researcher to use qualitative data analyses or statistical procedures to make meaning from the data collected, to determine the answers to the research questions, and to test hypotheses (Fain, 2021). Step five is utilizing research results (Fain, 2021). This requires researchers to share their findings with other members of the discipline and with the larger scientific community. Generally, this is accomplished through publications and public presentations.

Different study designs use different measures of rigor. Quantitative research uses various types of validity and reliability to support study rigor.

- **Validity** refers to the closest approximation to the truth, whereas **reliability** refers to the consistency or repeatability of a measure (Fain, 2021).
- Qualitative research uses **confirmability** as a measure of reliability. Confirmability is supported through three mechanisms: auditability, credibility, and fittingness.
- **Auditability** refers to allowing the reader to track the researcher's decision-making path and arrive at the same or comparable findings.
- **Credibility** refers to findings that are reported as accurate by the participants used in the study.
- **Fittingness** refers to the degree to which the research outcomes fit the gathered data (Fain, 2021).

Study designs also have different levels of evidence. **Levels of evidence** refer to the strength and rigor of a study's findings based on the study design. See Figure 4-4. Study designs at the top of the pyramid are considered the strongest levels of evidence; study designs at the bottom of the pyramid are considered weaker levels of evidence. Thus, systematic reviews and meta-analyses are considered the strongest levels of evidence in research.

Ethical Conduct of Research

Ethics are the principles that guide research and research practices. Research, when conducted ethically, benefits people and populations. Historically, however, research has not been conducted ethically. For example, in Nazi Germany prior to and during World War II (WWII), primary providers and medical researchers conducted experiments on prisoners in concentration camps. Without their subjects' consent, researchers forced prisoners to endure hypothermia, high altitudes, poisoning, infectious disease,

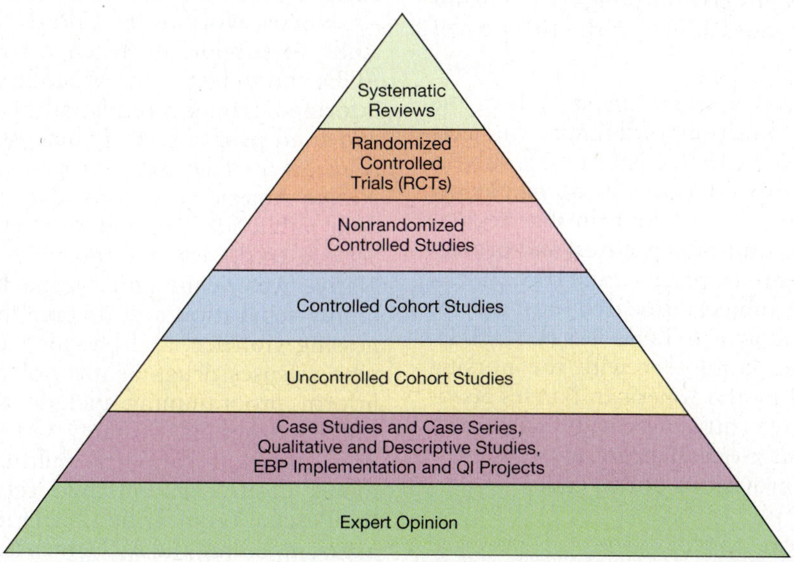

FIGURE 4-4 Levels of evidence. EBP, evidence-based practice; QI, quality improvement. (Adapted with permission from Melnyk, B. M., & Fineout-Overholt, E. (2023). *Evidence-based practice in nursing and healthcare* (5th ed., Fig. 6-2). Wolters Kluwer.)

consumption of seawater, bone, muscle, and joint transplantations, sterilization, artificial insemination, and eugenics (Tyson, 2000). Sadly, some of these practices were not uncommon research practices at the time (Roelcke, 2004).

At the end of WWII, the world's citizens were so outraged by the Nazi's conduct that the Nuremberg Trials were held to hold Nazi members accountable.

- In the Nuremberg Medical Trial, 23 doctors were charged with murder and torture (Shuster, 2018).
- The World Medical Association **Declaration of Helsinki** (originally adopted in 1964, amended in 1975, 1983, 1989, 1996, 2000, 2008, 2013) followed the Nuremberg Trials and outlined the ethical principles for medical research involving human subjects.
- The full text of the Declaration of Helsinki can be found at www.e-dmj.org/file/WMA-Declaration_of_Helsinki-2013.pdf.

Also, in 1932, the U.S. Public Health Service (USPHS) began the Tuskegee Syphilis Study. For the next 40 years, the USPHS studied the effects of untreated syphilis in approximately 600 men afflicted with the infection. When injectable penicillin became available in 1941, the men enrolled in the Tuskegee Syphilis Study were not offered treatment (Heller, 2017). Instead, they were monitored so the USPHS researchers could document the natural history of the disease (e.g., until the patient's death) (Gamble, 2014). The Tuskegee Syphilis Study marks one of the darkest chapters in the USPHS's history and is still cited as a reason why African American individuals may distrust medical and public health professionals (Heller, 2017).

- The public outrage about the Tuskegee Syphilis Study resulted in Congress passing the 1974 National Research Act and creating the National Commission for the Protection of Human Subjects of Biomedical and Behavioral Research (Centers for Disease Control and Prevention [CDC], 2021).
- In 1979, the **Belmont Report** was published, summarizing the ethical principles and guidelines for the protection of human subjects of research.
- Go to https://www.hhs.gov/ohrp/regulations-and-policy/belmont-report/index.html for the full text of the Belmont Report.

Today, human subjects' research must follow the Federal Policy for the Protection of Human Subjects (also known as the **Common Rule**). All human subject research now must be approved by **institutional review boards** (IRBs) whose purpose is to confirm that regulations, ethical standards, institutional policies, and protections for human subjects are in place (USDHHS, 2021). At a minimum, all human subjects' research must adhere to the ethical principles shown in Table 4-5 (USDHHS, 1979). These concepts are congruent with the nursing code of ethics articulated by the American Nurses Association (ANA, 2015); see https://www.nursingworld.org/practice-policy/nursing-excellence/ethics/code-of-ethics-for-nurses/ for the provisions of this code.

TABLE 4-5 Ethical Principles of Human Subject Research

Ethical Principle	Explanation
Respect for people	All people should be treated as autonomous and those with diminished autonomy are entitled to protection. This is demonstrated through informed consent, including the provision of information, assessment of comprehension, and notification of voluntariness.
Beneficence	Do no harm. Maximize possible benefits and minimize possible harms. This is expressed through disclosure of the nature and scope of risks and benefits.
Justice	All subjects should be treated equally. This is expressed through the selection of research subjects

Adapted from U.S. Department of Health & Human Services (USDHHS). (1979). *The Belmont Report: Ethical principles and guidelines for the protection of human subjects of research.*

C/PHN Using Research

Research validates that nursing care does matter and that you really can make a difference in the lives of your clients. For decades, nurses working in C/PHN have collected and analyzed data and used those data to justify funding for and outreach to vulnerable populations. For example, the Adverse Childhood Experiences (ACE) study was a joint project between the CDC and Kaiser Permanente. Originally, data were collected on those enrolled in the health maintenance organization from 1995 to 1997. Findings indicated that ACEs were strongly associated with health risk behaviors and the development of chronic disease later in life (Felitti et al., 1998). Based on the strength of the original study's findings, the CDC now collects ACE data as part of its ongoing Behavioral Risk Factor Surveillance System (BRFSS). More information about the ACE study and BRFSS can be accessed at www.cdc.gov/violenceprevention/aces/about.html.

Nurses working in C/PHN use data from the ACE study to support outreach for families at high risk for ACEs and to justify the broad implementation of trauma-informed care. Currently, all 50 states collect ACE data and fund programs to reduce ACEs in their populations (Centers for Disease Control & Prevention, 2023). Some Native American nations also use ACE data to inform their public health programming. The U.S. Indian Health Service (n.d.) reports the most common ACEs among Native Americans and Alaska Natives include poverty, family separation and divorce, being a victim of or witnessing violence, and having a person in the household who misuses drugs or alcohol. Examples of how ACEs inform programming include the Chickasaw Nation's (2024) program, Hofanti Chokma ("to grow well"). This program supports children and teens, and promotes positive parent/child relationships. Additionally, the Pascua Yaqui Tribe (2021) identified several priority areas, including the ACEs mentioned above in their 2021 Health Needs Assessment, and they employ C/PHNs to provide outreach to at-risk populations.

EVIDENCE-BASED PRACTICE

While not all nurses participate in research, every nurse is required to participate in **evidence-based practice** (EBP). In fact, the AACN (2021) nursing standards state that entry-level nurses "integrate best evidence into nursing practice" (Key Element 4.2, p. 43). There was a time when a systematic process for healthcare decision making was not the norm. So, how did this paradigm shift toward EBP occur? Dr. Archie Cochrane, a British epidemiologist, is widely regarded as the initial force behind evidence-based clinical practice in medicine (Brucker, 2016). Cochrane began the process of cataloging research, and the Cochrane Database of systematic literature reviews resulted from Dr. Cochrane's efforts. The Cochrane Database contains systematic reviews and guidelines for allied health professionals and nurse scholars seeking current research evidence on various topics.

Dr. David Sackett is also regarded as one of the founders of evidence-based medicine (EBM). Sackett led a group of clinical epidemiologists at McMaster University to publish a series of articles advising primary providers on how to appraise medical literature (Sackett, 1981). In 1996, Sackett and his primary provider colleagues disseminated the concept of EBM to standardize medical decision making (Sackett et al., 1997). As allied health disciplines adopted EBM, the term was changed to EBP for inclusivity. Today, EBP is normative for clinical decision making. It is widely accepted that higher education institutional libraries with allied health or medical education have dedicated EBP resource pages on their websites. Professional nursing organizations that support EBP include the ANA and Sigma, the international nursing honor society, both of whom have published position statements and guidance on the EBP process. The Johns Hopkins Center for Evidence-Based Practice describes EBP as the cornerstone of nursing practice (Johns Hopkins, 2024).

According to the ANA (n.d.), **evidence-based practice** (EBP) is defined as the provision of holistic quality care based on up-to-date research and knowledge as opposed to "the way it has always been done." According to Melnyk and Fineout-Overholt (2023), EBP in nursing is systematically searching for and critically appraising and synthesizing evidence (or research findings), along with consideration of expert clinical nursing judgment and patients' (or community's) wishes, in making healthcare decisions. EBP is represented visually as a triad of components: *the most current research, clinical acumen and experience*, and *patient (or community) preferences and values*. It is not a hierarchical process but an equitable process. As EBP has evolved, *healthcare resources* and *clinical state, setting, or circumstances* have been added (McMaster University, 2024). Incorporating setting and resources is relevant to the nurse working in C/PHN as often decisions are made using limited budgets and communities may be in areas with fewer resources. See Figure 4-5. Some of the most prominent resources are listed in Box 4-2.

Evidence-Based Practice Methods

Several models of the EBP methodology exist. Yet, all share the common goal of timeliness in clinical decision making. Nurses working in C/PHN are expected to develop clinical capacity to participate in or conduct EBP. Choosing a model and practicing the process of that model is one way to develop EBP clinical acumen.

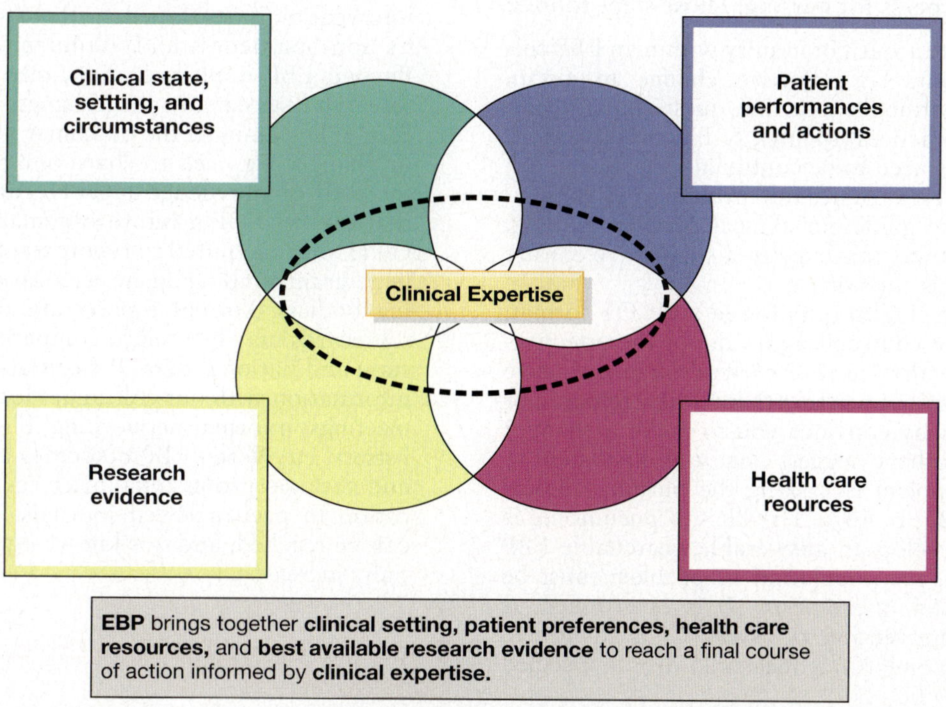

FIGURE 4-5 Evidence-based practice. (Reprinted with permission from McMaster University Health Sciences Library. *Evidence-based practice (EBP) at McMaster.* https://hslmcmaster.libguides.com/ebm/ebp)

BOX 4-2 Resources for Evidence-Based Practice Guidance or Toolkits

- The Centre for Evidence-Based Medicine at the University of Oxford EBM toolkit (https://www.cebm.ox.ac.uk/resources/ebm-tools)
- McMaster University Centre for Evidence-Based Medicine toolkits (https://hslmcmaster.libguides.com/ebm/ebp)
- Duke University Medical Center Library resources (https://guides.mclibrary.duke.edu/ebm#:~:text=Evidence%2Dbased%20practice%20is%20%22the,clinical%20evidence%20from%20systematic%20research.%22)
- Johns Hopkins Center for Evidence-Based Practice (https://www.hopkinsmedicine.org/evidence-based-practice/model-tools)
- American Nurses Association position on evidence-based practice (https://www.nursingworld.org/practice-policy/nursing-excellence/evidence-based-practice-in-nursing/)

The basic steps for EBM, based on Sackett et al. (1997), follow:

1. Pose a clinical question.
2. Find the best and most current evidence.
3. Evaluate the rigor of the evidence.
4. Apply information in combination with clinical expertise and patient values and priorities.
5. Evaluate outcomes.

Melnyk and Fineout-Overholt (2023) outline the steps of the EBP process for nursing. Those steps follow:

- Step 0: Cultivate a spirit of inquiry within an EBP culture/environment. For effective change to occur, nurses must continually examine, question, and challenge current practices (Melnyk & Fineout-Overholt, 2023). C/PHNs need to be continually curious about how we can best conduct our practice and the evidence needed to guide our clinical decision making; we also need to be immersed in a supportive culture that sustains this curiosity.
- Step 1: Ask the clinical question in a PICOT format. What if you or your colleagues doubt the effectiveness of some method in your current nursing practice and want to find out whether there is new research or evidence that may convince you to make a change? Melnyk and others suggest that the first step to solving the problem is "asking the burning clinical question" (2023, p. 467). The PICOT pneumonic is one way to develop an answerable, searchable EBP question. First, the population or problem must be specified (P). An intervention (I) is determined. A comparison intervention or issue (C) is identified. Finally, an outcome (O) is measured over a specified period of time (T).
- Step 2: Search for and collect the most relevant best evidence. Melnyk and Fineout-Overholt (2023) stress the importance of systematically searching for all relevant research on a clinical question of interest and critically analyzing the evidence while keeping in mind the unique needs of the clients served, as well as current practice standards, guidelines, and ethical considerations. Excellent places to begin are systematic, integrative, or scoping literature reviews.
- Step 3: Critically appraise the evidence for its validity, reliability, and applicability, and then synthesize that evidence. Collection and critical analysis of the best evidence in the literature constitute the second and third steps in the EBP process. Generally, it is helpful to generate a literature matrix so each article can be appraised for its level of evidence and its relevance to the phenomenon under investigation. Multiple methods exist for critical appraisals, including CASP (Critical Appraisal Skills Programme) Checklists for Research Papers, Johns Hopkins Nursing Evidence-Based Practice, Qualitative Evidence Synthesis Template, and PRISMA Transparent Reporting of Systematic Reviews and Meta-Analyses, among others (Downstate Health Sciences University, 2023).
- Step 4: Integrate the best evidence with one's clinical expertise, patient preferences, and values in making a practice decision or change. It is important to make a decision that incorporates your clinical expertise and your knowledge of your clients' values and preferences into your EBP practice (Melnyk & Fineout-Overholt, 2023). When examining population-based strategies, The Community Guide (n.d.) provides task force recommendations based on systematic reviews, along with additional resources on various topics of interest (https://www.thecommunityguide.org).
- Step 5: Evaluate outcomes of the practice decision or change based on evidence. A critical step of the EBP process is evaluating any practice change. Once an intervention is developed, further studies can evaluate its appropriateness and, ultimately, its effectiveness. Beyond EBP implementation, other clinically based research lines can also be designed.
- Step 6: Disseminate the outcomes of the EBP decision or change. We need to share our results to improve the body of knowledge in C/PHN and provide studies that can be used in future systematic reviews. Often, C/PHNs are required to report results to stakeholders (e.g., grant-funding agencies, local or county governing bodies). Formal reports are often required, or scorecards may be used to compare local results with state and national data. We can also share outcomes information with our colleagues locally, through staff meetings, informal networking, blogs, or a pertinent listserv, etc. When EBP outcomes are shared at state and national professional meetings or through publication in peer-reviewed journals, a wider audience can be reached, and our knowledge base is exponentially increased.

Evidence-Based Practice Ethical Considerations

The practice of EBP has demonstrated better patient health outcomes, but there are limits to EBP (Connor et al., 2023).

EBP has identified competencies that need to be developed and refined. If a deficit exists in the nurse's capacity to competently meet one or more of the steps in the EBP process, the process is impacted negatively. Nurses are ethically bound to develop competence in each area of EBP for implementation.

Constraints to ethical EBP also include the financial and policy limitations of the public health sector (see Box 4-3). The Institute for Healthcare Improvement (IHI) has a framework for calculating the return on investment (ROI) on an evidence-based intervention. The ROI is a ratio that divides the net profit or loss by the investment cost (Sadler et al., 2009). Implementation of EBP requires institutional time and money so nurses are provided with skilled mentors, education (e.g., workshops or webinars), and institutional commitments to the interdisciplinary process. If these factors are compromised, the EBP findings may be erroneous. Other constraints may include geographical locations. Rural or underserved healthcare areas may have limited material or human resources to allow nurses to develop EBP proficiencies. However, nurses can seek EBP mentors via memberships in professional organizations (e.g., Sigma Theta Tau) or via affiliations with area health education centers (AHECs) in their areas (AHEC, n.d.). See Box 4-4 for Spotlight on Essential Nursing Competencies.

Generally, EBP projects do not require IRB oversight or approval because they don't meet the federal definition of human subject protection. If an EBP project includes the use of an untested or new treatment or intervention, IRB approval and oversight is required. If the project includes protected health information of people, the standards of privacy and confidentiality apply. Even if an EBP project is exempt from IRB approval, ethics governing nursing practice (Table 4-5) still apply. Lastly, if EBP projects are to be disseminated (e.g., published in a journal), the author is still required to receive IRB approval prior to dissemination (Hockenberry, 2014).

C/PHNs Using EBP

Nurses use EBP across many C/PHN settings. For example, research has demonstrated the effectiveness of using the screening, brief intervention, and referral to treatment (SBIRT) method for substance misuse. SBIRT is widely recommended by governmental (CDC) and professional (American Academy of Pediatrics) organizations to help prevent disease, injury, and other negative consequences of substance misuse in people, families, and communities. Since 2016, SBIRT is required training among school nurses in Massachusetts public schools. For more information about SBIRT in Massachusetts schools, see https://shield.bu.edu/content/sbirt-schools-0 (School

BOX 4-3 LEVELS OF PREVENTION PYRAMID

Distributive Justice for People Experiencing Domestic Violence

SITUATION: Provide distributive justice for people experiencing domestic violence by changing a proposed state law that would eliminate funding for shelters for people experiencing domestic violence to a law that preserves resources for this population.
GOAL: Using the three levels of prevention, avoid or promptly diagnose and treat negative health conditions and restore the fullest possible potential.

Tertiary Prevention

Rehabilitation

If unable to stop the proposed law
- Seek volunteer services to fill the gaps in funding paid employees.
- Seek donations to support existing shelter buildings.

Prevention

Health Promotion and Education
- Educate the public regarding the need for lost/limited services using various forms of media and venues.

Health Protection
- Seek private resources or grants to fund shelters.
- Propose a new bill to match private funding for shelters at the next legislative session.

Secondary Prevention

Early Diagnosis
- Recognition that the proposed bill is going to pass

Prompt Treatment
- Advocate for amendments to the proposed bill to preserve limited funding for shelters.

Primary Prevention

Health Promotion and Education
- Advocacy
- Active lobbying against the bill
- Garnering community support in favor of the revised bill

Health Protection
- Community understands the impact of the potential loss
- Put a "human face" on the problem

BOX 4-4 **SPOTLIGHT ON ESSENTIAL NURSING COMPETENCIES**

Patient-Centered Care for EBP and Ethics

As a nurse, you have dealt with individual patients in acute care settings. Some of you have also worked closely with patient families. Now, you will be widening your lens to focus on larger groups of patients (e.g., aggregates) and communities (e.g., populations). How do your care practices apply to aggregates such as parents with substance use disorder or to population groups such as the older adults in your community?

As healthcare continues to evolve, nurses are being asked to shift to systems thinking rather than just focusing on an individual patient. The World Health Organization (2023) noted that systems thinking was needed to improve the quality of healthcare and that a quality health system was critical to the success of universal healthcare coverage around the world. We must solve the problems with quality and safety in healthcare. A systematic review of transitional care interventions that aimed to reduce hospital readmissions found that, to be successful, interventions needed to be flexible and individualized in response to patient needs, extend beyond the hospital stay, and include intensive discharge planning, coordination, and community referrals (Oyesanya et al., 2021). High-quality systems are patient centered and promote positive experiences for our clients. It is important that clients are treated with respect and courtesy, have their questions answered, be provided with education that they can understand, and have their needs addressed (Oyesanya et al., 2021).

We need to work with interdisciplinary teams to identify high-risk patients, prepare patients and their families for discharge, and then work with specialized programs that follow patients while they are at home to make sure they are continuing to adhere to medication and other intervention regimens (Oyesanya et al., 2021). Keeping care patient centered and demonstrating respect for our clients (people, families, aggregates, or populations) is a key to success.

1. *What other problems do you see that could benefit from a broader focus on quality and safety?*

Health Institute for Education and Leadership Development, 2024).

Nurses in Georgia employed EBP during the coronavirus (COVID-19) pandemic by using the Community Resiliency Model (CRM). The CRM model helps people understand stress reactions, distinguish between sensations of distress and well-being, and use sensory awareness skills to lessen the impact of stressful situations. Through their partnerships with community-based organizations, healthcare organizations, and the Georgia Nurses Association, these nurses were able to provide free virtual CRM classes across all of Georgia's 159 counties. Now that the pandemic has ended, the sustainability of this program includes engaging other C/PHNs in Georgia to become certified in CRM and continuing CRM training as part of their C/PHN practice (Duva et al., 2022).

QUALITY IMPROVEMENT

Like EBP, all nurses are expected to participate in QI. In fact, AACN's (2021) Domain 5 is specific to quality and safety and the roles of nursing across healthcare settings. **Quality improvement** (QI) is defined by the Agency for Healthcare Quality and Research (AHRQ, 2015) as a process by which the quality of care is continually assessed, and care is modified, where indicated, to produce better outcomes or to reduce cost. Unlike research, its results are not meant to be generalizable. QI processes are ongoing and potentially **transferable** across settings.

Quality Improvement Methods

The Public Health Foundation (n.d.), based in Washington, D.C., supports community-based and governmental organizations to improve community and public health outcomes. Its services include the provision of over 100 QI tools that can be accessed via https://www.phf.org/focusareas/qualityimprovement/Pages/Quality_Improvement.aspx. Two commonly used models used in C/PHN are Deming's Plan-Do-Study-Act (PDSA) cycles (The Deming Institute, 2024) and Green's PRECEDE-PROCEED model (Rural Health Information Hub [RHIH], 2024).

Deming's model is shown in Figure 4-6. The QI process begins with forming an interdisciplinary team so that diverse perspectives are offered with equity. Next, the team needs

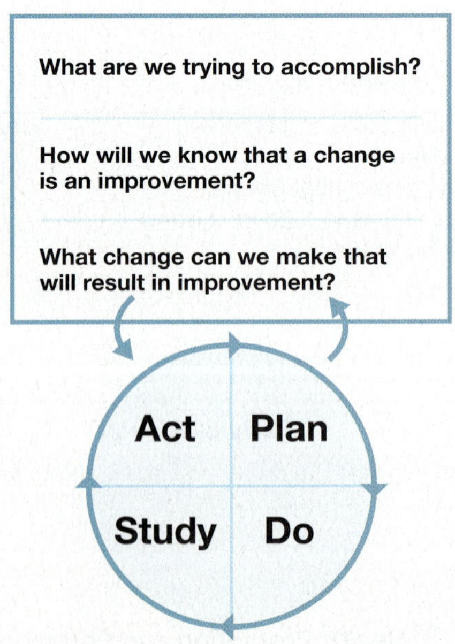

FIGURE 4-6 The model for Improvement. (Reprinted with permission from Institute for Healthcare Improvement. *How to improve: Model for Improvement,* https://www.ihi.org/resources/how-improve-model-improvement)

to define specific aims, including who, what, and where. Third, the team needs to define what constitutes a change from baseline. This requires the collection and evaluation of quantitative and qualitative data. To test for change, the team applies the PDSA cycle on a small scale in a real-world setting. After assessing for change on a small scale, changes can be implemented on larger scales through multiple PDSA cycles. If changes are positive, they can be implemented across other parts of the organization (IHI, 2023).

The PRECEDE-PROCEED model addresses health promotion and other public health needs. PRECEDE stands for predisposing, reinforcing, and enabling constructs in educational diagnosis and evaluation. Assessments associated with PRECEDE include social, epidemiologic, educational, ecologic, health program, and public policy domains. PROCEED stands for policy, regulatory, and organizational constructs in educational and environmental development. Evaluations included in PROCEED include process, short-term, intermediate, and long-term domains (RIRH, 2024). See Figure 4-7.

Quality Improvement Ethical Considerations

The ethics involved in QI are similar to those of EBP in that the formal definition of human subjects' research does not meet those defined by the federal government. Like with EBP, if a QI project includes the use of an untested or new treatment or intervention, IRB approval is required. Also, if the project includes protected health information of people, the standards of privacy and confidentiality apply. Finally, QI projects generally do not require IRB oversight prior to dissemination unless IRB approval and oversight is a condition of journal submission or an institutional requirement (Hockenberry, 2014).

C/PHNs Using QI

Nurses use QI to improve the public's health in a variety of ways. For instance, Thal and Jimenez (2019) used PDSA cycles to evaluate the job satisfaction of community health workers (CHWs) in the United States and abroad. Reaching out to CHWs in Lubbock, Texas, and Jinotega, Nicaragua, they sought to identify and explore characteristics and traits that might affect job satisfaction and, thus, improve the CHWs' services. Motivating characteristics included the desire to help people, to serve as change agents, and to be the voice of the people. CHWs identified teaching needs, allowing the nurses to provide

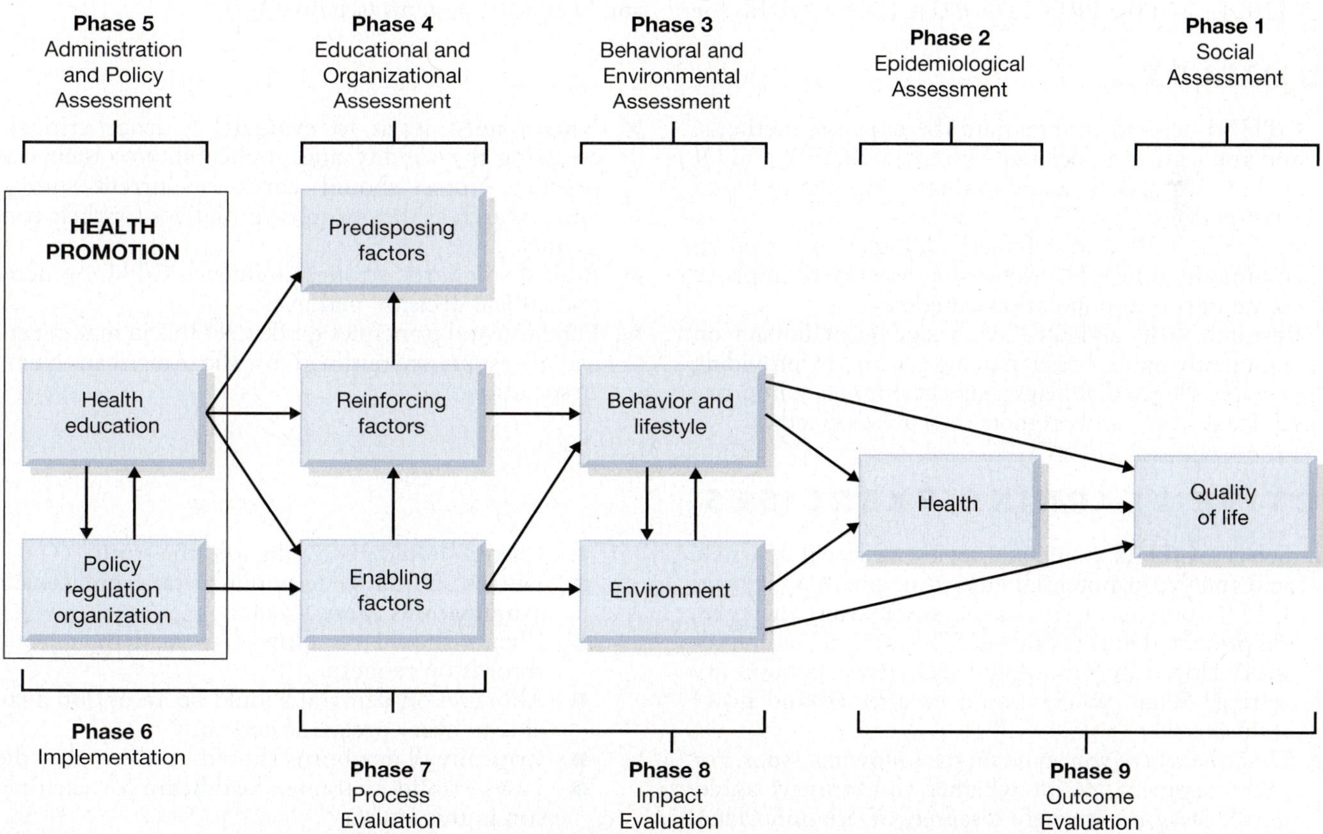

FIGURE 4-7 Applied PRECEDE-PROCEED Model. (Reprinted with permission from Korshus, E. (2015). *Weighing the evidence: One university takes a hard look at disordered eating among athletes.* Advanced Lesson Plan for Teachers. Harvard School of Public Health. Retrieved from https://www.hsph.harvard.edu/wp-content/uploads/sites/1267/2015/02/RevFINAL–Advanced–Teach–Note-Athletes-Case-Feb-20-15.pdf)

BOX 4-5 WHAT DO *YOU* THINK?

Neonatal Abstinence Syndrome (NAS)

Neonatal abstinence syndrome (NAS) is a set of conditions caused when a baby withdraws from drugs it was exposed to in utero. NAS can also be referred to as neonatal opioid withdrawal syndrome (March of Dimes, 2024). This can be caused by a person taking opioids during pregnancy. It can also be caused by antidepressants, barbiturates, or benzodiazepines. These drugs can pass through the placenta and expose the fetus. Public health nurses working with a local hospital in Indiana created a QI project addressing the prolonged hospitalization and medications required to treat NAS (Nicholson et al., 2023). Applying the eat, sleep, console (ESC) method, nurses hoped to influence length of stay and decrease morphine use when compared with a current scoring system (Finnegan Neonatal Abstinence Scoring System). Use of the ESC method decreased length of hospital stay and showed an 88% reduction in rate of scheduled morphine initiation. While further research on long-term neurodevelopment needs to be done, C/PHN can be part of broader interdisciplinary community change through QI projects. These projects can influence new processes improving the community's health.

1. *What issues do you see in your community setting that would benefit from quality improvement projects?*
2. *How can C/PHN partner with industry for change in your community?*
3. *How would you apply the PRECEDE-PROCEED model to this QI project?*

Source: March of Dimes (2024); Nicholson et al. (2023).

courses on chronic disease management and hands-on skill training.

Li et al. (2022) used the PRECEDE-PROCEED model to improve Chinese birthing parents' knowledge, skill, and sense of competence in caring for their preterm infants. Their results suggested that this model could help improve family caregiving among this population. Finally, Guevarra et al. (2021) used the PRECEDE-PROCEED MODEL for drowning prevention in the Philippines. The authors demonstrate that the model was effective not only for both planning drowning prevention interventions but also for evaluating the results of the implementation process, the capacity of the population, and outcomes for drowning prevention. Through standardized processes and structures, QI can improve health outcomes for patients, communities, and healthcare systems (see Box 4-5).

SUMMARY

- C/PHNs need to differentiate the purpose, methods, and application associated with research, EBP, and QI as they create, design, and evaluate community-based interventions.
- Research, EBP, and QI methodologies are used in community public health nursing practice to improve community and population outcomes.
- Research, EBP, and QI have a significant impact on community public health nursing practice by providing new knowledge that helps shape health policy, improve service delivery, and promote the public's health.
- Nurses must learn to evaluate evidence critically, assessing the validity and applicability to their own practice. Nurses should search for current evidence and research as they propose initiatives for their community.
- Ethical standards strongly influence C/PHN practice and ethical decision making.
- Fundamental principles guide C/PHNs in making ethical decisions as outlined by the American Nurses Association.

ACTIVE LEARNING EXERCISES

1. Select a C/PHN systematic review or research article and analyze its potential impact on health policy and C/PHN practice. Critique the article using the criteria presented in this chapter. What are the main findings? How can you apply this to your community setting? What policies could be affected and how? (Objective 1)
2. Describe where you stand on the following issues. For each statement, decide whether you strongly agree, agree, disagree, strongly disagree, or are undecided. Discuss your rationales and compare your results with a small group of classmates. (Objective 2):
   - Clients have the right to participate in all decisions related to their healthcare.
   - Continuing education should not be mandatory to maintain licensure.
   - Clients should always be told the truth.
   - Nurses should be required to take prelicensure examinations every 5 years.
   - Clients should be allowed to read their health records on request.
   - Abortion on demand should be an option available to every pregnant person.
   - Critically ill newborns should be allowed to die.
   - Laws should guarantee healthcare for each person in this country.
3. Search local or national news for stories involving ethical dilemmas. Pick one and describe which ethical principles were involved. How was the dilemma resolved? Or how would you go about deciding on an equitable resolution? (Objective 2)

4. As a C/PHN working in a big city, you encounter a large number of children with lead poisoning due to environmental contamination. You are interested in lead abatement programs. Where can you find evidence of successful programs/outcomes, cost-benefit analysis, and policies that have been implemented in other areas? Who would need to be involved in getting this type of program instituted? (Objective 3)
5. Find a community/public health study (research, EBP, or QI) that represents efforts to "Strengthen, Support, and Mobilize Communities and Partnerships" (one of the 10 Essential Public Health Services; see Box 2-2) (e.g., community-based participatory research study). How would you apply the methods, interventions, and findings of that study to an issue in your community? (Objective 3)
6. You have just completed an EBP implementation study on the effectiveness of a series of birth control classes in three high schools, and the results show a reduction in the number of pregnancies over the last year. Is this enough information to declare it a success? What else could you do to strengthen your case? Describe three ways that you could disseminate this information to your nursing colleagues and school officials. (Objective 4)

CHAPTER 5

Transcultural Nursing

"The beauty of the world lies in the diversity of its people."

—Author Unknown

KEY TERMS

Complementary and alternative medicine (CAM)
Cultural assessment
Cultural brokering
Cultural diversity
Cultural self-awareness
Culture
Culture shock
Dominant values
Enculturation
Ethnic group
Ethnicity
Ethnocentrism
Explicit bias
Home remedies
Indigenous
Intersectionality
Implicit bias
Majority—minority
Microcultures
Race
Subcultures
Transcultural nursing
Value

LEARNING OBJECTIVES

Upon mastery of this chapter, you should be able to:

1. Explain the concept of culture as it pertains to populations and care.
2. Discuss the meaning of cultural diversity and its significance for community/public health nursing.
3. Describe the meaning and effects of ethnocentrism and biases on community/public health nursing practices at the individual and agency level.
4. Identify ethnocultural health practices used to promote healing and treat illness.
5. Demonstrate culturally congruent actions for diverse groups and populations.
6. Apply principles of transcultural nursing in community/public health nursing practice.

INTRODUCTION

The United States is a country of immigrants. People of many different cultural groups and races built this nation. For hundreds of years, people have seen this land as a refuge from political, religious, or economic strife. **Indigenous** (native, endemic) people were present when the early settlers arrived on these shores and when people were brought here in slavery. Refugees fleeing poverty and hunger, as well as war and oppression, flocked to this country over the next two centuries. The citizenship of most countries around the world is an amalgamation of people who have different values, ideals, and behaviors. Many people have chosen to discover their ancestry through DNA testing as a means of drawing families closer together. Do you know the story of how your ancestors came to your country?

Although Americans have many differences, they also have much in common. In Western culture, a person's work and creative achievements are applauded. There is respect for one another's personal preferences about food, dress, or personal beliefs. The right to be oneself—and thereby to be different from others—is even protected by state and federal laws. Although individuality is a cherished American value, there are limits to the range of differences most Americans find acceptable. People with behavior outside the acceptable range may be labeled as socially nonconforming. For example, U.S. culture approves of moderate alcohol intake but not alcohol use disorder.

The beliefs and sanctions of the dominant or majority culture are called **dominant values**. In the United States, the majority culture is White people who are not Hispanic and whose dominant values have largely included work ethic, thrift, success, independence, initiative, privacy, cleanliness, attractive appearance, and a focus on the future. Dominant values reflect the cultural power differentials and the unearned, frequently unrecognized privileges held by Americans with White social identities (Krosch et al., 2022).

Following the 2020 U.S. census, the demographics of the United States reveal a change in size and distribution of the population. These changes reveal that the

U.S. population is more multiracial and diverse than in the past (United States Census Bureau, 2022). Changes noted from U.S. census data from 2010 to 2020 include the following:

- White alone, non-Hispanic is the most prevalent racial group in the United States at 57.8% of the population down from 63.7% in 2010.
- Hispanic/Latino population is the second largest racial or ethnic group comprising 18.7% of the population.
- Black or African American alone, non-Hispanic population is the third largest group at 12.1%.
- The remaining racial or ethnic groups combined make up 11.4% of the U.S. population.
- White alone, non-Hispanic population was the most prevalent racial or ethnic group for all states except California (Hispanic/Latino), New Mexico (Hispanic/Latino), Hawaii (Asian), and District of Columbia (Black/African American).
- Multiracial, non-Hispanic groups are the second most prevalent group in many counties throughout the United States (United States Census Bureau, 2022).

The rise within the United States in multiracial identity is measured by the diversity index which "measures the probability that two people chosen at random will be from different racial or ethnic groups" (United States Census Bureau, 2022, para 3). The states with the highest diversity scores include the following:

- States from the west include Hawaii, California, and Nevada.
- States from the east include Maryland, the District of Columbia, New York, and New Jersey.
- States from the southern region include Florida, Georgia, and Texas (United States Census Bureau, 2022).

The United States has become increasingly more blended, with a 276% rise in multiracial identification (two or more races) (Jones et al., 2021). Many people now identify with more than one racial or ethnic group. Coupled with the increase in mixed-race families, this has changed social dynamics, giving rise to multiracial identity (Mizrahi, 2020). However, despite this demographic shift, health disparities, structural inequality, and systemic racism does exist, influencing health disparities for vulnerable and underrepresented groups (see Chapter 23) (Berger & Miller, 2021). As the United States moves toward a **majority-minority**, defined as "racial minority Americans outnumbering non-Hispanic White" (Krosch et al., 2022), an understanding of diverse and cultural differences, inclusive and equitable practices for all people and the influence of SDOH on those practices, as well as power, privilege, and discriminatory actions, is necessary (Krosch et al., 2022; Santoro, 2023). As C/PHNs, awareness of our values as well as the values and beliefs of our clients is crucial. Values shape people's thoughts and behaviors; this awareness helps nurses answer questions such as the following:

- Why are some client behaviors acceptable to health professionals and others are not?
- Why do nurses have difficulty persuading certain clients to accept new ways of thinking and acting?
- What can I and community agencies do to support the needs of our diverse communities?

Explanations for such questions can be found by examining the concept of culture, especially its influence on health, health behaviors, and C/PHN practice. For example:

- An emphasis on the need for milk in the diet may reflect cultural blindness, considering that people from diverse ethnic groups are often lactose intolerant and that food allergies affecting the quality of life for underrepresented children appear to be understudied and undiagnosed (Warren et al., 2021).
- Regardless of their own cultural backgrounds, most healthcare providers are generally educated to believe that the biomedical model is the best framework, and dominant social values are often reinforced.

However, these dominant values can and do change as a result of changing demographics and population shifts (Fig. 5-1). Current research on this issue reveals areas of concern (Box 5-1).

Awareness of dominant culture and values helps us better understand political, socioeconomic, and healthcare outcomes.

- Because the powerful exert control over political, economic, and social structures that influence all members of society, laws are in place prohibiting discrimination based on "race, color, religion, national origin, and sex," as well as disability (U.S. Equal Employment Opportunity Commission, n.d.-a, para. 1). Governments' political decisions affecting the health of populations have led to discrimination, bias, inequality, incarceration, and other conditions tied to the health and well-being of the population (Supreme Court of the United States, 2022; U.S. Equal Employment Opportunity Commission, n.d.-b).
- Culture so strongly influences C/PHN practice that the Council of Public Health Nursing Organizations incorporated it into the competency domains for C/PHN practice. Domain 4, cultural competency skills, focuses on individual and community needs, actions to support a diverse workforce, an organization's cultural competence, and the effect of public health policies/programs on diverse populations (Council of Public Health Nursing Organizations, 2018).

THE CONCEPT OF CULTURE

Culture refers to the beliefs, values, and behaviors that are shared by members of a society and provide a template or "road map" for living.

- Culture tells people what is acceptable or unacceptable in a given situation.
- Culture dictates what to do, say, or believe.
- Culture is learned. As children grow up, they learn from their parents and others around them how to

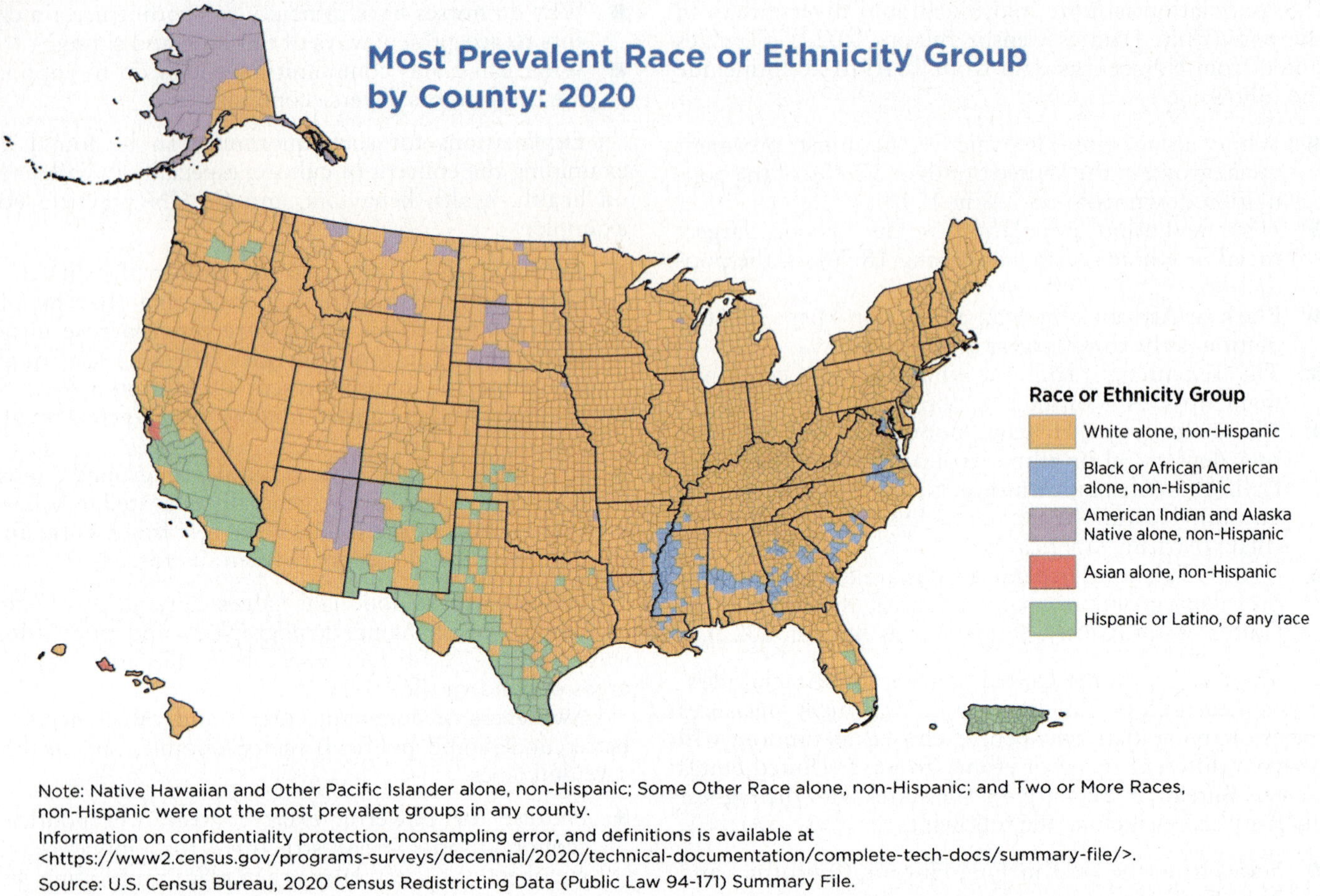

FIGURE 5-1 Most Prevalent Race or Ethnic Group by County: 2020. (Source: U.S. Census Bureau. (2022). *2020 U.S. population more racially and ethnically diverse than measured in 2010.* https://www.census.gov/library/stories/2021/08/2020-unitedstates-population-more-racially-ethnicallydiverse-than-2010.html)

BOX 5-1 WHAT DO *YOU* THINK?

Transition to a Majority—Minority Nation

According to projections from the U.S. Census Bureau, in a seminal article by Perez and Hirschman (2009), the United States will become a majority—minority nation in the 21st century. It is projected that by mid-century, the current underrepresented groups will gain in population while the existing majority non-Hispanic White population decreases as noted in trending from the last two decades (U.S. Census Bureau, 2022). This is manifesting across the 50 states with the growth of the Hispanic population and two or more races' groups (U.S. Census Bureau, 2022). Geographic areas are seeing a shift as well with majority demographics for some states and counties (U.S. Census Bureau, 2022). The shift to majority—minority standing may lead to anxiety and concern associated with beliefs in conspiracy theories regarding "White replacement" (Krosch et al., 2022, para 1). Additionally, this impending shift could lead to anger and fear toward underrepresented groups with implicit and explicit behaviors and attitudes as noted in actions and policies against those groups (Krosch et al., 2022). This phenomenon is not unique to one racial or ethnic group; researchers have found similar results with other groups who perceived a loss of status (socioeconomic or otherwise) as threatening to their position and perceived level of discrimination (Krosch et al., 2022).

1. *Have you noticed demographic changes in your area? How do you feel about these changes?*
2. *Do you see any signs of dominant group anxiety and perceived threats to group status? How might they affect healthcare in the coming decades?*
3. *Have you experienced or observed discrimination in healthcare settings?*

Source: Krosch et al. (2022); U.S. Census Bureau (2022); Perez and Hirschman (2009).

interpret the world. In turn, these assimilated beliefs and values prescribe desired behavior. We think of this as learned behavior, but can culture actually impact your neurobiology (Qu et al., 2019)? (Box 5-2).

Culture is a multifaceted concept, a way of organizing and thinking about life. Culture includes customs, law, morals, beliefs, knowledge, and habits practiced by members of a group or society. It is all the socially inherited characteristics of a group, comprising everything that one generation can tell, convey, or hand down to the next generation. Scholars from many disciplines have defined culture in the following ways:

- The characteristics or knowledge of a group of people encompassing their language, religion, social habits, food, art, and music (Pappas & McKelvie, 2022)
- The personal identification that is specific to race, religion, ethnicity, geographic region, or social groups (Agency for Healthcare Research and Quality [AHRQ], 2019)
- A mediating or moderating variable in business, human relations, psychology, and most human endeavors; culture is equivalent to our actions (Coyle, 2022).
- Shared standards as part of a group's socialization for interactions, behaviors, understanding, and beliefs (Les Elfes International, 2021).

Anthropologists describe culture as systems of beliefs, values, and norms of behavior found in all societies. More than simply custom or ritual, it is a way of organizing and thinking about life. It gives people a sense of security about their behavior; without having to consciously think about it, they know how to act. For example:

- Culture impacts the thinking process and one's perception of the world.
- It determines the value one places on family, work, religion, and independence.
- Culture influences current and past generations (Les Elfes International, 2021).

Every community and social or ethnic group has its own culture; individual members act based on what they have learned within their culture. As anthropologist Edward Hall (1959) noted over a half-century ago, culture controls our lives and influences even the smallest

BOX 5-2 EVIDENCE-BASED PRACTICE

Can Culture Affect Your Neurobiology?

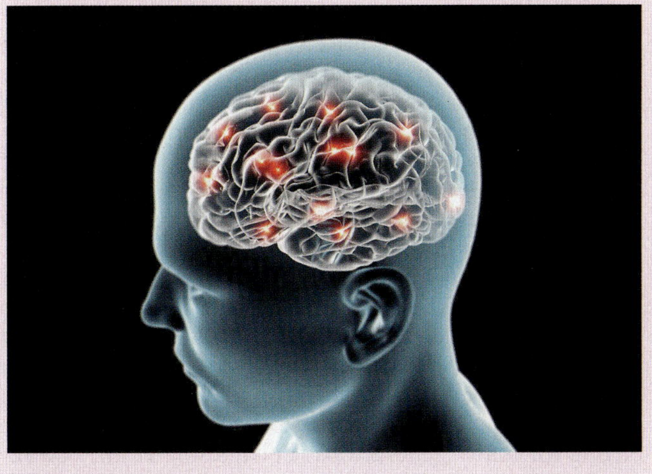

Research into the neuroscience of culture examines the interplay between culture, biologic factors, and physiologic processes.

Stress can affect our ability to make changes and to adapt to change. Chronic stress alters brain chemistry and can lead to poor decision making. As the brain senses anxiety, an innate sense of survival kicks in for greater performance; however, toxic stress (unmanaged stress) can influence our decision making, making everyday decisions more difficult while paradoxically increasing stress and fatigue. Prolonged or frequent activation of a stress response in the absence of buffering, protective, or supportive mechanisms impacts a lifetime of psychological, physical, and mental health issues (Shonkoff et al., 2021).

Racism has been identified as a source of toxic stress associated with poor health outcomes. Researchers examined 97 maternal–child dyads and the relationship between maternal experiences of racial discrimination and child indicators of toxic stress to determine if relational support by prior participation in a home-based early visiting intervention was a protective factor. Using the Experience of Discrimination Scale, birthing parents reported on racial discrimination as an indicator of toxic stress; child indicators included salivary biomarkers of inflammation (proinflammatory cytokines and C-reactive protein), maternal report of child behavioral issues, and body mass index. Black (33%) and Hispanic (64%) birthing parents' identification with racism were associated with their child's elevated tumor necrosis factor-α levels and salivary interleukin-6 but not body mass index. Interestingly, early home intervention mediated the child interleukin-6 levels (Condon et al., 2021).

A longitudinal study examined U.S. adults ages 71 to 80 years with heart disease and type 2 diabetes over 8 years. Participants self-identified their race. Stress along with a lifetime of discrimination were measured every 2 years using the Stressful Life Experiences survey. Of the 3004 adults in the study, lifetime discrimination was strongly associated with self-reported poorer health (negative health change over time) for Black and other race participants as compared with White. Having none versus two or more major experiences of lifetime discrimination were associated with 33% lower odds of poorer self-reported health (Nkwata et al., 2020).

1. *What are your impressions of these findings?*
2. *How can this information be useful to you as a nurse working with different cultural groups?*
3. *Can this research impart a risk of stereotyping people from different groups?*

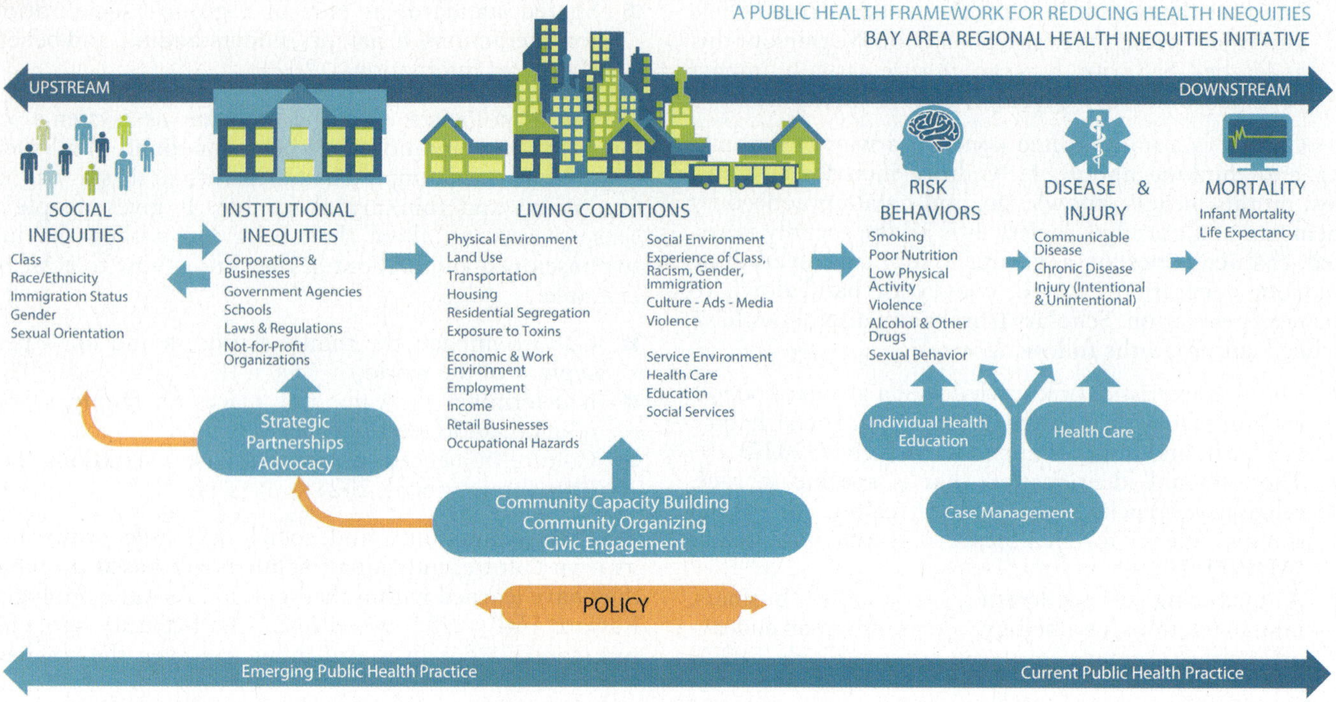

FIGURE 5-2 A public health framework for reducing health inequities. (Used with permission from Bay Area Regional Health Inequities Initiative, with updated graphics by California Department of Public Health. http://barhii.org/framework/)

elements of everyday living. It is the knowledge people use to design their own actions and, in turn, to interpret others' behavior (Pappas & McKelvie, 2022). For example, culture:

- Determines the appropriate comfortable distance for two people to stand when speaking to each other.
- Influences one's perception of time, such as whether time is considered to be a strict or more elastic construct (seen, for example, in whether individuals are on time or late for appointments).

The concept of culture must be distinguished from two other related but different concepts:

- **Race** is a social construct based on physical characteristics that cultures consider socially significant.
- An **ethnic group** is an assemblage of people with a shared **ethnicity** culture and identity; they may share a common geographic origin, race, language, religion, traditions, values, and food preferences (Ontology Search, 2023).

Race and ethnicity are factors influencing social inequality and, ultimately, morbidity and mortality. See Figure 5-2.

Cultural Diversity

Cultural diversity, or cultural plurality, refers to the coexistence of a variety of cultural patterns within a geographic area. This diversity can occur both between and within countries and communities. Cultural diversity within communities has unique advantages and challenges. Language barriers and misunderstanding of cultural values can occur, whereas cultural practices, celebrations, and food traditions can enrich the community.

A major driver of cultural diversity in the United States has been immigration. Cultural diversity in the United States began when Native Americans were challenged by early foreign settlements. Before the mid-20th century, settlers came primarily from European countries, peaking in numbers just after the turn of the 20th century, with about nine million immigrants admitted in the first decade. During much of that time, especially during the late 1600s through the early 1800s, Africans were brought to the United States against their will, mostly to Southern states, where they were sold to plantation owners as property to labor on large plantations and farms. Slavery and cultural oppression engendered profound effects for many generations (Bellagamba et al., 2020).

Immigration stayed high during the early 1900s and then dropped sharply from the 1950s to 1980s. It has risen more significantly since 2000. Immigration from regions such as Asia and South America steadily increased. In 2022, a record number of immigrants on the U.S. southern borders came from Cuba, Haiti, El Salvador, Guatemala, Nicaragua, Venezuela, and Mexico (Batalova et al., 2023). Ward and Batalova (2023) note that the total number of immigrants from all countries exceeded the number who arrived during the first decade of the 20th century, when immigration was formerly at its peak (Fig. 5-3).

Current trends in U.S. immigration include the following:

- The United States had nearly 51 million migrants in 2020 and has more international migrants than any

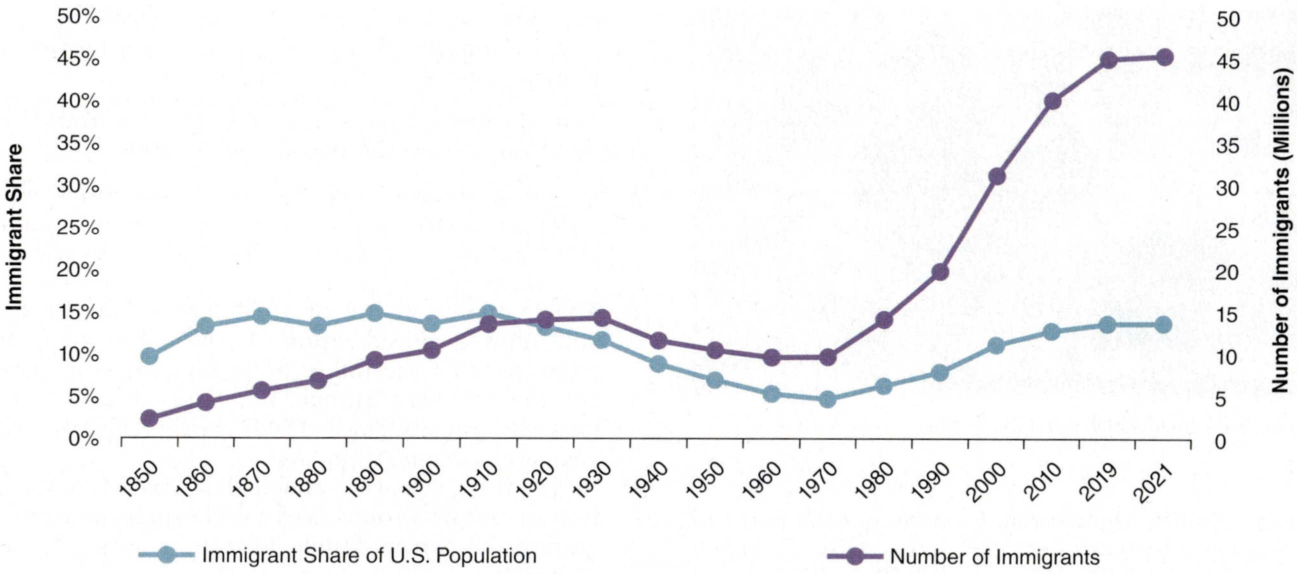

Sources: Migration Policy Institute (MPI) tabulation of data from U.S. Census Bureau, 2010-21 American Community Surveys (ACS), and 1970, 1990, and 2000 decennial census. All other data are from Campbell J. Gibson and Emily Lennon, "Historical Census Statistics on the Foreign-Born Population of the United States: 1850 to 1990" (Working Paper no. 29, U.S. Census Bureau, Washington, DC, 1999).

FIGURE 5-3 Size and share of the foreign-born population in the United States 1850–2021. (Originally published by the Migration Policy Institute in Nicole Ward and Jeanne Batalova, "Frequently Requested Statistics on Immigrants and Immigration in the United States," *Migration Information Source,* March 14, 2023, https://www.migrationpolicy.org/article/frequently-requested-statistics-immigrants-and-immigration-united-states. Reprinted with permission.)

other country due to displacement from conflict, violence, or disasters (Natarajan et al., 2022).

- Immigrants arrive from all regions of the world, in greater numbers from some areas than others (Fig. 5-4), becoming lawful permanent residents and, in due course, U.S. citizens (Homeland Security, 2022) (Fig. 5-5).
- Mexico/Latin America comprised the largest group of immigrants in 2021. India and China were the second largest immigration group (Ward & Batalova, 2023) (Fig. 5-4).
- The U.S. states with the most immigrants include California, Texas, Florida, New York, and New Jersey (Ward & Batalova, 2023).
- Rapid growth in the Hispanic/Latino population (Box 5-3; Table 5-1).

Undocumented or unauthorized immigration continues to be a controversial topic in the United States:

- Immigration backlog is at record levels; wait times for hearings now average 5 years.
- The Migrant Protection Protocols, also known as "Remain in Mexico," aimed to return thousands of immigrants on the U.S. southern Mexico border back to Mexico into dangerous and overcrowded shelters. The June 2022 Supreme Court ruling *Biden v. Texas* ended this practice.
- Unaccompanied minor crossings are at an all-time high on the southern U.S. Mexico border. Minors journey north to reunite with their families and to escape violence and poverty. Many minors cross the borders alone and are given asylum protection for unaccompanied minors.
- Temporary protected status (TPS) allows migrants from designated countries due to conflict to enter the United States for up to 18 months during which time they are eligible to work, have travel authorization, and are protected from deportation. Recent status

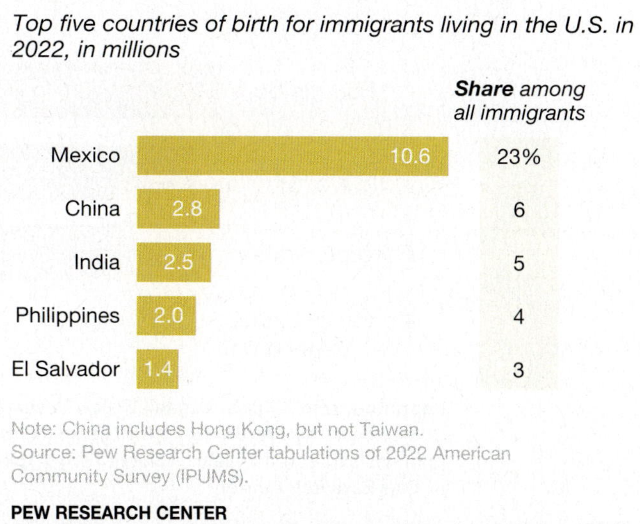

FIGURE 5-4 Mexico, China, and India are among the top birthplaces for immigrants in the United States. (Reprinted from "Key findings about U.S. immigrants." Pew Research Center, Washington, D.C. (2024). https://www.pewresearch.org/short-reads/2024/07/22/key-findings-about-us-immigrants/. Pew Research Center bears no responsibility for the analyses or interpretations of the data presented here. The opinions expressed herein, including any implications for policy, are those of the author and not of Pew Research Center.)

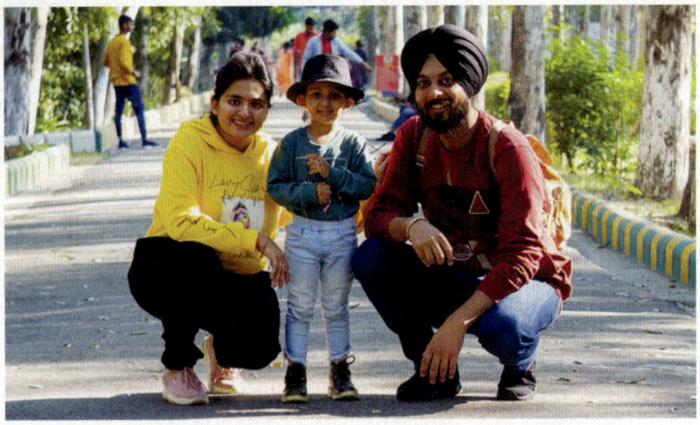

FIGURE 5-5 Sikh family, now U.S. citizens.

now includes Afghanistan, Cameroon, Ethiopia, and Ukraine; temporary protected status exists for many central American countries as well (Roy, 2022).

- Social justice is an important issue in community/public health nursing, and the national debate does not often consider the economic desperation and security concerns that drive people to put themselves in such jeopardy (see Chapter 23).

Immigration patterns are strongly influenced by immigration laws established since the 1800s:

- In 1891, medical and economic inspections were ordered at all major entry points as an influx of immigrants mostly from Europe led to fears of disease and contagion.
- The Immigration Act of 1924 limited immigration and allowed consideration of national origin in an effort to slow the influx of immigrants from Eastern and Southern Europe. Immigration has steadily trended upward since 1945, partly explained by changes in immigration laws.
- In 1965, quotas were ended that limited immigration of certain groups, and family-sponsored immigration, known as family migration, was officially endorsed.
- The Immigration Reform and Control Act of 1986 (Public Law 99-603) "legalized 2.7 million undocumented

BOX 5-3 Hispanic Population Trend in the United States

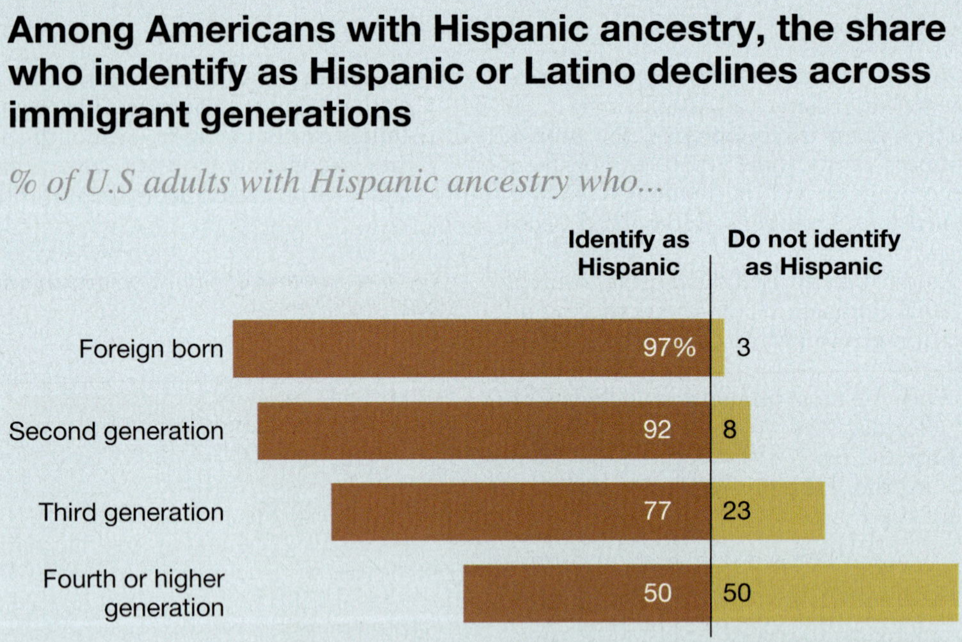

Reprinted from "Who Is Hispanic?" Pew Research Center, Washington, D.C. (2023). Pew Research Center bears no responsibility for the analyses or interpretations of the data presented here. The opinions expressed herein, including any implications for policy, are those of the author and not of Pew Research Center.

The U.S. Census Bureau identifies Hispanic as an ethnicity (not a race), and while the distinction surrounding race and ethnicity may seem unclear, identity is important. About 29% of Hispanics in the United States said being Hispanic was a matter of ancestry, 42% said it was a matter of culture, and 17% indicated being Hispanic was a matter of race. Many Hispanics/Latinos now define themselves (as noted in the 2020 census) as some other race, two or more races, or White. Generations of Hispanic/Latino families now live in the United States, with third and fourth generations of individuals as well as interracial marriage contributing to the percentage of adults with Hispanic ancestry who do not identify as Hispanic (as indicated in the figure in this box) but rather self-identify as multiracial or White.

Source: "Who Is Hispanic?" Pew Research Center, Washington, D.C. (2023).

TABLE 5-1 US Population by Race and Hispanic/Latino Origin, Census 2010 and 2020

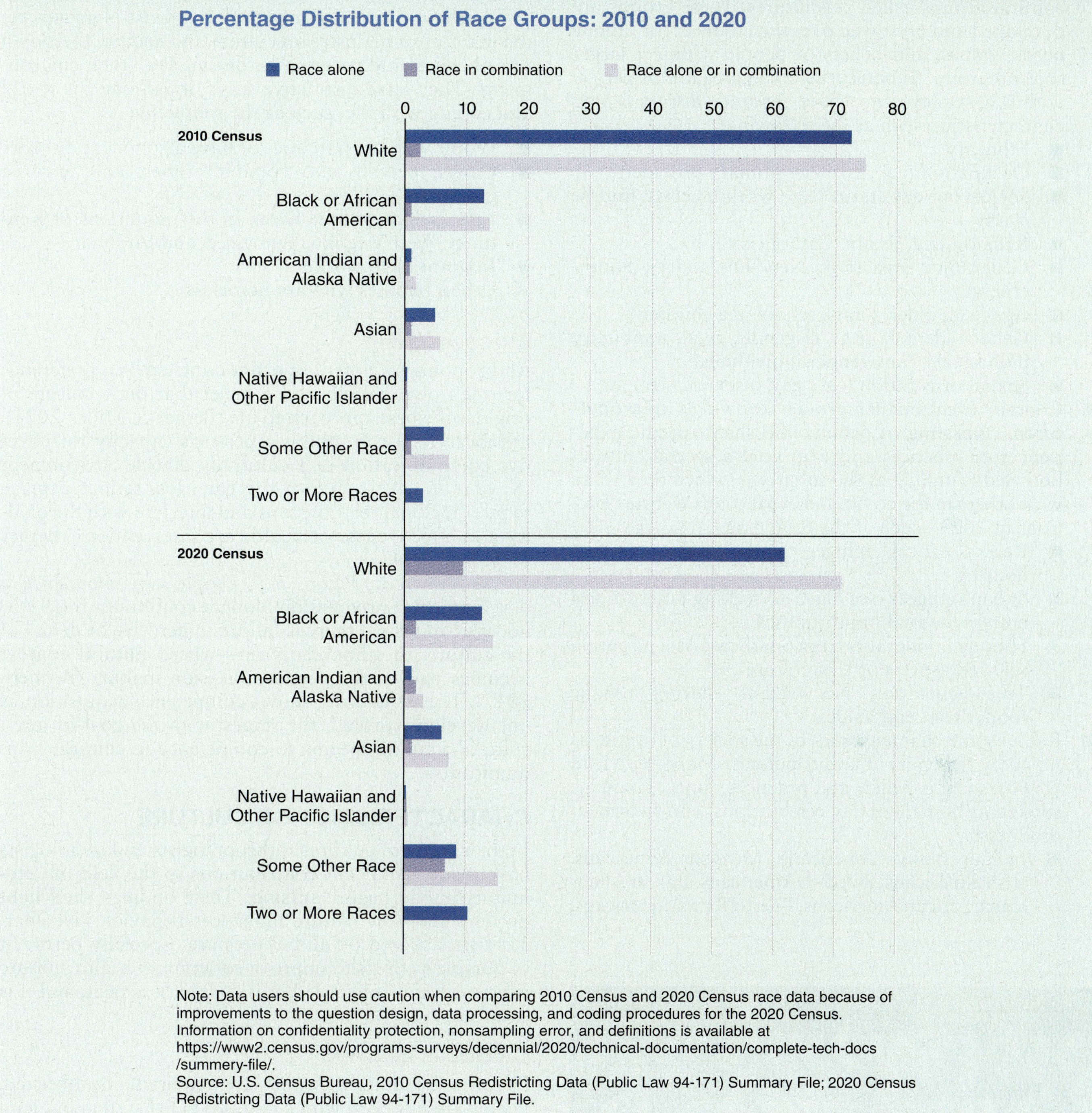

Source: U.S. Census (2022). *Improved race and ethnicity measures reveal U.S. population is much more multiracial.* https://www.census.gov/library/stories/2021/08/improved-race-ethnicity-measures-reveal-united-states-population-much-more-multiracial.html

immigrants," and the Immigration Act of 1990 (Public Law 101-649) set numerical ceilings on certain immigrant groups, in part due to the AIDS crisis, and authorized increases for highly skilled workers or specific family members of immigrants (Bolter, 2022).

The terrorist attacks in 2001 led U.S. President George W. Bush to suspend all immigration for 2 months. Suspicion about people from Middle Eastern countries permeated the nation—and worsened the social climate for immigrants. This social climate in the United States and other countries is often characterized by ambivalence about accepting refugees and immigrants and ambiguity about their status, such that newcomers find an environment that is both welcoming and hostile (Bolter, 2022).

- Although broad cultural values are shared by most large national societies, those societies contain smaller cultural groups called subcultures. These groups are developed and preserved over time to meet the unique needs, values, and beliefs of people within a larger societal group. **Subcultures** are aggregates of people within a society who share separate distinguishing characteristics, such as the following:
  - Ethnicity
  - Occupation (e.g., farmers, primary providers)
  - Socioeconomic status (e.g., working class, middle class)
  - Religion (e.g., Islam, Catholicism)
  - Geographic area (e.g., New Englanders, Southerners)
  - Age (e.g., older adults, school-age children)
  - Gender identity (e.g., cisgender, men, nonbinary individuals, transgender individuals)
  - Sexual orientation (e.g., gay, bisexual, straight)
- Contain even smaller groups known as **microcultures**, consisting of people who share specific experiences or practices and who hold a special cultural knowledge unique to the subgroup, which they share with others in the community (Merriam Webster Dictionary, 2023), such as the following:
  - Recent African refugees sharing resources and housing
  - Syrian refugees (see Fig. 5-6) seeking business and entrepreneurial opportunities
  - Hmong immigrants from Southeast Asia adopting selected aspects of U.S. culture
  - Third-generation Norwegians sharing unique food, dress, and values
- Retain some characteristics of the society of origin, as noted by the eminent anthropologist Margaret Mead (1960), such as beliefs and practices, foods, language spoken at home, holiday celebrations, and treatment of illness:
  - Include Native Americans, Mexican Americans, Irish Americans, Swedish Americans, Italian Americans, African Americans, Puerto Rican Americans, Chinese Americans, Japanese Americans, Vietnamese Americans, and many other ethnic groups

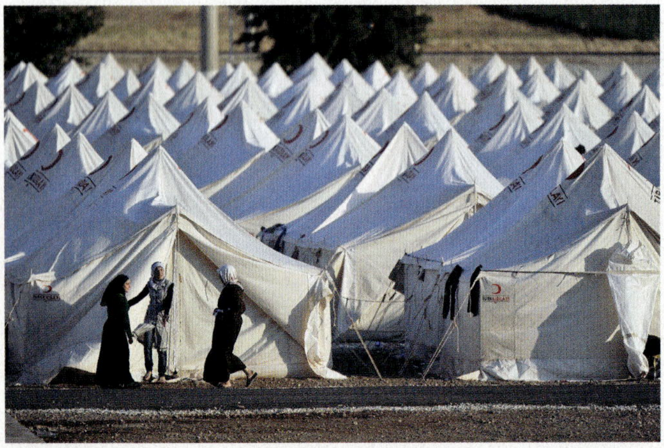

FIGURE 5-6 Syrian refugee camp.

Furthermore, many microcultures exist in groups on the margins of mainstream culture and acquire their own sets of beliefs and patterns for dealing with their environments. They have distinctive ways of defining the world and coping with life, such as the following:

- People who use narcotics or have alcohol use disorder
- Gangs, people who commit crimes, and terrorist groups
- Appalachian people living in the mountains of Kentucky, West Virginia, Tennessee, and Virginia
- Migrant farm workers
- Urban families who are homeless

Ethnocentrism

Anthropologists note that **ethnocentrism** is a preference for one's own culture and a belief that one's culture of origin is the best approach to life (Berger & Miller, 2021). Ethnocentrism can inhibit a person's capacity for effective communication in a culturally diverse environment (Kaya et al., 2021). In turn, this can cause serious damage to interpersonal relationships and interfere with the quality and effectiveness of healthcare interventions (Berger & Miller, 2021).

As shown in Figure 5-7, people can experience a developmental progression along a continuum from ethnocentrism, where there is failure to perceive or denial of the culture, to ethnorelativism—where cultural context becomes part of the person's decision making (Bennett, 2017). The sequencing shows competence acquisition as one develops through the stages, with the goal of intercultural training specific to competence in cultural communication.

CHARACTERISTICS OF CULTURE

In their study of culture, anthropologists and sociologists have made significant contributions to the field of community/public health nursing. Their findings shed light on why and how culture influences behavior. Five characteristics shared by all cultures are especially pertinent to nursing's efforts to improve community health: culture is learned, it is integrated, it is shared, it is tacit, and it is dynamic.

Culture Is Learned

Patterns of cultural behavior are acquired, not inherited. People are not born with a cultural belief system but gain it through **enculturation**, the process of learning one's culture (Fig. 5-8). Aspects one learns through enculturation include (Kottack, 2022) the following:

- Beliefs
- Dress
- Diet
- Language
- Expressions of emotions such as sadness, grief, joy, and happiness
- Smiling, laughter, and humor

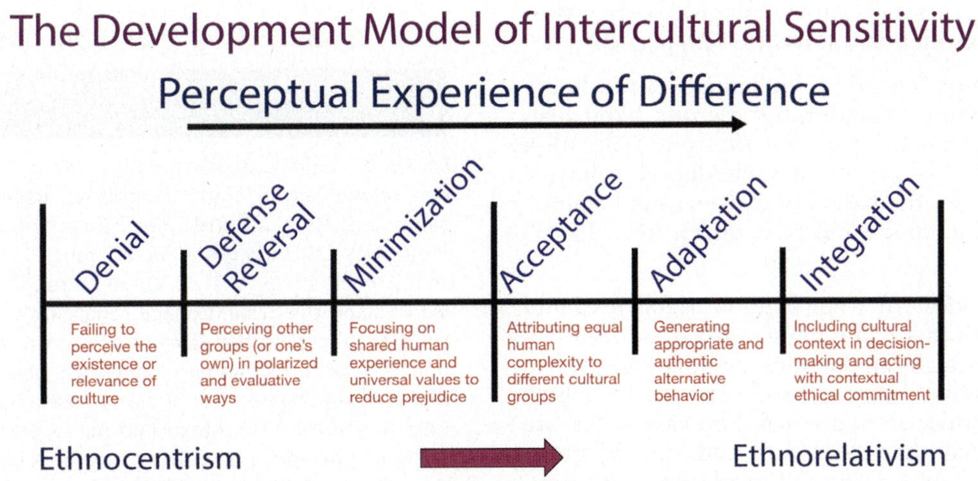

FIGURE 5-7 The development model of intercultural sensitivity. (Source: Bennett, M. (2017). Development model of intercultural sensitivity. In Kim, Y. (Ed.) *International encyclopedia of intercultural communication*. Wiley.)

Although culture is learned, each person may experience life in a singular way, which affects the process and results of that learning. Because culture is learned, parts of it can be relearned. People might change certain cultural elements or adopt new behaviors or values. Some individuals and groups are more willing and able than others to try new ways and thereby influence change.

Culture Is Integrated

Culture is a functional, integrated whole, not merely an assortment of customs and traits. As in any system, all parts of a culture are interrelated and interdependent. The components of a culture, such as its social norms or religious beliefs, perform separate functions but come into harmony with each other to form an operating and cohesive whole. Therefore, each component should be viewed considering its connection to other components and to the whole, not independently.

To provide effective nursing care, nurses may find their own cultural beliefs and practice systems need to be adjusted or reintegrated to accommodate the cultural beliefs and practices of others. For example, a nurse may promote the need for eating three balanced meals each day based on social and cultural beliefs and values that are related to good nutrition. This is necessary for health, and health is essential for productivity in work and career, quality of life, and achieving life goals. A client's beliefs and values in these areas may not be completely congruent with the nurse's (Box 5-4).

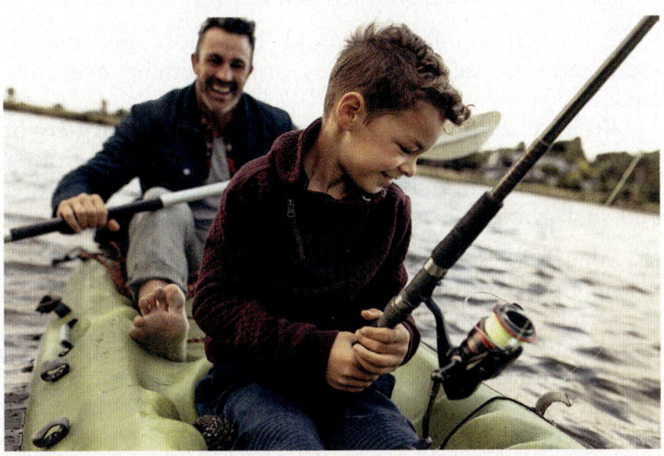

FIGURE 5-8 Family enculturation helps children acquire shared values and attitudes.

Culture Is Shared

Culture is the product of aggregate behavior, not individual habit. Certainly, individuals practice a culture, but customs are phenomena shared by all members of the

BOX 5-4 Recognizing and Respecting the Integrated Nature of Culture in Nursing

Below are some examples of clients whose beliefs and practices may prove challenging for the nurse to respect and accommodate if not viewed in the context of their culture:

- Parents who are Jehovah's Witnesses may refuse a blood transfusion for their child. This refusal may appear irrational or uninformed to those who do not understand their religious view of accepting blood and the need for bloodless procedures. The single behavior of refusing blood transfusions, when viewed in context, is part of a larger belief system and a basic component of the family's culture (Schuerger, 2022).
- A Muslim who is assigned female at birth may ask to be examined by a person of the same sex assigned at birth. Separation of people assigned male and female at birth is integral to her cultural beliefs, and it may be uncomfortable or even traumatic to receive care from a person of a different sex assigned at birth (Attum et al., 2023).

Source: American Psychiatric Association (2023); Attum, B., et al. (2023); Schuerger, B. (2022).

group. About 50 years ago, anthropologist George Murdock explained this idea as follows (1972), p. 258:

> Culture does not depend on individuals. An ordinary habit dies with its possessor, but a group habit lives on in the survivors... transmitted from generation to generation.... From earliest childhood behavior is conditioned by the habits of those around [them]. [A child] has no choice but to conform to ... [their] group.

Involving the ideas of what is good, right, just, and fair, a culture's values are among its most important elements. A **value** is a notion or idea designating relative worth or desirability. The normative criteria by which people justify their decisions are based on values that are more deeply rooted than behaviors and, consequently, more difficult to change. Each culture classifies phenomena into good and bad, desirable and undesirable, and right and wrong. When people respond in favor of or against some practice, they are reflecting their culture's values about that practice.

Examples of values include the following:

- Desirable traits: honesty, loyalty, and faithfulness
- Undesirable traits: lying, stealing, and cheating
- Eating meat: desirable and healthy versus sacrilegious or unhealthful
- Response to pain or grief: loud, vocal expressions versus silence and stoicism
- Speed and efficiency versus patience and thoughtfulness

No matter the culture, shared values give people in a specific culture stability and security and provide a standard for behavior, helping them know what to believe and how to act (Boyle et al., 2025). See Chapter 4 for more on values and ethics.

When C/PHNs know that culture is shared, their understanding of human behavior expands, and their ability to provide effective care to members of specific cultures increases. For example, it was found that people from the Hmong culture were reluctant to get a Pap test for cervical cancer because they had to be in the lithotomy position, which they perceived as immodest. Realizing that this impacts access to cancer screening, researchers have developed a urine test that can detect cervical cancer at early stages, similar to the Pap test, making screening more accessible to underserved populations (Gamelin et al., 2022; Novosanis, 2022). This demonstrates that focusing on one person's behavior may be less effective than working within the culture to promote well-being (Box 5-5).

BOX 5-5 STORIES FROM THE FIELD

Being Sensitive to Cultural Beliefs and Practices

In some Indigenous communities, the use of Mentholatum petroleum jelly in infant's nostrils was used to alleviate cold symptoms. Myra, a C/PHN, was concerned that the Mentholatum was too strong and would cause irritation. Realizing that culture is shared, Myra worked through a family member who was on the Tribal Council regarding their concerns. As the culture broker, this family member was able to share the concerns of the nurse and Indigenous community mothers. She proposed demonstrating how to use a bulb syringe at the next health fair. The nurse and nurse practitioner created handouts with pictures of tribal members demonstrating the correct use of the bulb syringe. The community health fair was held at the high school gym a month later. Myra brought her grandbaby to demonstrate how to use the bulb syringe to clear nasal mucous. The handouts were provided to reinforce teaching.

K. Bridget Marshall, DNP, APRN, CPNP-PC, PMHS

1. *Can you think of a similar cultural practice in your community that you may be able to approach in the same way as this C/PHN?*
2. *How would you go about researching the tradition and finding ways to incorporate the practice into your plan of care?*

Culture Is Tacit

As a guide for human interaction, culture can be tacit, mostly unspoken and unexpressed at the unconscious level. Members of a cultural group, without the need for discussion, know how to act and what to expect from one another. Culture provides an implicit set of cues for behavior, not a written set of rules. Culture often lies below a conscious level because it is such a regular and pervasive part of the daily environment (Miton & Dedeo, 2022). It is like a memory bank in which knowledge is stored for recall when the situation requires it, but this recall process is mostly unconscious.

Culture:

- Teaches the proper tone of voice to use for each occasion
- Prescribes how close to stand when talking with someone familiar or unfamiliar
- Guides how one should appropriately respond to older adults and based on one's gender, role, and status

All of these attitudes and behaviors become so ingrained—so tacit—that they are seldom, if ever, discussed.

Because culture is mostly tacit, realizing which of one's own behaviors may be offensive to people of other groups is difficult. It also is difficult to know the meaning and significance of other cultural practices.

- Silence is valued and expected in some cultures but may make others uncomfortable.
- Offering food to a guest in many cultures is not merely a social gesture but an important symbol of hospitality and acceptance; to refuse it, for any reason, may be an insult and a rejection.
- Touching or calling someone by their first name may be viewed as a demonstration of caring by some groups but could be seen as disrespectful and offensive to others.

Culture Is Dynamic

Every culture undergoes change; none is entirely static. Each culture is an amalgamation of ideas, values, and practices from many sources. This dynamic process is related to exposure to other cultural groups, and every culture is in a dynamic state of adding or deleting components. Functional aspects are retained; less functional ones are eliminated. Individuals may generate innovations within a culture, and some members see advantages to changing behaviors, being willing to adopt new practices. It is important when working with communities to use new resources, such as access to the yearly flu vaccine.

When people enter a new culture, such as Sudanese refugees resettling in the United States (see Fig. 5-9), anxiety and frustration can occur. Nothing may be familiar; foods, language, expectations for dress, gestures, and even facial expressions may be misunderstood. This lack of familiarity can result in conflicted feelings that have been termed **culture shock**, leading to difficulty with interactions in the new culture (McCluskey, 2020). Culture shock can develop with nurses providing care in unfamiliar countries and is known to affect international students studying in the United States or American students studying abroad. Serious difficulties can arise when members of a culture do not adapt to change or when culture shock is pervasive in a community (Box 5-6).

Cultural adaptation is the successful adjustment to cultural changes and often follows the process of culture shock. Examples of cultural adaptation can range from something as simple as learning to use a knife and fork to the complexities of becoming fluent in a new language. C/PHNs can facilitate cultural adaptation by explaining practices of the American healthcare system in the context of the original culture of their clients. C/PHNs must remember the dynamic nature of culture for several reasons.

- Cultures change as their members see greater advantages in adopting "new ways." Describing the changes in language and context acceptable to the culture is essential. Successful nurses understand their clients' culture when delivering culturally competent care (Boyle et al., 2025).

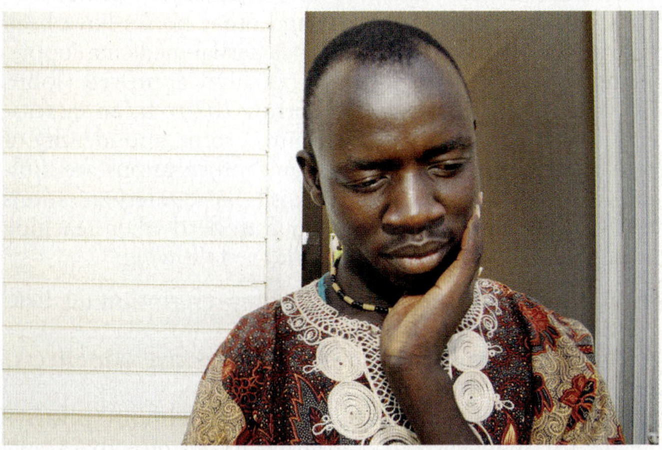

FIGURE 5-9 Sudanese man now living in the United States.

BOX 5-6 EVIDENCE-BASED PRACTICE

Cultural Identity and Outcomes

John Bul Dau's memoir titled *God Grew Tired of Us* recounts his experiences as a "Lost Boy" of Sudan, his stay in a refugee camp in Kenya, and his resettlement in the United States. He poignantly describes the culture shock he experienced upon his arrival in Syracuse, New York, as he began his life as a new American. His journey challenged him to adapt to his life ways in order to initially survive, and later, to fit in (Dau & Sweeney, 2008).

Cultural fit refers to the match between one's personal characteristics and values to that of the larger cultural group (Searle & Ward, 1990). It is also a dynamic psychological process whereby a person modifies their self-concept to adapt to a larger cultural context (West et al., 2018). For individuals such as Dau who identify with more than one culture, achieving a cultural fit can be complicated, particularly when the cultures vary dramatically. In order to thrive in dramatically different cultures, many people like Dau learn cultural frame switching (CFS). Cultural frame shifting refers to activating one's cultural knowledge structures in response to contextual cues (Hong et al., 2000). While CFS helps people achieve a cultural fit with positive social relationships (Garcha et al., 2023), it can have negative outcomes including a sense of inauthenticity (West et al., 2018) and identity conflict, guilt, and distress (Garcha et al., 2023).

Kathleen Hall, PhD, APRN, GNP-BC, AGPCNP-BC

1. *Can you identify refugee or immigrant populations in your community?*
2. *If you were a nurse working with a refugee or immigrant family, how would you facilitate them in achieving a cultural fit?*
3. *How would you help them with cultural frame switching so that the negative outcomes might be minimized?*

- The healthcare culture is dynamic; Westerners are beginning to appreciate the validity of practices such as acupuncture, meditation, and the use of therapeutic herbs and spices such as turmeric and fenugreek (Lee et al., 2022).
- The national health-related goals of the United States, the *Healthy People* initiative, change every 10 years. *Healthy People 2030* includes a focus on social determinants of health to eliminate health disparities and improve health for all (USDHHS, 2020). See Box 5-7.

ETHNOCULTURAL HEALTHCARE PRACTICES

Throughout history, people have relied on natural elements to treat misfortunes, illness, or injuries experienced by family, clan, tribe, or community members. Specialized knowledge about practices and substances (e.g., rituals, incantations, berries, plants, barks) is often held by one person in the group. This revered community

BOX 5-7 Healthy People and Social Determinants of Health

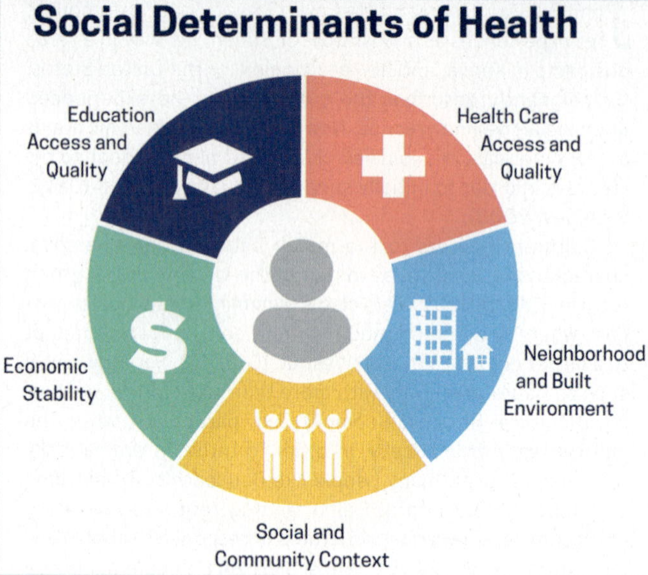
Social Determinants of Health
Education Access and Quality
Health Care Access and Quality
Neighborhood and Built Environment
Social and Community Context
Economic Stability

Reprinted from U.S. Department of Health and Human Services (USDHHS). (2020). *Social determinants of health.* https://health.gov/healthypeople/priority-areas/health-equity-healthy-people-2030. https://health.gov/healthypeople/priority-areas/social-determinants-health

leader, known as a medicine man/woman, healer, or shaman, may acquire the skills through apprenticeship or is believed to be born with them (Boyle et al., 2025; Lee et al., 2022).

Cultural practices may include the following:

- Practices based on one or more of the three views of healthcare: biomedical, magico-religious, and holistic
- Selected folk medicines and **home remedies**, such as herbs, teas, and poultices
- Over-the-counter (OTC) drugs and patent medications
- Complementary or alternative therapies
- Recently developed, expensive medications
- Various self-care practices

Biomedical View

Common in Western societies, the biomedical view theorizes that all aspects of health can be understood through the sciences of biology, chemistry, physics, and mathematics. Furthermore, there is the belief that life can be manipulated by humans through physical and biochemical processes (Boyle et al., 2025). Many healthcare professionals, including C/PHNs, believe the biomedical model is the only and best approach. As a result, they may have trouble understanding diverse cultures that incorporate the holistic or magico-religious views, and clients may not receive culturally competent care. To be effective with diverse clients, C/PHNs must be knowledgeable about and accepting of a range of cultural health practices (Shahzad et al., 2021).

Magico-religious View

Some cultural beliefs are grounded in the magico-religious approach, which focuses on control of health and illness by supernatural forces, where health is seen as a spiritual gift or reward and illness as an opportunity to be resigned to God's will (Boyle et al., 2025). Diseases are thought to originate from intrusion of a malevolent spirit, punishment for the deeds of ancestors, and other indications that God, the gods, or other supernatural forces are in control. Religious beliefs, a person's spirituality, and how these factors interface with wellness and healing practices are important to clients and cannot be separated from their culture.

Holistic View

In a holistic viewpoint, the world is viewed through harmonious balance; imbalance of natural forces can create chaos and disease. Many cultural groups use a holistic approach in tandem with other belief models. In this belief system, for a person to be healthy, all facets of the individual's nature—physical, mental, emotional, and spiritual—must be in balance (Meadows, 2023). The holistic viewpoint can be expressed by the use of specific foods, beverages, and herbs to balance hot or cold disease states (Boyle et al., 2025; Meadows, 2023).

Folk Medicine and Home Remedies

Home remedies are individualized caregiving practices. Treatments as part of folk medicine are verbally passed down from generation to generation and began when access to medical care was limited. For example, people who grew up in the United States may remember a caregiver giving them hot herbal tea with lemon or using ointments and extra blankets to relieve symptoms of a mild illness. Some clients may never plan to seek Western medical treatment but may share a practice they are using to treat a family member. Your response and actions may mean the difference between health and illness or injury because not all folk remedies may be safe.

Herbalism. Use of herbs to treat illness is a centuries-old practice that is gaining popularity in American culture (Fig. 5-10). Clients may not consider the use of herbs to be a "medical treatment" and may not tell healthcare professionals about their use. Textbooks and other books have been published on medicinal herbs; since herbal medicine supplements are not a drug, they are not FDA approved (Johns Hopkins, 2023; Pizzorno & Murray, 2020). In an increasingly multicultural society, the source, form, and identity of many herbs, roots, barks, and liquid preparations are difficult for most C/PHNs to distinguish. Basic safety questions that C/PHNs should answer about an herb when teaching or interacting with families include the following:

- Is the herb contraindicated with prescription medications the client is taking?
- Is the herb harmful? Does it have negative side effects? How often is it used?
- Is the client relying on the herb, without positive health changes, and neglecting to get effective treatment from a healthcare practitioner?

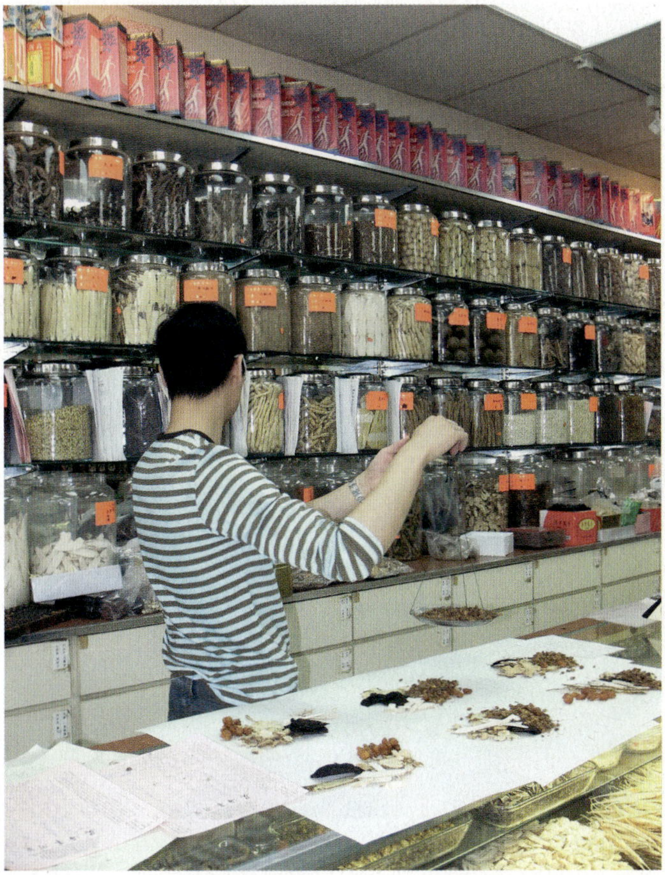

FIGURE 5-10 A Chinese herb store.

Just because herbs are not regulated as drugs, does not mean that they are risk-free. Variations in quality, strength, processing, storage, and purity may occur, leading to unpredictable effects. For these reasons, herbs must be used only in moderation and with caution, preferably with guidance by a healthcare practitioner (Johns Hopkins, 2023). Examples of potentially harmful herbal supplements include Ephedra, Ginko, and Goldenseal for those people with cardiac conditions, as these herbs can increase blood pressure and heart rate, as well as heighten the risk of bleeding (Cleveland Clinic, 2023).

Prescription and OTC Drugs

The cautions mentioned about herbs can also apply to most dietary supplements and OTC preparations. Additional concerns with these drugs include the following:

- Dietary supplements and OTC drugs undergo a less rigorous process of review and testing by the U.S. Food and Drug Administration than do prescription medications (USFDA, 2022a).
- Many OTC drugs were once available only by prescription and remain powerful medicines.
- Herbal or dietary supplements do not have to be FDA-approved before manufacturers can sell them (USFDA, 2022b).
- All drugs can have major side effects, may be contraindicated in people with certain conditions, and may not be safe to use in combination with certain other drugs.

C/PHNs who see clients over time can assist them through medication review and instruction, advocating for them to receive a less expensive form of the same medication and reporting on the effectiveness of newly prescribed medications. Many pharmaceutical companies now have low-cost prescription assistance programs for those in need (Needy Meds, 2020).

Integrated Healthcare and Self-Care Practices

Complementary and alternative medicine (CAM) includes a broad array of healing resources. Self-care activities may include CAM, other medications, and spiritual and cultural practices (USDHHS-NIH, 2023). These widely varied approaches are designed to promote comfort, health, and well-being and may include the following:

- Therapies and treatments (e.g., juice diets, fasting, coffee enemas, and biofeedback)
- Exercise activities (e.g., T'ai chi, yoga, and dance)
- Exposure (e.g., aromatherapy, music therapy, and light therapy)
- Manipulation (e.g., acupuncture, acupressure, chiropractic, cupping, and reflexology (Fig. 5-11)

Complementary therapies are often used in conjunction with Western medicine, an approach known as integrated healthcare, such as for pain relief during labor (Tabatabaeichehr & Mortazavi, 2020) and menopause (Abbaspoor et al., 2022). Complementary therapies have become so commonplace that some have suggested developing policies and guidelines for their use.

The C/PHN should be aware of the variety of therapies available and how to obtain information for clients while remaining objective and supportive of the client's choices. When a therapy contradicts the

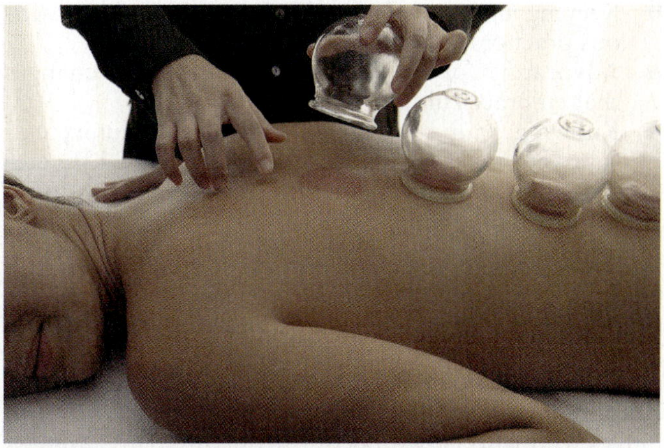

FIGURE 5-11 Cupping has been used by many cultures.

recommendations of the client's healthcare practitioner, the nurse may be able to provide the pros and cons of continuing the complementary therapy. Also, the nurse may be able to suggest therapy forms that would complement Western medicine for the client, such as music to promote relaxation and reduce stress or biofeedback for chronic pain management. Complementary and self-care practices should be uniquely chosen for each client within the context of their cultural group (Lindquist et al., 2022). The nurse practicing culturally congruent care respects these decisions, while promoting client health.

ROLE AND PREPARATION OF THE COMMUNITY/PUBLIC HEALTH NURSE

As a C/PHN, for you to be an effective healthcare advocate for clients from different cultural groups, you must be prepared to:

- Speak knowledgeably about healthcare practices and choices
- Assess the client or family adequately, to know what belief system motivates their choices
- Teach clients about the limits and benefits of cultural healthcare practices
- Individualize assessment and caregiving for the client within the client's culture, not generalize about the client based on cultural group norms

Preparation to work effectively with clients in the area of cultural healthcare involves developing cultural awareness and promoting sensitivity to the differences among people from diverse ethnocultural groups. You, the nurse, can prepare by:

- Performing a cultural self-assessment to identify your own beliefs and biases
- Learning from peers who are from the same cultural group as the clients
- Attending workshops or conferences on cultural topics, transcultural nursing, and cultural ethics
- Reading books on ethnocultural and alternative healthcare practices
- Talking with clients about their views and practices and learning from them
- Keeping an open mind and being curious about various practices
- Advocating for systems and organizational changes that embrace cultural awareness
- Knowing your community—attend community cultural events, such as ceremonies (Fig. 5-12), ethnic food and cultural festivals, and other cultural celebrations

There are textbooks, novels, and articles about cultures in the community in which one practices. For example, the classic book *The Spirit Catches You and You Fall Down* (Fadiman, 1998) describes a Hmong child, her American doctors, and the collision of two cultures in California. The experience of public health nurses who worked with people from different countries and cultures illustrates the benefits of being open-minded (Box 5-8).

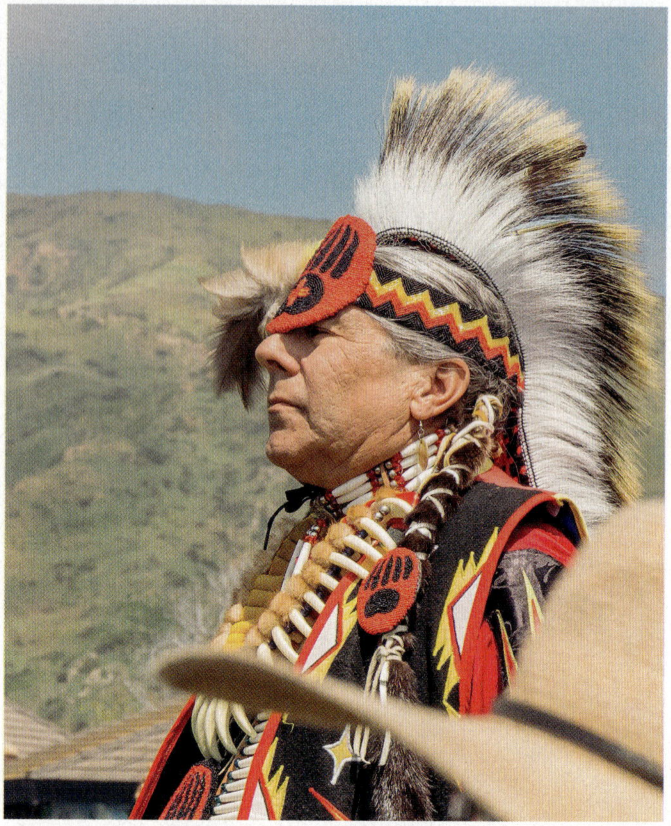

FIGURE 5-12 Indigenous tribal ceremony.

BOX 5-8 PERSPECTIVES

Learning About Other Cultures

I was always interested in learning about other countries and cultures. However, I didn't realize that an overseas assignment would teach me so much about myself in addition to other cultures and ways of living. The lessons were sometimes difficult but always rewarding. I knew that my expectations would not always be met, yet it did surprise me how different the experience was from what I had imagined it would be. My job assignment, location, and team members changed frequently. Flexibility, comfort with ambiguity, a sense of humor, a deeper reliance upon my faith, patience when results were not forthcoming, trust in others, and the ability to cross multiple cultures with some degree of ease were all skills that I developed over time. Most important to being successful at my job was to maintain the attitude of a "learner," not a "solver of problems" or "the person with all the answers." I made friends with people from all over the world who graciously accepted me into their lives, thus enriching mine. I learned that we all are different, but that every behavior has a reasonable explanation when you take the time to listen with your heart as well as with your ears. I found that I actually preferred other ways of doing and being while still maintaining those parts of my identity that were valuable to me. When I returned home, I found that my newly developed skills were still necessary—because I had changed and had to adjust to reentry into my home culture!

PHN

TRANSCULTURAL COMMUNITY/PUBLIC HEALTH NURSING PRINCIPLES

Community/public health nursing practice with cross-cultural groups, known as **transcultural nursing**, "focuses on people's culturally based beliefs, attitudes, values, behaviors, and practices related to health, illness, healing, and human caring" (Boyle et al., p. 4). Guiding principles for transcultural nursing practice can assist the C/PHNs (Box 5-9):

- Develop cultural self-awareness.
- Cultivate cultural sensitivity.
- Assess the client group's culture.
- Show respect and patience while learning about other cultures.
- Examine culturally derived health practices.

Culture profoundly influences thinking and behavior and has an enormous impact on the effectiveness of healthcare. Just as physical and psychological factors determine clients' needs and attitudes toward health and illness, so too can culture.

- About 50 years ago, Kark emphasized that "culture is perhaps the most relevant social determinant of community health" (1974, p. 149).
- Culture can determine how people rear their children, react to pain, cope with stress, deal with death, and value the past, present, and future.
- Culture influences diet and eating practices, thereby influencing health; these can be difficult to change due to culture's impact (Les Elfes International, 2021).

Despite its importance, the client's culture is often misunderstood or ignored in the delivery of healthcare (Les Elfes International, 2021). Cultural diversity is increasing in our world, and it is essential that healthcare professionals are prepared to effectively work with diverse healthcare team members and clients (Boyle et al., 2025). Avoiding ethnocentrism requires the nurse to be willing to carefully examine their own culture and to become aware that alternative viewpoints are possible. The nurse attempts to understand the meaning other people derive from their culture and appreciate their culture as important and useful to them (Kaya et al., 2021). Ignoring consideration of clients' different cultural origins often has negative results.

- Culture is a universal experience; each person is part of some group and that group helps to shape the values, beliefs, and behaviors that make up their culture. Even within fairly homogeneous cultural groups, subcultures and microcultures have distinctive characteristics.
- Further differences, often due to social class, socioeconomic status, age, or degree of acculturation, can be found within microcultures. These latter differences, called interethnic variations, underscore the range of culturally diverse clients served by C/PHNs.

BOX 5-9 Guidelines for Cultural Care

- Have knowledge of the culture
- Be educated in culturally competent care
- Critically reflect on your actions
- Be aware of verbal/nonverbal communication
- Employ culturally competent practices
- Systems and organizations must adopt culturally appropriate practices
- Advocate and empower the client
- Employ a cultural workforce including those in management and leadership roles
- Base nursing interventions on evidenced-based practice and research

Source: Transcultural Nursing Society. (2023). Standards. https://tcns.org/standards/

Develop Cultural Self-Awareness

To avoid stereotyping, prejudice and racism, ethnocentrism, cultural imposition, and cultural conflict (a perceived threat arising from a misunderstanding of expectations between clients and nurses when either group is not aware of cultural differences), self-awareness is crucial for the nurse working with people from other cultures (Boyle et al., 2025). **Cultural self-awareness** means recognizing the values, beliefs, and practices that make up one's own culture and becoming sensitive to the impact of one's culturally based responses.

Although C/PHNs may think they are being helpful when operating from their own sets of cultural values and practices, doing so may actually have negative consequences and even cause damage to relationships with clients when cultural values differ. The nurse who has expectations for prenatal weight gain and values actions to limit weight could cause damage to a therapeutic relationship if the nurse does not consider cultural expectations about diet during pregnancy to assure a healthy infant. To develop awareness, nurses can complete a cultural self-assessment by analyzing their own:

- Influences related to racial and ethnic background
- Verbal and nonverbal communication patterns
- Values and norms (expected cultural practices or behaviors)
- Health-related beliefs and practices

Because culture is mostly tacit, it takes conscious effort and hard work to develop true awareness of one's own cultural biases or influence. A nurse can ask selected clients to critique nursing actions in light of the clients' own culture. Developing this awareness will reward you with a more effective understanding of self and an enhanced ability to provide culturally relevant services to clients (Boyle et al., 2025). See Box 5-10 and Table 5-2.

Cultural Congruence and Intersectionality

Nurses should be aware of the significant impact of culture on behavior. Cultural competence requires recognizing that culturally based values, beliefs, and practices influence people's health and lifestyles and need to be considered in their plans for care (Mantyselka et al., 2019; Stubbe, 2020). It requires self-reflection about personally held stereotypes and biases, self-assessment of one's own cultural influences, personal cultural humility, and an

BOX 5-10 Cultural Self-Assessment

Think about the culture of your family (parents and grandparents). Answer the following questions about your own cultural background:

- Relationship to the dominant culture—Does the dominant culture have any stereotypes, misconceptions, suspicions, or historical issues related to your family's culture? If you are a member of an underrepresented group, what is your family's view of the dominant culture? What cultural stereotypes about the dominant culture does your family hold?
- Verbal—What is the dominant language of your family's culture? How does your family share information and feelings, explain the meaning of terms, use proverbs, and incorporate direct questioning versus silence and passivity?
- Nonverbal—Describe your family's use of eye contact, facial expressions, body movements, and touch.
- Perception of time—Is your family's culture future, present, or past oriented?
- Personal space—Describe your family's concepts of boundaries and interpersonal distance.
- Perception of family roles and organization—Who is responsible for care of the children in your family? Who makes financial and healthcare decisions? Describe gender roles.
- Physical characteristics—Describe your family's skin and hair color; susceptibility to disease; enzymes and metabolism; and typical growth and development.
- Diet—What are typical meals in your family? How is food used (celebrations, fasting, healing, etc.)?
- Education—Describe your family's typical learning style (visual, auditory, psychomotor; formal/informal education).
- Spirituality—What are your family's spiritual beliefs and values, spiritual practices and support, rituals and taboos?
- Health beliefs—Describe your family's understanding of the meaning of health and illness (e.g., cause, perception of symptoms/intensity, seriousness, expression of illness, need for medical attention); beliefs about death and dying; beliefs about pregnancy, labor and delivery, postpartum period, and childcare).
- Health behaviors—What activities does your family do to promote health and prevent disease? Describe your family's help-seeking behaviors and use of home remedies, traditional or folk healers, and magico-religious practitioners. What status is given to healthcare providers?

understanding of the interface of systems of oppression on groups and individuals due to race, class, or gender also known as **intersectionality** (Fitzgerald & Campinha-Bacote, 2019). Intersectionality acknowledges that the C/PHN is part of a larger system providing healthcare service, and the interplay of these entities require congruence for cultural understanding to be effective. Fitzgerald and Campinha-Bacote (2019) identify the gap between systems and individual health team levels, acknowledging the need for a structured and intentional joint approach for cultural competence. The American Nurses Association's (2021) *Nursing: Scope and Standards of Practice* outlines a set of competencies for culturally congruent practice identifying the need for healthcare organizations to provide structure and resources to support the culture and language needs of diverse clients and communities.

A client's cultural values and health practices may sharply contrast with those of the nurse. Failure to recognize this contrast can lead to a communication breakdown and ineffective care. Additionally, an institution may not recognize that their processes or policies are not culturally respectful. Once differences in culture are recognized, it is important to accept and appreciate them. Using an intersectional approach, a C/PHN working with community agencies and a migrant community can guide engagement in prevention programs, advocacy, outreach, and education. See Table 5-3 for culturally related competencies and an intersectional approach.

Implicit and Explicit Bias

The work toward culture congruency and addressing bias in healthcare was introduced well over 20 years ago (Berger & Miller, 2021). Institutions have provided guidance for culture competency such as the Culturally and Linguistic Appropriate Services Toolkit (Agency for Healthcare Research and Quality, 2022) and the *Nursing: Scope and Standards of Practice* (ANA, 2021). Recognition of explicit and implicit biases does affect health inequities and outcomes of care (CDC, 2022a). **Implicit bias** refers to behaviors or actions that occur automatically and unintentionally, while **explicit bias** is a conscious awareness of attitudes and beliefs; both affect judgment, decisions, and behaviors regarding healthcare resulting in diagnostic errors and poor patient outcomes (Sabin, 2022; Vela et al., 2022). Health disparities during COVID-19 were noted in many Black, Hispanic/Latino, Indigenous, and LGBTQ+ communities where a disproportionate number of underrepresented groups within the United States were affected (Andraska et al., 2021). Overestimation of arterial oxygenation of saturation levels by pulse oximetry during COVID-19 in patients in Black and Hispanic/Latino populations resulted in significant delays of therapeutic treatment for people in those groups as compared to White patients (Fawzy et al., 2022). Additionally, patients are not always included in their care, resulting in lack of information for informed decision making (e.g., as noted by people of color during pregnancy [Altman et al., 2019]). The C/PHN may not realize that they are providing information differently or not sharing information to all equally. Additionally, listening to the patient and hearing their concerns and perceptions of how they feel through an open, neutral lens provides respectful and culturally appropriate care.

Assess the Client Group's Culture

Learning the culture of the client first is critical to effective nursing practice. During a **cultural assessment** (Giger & Haddad, 2021), the nurse obtains health-related information about the values, beliefs, and practices of a the client's cultural group. There usually is a culturally based reason for clients to engage in (or avoid) certain actions. Instead of making assumptions or judging clients' behavior, the

TABLE 5-2 Cultural Assessment Guide

Category	Sample Data
Ethnic/racial background	Countries of origin Mostly native born or U.S. born? Reasons for emigrating if applicable Racial/ethnic identity Experience with racism or racial discrimination?
Language and communication patterns	Languages of origin Languages spoken in the home Preferred language for communication How verbal communication patterns are affected by age, sex assigned at birth, other? Preferences for use of interpreters Nonverbal communication patterns (e.g., eye contact, touching)
Cultural values and norms	Group beliefs and standards for gender roles and functions Standards for modesty and sexuality Family/extended family structures and functions Values regarding work, leisure, success, time Values regarding education and occupation Norms for child-rearing and socialization Norms for social networks and supports Values regarding aging and treatment of older adults Values regarding authority Norms for dress and appearance
Biocultural factors	Group genetic predisposition to health conditions (e.g., hypertension, anemia) Socioculturally associated illnesses (e.g., AIDS, alcohol use disorder) Group attitudes toward body parts and functions Group vulnerability or resistance to health threats? Does the group have any illnesses recognized by their group only? Group physical characteristics (e.g., bone mass, height, weight, longevity)
Religious beliefs and practices	Religious beliefs affecting roles, childbearing and child-rearing, health and illness? Recognized religious healers? Religious beliefs and practices for promoting health, preventing illness, or treatment of illness Beliefs and rituals regarding conception and birth Beliefs and rituals regarding death, dying, grief
Health beliefs and practices	Beliefs regarding causes of illness Beliefs regarding treatment of illness Beliefs regarding use of healers (traditional and Western) Health promotion and illness prevention practices Folk medicine practices Beliefs regarding mental health and illness Dietary, herbal, and other folk cures Food beliefs, preparation, consumption Experience with Western medicine

nurse first must learn about the culture that guides that behavior. For example, a client might severely limit the foods she allows her child to eat, believing that many people from her culture have food allergies (Warren et al., 2021).

Interviewing members of a subculture can provide valuable data to enhance understanding (Boyle et al., 2025). The concept of cultural diversity can be understood in a general way, but each group should be appreciated within its own cultural and historical context (see Table 5-4). Show respect and patience while learning about other cultures. Key behaviors to demonstrate include the following:

- Allow enough time for communication.
- Maintain a relaxed and unhurried attitude.
- Arrange for an interpreter when needed (Fig. 5-13).
- Speak to the client, not the interpreter.
- Use simple language and avoid slang and jargon.
- Watch for verbal and nonverbal cues.
- Ask open-ended questions.
- Validate feelings and understanding.

It is not practical to deeply study all cultural groups the nurse encounters. Instead, a general cultural assessment can be accomplished by questioning key informants, observing the cultural group, and reading current professional literature. Categories to explore in the assessment include values, beliefs, customs, and social structure components (see Table 5-2).

TABLE **5-3** Intersectionality and Cultural Competence: The ASKED Approach
Awareness—critical reflection of one's biases toward others' cultures and a self-examination of once's culture (organizational and individual).
Skill—cultural assessment of organization, employees, and community culture served.
Knowledge—shared educational baseline for both healthcare organizations and individuals of the cultural community in which they serve.
Encounters—healthcare organizations' and professionals' interaction with cultural community, diverse clients, and employees for authentic engagement.
Desires—the motivation for cultural competence through a lens of cultural humility and diffused throughout the ASKED process.

Adapted from Fitzgerald, E., & Campinha-Bacote, J. (2019, May). An intersectionality approach to the process of cultural competemility—part II. *OJIN, 24*(2). https://doi.org/10.3912/OJIN.Vol24No02PPT202

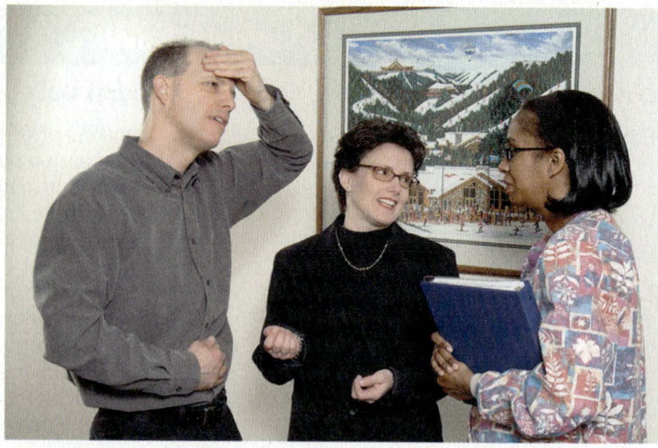

FIGURE 5-13 A client with hearing loss communicating through a sign language interpreter.

- When language is a barrier for effective communication, the nurse must make arrangements for an interpreter, including for those with hearing loss. Be patient; it takes time to establish the nurse–client relationship, especially when working with two different cultures. Trust must be earned, and that may take weeks, months, or years. Time must be allowed for both the nurse and the client to learn how to communicate with one another, to test one another's trustworthiness, and to learn about one another.

In the process of working with cultural groups, **cultural brokering** may be used. This involves mediating or building connections between those from different cultural backgrounds to promote change (Brar-Josan & Yohani, 2019). Aspects of both the nurse's and the clients' cultures can, and probably will, change. When working with a family from an unfamiliar cultural background, for example, you can explain your usual method of working with clients and may modify some usual practices to adapt them to the family's culture. The family, in turn, may begin to assume the nurse's recommended healthcare practices. This process of building trust and rapport with your client may take several months, but time, respect, and patience all help to break down cultural barriers (Fig. 5-14).

TABLE **5-4** Principles for Cultural Communication
1. Embrace Cultural Humility and Engagement ▪ Avoid any posturing, framing, and language of hierarchy, patriarchy, supremacy, saviorism, and colonialism ▪ Ensure communities are encouraged and have the opportunity to participate 2. Use a Global Health Equity Lens that considers Systemic Social and Health Inequities ▪ Demonstrate respect ▪ Be credible ▪ Avoid deficient perspective ▪ Use strength-based or asset-based approaches 3. Use Plain Language that is Culturally Relevant ▪ Avoid the use of technical language, jargon, and acronyms ▪ Regardless of communication method, insufficient consideration of culture may unintentionally result in misinformation, errors, confusion, and loss of credibility

Source: Centers for Disease Control and Prevention (CDC) (2023).

Consider Culturally Derived Health Practices

Some traditional practices, such as customary diet, birth rituals, and certain folk remedies, may promote both physical and psychological health. Other practices, neither harmful nor health promoting, are useful in preserving the culture, security, and sense of identity of a cultural group. Some traditional practices may be directly harmful to health.

Examples of harmful practices include the following:

- Sole use of herbal poultices to treat an infected wound when antibiotics are needed

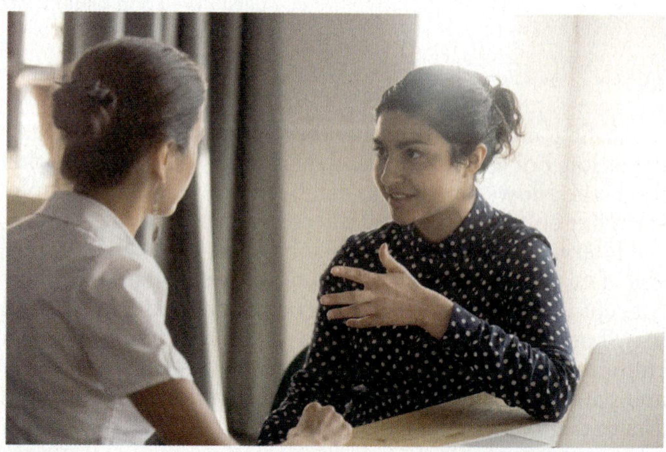

FIGURE 5-14 Building trust and rapport with your client is essential.

BOX **5-11** STORIES FROM THE FIELD

The Importance of Cultural Sensitivity

Although fetal alcohol spectrum disorder (FASD) is commonly associated with Native American people, data supports that FASD is prevalent in all ethnic groups within the United States (Soyeon et al., 2023). In a Native American community in North America, nurses worked as outreach members with a multidisciplinary team, including local community members, assessing for FASD. To increase understanding, the members of the multidisciplinary assessment team decided to destigmatize the work they were doing by writing and presenting a play to the local community about FASD using animals to represent the different roles in society. For the play, the owl represented medicine (or life and death), and the coyote was representative of something clever or mischievous. It is important to note that the Native American spirit animal is different than the animals represented in the play and were not meant to replicate someone's spirit animal. While the nurses were part of the interdisciplinary team and a member of the play, they respected the insight of the cultural insiders on how to write and present the play. Following the play, an increase in FASD referrals was received by the interdisciplinary team.

K. Bridget Marshall, DNP, APRN, CPNP-PC, PMHS

- "Burning" the abdomen to compensate for heat loss associated with diarrhea
- The use of Greta or Azarcon (common Hispanic home remedies for stomach discomfort), which contain lead (CDC, 2022b)

Cultural health practice and aggregate health assessment can be combined to determine appropriate treatment. If a group has a high incidence of low-birth-weight babies, pregnancy complications, skin infections, mental illness, or other health issues, it may be helpful to learn more about the group's cultural health practices. Practices clearly damaging to health can be discussed with group leaders and healers. Knowing the group's norms for authority and decision making can be helpful to achieve improvements while respecting traditional health practices. An example of the consequences of not clearly understanding cultural norms is found in Boxes 5-11 and 5-12.

BOX **5-12** STORIES FROM THE FIELD

Perception of Strength in Sub-Saharan Africa

The following is based on a true story yet compiles the experience, conversations, and reflection of multiple students into a single case study of a student named "Sammy."

As a senior in nursing school, Sammy spent 2 weeks in sub-Saharan Africa in an immersion nursing course to learn about the population's health needs. Sammy has a passion for international health and eliminating poverty. She prepared for the experience by learning health statistics on HIV, infant mortality rates, literacy, water quality, housing, and economic impacts on the community to name a few.

When Sammy was assigned to spend a day in the labor and delivery unit, she was excited she was able to see how the people and nurses experienced the tragic statistics she had researched. She immediately noticed the lack of resources as she observed laboring patients lined up on hallway benches waiting their turn for the labor and delivery room that barely had time for a surface clean before the next patient. She noticed nurses moving briskly from patient to patient doing quick assessments and vital signs with nothing but a stethoscope and BP cuff, shared by multiple nurses.

The unit was busy, and Sammy stood in awe of the laboring patients, the nurses, and the whole scene. She learned that the patients give birth "naturally" without any pain medications. One hundred percent of patients breastfeed after birth. The patients labor, birth, and recover as a community, with minimal privacy. Patients generally walk the halls during labor, offering each other support. After birth, they recover together in a large ward lined with single beds. They rely on each other when the nurses and medical staff are not available.

Sammy recalled her sister's "Birth Plan" in a Midwest suburb of the United States where she proudly chose natural birth, breastfeeding immediately after birth, and to be surrounded by her sisters. To a busy nurse, Sammy said with delight and respect, "Wow!! Your patients, are so strong. My sister chose a natural birth as well." The nurse looked directly at Sammy as she washed her hands without soap (it had run out) and said harshly, "They have no other choice." Sammy felt this harsh response in the pit of her stomach. She did not mean to offend anyone.

Sammy's assessment of the patients' strength and perceived resilience was based on a limited view. She did not see the day-to-day reality for these nurses and patients, including the persistent risk of maternal and child death. While indeed there is strength in the patients of this community, Sammy's statement came across to the nurse as naive and privileged in the face of suffering.

That evening, Sammy reflected in the debrief session with her team, "I learned to look around and take time to process beyond my original perception. It really hit me how important it is to not to make a comparative statement until I know enough to understand the full picture."

Kim Nuxoll, MSN, RN

CASE STUDY 10 ESSENTIAL PUBLIC HEALTH SERVICES

Hmong Youth

Southeast Asian Hmong teenagers from the late 1980s are among the first generation to be raised in the United States. Their parents had high hopes for them to restore honor and pride to a displaced people, but the teens struggle to balance their American lifestyle with Hmong traditions. They can feel overwhelming stress resulting from the generational and cultural gaps between themselves and their parents.

The youths' transition to adulthood in the last 20 years has identified a distinct bicultural identify as they become aware of "...the constraints of racism and their place in American racial hierarchies" (Swartz et al., 2022, p. 1197). A longitudinal study of Asian American youths (Youth Development Study-YDS) looked at patterns of incorporation from 1988–2019 focusing primarily on the domains of work, family, education, and mental health of Hmong immigrants from the St. Paul, Minnesota region. Early experiences of the immigrants make clear the need to attain education, which was reinforced by their parents and elders; the YDS survey indicated Hmong students spend more time on homework as compared with non-Hmong classmates (21 hours compared to 8 hours) and had lower drop-out rates as compared with non-Hmong students (5% compared to 9%) (Swartz et al., 2022). Education was viewed as assimilation into American culture, yet youth identified conflict related to social difference and co-ethnicities. Transition to adulthood for the Hmong youth led to refinement of understanding as it related to stereotypes and racial hierarchies, and an acceptance of a hybrid culture in which the old is preserved and a new perspective can be forged for the future.

Ci, a Hmong teenager who attends the high school where you are the school nurse, has seemed overly sad in her teachers' opinion and has been caught skipping classes. Ci was not always rebellious and until recently had good grades. You have witnessed a once outgoing middle school student transform into a quiet and withdrawn high schooler. Red marks on her arm indicate self-inflicted injures. In consultation with the school counselor and the family, a home visit was warranted.

You visit the home of Ci's family and note the multiple generations living within one house. You sense tension in the adult members of the family as they speak for the troubled teen.

1. ***Recognize Cues:*** *Which findings require immediate follow-up, are unexpected, or are most concerning?*
2. ***Analyze Cues:*** *What information is noted or needed for interpreting findings?*
3. ***Prioritize Hypotheses:*** *Based on the information that you have, what is happening?*
4. ***Generate Solutions:*** *What intervention(s) will achieve the desired outcome?*
5. ***Take Action:*** *What actions should you take or do first?*
6. ***Evaluate Outcomes:*** *Were outcomes achieved? Why or why not?*
7. *Which Essential Public Health Services influence this situation? (See Box 2-2.)*

Source: Swartz, T.T., Hartman, D. & Vue, P.L. (2022). Race, ethnicity, and the incorporation experiences of Hmong American youth adults: Insights from a mixed-methods, longitudinal study. Ethnic Racial studies, 45(7), 1197–1217. http://doi.org/10.1080/01419870.2021.1939091

SUMMARY

- The United States is a multicultural country and is founded on the varied beliefs and practices of immigrants, refuges, and native North American populations.
- U.S. Census Bureau data for the previous two decades recognizes a shift in dominant culture demographics toward increased multicultural and other self-identification as noted in diversity index percentages across the country.
- Culture refers to the beliefs, values, and behaviors that are shared by members of a society and provide a template or "road map" for living.
- Cultural diversity, or cultural plurality, refers to the coexistence of a variety of cultural patterns within a geographic area, either between cultures or within a given culture; smaller culturally distinctive groups may exist within a culture and are known as subcultures and microcultures.
- Nurses should be able to identify CAM treatments, such as folk medicine, home remedies, herbs, and other therapies; assess their clients' use of them; and, when appropriate, recommend their use.
- Use of transcultural nursing principles, drawn from an understanding of the concept of culture, can guide C/PHN practice.
- Understanding cultural diversity and being sensitive to the values and behaviors of cultural groups often is the key to effective community health intervention.
- C/PHNs should be aware of and respect cultural differences, striving to provide safe and effective nursing care in a manner consistent with clients' cultural values.
- Ethnocentrism, as well as implicit and explicit biases, both individually and at the systems level, can create serious barriers to effective nursing care.

ACTIVE LEARNING EXERCISES

1. Pair up with a student from a different culture. Have a conversation about your own cultural practices (e.g., food, health, values, holidays). Complete a cultural interview and assessment of each other using a guide from this chapter. What similar patterns or themes do you notice? What are the differences?

What was something new about this culture that you discovered? How does this apply to the C/PHN role? (Objective 2)

2. Complete a cultural assessment of one of your clients and share the findings with your class. How do cultural values influence health behaviors, parenting, diet, social interaction, and other areas of life? How can you incorporate this information into your plan of care? What ethnocultural health practices are used by the client or their family? (Objectives 1 and 4)
3. Consider health concerns or issues with a cultural group in your community. How could you apply 3 of the 10 Essential Public Health Services (see Box 2-2) in resolving this issue? Explain the rationale for your choices. What interventions would be most helpful? Are there ethnocultural practices that are used in your community? How would you ensure cultural competence and sensitivity? (Objectives 3 and 4)
4. Consider a recent high-profile event (e.g., hurricane, mass shooting) or a similar local event. Debate with other students whether ethnocentrism, stereotyping, and racism were influential factors, and give your rationale. What can be done at the systems level? (Objectives 3 and 5)
5. Find out if you have refugee populations in your area or state. Talk with program staff or the refugees themselves. Or, if this does not apply in your area, talk with two people from an unfamiliar cultural group. What caused them to move here? What assistance or resources are provided to them? If they do not know English at all or well, how are they learning it? How are they finding housing and jobs? What are their hopes for the future? Have they felt welcomed or experienced discrimination? Describe four ways that C/PHNs can provide care and assistance for refugee populations. (Objectives 5 and 6)

UNIT 2

Community/Public Health Essentials

CHAPTER 6

Structure and Economics of Community/ Public Health Services

"The success or failure of any government in the final analysis must be measured by the well-being of its citizens. Nothing can be more important to a state than its public health; the state's paramount concern should be the health of its people."

—Franklin Delano Roosevelt (1882–1945)

KEY TERMS

Adverse selection
Capitation
Cost sharing
Cost shifting
Cross subsidization
Diagnosis-related groups (DRGs)
Economics
Exclusive provider organization (EPO)
Fee-for-service (FFS)
Health maintenance organization (HMO)
Health reimbursement accounts (HRAs)
Health savings accounts (HSAs)
High-deductible health plans (HDHPs)
High-deductible health plans with a savings option (HDHP/SOs)
Macroeconomic theory
Managed care
Microeconomic theory
Moral hazard
Point-of-service (POS) plan
Preferred provider organization (PPO)
Risk averse
Supply and demand
Third-party payments
Underinsured
Uninsured

LEARNING OBJECTIVES

Upon mastery of this chapter, you should be able to:

1. Describe the current organizational structure of the United States' healthcare system, including public health.
2. Explain the influence of selected legislative acts in the United States on shaping current healthcare policy and practice.

3. Compare and contrast different payment systems for healthcare services, including managed care, fee-for-service, and single-payer systems.
4. Analyze the trends and issues influencing healthcare economics and delivery of public health services.
5. Discuss potential healthcare reform measures and the potential impact on community/public health nursing.
6. Describe how healthcare system funding and financing influences community/public health nursing practice.

INTRODUCTION

In the United States, two systems address the health of the people who live here: the healthcare system and the public health system (American Public Health Association [APHA], 2019). The United States' health system can be described as a "crazy quilt." This type of quilt is not planned; rather, it develops from scraps of fabric that are collected over many years. Similarly, healthcare and public health services in the United States are provided through a mix of private and public programs and institutions; each of these was created to meet specific needs at different times in history. The substantial gaps in both the healthcare and public health systems, or tears in the quilt, are intermittently patched with new programs, institutions, or funding streams. Each patch makes a complicated system even more difficult to navigate.

Our current public health system is not really a single entity but more of a loosely affiliated network of federal, state, and local health agencies that have been "chronically underfunded for decades" (Trust for America's Health [TFAH], 2022, para 6). Nurses preparing for population-based practice need to be familiar with both systems (healthcare and public health): their organization, operation, and financing. To understand financing, community/public health nurses must be familiar with the economics of healthcare and the influence of politics on health services. The structure and economics of community/public healthcare are intertwined.

This chapter begins with a review of significant events that influenced the current health system in the United States. It then provides an overview of healthcare economics, including different payment systems used in the United States and sources of public and private funding for healthcare and community health services.

DEVELOPMENT OF THE UNITED STATES' HEALTHCARE SYSTEM

Early healthcare in the American colonies consisted of private practices, with occasional (but infrequent) governmental action for the public good (Rosen, 2015). Primary providers had few tools at their disposal and could do little to change the course of illness (Hoffer, 2019b; Rosen, 2015).

- Until the mid-1800s, hospitals were places for people who lived in poverty to receive care, and the patients often died; those who could afford it had primary providers visit them at home (Kisacky, 2019).
- During the late 1800s, scientific advances, including germ theory and sterilization, made hospitals safer, whereas industrialization led to more people living in cities and away from family members who could provide care.
- An emphasis on improved sanitation, food handling, and working conditions stemmed from landmark reports (see Chapter 7).
- The professionalization of nursing care also occurred at this time, further contributing to the move from home-based to hospital-based care (see Chapters 2 and 3).

Early public health actions were isolated, local responses to specific problems (Birkhead, Morrow, & Pirani, 2021). The first *federal* public health action occurred in 1878, when the U.S. Congress created a federal quarantine system, enforced by the Marine Hospital Service (Edwards, C. (n.d.)). With increasing travel between cities and states, local quarantines became ineffective. The coordinated strategy was successful; epidemics were stopped more quickly, and communities recognized the benefits of federal government action, resulting in continued growth.

- The Marine Hospital Service eventually became the U.S. Public Health Service, one of the seven uniformed services of the United States (U.S. Department of Health and Human Services [USDHHS], n.d.-b).
- Their first lab in a New York hospital grew into the National Institutes of Health, headquartered in Bethesda, Maryland, which now includes more than 75 institutes supporting scientists conducting research activities in every state and globally (NIH, 2019).
- Since 1854, when President Pierce vetoed legislation to address "indigent insane," many presidents, from Theodore Roosevelt to Franklin D. Roosevelt and from Richard Nixon to William Clinton, have sought some type of universal health coverage (Commonwealth Fund, n.d.).
- In 1900, the average amount spent on healthcare by individual Americans was $5 a year (Blumberg & Davidson, 2009). This would equal just over $148 in 2023's economy (Saving.org, n.d.). Compare that to the $12,914 spent in 2021 (Centers for Medicare & Medicaid Services [CMS], 2022). In 1900, healthcare spending was just over 2% of gross domestic product (GDP), compared to more than 18% in 2021.

Over time, events and insights contributed to improved programs and services, along with a broader recognition that individual health was affected by the health of the wider community.

Early Health Insurance

- Starting in 1929 with Baylor University Hospital in Texas, hospitals offered prepayment plans for hospital services to teachers as a way to increase hospital use (Erickson, 2022).
- Soon after, primary provider groups developed similar plans. These became known as Blue Cross (hospital) and Blue Shield (primary provider) plans, the beginning of modern insurance companies.
- The first government involvement in health insurance was in 1965, when Medicare and Medicaid were created—providing insurance for older adults and families living in poverty (CMS, 2021a).

Over the next five decades, in addition to the prior public health actions, legislation passed addressing healthcare services for targeted groups. In recent years, healthcare reform has focused on regulating the health insurance industry, including the price for insurance and the services that are covered (Shi & Singh, 2019).

- The Patient Protection and Affordable Care Act (ACA) improved access to care by making insurance available to people who were considered "uninsurable" due to preexisting health conditions (USDHHS, 2022).
- The ACA expanded Medicaid in a number of states, extending coverage to people with low income and families not previously eligible.
- In addition, the ACA required insurance companies to cover preventative healthcare visits without a copay, improving access to care even for those with insurance.
- The percentage of **uninsured** (those lacking health insurance) had been 16.3% just before passage of the ACA but dropped to just 8.8% within 2 years (Sommers, 2020).
- In recent years, political disagreements about the ACA have led to weakening of some protections. States that have not implemented the Medicaid expansion, for example, have nearly double uninsured rates (15.4%) compared to expansion states (8.1%) (Rudowitz, Drake, et al., 2023).
- From 2016 to 2019, the number of uninsured Americans grew from 10.0% to 10.9% (Kaiser Family Foundation [KFF], 2022b). The uninsured rate dropped in 2021 to 10.2%; 1.5 million fewer people were uninsured in 2021 compared to 2019. This was, in part, due to the COVID-19 pandemic, as states were not permitted to disenroll people from Medicaid during the declared public health emergency (Lee et al., 2022).

HEALTHCARE ORGANIZATIONS IN THE UNITED STATES

A blend of private and public agencies provides oversight for both the healthcare and public health system in the United States. The actions of these agencies often complement each other, and, in recent years, the roles of private groups and government agencies have become increasingly interdependent (Birkhead, Morrow, & Pirani, 2021).

Private Health Sector Organizations

Private groups include professional associations and nongovernmental organizations (NGOs) focusing on health-related issues. Many health-related professional associations and health issues–focused NGOs have influenced the quality and type of community/public health services delivered in the United States (American Nurses Association, 2022).

Health-Related Professional Associations

Health-related professional associations influence the quality and type of community/public health services available in the United States through the promotion of standards, research, information, and programs. Many also lobby legislators. These organizations are funded primarily through membership dues, bequests, and contributions (U.S. Department of State, 2021). Some health-related professional associations include the following:

- American Public Health Association (APHA, n.d.-a), founded in 1872, maintains a prominent role in the dissemination of public health information, influence on health policy, and advocacy for the nation's health. APHA has a section focused on community/public health nursing.
- Council of Public Health Nursing Organizations (CPHNO, n.d.), a coalition of leading public health nursing organizations in the United States, works collaboratively with its partner organizations to strengthen the specialty of public health nursing by promoting research, education, and practice. The following are CPHNO organizations:
  - Alliance of Nurses for Health Environments.
  - Association of Public Health Nurses.
  - Association for Community Health Nursing Educators.
  - National Association of School Nurses.
  - Public Health Nursing Section, American Public Health Association (APHA).
  - Rural Nurse Organization.
  - Association of State and Territorial Health Officers (ASTHO, n.d.-a), established in 1942, supports the work of public health officials to promote excellence in public health policy in the United States.
  - National Association of County and City Health Officials (NACCHO, n.d.), founded in 1965, consists of almost 3000 local health departments in the United States. They focus on promoting leadership and being a catalyst for strengthening local health departments' services and programs.

Health Issues–Focused NGOs

Health issues–focused NGOs supply funds for research, lobby legislators, and educate the public. Funding is through private and corporate contributions.

- Some, such as the American Heart Association and American Diabetes Association, focus on particular health issues.

- Others, such as the National Society for Autistic Children, Planned Parenthood Federation of America, and the National Council on Aging, focus on the needs of special populations.
- Some NGOs provide services and healthcare. These include Habitat for Humanity, the American Red Cross, and the Public Health Institute (Yale School of Public Health, 2019).
- A few agencies focus on disease prevention, such as the Trust for America's Health and the Prevention Institute.
- Many foundations provide grant support for health programs, research, and professional education as part of their mission (e.g., Robert Wood Johnson Foundation, Bill and Melinda Gates Foundation) (National Philanthropic Trust, n.d.).

Public Health Agencies

Public health agencies perform a wide variety of activities, some requiring legal authority to ensure enforcement (e.g., environmental pollution, communicable disease control, food handling) (CDC, 2024). These agencies provide important data, including the collection and monitoring of vital statistics and communicable diseases. They also conduct research, provide consultation, and sometimes financially support other community/public health efforts. These activities can be grouped under one of the three core public health functions: assessment, policy development, and assurance. As discussed in Chapters 1 and 2, C/PHNs practice as partners with other public health professionals within these core functions.

Table 6-1 describes the actions of some federal agencies in relation to the three core functions. States retain the primary responsibility for their citizens' health and are responsible for implementing federal policies. At the local level, a city government health agency, a county agency, or a combination of both assess, plan, and serve the health needs of their community (Goldsteen et al., 2020). Table 6-2 compares the public health responsibilities of federal, state, and local governments related to the 10 Essentials Public Health Services. For more on the 10 essential services, see Chapter 2.

TABLE 6-1 Examples of Federal Government Agencies' Actions Related to the Three Core Public Health Functions

Core Public Health Function	Agency	Example of Action
Assessment	Centers for Disease Control and Prevention National Center for Health Statistics	Conducts surveillance for disease outbreaks Conducts national surveys that monitor health behaviors
Policy development	Substance Abuse and Mental Health Services Administration Health Resources and Services Administration	Uses data to educate policymakers about mental health and substance use disorders Analyzes potential effects of proposed policy
Assurance	Environmental Protection Agency Indian Health Service	Evaluates safety of water for drinking Funds or provides care for underserved populations living on tribal lands

Federal Public Health Agencies

The federal public health responsibilities include the following (CDC, 2014):

- Policymaking and implementing legislation
- Financing public health through healthcare services, grants, contracts, and reimbursements to states and local public health agencies
- Protection of public health and prevention activities through surveillance, research, and regulation
- Collecting and disseminating data (national data, health statistics, surveys, research)
- Acting to assist states in mounting effective responses during public health emergencies (e.g., natural disasters, bioterror events, emerging diseases)
- Developing public health goals in collaboration with state and local governments and other relevant stakeholders (e.g., Healthy People 2030)
- Building capacity for population health at federal, state, and local levels by providing resources and infrastructure
- Directly managing healthcare delivery through categorical grant programs (maternal–child health programs, Medicaid, Medicare, community health centers) and services (public health laboratories, health clinics on reservations for Native American tribes)

At the federal level, public health organizations can be clustered into four groups:

- U.S. Public Health Service (USPHS) is staffed by the Commissioned Corps, which consists of over 6700 uniformed health professionals. Employees of the USPHS work in many different federal agencies (USDHHS, n.d.-b).
- The U.S. Department of Health and Human Services (USDHHS), including the Centers for Disease Control and Prevention (CDC).
- Federal departments that oversee areas impacting health, such as the Departments of Labor, Education, Environmental Health, Agriculture, and Transportation, among others.
- Federal agencies that focus on international health concerns, such as the U.S. Agency for International Development and the Office of International Health Affairs, are under the auspices of the U.S. Department of State (Birkhead et al., 2021). See Chapter 16.

TABLE 6-2 Federal, State, and Local Activities Related to the 10 Essential Public Health Services

Essential Service	Federal	State	Local
Assess and monitor population health	Collect and disseminate information using national surveys	Collect and analyze data specific to the state	Complete community health assessments
Investigate, diagnose, and address health hazards and root causes	Maintain national surveillance systems and provide specialty laboratory services that state or local public health laboratories cannot perform	Monitor statewide health threats and report to the federal level when appropriate; perform laboratory testing to identify cause of health hazard	Identify people and groups who have conditions that threaten public health
Communicate effectively to inform and educate	Distribute national reports about health issues (Surgeon General examples)	Conduct media campaigns and programs on prevention; coordinate statewide health alerts	Provide educational materials supporting local programs
Strengthen, support, and mobilize communities and partnerships	Collaborate with national nongovernmental organizations	Coordinate efforts of state agencies	Establish relationships with community leaders and agencies
Create, champion, and implement policies, plans, and laws	Establish national public health goals, in collaboration with state and local health officials and public health experts	Set statewide health objectives and priorities	Implement programs to meet public health goals
Utilize legal and regulatory actions	Enforce public health regulations affecting interstate commerce	Develop statewide regulations for services and the environment	Assess compliance with regulations and take appropriate action
Enable equitable access	Establish and manage national health insurance programs and insurance marketplaces (U.S. Public Health Service)	Implement federal initiatives and equitably distribute funds to communities	Address unmet needs in the community through case management and clinics
Build a diverse and skilled workforce	Provide expertise or resources when public health needs exceed state capacity; promote diversity in health professions training	Set requirements and maintain records of licensure for public health professionals	Screen, hire, and train staff
Improve and innovate through evaluation, research, and quality improvement	Disseminate evidence-based practices for public health services	Gather data and compile results of program evaluations	Determine if existing services meet the community's needs and search for innovative solutions
Build and maintain a strong organizational infrastructure for public health	Promote adequate funding for public health programs and research	Determine solutions appropriate for specific state and provide adequate staffing for programs	Fund and implement new programs and report on effectiveness

Source: CDC (2024), Public Health Law Center (2015).

Table 6-3 provides a selected list of federal agencies related to public health and their main functions. Figure 6-1 represents the organizational chart for the USDHHS.

State Public Health Agencies

The state health department (SHD) is responsible for providing leadership in and monitoring of comprehensive public health needs and services in the state. SHDs promote population health, focusing on prevention and protection. They also administer federally funded programs.

General functions of SHDs include the following (CDC, 2014; Erwin & Brownson, 2017):

- Statewide health planning
- Intergovernmental and other agency relations
- Intrastate agency relations
- Certain statewide policy determinations
- Standards setting
- Health regulatory functions
- State laboratory services

TABLE 6-3 Selected Federal Public Health Agencies of the U.S. Department of Health and Human Services (USDHHS) and Other Public Health Agencies

Agency	Mission, Function, or Area of Focus
USDHHS Agencies	
Administration for Children and Families	Supports initiatives that empower families and people and improve access to services in order to create strong, healthy communities
Administration for Community Living	Funds services provided by community-based organizations that enable older adults and people with disabilities of all ages to live where they choose, with the people they choose, and with the ability to participate fully in their communities
Agency for Healthcare Research and Quality	Supports research on healthcare outcomes and costs, patient safety and medical errors, and access to effective services
Agency for Toxic Substances and Disease Registry	Prevents exposure and adverse human health effects and diminished quality of life associated with exposure to hazardous substances from waste sites, unplanned releases, and other sources of pollution present in the environment
Centers for Disease Control and Prevention	Promotes health and quality of life by preventing and controlling disease, injury, and disability
Centers for Medicare & Medicaid Services	Administers Medicare, Medicaid, and other major programs such as the State Children's Health Insurance Program; the Medicare Prescription Drug, Improvement, and Modernization Act; and the Health Insurance Portability and Accountability Act (HIPAA)
Food and Drug Administration (FDA)	Ensures the safety of foods and cosmetics and the safety and efficacy of pharmaceuticals, biologic products, and medical devices
Health Resources and Services Administration	Assures equitable access to comprehensive, quality healthcare for all
Indian Health Service	Is the principal federal healthcare advocate and provider for American Indians and Alaska Natives who belong to more than 550 federally recognized tribes in 35 states
National Institutes of Health	Provides leadership and financial support for research about ways to prevent disease, as well as the causes, treatments, and even cures for common and rare diseases
Substance Abuse and Mental Health Services Administration	Works to improve the quality and availability of prevention, treatment, and rehabilitative services in order to reduce illness, death, disability, and cost to society resulting from substance misuse and mental illnesses
Non-USDHHS Agencies	
U.S. Department of Labor, Occupational Safety and Health Administration	Workplace and worker safety
U.S. Department of Agriculture	▪ Dietary guidelines ▪ Food support programs (food stamps—Supplemental Nutrition Assistance Program) ▪ Farm-based food control (in contrast to control by the FDA, which is product-based)
Environmental Protection Agency	Pollution control
U.S. Department of Housing and Urban Development	Healthy Homes initiative (lead, etc.)
Federal Emergency Management Agency	Public health preparedness and disaster response
U.S. Department of Education	Safe and Healthy Students program

USDHHS, U.S. Department of Health and Human Services
Source: USDHHS (n.d.-d, n.d.-e)

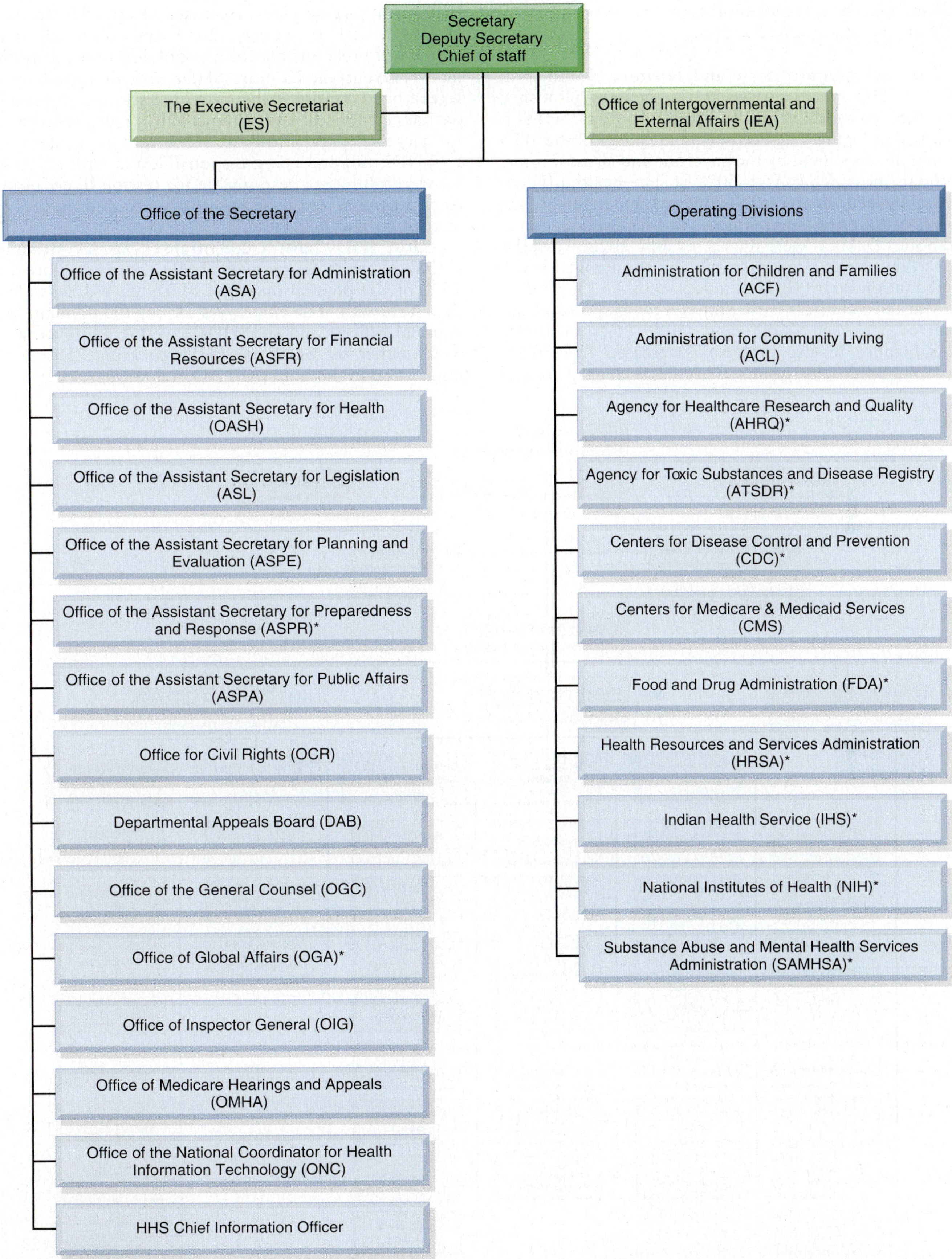

FIGURE 6-1 U.S. Department of Health and Human Services organizational chart: January (August 2023). *Components of the Public Health Service. (Reprinted from U.S. Department of Health & Human Services. (2023). *HHS organizational chart*. Content created by Assistant Secretary for Public Affairs (ASPA). Last reviewed August 17, 2023. https://www.hhs.gov/about/agencies/orgchart/index.html)

- Surveillance and epidemiology
- Training and technical support

The Association of State and Territory Health Officials (ASTHO, n.d.-c) surveys SHDs; the latest published data were collected in 2019. The structure of SHDs is described in Figure 6-2. The person in charge of the SHD is generally appointed by the governor and is, most often, a primary provider. In fact, 60% of state health officials have a medical degree (ASTHO, n.d.-b). In 2023, the leaders of four SHDs (Arkansas, New Jersey, Oklahoma, and South Dakota) were nurses. By July 2023, 41 SHDs had achieved initial accreditation by the Public Health Accreditation Board (PHAB, n.d.).

Marked changes in state-level responsibilities occurred between 2007 and 2016. Responsibility for substance misuse programs increased from 32% to 76%, while the number of SHDs that provided long-term care services decreased from 79% to 57% (ASTHO, 2017). Between 2016 and 2019, 20 more SHDs were responsible for alcohol and other drug primary prevention, 13 more SHDs provided prediabetes screening, 10 more SHDs provided syringe and needle exchange services, and 9 more SHDs were responsible for violence prevention (ASTHO, n.d.-c). In contrast, 29 SHDs stopped being responsible for vital statistics, 12 were no longer responsible for testing likely bioterrorism agents, and 4 SHDs stopped providing services in correctional facilities.

Most SHDs have a decentralized agency structure, with local health departments (LHDs) covering more than 75% of the population; eight SHDs have a centralized structure, with SHD employees serving the population in regional offices; and six SHDs have mixed governance, with neither the SHD nor LHDs covering 75% of the population in the state (ASTHO, n.d.-c).

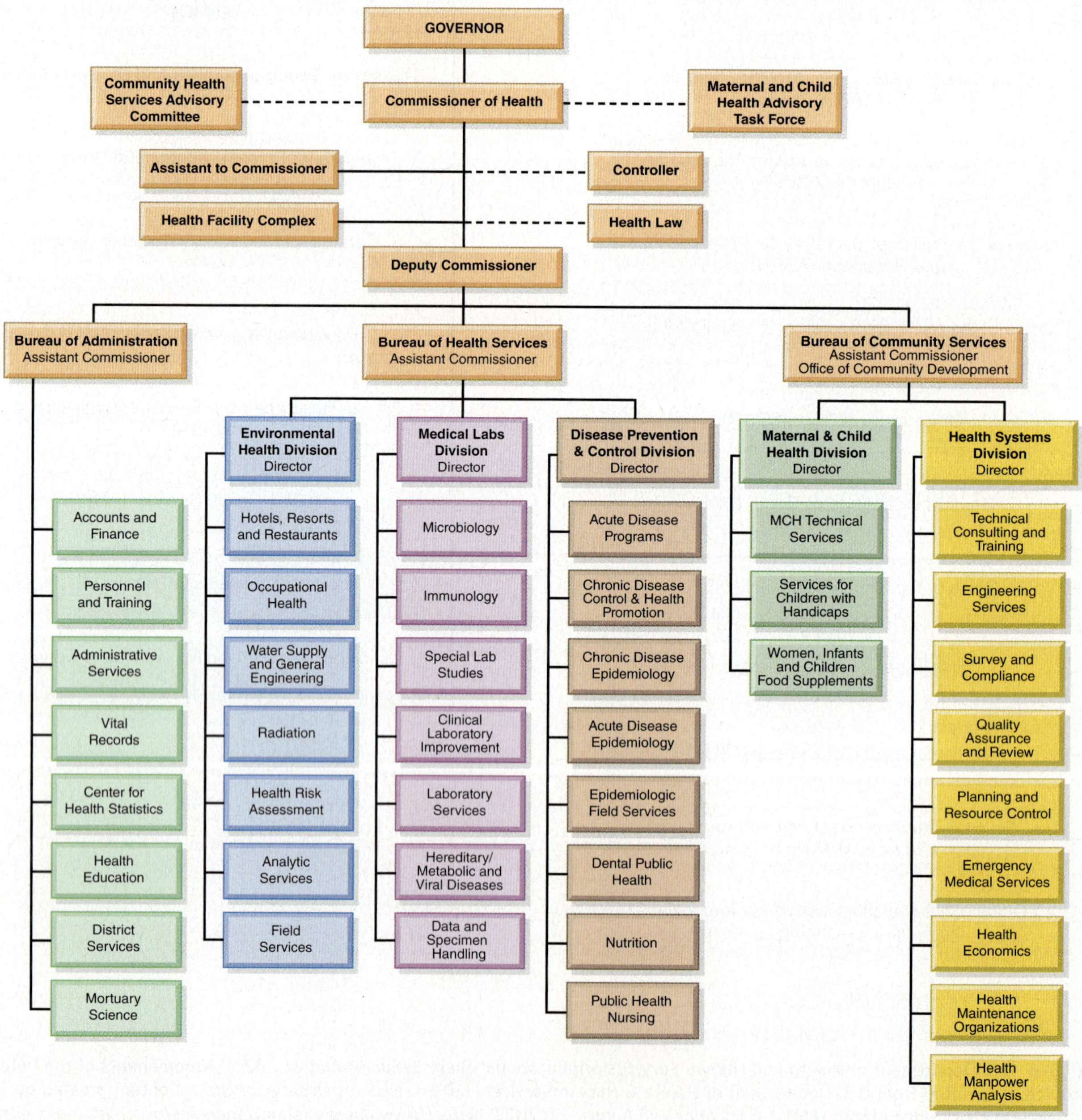

FIGURE 6-2 Organizational chart of a state public health department.

- Between 2012 and 2019, state health agency workforce dropped by 9.9%.
- The largest group of employees (35%) work within the financial/business and administrative categories and saw the largest losses in employees.
- Public health nurses comprise 7.8% of the state health agency workforce, compared to 0.7% of primary provider assistants and nurse practitioners and 0.6% of public health primary providers. Public health nurses had a small decrease in full-time equivalents (FTEs) between 2012 and 2019.
- Other employees include behavioral health specialists, epidemiologists/statisticians, environmental health and laboratory specialists, nutritionists, and dental health professionals, as well as informatics and public information specialists.

Local Public Health Agencies

The primary responsibilities of LHDs are to assess the local population's health status and needs, determine how well those needs are being met, and take action toward satisfying unmet needs. Specifically, they should fulfill these functions as follows (Erwin & Brownson, 2017):

- Monitor local health needs and the resources for addressing them.
- Develop policy and provide leadership in advocating equitable distribution of resources and services, both public and private.
- Evaluate availability, accessibility, and quality of health services for all members of the community.
- Keep the community informed about how to access public health services.

The National Association of City and County Health Officials (NACCHO, 2020) identified 2459 LHDs in the United States in 2019; about 77% of these had significant local governance, 16% were state-run agencies, and 7% had shared governance. Most LHDs (61%) serve populations of less than 50,000 people. A few (6%) serve over half of the U.S. population (each catchment area serves more than 500,000 people). Figure 6-3 shows a typical organizational chart for a LHD.

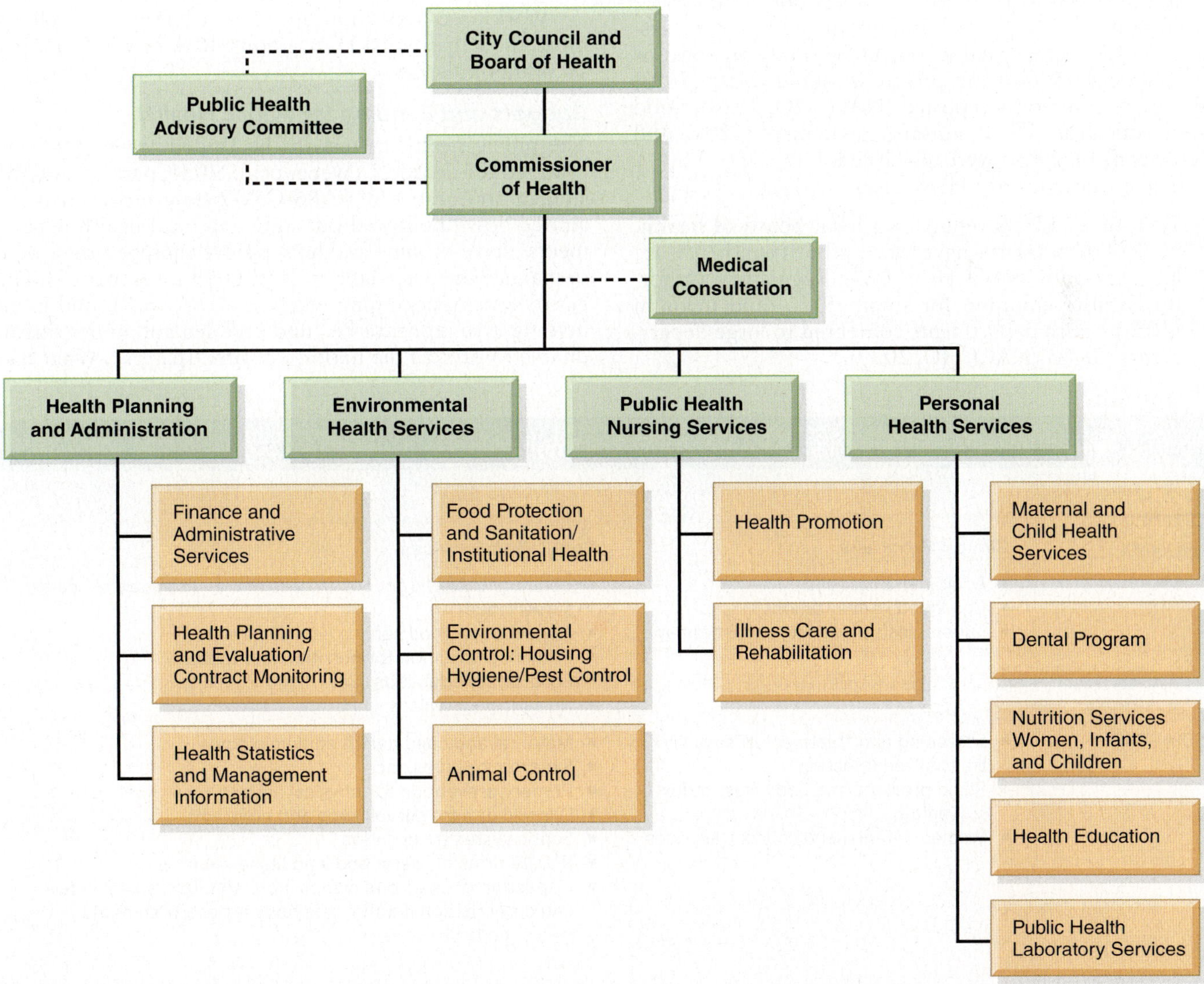

FIGURE 6-3 Organizational chart of a city public health department.

LHDs provide public health clinical services to help people lead healthy lives and specific population-based health programs within their jurisdictions. Table 6-4 lists clinical services and population-based programs reported by more than 50% of LHDs (NACCHO, 2020). The most commonly provided clinical services follow:

- Adult and childhood immunizations (88%)
- TB screening and services (86%, 83%)
- Women, Infants, and Children (WIC) services (68%)
- Screening for HIV and other STDs (62%, 70%)
- Home visits (60%)
- Screening for hypertension and BMI (56%, 52%)

The most common population-based health programs provided are (NACCHO, 2020) as follows:

- Communicable/infectious disease (90%)
- Environmental health (84%)
- Maternal and child health (70%)
- Syndromic surveillance (65%)
- Primary preventive programs for tobacco (78%), nutrition (75%), chronic disease programs (60%), and physical activity (59%)

In the area of regulations or inspections, food service establishments (78%), schools/day care (72%), septic systems (68%), recreational water (66%), body art (tattoos and piercings; 58%), and private drinking water (56%) were most commonly reported (NACCHO, 2020). Food safety education (78%), nuisance abatement (72%), and vector control (55%) were also listed.

The governance of LHDs varies:

- 70% of all LHDs report to a local board of health; 50% of these boards have legal authority and 20% are advisory only (NACCHO, 2020). Regulatory authority is more common for small (51%) and medium (50%) health departments compared to large departments (38%) (NACCHO, 2020).
- Unlike SHDs, nearly one quarter of directors of LHDs are nurses, including 30% of small LHDs and 33% of rural LHDs. Nurses are less likely to lead large (5%) and urban (16%) LHDs.
- Less than 10% of LHD chief executives are Hispanic/Latino or a race other than White; this has been stable since 2008.

LHDs can also achieve accreditation by the PHAB (n.d.). As of July 2023, 321 LHDs and 6 tribal health agencies had received initial accreditation by PHAB.

- Accredited SHDs and LHDs now serve more than 90% of the United States' population.
- In addition, a majority of nonaccredited LHDs were completing prerequisite activities required by the PHAB (i.e., community health assessments [78%], community health improvement plans [71%], and strategic plans [64%]) indicating continuing interest in accreditation (NACCHO, 2020).

As in SHDs, LHDs have also experienced a decrease in staffing in the past decade (NACCHO, 2020).

- Between 2008 and 2019, LHDs employed 17% fewer people and have 16% fewer FTEs.

Workforce reduction in large LHDs has declined more than in small LHDs, about 40% fewer FTEs per 10,000 population.

Budgets and Funding for Public Health

The public health system in the United States has been "starved for decades" (Weber et al., 2020, para 1), and the sudden appearance of SARS-CoV-2 only further demonstrated how "hollowed-out state and local health departments" have become and how poorly equipped they were to manage the onslaught of COVID-19 cases (para 7). The entire system, beginning with the CDC, was found in an investigative report to be "underfunded and under threat, unable to protect the nation's health" (para 5). What had

TABLE 6-4 Services Offered by Local Health Departments

% of LHDs Offering Services	Clinical Programs	Population Services
>75%	▪ Adult immunizations ▪ Childhood immunizations ▪ Tuberculosis screening and treatment	▪ Communicable/infectious disease and environmental health surveillance ▪ Inspection of food service establishments ▪ Primary prevention for nutrition and tobacco ▪ Food safety education ▪ Nuisance abatement
50%–74%	▪ Screening and treatment of sexually transmitted infections ▪ Blood pressure and body mass index screening ▪ Women, infants, and children services	▪ Maternal and child health epidemiology ▪ Syndromic surveillance ▪ Primary prevention for physical activity ▪ Chronic disease surveillance and programs ▪ Septic systems regulation ▪ Private drinking water and lead inspections ▪ Inspection of children's camps, hotels/motels, schools/day cares, recreational water, and body art establishments ▪ Vector control

Source: NACCHO (2020).

been considered a premier public health system, envied by other countries around the world, struggled to meet the crushing demands of a once-in-a-century pandemic on top of an already overworked and underfunded reality. Further, the degree to which the pandemic was politicized resulted in public health workers being "disrespected, ignored, and even vilified," leading to resignations, retirements, and occasional firings (para 8). In some states, as the pandemic worsened and the economy and tax revenues dwindled, workers were furloughed, had their hours cut, or their pay frozen—at a time when public health workers were most needed. See What Do You Think? (Box 6-1).

- Funding for public health was 2.8% of total health expenditures in 2019, increased to 5.8% in 2020 due to the COVID-19 pandemic emergency expenditures, and dropped to 4.4% in 2021 (Keehan et al., 2023). It is projected to decrease to 2.6% by 2031.
- While total health expenditures are expected to increase by 5.6% from 2025 to 2031, public health funding is expected to increase by only 1.8% over the same years (Keehan et al., 2023).
- In 2019, the CDC's budget was just $19 per person (DeSalvo et al., 2019). It is estimated that federal support of $32 per person is needed to achieve adequate foundational public health services.
- In 2021, total U.S. healthcare spending was $12,914 per person, or 18.3% of the GDP (CMS, 2022). This amount is projected to increase to $20,425 (19.6% of GDP) by 2031. When you compare this to the per person budget of the CDC and state public health agencies, you get a real sense of the very small percentage given to public health in comparison to overall health costs.

Determining the amount of government spending on public health is difficult as the sources of funding are varied and not coordinated across levels of government (TFAH, 2019). The numbers stated above for public health spending may actually be artificially overestimated. Research indicates that CMS inflates public health spending by including spending on behavioral healthcare, community health clinics, and disability-related services among other nonpublic health activities (Leider et al., 2020). While CMS estimated public health expenditures at 2.5% of total health expenditures in 2018, detailed analysis of the records showed that only 1.5% was spent on population health activities.

- Federal public health agencies are largely funded by the federal government, but about 75% of that funding ends up at the state and local levels, along with other private and public organizations (TFAH, 2019).
- At the state level, federal grants and monetary support, along with state tax dollars, fund programs.
- The majority of federal grant money is provided by the Prevention and Public Health Fund created by the ACA. From its 2018 budget, $586 million of the total $800 million budget went to state and LHDs (Johnson, 2019).
- The money that makes its way to LHDs often comes through competitive grants and block grants; it is supplemented by local taxes.

The lack of consistency and transparency limits public health officials' ability to defend public health programs when budget cuts are threatened (Bekemeier et al., 2018). Given that public health agencies are vital safety net services, the decreases in budgets and staffing are very challenging.

- The proposed 2024 budget allocates almost $11.6 billion in funding for the CDC, an increase of almost $2.4 billion from fiscal year 2023 (APHA, 2023).
- The senate funding bill for HHS, labor, and education keeps funding levels stable.
- However, the house funding bill for these same areas cuts current CDC funding by $1.6 billion and current Health Resources and Services Administration funding by $700 million below the FY 2023 level.

Both ASTHO and NACCHO collect information on public health spending by SHDs and LHDs. In 2018, federal dollars in SHD budgets totaled $12.9 billion, down from $14.3 billion in 2015 (ASTHO, 2020). The range of dollars per state was as small as $32.6 million and as high as $2.38 billion. In Alaska, Connecticut, Delaware, Hawaii, Illinois, Massachusetts, New York, and New Mexico state spending exceeds federal spending.

- More than 60% of SHDs derive 50% of their funding from federal sources.
- LHDs also receive federal funding, a portion of which are "pass through dollars," meaning that the state receives the funding from the federal government but sends the money on to LHDs who provide the services (CDC, 2014).
- In 2018, an average of 25% of LHD funding came from local taxes (NACCHO, 2020).

Figure 6-4 shows the percent of state health agencies' budgets derived from state and federal sources, while Figure 6-5 shows the sources of funding for LHDs.

BOX 6-1 WHAT DO *YOU* THINK?

Service Over Salaries

An investigative report found that 20% of public health employees (excluding large health departments) had salaries of $35,000 or less in 2017. Well-educated employees (i.e., those with bachelor's, master's, or PhDs) can earn substantially more working in the private sector. At times, some workers actually qualify for the very programs that they oversee, like WIC. For instance, a disease intervention specialist at the Kentucky state health department, tirelessly working to keep HIV and syphilis from spreading, found that her salary was so low that she and her three children qualified for Medicaid. Boston's 2018 budget for the police department was five times higher than its city public health department; Boston offered to move $3 million dollars from a police overtime fund to help with public health staffing and immunization clinics (Weber et al., 2020).

How can residents ensure that public health is adequately funded? What percentage of your city or county budget goes to public health compared to other services?

Source: Weber et al. (2020).

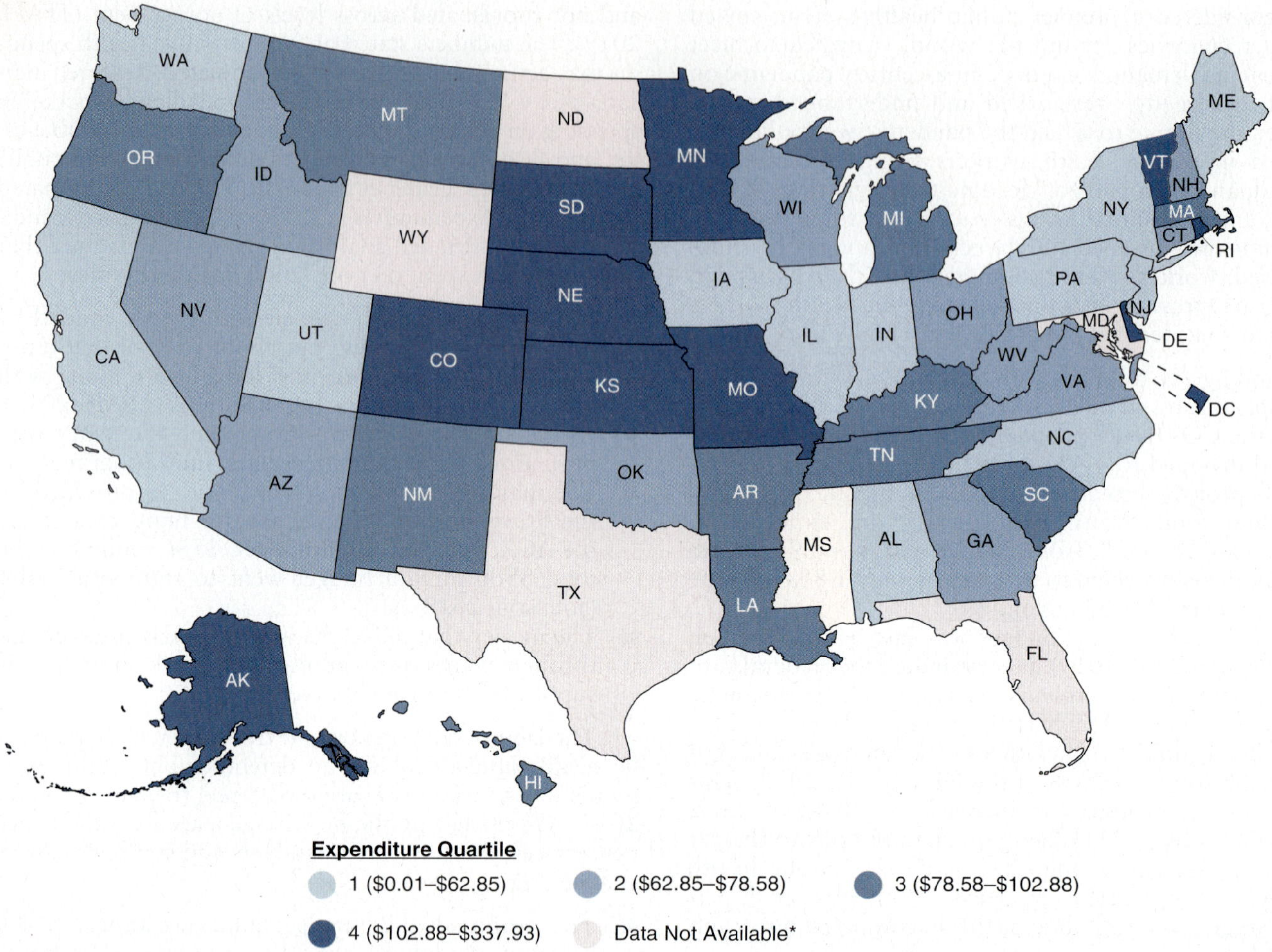

Source: Association of State and Territorial Health Officials (ASTHO) Profile of State and Territorial Public Health Survey.
Notes: *Data Not Available can mean that data were not reported, data were suppressed, or expenditures were $0 for a given expenditure category or from a specific funding source. (1) The fiscal year runs from July 1st through June 30th (e.g., FY2019 spans July 1, 2018 through June 30, 2019). (2) Agency structure or governance classification may affect categorical expenditures. (3) If a public health agency reported no expenditures in a category, it may be that a separate agency in the jurisdiction oversees that program. Thus, categorical expenditures do not reflect a state's total expenditures in a given category.

FIGURE 6-4 2021 per capita expenditures for federal spending, all expenditure categories, map of expenditures by year: all federal funding sources. (Data from the Association of State and Territorial Health Officials (ASTHO). (2021). *ASTHO profile of state and public health.* Retrieved from https://astho.shinyapps.io/profile/#finance)

For-Profit and Not-for-Profit Healthcare Organizations

Health agencies and hospitals may be for-profit or not-for-profit. For-profit agencies "can distribute their accounting profits to their founders, investors, and owners" (Moon & Shugan, 2020, p. 193). Not-for-profit agencies make money, but profits are used to offset the cost of other services that do not generate income or to improve the infrastructure of the agency's facilities. "Maintaining nonprofit tax status requires supplying often ill-defined community benefits (e.g., education, training, charity care)" (p. 193). Nonprofits use their money to expand services, fund research, or build capital projects. Nonprofit entities do not pay federal, state, or county taxes. Both for-profit and not-for-profit health agencies receive payments from Medicare, Medicaid, private insurance companies, and out-of-pocket payments from clients.

- There are 2978 nonprofit and 1235 for-profit hospitals in the United States (American Hospital Association, 2023).
- Private nonprofit hospitals provide more services and have higher prices and profits compared to for-profit hospitals.
- Definitive Healthcare (2023b) lists the top 50 hospitals by net patient revenue; all 50 are nonprofit entities.
- In a critical study of hospital profitability, Bai and Anderson (2016) found that 45% of hospitals were profitable, although the median hospital lost $82 per discharge.
- Hospitals with higher markups (higher prices compared to costs) had median earnings of $114 per patient discharge, while hospitals with lower markups lost a median of $243 per patient discharge.

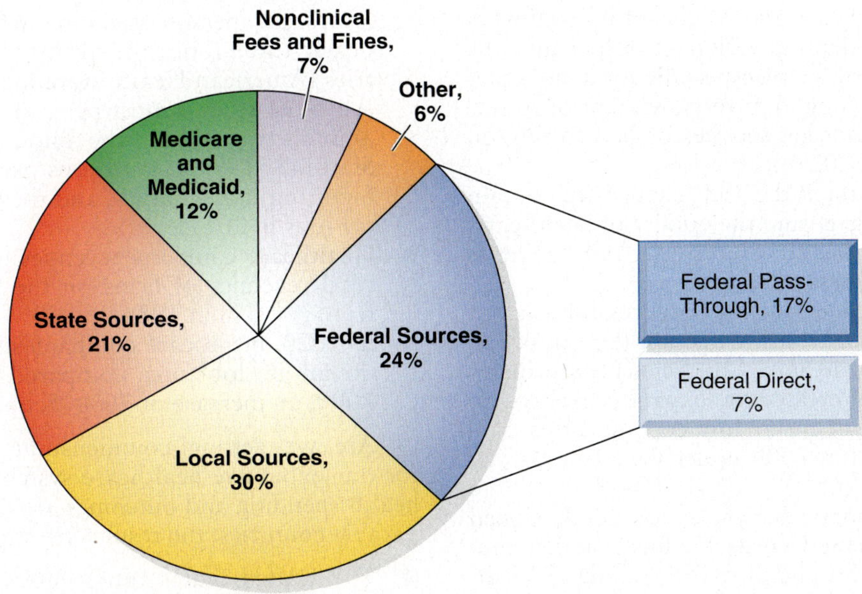

FIGURE 6-5 Funding sources for local health departments. (Data from National Association of County and City Health Officials (NACCHO). (2020). *2019 national profile of local health departments.*)

- Across the United States, the average hospital's net patient revenue is $210.4 million, while the average for the top 50 hospitals is $3.2 billion (Definitive Healthcare, 2023b).
- Hospital payment-to-cost ratios reveal that for private insurers, hospitals average about 145% of cost, but for Medicaid and Medicare, the ratios are 88.1% and 86.8%, respectively, of hospital cost (Gee, 2019).

INTERNATIONAL HEALTH ORGANIZATIONS

International cooperation in health dates back to early concerns for epidemics. Besides important humanitarian and moral concerns, there are pragmatic reasons for addressing health issues at the international level. Today, health—along with politics and economics—has become a global issue, as the COVID-19 pandemic exemplifies. The modern era of collaboration truly began with the development of the World Health Organization (WHO), an agency of the United Nations. Formed in 1948, in the aftermath of World War II, the WHO currently has 194 member nations (WHO, n.d.). International health agencies focus on issues of global concern, setting policy, developing standards, and monitoring health conditions and programs (see Chapter 16).

It may not seem possible that the health of a resident of a country 9000 miles away can affect anyone in the United States or vice versa. However, the reality of international air travel means that illness in one part of the world can quickly move to another. Over one billion people traveled internationally during 2014, with 80 million international visitors to the United States in 2018; travel and tourism accounted for 10.3% of global GDP in 2019 (World Travel & Tourism Council, n.d.). Despite close scrutiny of airline passengers for passports, visas, customs regulations, weapons, drugs, and even symptoms such as cough and fever, how can anyone know if someone sitting next to them on a plane or in an airport is carrying a deadly, communicable disease on their journey? As described in Chapters 7 and 8, during late 2019 and early 2020, travelers did bring a novel coronavirus (COVID-19) to the United States and a pandemic ensued (Gan et al., 2020; Lovelace, 2020; Schuchat, 2020).

DEVELOPMENT OF TODAY'S HEALTHCARE SYSTEM

Many of the historical influences on healthcare, public health, and advancements in health and social systems were brought about through legislative efforts and influenced by market forces.

Significant Legislation

In comparison to earlier history, more recent history demonstrates an ever-widening sense of responsibility for citizen's health leading to the passage of expanded health-related legislation. This legislation was not always focused on providing care but eventually promoted disease prevention. For example, the Sheppard–Towner Maternity and Infancy Act in 1921 funded education about prenatal and infant care (Shi & Singh, 2019).

- During the Great Depression, the U.S. government enacted the first significant legislation that affected the health and well-being of a wide range of citizens, the Social Security Act of 1935 (Social Security Administration [SSA], n.d.-a).
  - This law ensured greater public health programs and provided retirement income to participating workers aged 65 years and older.
  - The act included aid to dependent children, unemployment insurance, and supported educational programs.
- Later legislation (e.g., Hill-Burton) provided federal support for expansion of hospitals; care for people with developmental delays; research and support for heart disease, cancer, and stroke; and training for healthcare personnel.

- The landmark Medicare and Medicaid legislation in 1965 moved the federal government deeper into the role of financing healthcare, especially for many older adults and people living in poverty, who, prior to this time, either could not get services or had to rely on charity care (CMS, 2021a).
- Healthcare legislation in the 1980s sought to contain healthcare spending, ensure the quality of healthcare, promote national health objectives, and facilitate data collection and research.
- President Bill Clinton made an unsuccessful attempt at universal healthcare during his first term in office. However, in 1997, the State Children's Health Insurance Program was created to expand coverage to uninsured children at no or low cost, and this coverage was extended in 2009 under President Barack Obama (CMS, n.d.-a).
- The Medicare Modernization Act of 2003, signed into law by President George W. Bush, added prescription drug benefits and disease screening to Medicare and promoted health savings accounts.
- More recent laws have protected the confidentiality of health records and made it easier for workers to continue insurance coverage after being laid off.
- The ACA is the most recent legislation to impact healthcare financing in the United States (Knickman & Kovner, 2019), although efforts to repeal the act are ongoing as of 2023 (whitehouse.gov, 2023). The ACA provided expanded health insurance for Americans, in an effort to bring the United States more in line with other high-income countries. See Chapter 13 for more information on legislation, policy, and advocacy.

Cost and Quality of the U.S. Healthcare System

There has been much concern about the efficacy of the U.S. healthcare system; we have much to learn by examining what is done in other countries.

- Healthcare in the United States is very expensive and we do not have good outcomes compared to other countries. Health spending in 2021 was estimated at 18.3% of the U.S. GDP—the total amount of goods and services produced within a year (CMS, 2022). To put that in perspective, only 5.0% of GDP in 1960 was spent on healthcare.
- CMS (2022) predicts that healthcare spending will grow 0.8% faster than the U.S. GDP and increase to 19.6% of U.S. GDP by 2031—meaning that almost one fifth of all goods and services produced in the United States will go toward healthcare.
- Drug spending is one key driver of higher costs, with $350 billion spent in the United States in 2020, more than 25% of the $1.3 trillion spent globally on prescription drugs (Rajkumar, 2020).
- While the U.S. Veterans Administration has a 30% discounted rate for prescription medications, the federal government is not allowed to negotiate drug prices for Medicare or Medicaid programs (Cai et al., 2020). Total spending on healthcare services was $4.3 trillion in 2021 and is predicted to grow to more than $7 trillion in 2031 (CMS, 2022). The United States per person spending was $11,859 in 2020, nearly three times the average of comparable countries (American Health Rankings, 2022). Switzerland spent the second most per capita on healthcare; this amount was still 2/3 the amount spent in the United States ($7179). Health jobs grew faster than manufacturing jobs in 2008, and they surpassed retail sector jobs in 2017.
- Healthcare company revenues encompassed 16% of total revenues of firms on the S&P 500, increasing from just 4% in 1984.
- In 2020, healthcare companies spent $713.6 million dollars on lobbying, compared to $358.2 million in 2000, an increase of 70% (Schpero et al., 2022).

Are we getting commensurate value in exchange for our expensive healthcare system? When overall U.S. health spending and outcomes are matched against comparable countries, the results are startling:

- The United States ranks 33rd out of 38 countries on infant mortality rates, with 5.4 deaths/1000 live births compared to an average of 4.1 (America's Health Rankings, 2022).
- The maternal death rate in the United States in 2019 was 17.4/100,000 live births, about 5.5 times the rate of 3.2 in Germany and more than twice the rate of 7.5 in Canada (Schneider et al., 2021).
- Average life expectancy in the United States is 77 years, compared to an average of 80.5 years. The United States ranks 31st out of 38 countries (America's Health Rankings, 2022). Mississippi has the lowest life expectancy in the United States at 71.9 years, which is less than Lithuania (75.1 years), who ranks 38th of the 38 countries compared by the Organization for Economic Cooperation and Development (OECD) (Anderson et al., 2019).
- Spurred by substance misuse and injuries, disease burden (a measurement of quality of life and longevity) is 31% higher in the United States, also demonstrating a widening gap (Hoffer, 2019a).
- Rate of death responsive to healthcare is ranked on a scale from 0 to 100 (with 100 being the best). The United States falls behind at 88.7 compared to an average of 93.7.
- Preventable hospital admission rates are 143% higher for asthma, 55% higher for heart failure, and 38% higher for patients with diabetes in the United States versus comparable countries (Kamal et al., 2019).
- In 2015, the United States had 7.9/1000 practicing nurses versus a median of 9.9 when compared to other OECD countries (Anderson et al., 2019).
- The comparison for practicing primary providers was 2.6 versus a median of 3.2 per 1000 population.
- The United States ranks 11th out of 11 countries in health system effectiveness, a measure of access, equity, quality, efficiency, and healthy lives (Schneider et al., 2021; Fig. 6-6). You can examine the performance scores in more detail at https://www.commonwealthfund.org/international.
- Similarly, a Commonwealth Fund comparison of the United States and 10 other high-income countries (Box 6-2) noted that the United States ranked highest

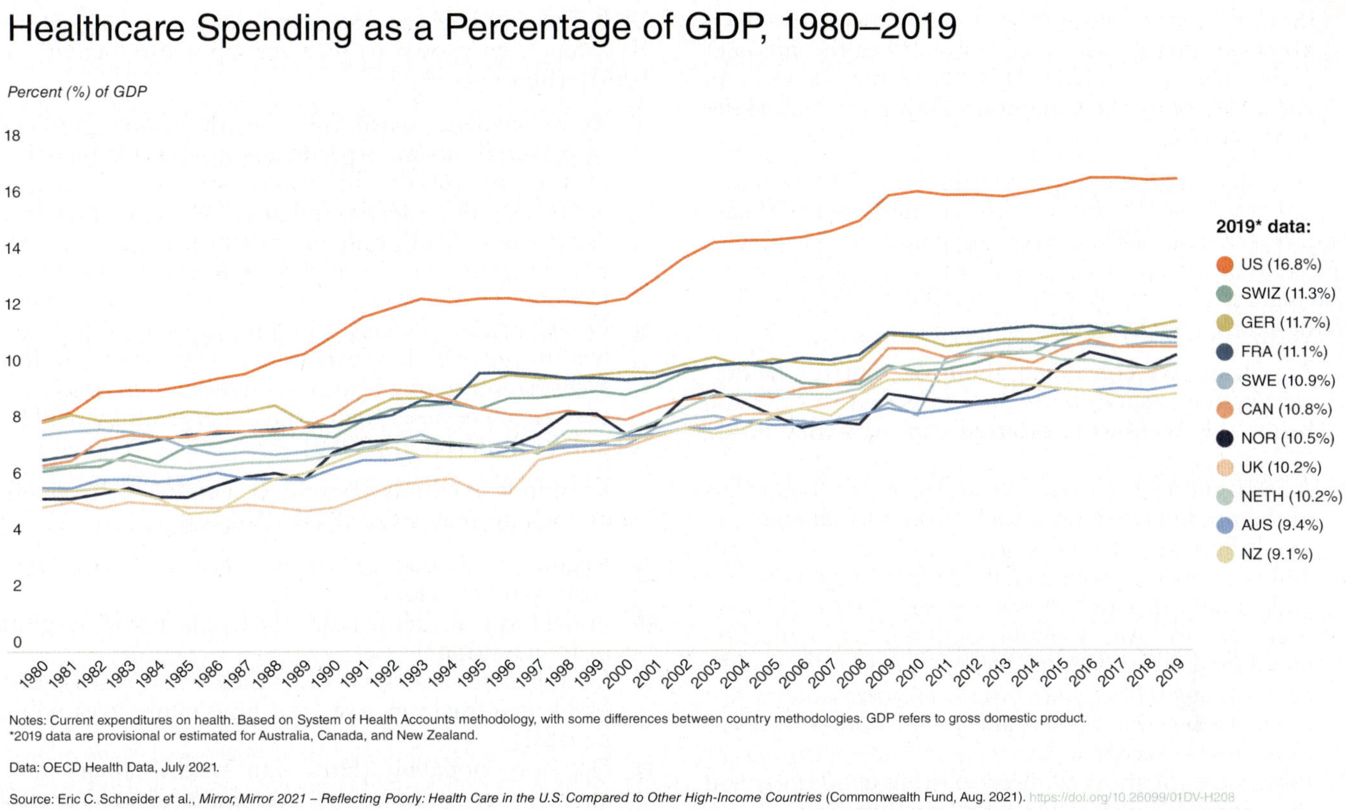

FIGURE 6-6 Healthcare spending as a percentage of gross domestic product, 1980–2019. (Reprinted with permission from The Commonwealth Fund (August 2021). Retrieved from Eric C. Schneider et al., 2021. *Mirror, Mirror 2021 — Reflecting Poorly: Health Care in the U.S. Compared to Other High-Income Countries*. https://doi.org/10.26099/01DV-H208)

BOX 6-2 Comparison of Health Systems in the United Kingdom, Australia, and The Netherlands

United Kingdom

National Health Service (NHS) began in 1948. Largely organized and care delivered by the national government, it is supported by taxes. Public hospitals and government staff employees are part of the NHS, but most primary care practices are independent and privately owned. Healthcare in the United Kingdom is more centrally managed, making accountability more governmentally driven than in the United States. About 10% of people purchase voluntary private health insurance, which excludes mental health, emergency care, and maternity care but does provide convenient and prompt access to care (Commonwealth Fund, n.d.; Schneider et al., 2021).

Australia

Medicare is the public insurance covering every citizen in Australia. It is paid for by taxes, and care is often available at private hospitals. About 50% of Australians also purchase private health insurance for access to care outside the Medicare system, but coverage is weighted higher among those with higher incomes. Coverage includes dental and vision care, along with other services. This system is similar to the U.S. Medicare system (Commonwealth Fund, n.d.; Schneider et al., 2021).

The Netherlands

Private health insurers cover the Dutch population. Funding is from payroll taxes and community-rated insurance premiums similar to the ACA insurance marketplaces. A standard benefit policy is available to everyone, with subsidies for low-income citizens, and those not enrolling in the plans being fined. The yearly deduction is around $500, and patients share some costs related to ambulance service and medical devices, for instance. Private providers are most common, and about 84% of people purchase additional voluntary insurance to cover dental, vision, and prescription drug copayments (Commonwealth Fund, n.d.; Schneider et al., 2021).

More comparisons of healthcare systems and statistics are available at https://international.commonwealthfund.org/countries/united_states/.

Source: Commonwealth Fund (n.d.); Schneider et al. (2021).

on healthcare spending (% of GDP) and last in overall performance, access, equity, and health outcomes (Schneider et al., 2021). This was also the case in an earlier study by the Commonwealth Fund (Schneider et al., 2017).

Out of 11 high-income countries in the OECD analysis, only the United States is without universal healthcare (Schneider et al., 2021). Even after increased access to care with the ACA, we remained last in access and equity. The highest-ranking countries overall were Norway, The Netherlands, and Australia.

- Americans are concerned about our current healthcare system, especially related to access to care and being able to afford preferred care (Crowley et al., 2020).
- A 2020 survey found that most Americans, regardless of their political views, want "substantial changes" to our healthcare system; goals include greater affordability, as well as coverage for preexisting conditions and long-term care (Public Agenda, 2020, para 4). Medicare for All, a public option plan, a market-based method, and a plan to give states wider healthcare responsibilities were offered as potential options; the market-based method and public option were the most widely accepted.
- Protection for those with preexisting conditions had the strongest support among all participants.

Dissatisfaction with the U.S. healthcare system has resulted in various proposals for national health plans (e.g., universal coverage, Medicare for All) and closer examination of issues such as competition, managed care, and healthcare rationing (Crowley et al., 2020). To gain a deeper understanding, an examination of some basic economic concepts can provide a broader perspective on healthcare financing and issues with healthcare access and coverage.

THE ECONOMICS OF HEALTHCARE

Economics is defined as the science of making decisions regarding scarce resources. It is concerned with the "production, distribution, and consumption of services" (Rambur, 2022, p. 8).

- Health economics is a specialized field of economics that examines problems faced in promoting health (Johns Hopkins, n.d.). It applies economic theories to try to understand how different health policies impact people's health and the behavior of healthcare consumers and providers (Henderson, 2022).
- The goal of healthcare economics, much like that of public health, is to overcome scarcity by making good choices while providing essential services.

Economics permeates our social structure—it affects and is affected by policies. Consequently, health is closely tied to economic growth and development, in that a healthy population is necessary for adequate national productivity. A nation with a healthy population has better worker productivity; longer life expectancies provide an incentive for investment in education and innovation. These factors encourage income growth and higher GDP. For instance, an increased adult survival rate of 10% has been shown to increase labor productivity by 10.6% (Bloom et al., 2022).

- Ample evidence exists for a health–income gradient, as personal income (specifically poverty) is linked to health status; studies have shown that social determinants of health affect as much as 50% of county-level variation in health outcomes (Whitman et al., 2022). For more on the social determinants of health, see Chapter 23.
- Public health policies and programs that promote health and wellness can impact economic development by improving health outcomes, often on a more cost-effective basis than other interventions (APHA, n.d.-b; Bloom et al., 2022).

Economic methods commonly employed by public health include analysis of (CDC, 2023c):

- Regulatory impact (How will this new law effect costs and behaviors?)
- Budget impact (How cost-effective is a new program or intervention?)
- Cost–benefit analysis (How much will a disease outbreak investigation cost, and how many lives will it benefit?)
- Decision modeling (How can mathematical models help determine cost-effectiveness of vaccine programs, pandemic spread, and disease management?)

Health economics can be better understood by examining the two basic theories underlying the science of economics: microeconomics and macroeconomics. In addition, concepts of healthcare payment must be understood.

Microeconomics

Microeconomic theory is concerned with supply and demand (Kramer, 2019).

- Supply is the quantity of goods or services that providers are willing to sell at a particular price.
- Demand denotes the consumer's willingness to purchase goods or services at a specified price.

In our free-market–driven economy, **supply and demand** is a key concept (Kramer, 2019). Economists use microeconomic theory to study the supply of goods and services: how we, as consumers, allocate and distribute our resources, and how those marketing goods and services compete. They also examine how allocation and distribution affect consumer demand for these goods and services.

- The concepts of supply and demand are influenced by each other and, in turn, affect prices.
- In a simplified example, an increase in, or oversupply of, certain products usually leads to less overall consumption (decreased demand) and lowered prices (Fig. 6-7). The opposite also is true. Limited availability of desired products means that supply does not meet demand, and when something needed is in short supply, prices usually increase.

As an example, let's look at the price of a gallon of gasoline. When demand for oil is high and supply begins

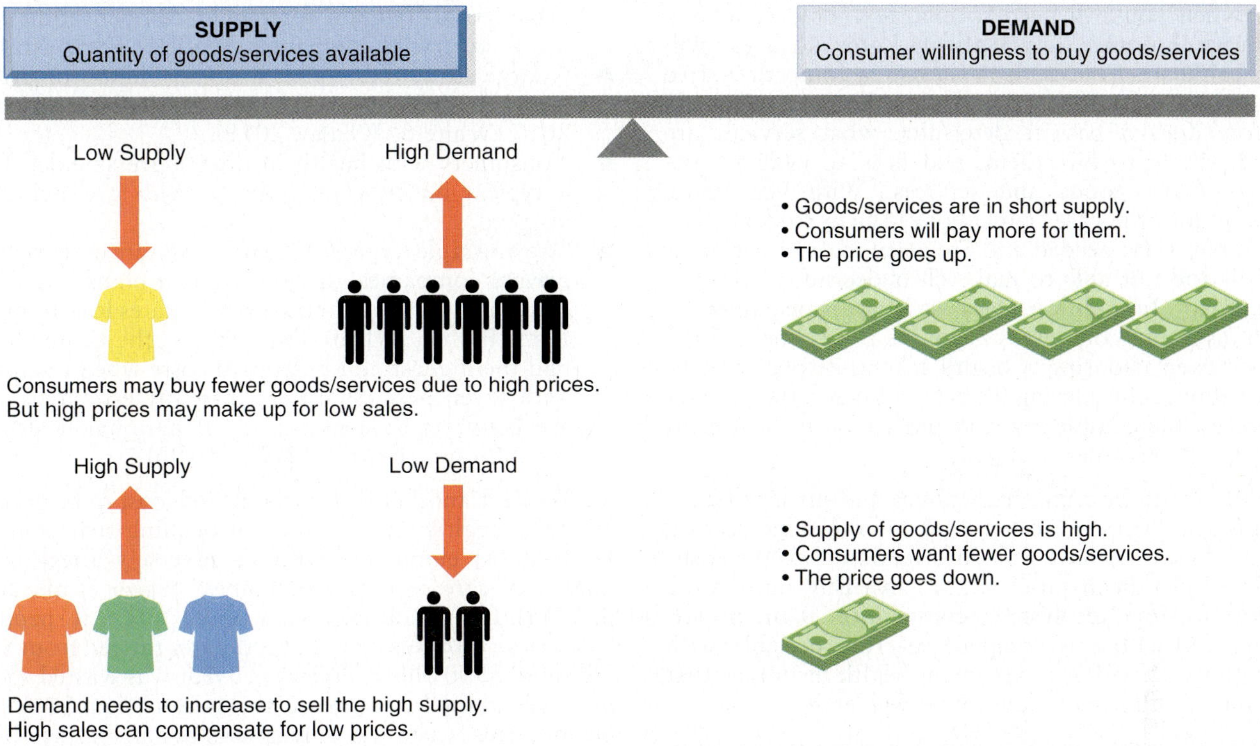

FIGURE 6-7 Supply and demand explained.

to dwindle, the prices go up. When demand drops and supplies become more plentiful, prices go down to attract more purchasers. This occurs as long as there are no monopolies to artificially control prices or only a few choices for goods and services that inhibit competition. Because most people need gasoline for their cars, they are more likely to continue to buy it even when the price is high. The same is true for healthcare.

- In healthcare economics, *demand-side policies* are enacted to increase or decrease the demand for healthcare (e.g., changing insurance deductibles and copayments to reduce or increase the cost of seeking care) (Parmar & Banerjee, 2019).
- *Supply-side policies* improve or restrict the supply of healthcare resources (e.g., increasing or decreasing the number of preferred providers for an insurance plan, denial of coverage for specific services).

Under the ACA, some traditional demand-side policies were removed to improve access to care. For example, preventive services must now be offered without deductibles or copayments, and insurance companies are limited in their ability to deny coverage for preexisting conditions (Healthcare.gov, 2019).

Issues such as cost containment, competition between providers, accessibility of services, quality, and need for accountability continue as areas of major concern. Several ACA provisions address these issues as well (Healthcare.gov, 2019):

- The law established the Centers for Medicare & Medicaid Innovation, which tests ways to improve quality and efficiency of care.
- Payments to hospitals and primary providers increase or decrease based on the quality of care provided, and all hospitals must publicly report several indicators of quality.

Evaluation of how these provisions affect the supply and demand for health services is ongoing. Search for projects in your state at their website https://innovation.cms.gov.

Macroeconomics

Macroeconomic theory is concerned with the broad variables that affect the status of the economy as a whole, such as production, consumption, investment, international trade, inflation, and recession or growth (Rodrigo, n.d.). The focus is on the big picture, the subject is usually an entire nation or region, or even the world.

The economics of healthcare encompasses both microeconomics and macroeconomics and an intricate and complex set of interacting variables. Healthcare economics is concerned with supply and demand, as well as the big picture: Are available resources sufficient to meet the demand by consumers and are the resources expended achieving the desired outcomes?

Supply and Demand in Healthcare Economics

We have all learned first-hand about supply-and-demand economics. For instance, when you buy textbooks, you—as the purchaser—are able to determine the best value for your money (generally based on price, availability, and condition of the book) and you have choices of vendors (e.g., college bookstore, online bookseller, other students) and formats (e.g., print book, e-book). As a student, you know when you will need specific textbooks, but as a healthcare consumer, do you always know when you will need healthcare services? Is healthcare a competitive free market?

How does a patient determine what services are needed, where to buy them, and how to evaluate the quality of the goods and services? With healthcare, this is seldom the case; patients need help to determine what services are needed and are often making decisions while ill and not able to make clear decisions (McPake et al., 2020). In addition, the cost is not transparent, as health insurance companies negotiate prices "behind the scenes." Even choosing a health insurance plan can be overwhelming considering the types of plans, the number of choices, the complexity, and one's level of health literacy (Colon-Morales et al., 2021).

- With health insurance companies and managed care, different prices are often paid for the same service, and consumers have little information as to the costs. Hence, healthcare purchases are not easily understood.
- In a free-market system, competition is an important factor, but is competition truly possible with employer-based or government health insurance that limits the choice of plans and providers?

In 1963, economist Kenneth Arrow wrote an influential article about healthcare economics detailing the lack of information in the medical marketplace (Arrow, 2004). The main points of the article still apply; Arrow noted that risk and uncertainty prohibit a true market economy in healthcare because consumers:

- Do not know when or if they will become ill, but they know they will need and want medical treatment when illness occurs—thus the demand for health insurance.
- Do not know what services will be needed and what works best for their condition—thus the need for healthcare providers.
- Do not know about the quality of healthcare good and services—thus the need for government regulation (e.g., licensing, certification) and malpractice lawsuits.
- Are subject to an asymmetric level of information, compared to the insurer, about the likely demand for healthcare services. This can result in **adverse selection** (e.g., high-risk patients are denied insurance or care, people who smoke have higher health insurance premiums) and market failure (e.g., inefficiencies, lack of appropriate competition)—although this is less severe in large group insurance plans that spread out the risk (Saltzman, 2021).

Healthcare is an "opaque market" that keeps consumers in the dark about actual costs of services and medications due to confidential negotiations, discounts, and rebates (Rao et al., 2022). For example, if you need an oil change for your car, the price is often clearly posted or advertised in advance, but are you aware of how much a chest x-ray or a vaccination will cost before you get one?

- Market consolidation (e.g., hospitals that monopolize a geographic area, buy up competitors) allows providers to bargain for higher compensation from health insurance companies (Wolfe & Pope, 2020).
- A large study found that hospital billing for private insurance patients was 241% of Medicare prices in 2017 (White & Whaley, 2019).
- Consumers with health insurance are shielded from a typical business relationship with a provider or hospital.
- The multiple types of health insurance (variety of private companies and government plans like Medicare and Medicaid) in the United States lead to higher costs (Hoffer, 2019b). For instance, the United States had the highest administrative costs when compared with seven peer countries; currently estimated costs are between 12% and 25% of national healthcare expenditures (Hoffer, 2019a, 2019b).

Waste is another factor in our high cost of healthcare. Wasteful healthcare spending is spending that could be "reduced or eliminated without adversely affecting the quality of care or health outcomes" (Speer et al., 2020, p. 1744). In a literature review about wasteful spending, Speer et al. (2020) found that estimates ranged from $600 billion to $900 billion dollars per year was wasted spending. Even at the low estimate, this is more than $1800 per person. This waste not only affects our healthcare but it also affects opportunities lost in other national priority areas.

As far as supply and demand are concerned, Zhang et al. (2020) noted that these factors are at play:

- Higher demand due to an aging population. The number of people over 65 years is roughly 52 million and is projected to almost double by 2060 (Mather et al., 2019). Older people are more likely to have chronic conditions requiring care: 94.9% have at least one chronic condition, and 78.7% have two or more (National Council on Aging, 2023a, 2023b).
- More people now have health insurance thanks to the ACA, estimated at about 35 million (USDHHS, 2022), and they have added to the demand.
- There is a projected primary provider shortage (estimated from 37,800 to 124,000 [Association of American Medical Colleges, 2021]), just as demand for healthcare services increases. Supply could be increased by hiring more nurse practitioners and increasing the number of medical residency slots available.
- Fully utilizing telemedicine would help extend care, especially into rural areas experiencing provider shortages, increasing supply in these areas (Mather et al., 2019).

Because traditional market forces of supply and demand work differently in healthcare, consumers are not solely responsible for prices, because government plays a substantial policy role in the provision of healthcare while insurance companies (and employers) control access to healthcare (Crowley et al., 2020). Some governments and employers have taken action to control costs. Examples of this are as follows:

1. Laws for price transparency in several states as well as a national requirement for providers to post list prices online (Zhang et al., 2020).

2. Medicare has changed from a fee-for-service model to one that holds providers accountable for high-quality, efficient care (Cheng et al., 2020).

Consumers seek value and convenience in healthcare. An example of this is the case of urgent care centers and retail clinics (Voran, 2023). Urgent care centers are more prevalent, although both services are numerous. There are more than 10,000 urgent care centers in the United States (Globalnewswire, 2020); most are located in urban areas (Voran, 2023). They earn more than $20 billion annually (Globalnewswire, 2020). Urgent care centers are generally staffed by primary providers with support from nurse practitioners and primary provider assistants, and offer a range of services for acute illness and injury care—things beyond what can be taken care of in a primary care office but also don't require the services of an ED.

As of March 2023, there were 1801 retail clinics located in 44 states (Definitive Healthcare, 2023a). Younger people, generally in good health, are most often using them, especially those without insurance, due to transparent costs and less expensive visits, as well as the ability to walk in without an appointment (Voran, 2023). The most common reasons for visits are immunizations and minor problems such as sinusitis; these make up 90% of visits.

Spurred by the COVID-19 pandemic, retail clinics grew 21.5% in 2020 and earned $3.4 billion in 2021, with a projected market of $4.22 billion by 2029 (Definitive Healthcare, 2023a). One study in New Jersey (Alexander et al., 2019) found that, if people lived close to an open retail clinic, ED use fell by "3.3% to 13.4% for preventable conditions and 5.7% to 12.0% for minor acute conditions" (para 1). This could lead to $70 million in annual savings from reduced ED use if such clinics were available across the state. There is also evidence, however, that inappropriate use of retail clinics, when an urgent care or ED is the better location for care, may negate these potential savings (Voran, 2023). There are, however, rare areas of healthcare where supply and demand works without any interference. These healthcare services are generally paid out-of-pocket, with direct interaction between the patient/consumer and the provider, as insurance does not cover them. Cosmetic procedures are a good example.

Elective cosmetic procedures are an area where prices are more transparent because costs are paid by the consumer and not usually by insurers. Therefore, consumers are cost conscious and providers operate in a competitive marketplace with more transparent pricing.

- Between 1998 and 2021, the average cost of 19 common cosmetic procedures and surgeries rose 31.3%, much less than the over 132% to 230% increases in medical and hospital services (Perry, 2022).
- The cost of three of the most popular nonsurgical cosmetic procedures Botox injections, laser skin resurfacing, and chemical peels actually dropped by 42.1%, 68.4%, and 54.8%, respectively.
- While elective procedures (e.g., cosmetic or LASIK surgery) demonstrate market influences, they are not typical of most healthcare expenditures. They also represent a select portion of the population—people who can afford them.

Health Insurance Concepts

Conventional economic theories hold that people will pay small premiums monthly to offset the risk of large medical bills should they become seriously ill (Roughley, 2023). This represents an *indemnity policy* (security against loss, much like car or homeowners' insurance), and this was the type of health insurance first offered in the United States.

- **Risk averse** is a label often applied to people to explain why they purchase life insurance; people do not like uncertainty and will pay monthly premiums to replace an uncertainty (how much money they may have saved when their life ends) with a certainty (the value of the life insurance policy) (Fels, 2019).
  - **Moral hazard**, on the other hand, is the term used by economists to explain how health insurance changes the behavior of people, resulting in more risk-taking and wasteful actions (Nickitas et al., 2020).
  - Economists liken it to fire insurance without a deductible, noting that a person may be less careful about clearing brush from a house or may even resort to arson if it costs the owner nothing to have the home replaced.
  - If a person has health insurance, many economists hypothesize, they are less likely to take good care of themselves, and if they do not pay for their healthcare (through premiums, copayments, and deductibles), they are more likely to overuse it, although empirical evidence of this is sparse.
  - In other words, economists theorize that insurance has a paradoxical effect and may lead to wasteful or risk-taking behaviors. In this scenario, patients will demand expensive healthcare, even if it provides only the smallest benefit. The concept of moral hazard is a driver for larger deductibles and copayments; these are used to control waste and overuse.

A more recent viewpoint notes that consumers purchase health insurance not to avoid risk but to earn a claim for additional income (i.e., insurance paying for medical care) when they become ill and that copayments and managed care actually work against the system by reducing the amount of income transferred to ill persons or limiting their access to needed services. Think about what would happen if you or your loved one were to suddenly need an expensive heart surgery or lengthy cancer treatment—without health insurance. You would want health insurance to protect against this possibility—to be able to pay medical bills without losing your assets (e.g., home, car).

- For instance, Rose-Jacobs et al. (2019) found that families of children with special healthcare needs who were without government-sponsored insurance had significantly greater odds of missing rent or mortgage payments, moving frequently, and homelessness than did similar families who had this insurance.
- Families may face a genuine risk of financial disaster when confronted with a serious medical emergency or long-term illness.

- Moral hazard alone doesn't easily apply to health insurance because its effects may not be as predictable as in other instances of indemnity. In healthcare, the cost of medical treatment can be quite large, and people may not be able to purchase it even if they consider it worth the cost (Fels, 2019).
- Health insurance overcomes this price barrier; by paying premiums on a monthly basis, the consumer has the ability to get medical treatment that would otherwise be unaffordable.
- People who gain access to health insurance will use it, but there are still constraints (e.g., high deductibles, high copays) that moderate use and can be harmful to families who may have to choose between buying medications and paying for food (Chandra et al., 2021).
- The case can also be made that even those with unlimited insurance coverage don't just "check into the hospital because it's free" as noted in a classic article by Gladwell (2005, para 11). For example, most people do not seek infinite numbers of colonoscopies, root canals, or other invasive procedures or surgeries just because they are well insured.
- Adverse selection, however, is a concern for health insurance companies when sick people seek insurance because they have an urgent need for healthcare, while healthy people do not want to buy it because they have no pressing health concerns (Saltzman, 2019).
- This imbalance is not cost-effective, yet a key feature of the ACA is for insurers to provide coverage for people with preexisting conditions (without charging them outrageous prices), which was formerly a common practice. This was initially balanced out by providing subsidies and requiring that everyone get insurance or face a penalty (Center on Budget & Policy Priorities, 2020; Saltzman, 2019).

Cost sharing, which includes copayments and deductibles, divides the cost of healthcare services between insurance companies and patients. Insurance companies use cost sharing to prevent overuse of health services. The amount of a copayment or deductible may change for some types of care, such as a visit to the ED.

- In a summary of "methodologically sophisticated studies," Mazurenko et al. (2019, p. 411) found that newer high-deductible health plans (HDHPs) did reduce costs, but they also led to a reduction in preventive care, particularly screening.
- A study examining uptake of the low-dose CT lung cancer screening for high-risk people who smoke found that people with insurance were more likely to participate in this screening (Kee et al., 2021). Generally, the earlier a health problem is found, the less expensive the treatment and the better the patient outcomes.
- A study examining control of hypertension found that the number of patients whose BP was under control was higher among those with private insurance (48.2%), Medicare (53.4%), or other government health insurance (43.2%) compared to patients without health insurance (24.2%) (Muntner et al., 2020).

Balancing the cost reduction against the lack of preventive care (that could eventually lead to more cost savings) is an important consideration. Also, the effect of cost sharing on use of services is not equal. People with low incomes decrease their use of medications and services more than those with higher incomes. The ACA limited cost sharing for people with low or moderate incomes, in plans offered by employers and plans purchased through the marketplace (Healthcare.gov, 2019).

For some people, the cost-sharing component of their health insurance is so high that they are considered **underinsured**. To be underinsured, one must have a deductible that is 5% of income or out-of-pocket costs in excess of 10% of income (not including premium costs). People and families often exhaust their savings, run up credit card debt, or else delay necessary medical care to avoid going into debt (KFF, 2022b). The numbers are rising:

- In 2018, 29% of American adults who reported having health insurance for the entire year were considered underinsured, compared to 23% in 2014 (Commonwealth Fund, 2019).
    - Of that group, 28% had employer-sponsored health insurance, up from 20% in 2014. But, people with individually purchased insurance were most likely to be inadequately covered (42%).
    - Delayed care (41%) and problems paying medical bills (47%) were more common among underinsured than the fully insured population (23%, 25%).
    - With the ending of the declared public health emergency in May of 2023, there could be new cost-sharing arrangements for receiving COVID-19 vaccines or getting tested (KFF, 2023c). People who are underinsured and uninsured "face the greatest risk of access challenges, including limited access to free vaccines and no coverage for treatment or tests" (para 19). This could lead to higher rates of COVID-19 in the United States in the future.
    - Yabroff et al. (2019) found that 46.9% of people 18-64 years old (as compared to those 65 or older) reported experiencing psychological effects of medical debt (i.e., distress). This was higher for the uninsured (71.4%), compared to those with private (43.4%) and public (42.6%) insurance.

Employer-Sponsored Health Insurance

Employer-sponsored health insurance is the leading source of coverage for nonelderly citizens in the United States. A total of 49% of Americans, almost 159 million workers, had this type of insurance in 2017 (KFF, 2019b, 2022a). Medicare, Medicaid, and other government plans provided coverage to 36%, while 7% purchased policies directly from insurers.

The flaws in this system were blatantly exposed during the COVID-19 pandemic, as millions of Americans filed for unemployment when businesses shut down, causing them to lose access to healthcare (Brown & Nanni, 2020). One example of the trickle-down effects of unemployment is the loss of reproductive healthcare for millions of women (Sonfield et al., 2020). About 56% of total jobs lost early on during the pandemic were among women, often those working in retail, education, and restaurant jobs. Black, Latina, and women with disabilities had the highest rates of unemployment. It is estimated that 40% of people losing employer-sponsored health insurance will continue to be uninsured; states without Medicaid expansion will be even harder hit. Loss of access to contraceptive and preventive healthcare for people assigned female at birth will place greater demands on publicly funded clinics that are continually underfunded and result in unplanned pregnancies or late diagnoses of cervical cancers and other health conditions.

How did the United States end up with this system of health insurance? Historically, employers became the leading source of coverage because of three policy decisions in the 1940s and 1950s (Rook, 2020).

1. During World War II, wage controls did not apply to health insurance, so employers used health insurance to lure workers from their competitors during wage freezes.
2. The U.S. government determined that health insurance could be part of collective bargaining with the Taft–Hartley Act in 1947.
3. In 1954, the internal revenue service exempted health insurance premiums paid by employers from federal income tax.

In 2022, 51% of employers offered at least some health benefits, a decrease from the prior year (59%), but similar to the percentage in 2017 (53%) (KFF, 2022a). Small businesses may not offer employee health insurance, however, because of the high cost and fewer employees (Fig. 6-8).

- The average annual costs for employees in 2019 were $7188 for a person and $20,576 for family health insurance coverage. This represents 4% and 5% increases, respectively, over 2018; however, family premiums are 22% higher than 5 years ago and 54% higher than 10 years ago. Wages increased only 1.4% above inflation from 2018 to 2019 (KFF, 2019b). Figure 6-9 shows the increases in annual costs over time.
- Keep in mind that the median U.S. income in 2019 was just over $63,179; the employee cost for a family policy would represent almost one third of that year's wages (Rothbaum & Edwards, 2019).

Employers are continuing to pass along some of the higher costs of health insurance to employees in the form of higher employee premiums, deductibles, copayments, and stricter enrollment requirements.

- The number of workers with insurance that includes an annual deductible has increased from 55% in 2006 to 88% in 2022 (KFF, 2022a).
- The percentage of covered workers enrolled in employer health plans with a deductible of $2000 or more for single coverage increased from 22% in 2017 to 32% in 2022 (KFF, 2022a).

Those people whose employers do not offer health insurance coverage or who are self-employed can purchase nongroup health insurance. However, premiums

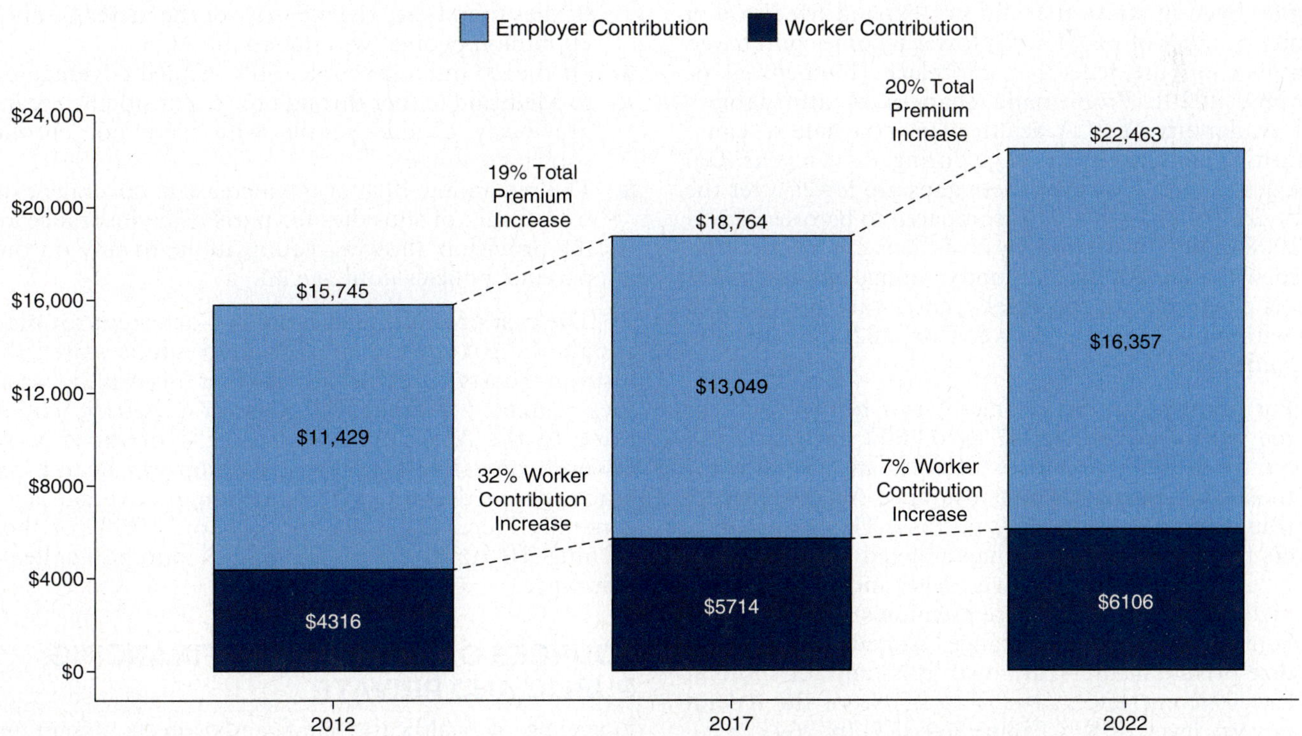

FIGURE 6-8 Average annual worker and employer contributions to premiums and total premiums for single and family coverage, by firm wage level, 2022. *Estimate is statistically different between All Small Firms and All Large Firms estimate ($p < .05$). (Reprinted with permission from Kaiser Family Foundation. (2022). *Employer health benefits 2022 annual survey*. https://www.kff.org/report-section/ehbs-2022-summary-of-findings/)

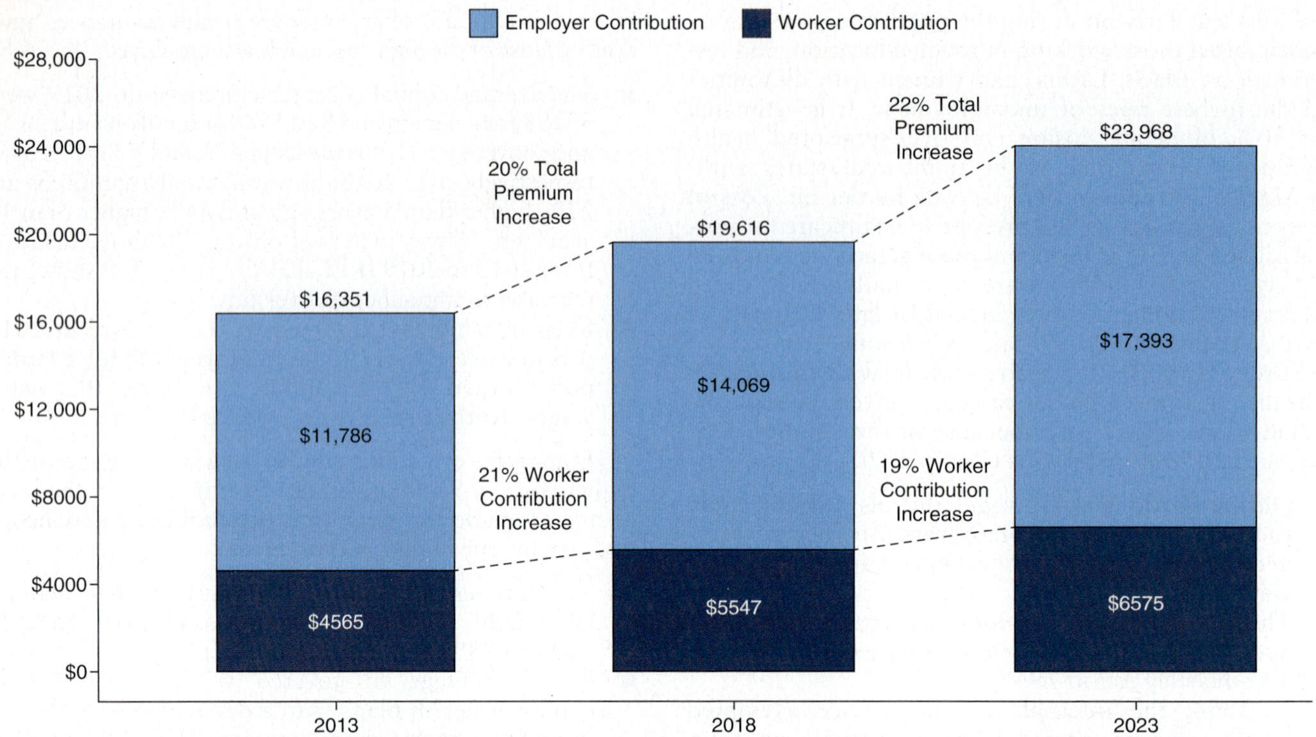

FIGURE 6-9 Average annual worker and employee premium contribution for family coverage, 2013, 2018, 2023. (Reprinted with permission from Kaiser Family Foundation. (2023). *2023 Employer health benefits survey.* https://www.kff.org/report-section/ehbs-2023-summary-of-findings/)

are greater than the worker's share of employer group coverage. The ACA has made purchasing a nongroup policy easier and subsidizes the premiums for eligible people. Even in states that did not expand Medicaid, a greater number of people with lower incomes purchased insurance on the federal marketplace (Blumenthal & Abrams, 2020). Problematic changes in affordability and availability of ACA health plans continue to cause "churning" or gaps in coverage during a given year (Gai & Jones, 2020). However, these gaps are fewer after the ACA (25.7% in 2015–2016) compared to before (34.6% in 2008–2009). Variation in costs has not been eliminated with the ACA's community rating, but the variation is geographical; specifically, costs vary by location, not within one location (Fehr & Cox, 2020; Healthcare.gov, n.d.-a).

- For persons earning incomes "at or below 400% of the federal poverty level" ($103,000 per year for a family of four), premium subsidies are provided for those purchasing on the insurance "marketplaces" (Blumenthal et al., 2020, p. 964). This keeps buyers from spending more than a "fixed percentage" of income (2.06% at the lowest level and 9.78% at the highest level) on healthcare premiums (p. 964).
- Some "cost-sharing assistance" is available to subsidize private insurers, although it is only for those at lower-income levels (100% to 250% of the federal poverty level, or $25,750 to $64,375) (p. 964).
- It is expected that about 94% of potential costs for a "moderately generous" plan will be covered for those receiving this benefit (Blumenthal et al., 2020, p. 964).
- Before the ACA became law in 2010, 16.3% of people in the United States were uninsured (Sommers, 2020). In 2016, the rate had fallen to 8.8%, representing 28.1 million more people insured. Some of this was due to an improving economy, but several research studies found that the majority of the increase (about 20 million people) was due to the ACA.
- Of the 20 million people, 60% gained coverage due to Medicaid (either through the expansion or because previously eligible people who were not enrolled sought coverage).
- The remaining 40% of the increase in coverage came from a mix of subsidies for purchasing insurance and the provision allowing young adults to stay on their parents' policies until age 26.

The cost of health insurance is a deterrent for many people. In 2018, 45% of uninsured adults stated that insurance costs were too high and that this was the reason they remained without it (Tolbert et al., 2019, para 4). Prior to the ACA, only 4% to 11% of those at the lower-income levels purchased nongroup health coverage (Bernard et al., 2009). Although coverage levels generally increase as income rises, only 25% of those earning 10 times the poverty level purchased health insurance.

SOURCES OF HEALTHCARE FINANCING: PUBLIC AND PRIVATE

Financing of healthcare significantly affects community/public health nursing practice. It influences the type and quality of services offered, as well as the ways in which those services are used. Sources of payment may be grouped into three categories: third-party payments, direct consumer payments, and private or philanthropic support.

Third-Party Payments

Third-party payments are monetary reimbursements made to providers of healthcare by someone other than the consumer who received the care. The organizations that administer these funds are called third-party payers because they are a third party, or external, to the consumer–provider relationship. Included in this category are four types of payment sources: private insurance companies, independent or self-insured health plans, government health programs, and claims payment agents (California Department of Insurance, n.d.).

Private Insurance Companies

Payments from private insurance companies make up approximately 34% of total healthcare spending (CMS, n.d.-b). They market and underwrite policies aimed at decreasing consumer risk of economic loss because of a need to use health services.

- There are three types of private insurers—commercial stock companies that maintain profit margins for stockholders (e.g., Anthem, Cigna), mutual companies owned by policyholders (e.g., MassMutual), and nonprofit plans (e.g., American Postal Workers Union) that must be approved by states (Firstquotehealth, n.d.).
- Today, about one third of Americans are covered by a health plan offered by the Blues (Blue Cross Blue Shield, n.d.). Parts of Blue Cross are nonprofit; others are for-profit (Firstquotehealth, n.d.).

The medical loss ratio is the amount spent on healthcare services and quality improvement initiatives compared to the amount spent on marketing, administrative costs, and profits (Hall & McCue, 2019; Healthcare.gov, n.d.). The ACA has an 80/20 rule requiring that at least 80% of every premium dollar must be spent on patient care, leaving 20% to pay for these other costs of business.

- Previously, insurers also resorted to *rescission of coverage*—or canceling coverage for failure to disclose a preexisting condition (often unrelated to the person's current healthcare problem) or some other means of disqualifying coverage after large medical claims have been filed (Healthcare.gov, n.d.-c). However, the ACA made this practice illegal, except in cases of consumer misrepresentation or fraud.
- A more recent trend in private insurance is the move to high-deductible health plans with a savings option (HDHP/SOs) such as **health savings accounts (HSAs)**—created and paid for by employees, or **health reimbursement accounts (HRAs)**—established and funded by employers (U.S. Office of Personal Management [USOPM], n.d.-b). The money put into these accounts is not taxed. About 28% of employers offered this type of plan in 2022 (KFF, 2022a).
- Six times more common than HRAs, HSAs tied to HDHPs can be rolled over yearly and move with the employee. The high deductibles in HDHPs (minimum of $1400 for a person and $2800 for a family) allow for lower premiums, but the attendant HSAs can only be used on medical expenses—nothing else—or tax-exempt status may be forfeited, and a penalty is incurred (KFF, 2019c; National Conference of State Legislation [NCSL], 2020).
- HRA funds are controlled by the employer, and as the employee turns in medical bills, funds are released for payment. Generally, remaining HRA funds carry over to the following year but do not go with the employee when they leave the company (KFF, 2019c).
- Most plans require employees to pay coinsurance, a percentage of their total health costs (often 20% of charges) rather than a fixed copayment per office visit or prescription as in many other plans.
- Most workers with employer-sponsored health insurance also have prescription drug coverage (98%) with the most comprehensive health plan offered, and 84% of those covered have a plan with three or more tiers of cost sharing, such as copayment or coinsurance (KFF, 2022a).
  - For instance, the average prescription copayment for tier one medications is $11, for second-tier medications is $37, for third-tier medications is $67, and for fourth-tier medications (specialty drugs such as biologics) is $116.
  - Only about 9% of large employers and 2% of small employers offer no cost sharing after deductibles are met.

While these copayments are used by insurance companies to reduce their costs, they can affect medication adherence. A systematic review of the literature concluded that lower (or no) copayments for medications improved adherence and patient outcomes (Gast & Mathes, 2019). Prescription coverage and lower medication cost sharing were associated with decreased use of healthcare services, including ED visits, outpatient visits, and hospital stays (Guindon et al., 2022).

Independent or Self-Insured Health Plans

Independent or self-insured health plans underwrite the remaining private health insurance in the United States. These plans have been offered through a limited number of organizations, such as large businesses, unions, school districts, consumer cooperatives, and medical groups. Employers with self-insured plans take on all or a major part of the risk for healthcare costs of their employees. These plans may be self-administered or utilize third-party claims administrators. Minimum premium plans are another form of self-insurance for which employers pay medical costs up to an agreed-upon limit, and insurers assume responsibility for the excess claims (Bureau of Labor Statistics, 2022).

- About 61% of employees receiving employer health insurance benefits were covered in full or partly by self-insured plans in 2018 (remained the same in 2019), up from 51% in 1999 (KFF, 2022b). Employees of large firms are more likely to have self-funded plans than small firms (81% vs. 13%).
- In 2022, only 21% of large firms offering employee health benefits extend that benefit to retirees, a decrease from 27% in 2021 (KFF, 2022b). In prior studies, benefits were extended to retires by 66% of employers in 1988 and 34% in 2006. There was an increase in employers extending benefits to retirees in 2019 because KFF changed how the question was asked.

Government Health Programs

The federal government is the largest payer of healthcare in the United States (CMS, 2023e). The U.S. government's four major health insurance programs are Medicare, Medicaid, the Federal Employees Health Benefits Plan, and the Civilian Health and Medical Program of the Uniformed Services. The VA (Veterans Administration) system is also part of the federal government, as are a few other specialized programs such as the Indian Health Service. The largest programs are Medicare and Medicaid. Federal sources comprised 34% of total payments from all sources in 2021. Spending for Medicaid rose by 9.2%, and growth in Medicare was 8.3% from 2020 (CMS, 2023e).

Medicare. Medicare, known as Title XVIII of the Social Security Act Amendments of 1965, has provided mandatory federal health insurance since July 1, 1966, for adults aged 65 years and older who have paid into the Social Security system (CMS, 2023b). It also covers certain people with disabilities (regardless of age). Medicare is administered by the Centers for Medicare & Medicaid Services (CMS) of the USDHHS.

- In 2021, Medicare covered more than 63.9 million people and paid healthcare costs of $900.8 billion (CMS, 2023d, 2023e).
- In 2018, 21% of total federal spending was for Medicare ($750.2 billion), and it is expected to increase 7.6% per year between 2019 and 2028 (CMS, 2021c).
- Financing of Medicare is through general tax revenues (43%), payroll taxes (36%), premiums from beneficiaries (15%), and other sources (KFF, 2019a).
- Out-of-pocket spending for Medicare beneficiaries was $5460 in 2016, almost equally divided between medical/long-term care and premiums (Cubanski et al., 2023).
- People with multiple chronic diseases and poor health spent more than their healthier counterparts (Cubanski et al., 2019).

About 85% of beneficiaries, 55.9 million people (CMS, 2023d), were over the age of 65; the remaining beneficiaries qualified for Medicare 24 months after they became eligible for Social Security Disability Insurance (SSDI). These recipients are younger than age 65 and have a permanent disability or chronic illness, including those with end-stage renal disease.

In 2020, 55.7 million Americans were aged 65 years and older; by 2060, that number is expected to almost double, at 94.7 million (Administration for Community Living, 2022a, 2022b).

- There are financial challenges facing Medicare and Social Security. The trust fund for Medicare Part A will have sufficient resources to pay full costs and benefits, without any adjustments, only through 2028, thanks to a recent extension due to pandemic relief funds (Kumar & Schulman, 2022).
- The disability insurance trust fund will be intact through 2035 (Button et al., 2022).

The parts of Medicare are funded by different funding streams (Kumar & Schulman, 2022). Hospital insurance is funded through payroll taxes (i.e., the Medicare trust fund), and medical insurance is funded through premium payments, as is insurance for prescription drugs. Premiums for drug coverage only account for 15% of the cost of the drug benefit, however. Nearly 75% of the cost of medical and drug insurance comes from general tax revenues or deficit spending. As these are the fastest growing parts of Medicare, and they require "significant annual public support," the solvency of the Medicare trust fund is only part of the picture (p. 132). There are four parts to Medicare (Fig. 6-10):

Part A of Medicare, the hospital insurance program, covers inpatient hospitals, limited-skilled nursing facilities, home health, and hospice services to participants eligible for SSDI (Medicare.gov, n.d.-a).

- The 2020 deductible per benefit period for inpatient hospitalization, including inpatient mental health, is $1408.
- Patients in a skilled nursing facility pay $200 per day after day 20 and assume all costs if care is needed longer than 100 days (Medicare.gov, n.d.-d).

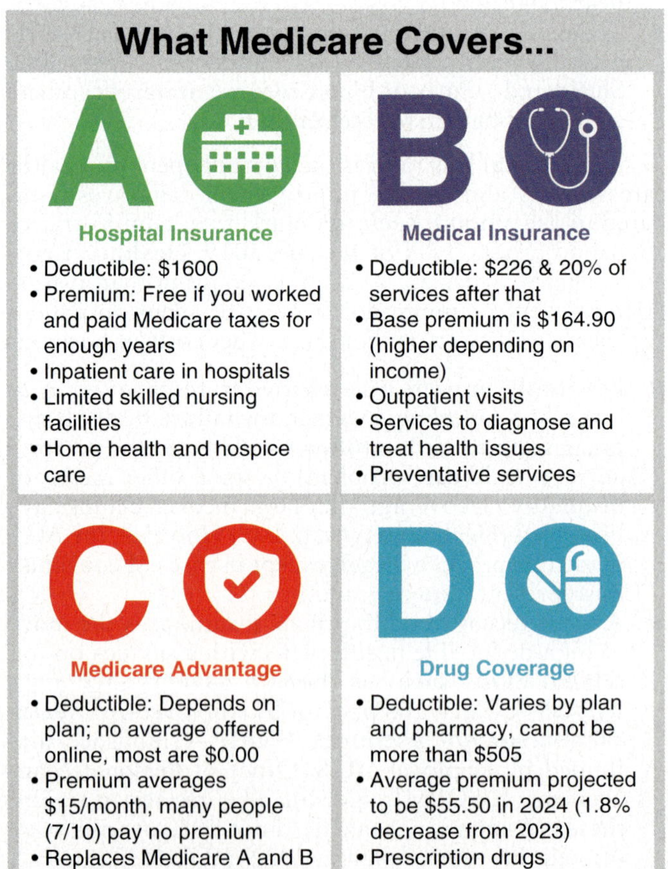

FIGURE 6-10 Medicare coverage: Parts A to D. (Figure concept by Claire Lindstrom; used with permission. Data from medicare.gov, 2023.)

- Information on hospice and home health can be found at https://www.medicare.gov/your-medicare-costs/medicare-costs-at-a-glance.

Part B of Medicare, the supplementary and voluntary medical insurance program, primarily covers necessary services to diagnosis or treat health issues and preventive services such as influenza vaccines (Medicare.gov, n.d.-a).

- The 2020 annual deductible is $197, and recipients pay 20% of services once the deductible is met. No out-of-pocket charges are applied for annual wellness visits or preventive services that are rated "A" or "B" by the U.S. Preventive Services Task Force.
- Monthly premiums vary depending on yearly income ranging from $164.90 to $560.50 (Medicare.gov, n.d.-e).

Part C Medicare plans, also called Medicare Advantage, are private plans subsidized by the federal government.

- Medicare Advantage plans are not supplemental to Part A and Part B—they take the place of Part A and Part B. Some may also cover vision, dental, and prescriptions (National Council on Aging [NCA], 2022a).
- Unlike traditional Medicare, Part C plans use provider networks, which limit the choice of primary providers or hospitals. They are regional, which may be problematic for older adults who want to spend winters in Florida and summers in Montana, for instance.

Older adults can change their Part C plan during open enrollment periods or revert to traditional Medicare Part A and Part B.

- In 2023, 30.8 million Medicare participants had Part C plans, which is 51% of the eligible Medicare population (KFF, 2023a).
- Other types of Medicare plans include Medicare Medical Savings Account plans, Medicare cost plans, Programs of All-Inclusive Care for the Elderly, and the Medication Therapy Management program; these are not available in all areas.

In 2023, 29.5 million Medicare beneficiaries had supplemental coverage through a private company or employer retiree health insurance plans—known as *Medigap* coverage—added to Medicare Part A and Part B (American Association for Medicare Supplement Insurance [AAMSI], 2020). Changes in Medigap coverage for new enrollees began at the start of 2020. Part B deductibles are no longer covered under Medigap, and Plans C and F are no longer allowed. However, these changes do not affect those enrolled prior to January 1, 2020 (Medicare.gov, n.d.-g).

- People with Medigap coverage through their employers' retiree health plan generally pay lower premiums than people with coverage through a private company (AAMSI, 2020).
- With rising costs of healthcare coverage, companies are increasing premium costs for retirees, offering new options, such as Medicare Advantage to replace traditional health plans, or paying only a set amount for health coverage and leaving retirees to purchase their own insurance.

Part D of Medicare is a volunteer prescription drug plan for those on Medicare or Medicare Advantage. The member can sign up for a Medicare Part D plan or an Advantage plan with medication coverage (KFF, 2019a; Medicare.gov, n.d.-f). Costs vary based on state of residence. Plans differ in coverage, so clients should be encouraged to research the plans to determine if their medications are included in the plan's formulary (see Box 6-3).

Supplemental Security Income and Social Security Disability Insurance. Supplemental Security Income (SSI) and SSDI are federally funded programs to assist older adults and those with disabilities who have financial needs. Older adults and people with disabilities, regardless of age, with limited incomes can receive SSI. SSDI, however, is only available for those with disabilities that "have a qualifying work history" (NCA, 2022b, para 3; SSA, 2023a, 2023b). Eligibility for healthcare benefits differs between the two programs as well (Fig. 6-11).

- Medicaid benefits are immediate for SSI recipients, whereas most people receiving SSDI can qualify for Medicare after 24 months (NCA, 2022b).
- To be eligible for SSI, a person's income must be less than $1260 a month (Social Security Administration, n.d.-b). In 2020, the highest amount individual SSI recipients receive is $783 a month.
- However, SSDI assistance is not based on income or severity of disability (Laurence, 2023). Rather, the monthly amount is based on the person's income prior to the disability. The average monthly income from SSDI is $800 to $1800 and a maximum monthly payment of $3011.

BOX 6-3 Deductibles and Copays

Deductible Phase

- While plans vary, most have an annual deductible that must be met before the prescription drug plan takes effect. Medicare caps the deductible at $435, and some plans do not have a deductible (Medicare.gov, n.d.-g; Social Security Administration [SSA], 2019).

Initial Coverage Phase

- When the deductible is met, members are responsible to pay a copayment (a set amount) or coinsurance (a percent of the price of the medication), with Medicare covering the rest of the cost (Medicare.gov, n.d.-h; SSA, 2023).
- The monthly premium depends on the type of plan chosen and the income of a person or family. People may pay nothing over their plan premium up to a monthly fee of $76.40 plus plan premium. Costs vary based on state of residence as well (Medicare.gov, n.d.-f).

Source: Medicare.gov (n.d.-c, n.d.-d, n.d.-e, n.d.-f, n.d.-g, n.d.-h); SSA (2023).

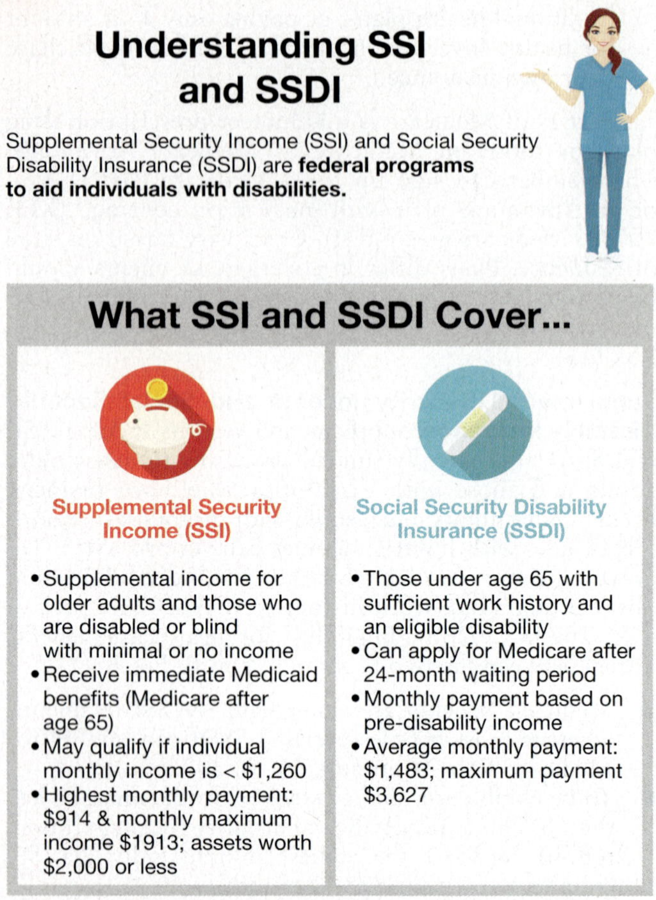

FIGURE 6-11 Supplemental Security Income and Social Security Disability Insurance coverage. (Figure concept by Claire Lindstrom; used with permission. Data from NCA (2023a, 2023b); Disability Secrets (n.d.). For additional information and updates, see https://www.ssa.gov/benefits/disability/)

Medicaid. Medicaid, known as Title XIX of the Social Security Amendments Act of 1965, provides medical assistance for children, pregnant people, parents with dependent children, older adults, and people with severe disabilities (Medicaid.gov, 2023).

- Medicaid is an optional program for states, but all states currently participate.
- Over time, the scope of Medicaid increased, and states opting to provide Medicaid were required to implement each increase—or lose their enhanced federal Medicaid funding (Tolbert & Ammula, 2023).
- Medicaid covered over 87 million people in April 2023 (Medicaid.gov, 2023). Between October 1, 2021, and September 30, 2022, Medicaid spending was over $728 billion (KFF, n.d.-d).
- As the importance of social determinants of health gains wider acceptance, more states are requiring Medicaid managed care organizations (MCOs) to screen for these determinants and provide social services, such as housing and nutrition assistance (Hinton et al., 2023).
- Because Medicaid covers so many people, many of whom have complex health needs, it represents a significant proportion of healthcare spending in the United States (Rudowitz, Burns, et al., 2023).

In 2018, Medicaid covered 35.7% of all children in the United States, a decrease from 37% in 2017 (Berchik et al., 2019). The uninsured rate for children rose from 5.0% to 5.5% during that same time (Haley et al., 2022). The situation improved in 2019 (5.1%) and 2020 (4.1%). Medicaid covered 72% of children living at or below 200% of the federal poverty level (KFF, n.d.-b). Medicare beneficiaries comprised 14% of Medicaid enrollment (Pena et al., 2023). Medicaid paid more than $415 billion on long-term support services: $131 billion for skilled nursing facilities and $284 billion for care in home- and community-based settings (including residential facilities) (Chidambaram & Burns, 2022).

- Prior to the ACA, childless adults without disabilities were not eligible for Medicaid. Under the ACA, Medicaid was expanded to all adults, including those under age 65, with incomes up to 138% of the federal poverty level or $17,236 for a person in 2019 (Garfield et al., 2020).
- Other changes made through the ACA were to extend Medicaid coverage for children in foster care until age 26—equal to the requirement that private plans allow dependent children to remain on a parent's plan until that age. States also needed to make the Medicaid application process easier (Manatt & Phillips, 2019).

The ACA initially required all states to expand Medicaid. This was legally challenged by several states, leading to a Supreme Court case—*National Federation of Independent Business v. Sebelius* (KFF, 2012). The Medicaid expansion was ruled to be unconstitutional because it was highly coercive and the Medicaid expansion became optional for states.

- Currently, 37 states have expanded Medicaid coverage (KFF, 2023c).
- A gap in coverage exists in states choosing not to expand Medicaid coverage (Fig. 6-12).
- Medicaid eligibility is 40% of the federal poverty level ($8532 for a family of three in 2019).
- According to the Center on Budget and Policy Priorities, since expanded Medicaid coverage was implemented, over 19,000 lives have been saved (Aron-Dine, 2019). Whereas in states that have not expanded Medicaid, roughly 15,500 lives have been lost.
- The largest portion of Medicaid spending goes toward people with disabilities (34%) and older adults (21%), but these two groups comprise only 21% of Medicaid enrollees (Rudowitz, Burns, et al., 2023).

Medicaid is jointly funded between federal and state governments to assist the states in providing adequate medical care to eligible persons (Schneider, 2019). The federal government matches state Medicaid spending, and this is the largest source of federal funding for states. The federal government pays a portion of the costs, called the Federal Medical Assistance Percentage (FMAP), at 50% to 76% (Hinton & Raphael, 2023). Historically, the FMAP was around 62%. In states with lower per capita income, there are higher federal matches.

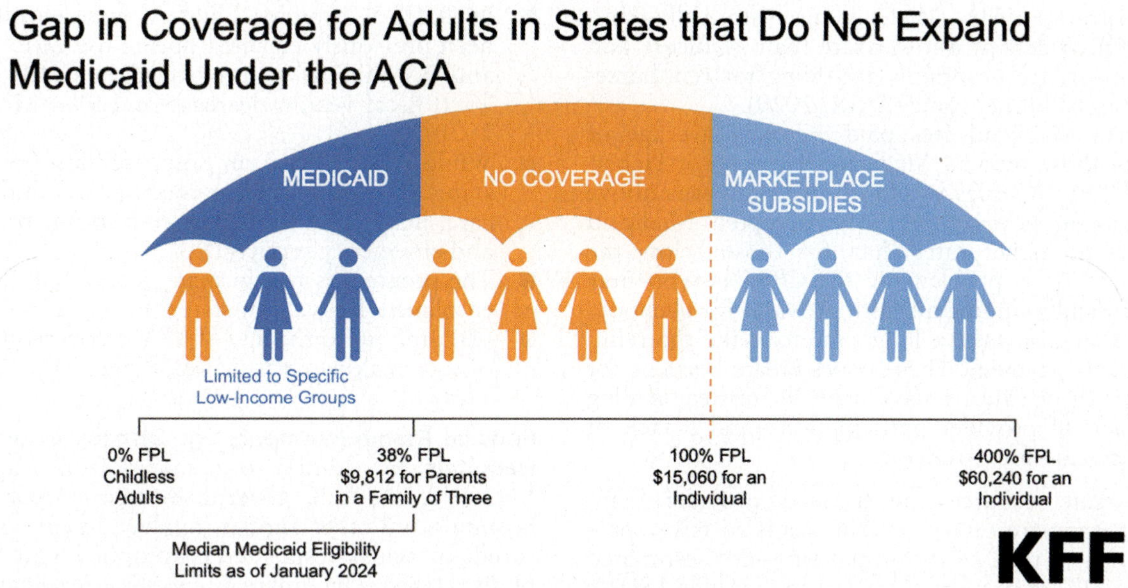

FIGURE 6-12 Gap in coverage for adults in states that do not expand Medicaid under the Patient Protection and Affordable Care Act. (Reprinted with permission from Rudowitz, Drake, et al. (2023). Figure 2: Gap in Coverage for Adults in States that Do Not Expand Medicaid Under the ACA. https://www.kff.org/medicaid/issue-brief/how-many-uninsured-are-in-the-coverage-gap-and-how-many-could-be-eligible-if-all-states-adopted-the-medicaid-expansion/)

The funding model for Medicaid has both benefits and problems. There isn't a limit on federal spending, so as states expand their Medicaid programs, more federal funding flows to states (Rudowitz, Burns, et al., 2023). This allows Medicaid to expand during epidemics or pandemics (e.g., COVID-19), natural or accidental disasters, or short economic downturns. At the same time, when the economy contracts, as in the 2008 recession, many more people become eligible for Medicaid at a time when state and federal funds are decreasing (Benitez et al., 2020). Eligibility varies by states, and Benitez and colleagues found that Medicaid enrollment grew more in states with "more generous" Medicaid programs than in states with a "more restrictive" program (p. 490).

The states have some discretion in determining what population groups their Medicaid programs cover and the financial criteria for Medicaid eligibility, as well as the scope of services, rate of payment, and how the program will be administered, so long as they meet the minimum requirements set by the federal government (Rudowitz, Burns, et al., 2023).

Medicaid mandatory services include the following (Medicaid.gov, n.d.):

- Outpatient and inpatient hospital services
- Early childhood screenings and well-child checkups (to age 21)
- Primary provider, nurse practitioner, and certified nurse midwife services
- Lab and x-ray services
- Family planning services
- Tobacco cessation counseling for pregnant people
- Home healthcare and nursing home services for those over age 21 (including rehabilitation centers)
- Federally qualified health centers and rural health clinic services
- Transportation to medical care

As with Medicare, Medicaid programs moved to a managed care concept following mandates within the Balanced Budget Act of 1997, in an attempt to restrain costs (Rudowitz, Burns, et al., 2023).

- In 2019, 69.5% of Medicaid beneficiaries were covered by managed care programs, compared to 40% in 2003 (Donohue et al., 2022), with 46% of the Medicaid budget going to managed care programs (Hinton & Raphael, 2023).
- In some states, a managed care plan is required.
- Medicaid beneficiaries are economically disadvantaged, frequently reside in medically underserved areas, and often have more complex health and social needs than other adults with higher incomes do.
- They often must choose between multiple plans, fewer providers, and may need to drive long distances to see specialists. Some managed care plans lack sufficient oversight, leading to fragmented services and poor health outcomes (Rudowitz, Burns, et al., 2023).

Medicaid is also a source of innovation in healthcare. States implemented medical homes, care coordination, integration of physical and mental healthcare, and other "new" services earlier than private health plans. The flexibility built into the federal requirements for Medicaid, Medicaid rule waivers to test ideas, and the new Innovation Center in CMS (part of the ACA) allow states to develop new models of healthcare delivery (CMS, 2023a).

Ensuring access and quality of care in a managed care environment will require fiscally solvent plans, established provider networks, and awareness of the unique needs of the Medicaid population (CMS, 2023a). Also, both providers and beneficiaries need more education about managed care.

- A key factor to Medicaid's future success is reimbursements to providers, both the amount of payments and administrative delays. Medicaid has historically reimbursed providers at a lower rate than Medicare and other insurance programs, and filing for reimbursement can be burdensome (AMA, 2020).

- In 2016, Medicaid fees paid were an average of 72% of those paid by Medicare (Holgash & Heberlein, 2019). In states where the fee ratio was above the median, primary providers accepted Medicaid patients at higher rates than for those below the median. This is problematic for C/PHNs who may have difficulty finding a health provider for clients.
- States may also take a long time to make the reimbursement payment. These issues create burdens for clinics and private primary provider offices, leading to a lack of provider participation—and a lack of access to care for enrollees.

When state resources are strained, provider reimbursement rates are often cut. This leads to fewer providers willing to take Medicaid patients—it is estimated that about 30% of primary providers in the United States will not accept new Medicaid patients; for specialty areas such as psychiatry, nearly 65% will not accept new Medicaid patients.

Despite these issues, Medicaid provides societal benefits. Medicaid coverage, including the Medicaid expansion under the ACA, is associated with reduced rates of infant mortality, especially in African American and Hispanic infants (Constantin & Wehby, 2023).

- In addition, providing coverage to children early in life leads to higher educational achievement, higher income, and decreased use of public programs (Manatt & Phillips, 2019).
- One large study examining differences between an uninsured population and those with Medicaid found that patients with Medicaid were more likely to see a primary provider at least once annually (Mondesir et al., 2019).
- Mondesir et al. (2019) found that hospitalizations for chronic conditions, especially short-term diabetes complications, decreased in states that expanded Medicaid and increased in states that did not expand Medicaid, indicating that people with Medicaid coverage are more likely to access preventive and primary care services.

Children's Health Insurance Plan. Enacted as part of the Balanced Budget Act in 1997, the Children's Health Insurance Plan (CHIP) provides health coverage to uninsured children under age 19 for families caught in the gap between Medicaid and affordable health insurance (Healthcare.gov, n.d.-d). Funding is provided from both federal and state budgets, and CHIP is a capped program; some states also offer the program to pregnant people (Medicaid and CHIP Payment and Access Commission [MACPAC], n.d.). In 2017, federal funding for this program lapsed, and it took 114 days to regain funding that was ensured, at that time, through 2027 (Park et al., 2023). In December of 2022, President Biden signed the Consolidated Appropriations Act, 2023, which extended funding for an additional 2 years.

- In 2019, 9.7 million children were enrolled or had been previously enrolled during the 2019 fiscal year, and 9.1 million were enrolled in CHIP during the 2020 fiscal year, a decrease of 1.9% (Medicaid.gov, 2020).
- While states differ on some services provided, all states must cover routine check-ups, dental and vision care, hospital services, immunizations, prescriptions, and emergency services.
- The program is free in many states, but premiums or enrollment fees vary by state (InsureKidsNow.gov, n.d.).
- Children up to the age of 19 are covered for families of four making up to $50,000 per year.

Federal Reimbursements for Disproportionate Share Hospitals. In addition to payments from Medicare and Medicaid, the U.S. government reimburses safety net hospitals and other entities involved in care of the uninsured, known as designated Disproportionate Share Hospitals (DSHs). The American Hospital Association (2022) reported a total of $42.7 billion in uncompensated care in 2020; increased from $21.6 billion in 2000. Although taxpayers help pay for uninsured patients through payments to DSHs, this does not fully cover costs of care.

- Zhang and Zhu (2021) examined national data on uncompensated care after the ACA Medicaid expansion and found significant reductions in the amount of uncompensated care for hospitals in states participating in expansion, although these reductions were offset by the reduced reimbursement rate from Medicaid compared to private insurance.
- Rhodes et al. (2020) found that public and rural hospitals saw improved financial performance after Medicaid expansion.
  - In states with ACA-related Medicaid expansion, early positive financial impacts continued in fiscal years 2016 and 2017, with lower rates of uncompensated care and higher rates of Medicaid payments (Blavin & Ramos, 2021). If Medicaid expansion were extended to the remaining 12 nonexpansion states, costs of uncompensated care are projected to drop by $4.3 billion (Buettgens & Ramchandani, 2022).

Other Government Programs. In addition to third-party reimbursement, the government offers some direct health services to selected populations, including Native Americans, military personnel, veterans, merchant marines, and federal employees. Government support, largely through grants administered through the CDC, provides free immunizations and well-child visits, as well as prenatal care and other programs at the state and local level.

Retrospective Payment

Reimbursement for healthcare services generally has been accomplished through one of two approaches: retrospective or prospective payment. A traditional form of reimbursement for any kind of service, including healthcare, is retrospective payment, which is reimbursement for a service after it has been rendered (Torrey, 2020). A fee may or may not be established in advance. However, payment of that fee occurs after the fact, or retrospectively, termed **fee-for-service (FFS)**. This type of system rewards "sick care" and more intensive interactions with healthcare (i.e., more laboratory or radiologic tests) (Fan et al., 2023).

Although retrospective payment worked well in other industries, from a cost-containment as well as a public health perspective, it has not worked well in healthcare and is now rarely used.

Surprise Medical Billing

"Surprise medical bills" occur when a person is caught unaware that a provider is not in-network and receives a large bill (Pollitz, 2021, para 1). For instance, a visit to an emergency department (ED) may be at an in-network hospital, but the ED primary providers are contracted employees and out-of-network. A scheduled surgery at a hospital may be covered under the plan yet the assistant surgeon, anesthesiologist, or radiologist is not part of the plan.

- More than 42% of patients hospitalized or seen in emergency rooms at in-network hospitals received surprise bills in a recent study, with bills doubling or tripling between 2010 and 2016 (Kaiser Health News, 2019).

Among insured adults who are under age 65, 39% reported an unexpected medical bill in the past year, half of these bills were less than $500, but 13% of bills were $2000 or more (Pollitz et al., 2020).

Prospective Payment

Prospective reimbursement, although not a new concept, was implemented for inpatient Medicare services in 1983, in response to the healthcare system's desperate need for cost containment (Rambur, 2022). It has since influenced the Medicaid program, as well as private health insurers. The prospective payment form of reimbursement has virtually eliminated the retrospective payment system (Nickitas et al., 2020). Prospective payment is a payment method based on rates derived from predictions of annual service costs that are set in advance of service delivery. Providers receive payment for services according to these fixed rates, set in advance. Payments may be in the form of premiums paid before receipt of service or in response to fixed-rate charges. To correct unlimited reimbursement patterns and counteract disincentives to contain costs, prospective payment involves four classic steps (Dowling, 1979; Meachum, 2020):

1. An external authority is empowered (by statute, market power, or voluntary compliance by providers) to set provider charges, third-party payment rates, or both.
2. Rates are set in advance of the prospective year during which they will apply and are considered fixed for the year (except for major, uncontrollable occurrences). The provider accepts the assignment of fees.
3. Patients, third-party payers, or both pay the prospective rates rather than the costs incurred by providers during the year (or charges adjusted to cover these costs).
4. Providers are at risk for losses or surpluses.

Prospective payment imposes constraints on spending and provides incentives for cutting costs. The federal government, as mentioned earlier, enacted a prospective payment plan (The Social Security Amendments Act of 1983; see the "Significant Legislation" section earlier in this chapter).

- The plan is a billing classification system known as **diagnosis-related groups (DRGs)**. The system is based on about 500 diagnosis and procedure groups. It provides fixed Medicare reimbursement to hospitals based on weighted formulas. Flat rates of payment are based on average national costs for a specific group, adjusted annually, with some regional variations accounting for higher wages and other costs (Meachum, 2020).
- This system was enacted to curb Medicare spending in hospitals and to extend the program's solvency period. It was designed to create incentives for hospitals to be more efficient in delivering services.
- The prospective payment system reduced Medicare's rate of increase for inpatient hospital spending and increased hospital productivity by reducing hospital stays and unnecessary admissions, according to classic studies by Clifton (2009) and Rambur (2022).
- The system, however, led to DRG creep or "upcoding" (i.e., classifying patients into more lucrative categories) and patient dumping (i.e., transferring patients whose reimbursement is expected to be lower than actual costs of services) in an effort to counteract the losses in revenue and in some circumstances make hefty profits.

In a classic article, Kinney (2013) calculated that the three major concerns faced by Medicare (and the ACA) are "cost and volume inflation, quality assurance, and fraud and abuse" (p. 253).

- Cost inflation was addressed by DRGs and other measures.
- Quality was addressed in October 2008, when Medicare began withholding payments to hospitals for preventable errors in an effort to provide an incentive to prevent avoidable mistakes and improve patient care. There are 29 preventable errors (often called "never events") grouped into 7 categories (Agency for Healthcare Research and Quality [AHRQ], 2019b).
- CMS has mechanisms in place to investigate fraud or abuse.
- Appropriate mechanisms must be in place to provide accountability and take action when needed—as when billing and other fraud is prosecuted (USDOJ, 2018, 2019). Speer et al. (2020) reviewed the literature and found a median value for wasteful spending due to fraud to be $185 billion, or $557 per person in the United States. This was enough to fund "the total annual estimated costs to provide free tuition at public colleges and universities ($79 billion), universal child care ($42 billion), universal pre-K ($26 billion), and partial wage replacement for up to 12 weeks of family leave ($28 billion)" (p. 1744–1745).

These changes were instituted at the request of Congress, and initially, many hospitals complained that their payments would be substantially reduced, especially for complicated patients.

"Never events" are medical errors or adverse events that never should happen and are largely preventable (AHRQ, 2019b; Patient Safety Network, 2019). An expanded list of 28 never events for hospitals—serious incidents that could have been prevented—was approved for nonpayment by Medicaid beginning in July 2012 for all states. The goal was to reduce serious medical errors and preventable infections that should reduce costs and improve patient care (AHRQ, 2019a). A frequently cited study from the AHRQ noted progress toward the goal of improved quality of care, estimating that a reduction in adverse events saved the lives of 8000 people and saved close to $3 billion from 2014 to 2016 (CMS, 2018). However, never events still occur. In October of 2018, 25% of Medicare patients experienced a harmful event, including 12% experiencing an adverse event and 13% experiencing temporary harm (Grimm, 2022). Medical errors account for 100,000 deaths and cost $20 billion a year (Rodziewicz, 2023a, 2023b). In addition, there are 4000 surgical errors reported yearly. The ACA includes incentive payments to primary care providers and hospitals who meet quality goals.

Debate continues about nonpayment outside of hospital settings and about which conditions should be included in the list of never events (Box 6-4).

Capitation

A more vigorous version of prospective payment is capitation. **Capitation** refers to a fixed fee per person that is paid to a MCO for a specified package of services (Nickitas et al., 2020). Fees remain in effect until renegotiated, regardless of the number of services provided. Because profit margins are very tight, utilization, quality, and costs are carefully monitored.

- The prospective payment concept has proved useful from a public health perspective. Prepaid services create incentives for providers to keep their enrollees healthy, thus reducing costs.
- A potential, indirect benefit from fixed rates and reduced costs is that prevention programs may capture a larger share of the healthcare dollar.

Claims Payment Agents

Claims payment agents administer the process for government third-party payments. That is, the government contracts with private fiscal agents to handle the claims payment process and function as an intermediary between them and the healthcare provider. As an example, Blue Cross Blue Shield, in addition to serving as a private insurance company, has also served as claims payment agent for Medicare since its inception (Blue Cross Blue Shield, n.d.).

Direct Consumer Reimbursement or Out-of-Pocket Payment

Another source of healthcare financing comes from direct fees paid by consumers. This refers to individual out-of-pocket payments made for several different reasons, such as:

- Payments made by people who have no insurance coverage (fees must be paid directly for health and medical services)
- Payments for limited coverage, insurance caps, and exclusions (services for which the consumer must bear the entire expense)
- Copayments or coinsurance for services

For example, some people carry only major medical insurance and must pay directly for primary provider office visits, prescriptions, eyeglasses, and dental care. In other instances, deductibles and coinsurance leave people and families with healthcare insurance out-of-pocket costs, with payments ranging from $360 to $1500; the highest being $7000 or more (Hayes et al., 2019). Roughly, 30% of Americans are worried about healthcare insurance premiums, deductibles, and out-of-pocket expenses (Kirzinger et al., 2019).

Two important factors to consider in healthcare costs are cost shifting and cross subsidization.

- **Cost shifting** consists of charging different prices for the same services, placing the burden of high cost of healthcare on others (Chernew et al., 2021). The idea is that healthcare agencies and providers are able to make up for the lower reimbursements from public sources, such as Medicare and Medicaid, by charging more to private payers.
- **Cross subsidization** is the practice of adjusting revenues from a central pool of funds to an area with higher healthcare needs to help cut site costs (Mathauer et al., 2020). The health risks of an area are calculated based on population's age, gender, poverty level, chronic diseases, and disabilities. This is used in many countries with decentralized healthcare such as Germany, Japan, Spain, and Switzerland.

Private and Philanthropic Support

Private or philanthropic support, a third funding source, contributes both directly and indirectly to healthcare

BOX 6-4 WHAT DO *YOU* THINK?

Nonpayment for Preventable Medical Errors

What if you were to hire a glass company to replace a broken windshield in your car, and while completing the repair, they accidentally broke off your rearview mirror. Would you expect them to pay for that mistake? Or would you just absorb the cost yourself?

In the past, we the taxpayers have been paying Medicare payments to hospitals and primary providers who have made serious errors that have led to adverse events, spiraling costs and resulting in poor patient outcomes. Congress and others feel that this is unfair and have enacted legislation to stop paying for these types of errors or preventable events.

Do you think this is fair? Can these conditions always be prevented? Are there extenuating circumstances that should be considered? Are there benefits to patients and taxpayers from holding healthcare providers accountable for errors and inadequate care?

financing. Charities in the United States received $499.3 billion in donations in 2022 (Giving USA, n.d.). Many private agencies fund programs, underwrite research, and provide benefits for people who otherwise would go without services. Nearly $25 billion was donated to health-related causes.

In addition, volunteerism, the efforts of numerous people and organizations that donate their time and services (e.g., hospital guild members), provides tremendous cost savings to healthcare institutions.

TRENDS AND ISSUES INFLUENCING HEALTHCARE ECONOMICS

The High Cost of Healthcare in the United States

As described earlier, the United States pays the most for what are often some of the worst health outcomes. Kurani and Wager (2021) reported healthcare comparisons across OECD countries and found that the United States ranked last on *amenable mortality levels* (deaths prior to age 75 that may be prevented through effective, timely healthcare). The United States was

- Among the lowest nations in the percentage of adults who smoke daily (OECD, 2019)
- Among the lowest third of nations in cancer deaths
- In the lower half of countries on childhood vaccination rates but third highest on influenza vaccination rates
- Among the highest among nations on the percentage of adults who are obese
- Among the lower third of countries for life expectancy at birth

Controlling Costs

The ACA has introduced many strategies to control the rise of healthcare costs, including increased funding for primary prevention strategies. A focus on primary prevention demands a paradigm shift in thinking about the practice and delivery of healthcare (see Chapter 1). It is one that fits more closely with the mission of public health. It expects that citizens are involved in their healthcare, are knowledgeable about their health status, can manage self-care practices, and can modify lifestyle behaviors to promote wellness. Our focus on illness and not health promotion or prevention has proven costly. Prevention should be at the forefront of a new era in healthcare. Trust for America's Health (TFAH, n.d.) has developed 10 top priorities for a National Prevention Strategy:

1. Fighting the Obesity Epidemic
2. Thwarting the Use of or Exposure to Tobacco
3. Preventing and Controlling Infectious Diseases
4. Preparing for Possible Health Emergencies or Bioterrorism Attacks
5. Acknowledging the Connection Between Health and U.S. Economic Competitiveness
6. Safeguarding Our Food Supply
7. Planning for Changing Senior Healthcare Needs
8. Improving the Health and Well-being of Low-Income and Underrepresented Communities
9. Diminishing Environmental Threats
10. Advancing Prevention of Diseases (para 1)

Access to Health Services: The Uninsured and Underinsured

Many services, preventive or illness focused, are not available to a large portion of our population.

- The U.S. Census Bureau (2023) shows that 47.2 million people (15.5% of the population) were uninsured in 2010; the percentage of uninsured (those lacking health insurance) had been as high as 18% before passage of the ACA (Congress.gov., 2010).
- The ACA (2010) improved access to care by making insurance available to people who were considered "uninsurable" due to preexisting health conditions. By 2015, the number of people who were uninsured decreased to 29.8 million or 9.4% of the population, and by 2020, the number of people who were uninsured dropped further to 28.1 million or 8.7% of the population (U.S. Census Bureau, 2023).
    - The rate of those lacking health insurance varies by age group (Fig. 6-13).
    - The uninsured rate in 2020 was highest for those living below the poverty level (15.7%) and higher for the Hispanic population (17.7%), the Black or African American population (9.9%), and similar for the Asian population (6.4%) compared to the non-Hispanic White population (5.9 %).
- The ACA expanded Medicaid in a number of states, extending coverage to low-income people and families. In addition, the ACA required insurance companies to cover preventative healthcare visits without a copay and to cover those with preexisting conditions.
- In recent years, political disagreements about the ACA have led to weakening of some protections. Despite this, federal surveys revealed an all-time low in the uninsured rate of 8.0% in 2022, in part due to the American Rescue Plan (Lee et al., 2022). Eighteen states had drops in uninsured rates from 2018 to 2020; 15 of these states had expanded Medicaid. Most states that did not expand Medicaid saw at least small increases in the uninsured rate in the low-income population, up to an 11.1% percentage-point increase in Wyoming. The average uninsured rate in low-income people in nonexpansion states was 32.4%.

Even those with Medicaid and Medicare can be underinsured or become uninsured.

- Among working-age adults, 43% were inadequately insured in 2022 (Collins et al., 2022). This included 23% underinsured, 11% with a gap in coverage in the past year, and 9% uninsured.
- A recent study found that 16% of Medicare participants delayed care due to cost or had problems paying medical bills (Madden et al., 2021). Near-poverty (income of $15,000 to <$25,000) Medicare participants were 3.4 times as likely to have difficulty paying medical bills and 2.5 times more likely to delay care.

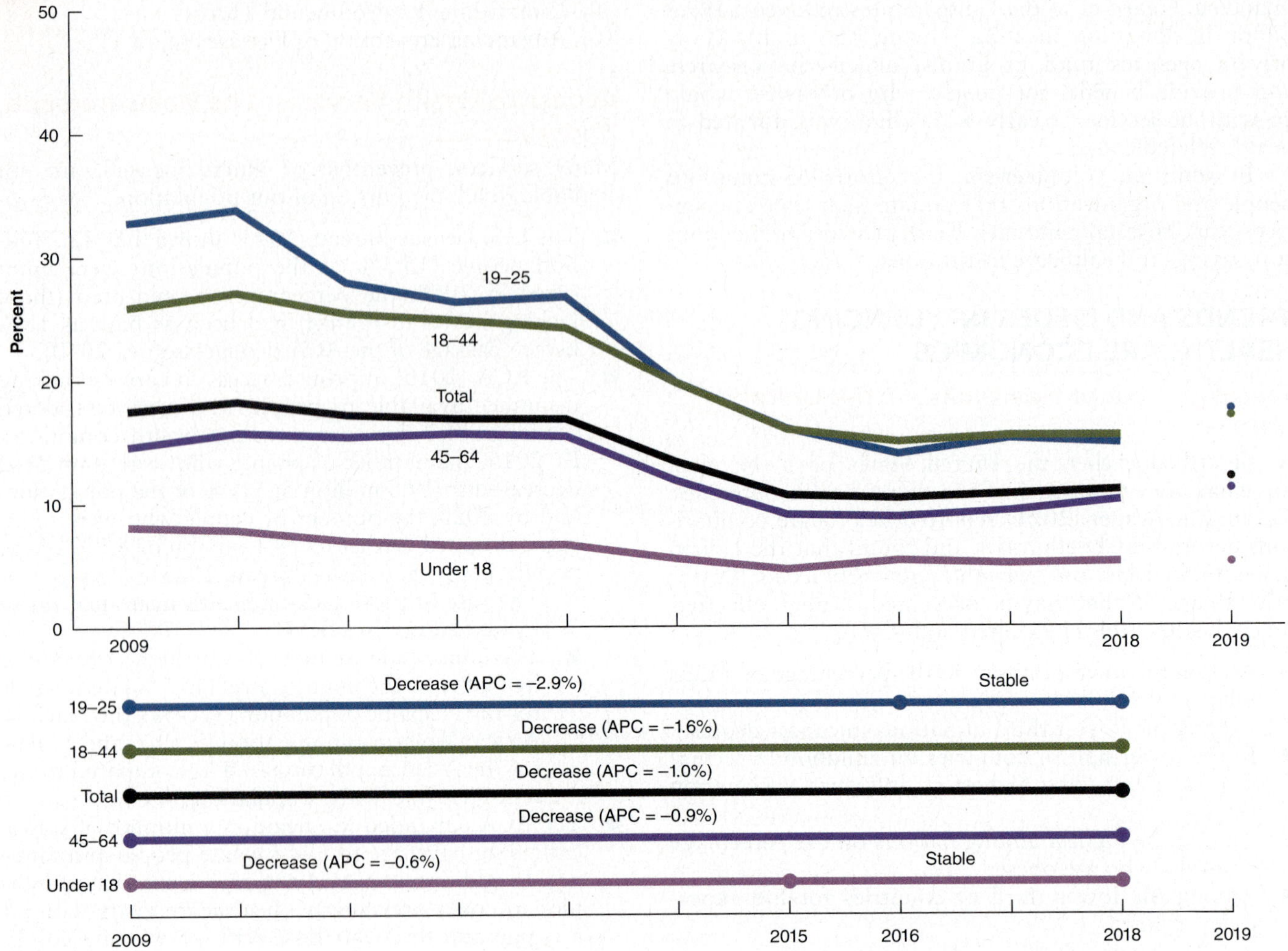

FIGURE 6-13 Lack of health insurance coverage by people under age 65, by age group: United States, 2009–2019. (From CDC, 2023b). Notes: APC is annual percentage change. "Stable" refers to no statistically significant trend during the period. (Source: National Center for Health Statistics, National Health Interview Survey. Retrieved from https://www.cdc.gov/nchs/hus/topics/health-insurance-coverage.htm#featured-charts)

- Approximately three million Medicaid recipients would lose their healthcare coverage in states where Medicaid work requirements are now being implemented (Zewde & Wimer, 2019; Fig. 6-14).
- The KFF estimated that between 62% and 91% will be disenrolled for not correctly reporting work hours or exemptions and between 9% and 38% for not meeting the work requirements (Garfield et al., 2018).

Before the work requirements, Sneed et al. (2022) found that adults aged 51 to 64 years who worked less than 20 hours a week, thus facing disenrollment, were more likely to have chronic disease and functional limitations.

Medical Bankruptcies

A wide variety of medical issues can lead to financial insecurity and bankruptcy. If you don't have health insurance and you undergo emergency surgery for appendicitis, it may take a great effort to pay off your medical debt (or you may turn to high-interest credit cards). Even if you have health insurance, long-term cancer treatments will likely mean large out-of-pocket costs—and your inability to work may lead to further financial problems. Bankruptcy can provide debt relief.

- Bankruptcy filings reached their peak in 2010; about 93% fewer filings were noted by 2021 (United States Courts, 2023). However, while the number of bankruptcies is down, the percent of bankruptcies due to medical costs was estimated to be 65.5% before full implementation of the ACA in 2014 and 67.5% of all bankruptcies in 2015 and 2016 (Himmelstein et al., 2019).
- Medical bankruptcies are uncommon in most developed countries, but GoFundMe efforts to help families with unexpected, crushing medical bills are commonplace in the United States, with over a quarter million requests for assistance annually, raising over $650 million annually (Hiltzik, 2019). Medical debt that doesn't lead to bankruptcy is still problematic. Himmelstein et al. (2022) studied changes in social determinants of health. They found that, from 2017 to 2019, 10.8% of all adults carried medical debt, with associations between medical debt and

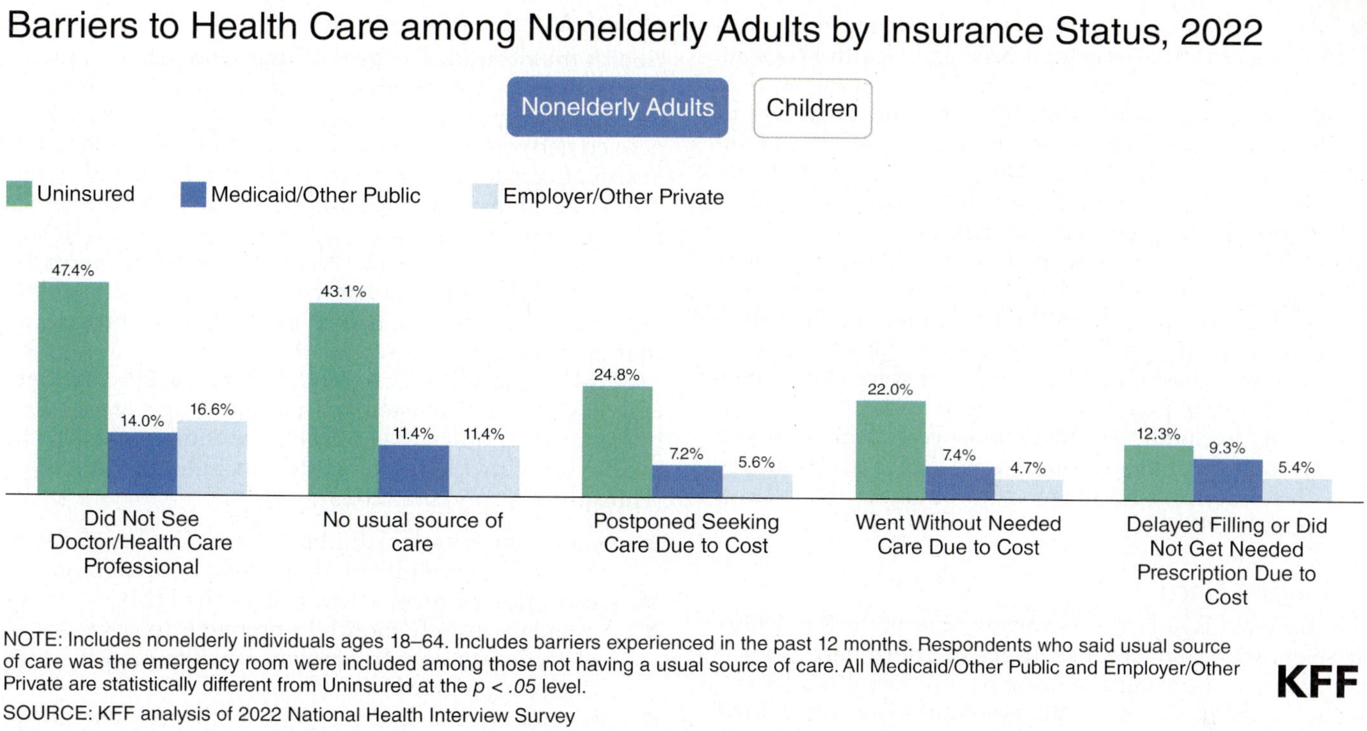

FIGURE 6-14 Barriers to healthcare among nonelderly adults by insurance status, 2022. (Reprinted with permission from Kaiser Family Foundation. (December 19, 2022). *Key facts about the uninsured population*, Figure 8. Retrieved from https://www.kff.org/uninsured/issue-brief/key-facts-about-the-uninsured-population/)

reporting poor health and being hospitalized. They also had higher odds of food insecurity, being unable to pay rent or mortgage and utilities, and experiencing eviction or foreclosure.

- Residents in Medicaid-expansion states had lower odds of being in medical debt.
- About 19% of people with employer-sponsored health insurance reported having been contacted by a collection agency within the last year because of unpaid healthcare expenses in a representative survey conducted by the KFF and the Los Angeles Times (Hamel et al., 2019). Over half of respondents reported skipping or postponing care.
- This is further evidence that the people who are underinsured, along with those people without health insurance, are in danger of financial disaster when confronted with a serious medical emergency or long-term illness (Ali et al., 2022).
- Those with chronic health conditions, insured (public or private) and uninsured, have even higher financial burdens from out-of-pocket healthcare expenses.

Healthcare Rationing

Healthcare in the United States is allocated based on price and the willingness and ability of patients to pay (APHA, n.d.-b). In other words, patients are entitled to purchase a share of the medical services that they value. Social justice, in contrast, emphasizes the well-being of the community over the person. Under this view, healthcare is regarded as a social good (as opposed to an economic good) that should be collectively financed and available to everyone regardless of ability to pay.

- Rationing implies that resources are fixed or limited and, therefore, cannot meet every need. This is the case in healthcare—the need will always be greater than the resources (Moosa & Luyckx, 2021).
- Although Americans may not consider our current system as rationing, when a person cannot afford healthcare or delays treatment because of copays, we begin to realize our current system actually is a form of rationing (Tikkanen & Osborn, 2019).
- Often insurance companies require preapproval prior to agreeing to cover an examination or procedure; this is also a form of rationing (Bihari, 2023).
- The United States rations healthcare chiefly by the high cost of healthcare and the lack of comprehensive insurance for all (Tikkanen & Osborn, 2019).
- Rationing also occurs in deferring care by requiring referrals for specialist care and waiting lists for elective surgery (Bhatia, 2020).

When rationing is based on social justice principles, it is considered a rational, fair, and equal distribution of resources according to a clinical need or potential for effectiveness and is not based on income or where one lives (Bowser, 2015). In this way, rationing focuses on the needs of the population more than the person.

- Rationing may occur by restricting people's choices, by denying access to services, or by limiting the supply of services or personnel. It may be overt, as in the oft-cited government health system of the United Kingdom, or more covert, as practiced by some health plans in the United States. When rationing is based on market justice principles, limited resources are distributed based on the ability to pay (Bowser, 2015).

- Rationing may jeopardize the well-being of groups of people (Physicians for a National Health Program, n.d.). With limited resources for health services delivery, the government, insurers, and providers of healthcare services make rationing decisions to contain costs (Bihari, 2023). This has included strict eligibility levels or monitoring the use of resources to ensure the most equitable distribution.
- In 2014, companies were no longer allowed to deny health coverage based on preexisting health issues (CMS, n.d.-c). Prior to the ACA, millions of Americans were at risk for being charged higher rates for insurance, had limited coverage, or were denied coverage. In the past, private insurers engaged in rationing by excluding enrollees who were at greatest risk for health problems—and, thus, higher expenditures. This practice is no longer allowed under the rules of the ACA (Box 6-5).

Managed Care

The term managed care became popular in the late 1980s. It refers to systems that contract to coordinate medical care for specific groups in order to promote provider efficiency and control costs. **Managed care** is a cost-control strategy used in both public and private sectors of healthcare. Care is *managed* by regulating the use of services and levels of provider payment. This approach is utilized in health maintenance organizations (HMOs), accountable care organizations, exclusive provider organizations (EPOs), and preferred provider organizations (PPOs). Among people with employer-based insurance, 49% are in PPOs and 12% are in HMOs (KFF, 2022a).

Managed care plans operate on a prospective payment basis and control costs by managing utilization and provider payments. Because costs are tight, preventive services are generally encouraged, so that more expensive tertiary care costs can be avoided if possible (Hinton & Raphael, 2023).

BOX **6-5** WHAT DO *YOU* THINK?

Rationing of Healthcare Services

When several people need an organ transplant and only one organ is available, what criteria should be used to select the recipient? It is now commonly accepted that certain lifestyle behaviors, such as smoking, alcohol consumption, or driving without restraints, create health risks. Should people who engage in these activities pay a higher price for healthcare or be excluded from certain services? Should a younger person needing specialized surgery take priority over an older person needing similar care?

There are no easy answers. At the height of the COVID-19 pandemic, healthcare systems in several countries were stretched beyond their means, and a form of triaging evolved out of necessity. Was this form of rationing used in your area? Or was it used in other areas of our country? Which strategies do you feel are the most effective for the United States in controlling costs and improving health outcomes?

Health Maintenance Organizations

Health maintenance organizations (HMOs) are systems in which participants prepay a fixed monthly premium to receive comprehensive health services delivered by a defined network of providers. In 2022, costs for employee health coverage were similar for HMO, PPO, and point-of-service plans with approximately a $300 difference for a person and $1000 for a family (KFF, 2022a). Insurance premiums, in general, rise more than wage increases. However, they remained flat from 2021 to 2022, possibly because rates were set before the extent of inflation in that year was known.

HMOs are the oldest model of managed care. Several HMOs have existed for decades (e.g., Kaiser Permanente), but others have developed more recently. The unique set of properties of HMOs includes the following (Falkson & Srinivasan, 2023):

- A contract between the HMO and the beneficiaries (or their representative), the enrolled population.
- Absorption of prospective risk by the HMO.
- A regular (usually monthly) premium to cover specified (typically comprehensive) benefits paid by each enrollee of the HMO.
- An integrated delivery system with provider incentives for efficiency, particularly a focus on preventive care. Some HMOs follow the traditional model, employing health professionals (e.g., primary providers, nurses), building their own hospital and clinic facilities, and serving only their own enrollees (Shi & Singh, 2019). Other HMOs provide some services while contracting for the rest.
- In response to concerns from managed care clients, a patient bill of rights stipulating the patient's right to timely emergency services, respect and nondiscrimination, as well as participation in treatment decisions and a more consumer-friendly appeals process was developed (California Department of Managed Care, 2020).

Preferred Provider Organizations

A **preferred provider organization (PPO)** is a network of primary providers, hospitals, and other health-related services that contract with a third-party payer organization (health insurer) to provide health services to subscribers at a reduced rate. Employers with these plans offer medical services to their employees at discounted rates.

- In PPOs, consumer choice exists. Enrollees have a choice among providers within the plan and contracted providers out of the plan. PPOs practice utilization review and often use formal standards for selecting providers (Pestaina, 2024).
- In 2022, PPOs were the most common form of health insurance offered by employers—with 49% of workers enrolled; companies with over 200 employees have the highest rate of PPO usage at 51% (KFF, 2022a).
- However, enrollment in PPOs began to decline, and increases were noted in HDHP/SO policies.

Point-of-Service Plans

A variation on the plans described above is the **point-of-service (POS) plan**, which permits more freedom of choice than a standard HMO or PPO. Enrollees choose a primary provider from within the POS plan who monitors their care and makes outside referrals when necessary. At an extra cost, enrollees can go outside the HMO or PPO network of contracted providers unless their primary provider has made a specific referral (Aetna, n.d.). POS is a type of hybrid or combination of an HMO and PPO. In 2022, about 9% of employees were enrolled in POS plans (KFF, 2022a). See Figure 6-15 for trends in types of health plan enrollment.

High-Deductible Health Plans

The **high-deductible health plan (HDHP)** is growing in popularity. Among employees in small and large size companies, a **high-deductible health plan with a savings option (HDHP/SO)** is often favored over HMOs and has grown in popularity, covering 19% of workers with insurance in 2012 and 29% in 2022 (KFF, 2022a). The plan has higher deductibles and out-of-pocket maximum limits. However, once these deductibles are met, the plan pays 100% of in-network healthcare. In addition, the HDHP plan is the only health plan that allows for money to be put aside pretax to be used to pay for deductibles and out-of-pocket expenses (USOPM, n.d.-a).

- The average annual out-of-pocket maximum in 2022 for HDHP plans with an HSA was $4422 for single coverage (KFF, 2022a).
- Deductibles have risen 61% between 2012 and 2022, and nearly a third of covered employees have plans with $2000 deductibles (or more). For employers with less than 200 employees, 49% of covered employees have at least $2000 deductibles for single coverage (KFF, 2022a).
- HDHPs are more often available with large firms than with small ones, 57% versus 27% (KFF, 2022a).

Exclusive Provider Organizations

Other than for medical emergencies, an **exclusive provider organization (EPO)** plan only covers services and providers within the network. Benefits of this type of plan are lower prices than an HMO and not needing a referral from a primary healthcare provider (O'Day, 2021). However, if a person goes out of network, 100% of the medical bill is owed by that person. A provider that was

Distribution of Health Plan Enrollment for Covered Workers, by Plan Type, 1988–2022

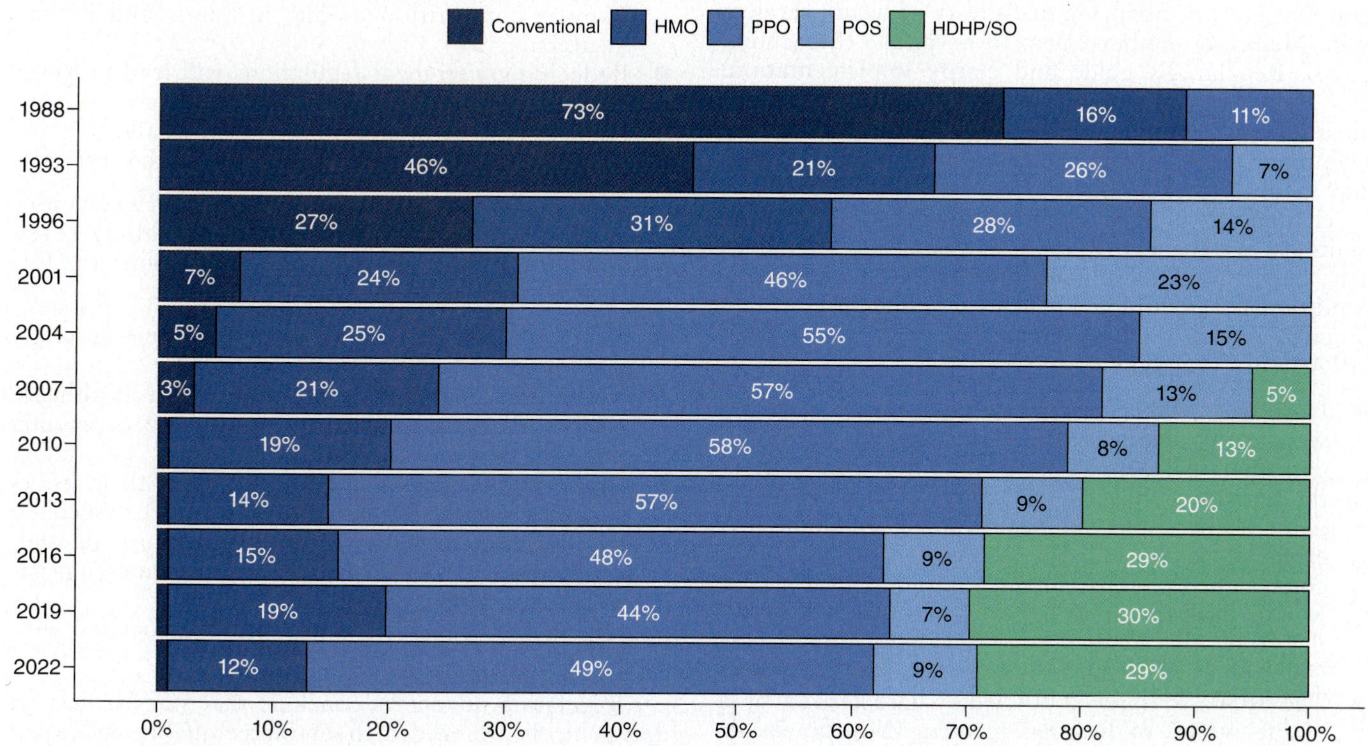

NOTE: Information was not obtained for POS plans in 1988 or for HDHP/SO plans until 2006. See the Survey Design and Methods section from the 2005 Kaiser/HRET Survey and the 2021 KFF Survey for a discussion of weighting changes.

SOURCE: KFF Employer Health Benefits Survey, 2018-2022; Kaiser/HRET Survey of Employer-Sponsored Health Benefits, 1999-2017; KPMG Survey of Employer-Sponsored Health Benefits, 1993 and 1996; The Health Insurance Association of America (HIAA), 1988.

FIGURE 6-15 Distribution of health plan enrollment for covered workers, by plan type, 1988–2022. (Reprinted with permission from Kaiser Family Foundation. (2022, October 27). Figure 10. *Employer health benefits: 2022 annual survey.* https://www.kff.org/mental-health/report/2022-employer-health-benefits-survey/)

covered when you bought your policy may no longer be part of the plan the following year, and you will not necessarily know this until you are billed for the visit.

Overall, EPOs account for less than 20% of all plans offered through healthcare.gov.

Competition and Regulation

Often, competition and regulation in health economics have been viewed as antagonistic and incompatible concepts.

- Competition describes a contest between rival healthcare organizations for resources and clients.
- Regulation refers to mandated procedures and practices affecting health services delivery that are enforced by law.

In a society in which there are long-held values of freedom of choice and individualism, competition provides opportunities for entrepreneurial endeavor, free enterprise, and scientific advancement. Yet, regulation also serves an important role in promoting the public good, overseeing equitable distribution of health services, and fostering community-wide participation.

Healthcare incorporates four major types of regulation—laws, regulations, programs, and policies (Johnson et al., 2022; Meachum, 2020).

Laws that regulate healthcare include any legislation that governs financing or delivery of health services (e.g., Medicare reimbursement to hospitals) (Meachum, 2020). Regulations guide and clarify implementation; they are issued under the authority of law and are part of most federal healthcare programs (e.g., CHIP eligibility requirements). Regulatory policies have a broader focus and involve decisions that shape the healthcare system by channeling the flow of resources into it and setting limits on key players' actions (e.g., state nurse practice acts, health worker training, ACA rules on preexisting conditions). Programs and policies are often developed in order to control costs and improve quality (e.g., HRRP, HIPAA). See Chapter 13.

- In the early 1980s, government cost-control measures were greatly diminished as the Reagan era ushered in deregulation (Johnson et al., 2022). The passage of the Omnibus Budget Reconciliation Act caused dramatic changes affecting healthcare. The federal government, having failed to contain rising healthcare costs, shifted responsibility for the public's health and welfare back to state and local governments. From all this grew the competition-versus-regulation debate (Johnson et al., 2022; KFF, n.d.-a).
- The 1990s to early 2000s were characterized by a "large wave" of hospital mergers (Morton et al., 2022).
    - Managed care became more popular, but by the late 1990s, fears were raised about MCOs withholding necessary care and a consumer "backlash" resulted (Morenz et al., 2023).
- Many states and the federal government enacted benefit laws between 1990 and 2008, in response to these concerns (KFF, n.d.-a). The ACA was passed into law in 2010. However, we still feel the results of decades of disjointed policies, and one of the most obvious consequences deals with competition in healthcare.
- Competition, its proponents say, offers wider consumer choice and positive incentives for cost containment and enhanced efficiency (Johnson et al., 2022). That is, consumers are free to select among various health plans on the basis of cost, quality, and range of services.
- Regulation advocates for almost 20 years have argued that there are at least four problems associated with the competition model (Johnson et al., 2022):

1. Consumers often do not make proper healthcare choices because they have limited knowledge of health services.
2. Competition may discriminate against enrolling certain consumers, especially high-risk, high-cost patients, thus excluding those who may need services the most.
3. The competition model may not encourage enough teaching and research—expensive elements of our present system.
4. Quality may be sacrificed to keep costs down.

The following tenets often guide discussions on healthcare reform efforts (Fitzgerald & Yencha, 2019):

- Reduction in healthcare prices occurs when there is more competition among hospitals and among insurers.
- Reducing government regulations will lead to lower healthcare prices.
- Higher prices can reflect higher-quality care.
- Higher provider costs are reflected in higher prices.

A study by Fitzgerald and Yencha (2019) examining outcome measures for those tenets among seven million hospital and patient interactions found the following:

- Generally, the greater the competition among hospitals (more choice), the lower the prices.
- Regulation does not consistently affect healthcare prices; prices can increase or decrease depending upon the cost measure used.
- As hospitals gain in quality measures, their prices generally rise; higher mortality rates were associated with lower prices. However, on two measures of quality, patient experiences and readmission rates, a negative relationship was found.
- Higher provider costs are generally associated with higher prices.

Regulation advocates conclude that standardization and controls are needed to guarantee quality and equal access (Meachum, 2020). But regulations are also often viewed as excessively restrictive and costly. For instance, the American Hospital Association claims that $39 billion per year is spent by hospitals, health systems, and postacute care providers on administrative costs involved in meeting regulatory requirements (AHA, n.d.). However, in a study of 2783 hospitals across the United States, Jenkins and Ho (2023) found that profits had increased 26.6% for both nonprofit and for-profit hospitals from 2012 to 2019.

Our capitalist system is driven by profits, and the profit motive in healthcare can lead to excesses and higher costs for taxpayers and patients.

- In 2019 first quarter reporting, more than half of all profits in the healthcare sector went to the top 10 companies, and 90% of those were large pharmaceutical companies like Pfizer ($3.9 billion), Eli Lilly ($4.2 billion), and Johnson & Johnson ($3.7 billion) (Jaggannathan, 2019).
- These high profits are occurring at a time when drug prices are escalating, with almost half of the population of the United States reporting use of a prescription medication in the last month.
- In 2020, 46 states, the District of Columbia, and 4 territories sued 26 drug manufacturing companies, accusing them of "conspiring to reduce competition and drive up generic drug prices" (Bartz & Stempel, 2020, para 1). As of October 2022, five states had settled their claims with one company, Teva Pharmaceuticals; the company paid each state a different sum, and it was estimated that they would spend $100 million if they continued to settle with individual states (Sullivan, 2022). In 2023, the U.S. Department of Justice announced that they would not prosecute criminal antitrust charges against these companies, with settlements that included paying fines of more than $250 million.
- The argument often made by pharmaceutical firms that more money is needed for research and development of new drugs was recently invalidated by examining the costs for 10 pharmaceutical companies introducing newly developed cancer drugs (cost = $9 billion) while their revenues reached over $67 billion (Anderson et al., 2019).

As the ACA was enacted, concerns arose about the continued financial stability of health insurers participating in the ACA marketplace exchanges, but the five largest health insurers have continued to be profitable, with increases as high as 24% in 2022 compared to 2021 net earnings (Emerson, 2023). These five companies represent about 46% of the nation's insured population (Guinan, 2023).

Leaders in the field have concluded that both competition and regulation are needed (Johnson et al., 2022; Meachum, 2020). With foresight, McNerney (1980) wrote, "It is rapidly becoming apparent that what we need is a proper balance between competition and regulation with more effective links [and] regulation [should be] used as a force to keep the market honest" (p. 1091).

Two plans that deal with balancing competition and regulation that are worth further review are managed competition and universal coverage, with and without a single-payer system.

Changing Our Healthcare System

The cry for healthcare reform is not new. In a classic study, Perkins (1998) examined the work of the 1927 to 1932 Committee on the Costs of Medical Care. Almost 100 years ago, the committee defined *costs* as the major problem and *business models of organization* as the major solution.

An important healthcare reform element is a standard set of benefits, set by law and enjoyed by the entire population, regardless of age, health status, income level, and employment. Many countries have successfully implemented such a package under a plan called the *statutory model* (Edwards & Dunn, 2019). Various versions of this model have worked well in Austria, France, Belgium, Japan, Germany, Israel, Poland, The Netherlands, and Switzerland. In this model, health insurance falls under the rubric of social security and is funded through government-mandated payroll premiums or taxes. Payment is made to private sector health insurers, from a fund known in some countries as a *sickness fund*. The ACA was a start toward this process in the United States, with 10 categories of services that health insurance plans must cover and specific services that must be offered without a copay. Health reform must focus on the central question: Is there coverage for the promotion of health and prevention of illness or simply payment for the diagnosis and treatment of those who are already ill?

- Research has shown that public health interventions are consistently more cost-effective than medical services, yet past health reform has often paid minimal attention to this critical issue (Owen et al., 2019; Smith et al., 2019).
- In addition, our frequent emphasis on medical care cost containment does not take into account the social determinants of health that need to be addressed outside the healthcare system (NASEM, 2019). C/PHNs can play an influential role in emphasizing health promotion services as being central to future health reform efforts through political involvement and policy development.
- With the successful passage of HR 3590 (Public Law [PL] 111–148), *The Patient Protection and Affordable Care Act*, on March 23, 2010, and the March 25 passage of HR 4872 (PL 111–152), *Health Care and Education Affordability Reconciliation Act of 2010*, amending HR 3590, the long journey toward healthcare system reform crossed a threshold. Both pieces of legislation are referred to as the *Affordable Care Act* (ACA).
- Although by no means a grand vision for change with its incremental implementation, it has been noted to be a significantly consequential achievement in reducing the number of uninsured Americans (Dillon, 2021).
- The ACA has been described as "consumer friendly" with coordination and seamless transition between programs as the goal, with exchanges given the power to remove insurers who abuse the system or provide inadequate service. Coordination between insurance exchanges, Medicaid, and CHIP provides for better coverage (MACPAC, n.d.).

The ACA encourages comprehensive case management of chronic disease as one way to decrease hospitalizations and the cost of care. Another component of the ACA, the Patient-Centered Outcomes Research Institute (PCORI) provides additional information on effectiveness of treatments and interventions, and the Innovation Center at CMS develops, evaluates, and tests new programs and policies that reduce cost and enhance care for Medicaid and Medicare patients (CMS, 2023a; Hoagland & Parekh, 2019; PCORI, n.d.). Improved value and quality outcomes are the proposed benefits of these programs. For a summary of the ACA, see http://kff.org/health-reform/fact-sheet/summary-of-the-affordable-care-act/.

Finally, with the lack of quality health outcomes in the United States, as described above, even if everyone received health insurance, how could quality be assured? Some believe that the overall performance of the healthcare system should improve as everyone gains access to care. Medicare currently has three programs that incentivize hospitals to provide higher quality care: The Hospital Value-Based Purchasing Program, the Hospital-Acquired Conditions Reduction Program, and the Hospital Readmissions Reduction Program (HRRP) (Yakusheva et al., 2022). A well-performing hospital can earn up to 2% more per Medicare discharge and a poor-performing hospital can lose up to 6%. However, each year, nearly 75% of hospitals are penalized for low performance by at least one of the three programs. Another factor that may also improve outcomes is a means of providing healthcare consumers with pertinent, timely information so that they can be more active participants in their care.

EFFECTS OF HEALTH ECONOMICS ON COMMUNITY/PUBLIC HEALTH PRACTICE

Health economics has significantly affected community/public health practice by advancing disincentives for efficient use of resources, incentives for illness care, and conflicts with public health values.

Overcoming Disincentives for the Efficient Use of Resources

Public health has been affected in several ways. The trend of diminished federal and state allocations has had profound effects on community/public health programs, and severe budget cuts have affected even basic public health services, especially during the coronavirus pandemic.

Public health agencies and providers in Accountable Care Organizations are joining together for initiatives to improve quality along with cutting costs (e.g., Triple Aim, outcome accountable care). Public health professionals can offer their expertise in community assessment and design of population-based interventions. The 6/18 initiative follows the format of promoting population health by accelerating collaborative partnerships to implement 18 evidence-based interventions that target 6 "common and costly health conditions" in a community-integrated healthcare program (CDC, 2018, para 1).

Managed Care and the Future of Public Health

Initially, managed care focused on event-driven cost avoidance (e.g., decreasing inpatient days and specialty primary provider use, using primary provider extenders) (Mendelson, 2019). This evolved into a second stage, in which the principal objective was to control resource intensity and improve the delivery process. Now, emphasis has shifted to a focus on health promotion and population health. Community assessments are an important part of this approach, so that high-risk groups can be identified and provided early interventions (CDC, 2024).

- Community health assessments could become standard quality tools for not only public health interventions but also healthcare in general. The ACA requires hospitals to conduct regular community assessments, and many have partnered with LHDs to do so (Allan & Lakey, n.d.). This provides an opportunity for the collaborative partnerships needed to improve population health and reach more community members.
- Healthcare reform legislation includes a requirement for community needs assessment every 3 years for state-licensed, tax-exempt health organizations such as hospitals and imposes a $50,000 annual penalty if this is not done. Prioritization of health needs and a description of community resources are to be included, as is input from those with expertise in public health (Lopez et al., 2021).
- While hospitals are required by the ACA to complete community health assessments, more research is needed to discover if intervention programs have been implemented to improve population health as a result (Lopez et al., 2021). See Chapter 15 for more on Community Assessment.

Improving the health status of a community mandates that healthcare agencies be actively involved in health teaching and health promotion, as well as developing community action plans to promote collaboration and focus on early intervention and treatment to improve health equity and health outcomes (NASEM, 2017). These are the proposals that public health advocates have been making for more than a century.

By partnering with hospitals on community assessment and research, these things, along with public health accreditation, may further improve the public health system (Yeager et al., 2020).

- Naik et al. (2019) described macro trends that will influence the future of public health. These include promoting employment and improving working conditions and regulating tobacco, alcohol, and food.
- The influences of Health in All Policies (described in Chapters 13 and 16), informatics and social media, demographic trends (e.g., increased older and racial/underrepresented populations), and global travel will encourage C/PHNs to become more adept in these areas in order to meet the needs of their clients and communities. However, across the country, there is a decline in recruitment and retention of C/PHNs, making it difficult to meet the coming challenges (Pittman & Park, 2021). Indeed, the decline in C/PHNs has been faster than the decline in other professions involved in public health work.
- Public Health 3.0 is an initiative promoted by the USDHHS (n.d.-b) and amplified by leaders in the field of public health (Balio et al., 2019).
  - Eight "strategic skill domains" were identified: "effective communication, data for decision

making, cultural competence, budget and financial management, change management, systems and strategic thinking, developing a vision for a healthy community, and cross-sector partnerships" (Resnick et al., 2019, p. 10).

Frieden (2015) called upon public health to join with clinical medicine, government agencies, health NGOs, private sector groups, and our communities to make our population healthier. The author shared a powerful example from the United Kingdom.

- Knowing that decreasing sodium intake would have great benefits for health outcomes (reduced hypertension, stroke, heart attacks), but recognizing that individual efforts are difficult due to the use of processed foods, the government partnered with the food industry to cut sodium in breakfast cereals by 57% and bread by 20%, along with many other foods.
- This caused a drop in the population average for sodium intake by 15% over 8 years and a 40% reduction in heart attack deaths and a 42% drop in strokes.

IMPLICATIONS FOR COMMUNITY/PUBLIC HEALTH NURSING

Kub et al. (2017) estimated that there were more than 47,000 public health nurses working in federal, state, and local public health agencies. This number has likely decreased since that time (Pittman, 2021). A large number of nurses also work in educational community organizations. Together, they strive to promote and protect the health of people, families, and populations.

C/PHNs have had to adapt to a constantly changing system. They need the ability to assist their clients in accessing programs and services. Some of your clients may be able to access healthcare services through your LHD (e.g., immunizations, school physicals), but others may need help in finding some type of health insurance to help pay for private healthcare services. Where do you begin? You will need the following information:

- What type of care is needed (e.g., primary provider, specialist)?
- Who needs the care (e.g., child, older adult, family)?
- Employment/finances (e.g., unemployed/laid off, intermittent or steady employment without health insurance/income level, sources of income)?

See Box 6-6 for online resources for accessing programs and services.

Nurses working within the public health system have, for a long time, developed innovative modes of service delivery (Muir, 2019). Some recent examples of innovation are as follows:

- The Sonoma County (California) Field Nursing Team developed the Trauma Informed Approach in Public Health Nursing (TIA PHN) Home Visiting program to meet the needs of clients who do not qualify for other programs, such as Nurse Family Partnership (Ballard et al., 2019). The model acknowledges parental exposure to Adverse Childhood Experiences (ACEs), with a goal of mitigating toxic stress, improving resilience, and optimizing health among families at high risk for trauma and experiencing medical or social challenges (Ballard et al., 2022).
- PHNs created an RN-led wellness clinic to serve people who are incarcerated currently in community correctional centers (these facilities lack on-site medical services that would be found in prisons), providing chronic disease management, healthcare navigation, and health education (Johnson et al., 2023).

Nurses in Portland, Oregon, established a "nurse-owned and fully nurse-operated" primary care clinic serving people experiencing homelessness (Fox et al., 2022, p. 1115). The "clinic attributes much of its success to registered nurses and nurse practitioners operating at the top of their scope of practice" (p. 1115).

Utilizing collaborative skills and knowledge of their communities, PHNs can continue to work with partners to meet the challenges of Public Health 3.0 and provide services needed for the vulnerable populations in our future healthcare system (Harmon et al., 2020).

BOX 6-6 Online Resources for Accessing Programs and Services

Basic Information on Paying for Medical Care and Prescriptions

- https://www.usa.gov/paying-for-medical
- https://www.verywellhealth.com/how-to-get-help-paying-for-health-insurance-1738500
- https://www.thebalance.com/save-money-health-care-insurance-4124456
- https://www.livestrong.org/we-can-help/insurance-and-financial-assistance/health-care-assistance-for-uninsured

Information Based on Income Levels

- If incomes are low, check for Medicaid and CHIP eligibility at https://www.healthcare.gov/medicaid-chip/getting-medicaid-chip/
- For those with higher-income levels, check your state's health insurance marketplace at:
  - https://www.healthcare.gov/apply-and-enroll/get-help-applying/
  - https://www.npr.org/sections/health-shots/2020/04/03/826316458/coronavirus-reset-how-to-get-health-insurance-now

Information for Older Adults

- https://www.nia.nih.gov/health/paying-care
- https://www.payingforseniorcare.com/homecare/paying-for-home-care
- https://www.caring.com/senior-living/nursing-homes/how-to-pay/

SUMMARY

- Many factors and events have influenced the current structure, function, and financing of community/public health services. Understanding this background gives the C/PHN a stronger base for planning for population health.
- Historically, healthcare has progressed unevenly, marked by numerous influences. The Middle Ages saw a serious health decline in Europe, with raging epidemics leading to extensive 19th century reform efforts in England and, later, in the United States.
- Public health problems prompted the gradual development of official interventions. Quarantines to control the spread of communicable disease, sanitary reforms, and establishment of public health departments were discussed.
- By the early 1900s, the federal government had assumed a more active role in public health, with a proliferation of health, education, and welfare services.
- Efforts to address community/public health needs have been made by public agencies and private individuals. They work together to promote an emerging healthcare system.
    - The public arm includes all government, tax-supported health agencies and occurs at local, state, national, and international levels. A different structure and set of functions are found at each level.
        - Public health services include three core public health functions: assessment, policy development, and assurance.
        - Inadequate funding has been problematic for the public health system, especially during the recent pandemic.
    - Private health services are the unofficial arm. They include voluntary nonprofit agencies as well as privately owned (proprietary) and for-profit agencies. They often supplement and complement the work of official agencies.
- The delivery and financing of community/public health services have been significantly affected by various legislative acts.
    - These include such innovations as health insurance and assistance for people who are older, have a disability, or have a low income; money to train health personnel and conduct health research; standards for health planning and delivery; health protection for workers on the job; and the financing of health services.
- Healthcare economics studies the production, distribution, and consumption of healthcare goods and services to maximize the use of scarce resources to benefit the most people.
    - The healthcare system is influenced by microeconomics (supply and demand) as well as macroeconomics.
- Healthcare is funded through public and private sources, which fall into three categories: third-party payers, direct consumer payment, and private support. Healthcare services have been reimbursed either retrospectively, typical of FFS plans, or prospectively, typical of most managed care plans.
- Several trends and issues have influenced community/public healthcare financing and delivery, including cost control, financial access, managed care, healthcare rationing, competition and regulation, managed competition, universal coverage, calls for a single-payer system, and healthcare reform.
- The changing nature of healthcare financing has adversely affected community/public health by promoting incentives to focus on illness care, and the competition model has generated a conflict with the basic public health values of health promotion and disease prevention for all persons.
- Healthcare reform has reduced the number of uninsured Americans, but access for many people is still difficult.
    - The United States remains the only industrialized nation without some type of universal health coverage.
    - It also ranks significantly lower than most other developed countries on health indicators, such as infant mortality and life expectancy, and we spend the highest percentage of GDP on healthcare.
- C/PHNs can lead the effort in making healthcare more accessible to all citizens and encourage policies and practices that promote health. C/PHNs should prepare for future changes in public health.

ACTIVE LEARNING EXERCISES

1. Explain how social, economic (e.g., Great Depression), political (e.g., WWII), and legislative actions have shaped our current healthcare system, public health system, policies, and practices. Give examples of legislation or policy that incorporates each of the three core public health functions (assessment, policy, and assurance) and identify which of the 10 Essential Public Health Services (see Box 2-2) are implicated. (Objectives 1 and 2)
2. Describe an everyday life example of supply and demand. Summarize three exceptions to the law of supply and demand in healthcare economics. How can this promote rising healthcare costs? Form two teams and debate the advantages and disadvantages of managed competition as opposed to mandatory universal coverage. (Objective 3)
3. Compare the United States with other similar countries. Where do we rank in spending on healthcare? Identify five measures (e.g., life expectancy) in which the United States has more negative outcomes. What healthcare system approach, that is common in all other high-income countries, does the United States lack? What are the advantages and disadvantages of a single-payer system? Debate

with a classmate if further healthcare reform is feasible in the United States. What is the most efficient way of ensuring universal coverage, as evidenced by examples from other countries outlined in this chapter? (Objective 4)

4. Debate the pros and cons of universal healthcare. Describe three key potential benefits and the three most serious potential negative consequences. Talk with your classmates and other students at your university about their access to healthcare and if they have some type of health insurance. If they do not, explore the reasons for this. Does your campus have a student health center? What services are offered there? What are the average costs to students? (Objective 5)
5. Interview two consumers about their perception of the problems and strengths of our healthcare system. What are their thoughts and feelings about our current healthcare system and availability of health insurance? Have they, or others they know, had problems with healthcare or health insurance coverage during the pandemic? Select people who represent distinctly different age groups and life situations, such as a single 25-year-old parent of three children making minimum wage and a 75-year-old person whose spouse has passed away; compare and contrast their responses. (Objective 6)

CHAPTER 7

Epidemiology in the Community*

"Epidemiology dates back to the Age of Pericles in 5th Century B.C., but its standing as a 'true' science in [the] 21st century is often questioned. This is unexpected, given that epidemiology directly impacts lives and our reliance on it will only increase in a changing world."

—Epidemiology is a science of high importance [Editorial]. (2018). *Nature Communications, 9*(1703), 1–2.

KEY TERMS

Causal matrix
Causality
Chain of causation
Endemic
Epidemic
Epidemiologic triangle
Epidemiology
Immunity
Incidence
Morbidity rate
Mortality rate
Natural history
Pandemic
Prevalence study
Reservoir
Risk
Vectors
Web of causation

LEARNING OBJECTIVES

Upon mastery of this chapter, you should be able to:

1. Discuss key highlights of the history of epidemiology.
2. Apply the epidemiologic triangle (host, agent, and environment model) to a common public health problem.
3. Describe theories of causality in health and illness.
4. Define immunity and compare and contrast passive, active, cross-, hybrid, and herd immunity.
5. Explain how epidemiologists determine populations at risk.
6. Describe sources of information for epidemiologic study, including existing data, informational observational studies, and scientific studies.
7. Discuss the types of epidemiologic studies that are useful for researching aggregate health and the process for conducting epidemiologic research.

INTRODUCTION

Epidemiology is the scientific discipline that seeks to describe, quantify, and determine how diseases occur in populations and aid in developing methods of controlling those diseases (Friis, 2018). The term is derived from the "Greek words *epi* (upon), *demos* (the people), and *logy* (study of)"; the knowledge or study of what happens to people (Friis, 2018, p. 6).

Purposes of epidemiology include the following:

- To examine determinants and distribution of diseases, disabilities, morbidity, and mortality, as well as health
- To provide a body of knowledge through research on which to base practice and methods for studying new and existing problems
- To provide C/PHNs with a methodology for assessing the health of aggregates
- To offer a frame of reference for investigating and improving clinical practice in any setting

Characteristics of epidemiology include the following:

- Is data driven
- Relies on an unbiased and systematic approach to collecting, analyzing, and interpreting data

*In this chapter, "male" means a person assigned male at birth, and "female" means a person assigned female at birth.

- Draws on methods and principles from biostatistics, informatics, biology, and the social, economic, and behavioral sciences

Epidemiologists are considered "disease detectives" as they search for causes of illness and outbreak (Centers for Disease Control and Prevention [CDC], 2023a). Epidemiologists ask such questions as:

- What is the occurrence of health and disease in a population?
- Has there been an increase or decrease in the state of health over the years?
- Does one geographic area have a higher frequency of disease than another?
- What characteristics of people with a particular condition distinguish them from those without the condition?
- What factors need to be present to cause disease or injury?
- Is one treatment or program more effective than another in changing the health of affected people?
- Why do some people recover from a disease and others do not?

As an example of epidemiology serving as a frame of reference, imagine that a county health department public health nurse's (PHN's) goal is to lower the incidence of sexually transmitted diseases (also referred to as sexually transmitted infections [STIs]) in a given community. Such a prevention plan would require information about population groups. The nurse would need to ask questions such as:

- How many STI cases have been reported in this community over the past year? What percentage of these are drug resistant (e.g., drug-resistant gonorrhea)?
- What is the expected number of STI cases (the morbidity rate)?
- Which members of the community are at highest risk for contracting STIs?

In fact, to be effective, any program of screening, treatment, or health promotion regarding STIs must be based on this kind of information about population groups.

Whether the PHN's goals are to improve a population's nutrition, control the spread of tuberculosis (TB), deal with health problems created by a flood, protect and promote the health of people experiencing intimate partner violence, or reduce the number of automobile crash injuries and fatalities at a specific intersection, epidemiologic data are essential.

HOW EPIDEMIOLOGY SUPPORTS THE 10 ESSENTIAL PUBLIC HEALTH SERVICES

- Assessment
  - *Monitor Health:* by gathering vital and disease statistics to provide data necessary to define the scope of disease and health and visually trend disease spread
  - *Diagnose and Investigate:* by providing population health and disease data to determine whether new diseases are spreading into new segments of the population and providing the basis for launching epidemiologic investigations
- Policy Development
  - *Inform, Educate, and Empower:* by providing statistical reports of the status of disease spread, investigations, and their progress so policymakers can inform and educate the public about health factors and empower the public to address them
  - *Mobilize Community Partnerships:* by sharing community epidemiologic data so stakeholders can collaborate in addressing health issues that affect their constituents
  - *Develop Policies:* by providing health data to community planning agencies and organizations so policymakers can develop more informed strategies to address issues affecting the community
- Assurance
  - *Evaluate:* by providing population health data that can be used as objective measures to evaluate the effectiveness of health programs in reducing morbidity and mortality (CDC, 2023b)

HISTORICAL ROOTS OF EPIDEMIOLOGY

Most of the early contributions to epidemiology were made by primary providers who sought the cause of disease through methodical observation and conducting experiments to test their theories of new treatment methodologies. The work of these primary providers formed the basic concepts that served as a foundation for the science of epidemiology.

Early Primary Provider–Epidemiologists

The roots of epidemiology can be traced to Hippocrates (460–375 BCE), a Greek primary provider who is sometimes referred to as the first epidemiologist.

Hippocrates:

- Explained disease occurrences from a rational, rather than a supernatural, viewpoint.
- In his essay, "On Airs, Waters, and Places," suggested that environmental and host factors (e.g., lifestyle behaviors) influence disease development (Bryant & Rhodes, 2023).
- Introduced observations of how diseases spread and affect populations.
- Considered diseases in relation to time and season, place, environmental conditions, and disease control.

Table 7-1 summarizes the contributions of the early primary provider–epidemiologists to the field of public health. Figure 7-1 shows an example of a spot map early epidemiologist John Snow used in tracking cholera cases.

Florence Nightingale: Nurse Epidemiologist

Nursing's epidemiologic roots can be traced to Florence Nightingale (1820–1910). Named after the Italian

TABLE 7-1 Physician–Epidemiologists—Their Contributions to Epidemiology

Physician–Epidemiologist	Contribution to Epidemiology
Thomas Sydenham (1624–1689)	Importance of close observations of disease. Classified London's fevers of 1660s and 1670s. Advocated for exercise, fresh air, and healthy diet as treatments and remedies.
James Lind (1716–1794)	Used clinical observations and experimental design to identify the effect of diet on disease. Identified scurvy among British naval seamen that was effectively addressed by eating oranges and limes. This practice gave rise to the use of the term "limeys" for British seamen.
Edward Jenner (1749–1823)	Based on observations and experiments by Benjamin Jesty, a farmer/dairyman, Jenner invented a vaccine for smallpox. Dairymaids never got smallpox but did get cowpox from the cows they milked. He theorized that getting cowpox would protect one from developing smallpox.
Ignaz Semmelweis (1818–1865)	As clinical director of the Viennese Maternity Hospital in the mid-1800s, he observed many patients die from childbed (puerperal) fever shortly after giving birth. Based on an introspective study and maternal death data, he concluded that these deaths were due to bacterial contamination from doctors who didn't wash their hands before conducting pelvic examinations on postpartum patients after performing autopsies of infected and decaying bodies. Semmelweis instituted the use of chlorinated lime in handwashing between patient examinations. As a result, maternal deaths dropped to 1.3% in 1848 from a high of 12.1% in 1842.
John Snow (1813–1858)	Approaches, concepts, and methods used to identify the cause of cholera in 1800s London were his greatest contributions to the field of epidemiology. He conducted a descriptive epidemiologic investigation of a cholera outbreak in London's Soho district and an analytic epidemiologic investigation of a cholera epidemic by comparing death rates of those getting their water from either the Lambeth Water Company or the Southward and Vauxhall Water Company. His spot (or dot) mapping of cholera cases plotted where cholera deaths were occurring, which helped to characterize when the epidemic started, peaked, and subsided. The removal of the handle from the Broad Street pump (so people could not get water from that public water pump) was the control measure that finally stopped the epidemic. Because of Snow's many contributions to epidemiology, he became known as the Father of Epidemiology (see Figs. 7-1 and 7-2).

Source: Merrill (2021).

city she was born in, Nightingale advocated training in science, strict discipline, attention to cleanliness, and the development of empathy for patients.

She also established a nursing school at London's St. Thomas Hospital and is commonly referred to as "The Lady with the Lamp," a designation given to her by soldiers during the Crimean War (1854–1856) as she ministered to them during the night. The unsanitary conditions at the army base hospital at Scutari in Constantinople (now known as Istanbul) shocked her into campaigning to improve the quality of nursing in military hospitals.

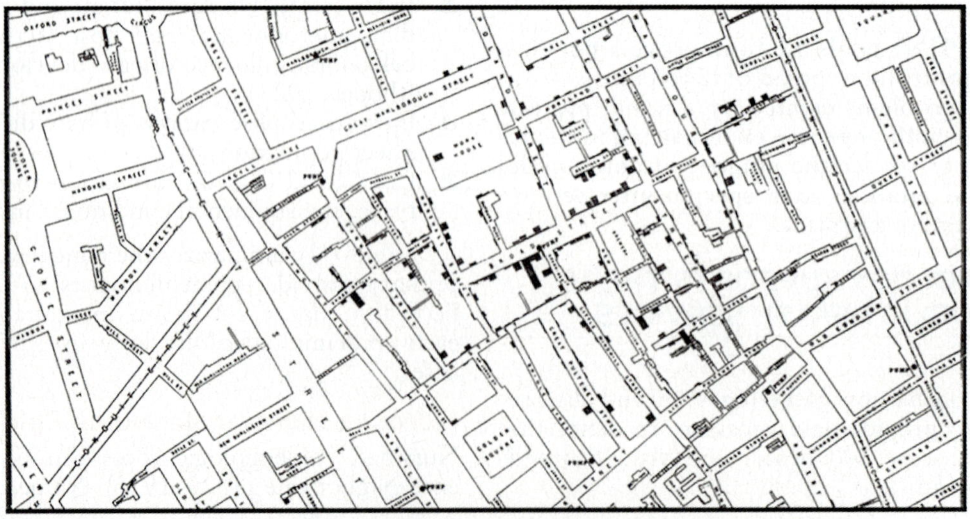

FIGURE 7-1 Map of cholera cases in Soho, London, 1854. (Source: Wikimedia Commons. https://blogs.cdc.gov/publichealthmatters/2017/03/a-legacy-of-disease-detectives/)

Queen Victoria recognized Nightingale's contributions to nursing and epidemiology. She was awarded the highest civilian medal, the Order of Merit, and was the first woman to receive it (The National Archives, n.d.).

Her contributions include the following:

- Monitoring disease *mortality rates* to improve hospital sanitary methods that decreased death rates
- Using a research perspective to conducting systematic descriptive studies of the distribution and patterns of disease in a population (detailed records and descriptions of health conditions, morbidity [sickness] statistics)
- Using applied statistical methods to visualize data (shaded and colored wedge-shaped graphs) as a new way to improve medical and surgical practices
- Using published statistical reports to gain the attention of politicians and powerful people (e.g., William Farr) to bring about hospital and public health reforms that created changes in hygiene and overall treatment of patients (Schiotz, 2015)

Nightingale's contributions to nursing are further explored in Chapter 3.

Eras in the Evolution of Modern Epidemiology

Modern epidemiology can be described as having four distinct eras, each based on causal thinking: (1) sanitary statistics, (2) infectious disease epidemiology, (3) chronic disease epidemiology, and (4) eco-epidemiology. Table 7-2 summarizes these four eras in the evolution of modern epidemiology. Below, each is described in detail.

Sanitary Statistics

Early causal thinking was dominated by the *miasma theory*, which had its origins in the work of the Hippocratic School and was formally developed in the early 1700s. This theory held that a substance called *miasma* was composed of malodorous and poisonous particles generated by the decomposition of organic matter and was the cause of disease. Prevention based on this theory attempted to eliminate the sources of the miasma or polluted vapors.

Despite the faulty reasoning, this type of prevention had positive consequences because it made people aware that decaying organic matter can be a source of infectious diseases. This theory dominated until the first half of the 19th century, when environmental sources and the idea that sanitary conditions were linked to disease led John Snow to identify the source of cholera (Tulchinsky, 2018).

Infectious Disease Epidemiology

The era of *infectious disease epidemiology* was dominated by the *contagion theory of disease*, which developed during the mid-19th century. Due to development of increasingly sophisticated microscopes, this theory attempted to identify the microorganisms that cause diseases as a first step in prevention. It inspired various theories of immunity and even prompted some initial attempts at vaccination against smallpox.

Additionally, once an agent had been identified, measures were taken to contain its spread. Fumigating ships to kill rats, protecting wharf buildings and human habitations from rats, and removing rat food supplies from easy access were all measures taken to protect the public by further preventing the spread of plague bacilli. Based on the work of Louis Pasteur, Jakob Henle, and Robert Koch (Box 7-1), the contagion theory was refined and became best known as the *germ theory of disease*, which was predominant from the late 19th century through the first half of the 20th century (Merrill, 2021; Seabert et al., 2021; Tulchinsky, 2018).

In the era of *infectious disease epidemiology*, scientists viewed disease in terms of a simple cause-and-effect relationship. Finding a single cause (e.g., plague bacilli) and attacking it (e.g., eliminating rats) seemed to be the solution for preventing many diseases. In the case of bubonic plague, this approach appeared to be quite effective (Merrill, 2021).

However, scientific research eventually revealed that disease causation was much more complex than first suspected. For example, although most members of a group might be exposed to the plague, many did not contract it. With bubonic plague, as with many other infectious diseases, host characteristics can determine both the spread

TABLE 7-2 Eras in the Evolution of Modern Epidemiology

Era	Paradigm	Analytic Approach	Prevention Approach
Sanitary statistics (1800–1850)	Miasma: poisoning from foul emanations	Clustering of morbidity and mortality	Drainage, sewage, sanitation
Infectious disease epidemiology (1850–1950)	Germ theory: single agent related to specific disease	Laboratory isolation and culture from disease sites and experimental transmission/reproduction of lesions	Interrupt transmission (vaccines, isolation, and antibiotics)
Chronic disease epidemiology (1950–2000)	Exposure related to outcome	Risk ratio of exposure to outcome at person level in populations	Control risk factors by modifying lifestyle (diet), agent (guns), or environment (pollution)
Eco-epidemiology (2000–present)	Ecological influences on human health: molecular, societal, and population-based	Analysis using new information systems and biomedical techniques	Modifying molecular, societal, and population factors

Source: Susser and Susser (1996a, 1996b); Susser and Stein (2009).

BOX 7-1 Koch's Postulates

1. The microorganism must be observed in every case of the disease.
2. It must be isolated and grown in pure culture.
3. The pure culture must, when inoculated into a susceptible animal, reproduce the disease.
4. The microorganism must be observed in, and recovered from, the experimentally diseased animal.

Source: King, L. S. (1952). Dr. Koch's postulates. *Journal of Historical Medicine*, 350–361. As cited in Friis, R. H., & Sellers, T. A. (2021). *Epidemiology for public health practice* (6th ed.). Jones and Bartlett Learning.

of the disease and its individual impact. Lessons learned from the bubonic plague include the following:

- Not everyone in a population is at equal risk; it is now known that untreated bubonic plague has a case fatality rate of 40% to 70%, meaning that about half of those who contract the disease and are not treated will eventually die.
- The agent and course of transmission can be quite complex. Although a flea carries the bacilli from rats to humans in bubonic plague, many infectious diseases spread directly from one human being to another.
- The environment must be considered as part of the cause of disease. Evidence suggests that the plague originated in the high plains of Asia and spread to other parts of the world. However, questions remain as to whether the bacillus spread from rats to ground squirrels or had always been part of the squirrels' ecology (CDC, 2021a).

After World War II, the causative agents of major infectious diseases were identified, methods of prevention were recognized, and antibiotics were added to the arsenal to fight communicable diseases.

Chronic Disease Epidemiology

The focus then became understanding and controlling the new chronic disease epidemics, ushering in the era of *chronic disease epidemiology*. Researchers completed case–control and cohort studies, to be discussed more fully later, that linked the causative factors of cholesterol levels and smoking with coronary heart disease and associated smoking with lung cancer.

According to the CDC, noninfectious diseases are the major causes of mortality in the United States (Fig. 7-2). Heart disease and cancer are the leading causes of death for those 45 years and older, while unintentional injuries are the main causes of death for those younger. In 2020,

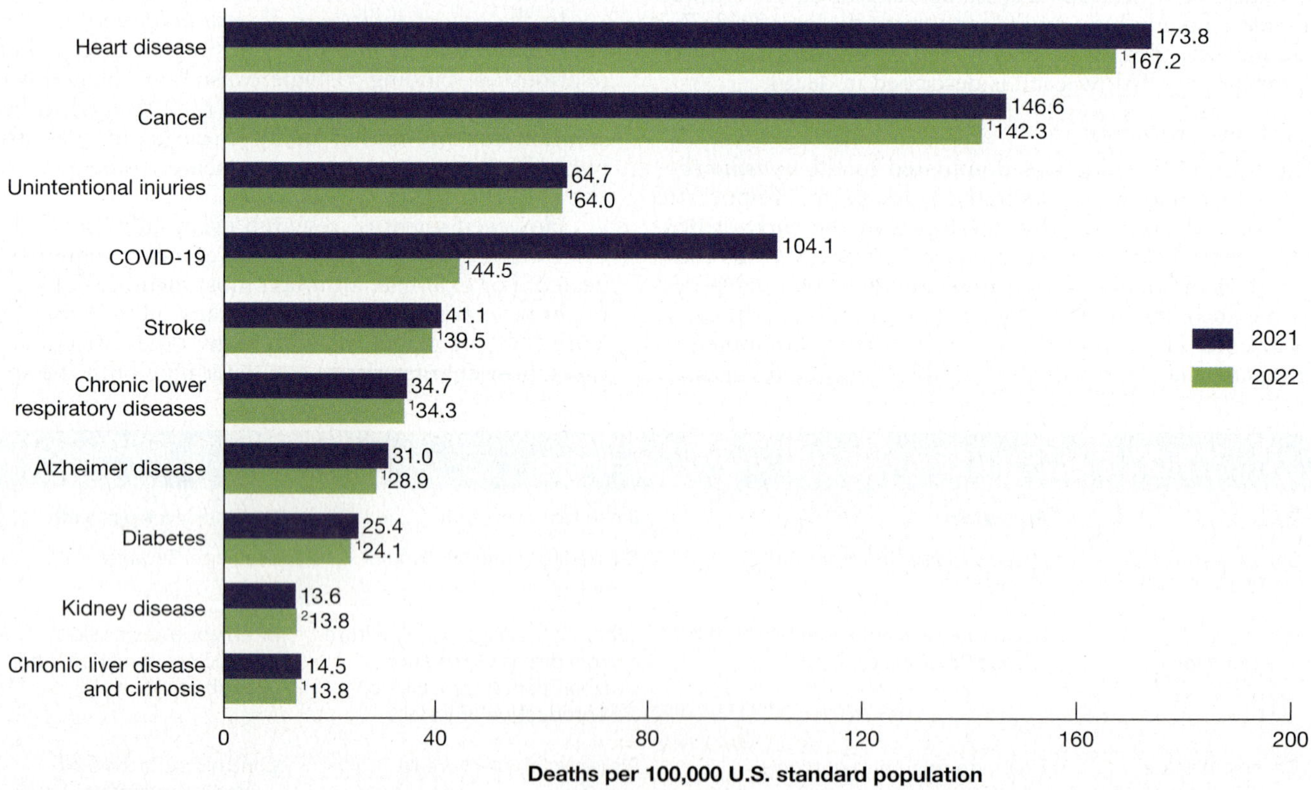

[1]Statistically significant decrease from 2021 to 2022 ($p < 0.05$).
[2]Statistically significant increase from 2021 to 2022 ($p < 0.05$).
NOTES: A total of 3,279,857 resident deaths were registered in the United States in 2022. The 10 leading causes of death accounted for 72.3% of all U.S. deaths in 2022. Causes of death are ranked according to number of deaths. Rankings for 2021 data are not shown. Data table for Figure 4 includes the number of deaths for leading causes and the percentage of total deaths. Access data table for Figure 4 at: https://www.cdc.gov/nchs/data/databriefs/db492-tables.pdf#4.
SOURCE: National Center for Health Statistics, National Vital Statistics System, mortality data file.

FIGURE 7-2 Age-adjusted death rate for the 10 leading causes of death in the United States, 2021 and 2022. (Reprinted from Centers for Disease Control and Prevention. (March 2024). https://www.cdc.gov/nchs/products/databriefs/db492.htm#section_4)

COVID-19 became the third leading cause of death for those 45 years and older. See more in Chapters 21 and 22.

Eco-epidemiology

We are now in the new era of *eco-epidemiology*, distinguished by transforming global health patterns and technological advances. New and emerging global infections, such as the COVID-19 pandemic in 2020, are now a concern, as is the spread of medication-resistant diseases (see more in Chapters 8, 9, and 16). The West Nile virus (WNV), sudden acute respiratory syndrome (SARS), influenza A (H1N1), multidrug-resistant TB, HIV, Zika, and Ebola virus disease illustrate this transformation.

In most cases, causative organisms and critical **risk** factors are known, yet diseases occur, spread, and suddenly appear in countries or regions previously free of them (Abubakar et al., 2016; Bain & Awah, 2014). For example, we know how to prevent the transmission of HIV, yet 1.5 million new cases worldwide were reported in 2021 (HIV.gov, 2022). How can preventive practices be promoted among populations at risk for communicable diseases? The same situation is true for many current chronic diseases. For instance, how many nurses smoke? Do you exercise as often as you know you should? Do you know your cholesterol level and eat healthy foods? Do you regularly use sunscreen? What are we missing to effectively change social behaviors? See Chapter 11.

Technological developments drive research, primarily in biology and biomedical techniques and in information system capabilities. The science of *genetics* is useful in modern *epidemiology*. For example, *genetic influence* in some cases of insulin-dependent diabetes is linked to human leukocyte antigens, and particular combinations of this gene variant can predict risk of type 1 diabetes, whereas other combinations either cause no problems or may be protective (American Diabetes Association, 2023). HIV, TB, and other infections can be tracked from person to person through identifying the molecular specificity of the organisms.

Among people assigned female at birth, in the general population about 13% will develop breast cancer sometime during their lives, whereas 55% to 72% who inherit a harmful *BRCA1* mutation and 45% to 69% who inherit a harmful *BRCA2* mutation will develop breast cancer by the age of 80 years. Among people assigned female at birth, in the general population about 1.2% will develop ovarian cancer sometime during their lives, whereas 39% to 44% who inherit a harmful *BRCA1* mutation and 11% to 17% who inherit a harmful *BRCA2* mutation will develop ovarian cancer by the age of 70 to 80 years (National Cancer Institute [NCI], 2020).

On a broader scale, using new technology, we can examine the *geographic distribution of* disease and correlate those data with other important health risks. For instance, using these geocoding systems, overweight and obesity in children can be correlated with other factors, such as after-school recreation opportunities, distribution of fast-food restaurants, access to farmer's markets, or socioeconomic status (see Chapter 10 for more on technology in public health). The possibilities of learning through technology have just begun in this current epidemiologic era.

Epidemics

An **epidemic** refers to a disease occurrence that clearly exceeds the normal or expected frequency in a community or region. When an epidemic, such as the bubonic plague (also called pneumonic plague or the Black Death) or HIV/AIDS, is worldwide in distribution, it is known as a **pandemic**. When a disease or infectious agent is continually found in a particular area or population, it is considered to be **endemic** (American Academy of Pediatrics, 2021).

Epidemic and pandemic diseases prompted the development of epidemiology as a science. Epidemiology became a distinct branch of medical science and provides

BOX 7-2 Epidemiology and COVID-19

To control the spread of epidemics or pandemics, the following measures and terminology are useful to consider:

- **The S-I-R model**—This model is a mathematical model of spread that places the population into three categories: (1) "susceptibles"—those who do not have the disease yet; (2) "infectives"—those have contracted the disease; (3) "removed"—those who have had the disease and recovered and are now immune, or those who have died, and no longer spread the disease. The model supports the importance of social isolation of those infected to prevent the spread to those susceptible (Smith & Moore, 2020; Yates, 2020).
- **R_0 (pronounced "R-naught" or "R-zero")**—Whether an outbreak spreads or dies depends on the basic reproduction number. This is the average number of previously unexposed people infected by a single, freshly introduced disease. If a disease has an R_0 less than 1 (each infected person on average gives it to less than one other person), then the infection will die out quickly. The outbreak cannot sustain its own spread. If R_0 is larger than one, then the outbreak will grow exponentially (Yates, 2020).
  - The early estimates of the R_0 for COVID-19 was at least two (varying between 1.5 and 4). This means that the first person with the disease spreads it to two others, who each, on average, is spreading the disease to two others and then to two others each, and so on.
  - The rate at which "susceptibles" become infected (the force of infection) and the rate of recovery or death from the disease can increase the R_0, while increasing recovery rate will reduce it.
  - The bigger the population and the faster the disease spreads between people, the larger the outbreak is likely to be. The quicker people recover, the less time they

(Continued)

BOX 7-2 Epidemiology and COVID-19 (*Continued*)

have to pass on the disease to others and, the easier it will be to bring an outbreak under control.

- The "effective reproduction number" is the average number of secondary infections caused by an infectious person at a given point in the outbreak's progression. If, by intervention, the effective reproduction number can be brought to below one, then the disease will die out (Yates, 2020, para. 19).
- The fraction of the population that needs to be immune to protect the rest depends on how infectious the disease is. The basic reproduction number, R_0, can be used to determine the proportion of the population that will need to be immune. The higher the R_0, the higher the immune proportion of the population needs to be. If the R_0 is 4, then three quarters of the population must be immune. If R_0 is 1.5, then only one third of the population must be immunized to protect the remaining two thirds (Yates, 2020).

- **Case fatality rate**—R_0 does not capture the seriousness of the disease for an infected person. The proportion of infected people who ultimately die from a disease is known as the case fatality rate. A high case fatality rate means that a high number of those who get the disease usually die from the disease. Diseases with high fatality rates are less infectious because those who are ill die quickly, thus reducing the chances of infecting others (Yates, 2020).
  - Early estimates indicate that the case fatality rate of COVID-19 is between 0.25% and 3.5%. This low fatality rate can end up killing more people because more people can become infected from those who are presymptomatic or have mild cases of the disease.
  - Case fatality rates for COVID-19 vary significantly with the age of the patient, with the older adults being worst affected. Older people are more likely to die from COVID-19 than the population as a whole (Yates, 2020).
  - Current estimates of the death rate of COVID-19 found that globally, the case fatality rate for those under age 60 was 1.4%. For those over age 60, it was 4.5%. For hose 80 and over, the case fatality rate was 13.4% (Resnick, 2020).

Source: Resnick (2020); Smith and Moore (2020); Yates (2020).

public health with the tools to investigate disease outbreaks, as well as controlling disease to prevent future outbreaks. Despite hundreds of years of experience with disease outbreaks, new diseases arise all the time, such as COVID-19; see Box 7-2 for its epidemiology and information on its background, transmission, symptoms, and testing. New diseases challenge us to come up with new methods. Eradication would be ideal, but sometimes, it may take a long time, or it may not happen at all. Read about smallpox eradication in Chapter 8.

Historically, as the threat of the great epidemic diseases declined, epidemiologists began to focus on other infectious diseases, such as diphtheria, infant diarrhea, typhoid, TB, and syphilis. According to the World Health Organization data for 2000–2019, noncommunicable diseases make up 7 of the world's top 10 causes of death. The global focus now is on preventing and treating cardiovascular diseases, cancer, diabetes, and chronic respiratory diseases as well as addressing injuries (World Health Organization, 2020).

Opioid Epidemic: A 21st Century Public Health Epidemic

The current, ongoing opioid epidemic is an example of how epidemiology has helped define the scope of the problem and how this knowledge impacts public health policies in addressing the epidemic. Public health surveillance of drug use and drug-related deaths has helped to better define who are most affected by the opioid epidemic.

In mapping drug overdose deaths in the United States for 2020, the number and age-adjusted rates varied by state (Fig. 7-3). Demographic analyses of age-adjusted rate of drug overdose deaths show that between 2001 and 2021, more males died from overdoses than did females (CDC/NCHS, 2022; Fig. 7-4).

Differences in Drug Overdose Deaths

In June 2023, researchers reported that overdose mortality rates for opioids and stimulant drugs were substantially higher in males than in females. There was an increase in drug-related deaths during the COVID-19 pandemic (March 2020 and thereafter) for fentanyl and its analogs and stimulants (methamphetamine, but not heroin), prescription opioids, and methadone. This was due to increases in the distribution of synthetic opioids such as fentanyl and their use to lace other drugs (illicit preparations disguised as prescription opioid analgesics, stimulant medications, or benzodiazepines).

Epidemiologic studies show that males experience greater overdose mortality than do females. This has been attributed to males having a greater propensity for risky behaviors associated with morbidity and mortality, such as speeding while driving.

For specific drugs, and after controlling for the sex-specific rate of drug misuse, the overall rates of drug overdose death by sex assigned at birth from 2020 to 2021 were as follows (Butelman et al., 2023; NIH, 2023):

- **Synthetic opioids (e.g., fentanyl):** 29.0 deaths per 100,000 people for males and 11.1 for females
- **Heroin:** 5.5 deaths per 100,000 people for males and 2.0 for females

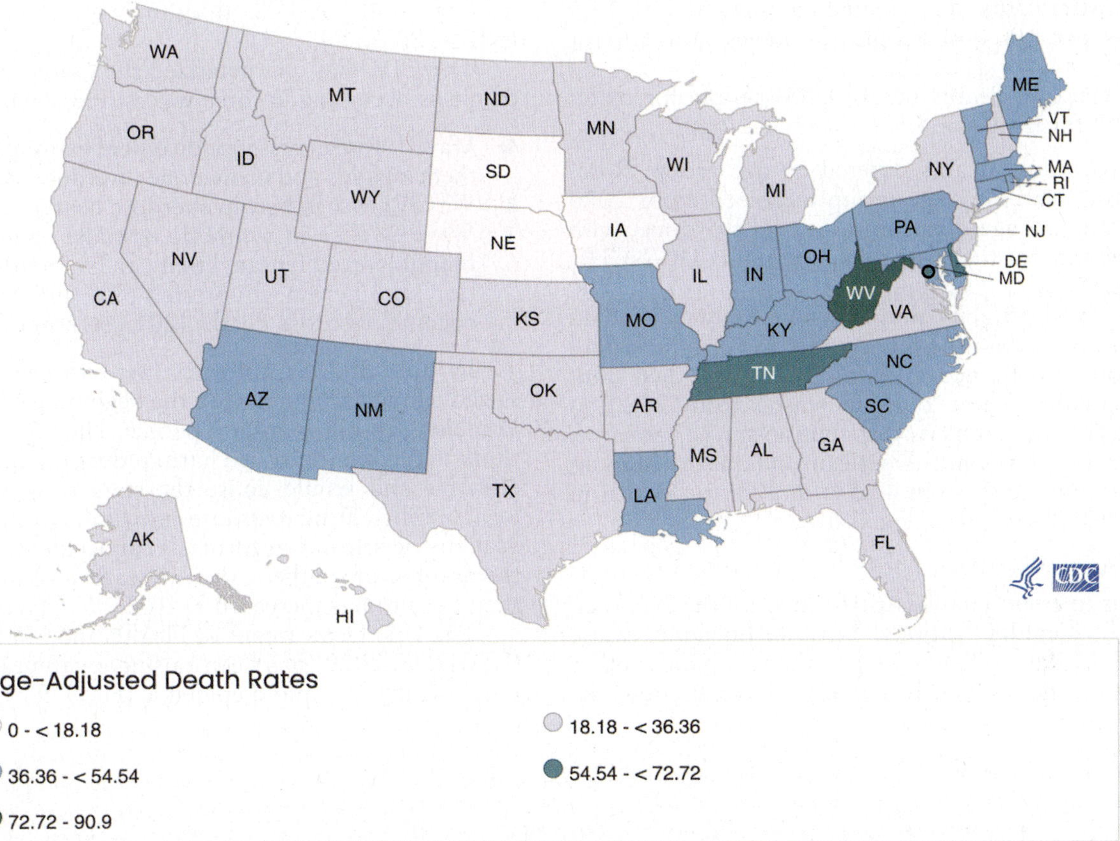

FIGURE 7-3 Drug overdose death rates in 2022: Number and age-adjusted rates of overdose deaths by state. (Reprinted from Centers for Disease Control and Prevention. (March 2022). https://www.cdc.gov/nchs/pressroom/sosmap/drug_poisoning_mortality/drug_poisoning.htm)

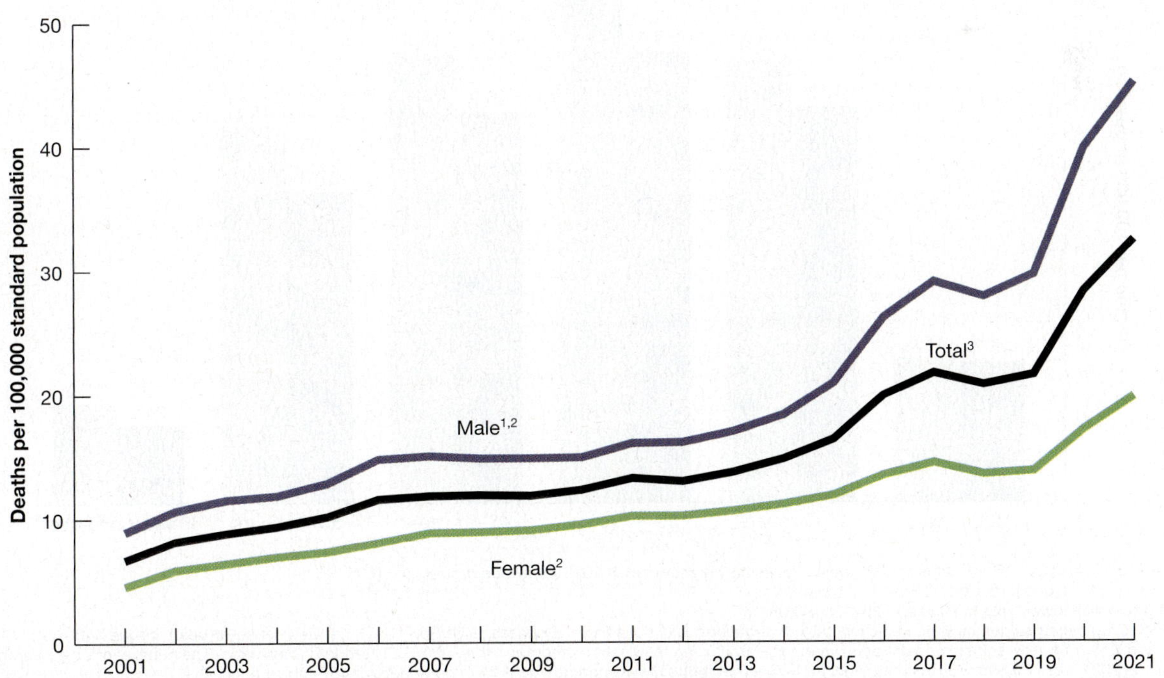

[1]Rate for males is significantly higher than for females for all years, $p < 0.05$.
[2]Significant increasing trend from 2001 through 2021, with different rates of change over time, $p < 0.05$.
[3]Significant increasing trend from 2001 through 2006, stable trend from 2006 through 2013, then significant increasing trend from 2013 through 2021, $p < 0.05$.
NOTES: Drug overdose deaths were identified using *International Classification of Diseases, 10th Revision* underlying cause-of-death codes X40–X44, X60–X64, X85, and Y10–Y14. Age-adjusted death rates were calculated using the direct method and the 2000 U.S. standard population. The number of drug overdose deaths in 2021 was 106,699. Access data table for Figure 1 at: https://www.cdc.gov/nchs/data/databriefs/db457-tables.pdf#1.
SOURCE: National Center for Health Statistics, National Vital Statistics System, Mortality File.

FIGURE 7-4 Age-adjusted rate of drug overdose deaths, by sex assigned at birth. United States, 2001–2021. (Reprinted from Centers for Disease Control and Prevention/National Center for Health Statistics (NCHS). (December 2022). https://www.cdc.gov/nchs/products/databriefs/db457.htm)

- **Psychostimulants (e.g., methamphetamine):** 13.0 deaths per 100,000 people for males and 5.6 for females
- **Cocaine:** 10.6 deaths per 100,000 people for males and 4.2 for females

Drug overdose deaths differed by age group. Rates of overdose deaths by age group increased from 2020 to 2021, but the age distribution stayed the same, with the highest rate for the 35 to 44 age group (CDC/NCHS, 2022; Fig. 7-5).

By race and ethnicity, non-Hispanic American Indian or Alaska Native had the highest rate for drug overdose deaths, followed by non-Hispanic Black and then non-Hispanic White. These rates increased from 2020 to 2021, but the race/ethnicity distribution stayed the same. Rates for non-Hispanic American Indian or Alaskan Native rose the most, from 42.5% in 2020 to 56.6% in 2021 (CDC/NCHS, 2022; Fig. 7-6).

Opioid Overdose Waves

According to trend analyses performed by the National Institute of Health's National Institute on Drug Abuse (NIH/NIDA) for 1999–2021, synthetic opioids other than methadone (primarily fentanyl) have become the leading cause of U.S. drug-involved overdose deaths (NIDA, 2023; Fig. 7-7).

The CDC has characterized the opioid overdose epidemic as occurring in three waves (Fig. 7-8).

- Wave 1: Rise in prescription opioid (natural and semisynthetic opioids and methadone) overdose deaths (1990s)
- Wave 2: Rise in heroin overdose deaths (2010 to now)
- Wave 3: Rise in synthetic opioids, involving illicitly manufactured fentanyl that can be found in combination with heroin, counterfeit pills, and contributed to cocaine overdose deaths (2013 to now)

In June 2023, California law enforcement officials seized enough fentanyl since the beginning of May, in San Francisco, to kill 2 million people. The governor did not think that community-led harm reduction initiatives were effective and would cause the state to bear significant legal liability. Drug overdoses now kill two to three times as many people in California as car accidents. Since 2017, the number of synthetic opioid deaths (50 times stronger than heroin) has increased by 1027% (Clayton, 2023).

The U.S. Department of Health and Human Services (USDHHS, 2022) has been raising awareness about fentanyl fueling the opioid epidemic (Fig. 7-9). The National

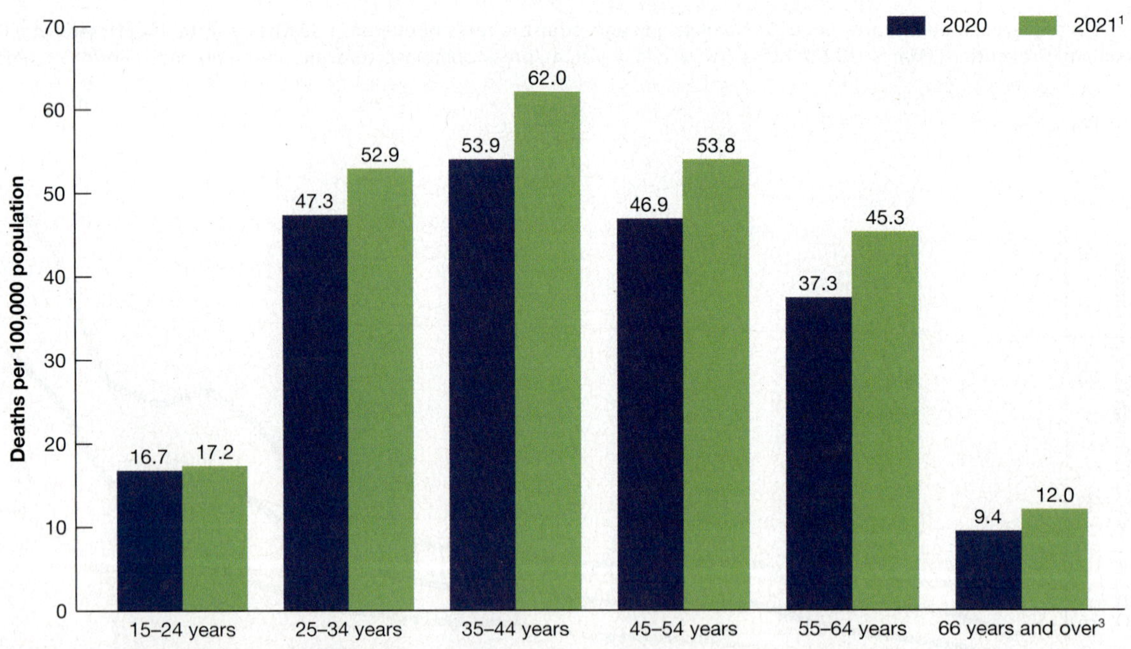

¹Except for those aged 15–24, rates in 2021 were significantly higher than in 2020 for all age groups, $p < 0.05$.
²Age group with highest rate in 2020 and 2021, $p < 0.05$.
³Age group with lowest rate in 2020 and 2021, $p < 0.05$.
NOTES: Drug overdose deaths were identified using *International Classification of Diseases, 10th Revision* underlying cause-of-death codes X40–X44, X60–X64, X85, and Y10–Y14. Age-adjusted death rates were calculated using the direct method and the 2000 U.S. standard population. The number of drug overdose deaths in 2021 was 106,699. Access data table for Figure 2 at: https://www.cdc.gov/nchs/data/databriefs/db457-tables.pdf#2.
SOURCE: National Center for Health Statistics, National Vital Statistics System, Mortality File.

FIGURE 7-5 Rate of drug overdose deaths, by selected age groups, 15 and over, United States, 2020–2021. (Reprinted from Centers for Disease Control and Prevention/National Center for Health Statistics (NCHS). (December 2022). https://www.cdc.gov/nchs/products/databriefs/db457.htm)

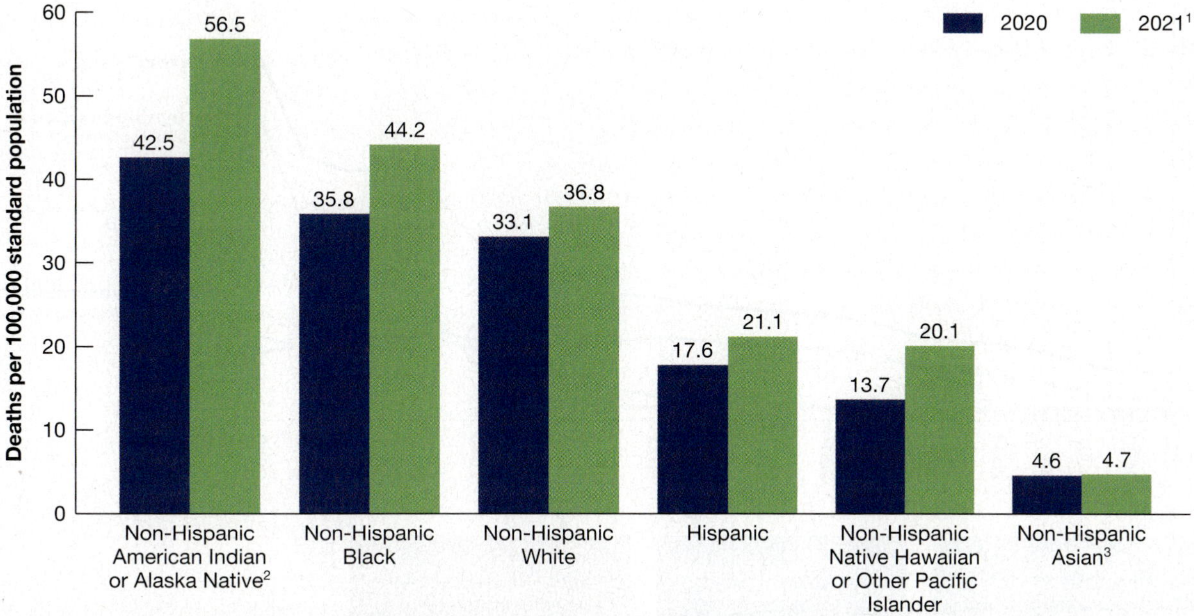

[1]Except for Non-Hispanic Asian people, rates in 2021 were significantly higher than 2020 for all race and Hispanic-origin groups, $p < 0.05$.
[2]Race and Hispanic-origin group with highest rate in 2020 and 2021, $p < 0.05$.
[3]Race and Hispanic-origin group with lowest rate in 2020 and 2021, $p < 0.05$.
NOTES: Misclassification of race and Hispanic origin on death certificates results in the underestimate of death rates by as much as 34% for American Indian or Alaska Native people and 3% for non-Hispanic Asian and Hispanic people. Drug overdose deaths were identified using *International Classification of Diseases, 10th Revision* underlying cause-of-death codes X40–X44, X60–X64, X85, and Y10–Y14. Age-adjusted death rates were calculated using the direct method and the 2000 U.S. standard population. Access data table for Figure 3 at: https://www.cdc.gov/nchs/data/databriefs/db457-tables.pdf#3.
SOURCE: National Center for Health Statistics, National Vital Statistics System, Mortality File.

FIGURE 7-6 Age-adjusted rate of drug overdose deaths, by race and Hispanic origin, United States, 2020–2021. (Reprinted from Centers for Disease Control and Prevention/National Center for Health Statistics (NCHS). (December 2022). https://www.cdc.gov/nchs/products/databriefs/db457.htm)

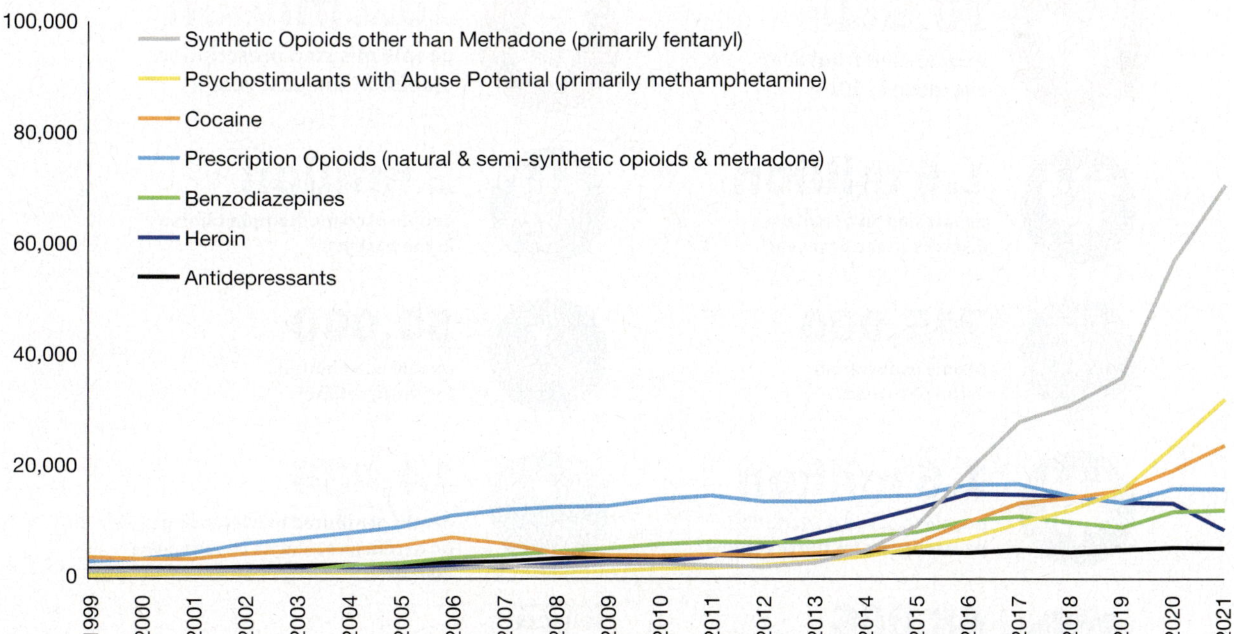

*Includes deaths with underlying causes of unintentional drug poisoning (X40–X44), suicide drug poisoning (X60–X64), homicide drug poisoning (X85), or drug poisoning of underestimated intent (Y10–Y14), as coded in the International Classification of Diseases, 10th Revision. Source: Centers for Disease Control and Prevention, National Center for Health Statistics. Multiple Cause of Death 199–2021 on CDD WONDER Online Database, released 1/2023.

FIGURE 7-7 National drug-involved overdose deaths by specific category—number among all ages, 1999–2021. (Reprinted from National Institute on Drug Abuse. (May 2024). https://nida.nih.gov/research-topics/trends-statistics/overdose-death-rates)

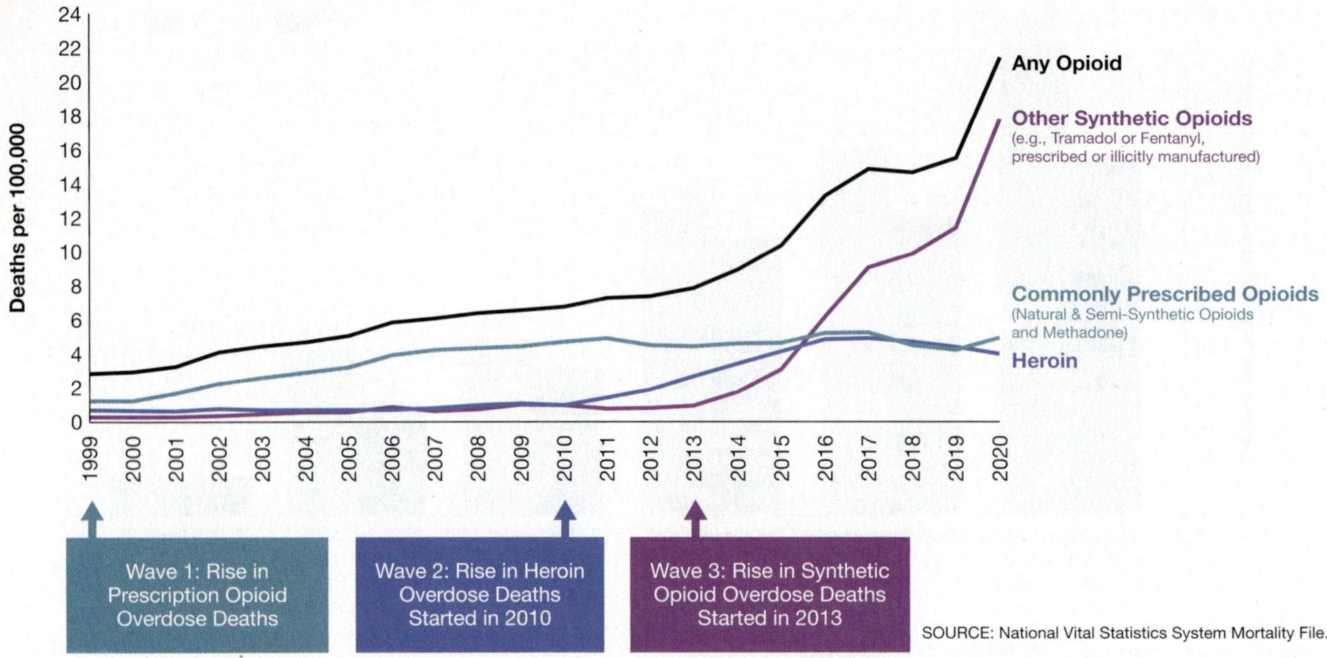

FIGURE 7-8 Three waves of opioid overdose deaths. (Reprinted from Centers for Disease Control and Prevention. (April 2024). https://www.cdc.gov/overdose-prevention/about/understanding-the-opioid-overdose-epidemic.html)

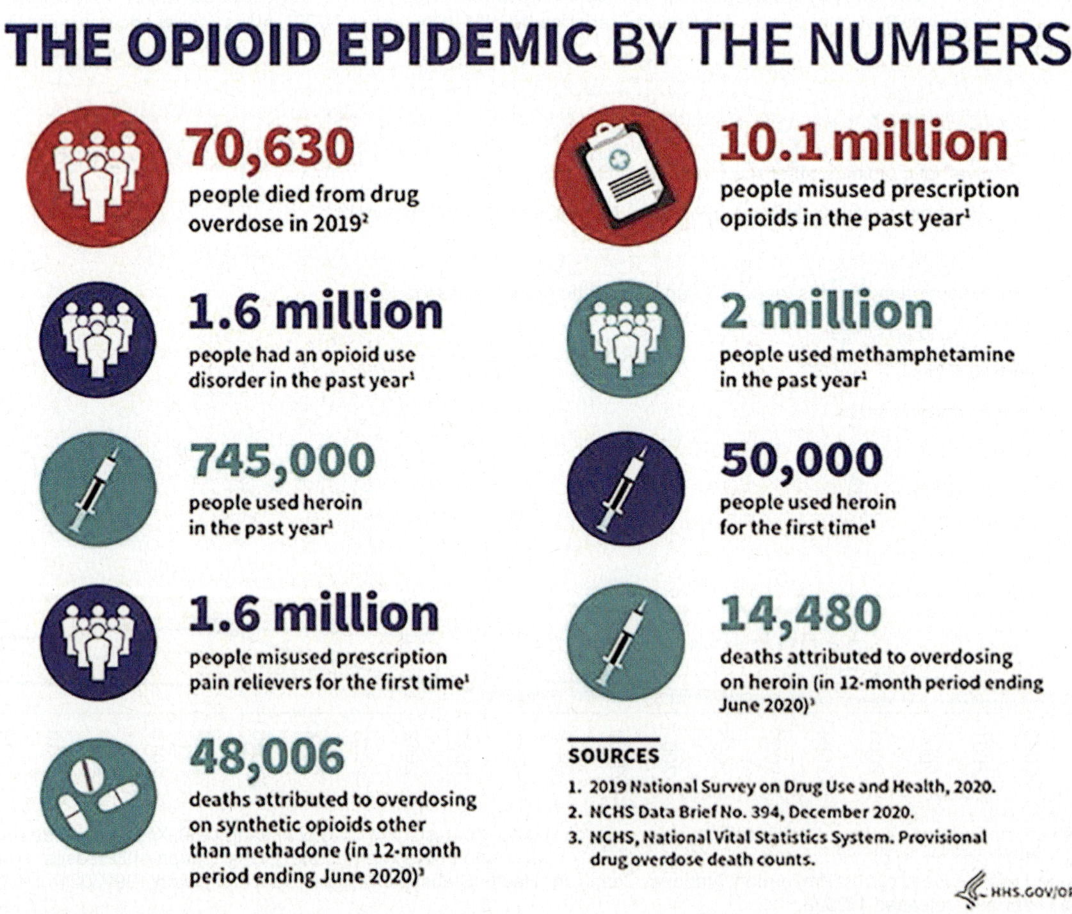

FIGURE 7-9 The opioid epidemic by the numbers, as of December 16, 2022. (Reprinted from U.S. Department of Health and Human Services. (2022). https://www.hhs.gov/opioids/statistics/index.html)

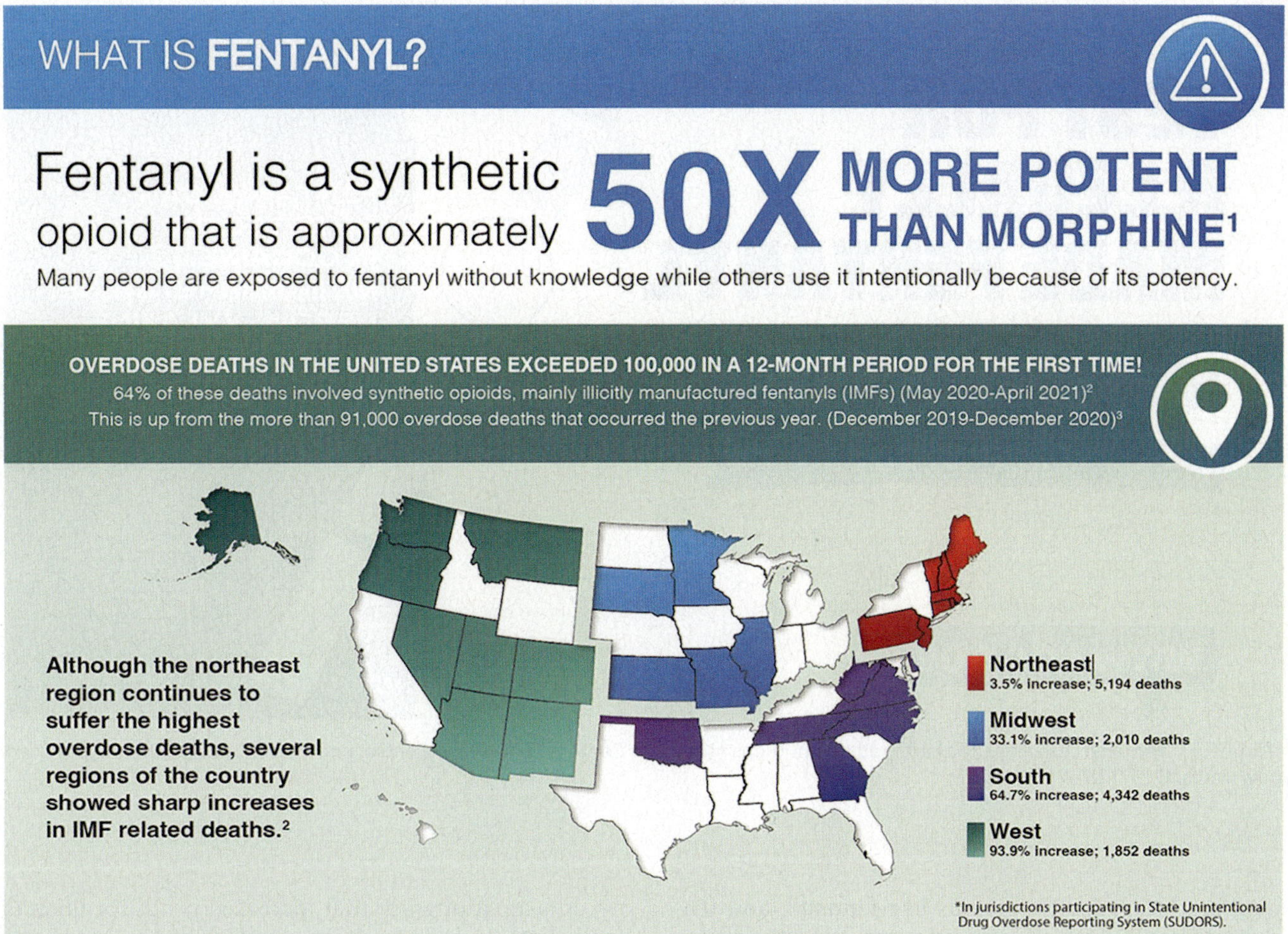

FIGURE 7-10 What is fentanyl? (Reprinted from National Institute on Drug Abuse. (May 2022). https://nida.nih.gov/research-topics/trends-statistics/infographics/what-fentanyl)

Institute on Drug Abuse provides online information about fentanyl (Fig. 7-10), and the CDC has a webpage of fentanyl facts (CDC, 2019a). The CDC has also been publicizing the use of fentanyl test strips as a harm reduction strategy for addressing fentanyl overdoses (Figs. 7-11 and 7-12).

Rise of Polysubstance Overdoses

Daniel Ciccarone, MD, MPH, published a 2021 review of the rise of illicit fentanyl, risks for overdose, in combination with other substances. He notes that fentanyl-related overdoses are rising in new geographic areas. Stimulant-related overdoses are also rising nationally due to methamphetamine and cocaine. Polysubstance use (stimulant along with an opioid) is driving stimulant-related overdoses. He sees a "fourth wave" of high mortality involving methamphetamine and cocaine entwining with the availability and use of illicit fentanyl as major drivers of overdose deaths (Ciccarone, 2021).

A June 10, 2022, Morbidity and Mortality Weekly Report (MMWR) noted that of those U.S. adults assessed for substance use treatment in 2019, 35.8% used alcohol during the past 30 days and 32.6% used multiple substances along with those with severe problems (e.g., psychiatric, medical, or family) across multiple biopsychosocial domains (CDC, 2022a; Fig. 7-13).

Researchers noted that there is a need to enhance comprehensive substance use programs that incorporate polysubstance use and co-occurring mental health problems into strategies for prevention and treatment (Kacha-Ochana et al., 2022).

In June 2023, the Substance Abuse and Mental Health Services Administration (SAMHSA) reported on the frequency of polysubstance-related emergency department (ED) visits for 2022 and noted that 43.1% of heroin and 54.2% of fentanyl ED visits were polysubstance related (SAMHSA, 2023; Fig. 7-14).

Polysubstance use is impacting the opioid epidemic in significant ways with the introduction of xylazine in the illegal synthetic opioid supply. In October 2022, the U.S. Department of Justice's Drug Enforcement Administration issued its report "The Growing Threat of Xylazine and its Mixture with Illicit Drugs" (USDOJ/DEA, 2022) describing xylazine's role in the opioid epidemic.

According to White House Domestic Policy Advisor Neera Tanden, JD, "Almost 7 in 10 overdose deaths can

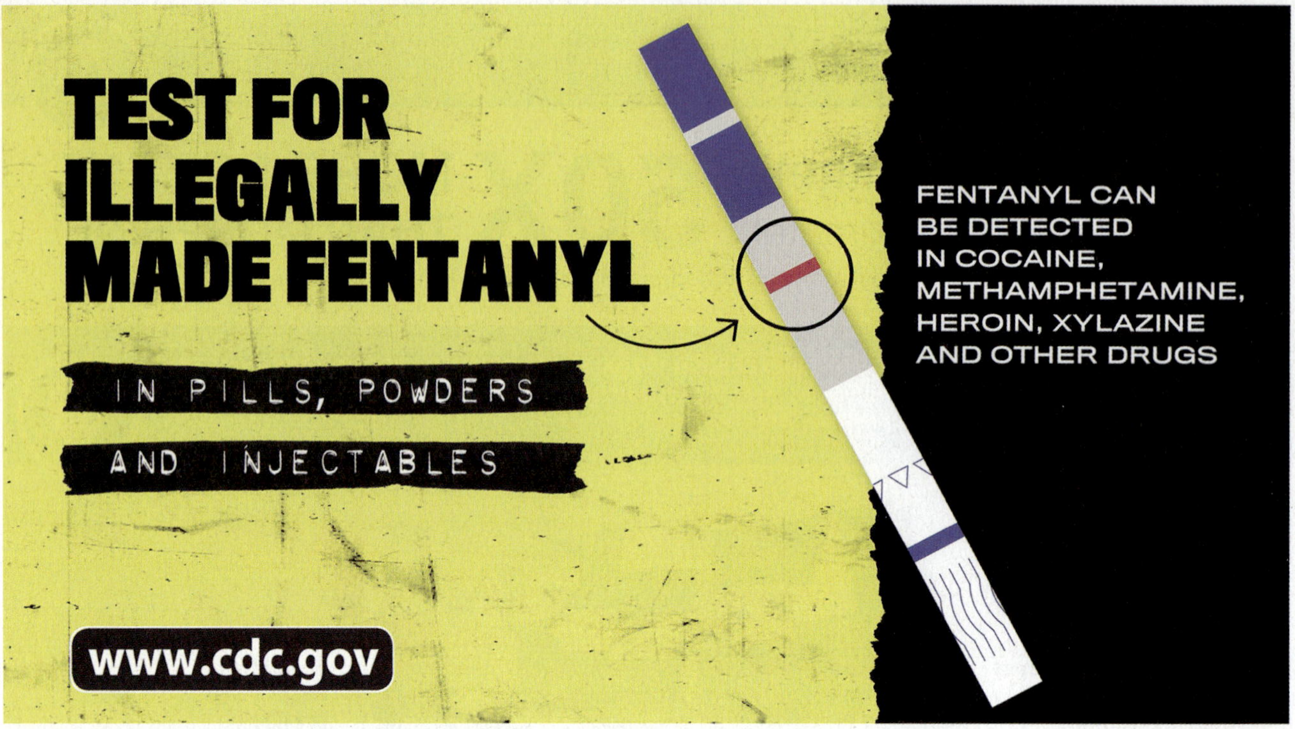
TEST FOR ILLEGALLY MADE FENTANYL
IN PILLS, POWDERS
AND INJECTABLES
FENTANYL CAN BE DETECTED IN COCAINE, METHAMPHETAMINE, HEROIN, XYLAZINE AND OTHER DRUGS
www.cdc.gov

FIGURE 7-11 Fentanyl test strips for harm reduction. (Reprinted from Centers for Disease Control and Prevention. (2023). https://x.com/CDCgov/status/1719772817158246521)

be attributed to synthetic opioids like fentanyl, and fentanyl adulterated with xylazine presents another rising threat." Xylazine was detected in nearly 11% of fentanyl-involved deaths (Frieden, 2023).

Xylazine (AKA "tranq") is a nonopiate sedative, analgesic, and muscle relaxant only authorized in the United States for veterinary use by the U.S. Food and Drug Administration. It is not a controlled substance under the U.S. Controlled Substances Act. It is inexpensive, and its psychoactive effects allow drug traffickers to reduce the amount of fentanyl or heroin used in a mixture.

It is an adulterant that increased profit for illicit drug traffickers and found in many illicit drug mixtures with cocaine, heroin, fentanyl, and other drugs, usually in combination with two or more substances present, and has been detected in fatal overdoses. It can lead to central nervous system depression. It is attractive to fentanyl users looking for a longer high than fentanyl alone, but it reduces the euphoria experienced with heroin or a heroin–fentanyl mix.

Users who inject xylazine or drug mixtures with xylazine often develop soft tissue injuries that can lead to

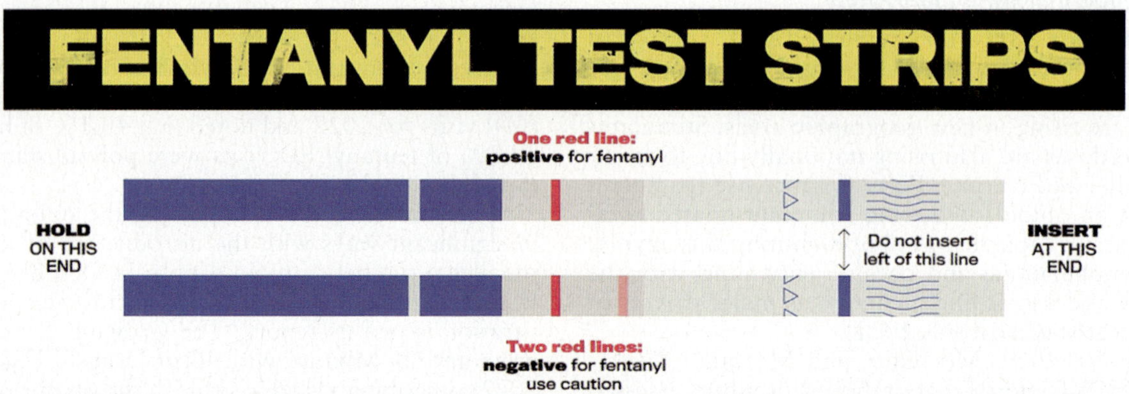

FIGURE 7-12 Fentanyl test strips. (Reprinted from Centers for Disease Control and Prevention. (April 2024). https://www.cdc.gov/stop-overdose/safety/index.html#cdc_preparedness_risks-fentanyl-test-strips-a-harm-reduction-strategy)

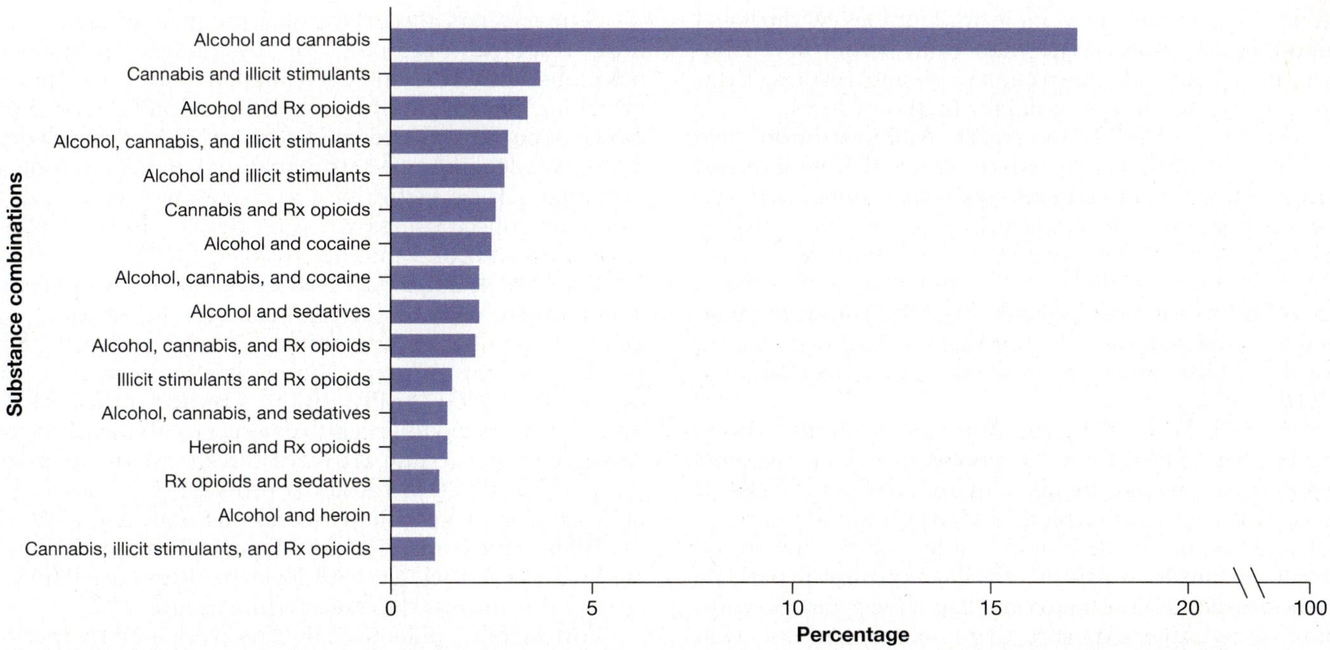

FIGURE 7-13 Most common substance combinations reported among past 30-day polysubstance users aged ≥18 years (*N* = 16,033)—United States, 2019. (Reprinted from Centers for Disease Control and Prevention. (June 2022). https://www.cdc.gov/mmwr/volumes/71/wr/mm7123a1.htm)

Substance	Polysubstance weighted frequency (n)	Lower 95 CI	Upper 95 CI	Proportion that are polysubstance (%)
Alcohol	653,310	469,092	837,528	20.2
Cannabis	407,995	285,962	530,027	47.6
Cocaine	311,945	157,552	466,338	74.7
Methamphetamine	248,817	138,679	358,954	42.5
Heroin	173,307	67,655	278,960	43.1
Rx or other opioid	160,169	121,596	198,743	44.5
Benzodiazepine	138,829	112,705	164,953	72.8
Fentanyl	103,184	49,745	156,622	54.2

Alcohol had the highest number of polysubstance-related ED visits (n=653,310) but the lowest proportion of visits involving polysubstance (20.2%). Approximately four out of five alcohol-related ED visits involved alcohol only. Cocaine had the third highest frequency of polysubstance ED visits (n=311,945) but the highest proportion (74.7%) involving additional substances.

FIGURE 7-14 Frequency of polysubstance-related ED visits and proportion of visits that were polysubstance for each drug (2022). (Reprinted from Substance Abuse and Mental Health Services Administration. (2023). https://store.samhsa.gov/sites/default/files/pep23-07-03-001.pdf)

necrotic tissue that may result in amputations. Withdrawal symptoms are more severe than from heroin or methadone and can include sharp chest pains and seizures. Xylazine can increase the potential for fatal overdoses.

The U.S. Drug Enforcement Administration also released a Public Safety Alert about the widespread threat of fentanyl mixed with xylazine. It noted that xylazine and fentanyl drug mixtures place users at a higher risk for suffering a fatal drug overdose. Because xylazine is not an opioid, naloxone does not reverse its effects. According to the CDC, of the 107,735 Americans who died between August 2021 and August 2022 from a drug overdose, 66% involved synthetic opioids like fentanyl (USDEA, n.d.).

The U.S. Food and Drug Administration also issued an alert for healthcare professionals of risks to patients exposed to xylazine in illicit drugs (USFDA, 2022). It noted that routine toxicology screens do not detect xylazine and that naloxone should be administered for opioid overdoses and to consider xylazine exposure if patients are not responding to naloxone and have signs or symptoms of xylazine exposure (e.g., severe, necrotic skin ulcerations).

Harm reduction groups have reported that overdoses are becoming more difficult to reverse for those experiencing overdoses from a combination of opioids and xylazine. Instead of just administering naloxone, oxygen is being given because xylazine is a sedative and not an opioid that would respond to naloxone.

It can also involve giving rescue breathing, avoiding direct mouth-to-mouth contact by using a barrier, providing supplemental oxygen and employing airway management techniques—manipulating head, neck, and body to ensure breathing is not blocked. Other tools include pulse oximeters and oxygen tanks.

Xylazine has forced the development of new overdose response protocols for bystanders: Administer naloxone, call 911, and then immediately start "rescue breathing" to ensure overdose victims don't die or experience hypoxic brain injury before emergency responders arrive. While naloxone acts quickly, it can take as long as 20 minutes for a victim of a xylazine-involved overdose to regain consciousness when an opioid-alone overdose reversal takes 3 or 5 minutes (Facher, 2023).

On April 4, 2022, Xavier Becerra, Secretary of Health and Human Services (HHS), renewed the October 26, 2017 determination by former Acting Secretary Eric D. Hargan that an opioid public health emergency still exists nationwide (ASPR, 2022). The declaration of the opioid crisis as a public health emergency allows HHS leeway to conduct certain activities in response to the opioid crisis (USGAO, 2018). And the problem of fentanyl contaminated with xylazine is so serious that in July 2023, the White House released the 15-page "Fentanyl Adulterated with or Associated with Xylazine Response Plan" to holistically address the issue (White House, 2023).

Fortunately, epidemiologic data were used to develop new guidelines for treating those who are brought in for treatment and provide data to drug enforcement agencies to develop strategies to reduce the trafficking of illegal drugs that will save lives in the long run.

As the United States continues to grapple with the opioid epidemic as it becomes more complex with polysubstance use, the world is still dealing with the COVID-19 pandemic that started in Wuhan, China, in 2019. Although the World Health Organization and the United States declared an end to the public health emergency phase of COVID-19 in May of 2023, the virus continues to mutate and remains unchecked, and the development of other pandemics is possible (see Box 7-3).

BOX 7-3 POPULATION FOCUS

Epidemiology and the Avian Influenza Pandemic

Pandemic Planning

Over the course of the Barack Obama presidency (2009–2017), a pandemic infrastructure was put in place to respond to emerging infection threats, including a potential avian influenza pandemic. Called the "Playbook for early response to high-consequence emerging infectious disease threats and biological incidents," it was used with relative success to address swine flu in 2009 and the Ebola outbreak of 2014. After Donald Trump became president in 2017, his administration systematically dismantled the executive branch's science infrastructure and rejected the role of science to inform policy.

COVID-19

By the time the first cases of COVID-19 were reported, no meaningful science policy infrastructure was in place to advise President Trump. As a result, the responses to the pandemic were largely ineffectual and inconsistent (Karlawish, 2020). People were confused by the misinformation and disinformation spread on social media, etc. And this lack of a structured approach to addressing the pandemic continued even as the ending of the public health emergency was issued in May 2023.

The virus responsible for COVID-19 continues to mutate and remains unchecked. Although vaccines have been developed and have shown success in preventing hospitalizations and deaths among the older populations, vaccination rates have been low, and reinfections are occurring, placing those with underlying diseases at risk for dying or developing long COVID.

Disease surveillance has become spotty, with funding for such public health activities having disappeared and mandates for reporting COVID-19 data having ceased with the ending of the public health emergency. Because results of home testing are not consistently reported by people to proper authorities, no one knows how much testing is going on and how many have tested positive, so new case counts are missing, which prevents understanding of the extent transmission is occurring.

BOX **7-3** POPULATION FOCUS (*Continued*)

Epidemiology and the Avian Influenza Pandemic

The SARS-CoV-2 virus responsible for COVID-19 is a novel virus. Although it is part of the coronavirus family, and even after 3 years, we do not know enough about it to predict its pathogenicity or transmission trends. It does not follow a seasonal course, making it hard to prepare for the next outbreak (Jung, 2023a). We are still learning new things about the damage it is doing to various organs of the body. Much of the damage done is more from the inflammation the immune system causes than from the virus itself.

Avian Influenza

Unlike the SARS-CoV-2 virus, public health experts are familiar with the bird flu virus and are aware that several outbreaks have occurred (see Fig. 7-15). Right now, we are experiencing the largest avian influenza outbreak in U.S. history; 58 million poultry died since it began in 2022 (McGlone, 2023). Researchers know that exposure to infected backyard poultry could result in humans becoming infected. One current solution is to cull infected flocks to prevent spread (see Fig. 7-16).

The most worrisome trend is the number of different types of animals contracting the flu virus and then transmitting it to the same or other animal species (see Fig. 7-17). Numerous animals have died. In December 2022, a domestic cat that was infected with H5N1 from exposure to a duck farm in which 8000 ducks were infected, became so ill that it was euthanized (Dutta, 2023). In July 2023, 20 cats were confirmed with bird flu in Poland, with deaths of 70 domestic cats under investigation by the European Centre for Disease Control and Prevention. The concern was whether there was any feline-to-feline or feline-to-human transmission (Hackett, 2023).

The other concern is the growing number of mutations of H5N1 that could make it possible to infect humans and result in human-to-human transmission. Butyrophilin, the human immune system protein that stops bird flu from infecting people, could be overcome by some viruses that have mutated that are currently causing outbreaks in wild birds, although more genetic changes would be needed to result in a pandemic among people (Wilson, 2023). Government organizations are monitoring the spread of H5N1 on such sites as USDA's 2022–2023 Detections of Highly Pathogenic Avian Influenza in Mammals, the Wildlife Health.org's links to USDA's 2022–2023 Detections of Highly Pathogenic Avian Influenza in Wild Birds, and the USDA's Confirmations of Highly Pathogenic Avian Influenza in Commercial and Backyard Flocks.

Although a vaccine is available, supply chain issues may hinder the rapid dissemination of vaccines to various populations, should the need arise. An additional possible issue is vaccine hesitancy, which has been seen with the COVID-19 vaccines. It is possible that the high fatality rate for avian influenza (53%) (CDC, 2023c) may motivate vaccine compliance.

CONCEPTS BASIC TO EPIDEMIOLOGY

The science of epidemiology draws on certain basic concepts and principles to analyze and understand patterns of occurrence among aggregate health conditions.

Disease Etiology

In 1856, John Stuart Mill formed three methods of hypothesis formulation for determining disease etiology. These methods include method of difference, method of agreement, and method of concomitant variation.

In 1965, Sir Austin Bradford Hill proposed expanding on Mill's postulates about causality by developing nine criteria to evaluate the relationship between environmental exposure and potential health outcomes. The criteria can be used with infectious disease as well as noninfectious disease. These elements are as follows:

1. *Strength of Association*: The ratio of the rate of a disease in those with a suspected causal factor to the rate of the disease in those without it: a higher rate in the group with the factor than in the group without it indicates a strong association.
2. *Consistency of Association*: An association is demonstrated in varying types of studies among diverse study groups (i.e., replication).
3. *Specificity*: A cause leads to one effect (not always the case in noninfectious diseases).
4. *Temporality*: Exposure to the suspected factor must precede the onset of disease (i.e., time order or time sequence).
5. *Biological Gradient*: This relationship is demonstrated if, with increasing levels of exposure to the factor, there is a corresponding increase in occurrence of the disease (i.e., dose–response relationship).
6. *Biological Plausibility*: The hypothesized cause makes sense based on current biologic or social models (i.e., it is possible).
7. *Coherence of Explanation*: The hypothesized cause makes sense based on current knowledge about the natural history or biology of the disease (i.e., scientific knowledge).
8. *Analogy*: Similarities between the association of interest and others (e.g., potential links to birth defects from new drugs is a concern because we already recognize this potential from the use of the drug thalidomide during the 1950s and early 1960s).
9. *Experimental Evidence*: Experimental and nonexperimental studies support the association (e.g., reduced tobacco use in a population should lead to reduced lung cancer rates; Merrill, 2021).

The elements described by Hill are still used by epidemiologists and provide the fundamental principles C/PHNs can use to evaluate evidence of disease causation in all types of published reports, both scientific and lay.

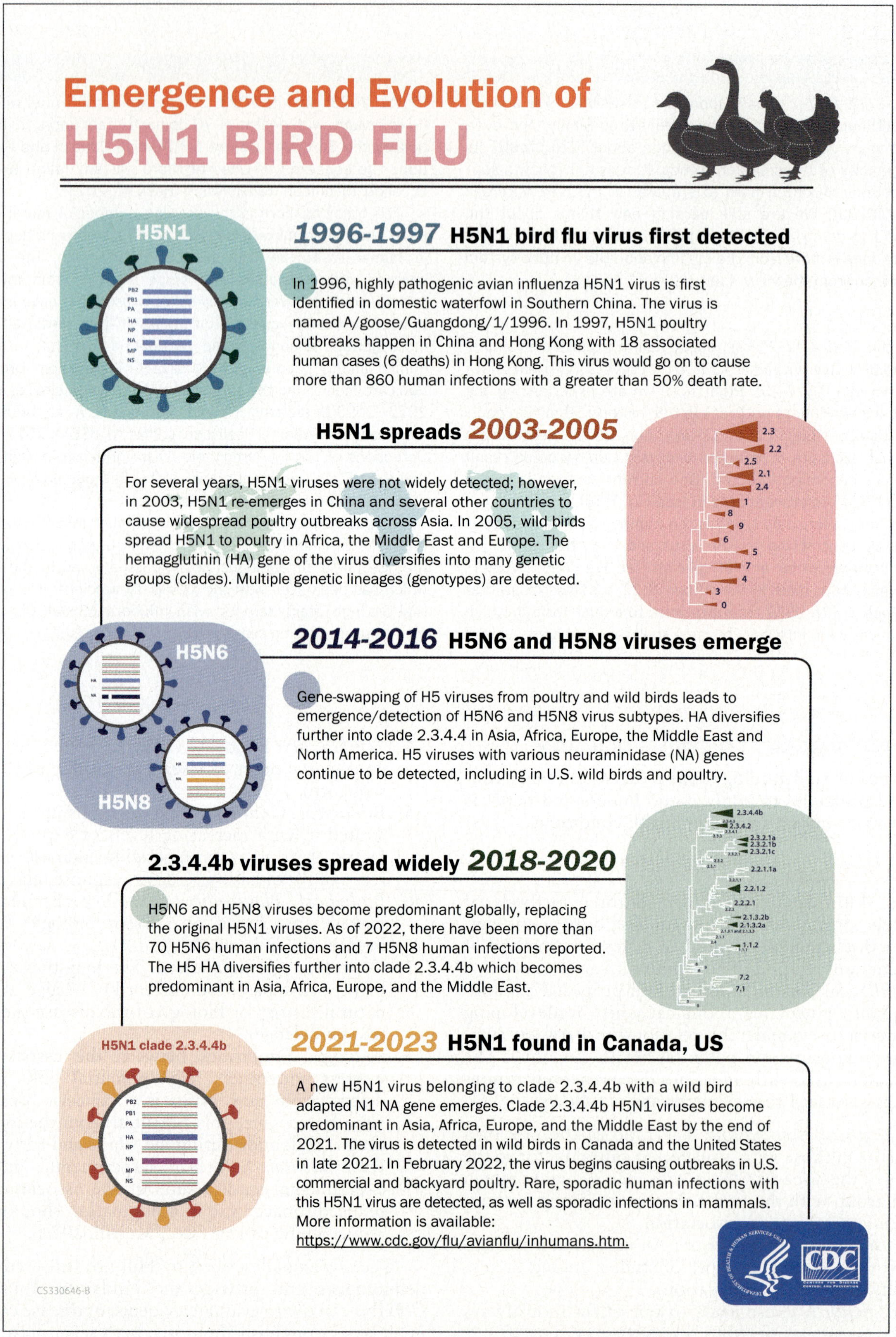

FIGURE 7-15 Emergence and evolution of H5N1 Bird Flu. (Reprinted from Centers for Disease Control and Prevention. (June 2022). https://www.cdc.gov/flu/pdf/avianflu/bird-flu-origin-graphic.pdf)

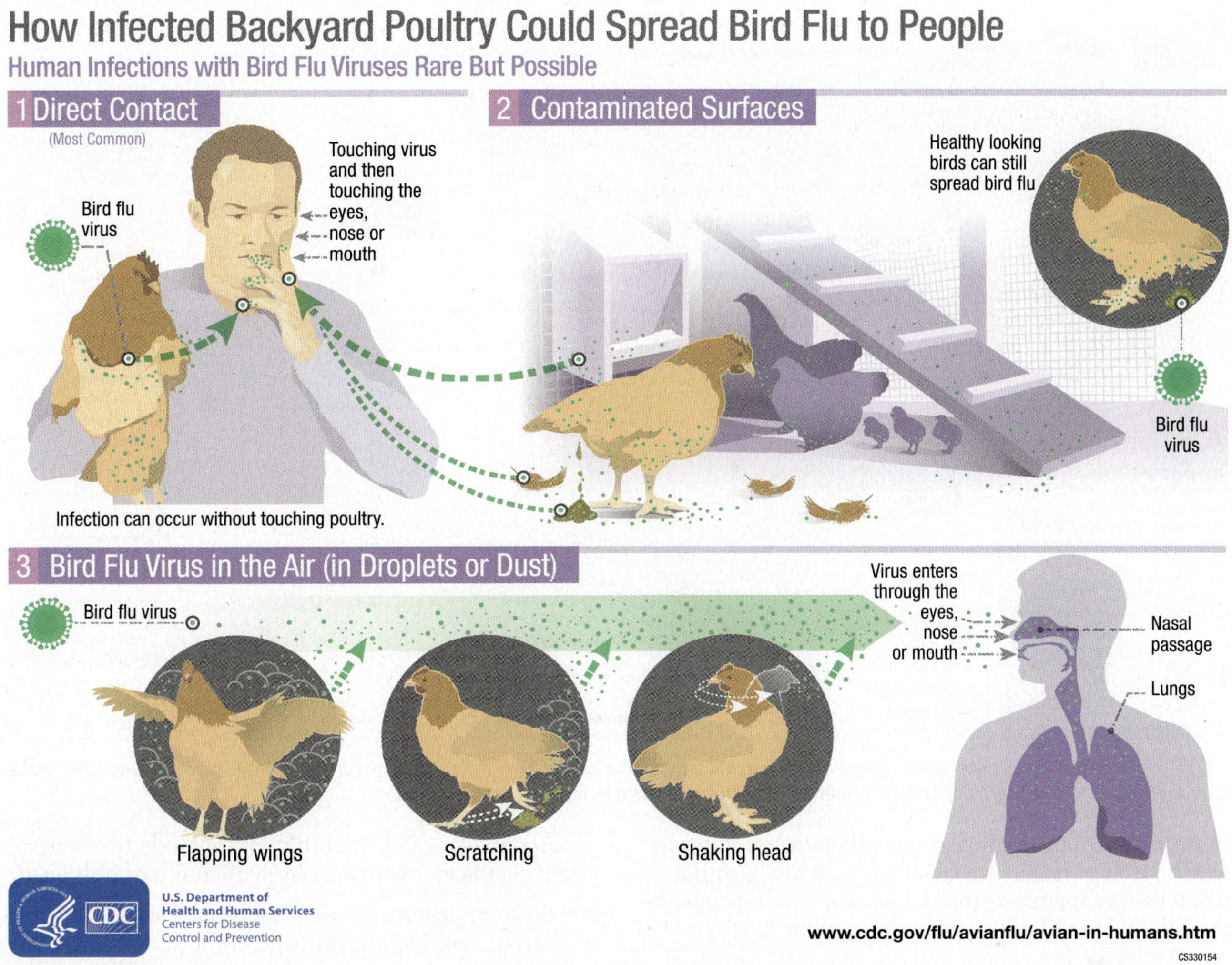

FIGURE 7-16 How infected backyard poultry could spread bird flu to people. (Reprinted from the CDC. https://www.cdc.gov/flu/pdf/avianflu/avian-flu-transmission.pdf)

Epidemiologic Triangle or Host, Agent, and Environment Model

Through their early study of infectious diseases, epidemiologists began to consider disease states in terms of the **epidemiologic triangle**, or the *host, agent, and environment model*, shown in Figure 7-18. Interactions among these three elements explained infectious and other disease patterns.

Host

The *host* is a susceptible human or animal who harbors and nourishes a disease-causing agent. Many physical, psychological, and lifestyle factors influence the host's susceptibility and response to an agent (Friis, 2018):

- Physical factors: age, sex, race, socioeconomic status, and genetic influences
- Psychological factors: outlook and response to stress
- Lifestyle factors: diet, exercise, and other healthy or unhealthy habits

The concept of resistance is important for community/public health nursing practice. People sometimes have an ability to resist pathogens, which is called *inherent resistance*. Typically, these people have inherited or acquired characteristics, such as the various factors mentioned earlier, that make them less vulnerable. For instance, people who maintain a healthful lifestyle may not contract influenza even if exposed to the flu virus. Resistance can be promoted through preventive interventions that improve one's immunity system and support a healthy lifestyle.

Such healthy habits include not smoking, eating more fruits and vegetables, exercising regularly, maintaining a healthy weight, drinking alcohol in moderation, getting adequate sleep, washing hands frequently, cooking meals thoroughly, and minimizing stress (HHP, 2018). Preventive practices such as being up to date with immunizations and seeing your healthcare provider for appropriate screenings can also help to keep the immune system strong.

Agent

An *agent* is a factor that causes or contributes to a health problem or condition (Friis, 2018). Causative agents can be factors that are present (e.g., bacteria that cause TB,

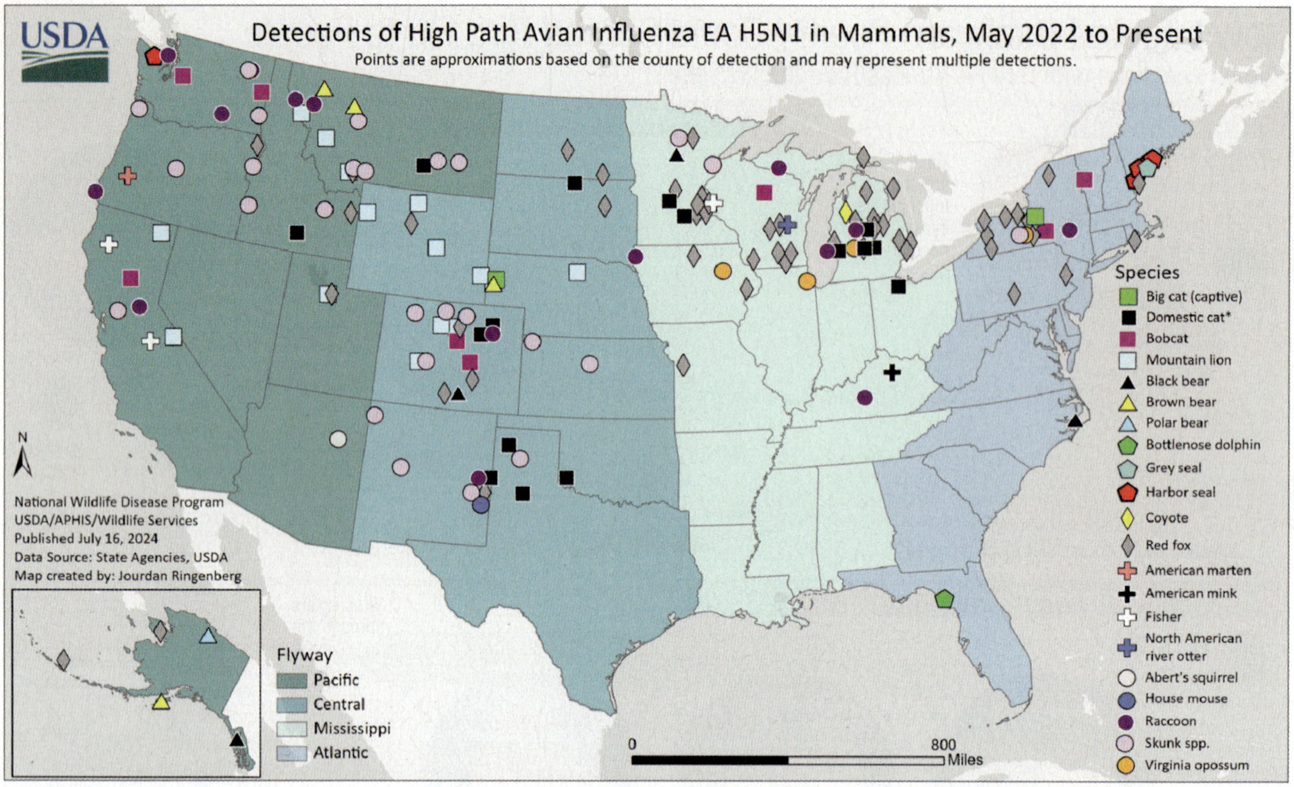

FIGURE 7-17 2022–2023 detections of highly pathogenic avian influenza in mammals. (Reprinted from USDA. https://www.aphis.usda.gov/livestock-poultry-disease/avian/avian-influenza/hpai-detections/mammals)

rocks on a mountain road that contribute to an automobile crash) or factors that are lacking (e.g., a low serum iron level that causes anemia or the lack of seat belt use contributing to the extent of injury in an automobile crash).

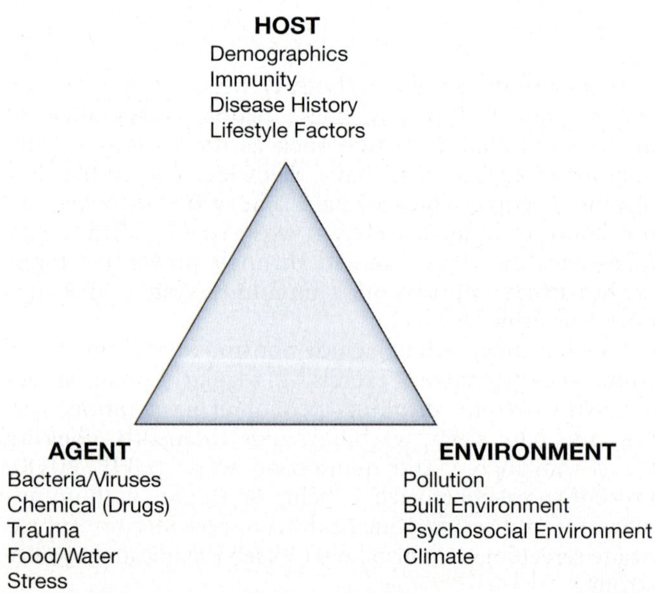

FIGURE 7-18 Epidemiologic triad. Epidemiologists study the causal agent, the susceptible host, and environmental factors that contribute to an illness, an injury, or a wellness state. Intervention may focus on any of these three to prevent the spread of illness or to improve health in a population.

Agents vary considerably and include five types: biologic, chemical, nutrient, physical, and psychological:

- *Biologic* agents include bacteria, viruses, fungi, protozoa, worms, and insects. Some biologic agents are infectious, such as influenza virus or HIV.
- *Chemical* agents may be in the form of liquids, solids, gases, dusts, or fumes. Examples are poisonous sprays used on garden pests and industrial chemical wastes. The degree of toxicity of the chemical agent influences its impact on health.
- *Nutrient* agents include essential dietary components that can produce illness conditions if they are deficient or are taken in excess. For example, a deficiency of niacin can cause pellagra, and too much vitamin A can be toxic.
- *Physical* agents include anything mechanical (e.g., chainsaw, automobile), material (e.g., rockslide), atmospheric (e.g., ultraviolet radiation), geologic (e.g., earthquake), or genetically transmitted that causes injury to humans. The shape, size, and force of physical agents influence the degree of harm to the host.
- *Psychological* agents are events that produce stress leading to health problems (e.g., war, terrorism).

Agents may also be classified as infectious or noninfectious. Infectious agents cause communicable diseases, such as influenza or TB—that is, the disease can be spread from one person to another. Certain characteristics of infectious agents are important for C/PHNs to understand:

- *Exposure* to the agent
- *Pathogenicity* (capacity to cause disease in the host)

- *Infectivity* (capacity to enter the host and multiply)
- *Virulence* (severity of disease)
- *Toxigenicity* (capacity to produce a toxin or poison)
- *Resistance* (ability of the agent to survive environmental conditions)
- *Antigenicity* (ability to induce an antibody response in the host)
- *Structure and chemical composition* (Friis, 2018)

Chapter 8 examines the subject of communicable disease in greater depth. Noninfectious agents have similar characteristics in that their relative abilities to harm the host vary with type of agent and intensity and duration of exposure (Szklo & Nieto, 2019).

Environment

The *environment* refers to all the external factors surrounding the host that might influence vulnerability or resistance and includes physical and psychosocial elements (Friis, 2018):

- The *physical environment* includes factors such as geography, climate and weather, safety of buildings, water and food supply, and presence of animals, plants, insects, and microorganisms that have the capacity to serve as reservoirs (storage sites for disease-causing agents) or **vectors** (carriers) for transmitting disease.
- The *psychosocial environment* refers to social, cultural, economic, and psychological influences and conditions that affect health, such as access to healthcare, cultural health practices, poverty, and work stressors, which can all contribute to disease or health (Szklo & Nieto, 2019).

Interaction of the Host, Agent, and Environment

Host, agent, and environment interact to cause a disease or health condition. For example, WNV is spread to people by mosquito bites and occurs during mosquito season (summer through fall). There are no vaccines to prevent or medications to treat WNV.

Most people infected with WNV do not feel sick. About one in five people who are infected develop a fever and other symptoms. About 1 out of 150 infected people develop a serious, sometimes fatal, illness. The risk of WNV can be reduced by using insect repellent and wearing long-sleeved shirts and long pants to prevent mosquito bites (CDC, 2023d). WNV, which was widespread in Africa and the Middle East, arrived in the United States in 1999 and spread throughout the continental United States. Mapping the distribution of infectious diseases (Fig. 7-19) helps authorities know where to make resources and aid available.

Causality

Causality refers to the relationship between a cause and its effect. As scientific knowledge of health and disease has expanded, epidemiology has changed its view of

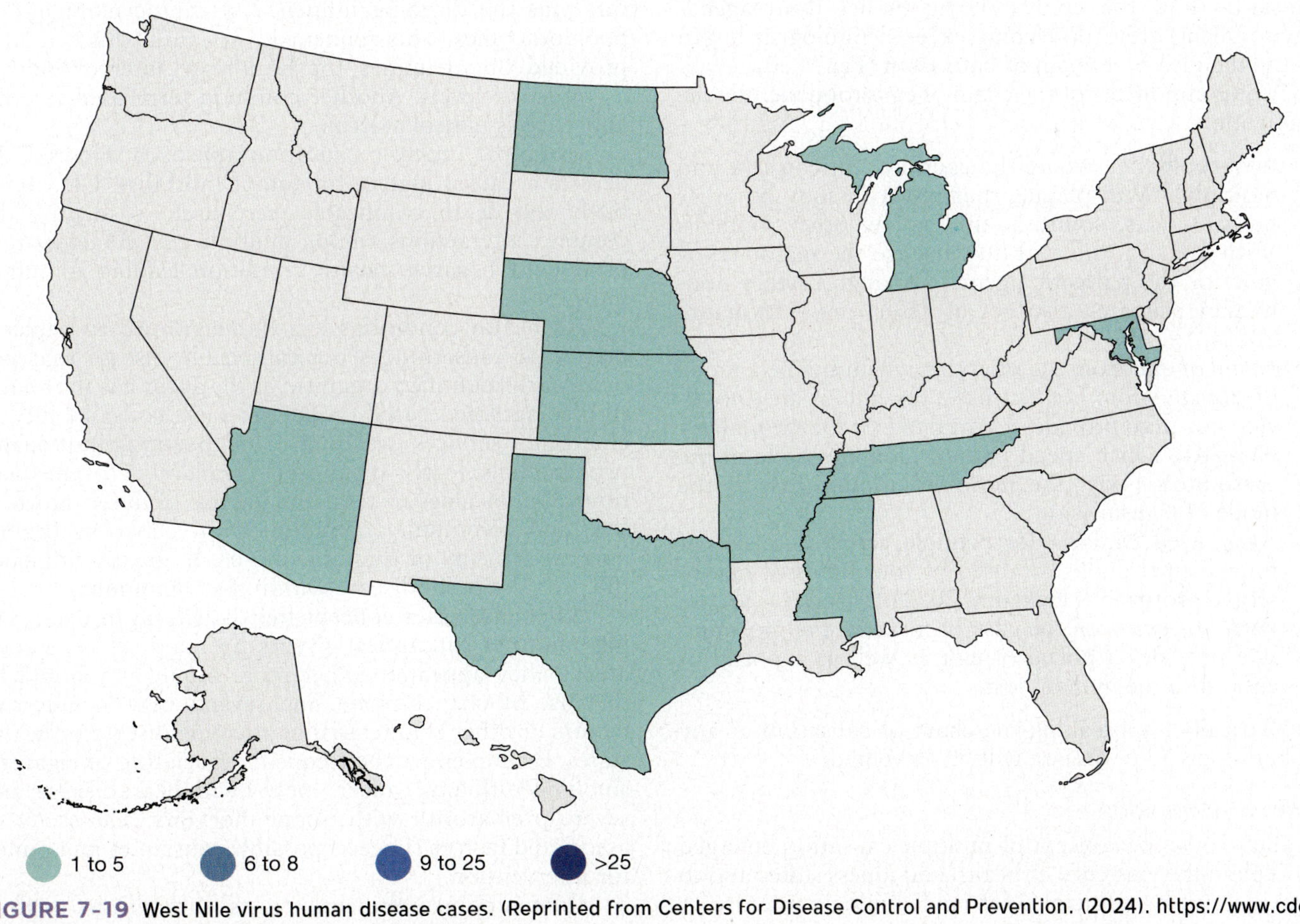

FIGURE 7-19 West Nile virus human disease cases. (Reprinted from Centers for Disease Control and Prevention. (2024). https://www.cdc.gov/west-nile-virus/data-maps/current-year-data.html)

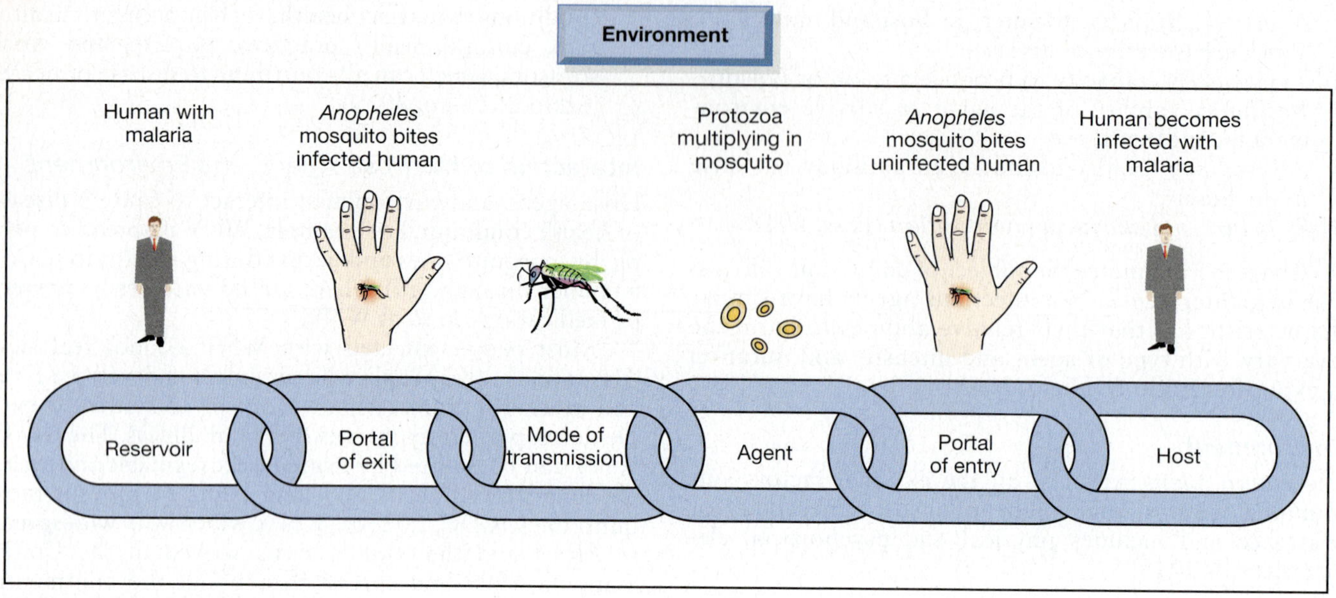

FIGURE 7-20 Chain of causation.

causality. The following section discusses some of those changes in thinking, which began in the 1960s and continue today.

Chain of Causation

As the scientific community thought about disease causation and the epidemiologic model (host–agent–environment) grew more complex, epidemiologists began to use the idea of a **chain of causation** (Fig. 7-20).

The components of the chain of causation include the following:

- **Reservoir** (i.e., where the causal agent can live and multiply). With plague, that reservoir may be other humans, rats, squirrels, and a few other animals. With malaria, infected humans are the major reservoir for the parasitic agents, although certain nonhuman primates also act as reservoirs (Heymann, 2022).
- *Portal of exit* from the reservoir, which can be a mode of transmission. For example, the bite of an *Anopheles* mosquito provides a portal of exit for the malaria parasites, which spend part of their life cycle in the mosquito's body; the mosquito in this case is the mode of transmission.
- *Agent* itself. Malaria, for example, actually consists of four distinct diseases caused by four kinds of microscopic protozoa (Heymann, 2022).
- *Portal of entry*. In the case of malaria, the mosquito bite provides a portal of exit as well as a portal of entry into the human host.

Basically, by breaking the chain of causation at any link, the spread of disease will be prevented.

Web of Causation

In the 1960s, the concept of multiple causation emerged to explain the existence of health and illness states and to provide guiding principles for epidemiologic practice. A causal paradigm that gained attention was referred to as the **web of causation**. The implication was that an intervention (or breaking of the web at any point nearest to the disease) could profoundly impact the development of that disease (Merrill, 2021; Szklo & Nieto, 2019).

This was a significant shift in thinking about disease and health, positing that the combination of multiple factors was the deciding influence in the development of poor outcomes. This refinement in causal thinking also provided opportunities for healthcare interventions at a variety of levels. Another common term used for this approach is **causal matrix**.

Using the multiple causation approach, Figure 7-21 depicts a causal matrix for infant mortality. Data from birth and death certificates were used to identify the complex interactions among multiple causal factors that produce a negative health condition leading to infant mortality.

All health conditions can be diagramed to depict a matrix of causation. A communicable disease that has one clearly identified organism as the agent has the ability to be diagramed based on factors such as availability of emergency services (treatment), diagnostic skill of health professionals (early diagnosis), availability of medications and vaccines to treat the disease (reduced morbidity), and community communication networks (public awareness). Any of these factors could greatly influence the progression of disease within the community.

Association is a concept that is helpful in determining multiple causalities. Events are said to be associated if they appear together more often than would be the case by chance alone. Such events may include risk factors or other characteristics affecting disease or health states. Examples are the frequent association of cigarette smoking with lung cancer, obesity with heart disease, and severe prematurity with infant mortality. The study of associated factors suggests possible causalities and points for intervention.

Contemporary epidemiologists continue to explore new and more comprehensive ways of viewing health and

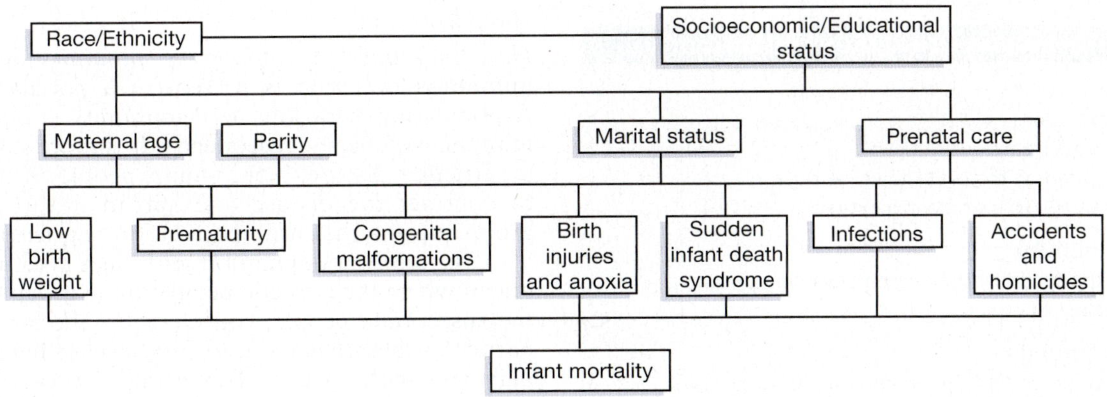

FIGURE 7-21 Web of causation for infant mortality.

illness. The associations among lifestyle, behavior, environment, and stress of all kinds and the ways in which they affect health states are gaining importance in epidemiology (Szklo & Nieto, 2019).

Causation in Noninfectious (Noncommunicable) Disease

With the availability of vaccines and antibiotics by the mid-20th century to thwart most infectious diseases in the United States and the developed world, attention shifted to the causes of noninfectious diseases such as cancer and diabetes. A new causal paradigm was clearly needed. The linear thinking embodied in models such as the *chain of causation* was insufficient in understanding the causes of these emerging health threats.

The web of causation model, which previously was used to study infectious diseases and which encompasses multifactorial causes of health problems and issues, has therefore been adapted to study the causation of noninfectious (noncommunicable) diseases. One such adaptation of this model, proposed by Egger (2012), explains the rise of chronic, noncommunicable diseases, for which there is no single underlying etiology, as the result of the body's reaction to its surrounding ecologic environment. According to this model, the body develops systemic and chronic inflammation (*metaflammation*) at the molecular level to inducers (*anthropogens*) that are associated with lifestyles and modern built environments (Fig. 7-22).

Thus, preventive approaches to improving the health of those with chronic disease that are based on this model focus on reducing this inflammatory process through lifestyle changes (Straub & Schradin, 2016). Such preventive approaches are being taken today to address the top two leading causes of death—heart disease and cancer—and include modifying lifestyle and addressing environmental factors.

Examples of disease that can be studied using this model include the following:

- Environmental Protection Agency (EPA) research has found that exposure to increased concentrations of PM2.5 over a period of time (few hours to weeks) can trigger cardiovascular disease–related heart attacks and deaths. Long-term exposure can result in cardiovascular mortality and decrease life expectancy (EPA, 2022).
- Another example is how gene changes that alter cell function cause cancer. Genetic changes can occur naturally during the process of cell division, while others are the result of environmental exposures that damage the DNA. Such environmental exposures include tobacco smoke chemicals and ultraviolet radiation (NCI, 2020).

Another aspect of this transition in focus from infectious to noninfectious disease is a shift from concern with individual susceptibility to the vulnerability of an entire population to chronic disease as a result of exposure to common environmental factors. Increasingly, public health workers came to realize the limitations imposed on individual control of health. After all, even people who are in the best of health may not withstand toxic agents in the workplace—for example, nuclear waste in the atmosphere from power plant accidents—or other debilitating conditions created by modern society. Therefore, more and more public health professionals are studying the environment and looking for methods to change conditions that contribute to illness in populations rather than just in people (see Chapter 9).

Immunity

Immunity refers to a host's ability to resist a particular infectious disease–causing agent. This occurs when the body forms antibodies and lymphocytes that react with the foreign antigenic molecules and render them harmless (Friis, 2018).

For community/public health nursing, this concept has significance in determining which people and groups are protected against disease and which may be vulnerable. Principles of immunity are shown in Box 7-4, are important in community health: passive, active, cross, hybrid, and herd. Herd immunity is covered in greater detail in Chapter 8.

BOX 7-4 Basic Principles of Immunity

Immunity
Self versus nonself
Protection from infectious disease
Usually indicated by the presence of antibody
Generally specific to a single organism

Active Immunity
Protection produced by the person's own immune system
Often lifetime

Passive Immunity
Protection transferred from another animal or human
Effective protection that wanes with time

Cross Immunity
Immunity to one bacteria or virus is effective in protecting the person against an antigenically similar but different organism (e.g., cowpox vaccination protects against smallpox).

Hybrid Immunity
Hybrid immunity occurs in those who have been both infected with and vaccinated against SARS-CoV-2.

Antigen
A live (e.g., viruses and bacteria) or inactivated substance capable of producing an immune response

Antibody
Protein molecules (immunoglobulins) produced by B lymphocytes to help eliminate an antigen

Source: Wodi and Morelli (2021); Merriam Webster Dictionary (n.d.); Suryawanshi and Ott (2022).

Herd Immunity

Herd immunity or *community immunity* describes the immunity level that is present in a population group. A population with low herd immunity is one with few immune members; consequently, it is more susceptible to a particular disease. Nonimmune people are more likely to contract the disease and spread it throughout the group, placing the entire population at greater risk.

Conversely, a population with high herd immunity is one in which the immune people in the group outnumber the susceptible people; consequently, the *incidence* of a particular disease is reduced. The level of herd immunity may vary with diseases. For instance, a level of community immunity of between 83% and 85% may be necessary for rubella, but for pertussis (whooping cough), 92% to 94% may be needed to be effective (Merrill, 2021). Mandatory preschool immunizations and required travel vaccinations are applications of the herd immunity concept (Fig. 7-23).

Risk

Epidemiologists are concerned with risk, or the probability that a disease or other unfavorable health condition will develop. For any given group of people, the risk of developing a health problem is directly influenced, either positively or negatively, by such factors as their biology or inherited health capacity, living environment, lifestyle choices, and system of healthcare (Seabert et al., 2021). When such factors are negative influences, they are called *risk factors*. The degree of risk is directly linked to susceptibility or vulnerability to a given health problem (Box 7-5).

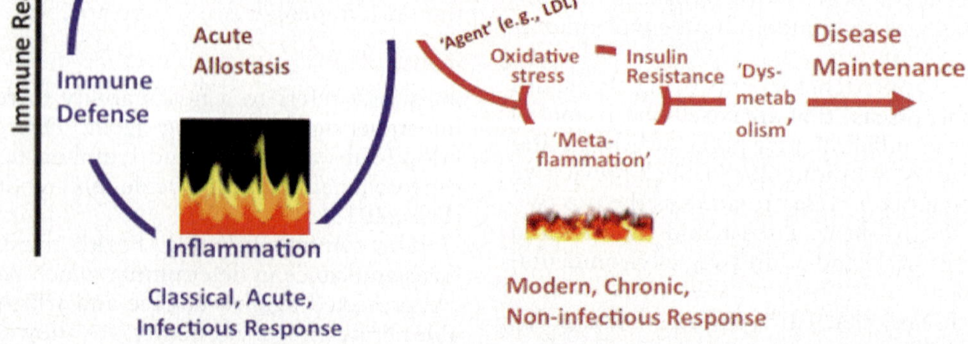

FIGURE 7-22 Anthropogen-induced metaflammation as the cause of chronic diseases. (Reprinted with permission from Egger, G. (2012). In search of a germ theory equivalent for chronic disease. *Preventing Chronic Disease, 9*, e110301. https://www.cdc.gov/pcd/issues/2012/11_0301.htm)

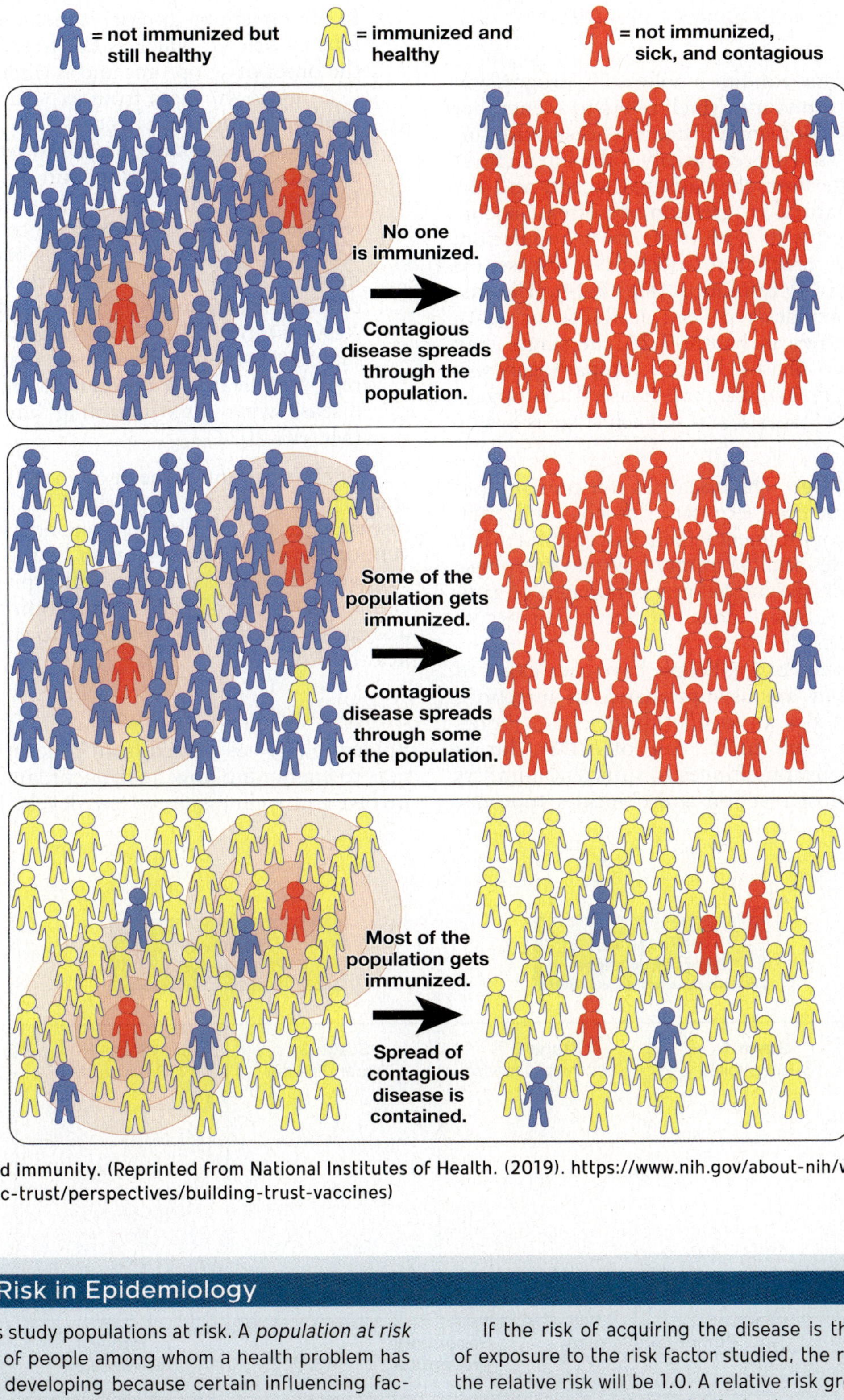

FIGURE 7-23 Herd immunity. (Reprinted from National Institutes of Health. (2019). https://www.nih.gov/about-nih/what-we-do/science-health-public-trust/perspectives/building-trust-vaccines)

BOX 7-5 Risk in Epidemiology

Epidemiologists study populations at risk. A *population at risk* is a collection of people among whom a health problem has the possibility of developing because certain influencing factors are present (e.g., exposure to HIV) or absent (e.g., lack of childhood immunizations, lack of specific vitamins in the diet), or because there are modifiable risk factors present (e.g., cardiovascular disease). Epidemiologists measure this difference using the *relative risk ratio*, which statistically compares the disease occurrence in the population at risk with the occurrence of the same disease in people without that risk factor.

$$\textit{Relative risk ratio} = \frac{\textit{Incidence in exposed group}}{\textit{Incidence rate in unexposed group}}$$

If the risk of acquiring the disease is the same regardless of exposure to the risk factor studied, the ratio will be 1:1, and the relative risk will be 1.0. A relative risk greater than 1.0 indicates that those with the risk factor have a greater likelihood of acquiring the disease than do those without it; for instance, a relative risk of 2.54 means that the exposed group is 2.54 times more likely to acquire the disease than the unexposed group (Merrill, 2021).

Natural History of a Disease or Health Condition

Any disease or health condition follows a progression known as its **natural history**, which refers to events that occur before its development, during its course, and during its conclusion. This process involves the interactions among a susceptible host, the causative agent, and the environment. The natural progression of a disease occurs in four stages in terms of how it affects a population: (1) susceptibility, (2) preclinical (subclinical) disease, (3) clinical disease, and (4) resolution (Fig. 7-24). The last stage, resolution, includes recovery, disability, or death (Friis, 2018). As shown in Figure 7-24, the stages may be grouped into two phases: Phase I (prepathogenesis), which includes Stages 1 and 2, and Phase II (pathogenesis), which includes Stages 3 and 4. Each stage is briefly described below.

1. *Susceptibility Stage*: The disease is not present, and people have not been exposed, but host and environmental factors influence their susceptibility. If a pathogen invades and the immune system's response is effective, then the infection is eliminated or contained, and the disease does not occur (History of Vaccines, 2022).
2. *Subclinical Disease Stage*: People have been exposed to a disease but are asymptomatic. In infectious diseases, it includes an *incubation period* of hours to months (or years, in the case of AIDS), during which the organism multiplies to sufficient numbers to produce a host reaction and clinical symptoms. In noninfectious disease, it includes an *induction* or *latency period*, which is the time from exposure to the onset of symptoms and is often years to decades (e.g., up to 40 years from exposure to asbestos and development of lung cancer).
3. *Clinical Disease Stage*: Signs and symptoms of the disease or condition develop, and diagnosis may occur. Early signs may be evident only through laboratory test findings (e.g., premalignant cervical changes evident on Papanicolaou smears), whereas later signs are more likely to be acute and clearly visible (e.g., enterocolitis in a salmonellosis outbreak; Heymann, 2022).
4. *Resolution or Advanced Disease Stage*: Depending on its severity, the disease may conclude with a return to health, a residual or chronic form of the disease with some disabling limitations, or death (Merrill, 2021).

C/PHNs can intervene at any point during these four stages to delay, arrest, or prevent the progression of the disease or condition. Primary, secondary, and tertiary prevention can be applied to each of the stages. However, primary prevention through health promotion and education strategies and health protection policies is the best and most cost-effective approach to ensuring population health (Box 7-6).

Epidemiology of Wellness

Epidemiology has moved from concentrating only on illness to examining how host, agent, and environment are involved in wellness at various levels. In response to an

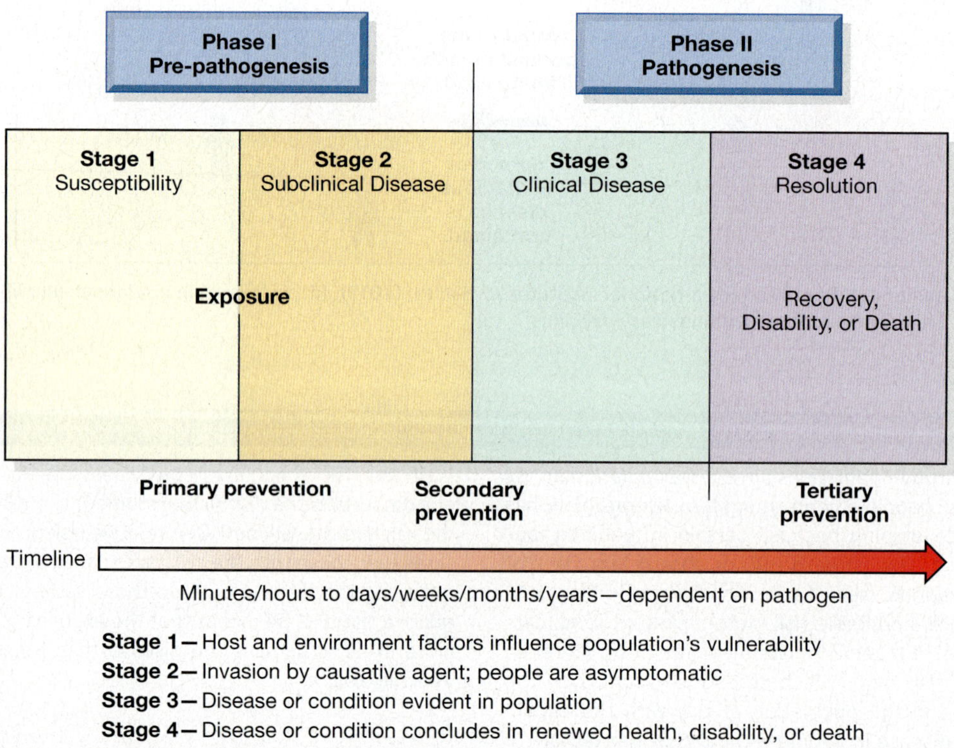

FIGURE 7-24 Natural history stages of a disease. (Source: CDC. (n.d.). Lesson 1: Introduction to epidemiology. In *Principles of epidemiology in public health practice* (3rd ed.). https://stacks.cdc.gov/view/cdc/6914/cdc_6914_DS1.pdf)

BOX 7-6 LEVELS OF PREVENTION PYRAMID

Application to the Four Stages of the Natural History of a Disease

SITUATION: Apply the levels of prevention during the four stages of the natural history of a disease to eradicate or reduce risk factors (examples of possible conditions provided).

GOAL: Using the three levels of prevention, negative health conditions are avoided, or promptly diagnosed and treated, and the fullest possible potential is restored.

Tertiary Prevention

Rehabilitation	*Primary Prevention*	
	Health Promotion and Education	*Health Protection*
▪ Reduce the extent and severity of a health problem to minimize disability ▪ Restore or preserve function	▪ Training for employment—people who are experiencing homelessness ▪ Group treatment and rehabilitation—adolescents with substance use disorder ▪ Food, shelter, rest/sleep, exercise	▪ Health services ▪ Immunizations as needed

Secondary Prevention

Early Diagnosis	*Prompt Treatment*
The third stage in the natural history of disease, the early pathogenesis or onset stage: ▪ Screening programs—breast and testicular cancer, vision and hearing loss, hypertension, TB, diabetes	▪ Initiate prompt treatment ▪ Arrest progression ▪ Prevent associated disability

Primary Prevention

Health Promotion and Education	*Health Protection*
May include ▪ Nutrition counseling—diabetes ▪ Sex education—pregnancy ▪ Smoking cessation—lung cancer	May include ▪ Improved housing and sanitation—waterborne diseases ▪ Immunizations—communicable diseases ▪ Removal of environmental hazards—accidents

escalating need for improved methods of health planning and health policy analysis, epidemiology has developed more holistic models of health (Marks, 2022).

These evolving epidemiologic models are organized around four attributes that influence health:

1. The physical, social, and psychological environment
2. Lifestyle, with its self-created risks
3. Human biology and genetic influences
4. The healthcare system

In the United States, *Healthy People 2030* (USDHHS, 2023a) and greater recognition of the importance and cost-effectiveness of illness prevention and health promotion are driving new efforts to develop policy and research initiatives that can improve the public's health (Box 7-7). There is also growing recognition of the impact of *social determinants of health* on health outcomes and conditions, not merely a person role in one's health. Population disparities result when these social determinants disproportionately impact people owing to race/ethnicity, socioeconomic status, gender, age, disability status, sexual orientation, and geographic location (USDHHS, 2023b). See Chapter 11 on health promotion and Chapters 15, 23, and 25 for more on this.

Wellness models that at first focused on person behavior now include approaches that encompass aggregates, including:

- Older adults (see Chapter 22)
- Workers (i.e., in occupational health settings; see Chapter 2)
- Students (i.e., children and teens at schools with wellness programs; see Chapter 20)
- Beginning and growing families (see Chapter 19)

Programs designed for aggregates focus on a wellness approach to growth and development, such as programs for teens who are pregnant and programs for infant and child development (e.g., Healthy Start, Head Start). Societal changes, such as the aging population, the technological revolution, the global economy, environmental threats, healthcare reform with its focus on prevention, and the health and wellness movements, are driving these new approaches (see Chapter 6).

Another approach to wellness is applying the four stages of the natural history of disease to wellness states:

- *Susceptibility*: People are amenable ("vulnerable") to healthier practices and improved health system organization.

BOX 7-7 SELECTED HEALTHY PEOPLE 2030 OBJECTIVES

Plan of Action

- Set national goals and measurable objectives to guide evidence-based policies, programs, and other actions to improve health and well-being.
- Provide accurate, timely, and accessible data that can drive targeted actions to address regions and populations that have poor health or are at high risk for poor health.
- Provide tools for the public, programs, policymakers, and others to evaluate progress toward improving health and well-being.
- Share and support the implementation of evidence-based programs and policies that are replicable, scalable, and sustainable.
- Report biennially on progress throughout the decade from 2020 to 2030.
- Stimulate research and innovation toward meeting Healthy People 2030 goals and highlight critical research, data, and evaluation needs.

Public Health Infrastructure Objectives

PHI-D03	Increase the proportion of vital records/health statistics programs that are nationally accredited
PHI-R06	Enhance the use and capabilities of informatics in public health

Community Objectives

PHI-04	Increase the proportion of state and territorial jurisdictions that have a health improvement plan
PHI-05	Increase the proportion of local jurisdictions that have a health improvement plan
PHI-08	Increase the proportion of tribal communities that have a health improvement plan
PHI-R09	Explore the impact of community health assessment and improvement planning efforts
PHI-R10	Explore the impact of public health accreditation and national standards

Reprinted from U.S. Department of Health and Human Services (USDHHS). (2023a). *Healthy People 2030 framework*. https://health.gov/healthypeople/about/healthy-people-2030-framework; USDHHS. (2023b). *Browse objectives: Community*. https://health.gov/healthypeople/objectives-and-data/browse-objectives/community; USDHHS. (2023c). *Browse objectives: Public health infrastructure*. https://health.gov/healthypeople/objectives-and-data/browse-objectives/public-health-infrastructure

- *Subclinical*: A community is exposed to these health-promoting behaviors.
- *Clinical:* Signs of adoption of beneficial policies and activities are evident in the community.
- *Resolution:* The community fully adopts the beneficial policies and activities and achieves a higher level of well-being.

This approach has important implications for preventive and health promotion practices in community/public health nursing as it can play a primary role in the investigation and identification of factors that not only prevent illness but also promote health. This means sharpening skills in epidemiologic research to uncover the factors that contribute to a full measure of healthful living. The time for an epidemiology of wellness has come (Merrill, 2021).

Causal Relationships

One of the main challenges to epidemiology is to identify causal relationships in disease and health conditions among populations. Causal inference is based on consistent results obtained from many studies. Frequently, the accumulation of evidence begins with a clinical observation or an educated guess that a certain factor may be causally related to a health problem (Friis, 2018). In epidemiologic research, the types of studies to research causal relationships include the following:

- *Cross-sectional study:* Explores a health condition's relation to other variables in a specified population at a specific point in time and can show that the factor and the problem coexist (e.g., using the "broken window index" to correlate poor housing quality, public school deterioration, and the presence of abandoned cars, graffiti, and trash with crime and social isolation in neighborhoods [Aiyer et al., 2015] and, by extension, perceived sexual partner risk level or other risk behaviors [Haley et al., 2018])
- *Retrospective study:* Looks backward in time to find a causal relationship, allowing a fairly quick assessment of whether an association exists. Such studies use existing data that have been recorded for reasons other than research and are generally less expensive and less labor intensive. One disadvantage is that the data may not be collected with a research outcome in mind (Nickson, 2020).
- *Prospective study:* Looks forward in time to find a causal relationship that is crucial to ensure that the presumed causal factor actually precedes the onset of

the health problem (e.g., The Nurses' Health Study, with over 280,000 participants, related to female health; NHS, 2021).

- *Experimental study:* The key to an experimental study is that the investigator controls the assignment of the exposure or of the treatment. Potential unknown confounders are addressed through randomization. Properly executed experimental studies provide the strongest empirical evidence. The randomization provides a better foundation for statistical procedures than do observational studies (Madigan Library, 2023).

Epidemiologically, a causal relationship may be said to exist if two major conditions are met: (1) the factor of interest (causal agent) is shown to increase the probability of occurrence of the disease or condition as observed in many studies in different populations and (2) evidence suggests that a reduction in the factor decreases the frequency of the given disease.

The synthesis of data begins by selecting as many of the various types of epidemiologic studies of the problem as possible and reviewing those that are sound. The goal of any epidemiologic investigation is to identify causal mechanisms that meet Hill's nine criteria for disease causation and to develop measures for preventing illness and promoting health (Celentano & Szklo, 2019). The C/PHN may need to gather new data for this type of investigation but should thoroughly examine pertinent existing data first.

SOURCES OF INFORMATION FOR EPIDEMIOLOGIC STUDY

Epidemiologic investigators may draw data from any of three major sources: existing data, informal investigations, and scientific studies. The C/PHN will find all three sources useful in efforts to improve the health of aggregates. See Chapter 15 on community assessment for more on sources of data.

Existing Data

A variety of epidemiologic information is available nationally, by state, and by section (e.g., county, region, census tract, metropolitan statistical area). This information includes vital statistics, census data, and morbidity statistics on certain communicable or infectious diseases. Local health departments often can provide these data on request.

C/PHNs seeking information on communities may find local health agencies helpful. These agencies collect health information for groups of counties within states and interact with health planning authorities at the state level. They have access to many types of information and can give advice on specific problems. A good place to start is at the National Center for Health Statistics website (https://www.cdc.gov/nchs/index.htm).

Vital Statistics

Vital statistics refers to the information gathered from the ongoing registration of births, deaths, adoptions, divorces, and marriages. Certified births, deaths, and fetal deaths are the most useful vital statistics in epidemiologic studies.

The PHN can obtain blank copies of a state's birth and death certificates to become familiar with the information contained in each. Death certificates report the fact and cause of death along with much more pertinent information. Birth certificates also can provide helpful information (e.g., weight of the infant, amount of prenatal care received by the birthing parent), which can be used to identify people in those populations who are at high risk.

However, nurses should note that the lack of standardization in collecting and reporting vital statistics data can lead to threats to reliability and validity. For example, if an agency changes the definitions for the categories used in grouping the data (reclassification), an inflation or deflation of the total of those affected can occur. Trending data over time would not be possible without including an explanation about the redefinitions used.

Sources for vital statistical information include state websites, local and state health departments, city halls, and county halls of records. Statistics regarding general aggregate morbidity and mortality for specific states are available from the CDC and at the national level from the National Center for Health Statistics (NCHS). State statistics are obtained from state health departments, and county information (regarding specific cities or census tracts) can be obtained from either the state or the county health department.

Census Data

Data from population censuses taken every 10 years in many countries are the main source of population statistics. This information can be a valuable assessment tool for the C/PHN who is taking part in health planning for aggregates. Population statistics can be analyzed by age, sex, race, ethnic background, type of occupation, income gradient, marital status, educational level, or other standards, such as housing quality.

Analysis of population statistics can provide the C/PHN with a better understanding of the community and help identify specific areas that may warrant further epidemiologic investigation. Data from the 2020 Census can be found on the U.S. Census Bureau website (https://www.census.gov/) and is an easily accessed source of population-level data.

Reportable Diseases

Each state has developed laws or regulations that require health organizations and practitioners to report to their local health authority cases of certain communicable and infectious diseases that can be spread through the community (Heymann, 2022). This reporting enables the health department to take the most appropriate and efficient action, for instance, in the case of foodborne illnesses. All states require that diseases subject to international quarantine regulations be reported immediately.

The World Health Organization has numerous diseases under surveillance (e.g., TB, malaria, viral influenza) globally, and these must also be reported. Other reportable diseases (numbering between 20 and 40 in each state) are usually classified according to the speed with which the health department should be notified. Some should be reported by phone or e-mail, others weekly by regular mail. They vary in potential severity from varicella (chickenpox) to rabies and include AIDS, encephalitis, measles, meningitis, pertussis (whooping cough), syphilis, and toxic shock syndrome (MedlinePlus, 2021). The Laboratory Response Network provides early response to biologic and chemical agents involved in public health emergencies or bioterrorism (CDC, 2019b; see Chapter 16).

C/PHNs should obtain the list of reportable diseases from their local or state health department office. Following up on occurrences of these diseases is a task frequently assigned to PHNs working for local health departments. Chapter 8 includes more information on reporting and tracking communicable diseases at the local, regional, and national levels.

Disease Registries

Some areas or states have disease registries or rosters for conditions with major public health impact. TB and rheumatic fever registries were more common when these diseases occurred more frequently. Cancer registries provide useful incidence, prevalence, and survival data and assist the C/PHN in monitoring cancer patterns within a community. Nurses can access these registries through federal and state health department websites.

Federal registries include the following:

- Agency for Toxic Substances and Disease Registry (ATSDR, 2019) maintains three registries of major public concern:
  - *National Amyotrophic Lateral Sclerosis (ALS) Registry*: A congressionally mandated registry for people in the United States with ALS (Lou Gehrig's Disease). It is the only population-based registry in the United States that collects information to help scientists learn more about who gets ALS and its causes.
  - *Rapid Response Registry*: A registry of people who are exposed or potentially exposed to chemical and other harmful substances during catastrophic events to help local, state, and federal public health and disaster response agencies.
  - *World Trade Center Health Registry*: A comprehensive and confidential health survey of those directly exposed to fallout and debris on September 11, 2001.
- *Surveillance, Epidemiology, and End Results Program of the NCI:* An organization that collects and publishes cancer incidence and survival data from population-based cancer registries that cover a portion of the U.S. population (NCI, n.d.).

Surveillance Systems

The CDC maintains various surveillance systems to monitor diseases so it can develop and evaluate control strategies, including:

- The *Behavioral Risk Factor Surveillance System* conducts an ongoing state-based telephone survey of the civilian, noninstitutional adult population. Data collected indicates the prevalence of high-risk behaviors, such as excessive alcohol consumption, cigarette smoking, physical inactivity, and lack of preventive healthcare, such as screening for cancer. Results are published on a periodic basis in the *Morbidity and Mortality Weekly Report's* CDC Surveillance Summaries and are available online at https://www.cdc.gov/brfss/.
- The *Youth Risk Behavior Surveillance System* monitors unintentional injuries and violence, tobacco use, alcohol and other drug use, sexual behaviors that contribute to unintended pregnancy and STIs, unhealthy dietary behaviors, and physical inactivity, as well as the prevalence of obesity and asthma, in the national *Youth Risk Behavior Survey*. Results are available online at https://www.cdc.gov/healthyyouth/data/yrbs/index.htm (Seabert et al., 2021).
- The *National Wastewater Surveillance System* was created in response to the COVID-19 pandemic in September 2020 (CDC, 2023e). Whatever substances and pathogens we inhale or ingest eventually get eliminated in our stool, which ends up in wastewater. By analyzing the content of wastewater, epidemiologists can help communities detect and prepare for disease outbreaks. It also can detect substances that are legally and illegally used by community residents, which helps local health professionals to identify and focus on areas in their communities in need of health education and services to address substance misuse. During the COVID-19 pandemic, it helped to identify pockets in the community with the highest number of infections in need of intervention for testing and treatment. When the public health emergency ended in May 2023, wastewater surveillance became one of the most important community tools to monitor and detect ongoing COVID-19 infections when testing dropped, and transmission data became unavailable due to the ending of disease surveillance activities (Fig. 7-25).
- The *Pregnancy Risk Assessment Monitoring System* (PRAMS) collects state-specific, population-based data on maternal attitudes and experiences before, during, and shortly after pregnancy (CDC, 2023f). PRAMS surveillance currently covers about 83% of all U.S. births, and the data can be used to identify groups of birthing parents and infants at high risk for health problems, to monitor changes in health status, and to measure progress toward goals in improving the health of people in this population (CDC, 2023b).
- The *Traveler-based Genomic Surveillance program* is operated by the CDC's Travelers' Health Branch in partnership with Ginkgo Bioworks and XpresCheck (CDC, 2023g). Begun in September 2021, this voluntary program tests travelers anonymously to detect new COVID-19 variants entering the country (Fig. 7-26).
- The *U.S. Zika Pregnancy & Infant Registry* was created in 2018 and is a collaborative system to learn about Zika virus infection during pregnancy and after birth. Information from the Registry is used to make recommendations for healthcare providers caring for families affected by Zika virus and plan for needed services (CDC, 2022b).

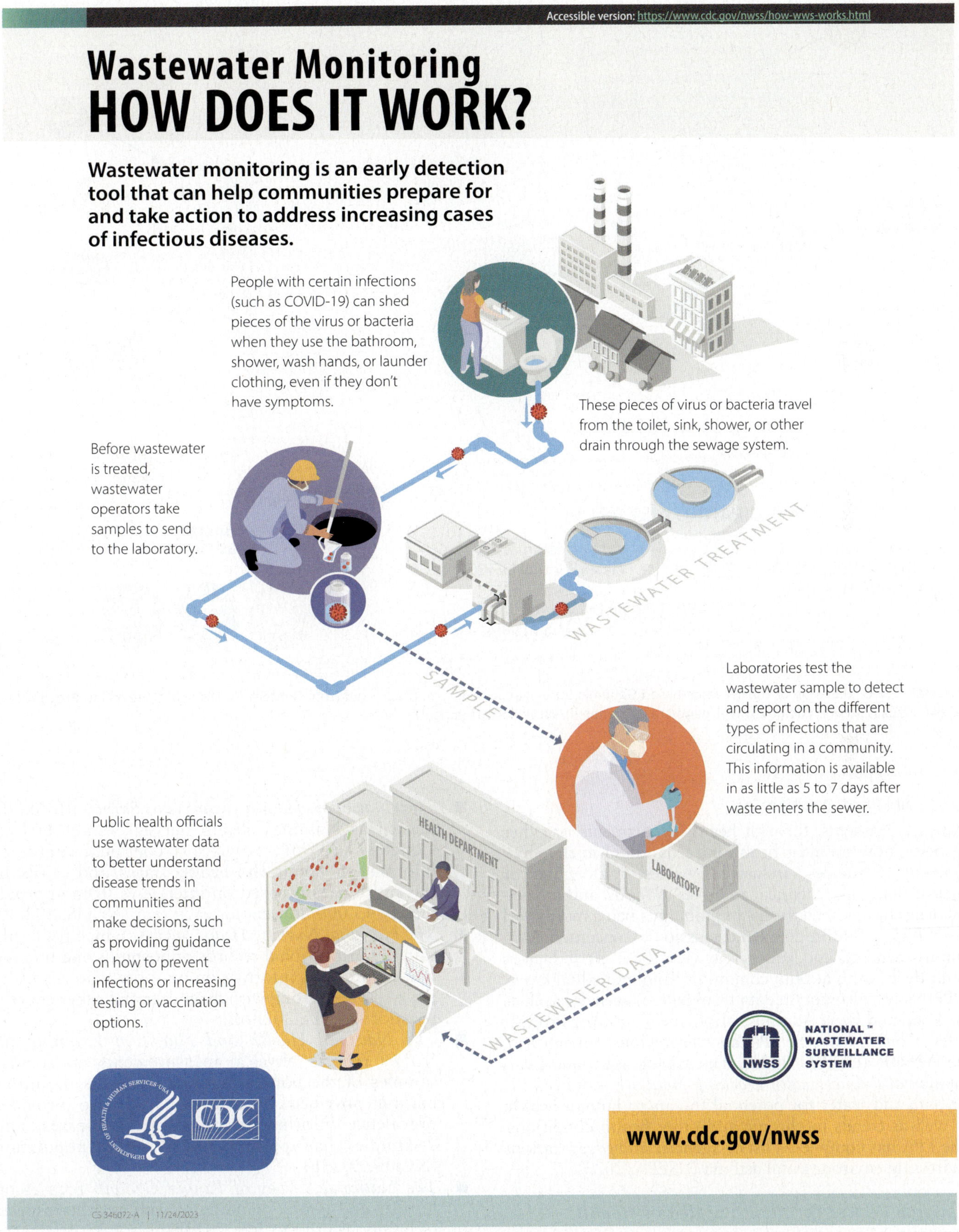

FIGURE 7-25 National Wastewater Surveillance System—How does it work? (Reprinted from Centers for Disease Control and Prevention. (2023). https://www.cdc.gov/nwss/pdf/Wastewater-COVID-infographic-h.pdf)

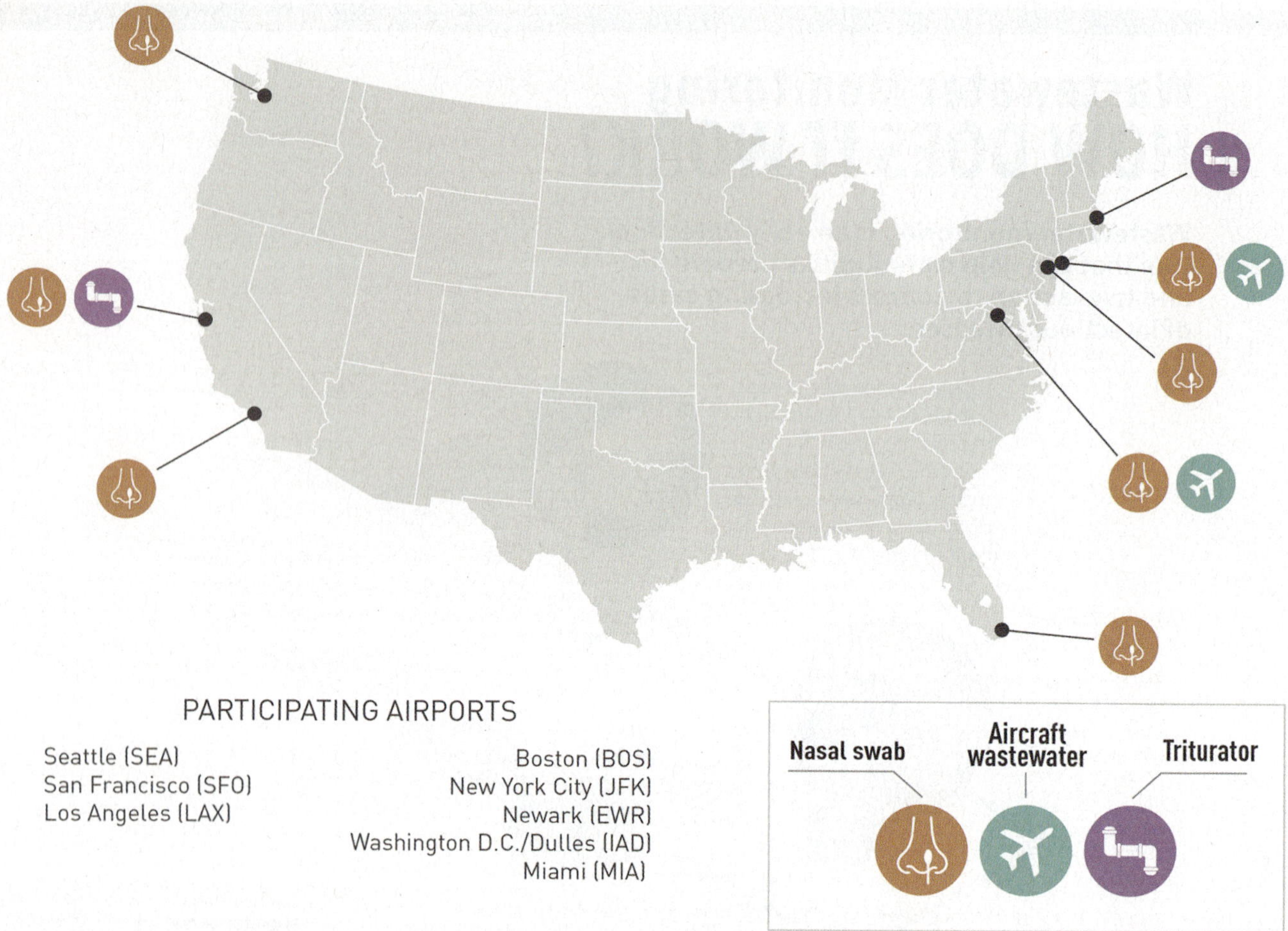

FIGURE 7-26 U.S. Map of the Traveler-based Genomic Surveillance program. (Reprinted from Centers for Disease Control and Prevention. (2024). https://wwwnc.cdc.gov/travel/page/travel-genomic-surveillance#impact)

Environmental Monitoring

State governments, through health departments or other agencies, now monitor health hazards found in the environment. Pesticides, industrial wastes, radioactive or nuclear materials, chemical additives in foods, and medicinal drugs have joined the list of pollutants being monitored (see Chapter 9 for a detailed discussion). Concerned community members and leaders may view these as risk factors that affect health at both community and individual levels. C/PHNs can also obtain data from federal agencies such as the Food and Drug Administration, the Consumer Product Safety Commission, the EPA, and, as previously mentioned, the ATSDR (USEPA, 2023). The CDC's *National Environmental Public Health Tracking Network* monitors the air, soil, and water for potential threats to human health, as well as trends in chronic and other health conditions. The EPA has compiled a list of agencies and organizations addressing environmental asthma (USEPA, 2023).

National Center for Health Statistics Health Surveys

The NCHS furnishes valuable health prevalence data from surveys of Americans. Published data are also frequently available for regions. Examples are as follows:

- *The National Health Interview Survey* (formerly known as National Health Survey), established by Congress in 1956, provides a continual source of information about the health status and needs of the entire nation based on interviews from approximately 43,000 households each year (NCHS, 2023a).
- *The National Nursing Home Survey*, which primarily samples institutional records of hospitals and nursing homes, provides information on those who are using these services, along with diagnoses and other characteristics (NCHS, 2023b).
- *The National Health and Nutrition Examination Survey* reports physical measurements on smaller samples of the population and augments the information provided by interviews. It also provides prevalence information on injuries, diseases, and disabilities that appear frequently in the population (NCHS, 2023b).
- *The National Survey of Family Growth* focuses on fertility and family planning as well as other aspects of family health (NCHS, 2023b).

Other studies investigate vital statistics events and characteristics of ambulatory patients in primary providers' community practices. Each of these nationally

BOX 7-8 STORIES FROM THE FIELD

How Public Health Nurses Make the Case

PHNs working for a local or county health department often find themselves more involved with program planning than direct patient care. Often, they are asked to help develop a health education program based on what is affecting the community the most, limited by budgetary constraints while still meeting reporting requirements of grant funders.

Let's say your health department has been given the opportunity to apply for funding from three sponsoring organizations. The choices are to develop public health education programs about alcohol consumption, smoking cessation, or community HIV testing. In an upcoming department meeting, you are asked to make a case for and against applying for funding of each of these programs.

1. *In preparing for this presentation, which specific types of data would you recommend to the department?*
2. *What would be the sources of these data? Are those sources from local, state, or national resources?*
3. *How could Healthy People 2030 help frame this presentation?*

sponsored efforts suggests ways in which nurses can examine health problems or concerns affecting their communities (see Box 7-8). Interviews, physical examinations of subsets of community members, and surveillance of institutions, clinics, and private primary providers' practices can be carried out locally after needs are identified and funds made available. Other sources may be found in data kept routinely, but not centrally, on the health problems of workers in local industries or the health problems of schoolchildren, a key issue for many C/PHNs. Existing epidemiologic data can be used to plan parent education programs, health promotion among students, and almost any other type of service.

Federal Public Health Agency Reports

The CDC issues the *Mortality and Morbidity Weekly Report*. This publication presents weekly summaries of disease and death data trends for the nation. It includes reports on outbreaks or occurrences of diseases in specific regions of the country and international trends in disease occurrences that may affect the U.S. population.

Most health departments subscribe to this publication, which provides important information both for epidemiologists and PHNs. It is also available free online from the CDC at https://www.cdc.gov/mmwr/index.html.

The Community Preventive Services Task Force (CPSTF) maintains the *Guide to Community Preventive Services* website. It houses the official collection of all the CPSTF findings, and the systematic reviews on which they are based are offered as a free resource to help C/PHNs, and other public health professionals choose programs and policies to improve health and prevent disease within the communities with whom they work (CPSTF, 2023).

Informal Observational Studies

In addition to perusing existing data, the C/PHN can also gain epidemiologic data by engaging in informal observation and description. The C/PHN can perform such study on almost any client group the nurse encounters.

If, for example, if a nurse at a clinic encounters a child experiencing abuse, a study of the clinic's records to screen for additional possible instances of child abuse and neglect could lead to more case findings. If several cases of diabetes come to the attention of a nurse serving on a Navajo reservation, a widespread problem might come to light through informal inquiries about the incidence and age at onset of the disease among this Native American population. Informal observational study often raises questions and suggests hypotheses that form the basis for designing larger-scale epidemiologic investigations.

Scientific Studies

A third source of information used in epidemiologic inquiry involves carefully designed scientific studies. The nursing profession has recognized the need to develop a systematic body of knowledge on which to base nursing practice. Systematic research is becoming an accepted part of the C/PHN's role.

Findings from epidemiologic studies conducted by or involving nurses are appearing more frequently in the literature. The *Cochrane Database of Systematic Reviews* is the most popular resource for systematic reviews in healthcare and includes a section on public health. Its website is searchable by topic or Cochrane Review Group. Additionally, the website includes reviews, methods studies, technology assessments, and economic evaluations (Wiley Online Library, 2023; see Chapter 4). Systematic reviews can routinely be found in many professional journals and the aforementioned Community Guide. These can provide the C/PHN with valuable information that can be used to positively affect aggregate health.

METHODS IN THE EPIDEMIOLOGIC INVESTIGATIVE PROCESS

The goals of an epidemiologic investigation are to identify the causal mechanisms of health and illness states and to develop measures for preventing illness and promoting health. Epidemiologists use an investigative process that involves a sequence of three approaches that build on one another: descriptive, analytic, and experimental studies. All three approaches have relevance for community/public health nursing (see Chapter 4 for a more detailed description).

Descriptive Epidemiology

Descriptive epidemiology includes investigations that seek to observe and describe patterns of health-related conditions that occur naturally in a population. At this stage, in the epidemiologic investigation, the researcher seeks to establish the occurrence of a problem. Data from descriptive studies suggest hypotheses for further testing. Descriptive studies almost always involve some form of broad-based quantification and statistical analysis (Celentano & Szklo, 2019).

Descriptive studies can be *retrospective* (identify cases and controls and then go back to review existing data) or *prospective* (identify groups and exposure factors and then follow them forward in time). In a descriptive study of child abuse, for example, the investigator would note the age, gender, race or ethnic group, and physical and emotional conditions of the children affected. In addition, the investigator would collect data that describe the economic status and occupation of the parents, the location and setting of the abusive behavior, and the time of year when the abuse occurred. In a retrospective study on reported varicella deaths, the investigators would describe the age, sex, ethnic background, and birthplace of victims and other information. Describing facets of these deaths provides information for further study and suggests avenues for intervention or prevention (Celentano & Szklo, 2019).

Counts

The simplest measure of description is a *count*. "Frequency of disease" should be interpreted to include any health outcome of interest (e.g., diseases, congenital defects, injuries, deaths, mental health problems; LaMorte, 2021).

Obtaining a count of this type always depends on the definition of what is being counted and when it was counted. This particular count, for example, uses a large database that takes time to be made public and therefore may not provide a current picture of actual deaths. When using this type of data, the C/PHN should always consider the time delay involved. If a C/PHN needs more current information within a specific community or state, hospital records or death certificates may be another source.

Rates

Rates are statistical measures expressing the proportion of people with a given health problem among a population at risk. The total number of people in the group serves as the denominator for various types of rates. To express a count as a proportion, or rate, the population to be studied must first be identified. If those deaths are considered in relation to the total number of cases in the country, there will be one rate; if, however, those fatalities are considered in relation to the total population, there will be a quite different rate. It is important when reviewing rates that you understand which measures are being compared.

In epidemiology, the population represents the universe of people defined as the objects of a study. Because it is often difficult, if not impossible, to study an entire population, most epidemiologic studies draw a sample to represent that group.

Sometimes, it is important to seek a random sample (in which everyone in the population has an equal chance of selection for study and choice is made without bias). At other times, a sample of convenience (in which study subjects are selected because of their availability) is sufficient. In many small epidemiologic studies, it may be possible to study almost every person in the population, eliminating the need for a sample. Several rates have wide use in epidemiology (Merrill, 2021). The most important for the C/PHN to understand are the incidence rate, the prevalence rate, and the period prevalence rate (see Box 7-9).

BOX 7-9 Incidence, Attack Rate, and Prevalence

Incidence

Not everyone in a population is at risk for developing a disease, incurring an injury, or having some other health-related characteristic. The *incidence rate* recognizes this fact. **Incidence** refers to *all new cases* of a disease or health condition appearing *during a given time*. Incidence rate describes a proportion in which the numerator is all new cases appearing during a given period of time and the denominator is the population at risk during the same period (Merrill, 2021).

$$\text{Incidence rate} = \frac{\text{Number of persons developing a disease}}{\text{Total number at risk per unit of time}}$$

Attack Rate

An *attack rate* describes the proportion of a group or population that develops a disease among all those exposed to a particular risk. This term is used frequently in investigations of outbreaks of infectious diseases such as influenza. If the attack rate changes, it may suggest an alteration in the population's immune status or that the disease-causing organism is present in a more or less virulent strain (Celentano & Szklo, 2019).

$$\text{Rate} = \frac{\text{Number of new cases in the population at risk}}{\text{Number of persons at risk in the population}}$$

Prevalence

Prevalence refers to all of the people with a particular health condition existing in a given population at a given point in time. The *prevalence rate* describes a situation at a specific point in time (McKenzie et al., 2018). If a nurse discovers 50 cases of measles in an elementary school, that is a simple count. When this number is divided by the total number of students in the school, the result is the prevalence of measles. For instance, if the school has 500 students, the prevalence of measles on that day would be 10% (50 measles/500 population).

$$\text{Prevalence rate} = \frac{\text{Number of persons with a characteristic}}{\text{Total number in population}}$$

The prevalence rate over a defined period of time is called a *period prevalence rate*:

$$\text{Period prevalence rate} = \frac{\text{Number of persons with a characteristic during a period of time}}{\text{Total number in population}}$$

Source: Celentano and Szklo (2019); Merrill (2017).

Computing Rates

To make comparisons between populations, epidemiologists often use a common base population in computing rates. For example, instead of merely saying that the rate of an illness is 13% in one city and 25% in another, the comparison is made per 100,000 people in the population. This population base can vary for different purposes from 100 to 100,000. However, in order to make valid comparisons, the same denominator would need to be used.

To describe the **morbidity rate**, which is the relative incidence of disease in a population, the ratio of the number of sick people to the total population is determined. The **mortality rate** refers to the relative death rate or the sum of deaths in a given population at a given time (Celentano & Szklo, 2019). Table 7-3 includes formulas for morbidity rates, and Box 7-10 includes formulas for computing mortality and other rates used frequently in community/public health.

Analytic Epidemiology

A second type of investigation, *analytic epidemiology*, goes beyond simple description or observation and seeks to identify associations between a particular human disease or health problem and its possible causes. Analytic studies tend to be more specific than descriptive studies in their focus. They test hypotheses or seek to answer specific questions and can be retrospective or prospective in design (Merrill, 2021). Analytic studies fall into three types: prevalence studies, case–control studies, and cohort studies.

Prevalence Studies

When examining prevalence, it is helpful to remember that the health condition may be new or may have affected some people for many years. A **prevalence study** describes patterns of occurrence, as in the study of varicella-related deaths. It may examine causal factors, but a prevalence study always looks at factors from the same point in time and in the same population. Hypothesized causal factors are based on inferences from a single examination and most likely need further testing for validation. Intervening or confounding variables can lead to inaccurate assumptions about results, and studies must be carefully designed to avoid both falsely positive and falsely negative outcomes (Merrill, 2021). A recent international prevalence study found that sociodemographic factors (e.g., education, gender) were moderators of the built environment (safety from crime) in meeting physical activity goals (Perez et al., 2018).

Case–Control Studies

A *case–control study* compares people who have a health or illness condition (number of cases with the condition) with those who lack this condition (controls). These studies begin with the cases and look back over time (retrospectively) for the presence or absence of the suspected causal factor in both cases and controls (Celentano & Szklo, 2019).

One of the more successful case–control studies showed the relationship between smoking and bladder cancer in 2008. The connection was further supported by a 2022 meta-analysis looking at the same connection, which found a nonlinear dose–response relationship between smoking and bladder cancer (Zhao et al., 2022).

Cohort Studies

A *cohort* is a group of people who share a common experience in a specific time period. In epidemiology, a cohort of people often becomes a focus of study. Cohort studies, rather than measuring the relationship of variables in existing conditions, study the development of a condition over time.

A cohort study begins by selecting a group of people who display certain defined characteristics before the onset of the condition being investigated (Merrill, 2021). In studying a disease, the cohort might include people who are initially free of the disease but were known to have been exposed to a particular substance or risk factor. They would be observed over time to evaluate which variables were associated with the development or nondevelopment of the disease. These types of studies are often used with environmental hazard exposures, as with

TABLE **7-3** Frequently Used Measures of Morbidity

Measure	Numerator	Denominator
Incidence[a] proportion (or attack rate or risk)	Number of new cases of disease during specified time interval	Population at start of time interval
Secondary attack rate	Number of new cases among contacts	Total number of contacts
Incidence rate (or person-time rate)	Number of new cases of disease during specified time interval	Summed person-years of observation or average population during time interval
Point prevalence	Number of current cases (new and preexisting) at a specified point in time	Population at the same specified point in time
Period prevalence	Number of current cases (new and preexisting) over a specified period of time	Average or mid-interval population

[a]Incidence refers to the occurrence of new cases of disease or injury in a population over a specified period of time. Although some epidemiologists use incidence to mean the number of new cases in a community, others use incidence to mean the number of new cases per unit of population. Reprinted from CDC. (n.d.). *Lesson 3: Measures of risk*. https://www.cdc.gov/csels/dsepd/ss1978/lesson3/section2.html

BOX 7-10 Common Epidemiologic Mortality Rates

Mortality Rate

A mortality rate is a measure of the frequency of occurrence of death in a defined population during a specified interval. Morbidity and mortality measures are often the same mathematically; it's just a matter of what you choose to measure, illness or death. The formula for the mortality of a defined population, over a specified period of time, is:

$$\frac{\text{Deaths occurring during a given time period}}{\text{Size of the population among which the deaths occurred} \times 10^n}$$

When mortality rates are based on vital statistics (e.g., counts of death certificates), the denominator most commonly used is the size of the population at the middle of the time period. In the United States, values of 1000 and 100,000 are both used for 10^n for most types of mortality rates.

General Mortality Rates

$$\text{Crude mortality rate} = \frac{\text{Number of reported deaths during 1 year}}{\text{Estimated population as of July 1 of same year}} \times 100{,}000$$

$$\text{Cause-specific mortality rate} = \frac{\text{Number of deaths from a specified cause during 1 year}}{\text{Estimated population as of July 1 of same year}} \times 100{,}000$$

$$\text{Case fatality rate} = \frac{\text{Number of deaths from a particular disease}}{\text{Total number with the same disease}} \times 100$$

$$\text{Proportional mortality ratio} = \frac{\text{Number of deaths from a specific cause within a given time period}}{\text{Total deaths in the same time period}} \times 100$$

$$\text{Age-specific mortality rate} = \frac{\text{Number of persons in a specific age group dying during 1 year}}{\text{Estimated population of the specific age group as of July 1 of same year}} \times 100{,}000$$

Specific Rates for Maternal and Infant Populations

$$\text{Crude birth rate} = \frac{\text{Number of live births during 1 year}}{\text{Estimated population as of July of same year}} \times 1000$$

$$\text{General fertility rate} = \frac{\text{Number of live births during 1 year}}{\text{Number of females ages 15} - \text{44 as of July of same year}} \times 1000$$

$$\text{Maternal mortality rate} = \frac{\text{Number of deaths from puerperal causes during 1 year}}{\text{Number of live births during same year}} \times 100{,}000$$

$$\text{Infant mortality rate} = \frac{\text{Number of deaths under 1 year of age for given year}}{\text{Number of live births reported for same year}} \times 1000$$

$$\text{Perinatal mortality rate} = \frac{\text{Number of fatal deaths plus infant deaths under 7 days of age during 1 year}}{\text{Number of live births plus fetal deaths during same year}} \times 1000$$

Source: Centers for Disease Control (CDC) (2006).

the Health Registry and the National Toxic Substance Incidents Program discussed earlier (ATSDR, 2019).

In 1993, the Women's Health Study, a 10-year national longitudinal, experimental, cohort study involving nearly 40,000 female health professionals was initiated (Harvard Medical School & Brigham and Women's Hospital, n.d.). Over the course of many years, significant findings regarding female health issues were published (600+) and implemented to improve health outcomes.

In practice, the various types of studies just discussed are frequently mixed. A case–control study may include description and analysis with a retrospective focus; a cohort study may be conducted prospectively or retrospectively. The Women's Health Study is an example of a case–control study, a cohort study, and an experimental study. Flexibility is essential to allow the investigator as much freedom as possible in choosing the most useful methodology.

Experimental Epidemiology

Experimental epidemiology follows and builds on information gathered from descriptive and analytic approaches. In an experimental study, the investigator actually controls or changes the factors suspected of causing the health condition under study and then observes what happens to the health state (Merrill, 2021).

In human populations, experimental studies should focus on disease prevention or health promotion rather than testing the causes of disease, which is done primarily on animals. Experimental studies are carried out under carefully controlled conditions and must be approved by an Institutional Review Board. The investigator exposes an experimental group to some factor thought to cause disease, improve health, prevent disease, or influence health in some way (as in the Women's Health Study). Simultaneously, the investigator observes a control group that is similar in characteristics to the experimental group but without the exposure factor. See Chapter 4 for more on experimental research studies.

The C/PHN should be alert for opportunities to conduct experimental studies in the course of working with groups. A study need not be elaborate to provide important data for future nursing practice. For example, a C/PHN can provide focused instruction to 20 new birthing parents, encouraging them to breastfeed, and then compare the health outcomes of their infants with infants of 20 birthing parents in the same service area who use formula.

An expanding area of experimental epidemiology involves the use of computers to simulate epidemics. The National Science Teaching Association reported on an 8-day unit in which students developed epidemic simulations and used them to investigate how individual human behaviors and interactions impacted epidemic dynamics at the population level (Xiang & Diamond, 2022).

Occasionally, an experiment occurs naturally, thus affording the researcher a chance to make important discoveries. John Snow discovered such a "natural experiment" in London in 1854 (as discussed earlier in the chapter). In his seminal study of an epidemic of cholera, he observed one group that contracted the disease and another that did not. Closer inspection revealed that the major difference between these groups was their water supply. See Chapter 9 for more information on environmental health.

A *community trial* is a type of experimental study done at the community level. Geographic communities are assigned to intervention (experimental) or nonintervention (control) groups and compared to determine whether the intervention produces a positive change in the community (Merrill, 2021).

Community trials can be extremely expensive and are not undertaken unless there is substantial evidence that the intervention will make a difference at the aggregate level. There are times when these community trials occur spontaneously, and it is important for the C/PHN to recognize these opportunities. For instance, one local public health department institutes an aggressive campaign to educate healthcare workers on the signs of abuse of older adults. Selecting a similar community where that level of training is not available, the PHN can then compare the rates of abuse reporting between these two communities. If you were conducting this research, what outcome would you expect in the community with the enhanced training? Where could you obtain this information? Think about what other measures you might also want to compare between these two communities.

CONDUCTING EPIDEMIOLOGIC RESEARCH

The C/PHN who engages in an epidemiologic investigation becomes a kind of detective. First, there is a problem to solve, a puzzle to unravel, or a question to answer. The nurse begins to search for basic information, for clues that might help answer the question.

Information is never self-explanatory, and, like a detective, the nurse must analyze and interpret every additional clue. Slowly, there is a narrowing of possible suspects until the causes of a particular disease, the consequences of a prevention plan, or the results of treatment are identified. On the basis of this investigation, the nurse can draw further conclusions and make new applications to improve health services.

Epidemiologic studies are a form of research. The steps outlined here are similar to those discussed in Chapter 4. Epidemiologic research involves seven steps (Table 7-4). Everything from an informal study in the course of nursing practice to the most comprehensive epidemiologic research project can be undertaken with these steps. Box 7-11 discusses conducting an epidemiologic investigation of lead poisoning from an herbal remedy, and Table 7-4 describes examples for each step of the investigation discussed in Box 7-11.

Findings from epidemiologic investigations should be disseminated in forms that are easily understood by the general public, such as the flow chart developed during an outbreak investigation of coccidioidomycosis among solar farm workers (Wilkin et al., 2015). See Figure 7-27 for a flowchart of the sequence of investigation that took place and how cases were identified, as well as what was done.

Figure 7-28 shows the impact of conducting investigations of multistate food outbreaks. Such outbreaks are becoming quite common because the manufacturing process of food products can affect people living in many states. It is vital that collaborative processes are in place in which all levels of public health agencies and health systems can communicate findings efficiently to prevent outbreaks as well as reduce morbidity and mortality.

TABLE 7-4 Steps in Epidemiologic Research

Step	Description
Identify the problem	Any threat to the health of a group offers fertile ground for epidemiologic investigation. Issues can be identified by looking at local health statistics and trending data over time, defined by funding agencies, or unusual cases identified through screening and intervention activities. (Example: Why did the woman discussed in Box 7-11 have an elevated lead level?")
Review the literature	Find out what has already been done to address the problem identified. Every epidemiologic investigation should begin with a review of the literature. Even discovering that little research has been done on the problem can be valuable information, a good source for conducting a literature review is the Community Guide website. Conversely, if many studies have already been conducted in the area, this information can help narrow the study to areas that have not previously been investigated or allow researchers to replicate earlier studies to confirm findings in a different setting. A valuable source is the systematic review, which evaluates research studies done on specific topics. (Example: Are the Koo Sar pills taken by the woman discussed in Box 7-11 known to contain lead?)
Design the study	The first step in designing a study is to formulate one or more specific questions to answer or hypotheses to test. Sometimes, the question or hypothesis emerges from the literature review, or from the researcher's own analysis and hunches. Come up with one or more hypotheses to test or questions to answer. Then plan what study type (descriptive, analytic, or experimental) or combination of study types best suits the goals of the research and how the study will be conducted. Will the data be collected retrospectively from existing records, or will new data be collected? Who will conduct interviews? What kinds of data will be needed to measure the outcomes of intervention? (Example (see Box 7-11): Who else may be affected? The pills were bought at several locations. Did those other pills have lead also?)
Collect the data	Use available online sources (e.g., U.S. census demographic data; NCHS health-related data; CDC BRFSS risk factor data; geographic data from CDC's GIS, U.S. Geological Survey, and the Environmental Protection Agency), as well as data from state and local agencies and nongovernmental organizations. Data about a particular community may be available from the state, county, or local health departments, upon request. The Community Guide website may provide ideas about how to collect data for a particular purpose (e.g., assessment, evaluation, pilot testing) and what works and doesn't work. Development of data collection tools should start with why the data are being collected and what data are needed at the end of the study. This will help determine what kinds of data collection are most suited (e.g., mail surveys, telephone surveys, online surveys, face-to-face surveys, focus groups, etc.) in order to gather the data. There are many freely available data collection tools online. All methods of collection have pros and cons (DJS, 2015) that should be considered. (Example (see Box 7-11): Gather samples of pills from cities where the person bought them and test them for lead content.)
Analyze the findings	In most epidemiologic studies, data analysis consists of summarizing the findings, computing rates and ratios, and displaying the findings in tables and graphs. At this stage, the data are used to address the original question or test the original hypothesis. Was the hypothesis supported or not supported by the data? Summarized data can also generate more questions or indicate areas that warrant further investigation. (Example (see Box 7-11): Lead was found in three different sources, from three different cities, and each specimen contained different lead levels.)
Develop conclusions and applications	Stating conclusions is an outcome of analysis and interpretation. The investigators summarize the results and their meaning for the purpose of making this information useful to the public and other public health and health services providers. Many times, research has direct practical application for improving health services, continuing or discontinuing services, or conducting future research. It is also important to describe mistakes made and lessons learned about study design and other aspects of the research and to propose further areas of study, to assist future investigators. (Example (see Box 7-11): Laboratory findings indicated that lead was a contaminant during the manufacturing process.)
Disseminate the findings	Finally, research findings should be shared. The audience for the reporting of findings should be considered during the development of the study to ensure that the concerns and questions of the audience will be addressed by the study. Of course, if the study is being sponsored, then the purpose for the study is clear, making the dissemination of the findings easier. Sponsorship, however, can affect how the findings are perceived. In medical research, financial conflicts of interest (e.g., pharmaceutical-funded studies) can negatively impact the value of the findings (Johnston, 2015). Nevertheless, information gained from epidemiologic studies must be disseminated throughout the professional community to strengthen the knowledge base for improved practice and to promote future research. (Example (see Box 7-11): Findings from the three-state investigation were reported to the CDC and published in the MMWR. As a result of the report, California and other environmental entities issued an alert that people can be poisoned by taking Koo Sar pills.)

BOX 7-11 PERSPECTIVES

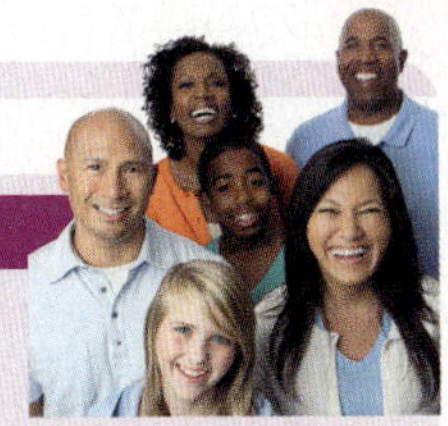

Conducting an Epidemiologic Investigation into Adult Lead Poisoning

During a free lead-screening event, sponsored by a nursing school community health promotion center, a 33-year-old Cambodian woman who brought her two children to the center to be tested for lead poisoning also participated in being tested. She was found to have an elevated blood lead level (BLL) of 44 µg/dL and a confirmatory BLL 1 month later of 42 µg/dL. Any level above 10 µg/dL is considered abnormal. The children and her husband were found to have normal BLLs. This woman was referred by the director of the health promotion center for follow-up to the Connecticut Department of Public Health.

As the Connecticut Adult Blood Lead Surveillance Program's Adult Lead Registry and Case Management Coordinator, I was responsible for compiling and analyzing BLL data from Connecticut laboratories performing these tests and to follow-up on any reports of elevated lead levels, such as this woman, who was identified through a community screening event sponsored by a nursing school.

The woman mentioned she took Koo Sar pills for menstrual cramps. After finding lead in the Koo Sar pills the woman purchased in Connecticut, New York City, and San Francisco, public health department follow-up was conducted with the New York City and California health departments. Eventually, it was determined by state laboratories in three states that lead was not a listed ingredient of these pills but a contaminant during the manufacturing process.

The investigation was considered significant and was reported in an issue of the CDC's *Morbidity and Mortality Weekly Report* (CDC, 1999). As a result of this report, this case was further reported by various public health agencies to the public and their constituencies, including the World Health Organization's International Agency for Research on Cancer (IARC) Monograph of Inorganic and Organic Lead Compounds (Jung, 2023b).

Lessons learned from this investigation:

- Collaboration between healthcare providers and public health entities allowed for a broader approach to addressing health and environmental issues, such as lead poisoning.
- Detailed follow-up at various points of an epidemiologic investigation allowed for cross-state efforts to identify new sources of exposure.
- Dissemination of findings by the CDC (via MMWR) provided scientific evidence that enabled the implementation of legislation in other states other than where the exposure initially occurred.
- Public health education regarding lead contamination of consumer products was expanded to include unusual sources of exposures.

BC Jung, MPH, RN, MCHES(R)

Source: Centers for Disease Control and Prevention (1999); Jung (2023b); Poison Control (2023).

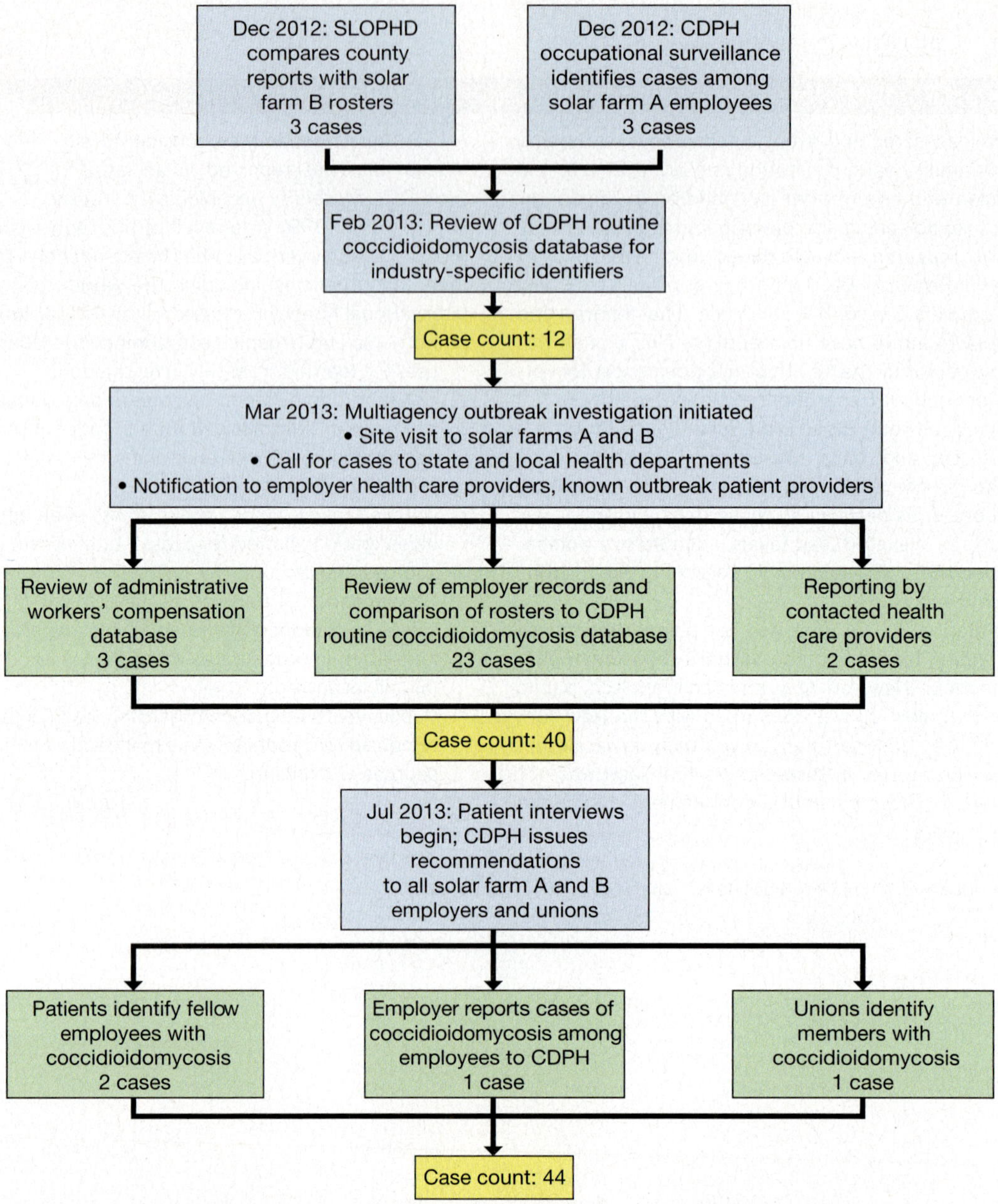

FIGURE 7-27 Flowchart of outbreak investigation of coccidioidomycosis among solar farm workers, San Luis Obispo County, California, United States, October 2011 to April 2014. CDPH, California Department of Public Health; SLOPHD, County of San Luis Obispo Public Health Department. (Adapted from Wilkin, J. A., Sondermeyer, G., Shusterman, D., McNary, J., Vugia, D., McDowell, A., Borenstein, P., Gilliss, D., Ancock, B., Prudhomme, J., Gold, D., Windham, G. C., Lee, L., & Materna, B. L. (2015). Coccidioidomycosis among workers constructing solar power farms, California, USA, 2011–2014. *Emerging Infectious Diseases, 21*(11). https://wwwnc.cdc.gov/eid/syn/en/article/21/11/15-0129.htm)

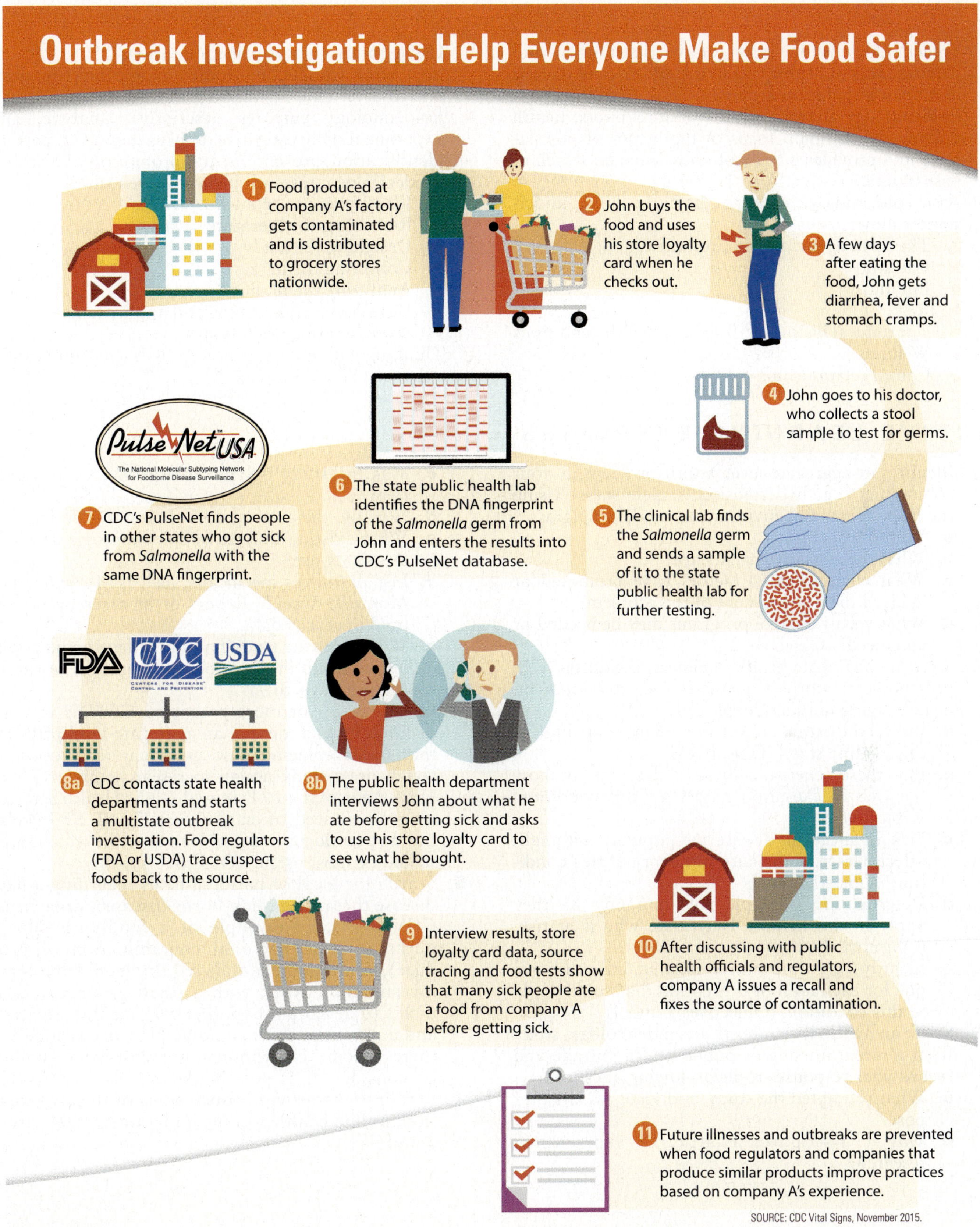

Outbreak Investigations Help Everyone Make Food Safer
1 Food produced at company A's factory gets contaminated and is distributed to grocery stores nationwide.
2 John buys the food and uses his store loyalty card when he checks out.
3 A few days after eating the food, John gets diarrhea, fever and stomach cramps.
4 John goes to his doctor, who collects a stool sample to test for germs.
5 The clinical lab finds the *Salmonella* germ and sends a sample of it to the state public health lab for further testing.
6 The state public health lab identifies the DNA fingerprint of the *Salmonella* germ from John and enters the results into CDC's PulseNet database.
PulseNet USA
The National Molecular Subtyping Network for Foodborne Disease Surveillance
7 CDC's PulseNet finds people in other states who got sick from *Salmonella* with the same DNA fingerprint.
FDA
CDC
USDA
8a CDC contacts state health departments and starts a multistate outbreak investigation. Food regulators (FDA or USDA) trace suspect foods back to the source.
8b The public health department interviews John about what he ate before getting sick and asks to use his store loyalty card to see what he bought.
9 Interview results, store loyalty card data, source tracing and food tests show that many sick people ate a food from company A before getting sick.
10 After discussing with public health officials and regulators, company A issues a recall and fixes the source of contamination.
11 Future illnesses and outbreaks are prevented when food regulators and companies that produce similar products improve practices based on company A's experience.
SOURCE: CDC Vital Signs, November 2015.

FIGURE 7-28 Outbreak investigations help everyone make food safer. (Reprinted from CDC. (2015). *Safer food saves lives*. https://www.cdc.gov/vitalsigns/foodsafety-2015/index.html)

SUMMARY

- Epidemiology is the study of the distribution and determinants of health, health conditions, and disease in human population groups.
- Epidemiology shares with community/public health nursing the common focus of the health of populations and provides a body of knowledge on which to base practice.
- Basic epidemiologic concepts the nurse should understand follow:
  - The host, agent, and environment model
  - Causality
  - Immunity
  - Risk
  - The natural history of disease or health conditions
  - Wellness
  - Causal relationships
- Using epidemiologic principles, the C/PHNs can use data when conducting epidemiologic investigations and to determine populations at risk.
- Epidemiology employs descriptive, analytic, and experimental investigative approaches as a part of identification, prevention, and promotion of health.
- Epidemiologic research includes seven steps:
  - Identifying the problem
  - Reviewing the literature
  - Designing the study
  - Collecting the data
  - Analyzing the findings
  - Developing conclusions and applications
  - Disseminating the findings
- Thinking with an epidemiologic lens can significantly enhance C/PHN practice.

ACTIVE LEARNING EXERCISES

1. Identify an aggregate-level health problem in your community (e.g., hypertension, homelessness). Using the host, agent, and environment model, explain:
   a. Who the host is?
   b. What the causative agents are?
   c. What environmental factors have promoted or delayed the development of the problem?
   d. What vector control programs may be needed or enhanced? (Objective 2)
2. Select an aggregate health (wellness) condition (e.g., preschoolers' normal growth and development, healthy aging in older people) and:
   a. List all the causal factors that might contribute to this healthy state. (Objective 3)
   b. Plot these schematically in a diagram to show the web of causation model for this condition. (Objective 3)
   c. Pick an infectious disease and population it might affect. Describe the natural history of this condition. (Objective 1)
   d. Describe the principles of immunity as they apply to this disease. Determine who is at risk. (Objective 4)
   e. Identify three preventive nursing interventions, one for each level of prevention that could apply to this condition. (Objectives 1 and 4)
3. Select an article that reports an epidemiologic study from a recent nursing or public health journal, and record your responses to the following questions:
   a. What prompted the study, and what was its purpose?
   b. Was it descriptive, analytic, or experimental research?
   c. Was the study design retrospective or prospective?
   d. Why did the investigators choose this design?
   e. What existing sources of epidemiologic data did this study use?
   f. List all sources specifically, such as *Morbidity and Mortality Weekly Report* or incomes by household in census data.
   g. What were the study findings? Identify the population group that will benefit from this research. (Objectives 5 to 7)
4. Interview one or more practicing C/PHNs in your community and identify an aggregate-level problem that needs epidemiologic investigation. Propose a rough draft study design to research this problem. How many of the 10 Essential Public Health Services would you need to employ (see Box 2-2)? In relation to your identified problem, describe which three would be most useful. (Objective 7)
5. Search for local or national news regarding a new disease threat (e.g., tick-borne diseases, Zika virus, COVID-19), an example of a foodborne illness outbreak (e.g., bacterial contamination of produce), or another example requiring epidemiologic investigation. Work with a small group of classmates to develop a hypothetical case investigation and a potential epidemiologic plan for action. Are there specific environmental factors that should be considered? If possible, watch for the resolution of the issue (e.g., conclusions of the investigation, public health recommendations). (Objectives 5 and 7)

CHAPTER 8

Communicable Disease*

"There are only two things a child will share willingly: communicable diseases and its mother's age."

—Benjamin Spock (1903–1998), Pediatrician and Author

KEY TERMS

Active immunity
Antigenic drift
Antigenic shift
Communicable disease
Direct transmission
Epidemics
Fomites
Geographic information system (GIS)
Herd immunity
Incubation period
Indirect transmission
Infectious agent
Isolation
Novel
Pandemics
Passive immunity
Quarantine
Reservoir
Vaccine
Vaccine hesitancy
Vector

LEARNING OBJECTIVES

Upon mastery of this chapter, you should be able to:

1. Articulate the nurse's role in communicable disease control.
2. Describe the three general principles of modes of transmission for communicable diseases.
3. Identify four major communicable diseases in the United States.
4. Compare and contrast the strategies used for the levels of prevention in communicable disease control and how informatics and technology have been used effectively.
5. Explain the significance of immunization as a communicable disease control measure and the importance of interprofessional partnerships.
6. Identify strategies to address the major concerns of parents and individuals who choose not to vaccinate their children or themselves.
7. Explain the importance of herd immunity in controlling vaccine-preventable diseases and pandemics.
8. Incorporate knowledge from nursing and other disciplines to discuss the legal and ethical issues affecting communicable disease and infection control.

INTRODUCTION

Communicable diseases pose a major threat to public health and are of significant concern to community/public health nurses. A **communicable disease** is caused by an **infectious agent**, such as a virus or bacteria, and can be transmitted from one source to another. Transmission to a susceptible host can occur directly either from person to person or from animal to human, or transmission may occur indirectly through a **reservoir** such as contaminated water (Bloom & Cadarette, 2019). Some noncommunicable diseases can also be caused by infectious agents, such as tetanus, but cannot be transmitted from one source to another (CDC, 2020a).

Over the past century, public health programs have led the way in decreasing communicable diseases in the United States and are responsible for managing outbreaks, **epidemics** (an increase in cases or an increase of cases in a geographical area), **pandemics** (similar to an epidemic but has spread across international borders and continents and affects a large number of people),

*In this chapter, "male" means a person assigned male at birth, and "female" means a person assigned female at birth.

and emerging infections (Lederberg, 2000). Jurisdictional laws and regulations mandate that infectious and noninfectious diseases be reported to local, state, and territorial public health departments. The National Notifiable Diseases Surveillance System (NNDSS) allows the sharing of notifiable disease information nationally and between jurisdictions for surveillance, control, and prevention purposes (CDC, 2023u).

Knowledge of communicable diseases is fundamental to the practice of community/public health nursing because these diseases typically spread through communities of people. A nurse needs to understand the basic concepts of communicable disease control, such as teaching important and effective preventive measures to community members, advocating for those affected, protecting the well-being of uninfected people (including healthcare workers and nurses themselves), and controlling communicable disease in populations and groups (CDC, 2023s).

In the last century, numerous public health changes have occurred in the lives of people throughout the world. The CDC is charged with protecting Americans against threats of disease, both in the United States and abroad, and partners with the World Health Organization (WHO), foundations, nongovernmental organizations, business and private organizations, academic institutions, and foreign governments and ministries of health (CDC, 2021a, 2023t). The collaboration between the various entities has led to the near eradication of polio and the complete eradication of smallpox in 1980 (WHO, 2023a). Immunization campaigns from the WHO and Centers for Disease Control and Prevention (CDC) have resulted in the protection of children from 14 diseases due to routine vaccines. The CDC estimates that childhood immunizations can prevent more than 50 million deaths between 2021 and 2030 (CDC, 2023q). One of the big challenges to the prevention of communicable diseases comes from reemerging and *emerging infectious diseases*, which are defined as "infectious diseases that are newly recognized in a population or have existed but are rapidly increasing in incidence or geographic range" (Lederberg, 2000; McArthur, 2019). Human migration, modern transportation, and globalization have led to the spread of new pathogens and vectors such as the H1N1 influenza pandemic in 2009 and 2010 and Zika and Ebola virus outbreaks in West Africa in 2014 (CDC, 2023s; McArthur, 2019; WHO, 2023a). Current potential threats are as follows:

- Diseases with epidemic potential due to little or no countermeasures being in place, such as the Ebola virus and Middle East respiratory syndrome coronavirus (CDC, 2019b, 2023g).
- The COVID-19 (SARS-CoV-2) pandemic was responsible for an estimated 14.83 million deaths globally during the period of December 2019 through May 2023 (Msemburi et al., 2023).
- Post COVID-19 pandemic resurgence on communicable diseases (CDC, 2023c; Hamson et al., 2023), climate variability, and increased rate of urbanization affecting the transmission patterns of vector-borne diseases such as dengue and Zika virus diseases (Fouque & Reeder, 2019).
- Development of antibiotic-resistant strains of the bacteria *Neisseria Meningitides*, groups A and B *Streptococcus*, tuberculosis (TB), and gonorrhea that threaten the public's health and pose significant occupational health risks for health workers (CDC, 2022h, 2022k; Kuehn, 2020; WHO, 2019).
- The threat of bioterrorism, which involves the use of biologic agents with the intent to cause harm (CDC, 2020c); see Chapter 17 for more on emerging infections and bioterrorism.

This chapter provides information to help you better understand communicable diseases in communities and around the globe. It describes ways to plan and implement appropriate prevention interventions, including immunization of children and adults, environmental interventions, community education, screening programs, disease investigation, and case/contact finding. Ethical issues of communicable disease control are also discussed along with communicable disease information sources useful to the C/PHN.

BASIC CONCEPTS REGARDING COMMUNICABLE DISEASES

Communicable diseases have challenged healthcare providers for centuries. Exposure to infectious agents can occur in the community or within healthcare settings. The threat of these diseases has led to the development of important infection control measures over the last century (Rosner, 2010):

- Hand washing
- Use of personal protective equipment
- Safe handling of contaminated sharp equipment
- Appropriate disposal of potentially infectious materials
- Community sanitation
- Pest control
- Vaccines
- Antimicrobial medications

Evolution of Communicable Disease Control

Communicable diseases have been present since ancient times and continue to shape our society and medical practice (Sakai & Morimoto, 2022). The bubonic plague, caused by *Yersinia pestis*, is one example of how communicable diseases have changed the course of history. The disease is transmitted when humans are bitten by infected fleas, when they come in contact with infected tissue or body fluids of an infected animal, or when droplets from a person infected with plague pneumonia are inhaled by another person (CDC, 2021d). The first documented pandemic plague occurred in 541 AD. The next 200 years saw outbreaks in Africa, Egypt, Istanbul, Europe, and across the Middle East, with over 100 million deaths due to the plague (CDC, 2021d;

Frith, 2012). In 1347–1352, the great plague pandemic, known as the Black Death, killed 25% of the European population in the first plague and another 20% in the second one; it killed over 25 million people in Africa and Asia (Frith, 2012). The Black Plague introduced the control measures and the word **quarantine**. The origin of word the *quarantine* comes from the Italian word "quaranta giorni," meaning "40 days." It referred to the amount of time ships arriving from infected ports were expected to anchor and not disembark when arriving in Venice (CDC, 2020k).

Historically, as countries became industrialized, increased productivity, trade, and economic growth also brought on the four Ds of disruption, deprivation, disease, and death. Industrialization brings large numbers of people close together in condensed living conditions. Trade also brings populations together, exposing them to infectious agents they had not previously seen (Boyce et al., 2019). Control measures were started in the 19th century with the discovery of the microorganisms responsible for cholera and TB through disinfection and improved hygiene. The 20th century saw further improvements and control of diseases in the form of improved sanitation, hygiene, antibiotics, and childhood vaccination programs. Additionally, infections were targeted, and vaccines were created for influenza, human cytomegalovirus, hepatitis virus infections (hepatitis B and C), and respiratory syncytial virus (RSV) infections. As a result of the new control measures, surveillance, and scientific discoveries, the 20th century saw a decline in deaths from infectious diseases, and communicable diseases were no longer the leading cause of death in the United States (CDC, 2019b, 2022f; Hall & Wodi, 2021).

Challenges for controlling communicable diseases in the 21st century are as follows:

- Emerging infections as a result of interactions between humans and domestic and wild animals such as the monkeypox outbreak and the three coronavirus pandemics (SARS-CoV, MERS-CoV, and SARS-CoV-2) have occurred in the 21st century (Sakai & Morimoto, 2022). The last pandemic started in December 2019, and 3 years later, more than 7.3 million people worldwide were killed, making it one of the leading causes of death during this time (Troeger, 2023).

To address this threat, the CDC is tasked with health promotion and disease prevention (see Chapter 11). It is recognized globally for its partnerships in disease surveillance, research, data collection, and analysis, as well as for responding nationally and globally with peer agencies to disease outbreaks (CDC, 2023t; WHO, n.d.-a). The WHO addresses communicable and noncommunicable diseases, working on emergency preparedness, vaccine hesitancy, and response (WHO, n.d.-a). The COVID-19 pandemic highlighted the need for public health systems across the globe to examine their management of emerging infectious diseases, containment, protection, and dissemination of information in order to be better prepared to manage the next outbreak (Filip et al., 2022). See more on global health in Chapter 16.

Community/Public Health Nurse's Role: Process of Investigating Reportable Communicable Diseases

Healthcare providers, veterinarians, and laboratories are required to report certain diseases in humans to the local health authority and, in some cases, to the CDC. Each state has a State Health Department, and some states have local sites, such as a county or city health department. Such departments are typically staffed by a combination of nurses, epidemiologists, and communicable disease investigators (CDC, 2023u). See Chapter 6.

The local health department or agency is the initial point of notification of a communicable disease investigation. If a person is identified in one jurisdiction but was exposed in another, the health agency receiving the report should notify the health agency where the exposure occurred, so an investigation can be conducted in the originating region. In most states, reporting known or suspected cases of a reportable disease is considered to be an obligation of the following (CDC, 2022n):

- Physicians, dentists, nurses, veterinarians, pharmacists, and other health professionals
- Medical examiners
- Administrators of hospitals, clinics, nursing homes, schools, and nurseries

Some states also require or request reporting from the following:

- Laboratory directors
- Any person who knows of or suspects the existence of a reportable disease (County of Los Angeles Department of Public Health, n.d.)

Figure 8-1 outlines the Notifiable Disease Surveillance process. Each state has a disease report form, and the local health department or agency investigates a specific disease using a protocol set by the local, state, or federal public health official. Reportable diseases must be reported to the state health department. Notifiable diseases are voluntarily reported by the state to the CDC (CDC, 2020j). Individual citizens may also contact the CDC directly via mail, phone, or the internet. You can reach them at:

Centers for Disease Control and Prevention
800-CDC-INFO (800-232-4636); TTY: (888) 232–6348, 24 hours/every day
E-mail: cdcinfo@cdc.gov
Website: https://www.cdc.gov/

Disease investigation requires a systematic approach. The nurse may be assigned to work on individual cases of a disease or several cases that make up a cluster or outbreak. Whether it is a solitary case of illness in a small town or a

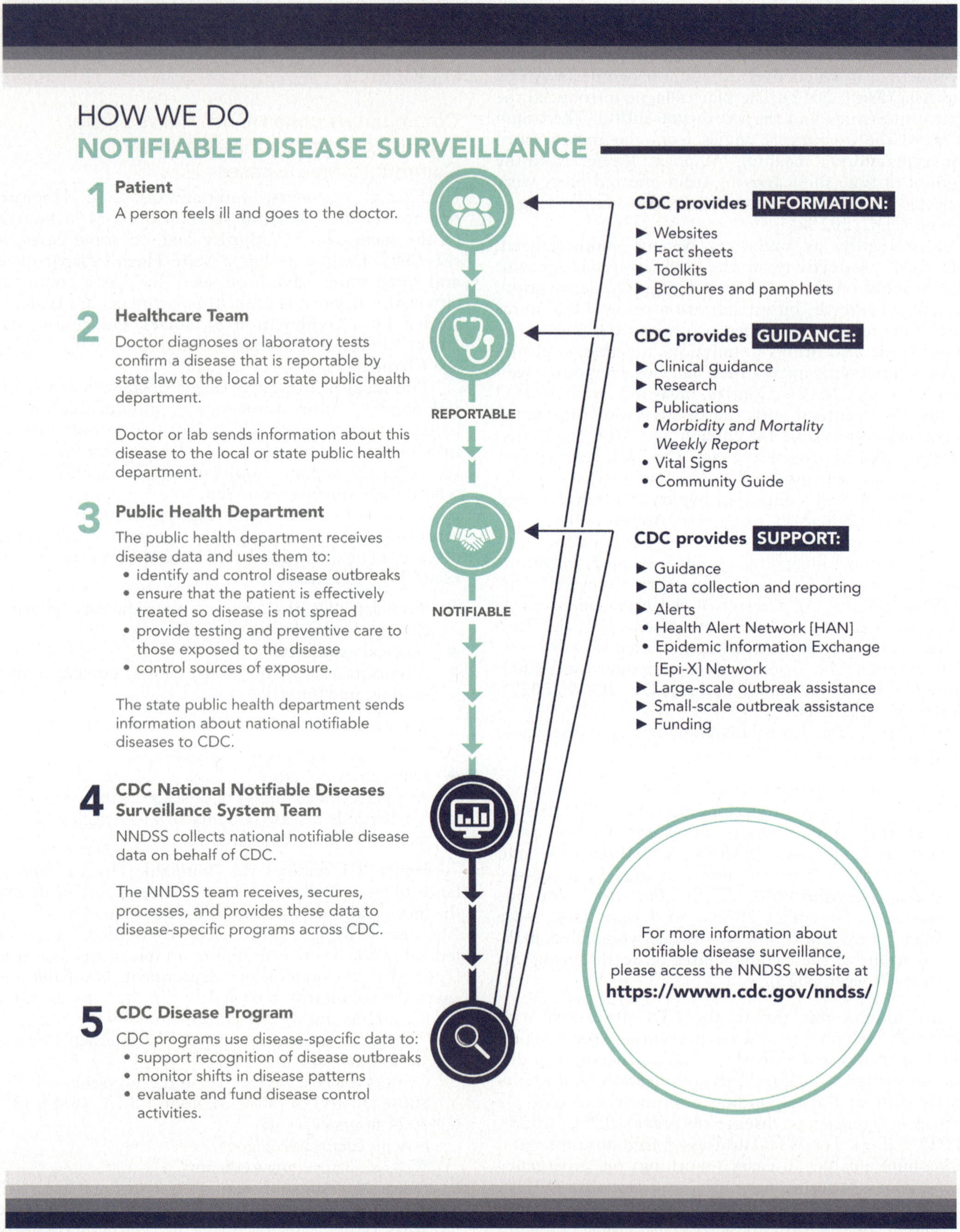

FIGURE 8-1 How we do notifiable disease surveillance. (Reprinted from Centers for Disease Control and Prevention. (2018). *Defending America from health threats.* https://wwwn.cdc.gov/nndss/how-we-do.html)

multijurisdictional outbreak, the nurse should follow similar steps (CDC, 2022n):

1. Identify additional people who might be infected (surveillance).
2. Determine the possible source of infection and means of transmission.
3. Identify others who are at risk so screening and prevention measures can be implemented.
4. Prevent further transmission.
5. Monitor the response to these interventions.

In the event of an outbreak, the response should also include confirming the outbreak, establishing a task force to serve as the command and control center of the response, communicating with the public, managing care for those who are ill, and conducting an outbreak investigation (CDC, 2022n).

When investigating a disease outbreak, before contacting a person for an interview:

- Review the information received from the mandated reporter for completeness and see if it meets the case definition (criteria a person must meet to be considered to have the disease).
- Understand whether the disease is suspected (meeting certain clinical criteria) or lab-confirmed.
- Review the disease information (reservoir, incubation and infectious periods, symptoms, and treatment), know the methods of control, and be prepared to provide education to the client while also conducting the investigation. See Chapter 7 to review the natural history of a disease or health condition.
- Review the disease-specific questionnaire, if applicable.
- If no questionnaire exists, prepare a narrative report including the information related to the onset of illness, symptoms, medical evaluation, treatment (if received), recovery state, and individuals the person has been in contact with, depending upon the nature of the disease (see for a sample disease investigation form https://www.cdc.gov/urdo/php/surveillance/data-collection.html?CDC_AAref_Val=https://www.cdc.gov/urdo/sampleforms.html)

When conducting the interview, do the following:

- Arrange to call or meet with the person (Fig. 8-2), depending on department protocol and disease being addressed.
- Introduce yourself, and explain the purpose and process as the confidential nature of the interview. Maintain a neutral and nonjudgmental attitude as this helps elicit information, especially during interviews involving sensitive topics, such as sexually transmitted infection (STI)
- Assess knowledge base to guide education.
- Gather information using a disease-specific questionnaire, if available, and note any sources of the disease or additional infected contacts.

After the interview, contact individuals identified as possibly infected, which may help establish whether an outbreak is occurring (Minnesota Department of Health, 2019).

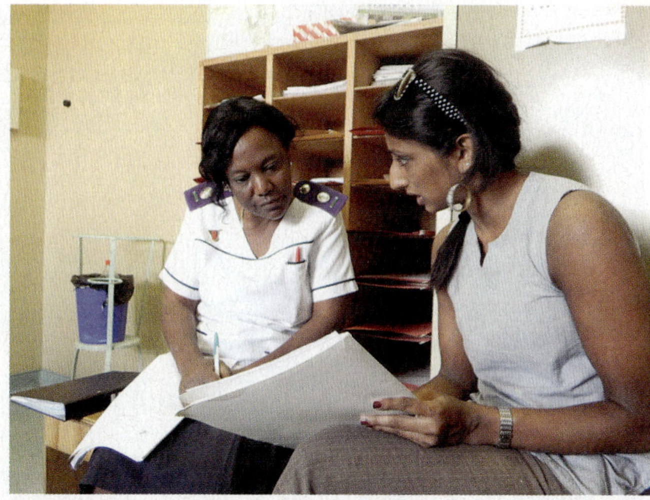

FIGURE 8-2 A PHN interviews a health center nurse during a TB/HIV investigation.

The next step is surveillance of communicable diseases. The WHO has defined surveillance as the ongoing and systematic collection, analysis, and interpretation of health data. Surveillance allows for early identification of public health emergencies and evaluation of the effectiveness of public health interventions and is used to help inform policy changes (WHO, n.d.-c). Contact tracing can identify additional people who are also affected. The C/PHN or other local investigator sends information obtained during the interview to the next highest level of government for analysis and interpretation. If an outbreak is occurring, properly addressing it may require assistance from the next level of government (Minnesota Department of Health, 2019).

COVID-19 brought about new ways for public health to conduct disease surveillance that used data attached to unique locations to create graphs and maps. John Hopkins Coronavirus Resource Center began on January 22, 2020 and was a "new standard for infectious disease tracking" and shared pandemic data in real-time (John Hopkins University & Medicine, 2023) (see Fig. 8-3). These type of data were collected by organizations and governments throughout the world during the pandemic and were used to trace the virus spread and vaccination status and to provide a picture of the disease. Geographic Information System (GIS) data proved to be a valuable tool especially early in the pandemic and can be a tool for monitoring future outbreaks, effectiveness of vaccines, and control measures (Ahasan et al., 2022; United States Geological Survey (USGS), 2021) (see Chapter 10 for more on GIS).

The next step is disease control. Disease control measures are determined by the characteristics specific to the disease. C/PHNs must understand the characteristics of the infectious agent so that appropriate control measures can be implemented. Prompt, appropriate action could minimize or even prevent an outbreak. Control measures may include testing, counseling, education, environmental modifications such as draining standing water, vaccination, treatment, or prophylaxis as appropriate (Minnesota Department of Health, 2019). Effective surveillance

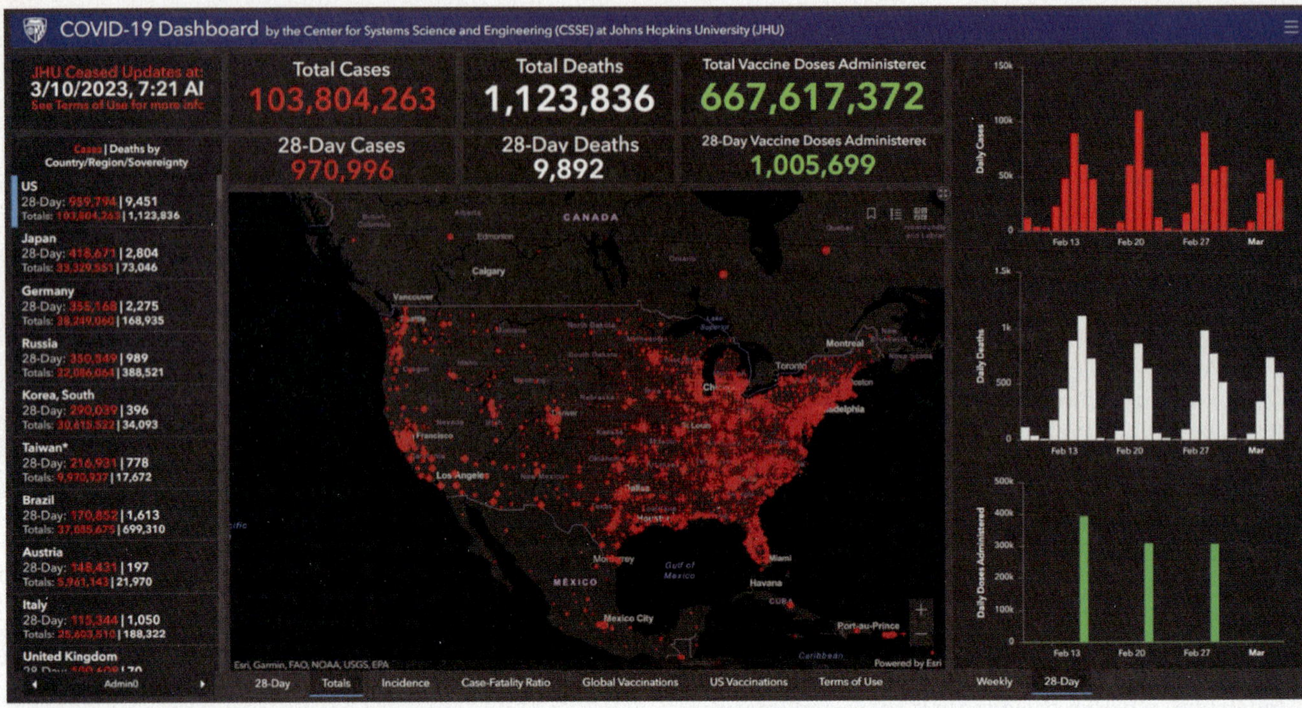

FIGURE 8-3 COVID-19 global dashboard. (Dong, E., Du, H., & Gardner, L. (2020). An interactive web-based dashboard to track COVID-19 in real time. *Lancet Infectious Diseases, 20*(5), 533–534. https://doi.org/10.1016/S1473-3099(20)30120-1. This data set is licensed under the Creative Commons Attribution 4.0 International (CC BY 4.0) by the Johns Hopkins University on behalf of its Center for Systems Science in Engineering. Copyright Johns Hopkins University 2020.)

and control can lead to the elimination and eradication of a disease in many cases. However, the COVID-19 pandemic caused significant damage to our societies due to miscommunication between states and federal agencies, policy differences, delays in implementing control measures (such as masking, testing, vaccinations, social distancing), and supply chain issues, which highlighted the limitations and inconsistencies of our current public health system (Dominquez et al., 2022). See Chapter 16 for more on the global eradication of infectious diseases.

Modes of Transmission

Transmission of a communicable disease describes how the disease is passed from person to person or from another source to a person. The spread can occur by **direct transmission** or **indirect transmission** methods. Refer to Table 8-1, which summarizes the modes of infectious disease transmission. Two indirect modes of transmission particularly important for C/PHNs, vector transmission and food and water transmission, are discussed in detail below (Minnesota Department of Health, 2019).

Vector Transmission

Vectors are living organisms that can transmit infectious diseases to humans. Insects, a common type of vector, carry diseases on their feet or expel them through their digestive tract. This *mechanical transmission* does not require the infectious organism to multiply. Insects can also transmit disease when the infectious agent has propagated within the insect, which is known as *biologic transmission* (Open Stax, 2019). This requires an **incubation period** for the infectious agent to be passed to the host. These modes of transmission, together known as vector-borne transmission, involve the bite of the infected insect (e.g., mosquito) or animal (e.g., rat) or some other form of exposure to the infected animal's body fluids, such as contact with the urine from the Hantavirus-infected rodent (CDC, 2020a, 2022g; Open Stax, 2019).

Food- and Water-Related Illness

Food- or water-related illness can be caused by bacteria (e.g., *Salmonella*, *Shigella*, *Escherichia coli* 0157, *Listeria monocytogenes*, and *Campylobacter*), viruses (e.g., norovirus, hepatitis A), or parasites (e.g., *Cryptosporidium*, *Giardia*; CDC, 2023i). Toxins released in response to bacteria in the intestines can also result in severe illness. Ingestion of the pathogenic organism sets in motion the events of a food- or water-related intestinal illness or even death.

The contamination can occur:

- At the source (e.g., animal waste being introduced into the food or water chain)
- Through unsanitary food handling or practices (e.g., ingestion of fecal material, fecal–oral route)
- Due to food storage at improper temperatures, allowing microorganisms to grow (CDC, 2023i)

Most commonly, exposure to contaminated food or water results in symptoms related to gastrointestinal function. These include diarrhea, nausea, vomiting, stomach cramps, and bloating. Fever may accompany these infections, as well. Depending on the microorganism, the

TABLE **8-1** Modes of Infectious Disease Transmission

Routes	Method of Transmission	Examples
Direct: reservoir → host by direct contact or droplet spread		
▪ **Direct contact**	Sexual contact, kissing, skin-to-skin contact, bites, contact with soil or vegetation contaminated with infectious organisms	Gonorrhea, herpes, rabies, hookworm
▪ **Droplet spread**	Large, short-range aerosols produced by sneezing, coughing, or even talking	Pertussis, meningococcal infection
Indirect: reservoir → host by suspended air particles, inanimate objects (vehicles), or animate intermediaries (vector)		
▪ **Airborne**	Infectious agents are carried by dust or droplet nuclei and suspended in air	Measles virus, tuberculosis
▪ **Vehicles**	Indirect transmission of an infectious agent may involve food, water, biologic products (blood), and fomites (inanimate objects such as handkerchiefs, bedding, surgical scalpels, or needles) or The vehicle may provide an environment in which the agent grows, multiplies, or produces toxin (e.g., improperly canned foods)	Hepatitis A virus Botulinum toxin by *Clostridium botulinum*

Source: CDC (2024). https://www.cdc.gov/infection-control/hcp/basics/transmission-based-precautions.html?CDC_AAref_Val=https://www.cdc.gov/infectioncontrol/basics/transmission-based-precautions.html

onset of symptoms may occur within a few hours after exposure or days or even weeks later. This time interval between exposure and the onset of symptoms is called the incubation period.

Microorganism contamination of food resulting in human illness occurs because of either infection or intoxication (CDC, 2022i):

- *Infection:* Ingestion of food contaminated with *Salmonella*, *Shigella*, *E. coli*, or another pathogen that has multiplied and grown in the food and that irritates the normal gastrointestinal mucosa
- *Intoxication:* Ingestion of food contaminated with a toxin, or byproduct of the normal bacterial life cycle, rather than the microbe itself (e.g., heat-stable *Staphylococcus* toxin; the neurotoxin botulinum, produced by the bacterium *Clostridium botulinum*), which may be introduced to the food by bacteria in the food (e.g., cooked food left at room temperature) or living on the skin of a food preparer

This distinction is relevant because, compared with bacteria, toxins (CDC, 2020i):

- Are difficult to isolate and identify, causing some foodborne illnesses to go unidentified
- Are stable at normal cooking temperatures and therefore can occur in thoroughly cooked food
- Typically require only supportive care to address, rather than medical treatment

Food- and water-related outbreaks can impact large numbers of people. A famous historical example is Typhoid Mary. Mary Mallon was the "first identified healthy carrier of typhoid fever" who spread the bacteria (*Salmonella typhi*) in 10 outbreaks, resulting in 51 typhoid fever cases and 3 deaths (The College of Physicians of Philadelphia, 2019, para. 2). Such outbreaks serve to remind all C/PHNs of the continuing need to teach and observe the most basic methods for preventing food and water contamination. Box 8-1 summarizes the correct methods for maintaining the safety and cleanliness of food.

Investigating outbreaks involves three types of data:

1. Epidemiologic data:
   - Patterns in the geographic distribution, time of onset, and past incidents of illnesses
   - Associated exposures to foods, infected people, or other sources of disease
   - Clusters of unrelated sick people who share a common event (e.g., eating at the same restaurant, shopping at the same store, attending the same concert; CDC, 2020d)
2. Traceback data:
   - Common points of contamination in the distribution chain, identified by reviewing records collected from restaurants and stores where sick people ate or shopped
   - Findings of environmental assessment in food production facilities, farms, and restaurants identifying food safety risks (CDC, 2022i)
   - Whole-genome sequencing (WGS) to help obtain detailed information of the bacteria (CDC, 2022o)
3. Food and environmental testing data:
   - Specimens collected from suspected food items and sent to the lab for processing and identification of the organism (CDC, 2023j)
   - Specimens processed through the CDC surveillance system, PulseNet, which is designed to identify organisms that may come from the same source, allowing outbreaks to be identified and sources to be eliminated (CDC, 2023v)

BOX 8-1 Correct Methods for Preserving the Safety and Cleanliness of Food

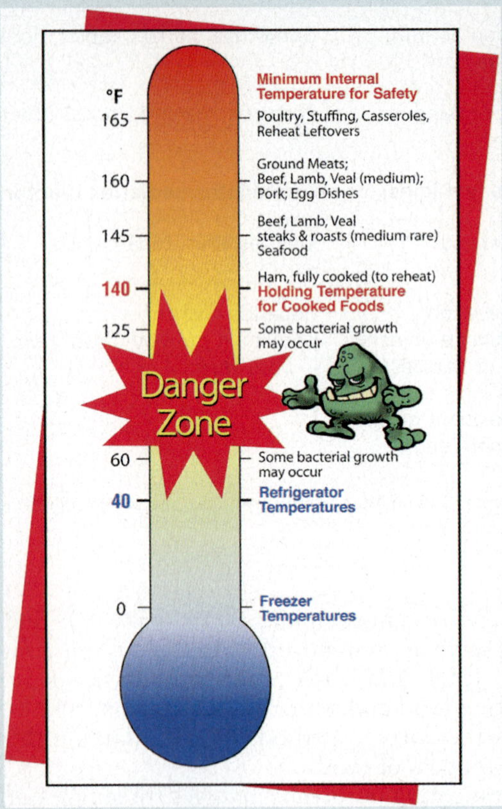

Before Handling Food

Wash hands and all food preparation surfaces and utensils thoroughly with soap and water.

When Preparing Food

- Wash foods that are to be eaten raw and uncooked thoroughly in clean water. This includes foods that are to be peeled that grow on the ground or come in contact with soil.
- Cook all meat products thoroughly.
- Do not allow cooked meats to come in contact with dishes, utensils, or containers used when the foods are raw and uncooked.

When Storing Leftover Foods

- Cool cooked foods quickly; store under refrigeration in clean, covered containers.

When Reheating Leftover Foods

- Heat foods thoroughly. Bacteria contaminating food grow and multiply in a temperature range between 39°F and 140°F.

Source: USDA (2015).

Since 2019, whole-genome sequencing (WGS) of pathogens is part of all foodborne outbreak investigations. WGS allows precise data on pathogens, allowing for quicker identification of outbreaks and tracking bacteria (CDC, 2022o). An example of the effectiveness of WGS was an August 2021 Salmonella Thompson outbreak that occurred in several states (Colorado, Missouri, Washington, and Wisconsin). Using WGS data, it was discovered that the 2021 isolates were genetically related to an isolate that was identified in 2020 and found in sushi-grade salmon and tuna. By October 2021, the outbreak had spread to a total of 15 states and affected 115 people. WGS data allowed the outbreak to be tracked, and with the help of investigations, the Salmonella Thompson strain was tracked to a seafood distributor and processor, and corrective measures were put in place with no further outbreaks detected (CDC, 2023j).

MAJOR COMMUNICABLE DISEASES IN THE UNITED STATES

C/PHNs encounter many communicable diseases in their practice, some reportable, some not, though equally transmittable. These diseases are frequently diagnosed and treated in the community care setting rather than the hospital. The following sections discuss some of the more common communicable diseases, excluding many that are reportable. Diseases are presented in groups by similarity rather than by virulence or prevalence.

Influenza

Influenza (flu) is an acute communicable viral disease of the respiratory tract and has been documented since 412 BC. It existed throughout the early centuries, and about 30 probable pandemics have been documented in the past 400 years. Three have occurred in the 20th century. The 1918 "Spanish flu" pandemic was the most devastating, with 20% to 40% of the world population affected and an estimated death toll of 50 million worldwide; in the United States, roughly 675,000 died (Jernigan, 2018). The last pandemic occurred in 2009, when the novel strain H1N1 emerged with infection rates ranging from 43 million to 89 million people and deaths from 8868 to 18,306 (Jernigan, 2018) in the United States. Symptoms included fever, headache, myalgia, prostration, coryza, sore throat, and cough. Influenza derives its importance from the rapidity with which epidemics evolve, the widespread morbidity, and the seriousness of complications, specifically pneumonias. The antigenic types of influenza virus are as follows (CDC, 2023aa):

- Influenza A virus causes the most severe and widespread disease (pandemic) and undergoes minor genetic mutations from year to year, referred to as **antigenic drift**, and drastic transformations periodically, referred to as **antigenic shift**. Subtype descriptions of proteins on the surface of the virus, hemagglutinin, and neuraminidase antigens are included in parentheses A(H1N1) and A(H3N2).
- Influenza B virus causes milder disease outbreaks, and they change or mutate at a slower rate.
- Influenza C virus relates to only sporadic cases of milder respiratory disease.
- Influenza D viruses do not cause illness in people but do affect cattle and can cross over to other species.

Influenza is usually seasonal, occurring in the winter months, but may be found year-round if testing is done.

Each year, a **vaccine** is developed based on what WHO identifies through global surveillance and then is prepared for the upcoming flu season. CDC recommends that flu vaccines be given yearly to protect from **novel** (new) strains related to influenza A and B only. The protection provided by the flu vaccine depends on two factors: (1) age and health of person and (2) if the vaccine produced for the particular year matches the current strain circulating (CDC, 2023aa). The injectable influenza vaccine is inactivated. The nasally inhaled version is a live attenuated vaccine and is licensed for use in people ages 2 to 49 years (CDC, 2022m). An adjuvanted and high-dose inactivated vaccine is recommended for those 65 years of age and older, whereas adults 18 to 64 years may receive a recombinant influenza vaccine (CDC, 2022l). The vaccine should be given every year before influenza is expected in the community. The season can begin as early as October, so vaccinating in September may be indicated, but it usually begins by the end of October in most of the United States. For those living or traveling outside the United States, the timing of the immunization should be based on the seasonal patterns of influenza in the area to which they are traveling (CDC, 2023z). Influenza immunization clinics are frequently planned and organized by or with the local public health agency, with the injections usually administered by C/PHNs. Flu shots are also available through major pharmacies.

SARS-CoV-2

Severe acute respiratory syndrome coronavirus 2 (SARS-CoV-2) is the virus name for COVID-19 and was first discovered in December, 2019 in Wuhan, China. The virus is spread when an infected person breaths out droplets containing the virus and then an uninfected person comes into contact with the droplets or particles via eyes, nose, mouth, or contaminated surfaces (CDC, 2023a). WHO declared a public health emergency of international concern from January 30, 2020 to May 5, 2023, with over 700 million globally confirmed cases (WHO, 2023b, 2023c). The most common symptoms are respiratory related similarities to the common cold, the flu, or pneumonia but could also include other parts of the body. In many cases, a person could be asymptomatic (CDC, 2022d). Individuals at high risk for severe illness from COVID-19 are older adults (over the age of 50 years), people who are immunocompromised, and those with underlying health conditions such as obesity, chronic diseases, mental health conditions, and pregnancy (CDC, 2023b). New variants of SARS-CoV-2 have occurred and will continue to occur and are being monitored (WHO, 2023j). Refer to Box 8-2 for more information on variants.

Protection against COVID-19 involves keeping up to date with vaccines and boosters, getting tested if needed, following recommendations for exposure, staying home if you suspect or have a confirmed positive test, avoiding contact with individuals who have COVID-19, and improving ventilation and filtration in your environment (CDC, 2023b).

BOX 8-2 Understanding How Variants Work

If you think about a virus like a tree growing and branching out, each branch on the tree is slightly different than the others. By comparing the branches, scientists can label them according to their differences. These minor differences, or variants, have been studied and identified since the beginning of the pandemic. Some variations allow the virus to spread more easily or make it resistant to treatments or vaccines.

Watch What You Need to Know About Variants on the CDC YouTube page (https://www.youtube.com/watch?v=p1BMvCBrYs8)

Source: www.cdc.gov/coronavirus

Pandemic Prevention and Surveillance

C/PHNs play a key role in pandemic prevention, preparedness, and surveillance through primary prevention (Brownson et al., 2020; Coccia, 2021). Universal immunization is recommended for all people 6 months of age and older. The WHO defines immunization as "the process whereby a person is made immune or resistant to an infectious disease, typically by administration of a vaccine" (WHO, 2020, para. 1). In older adults, immunization may be less effective in preventing illness but is still important because it may reduce the severity of disease. With immunization, the incidence of complications and death among older adults is reduced. Children younger than 6 months cannot receive the flu vaccine, so they need to be protected by immunization of the individuals surrounding them. C/PHNs must promote immunization of those who may have the poorest of outcomes and their caregivers, which include (CDC, 2020d, 2022a) the following:

- Healthcare workers and personal care providers
- Children younger than 5 years, but especially those younger than 2 years, as they have the highest rate of infection
- Adults 65 years and older, as they account for 90% of deaths related to influenza and pneumonia
- Pregnant people
- Individuals with asthma
- Those with chronic disease of any organ system or on long-term medication for an illness

SARS-Co-V-2 and variants are continually monitored through genomic surveillance through the CDC and public health partners. Influenza surveillance is through the WHO's Global Influenza Surveillance and Response System (GISRS) program. GISRS began in 1952 and now involves 144 institutions from 114 WHO member states. The mission of GISRS is to protect the world from the threat of influenza (CDC, 2022n; WHO, n.d.-c).

FluNet is an internet-based tool for worldwide influenza surveillance made up of 106 countries. This program allows for the electronic submission of influenza data from participating global laboratories. Real-time data can be accessed through this resource. As new data arrive and are verified, the maps and tables are revised to give users an up-to-date overview of the influenza situation. Data are provided remotely through the GISRS, the WHO regional databases, and other designated laboratories. Only designated users can submit data, but the results—graphics, maps, and tables of influenza activity on a global scale—are available to the public (WHO, n.d.-c) See more on global disease surveillance in Chapter 16.

Pandemic Lessons Learned and Preparedness

The pandemic exposed how underprepared our health departments, healthcare system, and society were for a pandemic. The United States experienced the most severe outcomes of any country. The pandemic also exposed inequalities; communities of color disproportionally experienced more infections, deaths, and financial strain (Dominquez et al., 2022). A review of research studying the pandemic showed the following:

- The United States Public Health Surveillance system has been underfunded for the last 20 years and as a result did not have the personnel or informatics and technology, such as geolocation, in place to manage and assist personnel in surveillance (Brownson et al., 2020). For example, the U.S. National Notifiable Disease Surveillance System (NNDSS) was still using technology from the 1980s to early 1990s. Early in the pandemic, other institutions such as Johns Hopkins University School of Medicine, along with other disciplines, created an interprofessional collaboration that quickly created the Coronavirus Resource Center (Donovan, 2023). Also, **Geographic Information Systems (GIS)**, a computer-based analyzer, was used along with spatial analysis to help guide public health decisions. Technology such as GIS and use of mobile data will be part of the tools used along with interprofessional collaboration to solve future pandemic problems.
- Public health's early response to COVID-19 was to focus on detection and contact tracing, but there were no public health mandates to reduce the transmission by travelers coming from countries with COVID-19, no limit on large social events, no protection for those in long-term facilities or restrictions of movements, or protection for high-density urban settings. The measures taken in the United States and other countries to shelter in place worked to flatten the curve but at a great economic burden that disproportionately affected certain demographics of society (Dominquez et al., 2022; Schuchat, 2020).
- Limited testing supplies and lack of testing and vaccine sites highlighted the healthcare disparity that impacts certain ethnic and racial groups (Fauci & Folkers, 2023).
- The lack of cohesive prevention mandates between the states resulted in states being at various stages of pandemic management. Research looking at COVID-19 transmission levels indicates that having uniform standards would have a positive impact on decreasing transmission and deaths (Fauci & Folkers, 2023).
- Prevention measures such as masking, distancing, washing hands, and staying home when sick was not enforced equally, and there was not a uniform message from public health, healthcare, and government. Countries that implemented the prevention measures early on had overall lower mortality rates. Research studies show that the precautions taken for COVID-19 saw influenza rates decrease from 92.4% to 99.9% in China, England, and the United States during the pandemic. Research using a population transmission model concluded that the use of face masks would reduce the number of flu cases and would be a useful tool along with the flu vaccine to avoid an influenza pandemic (CDC, 2023r; Han et al., 2023).
- The pandemic response to vaccine development was initially slow as COVID-19 was a novel coronavirus and research was limited (John Hopkins University & School of Medicine, 2020).
- Initial screening and testing were ineffective as it was based on symptoms and testing supplies were limited. As a result, new tests that worked faster, required less ingredients, and were more reliable were distributed by the government allowing for more access to testing.
- Misinformation and disinformation were prevalent, which undermined the efforts in vaccination and eroded the trust of the public in our public health institutions and science. Future pandemics will require the collaborative effort of all science and health agencies and the leveraging of partnerships with advocacy groups, clinicians, universities, and health systems (Califf, 2023).

Pneumonia

Pneumonia is a pulmonary infection that causes inflammation of the lobes of the lungs, bronchial tree, or interstitial space. People most susceptible to pneumonia are infants, older adults, and people with a history of chronic diseases, a compromised immune system, or any condition affecting the anatomic or physiologic integrity of the lower respiratory tract. Malnutrition and smoking also increase risk (CDC, 2023dd; MedlinePlus, 2020).

Key facts:

- Routes of transmission: droplet, direct oral contact, and **fomites** (inanimate objects freshly soiled with respiratory discharges)
- Most common viral causes: influenza, parainfluenza, and RSV
- Symptoms: sudden onset with a shaking chill, fever, pleural pain, dyspnea, a productive cough of "rusty" sputum, and tachypnea
- Symptoms in older adults: less abrupt, including fever, shortness of breath, and altered mental status
- Symptoms in infants and young children: initially fever, vomiting, and convulsions
- Diagnosis: may require confirmation by x-ray studies (MedlinePlus, 2020)

Community-acquired pneumonia is a significant cause of morbidity and mortality. The incidence of pneumonia is highest in winter. Viruses such as influenza, rhinovirus, and SARS-CoV are the common causes for viral pneumonia in adults. The virus responsible for pneumonia in children is RSV. In 2019, 2.5 million people died worldwide from pneumonia with almost a third of them children under the age of 5. Incidences are higher among people living in poverty or who have poor nutrition. Hospital admissions and mortality related to pneumonia are far more common among people older than age 65. Although this is not a reportable infectious disease, it can nevertheless have a significant impact upon the community (NHLBI, 2022).

The CDC recommends pneumococcal vaccination for children younger than 5 years of age and adults 65 years and older. PCV13 or PCV15 is recommended for children younger than 5 years old and children 5 through 18 years old with increased risk of pneumococcal disease due to underlying medical conditions. Individuals older than 65 years should talk to their healthcare provider to learn what pneumococcal conjugate vaccine would be appropriate. Adults between the ages of 19 to 65 years of age should consult their healthcare provider to see if they could benefit from the pneumococcal vaccine (CDC, 2023ff).

Education about risk factors, prevention measures, and pneumococcal vaccine information for at-risk groups is a major part of the C/PHN's role (Dadonaite & Roser, 2019).

Hepatitis

Of the five viral hepatitis infections that constitute serious liver disease, the three most reported types are hepatitis A, B, and C. Infection with hepatitis is an ongoing global epidemic. Substantial progress has occurred in the elimination of the viruses through the primary prevention practices of education and immunization with hepatitis A and B vaccines (CDC, 2020h).

Hepatitis A

Hepatitis A is caused by infection with the hepatitis A virus (HAV) and occurs around the world. Although high-income countries have seen a decrease in cases due to immunization, low- and middle-income countries are still burdened with the virus. HAV infection is highly contagious for an uninfected or unvaccinated person and is spread through oral–fecal contact via contaminated food, water, or through direct contact with an infected person. Typical symptoms for HAV are fever, malaise, anorexia, nausea, abdominal discomfort, and jaundice. HAV in children is asymptomatic. Age is a factor in the intensity and outcome of the infection with most making a full recovery and acquiring a lifelong immunity against HAV. The incubation period is usually 14 to 28 days, and diagnosis is made by the presence of immunoglobulin M antibodies against HAV in the serum of acutely or recently ill individuals. Recovery from HAV is usually around 2 months (CDC, 2020h; Gholizadeh, 2023; WHO, 2023f). Upon diagnosis, reporting: to the local health agency is mandatory for providers (Mayo Clinic, 2020; Minnesota Department of Health, 2019).

In the United States, cases tend to occur in the older population rather than children, in households of the infected, men who have sex with men (MSM), people who are unsheltered, those who use illegal drugs, and among travelers returning from countries where the disease is endemic. At times, common-source outbreaks are related to contaminated water, food contaminated by infected food handlers, raw or undercooked shellfish harvested from contaminated water, or contaminated produce. Outbreaks of hepatitis A may warrant mass vaccination outreach with either hepatitis A vaccine or postexposure immune globulin (CDC, 2020g; Hall & Wodi, 2021).

An inactivated hepatitis A vaccine is administered in a two-dose series, and these vaccines induce protective antibody levels in virtually all who are immunized. Ninety-five percent of immunized adults develop immunity after the first dose, and nearly 100% seroconvert after the second dose. The vaccine is recommended as a routine vaccine for 1 year and older. C/PHNs are vital to preventing and controlling this disease by offering hepatitis A vaccines to travelers, conducting case investigations, providing education, and identifying potential sources and exposed contacts who need referral or assistance in obtaining postexposure prophylaxis (PEP) and vaccination (Hall & Wodi, 2021).

Hepatitis B

Hepatitis B is both an acute and chronic serious disease and is a global problem. Approximately 296 million people are living with hepatitis B virus (HBV). Approximately 800,000 people die each year due to complications related to HBV. Rates are highest in China, Southeast Asia, most of Africa, most of the Pacific Islands, parts of the Middle East, and in the Amazon basin (WHO, 2023g). Transmission of HBV is through contact with blood or other body fluids that can occur during sexual contact, sharing of syringes or other drug injection equipment, and during pregnancy or delivery. Symptoms include fatigue, anorexia, abdominal pain, nausea, and jaundice; however, many cases are asymptomatic. HBV may be acute or chronic, and the severity of the disease is largely dependent on age and treatment. The younger a person gets infected with HBV, the greater the chance for developing chronic health issues such as liver disease or liver cancer. Diagnosis is confirmed by the presence of specific antigens to HBV in serum (CDC, 2023m).

Immunization and screening are the most effective ways of preventing HBV transmission. The hepatitis B vaccine has been available in the United States since 1981. Since then, rates of HBV infection in the United States have declined by 75% (CDC, 2023m). After receiving the recommended three doses of vaccine, 95% of infants and children develop immunity, whereas only 90% of adults become immune. Infants born to HBV carrier people are at an extremely high risk for developing hepatitis B. Receiving the hepatitis B vaccination and one dose of hepatitis B immunoglobulin within 24 hours after birth in combination with completing the three-dose series at 1 to 2 months and 6 months of age is 85% to 95% effective (Hall & Wodi, 2021). C/PHNs have an important role in the prevention and control of hepatitis B by encouraging immunization compliance, screening, and consistent adherence to universal precautions, especially for people in high-risk lifestyles or occupations.

Hepatitis C

Hepatitis C virus (HCV) causes a complex infection of the liver and is spread through contact with blood from an infected person. The most common method of transmission is through the sharing of needles or equipment used to prepare injected drugs. Individuals infected with hepatitis C often have no symptoms, and many individuals have "spontaneous clearance after acute infection." Fifty percent of the people with HCV develop symptoms when they are in the advanced stages of liver disease that can lead to life-threatening conditions such as cirrhosis and liver cancer. There is no vaccine for hepatitis C, so the best prevention is avoiding behaviors such as injecting drugs. Testing is also important as medical treatment can cure over 90% of HCV within 8 to 12 weeks (CDC, 2020i; Manns & Maasoumy, 2022; WHO, 2023d).

The C/PHN's role is primarily supportive, encouraging testing for people who identified as having HCV infection risk factors, referring individuals for care and treatment and to support/educational groups, and encouraging adherence to standard precautions in the home (CDC, 2020e).

HIV/AIDS

HIV is a retrovirus that attacks the body's immune system. HIV is a global health issue affecting an estimated 39 million people at the end of 2022 (WHO, 2023h). More than half of the new HIV cases were among gay and bisexual males. Black/African American populations and Hispanic/Latin American populations are disproportionately affected by HIV when compared to other racial and ethnic groups. The highest-risk groups are transgender women who have sex with males, and people who inject drugs. Risky behaviors are unprotected sex and sharing drug injection equipment (HIV.gov, 2023a). Other risk factors include having another STI and healthcare workers who experience needlestick injuries (CDC, 2019a).

Although there is no cure for HIV/AIDS, HIV infection is now treated with a combination of drugs collectively known as antiretroviral therapy (ART), which can reduce the viral load to the point that it is undetectable, thus reducing the risk of transmission of the virus provided the viral load remains undetectable (HIV.gov, 2023a). Antiretroviral (ARV) drugs are also being used for prevention of HIV. Pre-exposure prophylaxis (PrEP) drugs (e.g., ARVs) reduce the risk of infection by an HIV-negative partner when taken regularly. PEP is a type of ART medication that is taken only in an emergency situation and within 72 hours after possible exposure to HIV (CDC, 2022e, 2023o).

Acquired immune deficiency syndrome (AIDS) is a severe, life-threatening condition, representing the late clinical stage of infection with HIV. The immune system is badly damaged giving way to opportunistic infections. Individuals with AIDS typically survive around 3 years without HIV medicine intervention (HIV.gov, 2023b).

C/PHN interventions may include education about risk reduction behaviors for those who are at risk but not yet infected. For those who are infected, C/PHNs can provide education about treatment, noting that with early initiation of appropriate treatment, a person with HIV can expect to live almost as long as a person who is not infected. Nurses can also play a role in promoting good health for those who are infected, helping them access care and advising them on how to prevent transmitting the virus to others (CDC, 2021b).

Tuberculosis

TB is a disease primarily of the lungs and larynx, caused by the *Mycobacterium tuberculosis* (MTB) complex, *Mycobacterium africanum*, *M. tuberculosis*, and *Mycobacterium canettii*. These are all Gram-positive bacilli. Routes of transmission: airborne and spread of droplet nuclei (e.g., via coughing, sneezing, laughing, yelling, singing), in which one inhales the bacilli exhaled by a person with viable TB bacilli in the sputum. The areas affected by TB are apex of the lung (most common), kidney, brain, and spine (CDC, 2023i). Most individuals exposed to TB do not become infected, but if there are predisposing factors such as being HIV positive, young age, and close and prolonged contact, the chances increase. Other risk factors for contracting TB are comorbidities (e.g., diabetes, renal disease, immunocompromised or substance misuse disorder), employment or residence in a correctional facility or long-term facility, or experiencing homelessness (CDC, 2022r; Migliori et al., 2022; Reichler et al., 2020).

Most individuals exposed to people with TB do not become infected. Of those who do, approximately 90% are diagnosed with latent TB and are (CDC, 2020l; Migliori et al., 2022) as follows:

- Asymptomatic
- Cannot spread the TB bacteria to others
- Usually have either positive TB skin test reaction or blood test
- Represent a persistent pool of potential active TB cases if they do not receive TB preventive therapy (TPT)

Once almost eradicated, TB has reemerged as a serious public health problem, with around one quarter of the world's population being infected with latent TB (WHO, 2023e). A total of approximately 10.6 million cases of active TB were noted in 2021, and there were 1.5 billion deaths. TB is 1 of the 10 leading causes of death globally. The majority of new TB cases were found in South-East Asia (45%), Africa (23%), and the Western Pacific (18%) (WHO, 2022b). The United States had a rate of 2.5 TB cases per 100,000 people in 2022. There are up to 13 million people in the United States who have latent TB infection. There are sharply disparate rates among racial/ethnic underrepresented populations. In the United States, 84% of the reported TB cases in 2021 were among Hispanic, Black, and Asian individuals. In 2021, over 71% of reported TB cases were among individuals born outside the United States (CDC, 2022r). Figure 8-4 shows the geographic distribution of TB in the United States. The biggest challenges in eradicating TB are drug-resistant TB, screening, and providing preventative TB treatment to a quarter of the world who have latent TB. The COVID-19 pandemic delayed TB notifications, screening, and treatment. Other factors associated with the pandemic include changes in immigration, infection prevention strategies, and health service provision, which likely influenced TB epidemiology in 2021 and will likely continue in the future (WHO, 2022b) (see Fig. 8-5).

Multidrug-Resistant TB

TB is curable through treatment but not if it is drug-resistant TB (DR-TB). DR-TB is caused by the TB

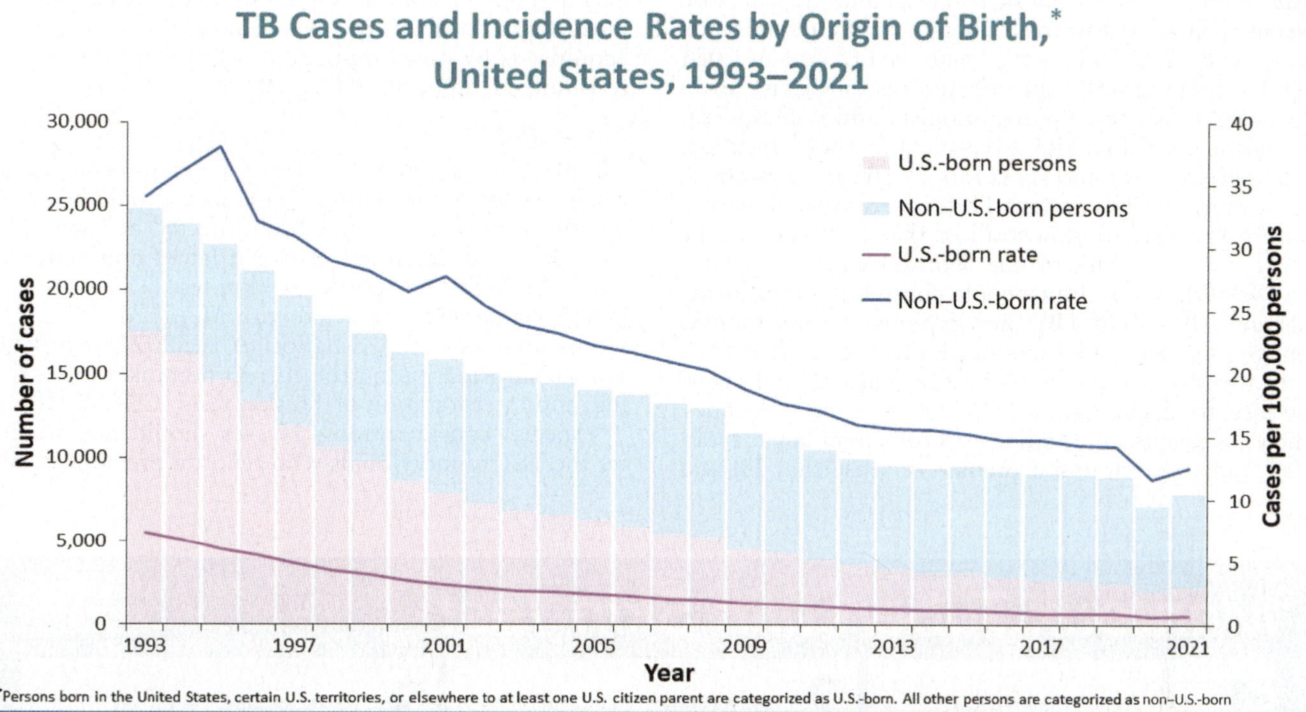

FIGURE 8-4 Reported tuberculosis (TB) case and incident rates by origin of birth, United States, 1993–2021. In 2021, the incidence rates among both non–U.S.-born and U.S.-born people increased. (Reprinted from Centers for Disease Control and Prevention. (2022, July 8). *Reported tuberculosis in the United States, 1993–2021 surveillance report.* https://www.cdc.gov/tb/statistics/reports/2021/default.htm)

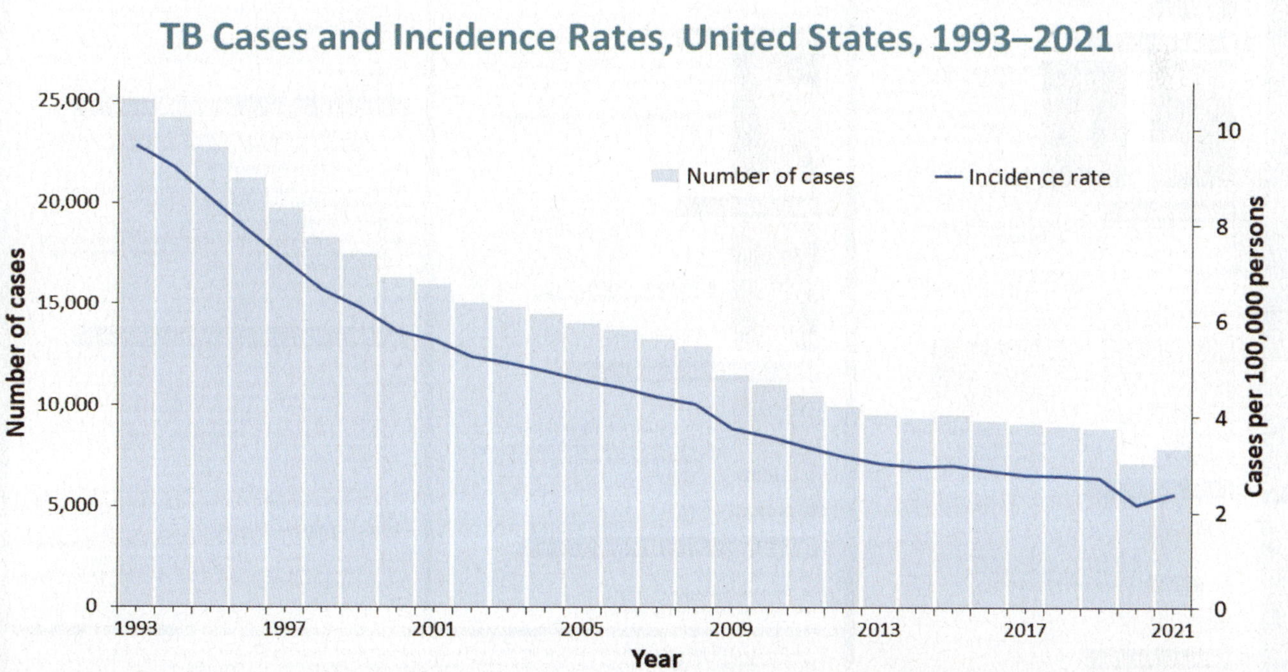

FIGURE 8-5 Reported tuberculosis (TB) cases and incidence rate, United States, 1993–2021. For the first time since 1993, there was an annual incidence rate increase of 9.8%. This increase might be partially explained by delayed detection of cases with symptom onset during 2020 that were not diagnosed until 2021 because of delayed healthcare-seeking behavior, interruptions in healthcare access, or disrupted TB services related to the COVID-19 pandemic. (Reprinted from Centers for Disease Control and Prevention. (2022, July 8). *Tuberculosis in the United States, 1993–2021. Surveillance report.* https://www.cdc.gov/tb/statistics/reports/2021/default.htm)

bacteria that have developed a resistance to the two first-line drugs used to treat TB, isoniazid and rifampin. The spread of DR-TB is the same as TB, and in 2021 WHO estimated 450,000 infected persons exist globally (WHO, 2022b). Epidemiologists and communicable disease specialists cite several factors that contribute to the development and spread of TB strains resistant to one or more of the standard TB drugs. Strains now exist that are resistant to almost all of the standard anti-TB drugs, and according to the World Health Organization (WHO), one in four people contracting multidrug-resistant TB (MDR-TB) dies rapidly, within months from the disease. Chief among the factors contributing to drug resistance seems to be the political and social response to declining rates of TB over past decades, which has resulted in funding cuts for surveillance, treatment, and research and a premature sense that TB was defeated (CDC, 2022q). On an individual case basis, the most common means by which resistant organisms are acquired is by noncompliance with therapy for the full, recommended period (CDC, 2023h).

Screening

TB infection can be detected by screening through either a skin test or blood testing. The tests can only be used to identify a person who has been infected at some point; they do not differentiate between latent and active disease. The Mantoux tuberculin skin test (TST) can detect whether a person is infected with *M. tuberculosis* 6 to 8 weeks after infection (Migliori et al., 2022). See Figure 8-6 for information on the correct administration, reading, and interpretation of TB skin tests (CDC, 2020m).

Special considerations: Nurses should not administer the TST to individuals who report a previous positive

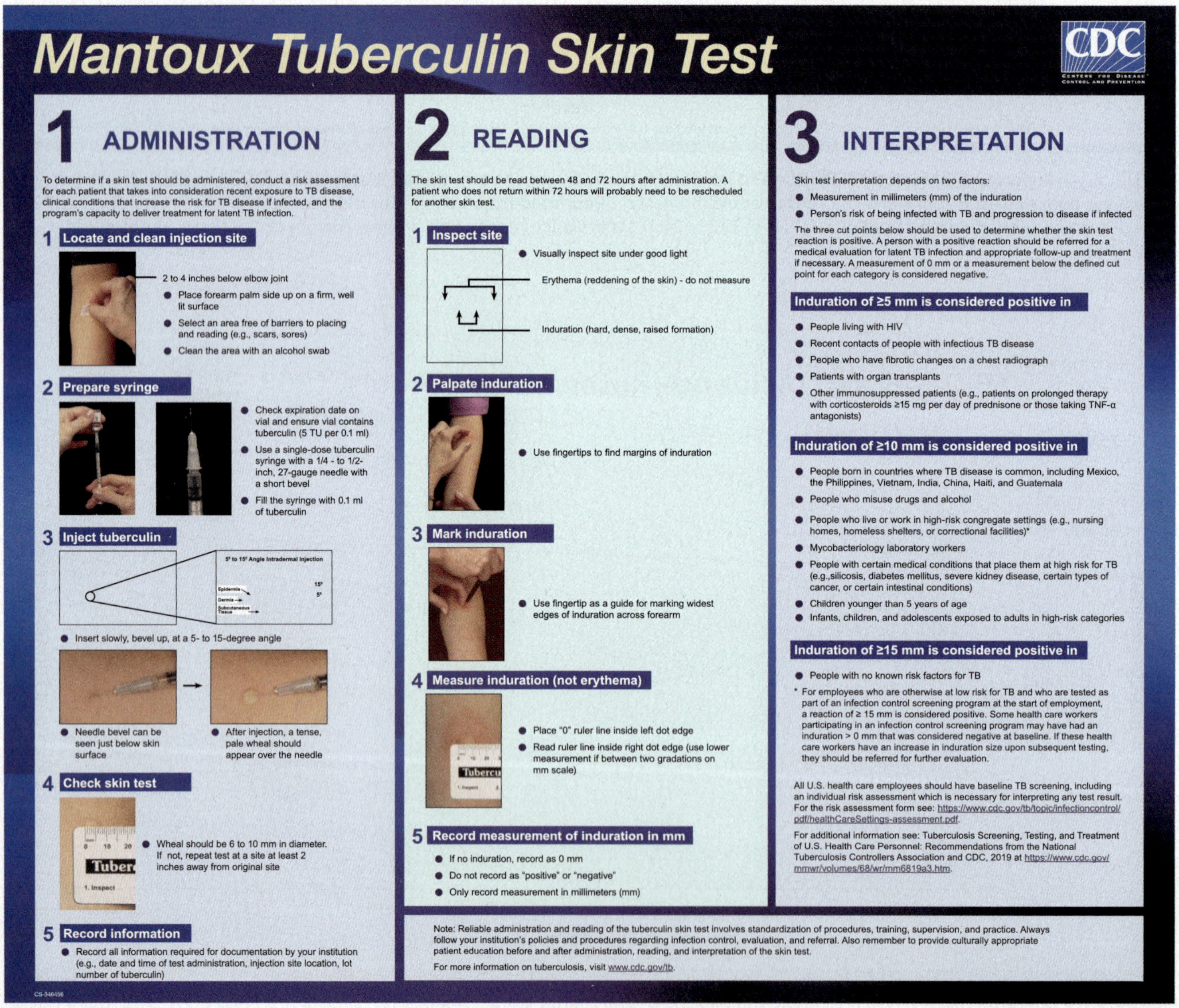

FIGURE 8-6 Mantoux tuberculin skin test wall chart. The chart provides a convenient reference for healthcare workers who administer and read the skin test. The first two panels of the wall chart list the key steps in administration and reading of the skin test and feature close-up photographs. The third panel describes how to interpret the skin test results. (Reprinted from Centers for Disease Control and Prevention (2023). https://npin.cdc.gov/publication/mantoux-tuberculin-skin-test-wall-chart)

TST or have been vaccinated with bacille Calmette-Guérin (BCG) vaccine. The BCG vaccine is used in TB-endemic countries to protect infants and young children from life-threatening TB illness and may cause a reaction to the TST. The TST approach allows the immune system to wake up and respond. Thus, the best test for previously positive TST or a person who received BCG vaccine is to do a blood test. Two different blood tests for interferon-gamma release assays (IGRAs), the QuantiFERON test and the T-spot test, detect the immune response to TB proteins in the blood (Migliori et al., 2022).

Advantages of using an IGRA (Migliori et al., 2022):

- Necessitates only one visit to be tested
- Allows a 24-hour turnaround time on results
- Does not boost responses measured by subsequent tests
- Is not affected by a healthcare provider's interpretation of the results
- Causes no false-positive results from past immunization with BCG vaccine

Disadvantages and limitations of using an IGRA:

- Requires the blood sample to be processed within 8 to 30 hours after collection
- Can be less accurate due to errors in collecting or transporting the blood specimens or in running and interpreting the assay
- Large volumes of blood needed from young children
- May be expensive

IGRAs are preferred for people who are not likely to return for reading of TST and people who have a history of receiving BCG vaccine. The TST is preferred for children under the age of 5 years (Migliori et al., 2022).

Diagnosis of Active TB

The diagnosis of suspected active TB disease is initially based on the presence of acid-fast bacilli in the sputum. Confirmation is determined by a culture that reveals MTB. The culture test also provides information about drug susceptibility that informs the decisions for treatment (Migliori et al., 2022). The nurse should conduct a full examination, including obtaining a chest x-ray and reviewing the person's history of risk factors and symptoms.

Prevention and Intervention

The clinical standards for TB prevention and treatment are based on the Global Plan to End TB 2023–2030 blueprint. The plan is focused on prevention and screening of contacts and high-risk groups, with a special consideration for screening for children as they make up approximately 49% of the new cases among non–U.S.-born people living in the United States (CDC, 2022r; Migliori et al., 2022). The plan is also focused on the treatment and diagnosis of active TB and latent TB individuals as well as patient-centered care and community support that includes healthcare providers, multidisciplinary services, and technology that will support adherence to treatment and prevention (Stop TB Partnership, 2022).

The C/PHN can apply all four levels of prevention when working with clients with TB and has integrated patient-centered care. The C/PHN must stay current with the latest research and technology and be willing to implement changes. According to the CDC Division of TB Elimination, a well-functioning TB control program must focus resources on those at risk for TB exposure and treating those with latent or active TB (CDC, 2020l; Stop TB Partnership, 2022). Refer to Box 8-3 for components of health education and counseling related to TB (Migliori et al., 2022).

BOX 8-3 Components of Health Education and Counseling Related to TB

General Principles

- All individuals (children and adults) undergoing TPT and TB treatment should have health education.
- Education should be used to motivate and elicit cooperation.
- Educational programs (including material) should be age- and gender-specific, culturally sensitive and delivered in the local language, and include all members of the household.
- Evaluation of learning outcomes is important.

Recommended Topics for Health Education

- Basic principles of TB: epidemiology and transmission routes
- Difference between TB disease and TB infection, role of TPT in reducing progression
- Importance of TPT (and treatment adherence/retention in care) to reduce the risk of developing TB disease in the presence of TB infection
- Simple concepts of infection control and safety procedures
- Advantages/importance of smoking cessation and risk of comorbidities (e.g., HIV coinfection and diabetes mellitus) in household/families
- Ensuring adequate nutrition and abstaining from alcohol consumption
- Importance of adhering to medical prescriptions for the management of comorbidities and vaccinations
- Recognition of drug adverse effects and the need to report to healthcare providers
- Information on how to contact the healthcare provider if needed
- Discussing with the person what potential barriers exist for TPT completion and how these can be addressed/overcome (adherence plan)

Source: Migliori, G. B., Wu, S. J., Matteelli, A., Zenner, D., Goletti, D., Ahmedov, S., Al-Abri, S., Allen, D. M., Balcells, M. E., Garcia-Basteiro, A. L., Cambau, E., Chaisson, R. E., Chee, C. B. E., Dalcolmo, M. P., Denholm, J. T., Erkens, C., Esposito, S., Farnia, P., Friedland, J. S., ... Ong, C. W. M. (2022). Clinical standards for the diagnosis, treatment and prevention of TB infection. *The International Journal of Tuberculosis and Lung Disease, 26*(3), 190–205. https://doi.org/10.5588/ijtld.21.0753

When candidates for drug therapy are identified, it is essential to provide program support to ensure that the maximum number of individuals comply with their medication regimen for the full duration of therapy. One of the most effective ways to achieve a high completion-of-therapy rate is through directly observed treatment (DOT) (CDC, 2023n). One variation of DOT is eDOT, which involves recording the patient taking the medication at home and is reviewed by trained staff. The vDOT uses a video-enabled device such as a smart phone, tablet, or computer and falls under eDOT. The eDOT method has a higher completion rate and is preferred over DOT because it costs 32% less than DOT and may be more convenient for the patient (it decreases travel and time away from work or dependents) (Migliori et al., 2022). eDOT and DOT are a public health strategy for delivering TB treatment and offer the benefits of timely completion of treatment, prevention of drug resistance, and prevention of further transmission. The eDOT program has a 95% completion rate as compared to 91% for in-person DOT. In addition, eDOT is cost saving and reduces the amount of staff time for travel and expense (CDC, 2023cc). It is not mandatory, but health officers may use the laws surrounding TB prevention and public protection to institute policy and statute to mandate its use. By using DOT with the client with active TB, providers can reduce ongoing potential sources of infection in the community (NTCA, n.d.).

It is important to assess the patient to see what form of DOT therapy would work the best. Clients who face challenges, such as those who misuse alcohol and drugs, those who are in transitional housing or are experiencing homelessness, and people stressed by socioeconomic problems, may benefit from DOT therapy, because it ensures that patients are often met where they are located (school, shelter, bar, or job). Implementation of an eDOT program requires input from information technology and legal representatives to ensure that it complies with both state and federal laws and that clients' Health Insurance Portability and Accountability Act (HIPAA) rights are protected (CDC, 2023cc).

Clients With HIV and TB

HIV infection is associated with an increased possibility of developing primary TB after exposure to a source. The person living with coinfection of latent TB infection and HIV infection have a higher risk of developing active TB than the person without HIV (CDC, 2023bb).

The client who is HIV-positive may not have the ability to react to a skin test for TB because of a weakened immune system. Therefore, other methods are needed to determine TB status. People with HIV infection and TB infection should be counseled about the benefit of preventive treatment and possibility of TB activation without treatment. These clients must be monitored closely for effectiveness of the preventive therapy and side effects (CDC, 2023bb).

TB Case Management

The functional aspect of the program should ideally strive for the following (CDC, 2023bb):

- Standardized public health practices for investigating, case and contact finding, as well as care and treatment.
- Case management of care and treatment of the person with TB to ensure medication compliance and barriers to treatment completion are dealt with so treatment completion will occur.
- Close monitoring for sputum conversion in people with active disease, to adjust medication as necessary.
- A high completion-of-therapy rate within 1 year after diagnosis.
- Assurance of adequate funding and a dedicated TB control infrastructure.

C/PHNs have a responsibility to build a relationship of trust with individuals who have TB or latent TB infection, which leads to seeking and adhering to treatment. It is also important to monitor for overall health and well-being, educating, and making referrals (Migliori et al., 2022).

Sexually Transmitted Diseases

Impact of COVID-19 on Sexually Transmitted Diseases

The COVID-19 pandemic resulted in the disruptions of screening, reporting, investigating, and sexually transmitted infection (STI) treatment with many of the resources diverted to COVID-19 activities during 2020 and likely 2021. Reported cases of chlamydia, syphilis, and gonorrhea dropped below 2019 levels during the shelter-in-place phase, but by the end of 2021, the numbers increased. Refer to Figures 8-7 to 8-9 for details. The data are difficult to interpret, and the best interpretation is that once clinics and health departments opened, many prioritized treatments of symptomatic STI such as syphilis and gonorrhea. Chlamydia is usually asymptomatic and identified through screenings and preventive care visits, and these types of visits were reduced due to the pandemic. The data highlight the impact the pandemic had on an already strained public health infrastructure and the underreporting that occurred, which should not be confused with a downward turn in STD infection. Likely, the impact of the COVID-19 pandemic's actual STD cases will never be known. What is certain is that prevention and control are even more important now (CDC, 2023w).

Chlamydia

Chlamydia trachomatis (CT) infections are the most commonly reported notifiable STI in the United States (CDC, 2023d). In 2021, more than 1.6 million cases of *Chlamydia* were reported in with the highest proportion found in those ages 15 to 24. Disparities exist, resulting in higher infection rates for males who are gay or bisexual, pregnant people, and racial and ethnic underrepresented groups (CDC, 2023w).

Key facts:

- Route of transmission: sexual contact and maternal transmission to a newborn (CDC, 2023d)
- Symptoms: often asymptomatic, resulting in a greater risk of going undetected, resulting in serious complications:
    - Pelvic inflammatory disease (PID)
    - Long-term damage to the fallopian tubes, uterus, and surrounding tissues

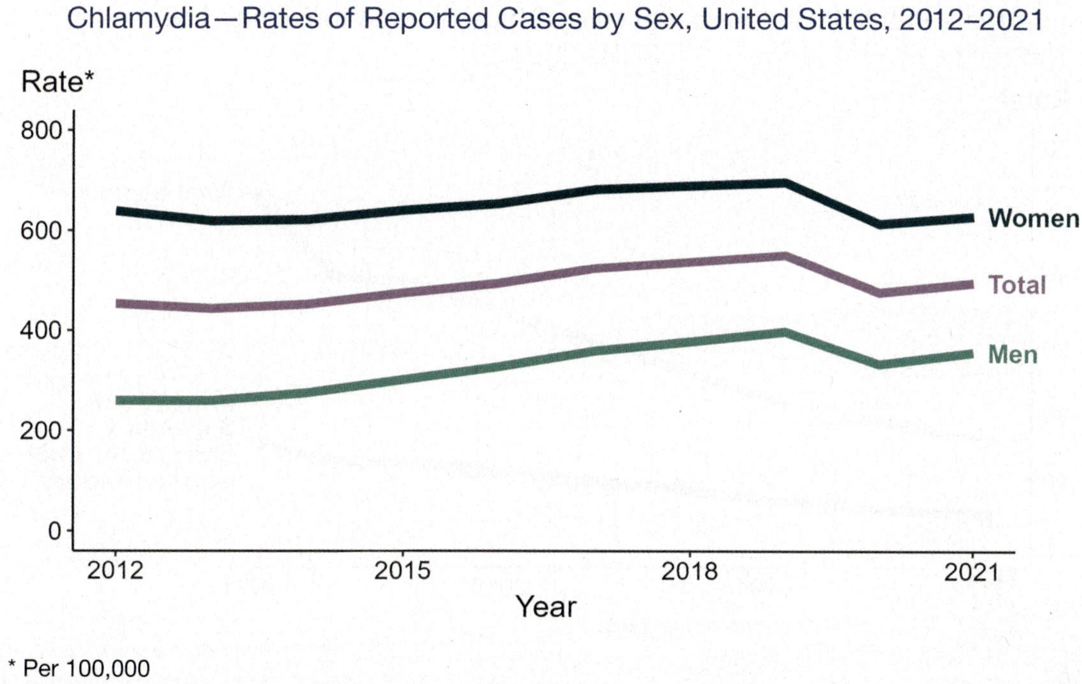

FIGURE 8-7 Chlamydia. Reported 2020 and 2021 cases as a percentage of 2019 by MMWR week, United States. (Reprinted from Centers for Disease Control and Prevention. (2023, April 11). *Sexually transmitted disease surveillance 2021*. https://www.cdc.gov/std/statistics/2021/impact.htm)

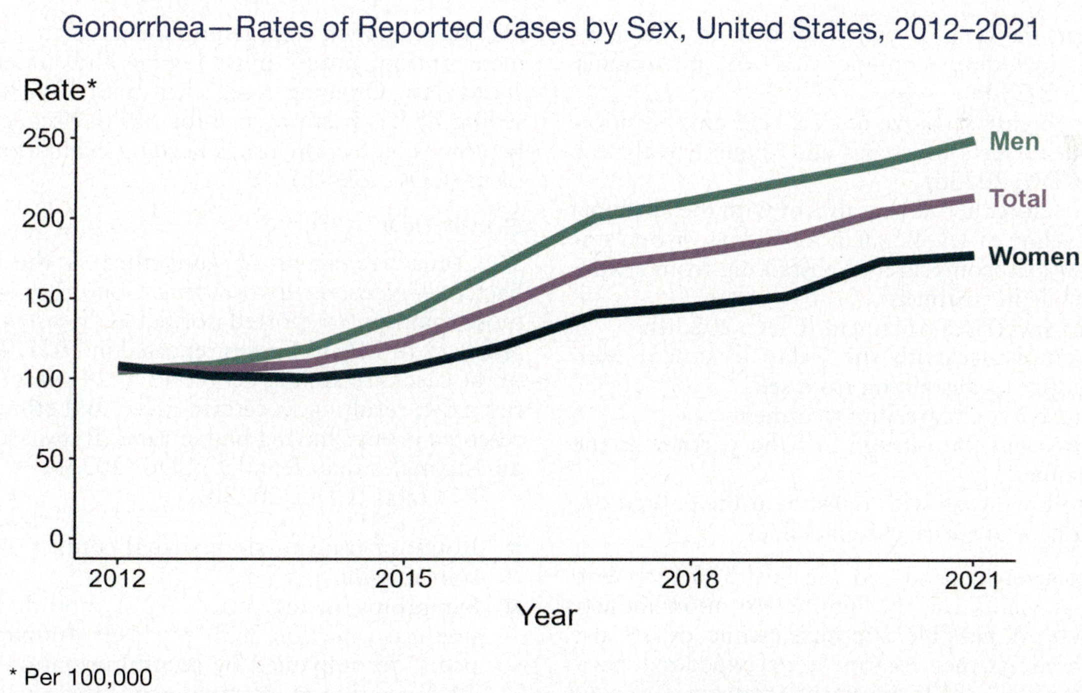

FIGURE 8-8 Gonorrhea. Reported 2020 and 2021 cases as a percentage of 2019 by MMWR week, United States. (Reprinted from Centers for Disease Control and Prevention. (2023, April 11). *Sexually transmitted disease surveillance 2021*. https://www.cdc.gov/std/statistics/2021/impact.htm)

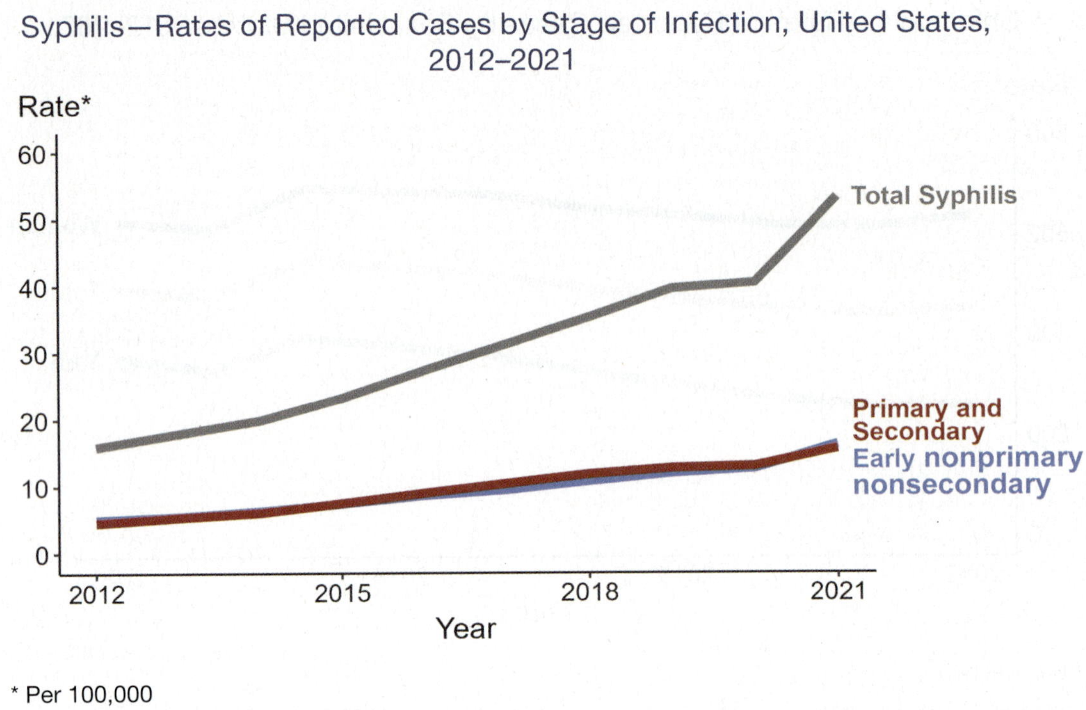

FIGURE 8-9 Syphilis. Reported 2020 and 2021 cases as a percentage of 2019 by MMWR week, United States. (Reprinted from Centers for Disease Control and Prevention. (2023, April 11). *Sexually Transmitted Disease Surveillance 2021.* https://www.cdc.gov/std/statistics/2021/impact.htm)

  - Preterm delivery or complications for the newborn, including conjunctivitis or pneumonia (CDC, 2023d)
- Diagnosis: highly sensitive nucleic acid amplification (NAAT) urine tests for males and vaginal swabs for females (CDC, 2023d)
- Treatment: either a 7-day treatment with the antibiotics doxycycline or levofloxacin for 7 days or one single dose of azithromycin and abstaining from sexual activity while in treatment
- Barriers to successful treatment (CDC, 2023d):
  - Noncompliance with the 7-day treatment with antibiotics or abstaining from sex
  - Stigma, costs of care, and treatment
  - Not treating the infection of the partner at the same time
  - Not following up with retesting if the patient did not adhere to treatment guidelines

STI notification depends on the health department, as some departments use the internet to anonymously notify partners of possible exposure, while others use patient-delivered partner treatment or expedited partner treatment (EPT). EPT treatment strategy is to give a prescription or medication to the infected patients to, in turn, give to their sex partners. This intervention is more effective than encouraging the patient to notify the partner(s) to seek testing and treatment. With EPT, it is important to provide very specific written instructions that include self-administration of the medication, warnings about pregnancy, allergic reactions, when to seek medical care, and how to prevent reinfection. Each state may have its own legal requirements related to this treatment option; nurses must review and understand their states' law. Ongoing research is mixed on whether providing EPT is best practice for MSM, because there may be other coinfection issues needing evaluation and treatment (CDC, 2021h).

Gonorrhea

The causative agent of gonorrhea is the gonococcus bacteria—*Neisseria gonorrhoeae*. Gonorrhea is the second-most commonly reported notifiable disease in the United States, with 710,151 cases reported in 2021. The majority of the cases are among people 15 to 24 years old. Disparities exist, resulting in certain racial and ethnic underrepresented groups having higher rates. Rates are also higher among males than females (CDC, 2023l).

Key facts (CDC, 2023l):

- Route of transmission: sexual contact and maternal transmission.
- Symptoms (males): many are asymptomatic or have a urethral infection with purulent drainage from the penis, accompanied by painful urination within 1 to 14 days after an infecting exposure.
- Symptoms (females): asymptomatic; mild vaginal discharge or bleeding after intercourse.
- Rectal infection may include discharge or anal itching, soreness, or bleeding with bowel movement. Pharyngeal infection is usually asymptomatic or sore throat.
- Diagnosis: urine analysis or urethral swabs for males and endocervical or vaginal swabs for females.

- Complications (females): if untreated, PID, infertility, or ectopic pregnancy.
- Complications (dissemination): petechial or pustular lesions, requiring hospitalization for treatment and evaluation for complications such as endocarditis and meningitis.

Antimicrobial resistance is a great concern when treating gonorrhea. Resistance to cefixime, a third-generation cephalosporin, appeared in Asia, Europe, South Africa, and Canada, causing further changes in dual treatment guidelines advising the exclusive use of only one recommended treatment, a third-generation ceftriaxone-ceftriaxone (CDC, 2022k). Medication will stop the infection but will not reverse any permanent damage caused by the disease. Gonorrhea transmitted to neonates during delivery presents 2 to 5 days after delivery. This can result in ophthalmia neonatorum and sepsis. As a result, most states have a law that requires a prophylactic agent be given to all infants after delivery. Treatment during pregnancy is the best way to prevent gonorrhea infection in the newborn (CDC, 2022k). Sex partners should be referred to a medical provider for testing and treatment, but if this is not possible, EPT can be used.

C/PHNs should remain vigilant in monitoring for suspected gonorrhea treatment failure and report suspected failure or resistance to GCFAILURE@cdc.gov (CDC, 2022j).

Syphilis

Syphilis is a systemic infection caused by the spirochete *Treponema pallidum*. Before 2014, the incidence rate of syphilis had been decreasing, but starting in 2014, the incidence rate has increased. In 2021, 176,713 new cases (all stages) were reported with 36% of the cases attributed to gay, bisexual, and other MSM (CDC, 2023x). The incidence rate of congenital syphilis has tripled, and in 2021, the number of cases were the highest since 1994. Mandatory testing for syphilis is determined by each state, but CDC recommends that testing should be done at the first prenatal visit and additional testing may be required based on history and medical provider advice (CDC, 2021g). Past historical data indicate a correlation between primary and secondary syphilis infectious rates of females in their reproductive years (CDC, 2023x).

Key facts (CDC, 2023x):

- Routes of transmission: direct contact with a lesion, blood transfusion during the primary or secondary stage of the disease, maternal transmission (CDC, 2021g)
- Process: Four distinct stages:
    1. Primary: A primary lesion called a *chancre* appears as a painless ulcer at the site where the infection entered the body, lasts 3 to 6 weeks, and heals regardless of medical treatment.
    2. Secondary: After 4 to 6 weeks, a more generalized secondary macular-to-papulosquamous skin eruption develops, classically appearing on the soles of the feet, palms of the hands, and trunk, often accompanied by fever, sore throat, lymphadenopathy, and fatigue. These secondary manifestations can resolve spontaneously within weeks or may persist up to 12 months.
    3. Latent: By this phase, the spirochete has invaded the central nervous system, but there may not be any signs or symptoms of infection for weeks to years.
    4. Tertiary: One third of those infected who do not receive treatment progress to tertiary syphilis, which is associated with recurring lesions, severe systemic involvement, disability, abnormalities in the cerebral spinal fluid, deafness, meningitis, cranial nerve palsy, or even death.
- Complications of congenital syphilis: fetal death, premature birth, death of the newborn, failure to thrive, anemia, lesions, and central nervous system symptoms (CDC, 2021g)
- Risk factors: MSM, HIV-positive, taking PrEP for HIV prevention, unprotected sex

Diagnosis is through a blood test. Penicillin is the treatment of choice for syphilis. The C/PHN instructs the patient to avoid sexual contact until the treatment is completed and the lesions have resolved and to encourage contacts to receive treatment. Contacts are defined as those with whom the patient had sex within the 3 months (for patients in the primary stage), 6 months (for patients in the secondary stage), or 1 year (for patients in the early latent stage) before the onset of symptoms or long-term sexual partners (for patients in the late latent stage) (New York City Department of Health & STD Prevention Training Center, 2019).

Genital Herpes

Genital herpes is an STI caused by the herpes simplex virus types 1 (HSV-1) and 2 (HSV-2) and is one of the most common STIs in the United States. Most genital herpes infections are caused by HSV-2; however, rates of HSV-1 genital herpes are increasing. HSV-1 is the virus that causes cold sores and spreads from the mouth to the genitals through oral sex. An estimated 87.4% of 14- to 49-year-olds infected with HSV-2 remain undiagnosed because of the symptoms being mild, causing the person to not recognize a need to seek medical care (CDC, 2021e).

Key facts (CDC, 2021e):

- Symptoms (initial): systemic, including fever and malaise, and bilateral lesions lasting 2 to 3 weeks on the cervix (females), external genitalia (males or females), or anus or rectum
- Symptoms (subsequent outbreaks): lesions in areas beyond the initial exposure site, which usually are unilateral, less severe, and less frequent and resolve more quickly than the primary lesion
- Diagnosis: by isolation of the virus, DNA detection through polymerase chain reaction (PCR) testing, or tests that detect HSV antigens, with viral isolates being typed to determine whether the infection is due to HSV-1 or HSV-2
- Prognosis: there is no cure for HSV, and the infection can remain in the body indefinitely; however, antiviral medications can prevent or reduce the duration of an outbreak and can reduce the risk of transmission to uninfected sexual partners

If a pregnant person becomes infected late in the pregnancy and has active lesions, delivery by cesarean section is often advised to reduce the risk of transmission to the neonate. Antiviral therapy can be given to the pregnant person at 36 weeks of gestation to suppress the virus to help reduce the need for a cesarean section birth.

Viral Warts

Condylomata acuminata, verruca vulgaris, papilloma venereum, and the common wart are all forms of a viral disease caused by the *human papillomavirus* (HPV). More than 120 HPV types have been identified, at least 40 of which are sexually transmitted. HPV is a common STD, with most sexually active people becoming infected with it at least once during their lifetime. It is estimated that around 42 million people in the United States have been infected with HPV (CDC, 2023p; Kombe et al., 2021).

Key facts (CDC, 2021f):

- Routes of transmission: direct contact with fomites; sexual (skin-to-skin) contact; or transmission by a birthing parent to a neonate during vaginal birth
- Symptoms: may include lesions on the skin or mucous membranes, including in the throat or respiratory tract (recurrent, respiratory papillomatosis) and the genital region (condylomata acuminata, or genital warts). Patients may be asymptomatic, putting them at increased risk for lack of detection and diagnosis, and ongoing transmission between or among sexual partners
- Prevention: condoms are not fully protective
- Prognosis: about 12,000 females are diagnosed with HPV-related cervical cancer each year, with oropharyngeal cancer being most common for males
- Vaccination: recommended for males and females against high-risk HPV (hrHPV) infection strains as follows:
  - Routine vaccination is recommended for children at age 11 or 12 years.
    - Patients 9 to 14 years old: 2 doses, with 6 to 12 months between doses.
  - Patients 15 to 26 years old: 3 doses, with at least 4 weeks between the first and second doses, 12 weeks between the second and third doses, and 5 months between the first and last doses.
  - Extended use up to the age of 45 years for males and females based on a shared clinical decision with healthcare provider (Meites et al., 2019).

The vaccine works best if given prior to being sexually active but can still be given to individuals already sexually active to protect against any hrHPV (high-risk) strains they have not yet acquired. The National Cancer Institute (NCI) stresses the importance of increasing the numbers of people vaccinated "to reduce the prevalence of the vaccine-targeted HPV types in the population, thereby providing some protection for individuals who are not vaccinated" (NCI, 2019, para. 15).

There is currently no routine recommended screening test for HPV-associated diseases other than cervical cancer. The USPSTF has issued the following recommendations for females 21 to 65 years of age, "regardless of sexual history, who have a cervix and show no signs or symptoms of cervical cancer" (USPSTF, 2018, para. 6):

- Females aged 21 to 29 years: cervical cytology screening alone every 3 years
- Females aged 30 to 65 years: cervical cytology screening alone every 3 years or hrHPV testing every 5 years or hrHPV testing in combination with cervical cytology screening (cotesting) every 5 years
- Females younger than 21 years: no screening recommended (USPSTF, 2018)

Treatment for HPV is for health problems as a result of the virus only and is for genital warts, cervical precancer, or HPV-related cancers (CDC, 2021f).

Sexually Transmitted Infection Prevention and Control

In general, underrepresented groups, low-income populations, the medically underserved, females, and children experience a disproportionate amount of the STI burden, and they also have a higher risk of serious complications from STIs, including PID, sterility, ectopic pregnancy, and cancer associated with HPV. Children can also be affected by exposure to maternal STIs, resulting in fetal and infant death, birth defects, blindness, and intellectual disability. Undiagnosed and untreated STIs may play a role in infertility (CDC, 2023y). C/PHNs need to be involved in accomplishing the *Healthy People 2030* goal of promoting healthy sexual behaviors, strengthening capacities within communities, and increasing access to quality services (ODPHP, 2020).

Infectious Diseases of Bioterrorism

The deliberate release of biologic agents into the environment with the intent to cause harm is a real risk and can occur as an overt or covert event (FDA, 2020). Although many disease-causing organisms can be weaponized, only anthrax and smallpox, two biologic agents that have a history of being used as terrorist weapons, are discussed here (see Chapter 17). In the event of such a terrorist attack, C/PHNs can allay fears, provide the public with correct information, and promote and carry out immunization.

Anthrax

The 2001 anthrax agent was disseminated through the U.S. mail. As a result, people were infected, five died, and 10,000 were identified as having been potentially exposed and were treated with antibiotics as a precaution. Anthrax spores are found in nature in the digestive tracks of herbivores and can be found in the soil. In humans, anthrax is an acute bacterial disease that mainly affects the skin or respiratory tract. Inhalation anthrax is nearly always fatal (Brock, 2022). The U.S. federal government have purchased and stored the vaccine that protects against anthrax and is part of the Strategic National Stockpile to be used in case of biologic warfare (FDA, 2023).

Smallpox and Mpox

Smallpox, also known as cowpox, is caused by the variola virus, which is part of the orthopoxvirus family. Smallpox was a deadly disease that was responsible for millions of deaths (CDC, 2022f). In 1980, the WHO declared a public health achievement when it declared that smallpox was eradicated. Before smallpox was eradicated, it spread via direct and close contact. Initial symptoms are fever and rash that transitions from macular to papular to vesicular to pustular. The infected person remains contagious through the initial symptoms and until the last scab falls off in 3 to 4 weeks (CDC, 2021i). Posteradication of smallpox research has continued, and vaccine and antivirals have been developed. The smallpox virus presently exists in only two places: the CDC in Atlanta and the State Research Centre of Virology and Biotechnology in Koltsovo, Novosibirsk Region, Russian Federation, in case of reemergence of the disease (WHO, n.d.-f).

Routine immunization against smallpox is no longer recommended for the general public. Laboratory workers who work in high-risk areas may still obtain the vaccine (CDC, 2022p).

The response plan for smallpox exposure includes vaccines that can either make people infected with the disease less sick or prevent the disease. Currently, there are enough smallpox vaccines available for every person in the United States. The second strategy is two antiviral drugs for the treatment of smallpox and for research for related diseases such as mpox (formerly known as monkeypox) (CDC, 2021i; WHO, n.d.-f).

Mpox is caused by monkeypox, a viral zoonotic disease caused by the orthopoxvirus genus, which is part of the Poxviridae family that includes smallpox. There are two strains of the virus, clade I and clade II. Mpox shares similarities to smallpox but with less severe symptoms and is less fatal (CDC, 2023t). In 1958, the first case of mpox was discovered in a colony of research monkeys in Denmark. The origin of the disease is unknown, but it has been associated with rodents and nonhuman primates (monkeys). Previously, most of the cases reported were in Africa with some cases occurring in other countries but always linked to Africa through international travel or exports of animals (WHO, 2023i).

The spread of mpox is through close or intimate contact, contaminated items, and infected animals. The symptoms usually start within a week but can also start between 1 and 21 days after exposure. See Figure 8-10. The symptoms include flu-like symptoms and a rash that starts as a flat sore but develops into small fluid-filled blisters that scab over within 2 to 4 weeks (WHO, 2023i; CDC, 2023t). People at risk for serious complications are children, pregnant people, and individuals that are immunocompromised (WHO, 2023i).

Outbreaks of the disease have occurred, including a 2003 outbreak in the United States that was linked to wild animals. Since that time there have been cases reported but largely relegated to Africa. On July 2022, the WHO declared a multicountry outbreak of mpox with the majority of the cases being clade II virus. The outbreaks spread quickly across the world. Refer to Figure 8-11 for countries affected. The outbreak spread through sexual networks and primarily affecting MSM (WHO, 2023i). Since the outbreak in 2022, there have been 106,310 laboratory-confirmed cases including 234 laboratory-confirmed deaths from 123 reporting countries

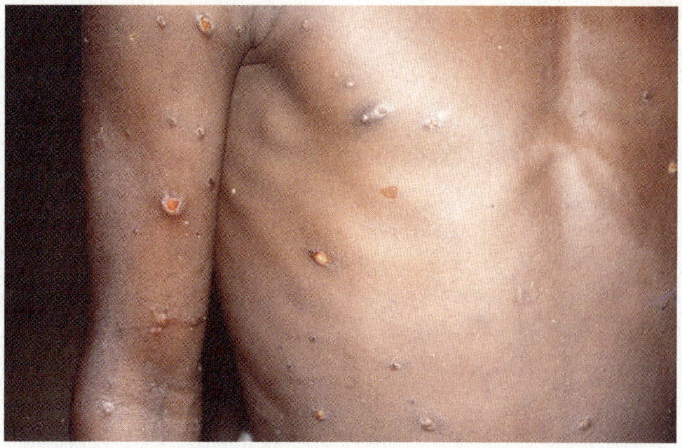

FIGURE 8-10 A patient with an active case of mpox. (Reprinted from Centers for Disease Control and Prevention. Public Health Image Library. https://phil.cdc.gov/Details.aspx?pid=12779)

(WHO, 2024a). The treatment for the mpox infection is antivirals approved for the treatment of smallpox because the two diseases are similar. The mpox vaccine was offered with a two-dose recommendation for at-risk populations (CDC, 2023t). The WHO declared the end of the mpox emergency on May 10, 2023 (PAHO, 2023).

PRIMARY PREVENTION

In the context of communicable disease control, two approaches are useful in achieving primary prevention: (1) education using mass media with targeted health messages to aggregates and (2) immunizations.

Education

Health education in primary prevention is directed both at helping individuals understand their risk and at promoting healthy behaviors. Chapter 11 deals more extensively with the concepts of learning theory and the variety of health education approaches and materials available to C/PHNs today.

Engaging With Communities/Populations of Focus

Engaging a community or population of focus is done through marketing of your health promotion or disease prevention message and educational outreach. The CDC recommends that messages and educational material be presented through a "health equity lens." A health equity lens is to look at the message you wish to deliver through the lens of the intended audience and look for positive and negative implications. It is also important to acknowledge historical and contemporary injustices that have created obstacles to care and have led to health disparities and look for ways to create positive change. Below are the Health Equity Guiding Principles from the CDC, 2023k):

1. Identify the intended audience who share common interests, needs, and behaviors.
2. Determine the educational level, view of the salience of the issue, involvement with the issue, and access to media channels.

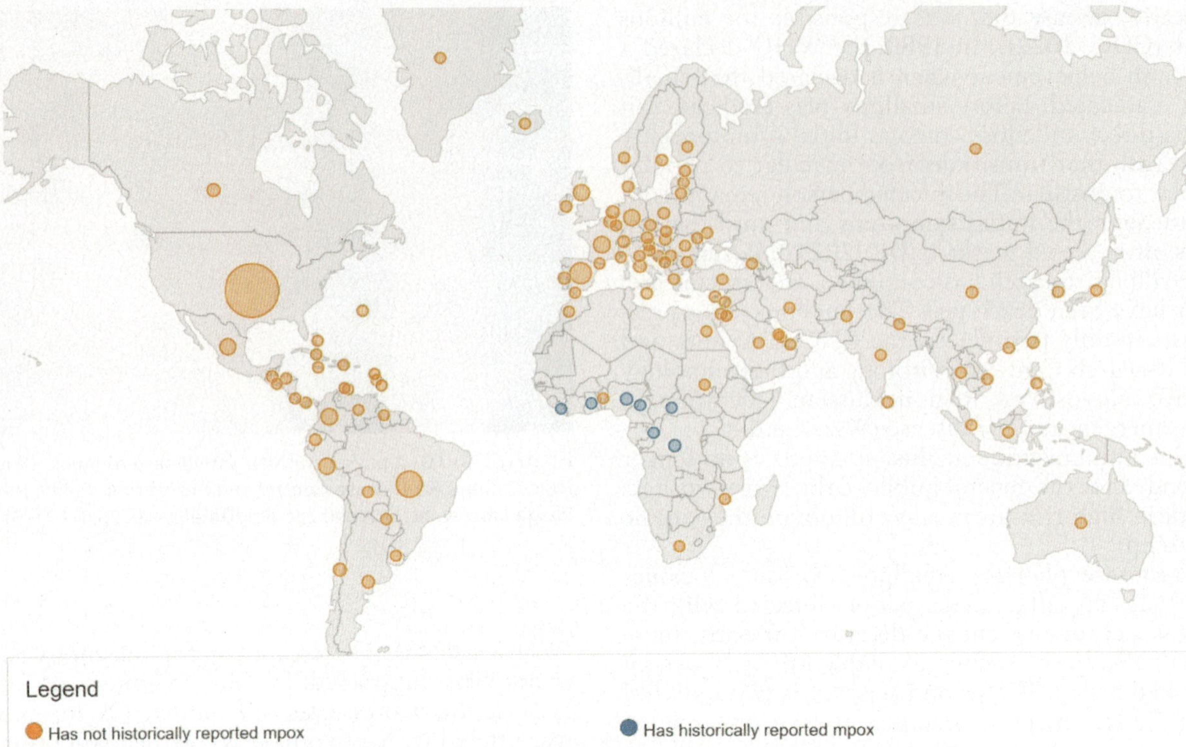

FIGURE 8-11 Mpox 2022 outbreak global case map (date as of August 16, 2023). (Reprinted from Centers for Disease Control and Prevention. https://www.cdc.gov/poxvirus/mpox/response/2022/world-map.html)

3. Consider the cultural, racial, and ethnic context of the target market and ensure that the message and educational materials are relevant to the needs and interests of the community and respect and reflect their values and traditions. In the example in Figure 8-12, social media platforms were used because 57% of Latino and Hispanic individuals were using social media as a primary source of information about COVID-19 (CDC, 2022c).
4. Select or develop materials that relate to the delivery of health services that are available, accessible, and acceptable to the intended population.
5. Pretest all materials and verify that they are attractive, comprehensible, acceptable, and persuasive to the target market and promote ownership.
6. Select or develop materials that are at the appropriate reading level for the intended audience.
7. Avoid using dehumanizing language and unintentional blaming and use person-first language.
8. Avoid saying target, tackle, combat, or other terms with violent connotation when referring to people, groups, or communities.

Ways to Communicate

Various types of social media—including Facebook, Instagram, YouTube, Snapchat, TikTok, and X (formerly Twitter)—offer the ability to engage a large number of participants in an interactive, collaborative, and synchronous manner. They allow practitioners to reach populations that are diverse and that they might not easily

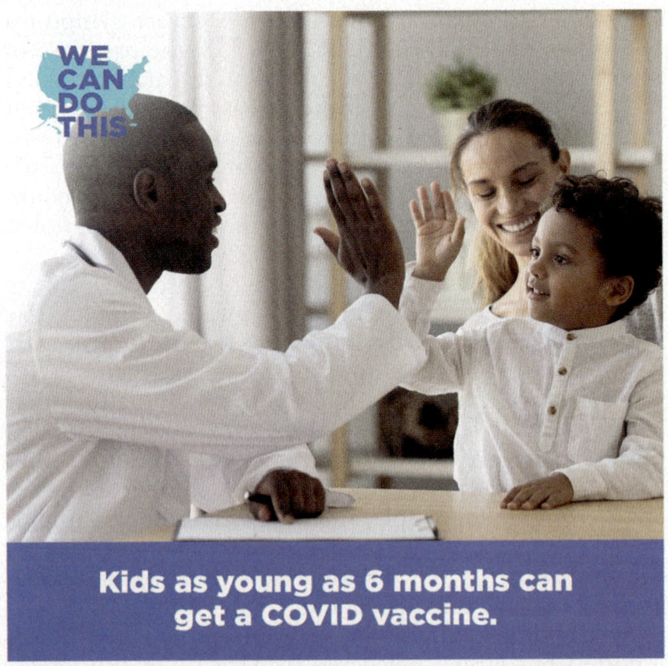
WE CAN DO THIS
Kids as young as 6 months can get a COVID vaccine.

FIGURE 8-12 A "We Can Do This" COVID-19 campaign graphic post for social media platforms. The photo shows the diversity within the Latin American population and seeks to emphasize the importance of vaccinating children 5 to 11 years of age because this is the age group parents/guardians in this population were most hesitant to vaccinate at the time of the campaign. (Reprinted from Centers for Disease Prevention and Control. *Social media graphic posts for parents.* https://wecandothis.hhs.gov/resource/social-media-graphic-posts-for-parents)

arrange to meet face-to-face. They also make sharing of information easier, through podcasts, YouTube, and blogs (CDC, 2020f); however, in using social media, nurses must take care to maintain patients' privacy. This approach can also be integrated with other public health communication strategies. Public health organizations need to use social media engagement to its full potential (Kanchan & Gaidhane, 2023). Nurses can explore ways that social media can be used to augment current public health communication approaches. See Chapters 10 and 12 for more information on social marketing and using technology to reach various populations.

Immunization

The extended life expectancy that has been enjoyed during the 20th century was largely due to the expansion of immunization programs. Immunizations are a cost-effective public health intervention that offer a high return on investment (see Fig. 8-13). Immunization and control of infectious diseases remain a national focus through *Healthy People 2030* (ODPHP, 2018). Box 8-4 highlights select objectives related to immunization and infectious diseases. A *Healthy People 2030* goal is to increase vaccination rates.

An example is the COVID-19 pandemic where with the guidance from the Advisory Committee on Immunization Practices (ACIP) provided vaccine and booster recommendations for the entire population (CDC, 2021j).

Although all states have established laws requiring immunizations in certain situations (such as for attendance in public schools and childcare facilities and employment in healthcare facilities), many allow for exempting immunizations for several reasons, whether religious, philosophical, or medical (Boxes 8-5 and 8-6). In 2019, 15 states allowed for personal, moral, or other beliefs exemption (National Conference of State Legislatures [NCSL], 2023). The C/PHN should look to immunization agency of the state of practice for the accepted exemption criteria (Immunization Action Coalition, 2023).

Barriers to Immunization Coverage

The majority of Americans have accepted immunizations as a part of overall healthcare. However, some that challenge the notion of immunizing their children oppose government mandates and the sheer number of vaccinations, and others want to veer from the recommended spacing schedule but plan to eventually complete the

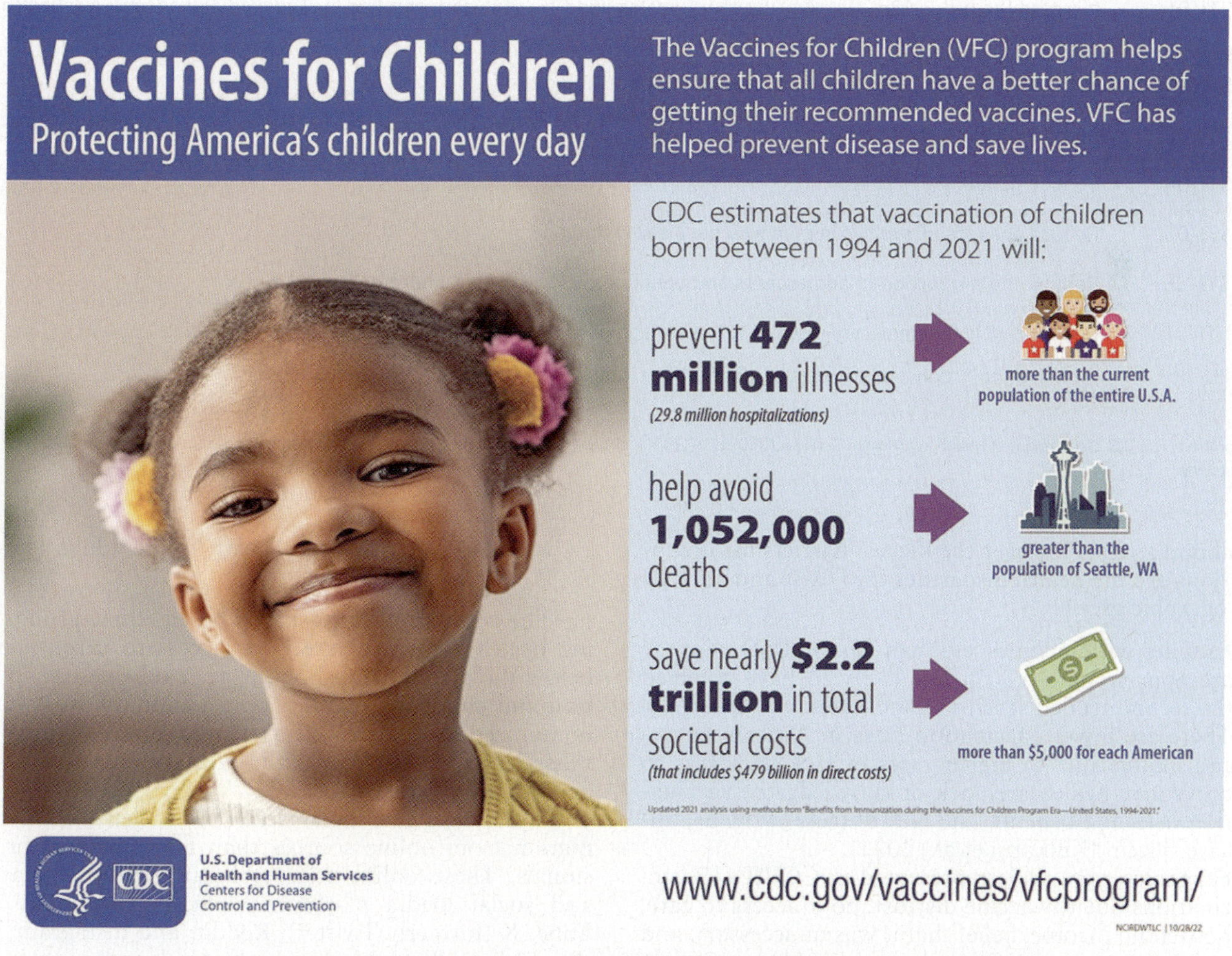

FIGURE 8-13 The Vaccines for Children (VCF) program ensures that children from all communities and income levels will be able to get recommended childhood vaccinations, preventing infectious diseases and their sequelae. (Reprinted from Centers for Disease Control and Prevention. (2019). https://www.cdc.gov/vaccines/programs/vfc/protecting-children.html)

BOX **8-4** *HEALTHY PEOPLE 2030*

Immunization and Infectious Diseases: Select 2030 Objectives

Core and Developmental Objectives

IID-02	Reduce the proportion of children who receive 0 doses of recommended vaccines by age 2 years
IID-03	Maintain the vaccination coverage level of 1 dose of the measles-mumps-rubella (MMR) vaccine among children by age 2 years
IID-04	Maintain the vaccination coverage level of 1 dose of measles-mumps-rubella vaccine (MMR) for children in kindergarten
IID-05	Reduce cases of pertussis among infants
IID-06	Increase the vaccination coverage level of 4 doses of the DTaP vaccine in children by age 2 years
IID-08	Increase the percentage of adolescents aged 13 through 15 years who get recommended doses of the HPV vaccine
IID-09	Increase the proportion of people who get the flu vaccine every year
IID-10	Reduce the rate of hepatitis A
IID-11,12	Reduce the rate of acute hepatitis B and C
IID-17	Reduce tuberculosis cases
STI-01	Increase the proportion of sexually active females aged 16–24 years enrolled in Medicaid and commercial health plans who are screened for chlamydial infections
STI-02	Reduce gonorrhea rates in male adolescents and young males
STI-03	Reduce the incidence of primary and secondary syphilis in rate in females
STI-04	Reduce congenital syphilis
STI-05	Reduce the rate of syphilis in men who have sex with men
STI-06	Reduce the proportion of adolescents and young adults with genital herpes
STI-07	Reduce pelvic inflammatory disease in female adolescents and young adult females
IID-D01	Increase the proportion of females who get the Tdap vaccine during pregnancy

Reprinted from U.S. Department of Health and Human Services (USDHHS). (2020). *Browse 2030 objectives.* https://health.gov/healthypeople/objectives-and-data/browse-objectives

childhood series. However, the biggest barriers for immunizations are the health disparities that exist and vary by demographic group:

- Families with incomes less than 75,000 USD per year are approximately 30% less likely to have received the recommended seven-vaccine series.
- There are lower vaccination rates in African American infants due to higher rates of lack of access to preventive healthcare, lack of knowledge of vaccination risks and benefits, and lack of trust of the healthcare system (Kulkarni et al., 2021).
- Hispanics were underrepresented in COVID-19 vaccinations due to vaccine distrust, poor access to care, household income, belief that it was unnecessary, and immigration status (Granade et al., 2022).
- Adult vaccination rates for influenza are lower in Black individuals (39%), Hispanic individuals (37.5%), and individuals who identify as other or multiple race (41.4%) when compared with White adults (49.3%) (Granade et al., 2022).

The common factors shared by all ethnic groups facing health disparities are poor access to care, incomes below the poverty threshold, lack of reliable transportation and childcare, inability to get time off work to get immunized, and a reliable system in place to notify for missed vaccinations (Granade et al., 2022; Kulkarni et al., 2021; Oliveira et al., 2022).

Individuals now more often obtain their medial information from online sources than from medical professionals. These online sources include internet searches and social media platforms such as Facebook, YouTube, X (formerly Twitter), Reddit, and Instagram. This change has allowed for users of social media to produce and disseminate their content directly, leading to widespread digital misinformation on vaccines and emerging diseases. The antivaccination movement has used

BOX 8-5 What Parents/Guardians Should Know When Signing a Personal Beliefs Affidavit Exemption of Immunization

1. Please educate yourself about the symptoms and complications that can arise from a vaccine-preventable disease (VPD). Information for parents/guardians about these diseases may be found by calling your local health department or by visiting the National Immunization Program site, http://www.cdc.gov/nip.
2. Have a plan of care coordinated with your healthcare provider, to act upon the mildest to most severe symptoms of the disease.
3. It is the parent/guardian's responsibility to ensure an approved copy of the exemption is filed with the child's school nurse.
4. An unimmunized child will be excluded from school by the County Health Officer when a VPD is identified in the school.
5. When a child is excluded from school, it is the responsibility of the parent/guardian to keep the child* isolated from the public at large to prevent spread of infection to the community.
6. VPDs are considered **reportable communicable diseases** under the Health and Safety Codes of **your local health department**. If your child contracts one of these diseases, a public health nurse will contact you. Be prepared to provide information about the illness to the investigator. **This information is confidential**.
7. The parent/guardian is also at risk for contracting any of these diseases when exposed to an ill child. If unimmunized, the parent or guardian will remain in isolation from the community through the incubation period.
8. The child who is exposed to the disease may be offered preventive medication or immunization to prevent the disease from occurring, either of which may keep the child from being excluded from school.

*The isolation time frame is determined by the county health officer. Isolation means that the exposed or ill child cannot leave home except for medical care. No social gatherings!

social media to spread misinformation and has increased vaccine hesitancy (Puri et al., 2020). "Echo chambers often appear on social media platforms where individuals gather and are surrounded by like-minded people in terms of political and ideological orientation" (Baines et al., 2021, para 5). They share information on social platforms and create content and more followers through hashtags. Social media platforms use algorithms to suggest similar content to viewers/followers and in search engines that hinder legitimate discussion (Puri et al., 2020; Swire-Thompson & Lazer, 2020). Research indicates that a lack of trust, perceived threat, and misinformation are common themes in the discussion of immunizations on social media (Jennings et al., 2021).

Frequent questions parents/guardians ask about vaccines and recommended responses by nurses are as follows:

- *Are the vaccines safe?* C/PHNs provide information after assessing knowledge base about the safety trials that the vaccines undergo prior to release to the public and advise parents/guardians of possible side effects and how to care for the child if side effects do arise. C/PHNs

BOX 8-6 PERSPECTIVES

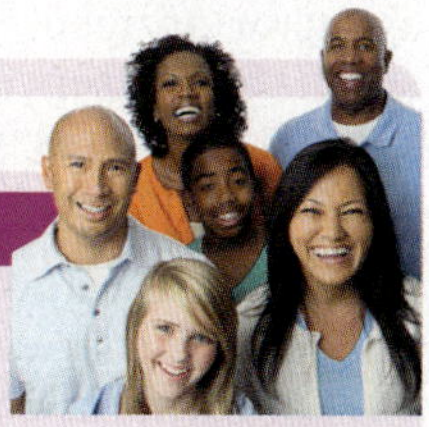

PHN: Personal Belief Exemption and Immunization

A whooping cough (pertussis) outbreak occurred in a small rural community. The outbreak of pertussis occurred in a small charter school, where most of the children were unvaccinated for reasons of parent/guardian personal belief objections. Unfortunately, with a large unvaccinated population and with many in the community against vaccinating children, 22 cases were reported among children and family members. The school closed early to stop the spread of the disease.

At a meeting with parents/guardians, members in the community, and C/PHNs and school nurses, it was discovered that not all parents/guardians signed the personal belief exemption out of true conviction; rather, some signed it to stop the school staff from pestering them for not having the time to vaccinate their high-risk children.

The county's immunization coordinator, the community's immunization coalition, and the school nurses determined that the school secretaries were the most common point of entrance to school registration. It was discovered that these individuals needed an in-service on how to properly offer the exemption to a family and what information parents/guardians would need to make an informed decision before signing the exemption.

The immunization coordinator developed an education tool that explained to parents/guardians their responsibility to the community at large if their child were to become ill with a vaccine-preventable illness. The Personal Beliefs Affidavit covered the points outlined in Box 8-5. The school secretaries were asked to give this document, as well as community resource information for families who may not have access to affordable immunizations, to parents/guardians who were interested in the exemption.

The parents/guardians at the charter school were very accepting of the information on what to do for an ill child, and the school secretaries expressed relief regarding dealing with parents who may want to request an exemption for convenience rather than conviction.

During the pertussis outbreak, as a C/PHN, what interventions would you direct to the parents/guardians who did not vaccinate their children due to true personal belief objections?

—*Ashley, PHN*

can also provide education on how to access reliable information sources (Opel et al., 2022).

- *I'm worried about giving so much at one time; how does that affect my child's immune system?* C/PHNs can assure parents/guardians that the small dose in the vaccine is not nearly as much as children are exposed to in everyday life. C/PHNs can explain that although incidences of diseases have declined, there are still VPDs, like pertussis and chickenpox that are common in the United States (CDC, 2023f).
- *Why are vaccines given at such a young age?* Nurses need to explain that vaccines are given as early as possible to provide the child with protection as early as possible and that declining an immunization at the time the child is eligible for it leaves the child vulnerable to the disease until the series is completed (CDC, 2023f).
- *Are preservatives or additives in the vaccine that will harm my baby?* The nurse could explain why the preservative is added to the vaccine (CDC, 2023f).

C/PHNs should be aware of any state law prohibiting the administration of a vaccine that contains thimerosal to a newborn (CDC, 2023f). Healthcare providers, C/PHNs, and school nurses are in positions to review records, educate families, and provide opportunities for a child and adult to obtain immunizations. Misinformation and health disparities present a real threat and should be a primary public health concern (Kulkarni et al., 2021; Opel et al., 2022).

Vaccine-Preventable Diseases

Hepatitis A and B, *Haemophilus influenzae* type b, measles, polio, diphtheria, pertussis, influenza, and chickenpox are examples of diseases that can be prevented through immunization, or VPDs. Immunization causes the body to become immune to an infectious agent by developing a defense against the invading infectious agent or antigen. The immunity allows the body to tolerate the presence of material that is foreign, such as a virus or bacterium (CDC, 2021c). Immunity may be either passive or active:

- **Passive immunity** is short-term resistance to a specific disease-causing organism; it may be acquired naturally (as with newborns through maternal antibody transfer) or artificially through inoculation with pooled human antibody (e.g., immunoglobulin) that gives temporary protection (CDC, 2021c).
- **Active immunity** is long-term (sometimes lifelong) resistance to a specific disease-causing organism; it also can be acquired naturally or artificially. Naturally acquired active immunity occurs when a person contracts a disease, whereas artificial immunity occurs when a person receives an inoculation of an antigen through a vaccine (CDC, 2021c).

Both prompt an immune response that stimulates the development of long-lasting antibodies that provide immunity against future exposure to that antigen (CDC, 2021c). See Chapter 7.

A vaccine is a preparation made from either a live organism or an inactivated form of the organism. Live attenuated vaccines are made from weakened wild virus organisms that can replicate but generally do not make the person ill. It only takes a small amount to initiate an immune response, and the organisms must replicate to be effective. Inactivated vaccines are made from a viral organism that has been inactivated by heat or chemicals. These vaccines cannot replicate in the recipient. Currently, measles, mumps, rubella, vaccinia, yellow fever, rotavirus, and intranasal influenza are all live attenuated vaccines (Iwasaki & Omer, 2020).

Schedule of Recommended Immunizations

A schedule for the administration of childhood vaccinations, based on recommendations by the ACIP, the American Academy of Pediatrics, the American Academy of Family Physicians, and the CDC, is published annually (see https://www.cdc.gov/vaccines/schedules/hcp/imz/child-adolescent.html). The CDC also provides "catch-up" schedules for children not receiving their first immunizations at birth, according to the standard schedule (CDC, 2023h). Current recommendations call for a child to receive 10 different vaccines or toxoids (many in combination form and all requiring more than one dose) in six or seven visits to a healthcare provider between birth and school entry, with boosters in the preteen to early teen years (Wodi et al., 2022).

Factors influencing the recommended age at which vaccines are administered include the following:

- Age-specific risks of the disease
- Age-specific risks of complications
- Ability of people of a given age to produce an adequate and lasting immune response
- Potential for interference with the immune response acquired from passively transferred maternal antibodies

Additional vaccines may be recommended based on public health outbreaks or pandemics as was the case during the COVID-19 pandemic. The ACIP provided guidance and booster recommendations for the entire population (CDC, 2021j; Wodi et al., 2022).

Herd Immunity

Herd immunity, or community immunity, is central to understanding immunization as a means of protecting community health. As described in Chapter 7, **herd immunity** is the immunity level present in a particular group or community of people. If only a few immune people exist within a community (i.e., if herd immunity is low), then the spread of disease is more likely (Fig. 8-14). However, if more individuals in the community are immunized (i.e., if herd immunity is high), this helps minimize the chance that an unvaccinated person will become ill (Desai & Majumder, 2020).

The level of required herd immunity (herd protection) varies. The percentage of people needed to reach herd immunity varies; 83% to 85% may need to be immune for rubella, but for pertussis (whooping cough), 92% to 94% may be needed to reach herd immunity (Merrill, 2021). An illustration of how herd immunity can cross all age groups is the Australian infant pneumococcal

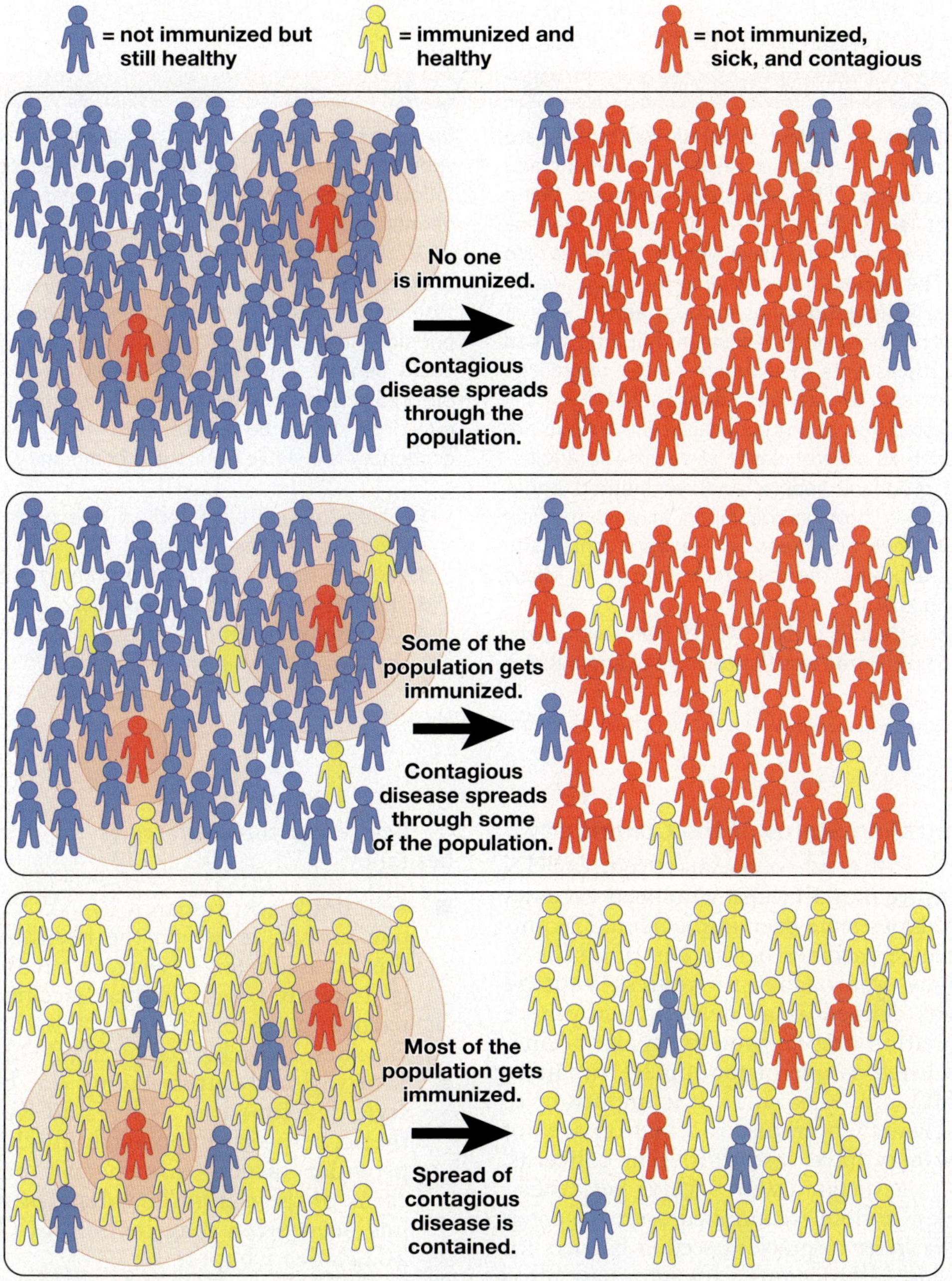

FIGURE 8-14 Herd immunity, or community immunity, is the result of a high immunization rate. (Reprinted from National Institutes of Health. (2019). https://www.nih.gov/about-nih/what-we-do/science-health-public-trust/perspectives/building-trust-vaccines)

vaccination program, which created a herd immunity resulting in a 50% decline in hospitalization and deaths across all age groups over 11 years (Chan et al., 2021). See Box 8-7. An informative animation explaining herd immunity and how it varies depending on infectious agent can be found at: https://www.youtube.com/watch?v=XJFoOCmJsdg

Herd immunity is not only important for limiting exposure of infection but also for reducing risks of cancer. A study looked at HPV-related cancers from 2001 to 2017 and found that cervical cancer rates have decreased 9.5% annually across all demographics since the vaccination approval. Before the approval of the HPV vaccine, cervical cancer rates had been decreasing at only 2.9% annually. The study showed a connection between increased vaccination rates of HPV with decreased HPV-related cancers among nonvaccinated females, thereby confirming the potential benefits of herd immunity in reducing HPV-related cancers (Liao et al., 2022).

Innovations are an important source of improved health-promoting practices and should not be discouraged, but, as always, solid research evidence is vital. With limited healthcare dollars, efforts must target the most cost-effective and proven methods available. Only time and research will show which strategy will be an effective tool in the public health arsenal.

BOX 8-7 EVIDENCE-BASED PRACTICE

New Preventive Strategies for an Old and New Disease

Despite high vaccination rates, pertussis outbreaks are occurring every 2 to 5 years in resource-abundant and resource-limited countries. The population primarily being affected are infants less than 6 months of age followed by children 10 to 14 years old who have yet to complete the vaccination series. The reasons may be due to the rising awareness of the disease, improved diagnostic tests, new strains of *Bordetella pertussis* not included in vaccine, asymptotic spread of *B. pertussis* in adolescents, and adults or the decreased protection time of vaccine (Decker and Edwards, 2021).

As a result, new strategies to protect against *B. pertussis* are under evaluation such as booster doses of vaccine to adolescents, adults, and pregnant people. Another method under evaluation is the practice known as cocooning, in which the goal is to immunize close family and friends or frequent contacts to reduce the risk of exposing the vulnerable person to these diseases (Decker and Edwards, 2021).

Cocooning is also effective with COVID-19 along with social distancing for not only children less than 5 years of age but also for adults greater than 65 years of age and other individuals at substantial risk for complications. Research shows that by following these two prevention measures, hospitalizations decrease as well as transmission of infections (Wang et al., 2020; Woodfield et al., 2021).

The C/PHN has an opportunity to evaluate the emerging research related to booster doses, immunization of pregnant people, and cocoon approach and determine if their community could benefit from any of these strategies in reducing VPD outbreaks and poor outcomes for the infant at risk. Several questions must be addressed when considering whether cocooning is a viable option in a community:

1. *Does the approach reduce infections in the population and where is the evidence?*
2. *What is the risk to the people being vaccinated?*
3. *What is the cost of this program?*
4. *Are there unintended consequences from this approach, such as delayed immunizations in the target population?*

Source: Di Mattia et al. (2018); Fernandes et al. (2019); CDC (2023d); Opel (2022).

Assessing Immunization Status of the Community

Immunization rates still need to be improved. C/PHN need to work to ensure that all those who need vaccines are receiving them. Laws have been implemented requiring students to receive vaccines before entering school. This section reviews approaches to address **vaccine hesitancy**, which is defined as a "delay in acceptance or refusal of vaccination despite availability of vaccination services" and listed as one of the top 10 threats to global health (WHO, n.d.-e, para. 1). It is important to recognize that all clients who refuse vaccination are not all the same. They may have vastly different concerns. Refer to Figure 8-15 associated with vaccine hesitancy.

Vaccine hesitancy is closely connected with the internet and social media (refer to previous section barriers for immunization and false information). False information has two sources: (1) occurs from misinformation and drawing conclusions based on wrong or incomplete facts or (2) disinformation where there is a deliberate intent to spread false information. As a C/PHN, you address misinformation with research supported research-based material while disinformation cannot. It can be challenging to change people's opinions, if vaccine hesitancy has become "enmeshed with people's worldview and cognitive biases" (Tuckerman et al., 2022). The best way to promote behavior change takes a coordinated effort between policymakers at all levels, leaders in the community (religious, healthcare professionals, and local business), and ensuring the source of the message and interventions are in agreement (Nuwarda et al., 2022). In addition, it is crucial to explore what barriers may be contributing to vaccination hesitancy and whether the hesitancy applies to all vaccines or only a particular vaccine. It is important to understand what barriers are present, such as difficulty accessing or affording care, and to understand if the hesitancy is group-specific (Tuckerman et al., 2022).

Below are three strategies for dealing with vaccine hesitancy:

- Tell, don't ask: research has shown that a presumptive format, in which the healthcare provider leads the discussion (e.g., "well, we have to do some shots"), is associated with higher vaccination rates than a participatory format (e.g., "How do you feel about vaccines?"; Tuckerman et al., 2022).
- Motivational interviewing (a brief intervention style developed by Miller and Rollnick): an empathetic, respectful approach in which the healthcare provider targets information based on the concerns of the parent/guardian only after permission has been given may be helpful (Tuckerman et al., 2022). See Chapter 10.
- "CASE" (Corroborate, About, Science, Explain) used by a health professional is one of the more promising methods (Nuwarda et al., 2022):
  - *Corroborate* the concerns and have a respectful conversation with the caregiver.
  - Tell the caregiver *about* yourself and your level of expertise.
  - Refer to the evidence from *science*.
  - *Explain* and advise, following the ACIP guidelines (CDC, 2023ee).

C/PHNs are viewed as one of the most trusted individuals in U.S. society and are considered as experts in immunizations and therefore are an important part ofachieving high vaccination rates in a community. The C/PHN must be up to date and knowledgeable on vaccinations and reasons behind vaccine hesitancy and be ready to speak and offer vaccine recommendations and share their decision to also be vaccinated (Nuwarda et al., 2022).

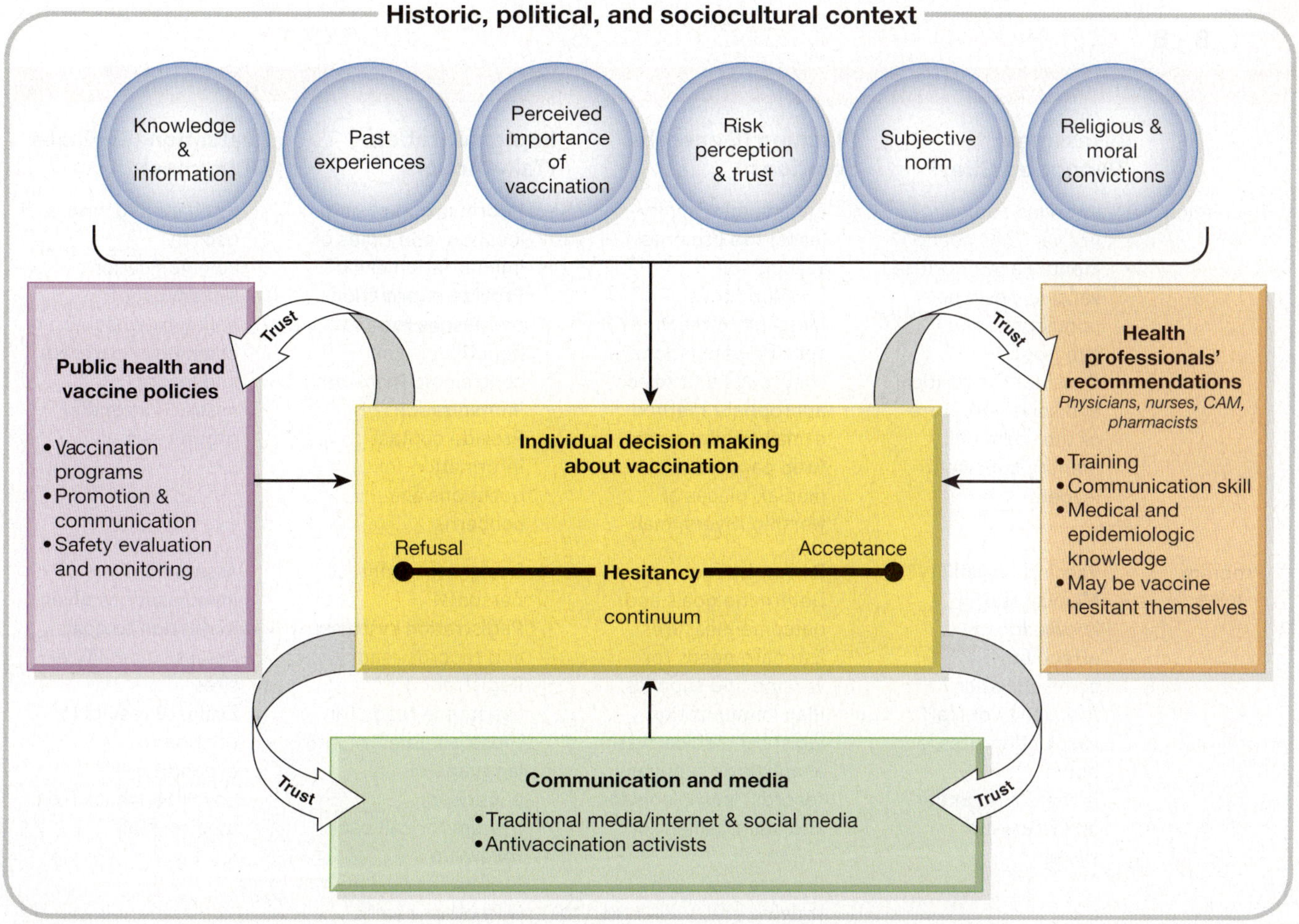

FIGURE 8-15 Conceptual model of vaccine hesitancy. (Adapted with permission from Dubé, E., Laberge, C., Guay, M., Bramadat, P., Roy, R., & Bettinger, J. (2013). Vaccine hesitancy: An overview. *Human Vaccines & Immunotherapeutic, 9*(8), 1763–1773.)

Planning and Implementing an Immunization Campaign

Immunization campaigns focusing on groups that have experienced economic and social inequities can increase effectiveness by including the following (CDC, 2023k):

- Use a health equity lens to formulate a plan.
- Messages should reflect the diversity of the community, and use strategies and language that works for the intended audience.
- Invite stakeholders and intended audience members to be part of the planning, and encourage shared responsibility for the success of the campaign.
- Leverage community influencers (clergy, local businesses) to be part of the campaign.
- Include plans for the following:
  - Transportation
  - Language interpreters
  - Childcare

Successful outreach efforts are motivated by the desire to reach the intended population, even if specific or unusual accommodations must be made. An online presence, with information about the benefits of vaccines and clinic locations, is helpful. Clinics can be scheduled and held at times and places specifically intended to make the service more accessible and convenient to the target group. Materials in multilingual form can be obtained through the state's immunization agency or the CDC. The CDC also has resources that include material and training on Health Equity Guiding Principles for Inclusive Communication and a Health Communication Playbook, and state immunization agencies have campaigns throughout the year for the C/PHN to participate in and provide to the public. Toolkits with materials and tips for planning and implementation are available through state immunization agencies. Box 8-8 outlines the process for administering an immunization campaign in a community setting. A 5-minute video on the importance of vaccines for older adults may be helpful for all age groups: https://www.youtube.com/watch?v=hodb65EkorM

Adult Immunization

Many people assume that vaccinations are for children only. However, ensuring all members in a community are fully vaccinated maximizes the protection of the community against VPD (Anderson et al., 2018). Adults are at risk for VPD if they are unimmunized or have immunizations that waned over time (e.g., tetanus, pertussis, influenza, and pneumococcal). Other vaccines are specific for adults, such as the varicella zoster, otherwise known as the shingles vaccine. The CDC provides an adult immunization schedule of recommendations. See Chapter 21 for adult vaccination schedule and adult screenings (CDC, 2020b).

BOX 8-8 C/PHN USE OF THE NURSING PROCESS/CLINICAL JUDGMENT

Administering an Immunization Campaign in a Community Setting

	Assessment (Recognize Cues)	Planning (Generate Solutions)	Implementation (Take Action)	Evaluation (Evaluate Outcomes)
Population level	• Intended audience? • Are vaccines needed? • Identify and prioritize vaccine-hesitant populations and subgroups? • Consider the political and social structure of the community • Identify important leaders	• Engage community leaders to promote vaccination • Develop focus of message to reach specific populations or subgroups and select appropriate method: e-mail, digital media (web pages, social media), places of worship, flyers, mail	• Inform group of date, location, and times of immunization clinic • Provide information on reasons for and benefits of (and contraindications to) immunization • Provide contact information for questions and concerns	• Evaluate and assess gaps in communication system used. • Solicit feedback from community partners and leaders. • Assess if intended group reached
Program level	• Vaccine availability? • Medical staff knowledge of effective communication? • Availability of staff, vaccination sites, and hours • Is there a reminder and follow-up system?	• Review budget • Determine goals and outcome measures • Estimate needs for vaccine and supplies • Plan immunization logistics: medical waste, anaphylaxis supplies, records, traffic control, and management of crowds. • Prepare staff with training and reinforcement of "herd immunity" message • Create or review reminder and follow-up system. • Plan on how to mitigate pain during immunization	• Designate a contact person(s) • Registration systems and records ready • Registration assistance ready for those not familiar with language of paperwork • System for call back, follow-up • System for dealing with other health issues and adverse events	• Assess numbers of immunizations given in relation to goals • Assess suitability of sites • Evaluate results in relation to expenditures • Solicit feedback from medical staff
Individual level	• Complete assessment (physical, health history, environmental) • Surveillance of communicable diseases • Is the vaccine wanted? • What are the reasons behind vaccine hesitancy (barriers and enablers)?	• Educate and have evidence-informed responses • Have a consistent message: • emphasize safety • Herd immunity • Remain free of signs and symptoms of disease • Complete vaccine (series)	• Education: informed consent, reporting of adverse reaction, and date next vaccine due. • Mitigate pain as much as possible • Reinforce message • Monitor for side effects • Provide opportunity for feedback	• Evaluate feedback • Evaluate the effectiveness of vaccine by confirming that the patient goals and expected outcomes have been met (see "Planning")

Source: MacDonald (2015); Martin (2018).

Substantial numbers of VPDs still occur among adults despite the availability of safe and effective vaccines. C/PHNs should be aware of factors that may contribute to low vaccination levels among adults (Cason & Williams, 2021):

1. Cost and reimbursement
2. Lack of a regular place to seek medical care
3. No reminder–recall system in place
4. Provider's lack of current knowledge of recommended immunizations or forgetting to ask about

vaccinations at the time of the visit, leading to missed opportunities to vaccinate
5. Need for training of healthcare staff on recommended immunizations for adults
6. Patient's lack of awareness of adult vaccination standards

International Travelers, Immigrants, and Refugees

As Americans interact more with people in other parts of the world, the incidence of Americans with tropical or imported diseases also rises. Within about 36 hours of boarding an airplane, one can reach almost any destination in the world. An average flight can equal the incubation period of some infectious diseases, and before the onset of symptoms is realized, microbial agents could be spread around the globe.

Travelers can take steps to protect themselves before embarking on their journey to new and exotic places by:

- Visiting the CDC Traveler Advice website to access recommendations for staying healthy during and on return from a trip (CDC, 2023z)
- Making an appointment for a consultation with a tropical medicine or travel clinic to prepare for international travel
- Being immunized with the recommended vaccines for the particular area of the world
- Having the necessary chemical prophylaxis on hand (e.g., antimalarial medications as prescribed)
- Learning about food and water hygiene precautions and basic first aid for simple injuries (CDC, 2023z)

Traveling internationally has grown over the past decade, with 1.2 billion worldwide tourist arrivals in 2015. Promoting a traveler's health is important to safeguard not only the individual's health but also the health of the individual's community (CDC, 2023z).

Refugees and international travelers who arrive in the United States may be unfamiliar with U.S. health systems, health precautions, and practices. Refugees and immigrants must follow prescribed guidelines, including extensive health screening mandated by U.S. immigration laws, immunizations, and treatment, as appropriate (CDC, 2023z). More than ever before, C/PHNs have professional contact with new Americans, whether close to their time of arrival or later, in schools, immunization clinics, or other locations. Visitors from other countries may also require assistance. For this reason, C/PHNs are encouraged to develop and maintain a global perspective on communicable diseases. See Chapter 16 for more information on global health.

SECONDARY PREVENTION

Two approaches to secondary prevention of communicable disease are possible: (1) screening and (2) disease case and contact investigation and notification (previously discussed).

Screening

Screening is a secondary prevention method because asymptomatic cases can be discovered and provided with prompt treatment (Kisling & Das, 2023).

The term screening is used in community/public health and disease prevention to describe programs that provide opportunities to detect disease in groups of apparently healthy individuals who are without symptoms. Common screening measures can include prenatal hepatitis B and syphilis screening, STI screens, and Mantoux TSTs for TB infection. C/PHNs working with clients in a screening setting must be prepared to clearly and correctly explain to individuals that screening tests are not definitive and that positive findings require subsequent investigation before diagnostic conclusions can be drawn.

Criteria for Screening Tests

Some important criteria are used in deciding whether to carry out a screening intervention in a community. They include validity and reliability and predictive value and yield.

Validity and Reliability

The screening test must be valid and dependable. *Validity* refers to the test's ability to accurately identify those with the disease. *Reliability* refers to the test's ability to give consistent results when administered on separate occasions by different technicians.

Predictive Value and Yield

The *predictive value* of a screening test is important for determining whether the screening intervention is justified. *Yield* refers to the number of positive results found per number tested. The predictive value and the yield of screening tests become important in planning screening programs for communicable disease detection and prevention because they can help planners locate screening efforts in areas or within population groups that are known to be at substantial risk for the disease. The predictive value of screening tests increases as the prevalence of the disease increases. For example, a screening test for TB among refugees would have a greater predictive value and yield than would TB screening in the population at large, owing to a higher endemicity of TB in many countries outside of the United States (CDC, 2022r).

See Chapter 7 for more on epidemiologic criteria for screening.

TERTIARY PREVENTION

The approaches to tertiary prevention of communicable disease include care and treatment of the infected person, isolation and quarantine of the infected person, and safe handling and control of infectious wastes.

Care and Treatment

Communicable diseases require care and treatment specific to the disease, and the nurse needs to:

- Understand the disease, the treatment, and follow-up requirements, and the educational component to discuss with the infected person
- Use information resources such as the CDC, state agency policies, and protocols provided by local public health agencies (Minnesota Department of Health, 2019).

Providing Services for Higher-Risk Populations

The lesbian, gay, bisexual, transgender, and queer (LGBTQ+) community has a disproportionate number of STIs, particularly among gay, bisexual, and other MSM, with HIV, syphilis, and gonorrhea rates higher than the general population. Transfeminine people are at 49 times greater risk of HIV infection than other adults (Mizock, et al., 2021). Although males are at a lower risk for cancer due to HPV, males who have anal sex are 17 times more at risk for anal cancer (CDC, 2023y).

C/PHNs can help alleviate the fear of bias that may be a barrier to accessing screening and treatment services by educating providers about LGBTQ+ care practices that include tailored education and client sexual health needs for those who are not cisgender as well as inclusion of mental health and substance use risk factors as part of the sexual history taking process (Mizock, et al., 2021).

Isolation and Quarantine

Communicable disease control includes two methods for keeping infected people and noninfected people apart to prevent the spread of a disease. **Isolation** refers to separation of the infected people (or animals) from others for the period of communicability to limit the transmission of the infectious agent to susceptible people. Quarantine refers to restrictions placed on healthy contacts of an infectious case for the duration of the incubation period to prevent disease transmission if infection should develop. The CDC has quarantine stations located at land-border crossings and ports of entry, where public health officials determine if international travelers who are ill may be admitted into the United States or held to prevent spreading infectious disease (CDC, 2020k).

Recent examples of U.S. isolation and quarantine took place during the COVID-19 pandemic in an effort to reduce the spread of the disease. On February 3, 2020, passengers on a flight from China were screened and monitored and subject to 14 days of mandatory quarantine. The following month, the CDC issued a "no sail order" for all cruise ships in all water that the United States holds jurisdiction over and a travel ban on non–U.S. citizens traveling from 26 European countries. Beginning in March 2020, some U.S. states began implementing shutdowns and social distancing mandates, which lasted until the end of August 2020 (CDC, 2023c). U.S. COVID-19 cases at the time of this writing (October 9, 2024) have reached 776,386,491, and deaths have totaled 7,067,260 (WHO, 2024b).

Safe Handling and Control of Infectious Wastes

The control of infection also relies on the proper disposal of contaminated wastes. The CDC and the Occupational Safety and Health Administration (OSHA) support and encourage *standard precautions* that stress that health-care workers think of all blood and body fluids and materials that they may encounter as potentially infectious (OSHA, n.d.). Although universal precaution observance is primarily considered while the nurse is giving hands-on treatment or care to a patient, keeping these principles in mind while making community health visits in the primary and secondary setting is paramount to the safety of both the client and the nurse (Carrico et al., 2018).

Infectious waste is waste capable of producing an infectious disease provided it contains pathogens with sufficient virulence and quantity so that exposure to the waste by a susceptible host could result in an infectious disease (OSHA, 2011). Requirements for medical waste disposal are for waste to be divided into the following categories:

- Used and unused sharps
- Cultures, specimens, and stocks of infectious agents
- Human blood and blood products
- Human pathologic, isolation, and animal waste

Four key elements of an infectious waste management program apply to community practice:

1. Health professionals must be able to distinguish waste that poses a significant infection hazard from waste that does not.
2. The waste management program must have administrative support and authority to institute practice guidelines and provide the containers and other resources needed for safe disposal of infectious waste.
3. Handling of the infectious waste must be minimized. Containers should be rigid, leak-resistant (sealed), impervious to moisture, rupture-resistant, and, for sharps, puncture-resistant.
4. An enforcement or evaluation mechanism must be in place to ensure that the goal of reducing the potential for exposure to infectious waste in the community is met.

LEGAL AND ETHICAL ISSUES IN COMMUNICABLE DISEASE CONTROL

The threats presented by communicable diseases can bring public safety and ethical considerations to a crossroad. Public health interventions to protect the public often overlap individual rights (Toebes, 2020). The communitarianism concept of what is good for the whole is good for the parts might be applied to public health practice. Considerations for ethical public health practice should include overall benefit to society, collective action, communitarianism, fairness in distribution of burden, harm principle, paternalism, liberty-limiting continua, social justice/fairness, and global justice. In addition, ethical issues of autonomy, beneficence, avoidance of maleficence, and justice also need to be taken into consideration (Meier et al., 2020).

C/PHNs must balance these ethical principles while working with the community to control the spread of infectious diseases. An example of this conflict might occur while conducting contact investigations for STIs among minors. The nurse must be mindful to conduct the investigation while maintaining confidentiality of the index case and be cognizant of the variations and complexities that exist across the United States (Nelson et al., 2023). Another example is mandating immunizations resulting in the exclusion of unvaccinated children from a school setting. Public health practitioners walk a fine line to protect the rights of the person while also protecting the health and safety of the community. Refer to Chapter 4 (ethical principles) for more details.

Enforced Compliance

Legally, the responsibilities of public health officials in communicable disease control include using police power to enforce compliance with treatment or restrict the activity of infectious people to protect the welfare of others (CDPH, 2020). Regulations that enforce compliance with disease prevention strategies are a justifiable restriction if the measures proposed are demonstrably effective and grounded in ethical principles (CDPH, 2020). However, during the recent Ebola epidemic, healthcare workers who treated Ebola victims in West Africa found themselves under 21-day quarantine once they returned to the United States even though they did not have symptoms, and some states took additional precautions not required by the CDC. As healthcare providers, it is important to be guided by scientific proof and not fear (Emrick et al., 2016; Jones, 2020). Due process is crucial to protect individuals from government intrusion, particularly ensuring that fundamental fairness has been implemented in situations requiring imprisonment (CDPH, 2020).

Confidentiality, Privacy, and Discrimination

While carrying out communicable disease interventions, nurses and other healthcare professionals must ensure clients' confidentiality and privacy. The HIPAA Privacy Rule, last revised in 2003, seeks to protect patients' confidentiality and privacy by establishing laws that govern how healthcare providers, insurance companies, and other "covered entities" may use and disclose patients' personal health information. Healthcare providers may only disclose when necessary to provide care for the patient and then must provide only the minimum amount of information needed to provide that care (USDHHS, n.d.-a). One exception is when disclosure of an individual's information is required to protect another person or people who are at risk for contracting an illness, but even then, the individual's identity is protected.

Society has a long-standing aversion to infectious diseases. Ostracism, which in the past targeted people with leprosy and other contagious conditions, has shifted to discrimination against people with TB or AIDS (Jones, 2020). An example of this occurred in 2007 when an Atlanta attorney caused an international health scare and found his medical and personal information in the media because of flying to Europe after a recent diagnosis of drug-resistant TB (Night, 2007). People are protected from discrimination under the Americans with Disability Act but not when they pose a public health threat, such as with the contagious state of TB (EEOC, n.d.).

CASE STUDY 10 ESSENTIAL PUBLIC HEALTH SERVICES

Tuberculosis Exposure

As a C/PHN, you are alerted to a person who has an active TB case. They present in the health department for an x-ray after they fail their tuberculin skin test. The person has recently arrived by plane from another state. They stayed for a few weeks with family members in a small house but now live with friends in a small apartment. When talking to the patient, you note that they cough often and do not cover their mouth.

1. ***Recognize Cues:*** *Which findings require immediate follow-up, are unexpected, or are most concerning?*
2. ***Analyze Cues:*** *What information is noted or needed for interpreting findings?*
3. ***Prioritize Hypotheses:*** *Based on the information that you have, what is happening?*
4. ***Generate Solutions:*** *What intervention(s) will achieve the desired outcome?*
5. ***Take Action:*** *What actions should you take or do first?*
6. ***Evaluate Outcomes:*** *Were outcomes achieved? Why or why not?*
7. *Which Essential Public Health Services influence this situation? (See Box 2-2.)*

SUMMARY

- Communicable diseases pose a major threat to the public's health and are transmitted globally as the result of mobile populations, increased urbanization, and international travel. They can be transmitted through direct contact from one person to another or indirectly through contaminated objects (air, water, food) or a vector (animal or insect).
- C/PHNs are concerned with communicable disease control and prevention and recognize environmental factors that promote communicable diseases, who is at risk, and what are the characteristics and vulnerability of community members and groups.
- Influenza and COVID-19 are evolving viruses that are responsible for widespread outbreaks and pandemics as most of the world population do not have the antibodies to protect them from novel (new) strains.
- TB is becoming more complicated to treat and manage due to the introduction of MDR strains, the increasing number of people diagnosed with TB and HIV/AIDS, the influx of refugees and increased travel, poverty, and inadequate access to healthcare.
- STIs threaten the health and lives of millions of people. Control of STIs can be accomplished through

effective screening, treatment, contact investigation, health campaigns, and the use of best practice strategies to facilitate behavioral change.

- The COVID-19 pandemic affected the prevention, screening, and treatment of communicable diseases.
- Primary prevention of communicable diseases includes methods such as using mass media education campaigns, one-on-one education, immunization promotion, and using the latest scientific information to inform best practices to reduce risk and help prevent diseases.
- Vaccine hesitancy is one of the 10 leading causes of death worldwide. C/PHNs need to understand the underlying causes of vaccine hesitancy and be able to provide education and strategies to assist the person.
- The COVID-19 pandemic highlighted the long-standing health disparities that exist in communities of color, and they need to be addressed to avoid similar outcomes in the future.
- Herd immunity, or community immunity, is central to understanding immunization as a means of protecting community health.
- Secondary prevention activities of screening and disease investigation are steps taken when primary prevention activities have failed.
- Tertiary prevention is needed to ensure additional people are not infected and those who are ill receive care and treatment. Ongoing disease transmission can be interrupted through treatment, isolation, or quarantine.
- Ethical issues in communicable disease control include enforced compliance, the justifiability of screening, preservation of confidentiality and privacy, and the avoidance of discrimination against infected people.

ACTIVE LEARNING EXERCISES

1. Visit your state and local public health website and evaluate a health prevention campaign (based on a major communicable disease in the United States) to see how health literacy, health disparity, and inclusive marketing is addressed. What would you do differently and would that improve the outcome desired in the campaign? Are your changes based on the latest scientifically based research? (Objectives 1 and 3)
2. How could social media be used by a C/PHN in the prevention of communicable diseases? Provide two examples—take into account the spread of disease and legal and ethical issues affecting disease and infection control. What are the advantages and disadvantages of using social media for disease prevention? (Objectives 2 and 8)
3. In the United States, TB cases are highest among foreign-born individuals. Review your local health department website and identify the measures and services provided for the at-risk population. Create a diagram of the service(s), and describe how it addresses complacency, confidence, and convenience. What would you do differently, and why would that change be significant to the screening and treatment of latent TB? (Objective 4)
4. Identify a WHO or CDC vaccination campaign/program and characterize the focused population. How can the nursing process be used to plan, execute, and evaluate the success of the campaign/program? Which of the 10 Essential Public Health Services is being used (Box 2-2)? (Objectives 4 and 7)
5. The antivaccine movement uses social media, websites, and blogs to spread antivaccine information. Find a website, social online group, or blog, and summarize who they are targeting and why. Create a response to one argument against antivaccination using evidence-based research that could be understood by a nonmedical person. (Objectives 5 and 6)

CHAPTER 9

Environmental Health and Safety

"When we try to pick out anything by itself, we find it hitched to everything else in the Universe."

—John Muir (1838–1914), Naturalist

KEY TERMS

Bioaccumulation
Biomonitoring
Brownfields
Built environment
Climate change
Cumulative risk assessment
Ecosystems
Endocrine-disrupting chemicals
Environmental epidemiology
Environmental justice
Epigenetics
Health risk assessment
Integrated pest management (IPM)
One Health
Planetary health
Precautionary principle
Structural determinants of health
Superfund
Sustainability
Sustainable Development Goals (SDGs)
Toxicology

LEARNING OBJECTIVES

Upon mastery of this chapter, you should be able to:

1. **Apply the ecologic perspective to human and environmental relationships.**
2. **Discuss concepts of prevention and upstream approaches to health impact and environmental health.**
3. **Discuss the community/public health nurse's role in reducing and managing environmental risk.**
4. **Discuss guiding documents for public health nursing that pertain to environmental health.**
5. **Discuss the influence of social and structural determinants of health on environmental health of a community.**
6. **Describe how nurses can collaborate with other professionals, government agencies, and communities to reduce environmental threats to health.**

INTRODUCTION

The air we breathe, the water we drink and bathe in, the food we eat, the buildings we occupy, the energy we rely on, and the products we use influence our health and the health of our communities. These potential areas of exposure fall under the public health domain of environmental health. This is an important area for all nurses to understand and address to promote safe and healthy populations. Additionally, with climate change, it is imperative that all nurses understand the relationship between the environment and our health.

The American Public Health Association (2023, para. 1) defines environmental health as "the branch of public health that: focuses on the relationships between people and their environment; promotes human health and well-being; and fosters healthy and safe communities" and "is a key part of any comprehensive public health system. The field works to advance policies and programs to reduce chemical and other environmental exposures in air, water, soil, and food to protect people and provide communities with healthier environments." The American Nurses Association (2021) has recognized the key role that nurses play in environmental health in the *Scope and Standards of Practice* with an environmental health standard that integrates addressing environmental issues while integrating nursing roles of advocacy and addressing the social determinants of health in the workplace and globally.

Historically, the nursing profession has recognized the significant relationship of our natural and built environments in influencing health. The natural environment includes all living and nonliving things that occur naturally, such as forests, grasslands, rivers, oceans, insects, animals, and rocks, while the **built environment** encompasses human-made structures such as housing, hospitals, clinics, office buildings, and roadways.

The ability to live in healthy natural and built environments increases not only the number of years of a healthy life but also one's quality of life. Thus, nurses, as the largest group of healthcare professionals globally, can play a key role in supporting environments that sustain health.

Florence Nightingale, the founder of professional nursing practice in the West, is credited for highlighting the importance of clean air and water, light, and noise to promote healing. Initially, Nightingale subscribed to the Miasma Hypothesis, which blames bad odors as the cause of disease. However, with an advanced understanding of science, Germ Theory, the paradigm of infectious disease transmission changed, and Nightingale's understanding changed with the evidence that supported factors beyond "bad odors" that influence health. With this knowledge, Nightingale gathered evidence regarding the patient care environment to change nursing practice (Gilber, 2020). Additionally, Nightingale addressed the social determinants that influenced health. This change in thinking and an understanding of nursing history is necessary to understand and embrace an environmental health lens in nursing practice. Nurses must be willing to address the scientific evidence related to environmental exposures and consider the social and regulatory factors to address and advocate for the needs of communities to restore and promote health.

ENVIRONMENTAL HEALTH IN GLOBAL AND NATIONAL CONTEXT

In 2015, the United Nations (UN) implemented a new set of global goals called the **Sustainable Development Goals (SDGs)**. The SDGs identify the need to care for the natural and built environments that support the health of our planet and its inhabitants (UN, 2020). See Chapter 16 on global health for more on SDGs. These goals and their targets address many environmental factors that influence human health. Furthermore, UN agencies have environmental programs that are valuable resources. Examples are UNICEF, WHO, and the UN Environment Program.

Increasingly, several factors have been recognized as detrimental to environmental health, including:

- Exposures to hazardous materials in air, water, food, and soil
- The rise in development and deforestation
- The use of synthetic chemicals not well tested for safety
- The adverse effects of natural and human-caused disasters
- The built environment
- Social determinants of health
- Structural determinants of health
- Consumerism
- Climate change

In the United States, *Healthy People 2030* is the framework for the nation's health. It addresses the social, economic, and physical factors, as well as behaviors, that can influence exposure to physical, chemical, and biologic environmental risks (Office of Disease Prevention and Health Promotion, 2019). Our national framework for health is, therefore, in line with global goals.

BOX 9-1 *HEALTHY PEOPLE 2030*

Objectives for Environmental Health

Core and Developmental Objectives

EH-01	Reduce the number of days people are exposed to unhealthy air
EH-02	Increase trips to work made by mass transit
EH-03	Increase the proportion of people whose water supply meets Sage Drinking Water Act regulations
EH-04	Reduce blood lead level in children aged 1–5 years
EH-05	Reduce health and environmental risks from hazardous sites
EH-06	Reduce the amount of toxic pollutants released into the environment
EH-07, 08, 10, 11	Reduce exposure to arsenic, lead, bisphenol A, and perchlorate in the population, as measured by blood or urine concentrations of the substance or its metabolites
EH-09	Reduce exposure to mercury in children
D02-13, 14, 15	Reduce diseases and deaths related to heat

Reprinted from U.S. Department of Health and Human Services (USDHHS). (2020). *Browse 2030 objectives.* https://health.gov/healthypeople/objectives-and-data/browse-objectives

In addition to guidelines for environmental health in nursing, there are federal guidelines from the Surgeon General Report on Healthy People and the core functions of public health (Centers for Disease Control and Prevention [CDC], 2023a) to support environmental health in nursing practice.

First released in 1990 as *Healthy People 2000*, *Healthy People* is the U.S. federal document produced every decade to set health goals to promote the health of the nation (Box 9-1). This document provides guidance for nurses to identify targets for health and is used for many public health nursing interventions. *Healthy People 2030* includes goals that support environmental health and policies to promote a healthier population. The environmental health section contains objectives that address major environmental health risks related to the natural and built environments in the United States. These objectives can be found in Chapter 1, Box 1-4.

ENVIRONMENTAL HEALTH AND NURSING

Historically, public health and occupational health nurses (OHNs) have been leaders in addressing the impact of the physical and natural environments through their work in homes, in communities, in industry, and with governmental organizations. As evidence of the environmental impact on our health continues to grow, nurses in all practice settings must be knowledgeable of environmental risks, the relationship of exposures to disease and illness, prevention measures, and growing scientific evidence to best protect and promote the health of the populations in the nurse's care. Professionally, nurses must be aware of the guiding documents that call for nurses to incorporate environmental health into all areas of practice:

- *Public Health Nursing: Scope and Standards of Practice*, 3rd ed. Standard 17: Environmental Health, Planetary Health, and Environmental Justice. American Nurses Association, 2022
- The ANA: *Nursing: Scope and Standards of Practice*, Standard 18 Environmental Health American Nurses Association, 2021 (Box 9-2)

Brief History of the Occupational and Environmental Health in Nursing

The specific role of nurses in occupational and environmental health first occurred in the workplace. Initially called industrial nurses, OHNs assess workers' health status and strive to ensure worker safety and prevent adverse health effects from workplace hazards. The American Association of Occupational Health Nurses (2020) cites the need for specific education and training in toxicology, epidemiology, workplace hazards, regulations, and prevention strategies. OHNs can be certified through the American Board of Occupational Health Nurses. Public health has included environmental health as a central aspect of health promotion and disease prevention. More recently, the nursing profession has responded to the call for nurses to establish environmental health competencies for nursing practice.

The work of public health nurses (PHNs) and leaders in occupational health nursing brought us to the advances in environmental health nursing we experience today. Significant historical milestones in environmental health nursing are as follows:

- 1995: The Institute of Medicine report *Nursing, Health, and the Environment* (Pope et al., 1995) identified the need for nursing environmental health knowledge, research, and interventions.
- 1995–2008: Many nursing programs incorporated environmental health into the curriculum. Nurses incorporated environmental health into their practice settings to reduce hazardous exposures for both health professionals and patients. Environmental health nursing advanced, and nurses became involved in a number of policy and advocacy efforts (Leffers et al., 2014).
- 2005: *Environmental Health Principles for Public Health Nursing* was published (APHA, 2005).
- 2007: *ANA Principles of Environmental Health for Nursing Practice* was published (ANA, 2007).
- 2008: The Alliance of Nurses for Healthy Environments (ANHE) was formed—the first professional nursing organization solely focused on environmental health (ANHE, 2019).
- 2008: International Council of Nurses adopted the position statement: nurses, climate change, and health. The statement was revised in 2018 to make the call for action stronger.
- 2010: ANA, Standard 16: Environmental Health was included in the second edition of *Nursing: Scope and Standards of Practice* (ANA, 2010) and revised for the 2015 and 2021 editions (ANA, 2021). Since the publication of the 2010 Standard 16: Environmental Health, all nurses must incorporate environmental health principles into nursing practice.
- 2022: National League of Nursing. Vision Statement: Climate Change and Health.
- 2023: ANA *The Nurse's Role in Addressing Global Climate Change and Human Health.*
- (Office of Disease Prevention and Health Promotion, 2020, para. 13.)

Importance of Environmental Health For Nursing

Nurses are essential to improve environmental health through nursing research, education, advocacy, and practice. We work with diverse populations in homes,

BOX 9-2 American Nurses Association, Public Health Nursing: Scope and Standards of Practice

Standard 18. Environmental Health: Below are selected competencies from Standard 18 that are related to the C/PHN. The competencies have been adapted for this text.

The registered nurse:

1. Forms a healthy and safe professional practice environment
2. Incorporates social determinants of health into environmental assessments
3. Includes environmental health concepts in all forms of nursing practice
4. Works to decrease environmental health risks for self, colleagues, patients, and wider community
5. Shares knowledge of environmental risk factors and strategies to reduce risk of exposure
6. Acts as an advocate for principles of environmental health within own community
7. Supports the utilization of technologies and products to ensure safe environments for nursing practice
8. Relies on a planetary health perspective of considering social, political, and economic factors when analyzing human and global health related to the environment
9. Promotes sustainable policies related to the natural environment globally

Adapted from American Nurses Association (ANA) (2021).

workplaces, and communities and are the largest group of healthcare providers in the United States, with 5.2 million registered nurses.

In addition, we are in one of the most trusted professions, are able to communicate complex information to our patients and communities, interact with many other healthcare organizations, and serve in policy-setting roles (Bender et al., 2021). Therefore, nurses are ideally situated to assess for and address environmental health risks.

CONCEPTS AND FRAMEWORKS FOR ENVIRONMENTAL HEALTH

Ecosystems

Ecosystems are dynamic, interdependent communities of plants, animals, microorganisms, and the nonliving environments in which they live. No organism, including humans, can live removed from its ecosystem or other species. Ecosystems help regulate water, gases, waste recycling, nutrient cycling, pollination, infectious disease, climate, and biology, as well as provide recreational and cultural opportunities for human use (Frumkin, 2016). Any change within an ecosystem, such as temperature or contamination of the water, can change the entire system (National Geographic, 2023).

The synergistic relationship between humans and the environment has been highlighted through the transdisciplinary framework of One Health. **One Health** relies on an ecologic approach to address the environmental interconnections of health between all living things (plants, animals, and insects) and their shared environment (CDC, 2023d). Through One Health, botanists, microbiologists, nurses, primary providers, and veterinarians have worked closely to understand and address the impact of an ecosystem on public health (see Chapter 16).

Community/public health nurses (C/PHNs) find that the interconnections found in the science of ecology have been applied to social–ecologic perspectives that identify not only the physical environment but also the social, political, economic, and cultural factors that exist for populations.

In public health, the ecologic model of population health (Fig. 9-1) is used to illustrate that determinants of health (biologic, behavioral, social, and environmental) interact to affect health (Friis, 2019). In addition, the framework of Planetary Health, which has been embraced by nursing, relies on an ecologic perspective to attain health, well-being, and equity through stewardship of the political, economic, and social systems as well as natural ecosystems (Haines, 2016; Leffers et al., 2017; Whitmee et al., 2015). Using the ecologic perspective of planetary health, nurses collaborate across disciplines to address social, political, economic, cultural, and natural environmental factors that influence human health within their practice setting (Kurth, 2017). The **Planetary Health** perspective calls on humans to examine their relationship with the natural environment, recognizing the significant impact of social, environmental, and economic systems on the health of all life on earth (LeClair & Potter, 2022).

APPROACH AND RATIONALE

A guide to thinking about the determinants of population health

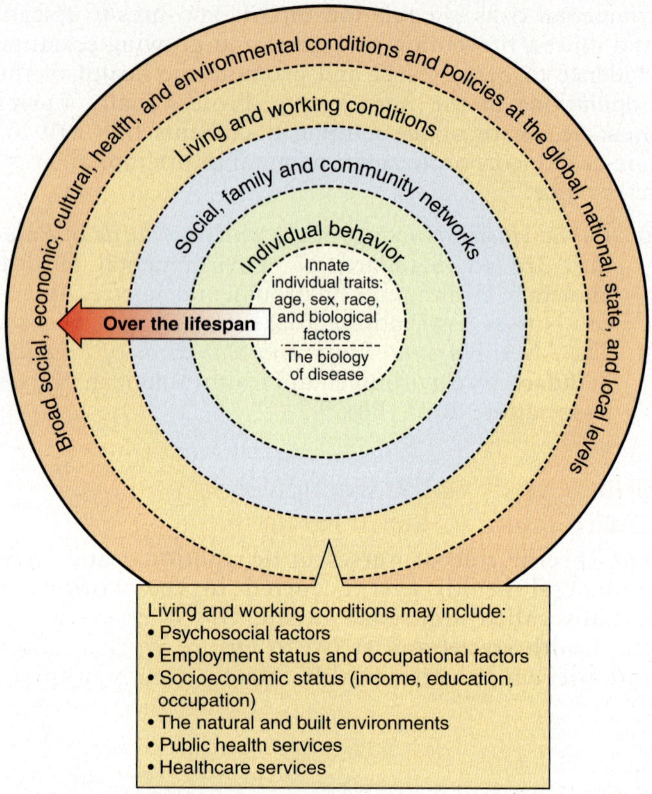

FIGURE 9-1 Ecological model for public health.

Sustainability

Sustainability relies on an ecologic approach and is based on the principle that human beings and the natural environment must coexist harmoniously for survival (U.S. Environmental Protection Agency [EPA], 2020b). When the concept of sustainability is applied to human systems, it is evident that the public must engage and respond to protect the environment and promote healthy characteristics in the population and in their communities.

Currently, many human/environment interactions are not sustainable. For example, our food production and energy use create pollution that threatens human life and ecosystems. Solutions to improve sustainability for humans and the environment include strategies that are socially desirable, economically feasible, and ecologically viable. These solutions will rely on the current science and existing and novel technologies (Wani et al., 2023).

One example of the importance of addressing sustainable practices is our use of single-use plastic (Chigwada & Tekere, 2023). Since the early 2000s, plastic waste has risen exponentially. According to the UN Environmental Programme (2023), about 400 tons of plastic waste is globally generated every year and most of this plastic is from single-use plastic that is produced from fossil fuels. This means that not only plastic waste is a problem but also plastic production adds to greenhouse gas (GHG) emissions that contribute to climate change. Furthermore, plastic enters the ecosystem as much of our plastic waste ends up in our oceans and breaks up into microplastics, which is taken up as food by aquatic life and birds (National Oceanic and Atmospheric Administration, 2023). Humans can consume microplastics in food or beverages. Although more research needs to be conducted, there is concern that microplastics can affect human immune and reproductive systems (Blackburn & Green, 2022).

Sustainability is an important concept in relationship to nursing practice and the healthcare setting. U.S. hospitals generate over 29 pounds of waste per patient bed each day, which generates millions of tons of waste annually and contributes to 8.5% of all GHGs, contributing to 25% of the global healthcare sector's GHG emissions (Dzau et al., 2021; Practice Green Health, 2023). Nurses working in patient care settings and administration are able to lead in addressing the environmental impact of delivering patient care.

Charlotte Brody, a nurse who identified the negative environmental impact of hospitals on the health of the communities they intend to serve, was a cofounder of Health Care Without Harm. This organization has become the leading international organization that promotes environmentally responsible healthcare (Health Care Without Harm, 2018). Sustainable practices within the health system have been supported by the ANA and EPA. For example, Beth Schenk, PhD, RN, FAAN, is the executive director of environmental stewardship for Providence St. Patrick Hospital in Montana. In this role, Dr. Schenk seeks to promote health system wide sustainability that includes decarbonization, waste management, and conservation programs.

Although this example highlights the work of a nurse leader for a large healthcare system, it also demonstrates the impact of health systems on public health. Nurses who work in community settings must comply with best practices for the conservation of resources, stewardship of supplies, and proper waste disposal. Pharmaceutical waste is another serious concern for nurses who work in home and school settings. This topic is more fully addressed in the section about water contaminants.

Upstream Focus

C/PHNs incorporate an "upstream" focus into their work with populations. This approach emerged from the seminal publication by John McKinley (1979), *A Case for Focusing Upstream*, which identified root causes of disease and the multiple factors that lead to illness. As the name implies, we are challenged to look upstream to determine the factors that led to pushing someone or a community into the river of illness. The C/PHN approach to prevention and health promotion relies on an upstream approach to address the root causes that influence health at the institutional, system, and the policy levels rather than looking solely at individual lifestyle issues (Butterfield, 2017).

For example, a C/PHN is taking an upstream approach to asthma prevention by working with legislators to strengthen ambient air quality polices. Thus, the nurse is moving up along the system to address a leading factor, outdoor air pollution that causes asthma (Fig. 9-2).

Dr. Butterfield's original work, the Butterfield Upstream Model for Population Health (BUMP), applies an upstream public health nursing approach to environmental risks by giving nurses the framework to address the determinants of health and health inequities that influence health outcomes across the life course of a population (Butterfield, 2017).

Specific points that are part of the BUMP framework follow:

- Assessing and analyzing the environmental exposures for the community or population
- Establishing health goals that include a multisector approach
- Determining where interventions will have the greatest impact
- Aligning with community partners to carry out the interventions
- Measuring effectiveness of interventions by process, outcome, and impact evaluations

With emphasis on data, it is estimated that as much as 25% to 33% of disease occurrences are globally attributable to environmental exposures, including environmentally linked health problems such as asthma, neurologic problems, certain cancers, poor birth outcomes, and early death (Smith et al., 1999). With the environmental impact of climate change, it is expected that this number will rise. A case can be made for nurses to use an upstream framework to assess, monitor, educate, advocate, and create policies to reduce environmental health risks. See Chapter 1, Figure 1-2.

Butterfield (2017) acknowledges that an upstream approach challenges nurses to consider the important root causes of illness in terms of the following:

- Etiologic pathways
- Social determinates of health
- Existing norms of our health system that focus on addressing disease instead of prevention

Health Disparities

Health disparities are a serious concern for overall health in the United States and globally. As noted in the discussion of upstream approaches to health, environmental factors are basic determinants of health and well-being. However, great inequities occur between the environments of people with higher incomes and those of resource-limited communities, people of color, and tribal and Indigenous populations. The CDC (2023b) defines health disparities as "preventable differences in the burden of disease, injury, violence, or opportunities to achieve optimal health that are experienced by socially disadvantaged populations" (CDC, line 1). Health disparities are the result of issues related to the structural and social determinants of health, which are discussed in more detail in the next section. Disparities that are directly correlated with environmental exposures include rates of asthma

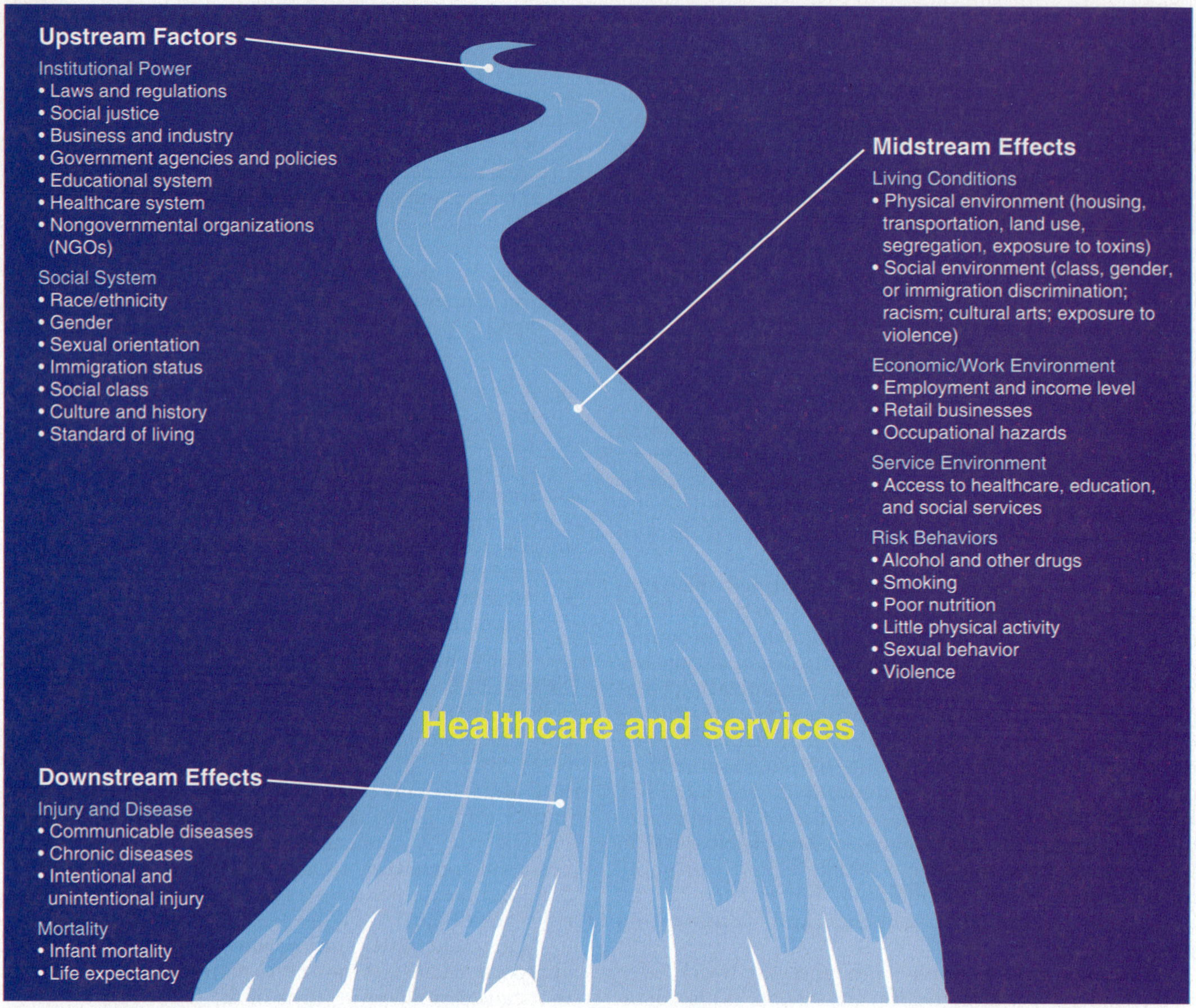

FIGURE 9-2 The influence of upstream factors on midstream and downstream effects. (Adapted from City of Richmond CA. (2013). *Health in all policies (HIAP) report*. http://www.ci.richmond.ca.us/2575/Health-in-All-Policies-HiAP; RAND Health. (2015). *Understanding the upstream social determinants of health*. https://www.rand.org/content/dam/rand/pubs/working_papers/WR1000/WR1096/RAND_WR1096.pdf)

among children, elevated blood lead levels (EBLLs), cancers that are linked to environmental exposures, and lung diseases among adults. Social and economic factors have created disproportionate exposures to pesticides, toxic chemicals in the workplace, poor indoor air quality in schools and homes, and ambient air pollution in communities.

Structural and Social Determinants of Health

Public health professionals have moved further upstream to better understand the social determinants of health and have identified **structural determinants of health**. These are the cultural norms, economic and social policies, institutions, and practices that influence the dissemination of social determinants of health across communities (Crear-Perry et al., 2021). Understanding the structural factors that influence the social determinants of health can support C/PHN community nursing practice. For example, understanding the distribution of resources for public education within communities provides the C/PHN context for addressing educational inequities that influence the health of a population. Social determinants of health are defined as "the conditions in the environments where people are born, live, learn, work, play, worship, and age that affect a wide range of health functioning, and quality-of-life outcomes and risks" (Healthy People, 2030, para. 1). These circumstances are shaped by the structural determinants of health (WHO, 2023, para. 1). More on the social and structural determinants of health can be found in Chapter 23 and Figure 9-3.

Environmental Justice

Closely related to structural and social determinants of health and health disparities is the issue of environmental justice. **Environmental justice** is a "principle that all people and communities have a right to equal protection

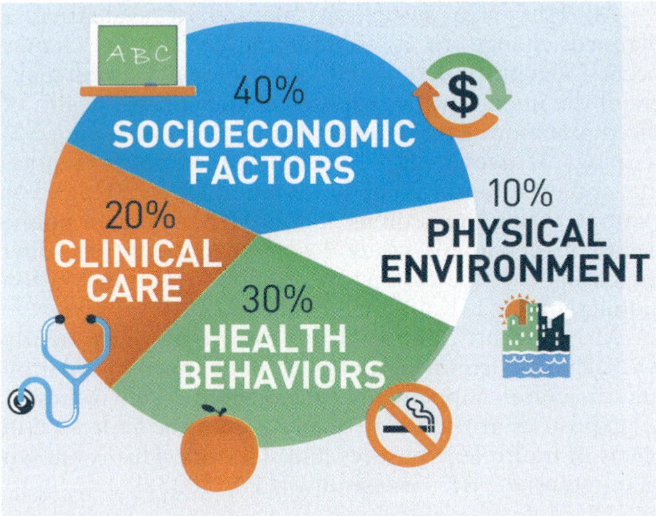

FIGURE 9-3 Infographic "What Affects Health." (Reprinted from https://www.cdc.gov/chinav/docs/chi_nav_infographic.pdf; data from www.countyhealthrankings.org.)

and equal enforcement of environmental laws and regulations" (Dr. Robert Bullard, 2023, para. 1). Recognition of unjust polluting practices in Black communities came from the work of sociologist, Robert Bullard, PhD, who found that Houston, Texas, municipal waste facilities, including landfills and incineration plants, were predominantly placed in Black communities. Dr. Bullard described the disproportionate placement of polluting industries in resource-limited Black communities as an affront to environmental justice.

The EPA defines environmental justice as "the fair treatment and meaningful involvement of all people regardless of race, color, national origin, or income with respect to the development, implementation, and enforcement of environmental laws, regulations, and policies" (EPA, 2020a, para. 1). The key difference between structural and social determinants and environmental justice is that the former addresses the factors that contribute to health disparities, whereas environmental justice is responsive to the inequities in the distribution of environmental hazards and exposure risks. The federal government took action to address environmental injustice through President Clinton's Executive Order 12898 in 1994 (EPA, 2020a, 2020b). In response to the obvious health disparities and injustices that were laid bare to the public during the COVID-19 pandemic and the Black Lives Matter movement, the EPA has shifted funding to support Black, Indigenous, and people of color communities (EPA, 2024; Taiwo et al., 2023).

In communities across the United States, Black, Indigenous, people of color, and people with low income bear a higher burden of exposures to environmental risks where they live (EPA, 2020a, 2021). Children are at particular risk in underrepresented communities, where they have cumulative risk from exposures in homes, schools, and neighborhoods. Developmental and behavioral factors make children more vulnerable to environmental contaminants, and they have little control over where they live, what they eat, or the socioeconomic factors of their lives (Chesney & Duderstadt, 2022).

C/PHN can support more just and healthier environments through a multifaceted and interdisciplinary approach to community development, community organizing, and community engagement by working with advocacy groups, networking, and educational programming. A valuable mapping tool when working in environmental justice is EJScreen. This tool can be used to identify areas of pollution such as hazardous waste, air pollution, and lead with consideration of socioeconomic status and proximity to important sites such as schools, hospitals, and tribal lands. It can be accessed at https://www.epa.gov/ejscreen. The Social Vulnerability Index (ATSDR, 2023d) can also be used to identify communities that require additional support. These tools can help the C/PHN move upstream to address environmental exposures at their source.

Nurses who work in communities that experience environmental injustice observe the impact of health disparities and health burdens on their clients who live in poverty or are people of color. Through community-based participatory research, translational research, partnering with local organizations, and collaborating with community members, nurses can build trusting relationships with community members that strengthen their voices to address the environmental exposures and risks they face. C/PHNs' skills in building relationships with community members, working collaboratively with community partners, and advocating for change through community and governmental programs make them important contributors to environmental justice work (McDermott-Levy et al., 2023). See Chapter 23 on vulnerable populations and Box 9-3 for further sources of environmental health information and for more in-depth resources.

Determining Risk

Merriam-Webster dictionary defines risk as "something that creates or suggests a hazard" (2023, para. 2). In the case of environmental health risks, exposure to a toxic substance within the environment creates a hazard to human health and thus increases the risk of illness or disease. C/PHN must rely on existing science to assess and determine environmental risk to communities. Nurses determine risk by relying on risk identification frameworks.

One such framework is the precautionary principle, which states, "When an activity raises threats of harm to human health or the environment, precautionary measures should be taken if some cause-and-effect relationships are not fully established scientifically. In this context, the proponent of an activity, rather than the public, should bear the burden of proof" (Science and Environmental Health Network [SEHN], 2023, para. 2). The **precautionary principle** relies on credible evidence to determine an action to protect the population from a potential environmental health risk and is rooted in precaution, scientific uncertainty, and human rights.

The ANA and the American Public Health Association adopted the precautionary principle in 2006 as a measure to protect public health. It is used when there is

BOX 9-3 Environmental Health Regulatory Agencies

Environmental Protection Agency (EPA)
This federal agency was established in December 1970 for the purpose of standard setting, monitoring, and enforcement of environmental protection in order to work for a cleaner and healthier environment for America. EPA is tasked with setting regulations based on scientific evidence that addresses environmental risks in homes, schools, workplaces, and natural environments (https://www.epa.gov/history).

Food and Drug Administration (FDA or USFDA)
This is an agency of the U.S. Department of Health and Human Services that regulates food safety, dietary supplements, prescription and over-the-counter pharmaceuticals, veterinary medications, cosmetics, biopharmaceuticals, blood transfusions, medical devices, products that emit radiation, and tobacco products (www.fda.gov/aboutfda/whatwedo/).

Consumer Product Safety Commission
Consumer Product Safety Commission was created in 1972 as an agency of the U.S. government to protect the public from risks of injury or death from consumer products. Commonly reported products are cribs, toys, household chemicals, and power tools but include any commercially traded product. As an independent agency, the CPSC does not report to any other agency of the U.S. government (https://www.cpsc.gov/About-CPSC/).

Occupational Safety and Health Administration
This agency was created in 1970 as a regulatory federal agency of the United States to assure safe working conditions. Occupational Safety and Health Administration sets and enforces standards for health and safety in work environments (https://www.osha.gov/about.html).

limited evidence to determine risk, but there are concerns of threats to human health. As scientific methods have advanced, public health practitioners, including nurses and policymakers, have sought to better understand the impact of the environment on the health of communities.

Health risk assessments and *health impact assessments* (HIA) provide a more comprehensive and systematic examination of a potential environmental health risk and thus address limitations of the evidence that result in the need to rely on the precautionary principle.

The **health risk assessment** is a systematic evaluation of the risk of a specific exposure. It involves four steps: (1) identification of the hazard; (2) dose–response assessment (quantifying the relationship between the identified exposure and the health effects); (3) exposure assessment (examining what is known about the risk, how the exposure presents in humans, and what the toxic levels of exposure are); and (4) risk characterization (estimate the level of exposure using an ecologic and One Health perspective and describe the risk and gaps in the data) if there is a health risk, identifying how it can be managed and reduced (EPA, 2023h).

An HIA is a systematic method of evaluating a planned change to a community *before* the change occurs. The purpose of an HIA is to inform decision makers of the impacts of a proposed change on the health of the population. An HIA has six steps: (1) screening, (2) scoping, (3) assessment, (4) recommendations, (5) reporting, and (6) monitoring and evaluation (EPA, 2023g). For example, using the findings of their HIA, a team of public health professionals made recommendations regarding increasing the tree canopy to promote health in Marion County, Indiana (Kampman et al., 2022).

More recently, public health researchers have rightly noted that environmental risks do not happen in isolation and they often happen over time. Therefore, environmental exposures are cumulative and need to be addressed in terms of multiple exposures and stressors. This is known as **cumulative risk assessment** (EPA, 2023e).

Specific Vulnerabilities

In addition to social vulnerabilities discussed in the social and structural determinants of health section, some groups are at greater risk during specific periods of physical development, due to existing health issues, or from social or environmental exposures related to where they live, work, or attend school. Exposures for people who are pregnant create a number of risks to both the pregnant person and fetus that can produce lifelong or intergenerational adverse outcomes. Some of these effects include fetal loss, low birth weight infants, menstrual abnormalities, recurrent miscarriage, malformations of the reproductive system, reduced fertility, hormonal changes, intrauterine growth restriction, altered semen quality, neurodevelopmental performance, and alterations in the onset of puberty (Gómez-Roig et al., 2021; Ramsay et al., 2023).

Children's exposures begin in utero, when many pollutants reach the developing fetus. Infants and children are at risk due to their stage of physical development, behavioral factors, and specific environments, such as neonatal intensive care units, schools, and homes.

Although breastfeeding is the best source of infant nutrition, many chemicals, such as per- and polyfluoroalkyl substances (PFAS), polychlorinated biphenyls, microplastics, dioxin, and benzene, have been identified in breast milk (Caba-Flores et al., 2023). The stage of physical development of the respiratory, neurologic, and excretory systems can also lead to an increased risk of exposure and decreased ability to metabolize toxins.

Childhood behaviors such as hand-to-mouth exploration, crawling and playing on or near the ground, and the use of toys all contribute to vulnerability to environmental hazards. Toxic materials on floors, in soil where children play, and in playthings (e.g., pressure-treated wood, toys, and paints) can increase the risk for childhood toxic exposures. Exposures to lead, mercury, and PFAS increase the risk for developmental disabilities. Studies suggest that the rise in attention deficit hyperactivity disorder, as well as antisocial and aggressive behavior diagnoses and possibly autism, can be attributed to the harmful effects of neurotoxic agents in the environment (Dórea, 2021).

One specific type of vulnerability involves a chronic disease arising from complex interactions between the environment and the genes. **Epigenetics** is the field of study that examines the gene–environment interaction to study the processes in which genes are expressed differently as a result of environmental influences (Hopkins & Zangrilli, 2023). **Endocrine-disrupting chemicals** mimic or block natural hormones in the human body and are linked to changes in genes inherited by offspring.

One example of epigenetic change was the use of diethylstilbestrol (DES) to treat patients at risk for miscarriage. Offspring assigned female at birth of patients who took DES showed increased rates of vaginal adenocarcinoma. Other cancers (breast, pancreatic) may now be linked to the estrogen taken by their birthing parents during pregnancy (Troisi et al., 2019). Further, a relationship between the DES-exposed granddaughters and their children born with heart and skeletal abnormalities has been noted (Titus, 2021).

Experts argue that the genetic changes that result from epigenetic processes because of developmental exposure to environmental stressors create negative effects on the health of future generations and contribute to rising rates of neurologic conditions, alterations in reproductive organ development, and cancer (Hopkins & Zangrilli, 2023).

Sciences for Environmental Health

Environmental health sciences include environmental epidemiology, toxicology, risk assessment, and risk management. In Chapter 7, you learned about the principles of epidemiology. **Environmental epidemiology** is a particular branch of epidemiology that examines the environmental determinants of disease. It is the study of environmental exposures and the risks that contribute to adverse health effects such as cancer, developmental disabilities, neurologic problems, reproductive health issues, or death. Environmental epidemiology seeks to understand the specific vulnerabilities of population groups and how toxic exposures adversely affect health and to contribute to public health policies that address risk and risk management (Bloom, 2020).

Toxicology is the study of the adverse effects of chemical, physical, or biologic agents on living organisms and the ecosystem. The study of toxicology enables us to understand the health effects of environmental exposures and address prevention of exposures (National Institute of Environmental Health Sciences, 2023). Toxicants are substances that are harmful and made by humans or result from human activities, in contrast to toxins that are naturally produced. By studying the physical properties of chemicals, scientists can examine the toxicity of chemicals as manifested by enzyme inhibition, cytotoxicity, inflammation, necrosis, immune hypersensitivity or immune suppression, neoplasia, and mutagenic reactions.

These processes should be familiar to nurses because they parallel the effects and adverse effects of pharmacotherapeutic chemicals. Chemicals are classified as alcohols, solvents, heavy metals, oxidants, and acids and may be found as industrial wastes, agricultural chemicals, waterborne toxicants, air pollutants, or food additives. Factors such as dose level and timing can make a difference in the efficacy or toxicity of a drug; dose and timing can also affect the toxicity of chemicals. The toxicity of a substance is affected by factors such as gender, age, lifestyle, diet, genetics, and disease states. A major difference when comparing pharmacology to toxicology is that we typically can identify the name, dose, and route of the administered drug; however, when dealing with environmental exposures, it can be challenging to determine the duration, amount, and route of exposure (McDermott-Levy, 2023).

Exposure pathways, or the routes by which a chemical enters the body, can affect toxicity, absorption, and metabolism. For example, children have less well-developed metabolic processes and are less able to detoxify chemical exposures. Likewise, older adults have reduced defense mechanisms in their lungs, skin, and other systems that make them more prone to adverse health effects (Leffers, 2023). Nurses can learn more about the toxicology and risk of specific toxicants through the Toxicological Profiles site at Agency of Toxic Substances Disease Registry of the CDC, available at https://www.atsdr.cdc.gov/toxprofiledocs/.

Although typical health screening does not test for most hazardous chemicals, biomonitoring may be necessary if there is concern about an environmental exposure. **Biomonitoring** refers to measuring environmental chemicals and their metabolites in human tissue, such as blood, hair, urine, or saliva (CDC, 2017). The CDC monitors and reports population exposures through the National Report on Human Exposure to Environmental Chemicals. Nurses can learn more about the CDC National Biomonitoring Program on their website: https://www.cdc.gov/biomonitoring/index.html.

Scientists identify health risks from epidemiology and toxicology, which provide information for government agencies to regulate hazards to human health. For example, the EPA uses human health risk assessments to "estimate the nature and probability of adverse health effects in humans who may be exposed to chemicals in contaminated environmental media, now or in the future" (EPA, 2023h, para. 1). As discussed earlier in the chapter, a health risk assessment is a systematic, step-wise process to estimate human health risk.

PUBLIC HEALTH NURSE'S ROLE

Addressing environmental health risks and exposures can be complex and involve many experts; consequently, C/PHNs work collaboratively with others in the community to promote health. Some of the most common areas of public health nursing practice to address environmental impacts on health are schools, homes, and the broader community (Box 9-4).

School nurses have been leaders in addressing indoor air quality in schools, particularly as rates of asthma in children rise (EPA, 2023c). School nurses have also served as advocates for **integrated pest management (IPM)** programs for pest prevention without increasing exposure to harmful toxins.

IPM uses data on life cycles and habitats of pests and their environmental impact, along with environmentally friendly, economical methods of pest control, to

BOX 9-4 **LEVELS OF PREVENTION PYRAMID**

Pesticides Exposures

SITUATION: Provide education, resources, and support to prevent and treat pesticide exposures and poisoning.
GOAL: Using the three levels of prevention, avoid or promptly diagnose and treat negative health conditions, and restore the fullest possible potential.

Tertiary Prevention	
Rehabilitation	***Prevention***
Call Poison Control Center at 1-800-222-1222 HAZMAT teams Disaster preparedness	Health education: Continue to educate employers and workers about common risks in their businesses and specific hazardous chemicals. Health protection: Advocate for safe use and storage of pesticides and how to proceed during emergencies.

Secondary Prevention	
Early Diagnosis	***Prompt Treatment***
Recognition of early signs of pesticide poisoning. Laboratory screening for pesticide toxicity (blood or urine samples)	Observe for symptoms as outlined on Data Safety Sheet. Follow exposure actions on Data Safety Sheet. Poisoning signs can be seen; for example, vomiting, sweating, or pinpoint pupils. Symptoms can also include functional changes in normal condition that can be described by the victim of poisoning (e.g., nausea, headache, weakness, dizziness, others). National Pesticide Information Center (http://npic.orst.edu/ingred/specchem.html)

Primary Prevention	
Health Promotion and Education	***Health Protection***
Educate community members to reduce exposures to pesticides in their homes and outdoor areas Educate employers and workers about Safety Data Sheets to understand hazardous chemicals	Advocate for: Clear product labeling with a package insert of warnings in multiple languages ■ Follow storage instructions on Data Safety Sheet ■ Community-level policy to restrict exposures to hazardous chemicals in pesticides in public places and use integrated pest management (IPM) for schools and playgrounds ■ Safe use of pesticides and preparation for emergencies Teaching parents, teachers, and caregivers about pesticide risk, exposure routes, and methods of pesticide exposure prevention

effectively manage damage done by pests with the least hazardous effects on humans and the environment (EPA, 2023k).

At the community level, C/PHNs are involved in many activities to promote and protect the health of the populations:

- Reducing pediatric obesity by participation in efforts to improve the built environment by advocating for safe walking paths, parks, and recreational areas
- Reducing exposure to pesticides in playgrounds (National Association of School Nurses, 2018)
- Educating about the health impacts of ambient air quality and wildfire smoke
- Organizing cooling centers for extreme heat

Assessment

The breadth of environmental health information available exceeds the scope of this chapter. Our discussion is organized around the settings where people live, work, recreate, and go to school and the routes of exposure, the types of hazards, and the health effects of environmental toxins (Box 9-5). It is important for nurses working in the community to identify priority environmental concerns where people spend the majority of their time (home, work, school). Although community assessment and epidemiology are essential skills for public health nursing, the ability to perform critical assessments for environmental health risks requires a background in the environmental health sciences.

Community/Public Health Nursing Assessments

In C/PHN practice, nurses routinely complete assessments for people, families, groups, and communities. There are many assessment tools available to help guide both C/PHNs and the people they serve to assess environmental health risks.

BOX 9-5 STORIES FROM THE FIELD

Chemical Exposure Risks in the Clinical Setting

How many chemicals do you come in contact with on a daily basis in your nursing practice? Of particular interest to nurses is the survey conducted by the National Institute for Occupational Safety and Health (NIOSH), which found that American nurses and other healthcare professionals are at risk for exposure to chemicals in the clinical setting. These chemicals are used to sterilize and disinfect equipment and are the medications, such as chemotherapeutic agents, that are used to treat patients. Exposure to these chemicals can place nurses, their patients, and others in the healthcare setting at risk for asthma, reproductive problems, and cancer (NIOSH, 2017, 2023). Another finding of the NIOSH survey was that healthcare workers do not know nor do they always follow the proper procedures to reduce the risk of chemical exposures in the workplace. These are important environmental health factors for the nurse practicing in the clinical setting to consider. A large-scale study of nurse workplace exposure during pregnancy to sterilizing agents, dangerous drugs, anesthetic gases, and chemicals used in housekeeping found an increase in birth defects among their offspring (Environmental Working Group, 2019). Higher incidences of asthma, contact dermatitis, cancer, and miscarriages were also noted in nurses who reported high exposure rates.

1. *How are decisions made about the products used in your facility?*
2. *Who determines policies and procedures for use of chemicals and medications that can affect the health of staff and patients?*
3. *Where would you find information about the cleaning chemicals used in your place of practice?*
4. *Where would you find information to reduce the risk of exposure to chemotherapeutic agents?*
5. *Develop a plan to share the information you found with other nurses within a healthcare setting.*

Individual Assessments

The *ecological model of public health* offers a framework to consider where to target public health nursing interventions (Fig. 9-1). The framework offers spheres of influence at the individual, social sphere or family, community, and national levels. The nurse must first identify the needs of the targeted sphere by assessing the environmental risk.

At the individual level, people should complete a personal environmental health exposure assessment. Ideally, this should be part of every health visit, workplace assessment, or other health history. Though there are some shared characteristics for environmental exposures, individual risks from work, home, school, and recreation all contribute to a person's overall risk.

In addition, there is an environmental exposure history card using the mnemonic "OCAREER" to support nurses and other health professionals in adding environmental health exposure questions to patient assessments (Table 9-1). This tool has assessment questions and ICD-10 codes that match possible health and exposure findings (Saberi & Becker, 2023). The use of ICD codes has the utility to document health impacts of the environment and climate change. These data can be used to gather population health data and develop evidence of the impacts of the environment on human health (McDermott-Levy et al., 2021).

While completing an individual assessment, it is important to consider those exposures specific to the workplace, school, or neighborhood. Workplace exposures are often addressed by OHNs and include not only physical hazards such as injuries from machinery, burns, falls, and crushing injuries but also hazardous exposure to toxic chemicals, particulate matter in the form of dust, volatile organic compounds (VOCs) and aerosols, heavy metals, and other chemicals that can contribute to poor indoor air quality (EPA, 2020c). Furthermore, chemical manufacturers, distributors, and importers are required to provide a Data Safety Sheet (Occupational Safety and Health Administration, 2012). The C/PHN can use the information on the product Data Safety Sheet to understand protection, toxicological, and safe disposal information of workplace chemical products such cleaning products, paint thinners, and lubricants for machinery.

School nurses often address students' exposures in school settings, but it is very important for C/PHNs to identify potential risks to educate parents about environmental hazards in schools. Similar to the workplace, many schools have issues of poor indoor air quality with the increased use of synthetics in building materials and reduced access to outdoor air (EPA, 2020c). Older schools may also have problems with asbestos, lead, and mold. Neighborhood exposures affect individual health and are discussed in the Community Assessment section of this chapter. It is especially important to assess hazards among school-aged children and the routes taken to school and playgrounds.

Home Assessments

C/PHNs frequently conduct home assessments for case finding, follow-up, screening, or other public health services. Home assessments often involve looking for safety hazards in the home but do not always include potential environmental exposures. During the home visit, C/PHNs must assess the home for environmental tobacco smoke; the possibility of asbestos, the presence of a carbon monoxide detector and heating sources; lead paint risk; mold, the water source, and the possibility of lead pipes; and other potential or actual hazardous materials (Table 9-2). Depending on the region of the country, C/PHNs should ensure that the family has their home tested for radon (EPA, 2023o).

Likewise, family members should be instructed to safely dispose of unused medication and old mercury thermometers. Cleaning products, paints, varnishes, strippers and other home remodeling materials, gardening fertilizers and pesticides (which can be carried into the home on shoes or pets; see Chapter 27), pest management insecticides and other materials, air fresheners, and mold and moisture can all be sources of exposure in the home and land around the home. C/PHNs must be well

TABLE 9-1 Physicians for Social Responsibility PA: OCAREER

Physicians for Social Responsibility PA: OCAREER

A practitioners' tool for evaluating climate and health

	Description	Questions to consider	ICD 10 Codes
		Primary Climate Code: Issues due to physical environment	**Z58**
O	Occupation and work	• What do you do professionally? • What is your workplace like (outdoor vs indoor, stationary vs mobile) Have you ever been in the military? worked on a farm? done volunteer or seasonal work? • How do you get to and from work?	• Z56.0 • Z56.1 • Z56.2 • Z56.89 • Z57.39 • Z57.6
C	Conditions/ Health: medications and mental health	• Do you have any chronic medical conditions? Are you currently being treated? If so, for what disease/symptoms? What medications do you take: prescribed, over the counter, and/or herbal? • Do you engage in any alternative healing or cultural practices? • *"What brings you here today?" "What do you think is going on?" "Can you trace your symptoms to a date, time, location or event?"*	• X30 • Z65.5 • Z75.3 • Z77.11 • Z77.118 • Z77.2
A	Activities: food and food access, transportation and travel, hobbies	• What activities do you and your family engage in? • What hobbies do you or your family have? • Do you garden, fish or hunt? Do you eat what you catch or grow? • How close are food/ grocery/pharmacy sources to you? • Do you use weed killer, bug killers, or foggers? • How do you get to work, or other places? What methods of transportation are available to you? How often do you travel by plane? Car? Other modes?	• Z59.4 • Z94.1
R	Residence: home, habitat, community, region	• In what kind of location do you live? • How far are necessary supplies and resources? What means do you have to access these places? • What is your current housing situation? When was your residence built? Have you done any remodeling or updating to your home? If so, when and for what purpose? How long have you lived there and what circumstances brought you there? Who owns or manages your residence? If not you, how responsive is that person to your needs? • What materials is your home primarily made up of? • Have you had problems with your home upkeep and maintenance? • Have you experienced frequent disruptions in your energy supply? What aspects of your medical care are dependent on a reliable energy source? • What systems in your home do you use for heating/cooling? What, if anything, stops you from using these systems when temperatures change? • What types of chemical products are stored in your residence? How are they stored? What steps do you take to limit your exposure to these chemicals?	• X01 • Z59.0 • Z59.4 • Z77.011 • Z77.11 • Z77.110 • Z77.111 • Z77.112 • Z77.118 • Z77.120 • Z77.2
E	Environmental concerns	• Do you live near a major highway, active or abandoned industrial site? a military base? a farm? Oil/gas well? How close is this to your home? • Do you have gas appliances or use a fireplace in the home? Any smokers at home? • Does your living space have a moisture or flooding problem? *For more residential questions, please see R-Residence.* • Where does your drinking water come from? Have you tested it? Does your water have any unusual taste, color, or odor? • Do you swim in your local water body? Do you eat fish caught in your local river/stream, etc.? • Does your area flood with extreme rain or snow?	• X31 • X37.8 • X38 • Z58.6 • Z77.110 • Z77.112 • Z57.4
E	Educate to Advocate and Communicate	Are materials available to educate the patient? Are alternatives available to minimize the risk of exposure?	
R	Referrals and Resources	Have prevention strategies been discussed? What is the plan for follow-up? What resources are available? What categories of referrals are appropriate?	

ICD Code	ICD Code Description	ICD Code	ICD Code Description
X01	*Exposure to uncontrolled fire, not in building or structure*	Z59.0	*Inadequate housing*
X30	*Exposure to excessive natural heat, initial encounter*	Z59.4	*Lack of adequate food*
X31	*Exposure to excessive natural cold*	Z59.9	*Problems related to housing and economic circumstances*
X37.8	*Other cataclysmic storms*	Z65.5	*Exposure to disaster, war and other hostilities*
X38	*Flood*	Z75.3	*Inaccessibility to healthcare*
Z56.0	*Unemployment, unspecified*	Z77.011	*Contact with and (suspected) exposure to lead*
Z56.1	*Change of job*	Z77.11	*Contact with and (suspected) exposure to environmental pollution*
Z56.2	*Threat of job loss*	Z77.110	*Contact with and (suspected) exposure to air pollution*
Z56.89	*Other problems related to employment*	Z77.111	*Contact with and (suspected) exposure to water pollution*
Z57.39	*Occupational exposure to other air contaminants*	Z77.112	*Contact with and (suspected) exposure to soil pollution*
Z57.4	*Occupational exposure to toxic agents in agriculture*	Z77.118	*Contact with and (suspected) exposure to other environmental pollution*
Z57.6	*Occupational exposure to extreme temperature*	Z77.120	*Contact with and (suspected) exposure to mold (toxic)*
Z58.6	*Inadequate drinking-water supply*	Z77.2	*Contact with and (suspected) exposure to other hazardous substances*

TABLE **9-2** Common Hazards in the Home Setting

Hazard	Source	Exposure Pathway	Risk Groups	Health Effects
Asbestos	Asbestos is a fiber that has been used for insulation and as a fire retardant Used in shipbuilding and other occupational exposures to metal work	Inhalation	Children of metal workers Home residents	Lung cancer (mesothelioma) and lung disease
Arsenic	Used in pressure-treated wood, was formerly used in industrial sites, can be present in soil and water	Drinking water Inhalation from indoor or outdoor air	Children playing in playgrounds with pressure-treated wood, those with contaminated water supply	High levels are lethal Exposure can cause decreased red and white blood cells
Carbon monoxide	Colorless and odorless gas that is a byproduct of combustion from home heating sources as well as automobiles housed in attached garage	Inhalation	People with respiratory and cardiovascular disease	Unconsciousness and death due to hypoxia
Environmental tobacco smoke	Cigarette smoking	Inhalation	Those people in areas where smoking occurs in indoor space/home	Lung disease; lung cancer; cardiovascular problems
Formaldehyde	Carpeting, particle board, glues, adhesives used in home construction, or decorating Also some personal care products	Inhalation		Cancer
Lead	Paint used prior to 1978; leaded gasoline prior to ban in 1970s; ceramics, pottery, pipes, soil; some alternative medical therapies	Ingestion from dust in home or soil	Children	Nervous system
Mold	Normal growth of fungi in and outside of home Can produce VOCs	Spores travel in the air Inhalation	Those people most sensitive to molds	Respiratory symptoms
Pests	Mites, cockroaches	Inhalation, physical contact with droppings	Children and those with asthma	Exacerbation of asthma
Per- and polyfluoroalkyl substances (PFAS)	Nonstick cookware, packaged food, contaminated water and food	Ingestion	Developing fetus All people exposed	Elevated cholesterol, changes in liver enzymes, kidney or testicular cancer, decreased response to childhood vaccinations, preeclampsia, and low-birth-weight infants
Pesticides	Used in homes and outside lawns and gardens to protect plants from pests, home from insects	Indoor or outdoor air; inhalation Dermal absorption	Children All people exposed	Specific types of pesticides have been linked to neurologic problems, others to cancer, and many as EDCs

(Continued)

TABLE 9-2 Common Hazards in the Home Setting (*Continued*)

Hazard	Source	Exposure Pathway	Risk Groups	Health Effects
Pharmaceutical waste	Unused, out-of-date prescriptions	If discarded by waste or water systems, may seep into aquifers	All people exposed	Possible health concerns (hormone disruption, antibiotic resistance) to humans
Radon	Naturally occurring radioactive gas	Seeps into homes through cracks in foundation of home; inhalation	Residents of home	Lung damage particularly lung cancer
Solvents such as paint thinners, varnishes, and resins (ethers)	Dry cleaning, home improvements	Inhalation Percutaneous absorption	Home residents	Neurologic problems, renal, liver, and reproductive effects
Personal care products	Shampoo, soaps, cosmetics	Percutaneous	People using them, children, adolescents	Varied EDCs, cancer, and neurologic effects
Volatile organic compounds (VOCs)	Alcohols, ketones, and esters that are present in thousands of products such as paint thinners, cleaning supplies, pesticides, building materials, office equipment, copiers, printers, glues, adhesives	Inhalation	Those exposed in indoor settings	Eye, nose, and throat irritation; headaches; kidney damage; and central nervous system disorders

EDC, endocrine-disrupting chemical.

versed in identifying potential environmental risks and existing hazardous materials and assess for them in their routine home visits, as noted in a classic, large, two-state study by Butterfield et al. (2011).

Additionally, the C/PHN must identify everyday products in clients' homes that contain hazardous materials, the risk they pose to health, and the importance of eliminating them or securing them to minimize the risk of exposure. The nurse should also direct families and others to the EPA Safer Choice program, which has lists and information about cleaning and other consumer products that have less health risk. See Safer Choice website: https://www.epa.gov/saferchoice.

Finally, a home assessment should address nearby environmental hazards or potential hazards such as coal-fired power plants, farms, industries, **brownfields** (properties where pollutants, contaminants, or hazardous substances may be present), toxic waste sites, highways, and contaminated waterways. Frequently, these hazards are visible in the neighborhood, but often, there are hidden routes of exposure from contaminated groundwater, ambient air, and contaminated soil. It is important that C/PHNs are aware of local industry and potential contaminations and the source of reliable data that can support the identification of families at risk in their home.

Community Assessments

A comprehensive community health assessment considers environmental factors in several ways. In Chapter 15, community health assessment is introduced with a focus on aspects of the community that promote health or provide risks to health. Environmental assessment refers to the natural and built environments.

Community assessment is central to public health nursing practice and to the core functions of public health. It is incumbent on the C/PHN to be aware of past, current, and emerging environmental health hazards within the community. For example, knowledge of actual or potential environmental exposures from new industries or past places of pollution such as Superfund sites within a community.

Various tools have been developed to help nurses and others assess environmental risks. The ANHE, the international environmental health nursing organization, and Environmental Protection Agency provide risk exposure assessment tools to use in a variety of settings. They can be accessed here:

- ANHE Environmental Assessment tools: https://envirn.org/resources/assessment-tools/
- EPA Exposure Assessment Tools by Approaches: https://www.epa.gov/expobox/exposure-assessment-tools-approaches

Furthermore, National Association on County and City Health Officials offers a Community Health Environmental Assessments Course; see their website (https://www.naccho.org/programs/environmental-health/assessment-tools), and ANHE offers many webinars to inform nurses about emerging environmental health issues. To learn about ANHE webinars, see their website (https://envirn.org/). Furthermore, the national Pediatric Environmental Health Network can support C/PHNs in identifying and addressing environmental health risks for young families (ATSDR, 2023c).

Though most community assessment tools address the environment, C/PHNs must also consider specific threats that may not be covered by general community assessments. To assess air quality, for instance, nurses should look for visible sources of air pollution from smokestacks, identify exhaust from vehicular traffic, and learn of significant industries, power sources, and incinerators in the community. The nurse must also consider the age and condition of the housing stock and the income of community members to fully understand the community's exposure and their ability to reduce environmental risk. The nurse can access real-time air quality data using the AirNow.gov and the Purple Air Map (https://community.purpleair.com/t/purpleair-map-guide/90). AirNow relies on the color-coded Air Quality Index (AQI) and has information about fine particulate (PM2.5), ozone, and smoke pollution. Purple Air provides hyperlocal data of PM2.5 pollution but does not measure hazardous air pollutants such as benzene and formaldehyde.

To assess water quality, C/PHNs must identify the source of drinking water as public or private, understand water treatment and quality, recognize evidence of pollution and whether there are fish alerts for local waterways, examine stagnant water and waterborne risks, and identify issues related to sewer function and possible contamination, as well as the likelihood of floods and other water emergencies (EPA, 2023f).

Soil contamination can occur from pesticides, nearby highways or airports, local industry, old buildings that use lead-based paint, or flooding. Soil contamination can be a risk:

- Indoors as people track the contaminated soil dust in the home
- When gardening and the contaminate gets into planted food
- Children playing in the soil and breathing or ingesting the contaminate

To assess land and soil, nurses must consider both current and former land use. **Superfund** refers to funding made possible by the Comprehensive Environmental Response, Compensation, and Liability Act of 1980 to address those contaminated areas of the United States that needed to be remediated; the EPA administers the funding and the authority to remediate the contamination. Scientists with the Agency for Toxic Substance Disease Registry (ATSDRb) will comment regarding the health risks of Superfund sites. Well-known examples of Superfund sites in which land contamination caused public health disasters are Love Canal in New York State and Times Beach, Missouri. Nurses must be aware of such sites in their communities, which are listed on the National Priorities List and can be located by searching on the EPA website (https://www.epa.gov/superfund/search-superfund-sites-where-you-live#map).

A brownfield site "is a property, the expansion, redevelopment, or reuse of which may be complicated by the presence or potential presence of a hazardous substance, pollutant, or contaminant" (EPA, 2023m, para. 1). In 2018, the Brownfields Utilization, Investment, and Local Development Act was ratified to bring more opportunities for sustainable local development and to redevelop brownfield sites that still required remediation (EPA, 2023m). Nurses should monitor the impact of the Brownfields Utilization, Investment, and Local Development Act of 2018 and advocate that the goals of this act serve their communities.

Built Environment. The built environment refers to all aspects of our environment that are not naturally occurring and includes not only the physical structures (e.g., homes, schools, workplaces, dams, roadways, buildings, energy sources) but also the features that contribute to social cohesiveness or disruption (Fig. 9-4). The impact of the built environment includes indoor and outdoor physical environments, which in turn affect the social environments where people live, work, and engage with others. Considering that most Americans spend upward of 90% of their time indoors, our built environment can have significant impact on our health (EPA, 2023c—indoor air quality).

Given the time spent indoors, the built environment is an environment that must be part of the C/PHN's consideration. This has gained additional attention as a result of the COVID-19 pandemic. Evidence suggests that many physical and mental health problems are related to the built environment, such as asthma, cardiovascular disease, lung conditions, obesity, and some cancers (Dovjak & Kukec, 2019).

Many U.S. cities are addressing issues related to community/public health and the built environment by implementing the UN SDGs. The UN Sustainable Development Solutions Network and the Sustainable Development Solutions Network USA produce a ranking of states in meeting the SDGs, which serves as an indication of the impacts of built and natural environments on community health (Lynch & Sachs, 2021).

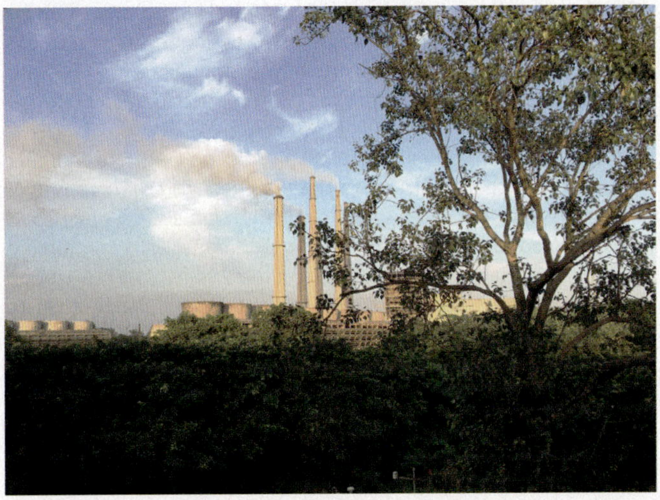

FIGURE 9-4 Neighborhoods, or the built environment, can contribute to population health or illness.

Another C/PHN role is to assess the quality of the housing. Buildings that were constructed prior to 1978 are likely to have lead-based paint, and homes built before 1987 may have lead soldering in the plumbing that delivers household drinking water (CDC, 2023e). Homes or buildings constructed between 1930 and 1950 are likely to have asbestos in the insulation, as well as in the hot water and steam pipes (ATSDR, 2023a).

The overall condition of the community indicates sanitation factors, safe waste disposal, and potential sources of contamination. The location of schools, playgrounds, and public transportation, and access to green spaces should be part of the community assessment. Examination of the overall community environment provides C/PHNs with essential information about how the environment is likely to impact the residents' health (Box 9-6).

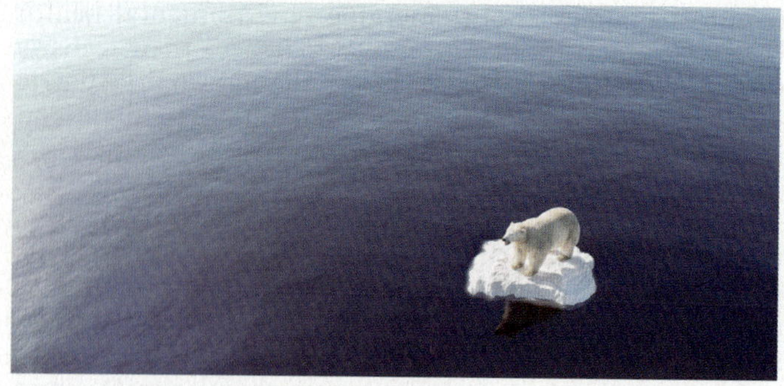

FIGURE 9-5 Climate change is related to melting ice caps, warming oceans, and increased volatile weather patterns.

Climate Change. Climate change is our greatest global public health threat (Costello et al., 2009, 2013; Desmond, 2016). **Climate change** "refers to significant changes in global temperature, precipitation, wind patterns and other measures of climate that occur over several decades or longer" (Fig. 9-5; UC Davis, n.d., para. 1).

In recent years, the reality of climate change has brought about engaged healthcare providers, communities, and policymakers including the U.S. rejoining the UN Paris Climate Agreement. The Paris Agreement is an international agreement of signatory countries to limit GHG emissions in an effort to keep global temperature rise below 2°C of preindustrial temperatures and to target temperature reduction to 1.5°C. The target of 1.5°C preindustrial temperatures has been further supported by a sobering report from the Intergovernmental Panel on Climate Change (IPCC, 2018), in which the world's leading climate scientist stated that to avoid severe impacts of climate change, the world must reduce carbon emissions by 45% now.

IPCC 6th Assessment Report stated that "it is unequivocal that human influence has warmed the atmosphere, ocean, and land. Widespread and rapid changes in the atmosphere, ocean, cryosphere, and biosphere have occurred (IPCC, 2021). The third part of the 6th Assessment Report further noted that major human activity that influenced climate change was the burning of fossil fuels (coal, gas, and oil) (IPCC, 2023). Temperature changes from climate change affect weather patterns that

BOX **9-6** PERSPECTIVES

A Student Viewpoint on Environmental Health in Health Systems

As a nursing student, I was bothered by the amount of waste I saw in the hospital during my clinical rotations. When we covered environmental health in class, I learned that while healing patients, health systems also contribute to GHGs and use toxic materials to maintain the patient care units. According to the American Hospital Association (2023), U.S. hospitals generate about 33.8 pounds per hospitalized patient each day! That's about 6 million tons of waste generated annually. I did not want to be part of a health system that was contributing to pollution and illness.

I spoke to my nursing professor, and we both agreed that education is the way to make the change. With the support of my professor and the nursing simulation lab staff, I developed a waste reduction program for the students within my nursing school's simulation lab. I started with the urinary catheterization lab and taught the sophomore students about hospital waste and what items can be recycled, reused, and must be discarded. By weighing the reusable, recycled, and discarded items from the urinary catheterization lab, I demonstrated the impact that education and end-use product management can have. The faculty, simulation lab staff, and students were excited to see that they could make a difference in the environment by being aware of end-use product management.

As I prepared for the educational session for my fellow nursing students, I learned where to find information about products that are used in the hospital. I looked first at the Practice Green Health website (https://practicegreenhealth.org/) to learn more about sustainable practices in hospital setting. I also looked at The Nurse's Drawdown (https://www.nursesdrawdown.org/) to learn about effective nurse-led programs. Through my research, I also learned about hospital Green Teams or Sustainability Teams that support institutional sustainability in purchasing, foods for dietary services, energy use, waste management, and product safety. Nurses can serve on these important hospital teams, support green practices on their units, and develop sustainable programs. I also learned about two organizations that support this important work:

- Practice Greenhealth (https://practicegreenhealth.org/)
- Health Care Without Harm (https://noharm.org)

When I look for my first staff nurse position, I am going to seek employment at a hospital where I can serve on the Green Team so I can continue to have an environmental health focus in my nursing career.

Marina, senior nursing student

Source: American Hospital Association (2023).

BOX **9-7** WHAT DO *YOU* THINK?

Climate Refugees

In addition to those already affected, it is estimated that by 2050, more that 216 million people around the globe will move within their countries due to climate change (World Bank, 2021). Approximately 21.5 million people have needed to migrate since 2008 (Elton, 2023). More climate migration will occur as slow-onset changes like rising sea levels and air pollution increase. Eight western Pacific islands have already submerged, with a projected 48 being under water by 2100 (Podesta, 2019).

One example in Louisiana highlights the dire circumstances. Isle de Jean Charles, about 50 miles southwest of New Orleans, was first settled by a Frenchman who described it not as an island but as a ridge covered with live oak trees and encircled by swampy marshlands. Native American tribes later settled there, hunting, trapping, fishing, raising domestic animals, and growing rice. In 1953, the marshland was linked to the mainland by a 2-mile causeway. Now, the island is 98% submerged into the Gulf of Mexico and is only a quarter-mile wide and two miles long. From a high of 300, now there are only 40 residents remaining. Over the last 20 years, six hurricanes have pummeled the island. Although residents are conflicted about being relocated to the mainland, they have been forced to leave their ancestral home and become climate refugees (Jarvie, 2019).

1. *Is climate change a driver for the increase in Central Americans requesting asylum at the U.S. southern border?*
2. *How should C/PHN address climate change migration for the people of Isle de Jean Charles?*

Source: Elton (2023); Jarvie (2019); Podesta (2019); World Bank (2021).

can result in more frequent extreme weather events, disease outbreaks, food and water shortages, and changing human migration patterns with an increase in refugees (see Boxes 9-7 and 9-8). Another valuable resource for nurses is the U.S. Global Change Research Program report, Fifth National Climate Assessment (2023). See Box 9-9 for a nurse's perspective on climate change and the experience of attending the UN climate change meeting, the Conference of the Parties (COP).

BOX **9-8** WHAT DO *YOU* THINK?

Pandemics and Pollution

Italy is considered a leader in lowering GHGs, having reduced GHGs 30% between 2004 and 2018. In mid-March 2020, satellite readings revealed a rapid drop in nitrogen dioxide levels since January. Because of the COVID-19 outbreak and isolation measures enacted in the northern part of Italy, fewer diesel-powered cars were being used as people remained in their homes. Time-lapse maps showed striking results, similar to even more dramatic results noted earlier in China, where the disease outbreak began (Mooney et al., 2020). Although these changes are temporary, they demonstrate how humans have an impact on their environment. What other changes might occur if the trend continued?

Nurses are in a position to take a lead in addressing the health impacts of climate change through individual, professional, local, national, and global mitigation, adaptation, and resilience strategies. When assessing communities, the nurse should note vulnerable groups such as people who are pregnant, infants, children, older adults, people with disabilities, non-English speakers, Indigenous populations and people of color, and people with limited resources. In addition, communities may experience risks related to food and water quality and availability, heat stress for those most vulnerable, increased air pollution, and severe weather-related events. Severe weather events such as flooding, droughts, hurricanes, tornados, sea level rise, and wildfires require emergency preparedness and disaster response from the public health sector.

It is incumbent that C/PHNs are knowledgeable of the regional impacts of climate change and have communicated those impacts with colleagues such as emergency services, food distribution, healthcare sector, and policymakers (Butterfield et al., 2021). Further, C/PHNs must be prepared for surge events by developing skills such as the following:

- Be personally prepared
- Communicate accurate information to colleagues and the community
- Respond to state and local disaster plans
- Perform public health triage
- Conduct a rapid needs assessment that includes mental health
- Investigate outbreaks
- Participate effectively in mass dispensing interventions
- Respond after the event to the debriefing and public health impact to climate change-related event

C/PHNs must work with communities and others to be prepared for inadequate resources and infrastructure, as well as the lack of electricity and technology (Federal Emergency Management Agency [FEMA], 2023) (see Chapter 17). C/PHNs must also disseminate timely and accurate information for nursing practice through resources and collaboration with nurse colleagues in other practice settings, healthcare systems, policymakers, and national organizations. All nurses must understand the implications of climate change on health, and C/PHNs are able to address the population impacts of climate change.

Land Use. Topics that must be considered when conducting community health assessment to address land use include zoning regulations and enforcement, industries and their toxic releases, types of transportation, sidewalks, bikeways, public transportation, recreational space including green space, what fertilizers or pesticides are applied to the fields, safe play areas for children, and information regarding a tree ordinance to promote healthy environments (EPA, 2020b).

School locations should be examined for accessibility by foot or bicycle, the safety of the surrounding area, artificial turf, and the use of pesticides on school fields.

BOX 9-9 PERSPECTIVES

A C/PHN's Viewpoint on Engaging in Climate Change and Health Advocacy

Having the opportunity to attend the 27th global Conference of Parties (COP) that was held in Sharm El-Sheikh, Egypt, as an observer was a transformative learning experience and a highlight of my nursing career. As part of the United Nations Framework Convention on Climate Change, the UN global climate change meeting, I had the opportunity to share space with delegates from countries all over the world as they discussed and negotiated strategies to address the growing climate crisis and efforts to work collectively to prepare for the worsening effects of climate change.

Attending COP27 was an eye-opening experience as I heard countless stories of devastating extreme weather events from other international observers. There were also inspiring presentations on community-led adaptation efforts and government pledges to invest in clean renewable energy. There was an overwhelming sense of urgency in relation to the climate crisis and the need to phase out fossil fuels throughout the entire 2-week conference. Beyond the walls of the meeting, people held demonstrations and painted murals—generations came together, as did cultures from opposite sides of the globe to advocate for climate action.

One of the larger negotiation discussions at COP27 was the commitment to "Loss and Damage" funding by resource-abundant countries that have made the greatest contribution to GHGs that are fueling the climate crisis. The loss and damage funding would be used to compensate resource-limited countries for damage caused by climate disasters and also help develop adaptation and mitigation plans for countries that may not have the ability to effectively address the climate crisis.

The health voice was unified at COP27 as nurses, doctors, health ministers, and community workers spoke about the impacts that climate change has on human health. I learned a lot by attending COP27; I feel the whole experience reshaped my worldview and expanded my appreciation of social determinants of health and my overall perspective as a PHN.

If I had the opportunity to attend another COP, I would return, and I am hopeful more nurses will attend with each passing conference. Nurses practice under a unique care model. We also have important messages to share directly from our patients with policymakers and we must share those messages on the international stage. Protecting health and wellness is a collective priority wherever you are in the world, and nurses attending future COPs can uphold that narrative as the world continues to find ways to address climate change.

Jessica M. Mengistab, BSN, RN
Program Manager, Climate & Clean Energy Advocacy
Alliance of Nurses for Healthy Environments

The community should be assessed for commercial lots, their safety and use, and vacant lots or unused property. Specific commercial businesses such as gas stations, auto repair shops, and dry cleaners are often common sources of toxic exposures (Amiri, 2023).

If the community has agricultural areas, these must be assessed for irrigation practices, use of pesticides, runoff, and land use practices. In addition, waste can be a source of environmental hazards. C/PHNs must assess for the presence of landfills or municipal waste incinerators, medical waste incinerators, and municipal trash collection or dumpsters throughout the community (Amiri, 2023).

Land use and transportation patterns and plans can influence the health of the community. The design of a city, community, or neighborhood affects physical activity, automobile dependence, the ability of those with age-related changes and physical disabilities to navigate the community, and opportunities for children to walk to school. Community design also highlights concerns for environmental justice when those who live in areas of low accessibility and high exposure to pollution are more likely to be in resource-limited areas and communities of color (Jackman-Murphy, 2023).

Studies of air quality exposures of bicyclists in urban settings have shown that they are exposed to higher levels of air pollution while biking in areas of heavy vehicular traffic (Adamiec et al., 2022). As communities transition to sustainable practices with more walking and biking areas, considerations should be made to reduce environmental risks for walkers and bikers in areas of high vehicular traffic.

Types of Toxic Exposures

Air

Air quality is a major variable in the health of populations. People living in areas that have poor air quality experience higher rates of disease and adverse health effects. Climate change contributes to air pollution and adversely affects health.

Our health is influenced by the air we breathe both indoors and outdoors. Ambient air, or outdoor air, is composed of gases such as nitrogen, oxygen, argon, carbon dioxide, hydrogen, neon, helium, and other gases, which are part of the atmosphere. It also contains moisture and particulate matter. The amount of hazardous material that is contained in ambient air is the reason that the Clean Air Act of 1970 was created (EPA, 2020e).

Ambient air can be affected by a number of air pollutants. Air pollution is composed of a variety of materials such as aerosols, criteria air pollutants (carbon monoxide, lead, ground-level ozone, nitrogen dioxide, sulfur dioxide, particulate matter), VOCs, and hydrofluorocarbons, as well as radon and other gases that contain harmful toxins (EPA, 2023a).

In response to the Clean Air Act of 1970, air quality is monitored by the EPA. In an effort to inform citizens about the air quality in their own communities, the EPA created the AQI, which is often reported in media sources on a daily basis. The AQI is calculated for four of the six criteria air pollutants (ground-level ozone, particle pollution, carbon monoxide, and sulfur dioxide) to determine if they exceed the national air quality standard set by the EPA, with an emphasis on effect of air pollution on health (EPA, 2023j).

The EPA's website presents a guide for the public to understand the importance of monitoring the ambient air, what the six criteria air pollutants are and how they affect health, and efforts to monitor air quality to provide public health advisories (EPA, 2023q). Additionally, the EPA offers the AirNow app, which can be used to monitor regional AQI readings and wildfire smoke. This is a useful resource for the C/PHN and community members.

The EPA publishes an annual report of *Our Nation's Air*. This report provides data and interactive graphs to visualize the trends in air quality. Through this monitoring, national air pollution has declined by 78% from 1990 to 2022 (EPA, 2023l). The American Lung Association also publishes an annual report, The *State of the Air*, and it rates air pollution at the county level while providing health data within each county (American Lung Association, 2023).

C/PHNs must understand the adverse effects of ambient air pollution to assess, monitor, and advocate for those most vulnerable, which includes children, people with lung disease, older adults, and healthy people who are active outdoors, such as outdoor workers and athletes (American Lung Association, 2023).

Health effects include irritation of the respiratory system with inflammation of the cell lining. This makes the lungs more susceptible to infection. Air pollution can also exacerbate asthma and cause chronic lung disease, reduce lung function, and lead to permanent lung damage. In addition, air pollution causes increased risk of stroke and cardiac disease, in particular acute myocardial infarctions and arrhythmias (American Lung Association, 2023; EPA, 2023l).

Indoor air quality is particularly important for home, school, and workplace assessments. When the AQI for outside air is high, in order to avoid pollutants, people are instructed to stay inside. However, indoor air quality may be poor and expose people to pollutants, microbials, and particulates that may also lead to adverse health conditions (EPA, 2023i, 2023j).

Air pollution in homes occurs from exposure to heating or combustion sources such as oil, coal, kerosene or wood; radon gas; secondhand smoke from cigarettes; building materials and furniture that contains pressed wood products; carpeting and adhesives that emit VOCs; asbestos in insulation; cleaning products; paints; varnishes, and paint removers; personal care products; and other sources used around the home such as pesticides (EPA, 2023c).

Mild health effects might be headaches and nausea; the more serious health effects include damage to the liver, kidneys, and central nervous system, as well as cancer. In addition, mold, dust, and known asthma triggers in the home can not only exacerbate asthma symptoms but also cause irritation to those with heart and lung conditions.

Air quality in school buildings is very important for staff, teachers, and students (Box 9-10). More than 56 million children and adults spend up to 6 to 8 hours in elementary and secondary school each day. In particular, children are at increased risk for a variety of reasons.

BOX 9-10 Indoor Air Quality in Schools

School environments can influence a child's health. This has been demonstrated in research studies. For example, environmental triggers have been shown to worsen asthma symptoms in children and affect student and staff absentee rates. The U.S. EPA offers a program, Healthy Schools, Healthy Kids. This program offers tools for schools regarding school air quality, building structure, transportation, and chemicals used in the building. The EPA (2023b) also offers webinars to address school indoor air quality. In addition, the EPA offers the "Air Quality Flag Program" that uses the flag colors that respond to the current local AQI to alert parents and the school community about ambient air quality. As wildfires increase, the Air Quality Flag Program can be helpful to share the effect of smoke on the local AQI. This supports parents, children, school nurses, and the wider school community to take proper precautions to reduce asthma symptoms in the student population. Nurse environmental health expert, Laura Anderko, PhD, RN, has worked with Washington, District of Columbia, school nurses on the flag program, and school officials have observed the parents respond to the air quality flags and take appropriate action to reduce asthmatic episodes for their children (Tomkins et al., 2016).

Source: EPA (2023b); Tomkins et al. (2016).

Young children are more likely to spend time on or near the floor where toxins are likely to settle, they use more hand-to-mouth behavior, and they take in more air per size than adults. Although exposures can be the same as in the home, those who attend or work in schools are in the same air environment for a large portion of their day where they are exposed to the toxins for long periods of time (EPA, 2023c).

Nurses who work in the school setting can access information through the EPA website to aid in assessments and interventions to improve air quality in schools. A comprehensive guide to healthier school environments is available at https://www.epa.gov/schools (EPA, 2023c).

Water

The human body is composed of 55% to 78% water, with, on average, newborn infants having the highest percentage of water, and adults assigned female at birth the lowest (U.S. Geological Survey [USGS], 2023a). Regardless, water is a necessary component of life. In public health, the concern is for access and safe water consumption; safe lakes, rivers, and streams for recreation; and safe waterways to support animal and plant life necessary for transport of nutrients, and ecology of the environment. The availability of clean water is becoming a very serious threat to human survival (USGS, 2023a).

Globally, over 2 billion people live in water-stressed countries and rely on drinking water that is contaminated with feces. Access to safe drinking water is expected to become more challenging with the impact of climate change (World Health Organization [WHO], 2023).

Poverty is linked with a lack of access to clean water and sanitation. Every day, approximately 1000 children die from water and sanitation-related diarrheal disease

(United Nations, 2023). The critical importance of this issue is highlighted by the UN including water and sanitation as one of its SDGs (see Chapter 16).

Drinking water is available in two forms: surface water and groundwater. Both are potential sources of contamination or pollution. Surface water sources include lakes, streams, and municipal reservoirs for water use. Underground sources, or groundwater, include aquifers that run beneath the ground level and are reached via wells and springs.

Many municipalities use reservoirs and other surface sources for their water supply, whereas in other areas, people must rely upon wells to provide their source of water. Safe drinking water is essential for human health. Public water systems provide water for community members. More than 90% of Americans are served by public water systems. Public water systems are monitored and regulated through the EPA. These regulations require that public water suppliers protect consumers from microorganisms and contaminants that are harmful to health (Box 9-11; EPA, 2023f).

The EPA does not regulate private sources of water from private wells. The individual users must be responsible for monitoring their own wells. Nurses can educate communities to review their annual water quality report if they have municipal water and those who have well water to test their water annually and any time there is an environmental change such as repair to the well system, local construction, or flooding (EPA, 2023f).

- Water can become contaminated from a number of sources, including point and nonpoint sources.
- *Point sources* are those that can be traced to one source, such as a wastewater facility release into municipal water or discharge from an industrial site.
- *Nonpoint sources* are contamination that comes from many sources and cannot be traced to a single source. Examples of nonpoint source pollution are runoff from agricultural areas, gasoline stations, and other contaminants carried by rain and waterways. Some common water contaminants are microbial (frequently *Cryptosporidium* and *Giardia*).

To rid public water systems of microorganisms, disinfection processes are used. Disinfectants that are chlorine-based can produce byproducts that can also be hazardous to health. Additionally, other inorganic (such as nitrogen derivatives, arsenic, lead, fluoride, cadmium, and mercury) and organic chemicals (commonly organophosphates, phthalates), as well as radionuclides, are frequent water contaminants (EPA, 2023f).

People can unknowingly contaminate the water supply. Between 2004 and 2009, the U.S. Geological Survey (USGS) identified that pharmaceutical manufacturing plants were a source of groundwater contamination. Further, pharmaceuticals have been found in the waterways from pharmaceuticals used by humans, excreted in their urine, and discarded into locations where they can reach water supplies but also animals are fed with hormones and antibiotics in animal feeding operations that can leach into water supplies (USGS, 2023b).

Another risk to community water supplies occurs in the communities where unconventional natural gas or oil extraction, also known as fracking, occurs. This is a process to extract natural gas or oil from deep underground for public use. Fracking has the potential to contaminate air and water from chemical sources such as methane, benzene, and other hydrocarbons, and it poses health risks to community members as well as the workers involved in extraction operations (Hill & Ma, 2022).

More recently, PFAS in drinking water have been a health concern. PFAS are a group of thousands of human-made chemicals that contain a carbon–fluorine bond that makes this group of chemicals strong enough to be used in manufacturing and consumer goods because they can withstand grease, heat, oil, and water. The carbon–fluorine bond also does not easily break down, thus PFAS are known as "forever chemicals" (ATSDR, 2023d). There are health implications of PFAS exposure. Studies have demonstrated a relationship between PFAS and elevated cholesterol, changes in liver enzymes, increased risk of kidney or testicular cancer, decreased response to childhood vaccinations, preeclampsia in people who are pregnant, and low-birth-weight infants (Anderko & Pennea, 2023; ATSDR, 2023e; Macheka et al., 2022). The science regarding PFAS and human health continues to evolve. C/PHNs should continue to monitor the health impacts and communities at greater risk for PFAS exposure. Proximity to airports, military bases, landfills, and Superfund sites could increase the risk of PFAS in the drinking water.

The Right to Know legislation and use of Safety Data Sheets provide some assurance and can be helpful in teaching clients how to better protect themselves. C/PHNs can direct community members to consult the EPA website to learn about their right to know. To locate local information, nurses and community members can visit the EPA website at www.epa.gov. Nurses can also teach their community partners how to access a consumer confidence report. Every public water system is required to provide information to consumers that identifies any detected contaminants or factors that affect the water quality for those customers that they serve. This responsibility to provide the public with information about public water systems is mandated through the Safe Drinking Water Act enacted in 1974, which established standards for safe drinking water. People can access information from their own water supplier or can visit the EPA website (EPA, 2020d).

Food

Food quality, quantity, and safety are essential to human health. Food quality refers to the relative nutritional value, cost, and variety of food available. The CDC estimates that each year more than 3000 people die from foodborne illness and 1 in 6 Americans becomes ill from food consumption (CDC, 2020).

C/PHNs frequently work closely with environmental sanitarians in state and local health departments who routinely monitor food establishments for their safety to prevent exposure to microbial agents that cause foodborne illness.

Environmental issues that affect food quality extend beyond the microbial exposures and include the availability of adequate nutritious food, chemical exposures through food additives and from agrichemicals and

BOX **9-11** STORIES FROM THE FIELD

Flint, Michigan

The public health of citizens in Flint, Michigan, was compromised in April 2014 when, in an attempt to save money, the city changed its water supply from Lake Huron water supplied by Detroit to the Flint River. Flint was once a booming automotive manufacturing area and the site of early labor strikes and conflicts. Now, the plants are closed, and jobs are scarce. Flint has some of the highest levels of violent crime, preterm birth/infant mortality, domestic violence, and illicit drug use in the state, as well as some of the poorest health outcomes (Hanna-Attisha et al., 2016). It is also marred by the effects of largely unrestrained industrial pollution from the industries that dominated the area for 80 years, as "huge amounts of lead and other toxins were pumped into the air, water, streams, and ground" (Rosner, 2016, p. 200).

After the water supply switch, residents noted changes in the taste, odor, and color of their drinking water. Flint's water system was old (with estimates of 10% to 80% of it with lead plumbing), and the city has struggled to maintain basic services in the face of declining tax revenues and high unemployment. City officials claimed that the water was fine. By August 2015, researchers had found high levels of lead in the Flint water supply, noting that the water was likely corroding the plumbing lines (Edwards, 2015). In October 2015, the Flint water supply was switched back to Detroit water from Lake Huron, but by then, Flint residents had been drinking and bathing in the tainted water for over a year. In January 2016, President Obama declared federal emergency status to help resolve the water issues (EPA, 2017).

In the meantime, researchers from Flint's Hurley Children's Hospital conducted a spatial analysis of risk and pre–/post–water system change blood lead levels for over 700 Flint children tested in their facility. They found statistically significant changes in EBLL in blood collected between the months of January to September 2014, compared to blood drawn from January to September 2015. Before the water system change, 2.4% of Flint children had EBLL, but after the change, the proportion increased to 4.9%; those children living outside Flint with no change in water source had no significant changes and low levels of lead in both samples. There were also statistically significant changes noted on demographic data, with higher proportions of African American children and greater levels for those with socioeconomic disadvantages. The "preexisting disparity in lead poisoning" broadened for those children living in Flint, especially for those with high levels of lead in their home water supply (Hanna-Attisha et al., 2016, p. 286). High blood lead levels (BLLs) can cause learning problems, lower IQ, behavioral issues, attention problems, aggression, and poor academic achievement, and the damage is irreversible (Keuhn, 2016; Wood, 2019).

By July 2018, the EPA had filed a report of the Flint water crisis and acknowledged lapses in EPA's, Michigan's, and Flint's oversight of water regulations (EPA, 2018a). The EPA agreed to improve the agency's oversight of the Safe Drinking Water Act and revise the Lead and Copper Rule to improve the effectiveness of drinking water monitoring requirements. Although this revision reduced the amount of lead required to trigger action from 15 to 10 parts per billion, critics note that enforcement requirements still appear weak and do not mandate removal of underground lead pipes (Dennis, 2019; EPA, 2018a, 2020e). Studies following the water crisis found that there was a 26% increase in White patients delivering low-birth-weight babies (there was no statistical significance for Black individuals) during that time (Abouk & Adams, 2018). Additionally, 40% of parents surveyed reported changes in their child's health and 65% reported changes in their own health (Heard-Garris et al., 2017). In 2016, criminal charges were filed against nine city and state officials for tampering with evidence, conspiracy, willful neglect of duty, and misconduct; these were dismissed but may be refiled (Kennedy, 2016). Residents are angry and no longer trust officials at any level of government to provide them with clean water (Wood, 2019).

A follow-up study regarding childhood BLL testing showed that despite the warnings of lead in water, Medicaid lead testing did not increase (Jenkins et al., 2022). This tells us that primary lead prevention is important to reduce lead exposure and that C/PHNs must support efforts to reduce lead exposure and BLL testing.

Other communities will be affected by this issue. In 2019, the city of Newark, New Jersey, finally admitted that the city's water had problems with lead levels and distributed water filters on a limited basis. The filters were ineffective; residents needed bottled water because of "ineffective corrosion treatment" at the water treatment plant that permitted lead to leach into the water supply (Fitzsimmons, 2019, para. 9).

It may be decades until we realize the full health impact of this crisis, as more cities with older buildings and infrastructure discover problems with their water. C/PHNs are among those who continue to be concerned about the current situation as well as the long-term consequences of lead exposure for the citizens of Flint, Michigan. Given the recent findings of the potential for multigenerational epigenetic changes in grandchildren linked to lead exposure in pregnant people, this environmental exposure has exponential potential for harm (Sen et al., 2015).

1. *What is the role of the community/public health nurse in addressing this issue? Which primary, secondary, and tertiary interventions could be applied?*
2. *Describe ethical issues, and potential health and social repercussions, related to this case.*
3. *List issues related to environmental justice in this case and describe how to address them.*

Source: Abouk & Adams (2018); Dennis (2019); Edwards (2015); Fitzsimmons (2019); Hanna-Attisha et al. (2016); Heard-Garris et al. (2017); Jenkins et al. (2022); Kennedy (2016); Keuhn (2016); Rosner (2016); Sen et al. (2015); U.S. Environmental Protection Agency (2017, 2018a, 2020e); Wood (2019).

antibiotics, contaminated food from diseased animals, and improper food handling. Pesticides are ubiquitous in the environment and are transmitted to humans through foods. Fresh fruits and vegetables must be thoroughly washed to remove pesticide residue (FDA, 2023a).

After production, many foods are processed for the market. Food additives such as dyes and flavors provide color and often improve the flavor of foods. Leavening and thickening agents improve consistency, while preservatives keep food from spoiling on the shelf. Many of these additives can be harmful to health with examples being linked to cancer and endocrine disruption.

There has been concern about genetically modified foods being marketed. These concerns not only address the safety of food for human consumption but also raise questions about the ecologic impact and sustainability. Like many public health policies and regulations, the U.S. Food and Drug Administration (FDA), EPA, and U.S. Department of Agriculture together monitor to ensure that the genetically modified foods are safe for humans, animals, and plants (FDA, 2023a, 2023b).

Microbial outbreaks are common from a variety of bacteria (*Shigella*, *Salmonella*, *Campylobacter*, *Escherichia coli*) and parasites (*Cryptosporidium parvum*, *Amoeba*; CDC, 2020). In 2023, for example, CDC reported a *Salmonella* outbreak linked to ground beef in the Northeastern United States (New York, New Jersey, Connecticut, Rhode Island, and Massachusetts) and another associated with raw cookie dough in the Northwestern United States (Oregon, Washington, Idaho, and Utah) (CDC, 2023c).

Although the public often hears about these outbreaks through the media, they may not be as aware of the risks from chemical contaminants. A great resource for families and community members is the Partnership for Food Safety Education (2023) that promotes safe food handling and education for both children and adults.

The FDA (2023a) is charged with the responsibility to ensure the safety of food produced, shipped, imported, and sold in the United States. This includes the monitoring of microbial toxins and chemicals such as lead and cadmium, pesticides, food additives, and packaging.

Fish and other seafood are an important part of food safety. Nurses should be aware and instruct communities to monitor fish advisories (EPA, 2019). The advisories warn consumers of contaminants (mercury, polychlorinated biphenyls, chlordane, dioxins, and DDT). Additionally, PFAS are an emerging hazard to our waterways that can contaminate seafood (FDA, 2022). These contaminants persist in the environment, particularly in river and lake sediments where fish consume them from bottom-feeding organisms (Fig. 9-6).

Bioaccumulation refers to the process where toxins accumulate in greater concentration in an organism than the rate of elimination. Toxins can accumulate from direct exposure or from eating contaminated food products. Through biomagnification, the toxins present at lower levels of the food chain are in greater concentration in those species further up the chain.

The Pesticide Action Network (2023) uses data from the USDA Pesticide Program to identify commonly applied pesticides for many foods. Consumers can consult their website, What's on my food?, to be informed of foods that pose the most serious threats to health, particularly for the most vulnerable groups.

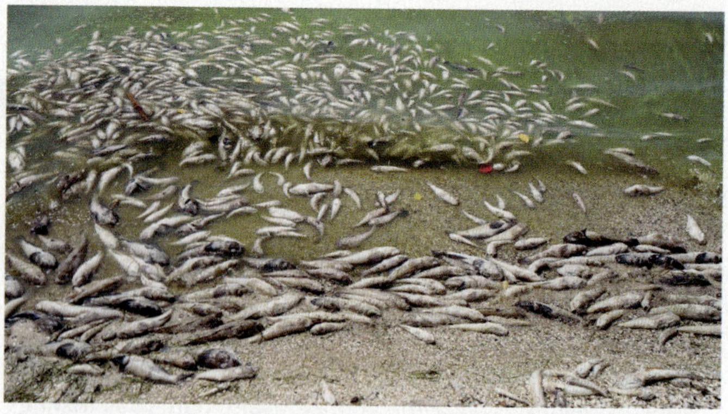

FIGURE 9-6 Fish contain valuable nutrients, but contaminated waterways can make fish a health risk.

In addition, the effect of climate change on weather extremes (droughts, floods, and storms), changes in rainfall and water supply for soil, rising atmospheric GHGs, soil salinization, and the ecology of microbial growth will have negative impacts on the food supply. Extreme weather events increase the likelihood of chemical contaminants and pesticide exposures from runoff that occurs with flooding.

Agriculture and fisheries industries are sensitive to climate conditions related to changes in temperature and levels of CO_2 in the atmosphere, which threaten food safety and security (Duchenne-Moutien & Neetoo, 2021). Additionally, our changing climate has led to loss of nutritional content (Zhu et al., 2018) and impact on water resources and crop production (De Pinto et al., 2020). Furthermore, agricultural workers are exposed to extreme weather events and pesticides.

Vulnerable Groups. C/PHNs must also be aware of the increased vulnerability of certain groups. For example, people who are pregnant are likely to transmit their exposure to chemicals, pesticides, and toxins to the unborn fetus. Children are more susceptible to hazards from food and waterborne pathogens because of their immature gastrointestinal systems and increased food and water intake per size compared to adults, and those with altered immunity due to cancer, diabetes, and other health conditions are more likely to be affected by food exposures. People living in resource-limited communities, people of color, and people who do not speak or read English are also vulnerable to environmental exposures.

Nurses can be a resource to ensure that community members learn about the specific local risks and identify ways to decrease their risk. Environmental health education must be targeted to the cultural, educational, economic, and language needs of the community. The EPA and CDC have a wealth of evidence-based information to educate and protect public health. The information is available to health professionals and the general public. Many of these tools and resources are available in different languages to meet the unique needs of diverse communities.

Toxic Waste

People, families, schools, governmental agencies, healthcare facilities, and industries all create waste that must be managed to minimize environmental impact and protect human health. The EPA reports that in 2018, Americans generated about 292.4 million tons of municipal solid waste. This comes to 4.9 lb of waste per person, per day (EPA, 2023d).

In an effort to minimize waste and environmental impact, local, state, and federal agencies have begun supporting sustainable practices that highlight the environmental value of reducing and reusing products and composting food and lawn waste. The EPA offers a waste management hierarchy that highlights the value of reducing and reusing materials as a priority and recycling is the second level, when the items are not able to be reused (EPA, 2023d).

In particular, our use of plastics and its ecologic impact on sea life highlights the importance of reducing and reusing products. The waste management hierarchy offers an upstream approach to reducing waste at the source of waste generation. For healthcare facilities, this can mean environmentally preferred purchasing of products that contain recycled materials and are more energy efficient, safer, and healthier for patients, healthcare workers, and the environment (Health Care Without Harm, 2023).

Although efforts are made to reduce health risks, hazardous wastes continue to be produced. These wastes include solvent wastes, dioxins, wastes from electroplating and other metal finishing operations, wastes from oil refineries, organic chemicals, pesticides, explosives, lead processing materials, and wood preservatives. We are exposed to these chemicals if they are aerosolized into the ambient air, leach into the ground or wells, and reach the soil where children play or crops are produced. What is particularly dangerous for human exposure is the fact that most community members are unaware of the hazards in their communities.

Communities may be burdened with many brownfield sites, as well as those listed on the National Priorities List of hazardous sites such as Superfund sites (EPA, 2018b). Popular media such as books, films, newspapers, television, and social media may be the first place that nurses become aware of communities affected by toxic waste. The Flint water crisis was played out in the news and chronicled in Dr. Mona Hanna-Attisha's (2019) book, *What the Eyes Don't See*.

Nurses should be knowledgeable about the toxic hazards in their own communities and those where the patients and families they care for reside. Through the EPA Superfund website (https://www.epa.gov/superfund/search-superfund-sites-where-you-live) and the EJScreen mapping tool (https://www.epa.gov/ejscreen), nurses can assist community members in learning about Superfund sites that impact their communities. Further, on the EPA Brownfields website, nurses and community members can learn about *Brownfields and Land Revitalization Near You* (https://www.epa.gov/brownfields/brownfields-near-you). It is important for the nurse to be alert for reports of toxic exposure risk, evaluate the science and toxicological risk, and advocate for community/public health. The nurse can support communities in petitioning ATSDR to evaluate possible contamination affecting human health (ATSDR, 2023b).

Radiation

Humans are exposed to radiation in a variety of forms. Risks and forms of radiation are generally categorized as ionizing and nonionizing radiation. Ionization refers to the process where the atomic particle (ion) breaks away from the nucleus of the atom. Ionizing radiation occurs in natural forms as radon gas and cosmic radiation from the atmosphere. Nonionizing radiation refers to radiation from sources such as infrared, microwave, and radio wave radiation (EPA, 2023o).

Radon is an odorless, naturally occurring, ionizing, radioactive gas. Radon can seep into the foundation of homes from the ground and expose residents to the radiation effects. Radon exposure is a leading cause of non–tobacco smoking lung cancer.

Nurses must be aware of areas with high radon risk and should be sure that community members are educated about the risks of radon. Community members can access the EPA's *A Citizen's Guide to Radon: The Guide to Protecting Yourself and Your Family from Radon* from their website (EPA, 2023n, 2023o). EPA map of radon zones is available at https://www.epa.gov/radon/epa-map-radon-zones.

Another form of radiation that has public health concerns is electromagnetic radiation (EMR). EMR can be ionizing or nonionizing radiation. Electricity creates low-frequency, nonionizing radiation (EPA, 2023p). There is emerging evidence of possible relationships between EMR and human health. Electromagnetic hypersensitivity or "microwave syndrome" has been noted to affect the neurologic, cognitive, and cardiovascular systems (Stein & Udasin, 2020). More research is needed to identify and confirm the effects of EMR on public health.

Policy Development

C/PHNs participate in the other core functions of public health for environmental health nursing. Policy development is the core function that addresses the need for legislation to protect human health. In addition, policy development also provides opportunities for nurses to engage with communities in addressing policies specific to their needs.

To advocate for change, C/PHN must be informed about the community hazards, existing legislation, and governmental and nongovernmental groups that can be partners in the efforts to protect health. C/PHNs must also partner and collaborate with community members and youth to amplify the environmental health concern (Cardarelli et al., 2021). C/PHNs provide a critical link in identifying the influence of the environment and social and structural determinants of health upon human health for policymakers.

Nurses can begin their environmental advocacy by writing letters to their legislators in support of health-protective laws such as sustainable energy choices, improved air quality, or ecologic agricultural practices. Important nursing actions related to environmental policy are to advocate for health-protective policies and to inform community members about the health risks related to the specific issue (Moyer, 2023).

Additionally, letters to local newspapers and periodicals can remind community members of safe practices in the home and personal environment. Nurses can also present testimony at public forums or hearings. As knowledgeable and trusted members of the community, C/PHNs help educate and empower community members to advocate for their environmental health concerns (American Nurses Association, 2022).

C/PHNs serve on local and national committees and boards to advocate for change. Examples of agencies where nurses play an advocacy role are the Children's Environmental Health Network, Just Green Partnership, local and country environmental and climate change groups, state nurses associations, environmental affairs committees, and Health Care Without Harm, to name just a few. Nurses engaged in environmental health research can share the findings of successful environmental health nursing interventions to promote policy change.

For nurses to function effectively as advocates for safer environments, it is essential to be aware of important legislation for environmental health. Nurses can also use the *EnviRN* website to follow current advocacy efforts in nursing practice. Finally, all eligible nurses should be registered to vote and consider the impact of the environment when voting at the local, state, and national levels. For more on policy development and advocacy, see Chapter 13. See ANHE (envirn.org) for a list of important legislation related to environmental protection.

Assurance

The public health regulatory function for policy ensures that appropriate services are provided. This demands that C/PHNs must incorporate environmental health principles into practice (ANA, 2021, 2022).

For example, a C/PHN will educate families to reduce their risks from environmental hazards in the home, an OHN will ensure that safety regulations are followed in work settings, or a school nurse will ensure that indoor air quality is monitored for the school setting. Assurance guarantees that policy and regulatory functions are followed through the provision of public health essential services. The following examples illustrate how community nurses fulfill the assurance function.

Home

People spend 90% of their time in their homes. To ensure that nurses are prepared to address environmental risks to health in home settings, competencies for nursing education include home assessment strategies. Nurses working with families and in communities participate in research programs and collaborative projects that impact home environments.

To address some of those health issues, particularly for children, the U.S. Department of Housing and Urban Development (USHUD, 2023) created the Healthy Homes Program to protect children and their families from health and safety hazards in their homes. The program targets multiple childhood diseases and injuries in the home by using a comprehensive approach. Some of the environmental health concerns addressed include lead, carbon monoxide, pesticides, radon, mold, home safety, and asthma. C/PHNs have led, collaborated, and found sustainable solutions to Healthy Homes projects.

Severe Weather Events

A second area for nurses to ensure that essential services are provided to community members is in response to severe weather events (Fig. 9-7). Although studies indicate that nurses are involved in disaster response, results indicate that nurses are not always prepared for their role in emergency response situations (Su et al., 2023).

The United States is experiencing more frequent and severe weather events. As of the end of the summer in 2023, the cost of these events had already exceeded past years, with the exception of 2005 ($202.7 billion) and 2017 ($184.4 billion). The expenses for the first 8 months of 2023 were over 57.6 billion U.S. dollars. Extreme weather events, such as flooding, heat, tornadoes, extreme cold, and wildfires caused damage and destruction across the United States (The Weather Chanel, 2023; Box 9-12).

Whereas Chapter 17 discusses disasters and the role of public health, this chapter covers some specific issues related to environmental risks that occur after severe weather events or disasters that are important for C/PHNs. These include power outages, safe water and food supply, wastewater, mold, toxic exposures, and poor air quality (EPA, 2020d).

For example, when there is a power outage, many families depend upon generators to supply electricity. These can be a source of carbon monoxide poisoning if they are not effectively functioning or properly ventilated. During cold weather, families may use wood or kerosene for heat that can pose a danger of fire, explosion, and asphyxiation from carbon monoxide, but kerosene heaters can also emit other pollutants including carbon dioxide, nitrogen dioxide, and sulfur dioxide.

In particular, people who are pregnant, people who have asthma, people with cardiovascular disease, older

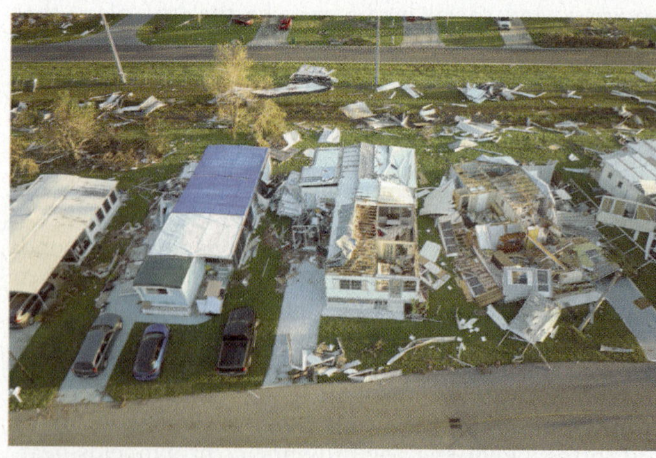

FIGURE 9-7 Severe weather, like tornadoes, can have a serious impact on the environment and population health.

BOX 9-12 PERSPECTIVES

A Nurse's Viewpoint on a California Wildfire

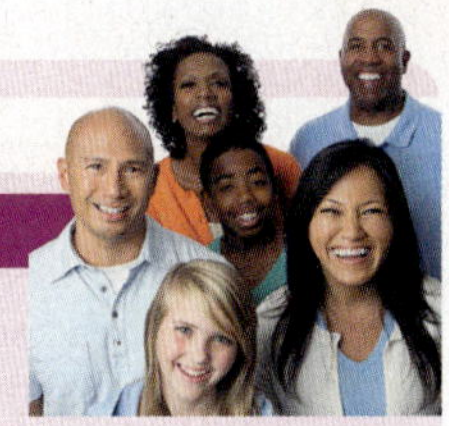

In November 2018, California experienced the worst wildfire in its history to date. Eighty-eight people lost their lives and 12,000 homes were destroyed. The town of Paradise, California, was engulfed in flames, and nurse manager, Allyn Pierce, was among the last to evacuate patients from the town's hospital. As they traveled through the evacuation route with heavy traffic and smoke fires burning on both sides of the road, Mr. Pierce knew that his family had already been evacuated to safety days earlier. After a harrowing evacuation, he returned to the hospital to assist first responders, primary providers, and other nurses to help smoke inhalation victims and those with more serious injuries. Afterward, Mr. Pierce reported that although he was frightened for his own safety, he did what nurses are trained to do, remain calm, work within the team, and address the situation. He also reported that following the wildfires, he has had unsettling moments where he sees fires in his sleep.

In addition to the loss of life and property, the air quality in the surrounding area had reached the "dangerously unhealthy" range for 10 consecutive days requiring San Francisco bay area (roughly 170 miles away) to close schools and issue warnings to limit outdoor activity.

Source: Santiago (2018).

adults, and young children are at particular risk from these toxic emissions. Nurses must inform community members of safety in the home when using alternate sources of heat or power.

If a home is without power, there is a risk for food storage and safety. If the home has a well and water pump, there may not be access to potable water during the power outage. Community members should be informed of issues related to the safe storage of food and the need to dispose of improperly refrigerated foods.

Homes that have septic systems may find that they have overflowed if there is any flooding from a severe storm. It is important to understand when it is safe to return to well or septic system use after ground-level flooding.

Floods also pose a problem to residents who have water that enters their homes. Standing water can cause mold and mildew, possibly harm home furnaces, pose a risk of fire, and release toxins into the water and air. Small children and older adults are at more risk of environmental exposures during and after a natural disaster, and the C/PHN must address not only emergency planning but also safe remediation strategies to avoid toxic exposures among community members (EPA, 2020d).

GLOBAL ENVIRONMENTAL HEALTH

Nurses must engage in strategies to protect human health in their communities through the core functions of public health: assessment, policy development, and assurance. To effectively do this, nurses must think globally in order to be effective locally. This means adopting an ecologic perspective related to impacts on human health.

By broadening our perspectives, consideration of foods imported from countries around the world, toys made in other countries and used in the United States, and the manufacture of products in locations where the regulations for safety are not as stringent (or in some cases more stringent) as in the United States is helpful for nurses in addressing environmental health knowledge and advocacy. See Chapter 9 for an example.

Nurses who endorse "green nursing" by promoting more ecologic and environmentally safe practices in their workplace are making an impact on global environmental health. The UN SDGs call on us to think more broadly as global citizens of the multiple factors that influence thriving communities and thus enhance human health. Also, nurses are engaging globally to collaborate in addressing environmental risks, climate change, and planetary health (see Chapter 16).

Climate change reinforces that we are one ecosystem. What is placed in the environment in the form of GHGs affects the entire planet and the human family. Although it is now illegal in most countries to dump waste into the ocean or to ship waste to resource-limited countries that have less stringent laws to protect their citizens from toxins, large quantities of toxic industrial waste, medical waste, toxic ash from incinerators, as well as the growing issue of e-waste from computers and other electronic products have found their way to ocean waters and resource-limited countries. In order to fully promote the health of populations, nurses must take personal action to reduce their use of products (particularly those with toxic chemicals), reuse as much as possible, and recycle (in safe processes) to decrease their personal environmental footprint (ANA, 2021; EPA, 2020c). Nurses must also incorporate the environmental health knowledge and skills mandated by the ANA *Scope and Standards of Nursing Practice* into their nursing practice (ANA, 2021). See Chapter 16 for more on global health issues.

CASE STUDY **10 ESSENTIAL PUBLIC HEALTH SERVICES**

Environmental Community Concerns

The citizens of Trenton, a small rural community in the Rocky Mountains, have become concerned about their drinking water because of fracking activities. In your work in the local community hospital, you have noticed more pediatric hospital admissions for asthma exacerbations, and a recent study pointed out that children exposed to newly drilled gas wells were more likely to be hospitalized for an asthma-related diagnosis (Bushong et al., 2022). Community members said they felt powerless; they reported health problems and concerns about the quality of their air and water (Black et al., 2021), but the elected officials and government agencies did not respond. Meanwhile, nurses and other health professionals in a nearby state were attending town halls and meetings with state and federal policymakers to prevent a proposed natural gas pipeline from being routed through their communities. These health professionals cited air quality, water quality, and safety concerns related to the required infrastructure to transport the gas through their region and to nearby states.

1. ***Recognize Cues:*** *Which findings require immediate follow-up, are unexpected, or are most concerning?*
2. ***Analyze Cues:*** *What information is noted or needed for interpreting findings?*
3. ***Prioritize Hypotheses:*** *Based on the information that you have, what is happening?*
4. ***Generate Solutions:*** *What intervention(s) will achieve the desired outcome?*
5. ***Take Action:*** *What actions should you take or do first?*
6. ***Evaluate Outcomes:*** *Were outcomes achieved? Why or why not?*
7. *Which Essential Public Health Services influence this situation? (See Box 2-2.)*

SUMMARY

- Environmental health is a discipline encompassing all the elements of the environment that influence the health and well-being of its inhabitants.
- C/PHNs include environmental health in their practice by:
  - Accessing environmental information from reliable resources
  - Relying on environmental frameworks such as HIA, the precautionary principle, and planetary health to determine and address risk
  - Utilizing an upstream approach to reduce environmental risk
  - Monitoring for causal links between people and their environments
  - Including an ecologic perspective by linking the human–environment relationship and how the health of one affects the health of the other
  - Addressing specific needs of groups that are vulnerable to environmental risk
  - Advocating for health-protective policies
  - Addressing climate change mitigation and adaptation
  - Understanding that what is done today may affect the health of future generations
- Both public and private sectors are involved in regulating, monitoring, and preventing environmental health problems.
- Utilizing the core functions for public health, the C/PHN recognizes the key role of assessment, assurance, and policy development to influence change in the health of people, families, communities, and the environment.
- The C/PHN should be a leader of the team of health professionals who promote and protect the reciprocal relationship between the environment and the public's health.

ACTIVE LEARNING EXERCISES

1. How important is engaging in climate mitigation and adaptation? This effort has met with resistance from a variety of people. There are several organizations that have examined messaging about climate and health risk.
   a. Examine the Yale Climate Opinion Map at https://climatecommunication.yale.edu/visualizations-data/ycom-us/
   b. Select your state and county or a state and county of interest.
   c. Choose five topics in the select topic response for the selected state and county. Look at the county-level response to the topic you selected. Were you surprised by the response? Why or why not? How does this fit with the ecological model for public health? How can you address this as a C/PHN? What preventative or upstream approaches might be considered? (Objectives 1 and 2)
2. Have you heard alerts on TV or radio or seen internet reports about unhealthy air quality? Do you know what toxic substances are in your community's air? How do these impact you and sensitive groups such as children, people who are pregnant, older adults, resource-limited communities, and immigrant groups?
   a. You can find out by examining AirNow websites (http://www.airnow.gov/). Other helpful sites may be found through the CDC, the EPA, and local air resources boards or agencies. Go on a computer scavenger hunt and see what you can find.

b. Look at the air quality index (AQI) in your community. Are there any air pollutants that could cause health problems? (Objective 3)
c. Look around your community. What are the most common environmental hazards? Look at the AQI and air facilities on the map on this site. Be sure to read about radon too. How might these impact the air you breathe?
d. Find the AirNow website and enter your zip code. For your city or area, which three companies have the highest amounts of emissions? Are there any VOCs, metals, or polycyclic aromatic hydrocarbons listed for the top company?
e. If you were a school nurse, what would be your concerns for the children's exposures to air pollution?
f. If you were a home care nurse, what would be your concerns for the older patients you care for?
g. How could you advocate for change? What professionals, government agencies, and institutions might assist in reducing environmental threats? (Objective 6)

3. As a nursing student, it is important to know about common community hazards in order to educate community members. Visit the EPA's MyEnvironment website, and enter your home zip code or that of the community where you work. The link for this site is https://enviro.epa.gov/myenvironment/.

   There you will find headings for MyMaps, MyAir, MyWater, MyEnergy, MyHealth, MyClimate, MyLand, MyEnvironmentReports, and MyCommunity.

   a. Look through these headings to identify the hazards in your community. What is the air quality? Are there particular industries, power plants, or high areas for auto emissions that affect health? What about water quality? Are there significant toxic waste sites? What types of exposures are there in the community?
   b. Can you identify possible risks from climate change and severe weather events? What might be ways to assure emergency preparedness for those most at risk?
   c. Using the framework for this chapter, the core public health functions, select a strategy that is most appropriate for your community for each area: assessment, policy development, and assurance (Objective 4)

4. Conduct a walking tour of a community. Consider housing stock, industry, the built environment, and open space.
   a. What do you observe that could be an environmental risk for this community?
   b. Do you observe specific vulnerable populations in the community?
   c. Use the resources at the EPA website, including MyEnvironment, and develop a list of five recommendations to reduce environmental health risks in the community you observed. Identify why these are an environmental health risk for this community.
   d. Describe which of the 10 Essential Public Health Services (Box 2-2) applies here. (Objective 5)

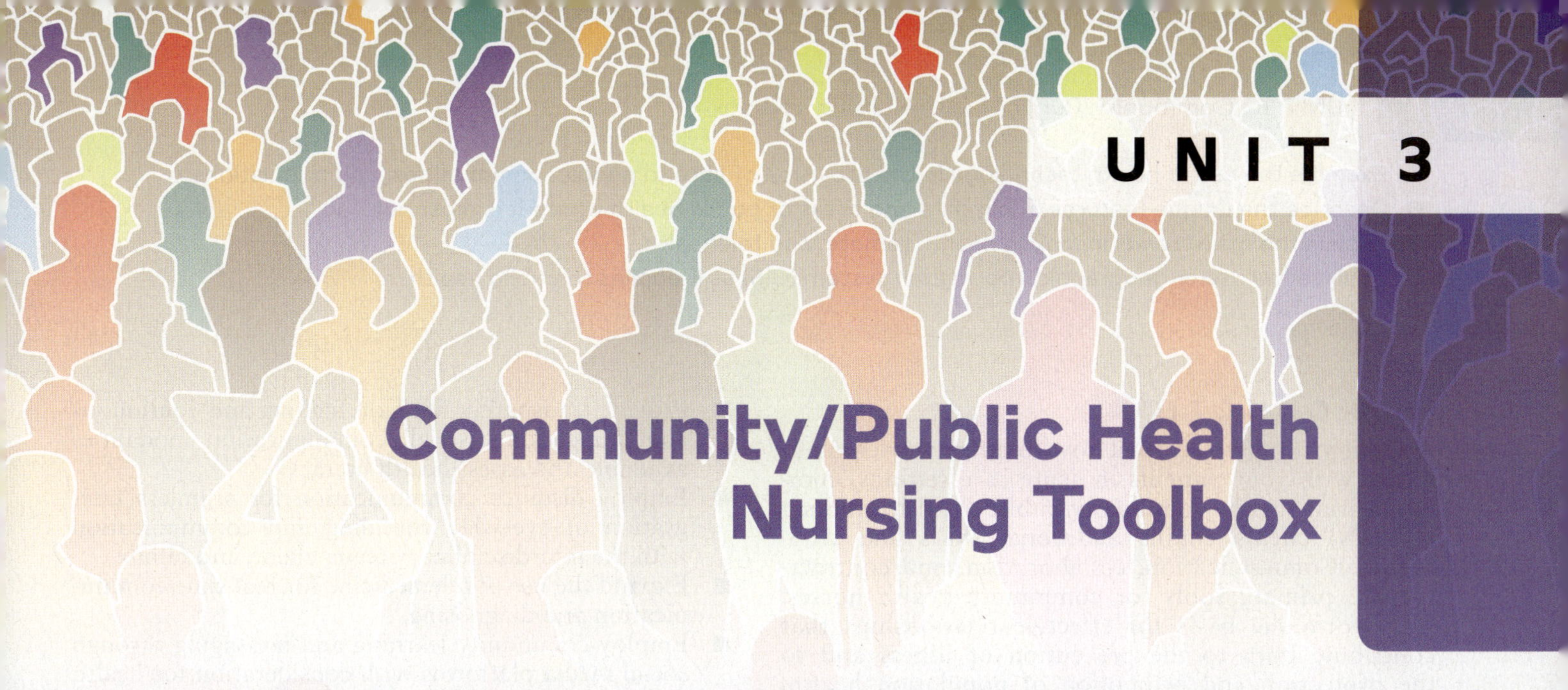

UNIT 3

Community/Public Health Nursing Toolbox

CHAPTER 10

Communication, Collaboration, and Technology

"To effectively communicate, we must realize that we are all different in the way we perceive the world and use this understanding as a guide to our communication with others."

—Tony Robbins

KEY TERMS

- Active listening
- Asset-based community development (ABCD)
- Big data
- Blogs/weblogs
- Brainstorming
- Community-based participatory research (CBPR)
- Contracting
- Critical pathway
- Digital health
- Electronic health records (EHRs)
- Feedback loop
- Geographic information system (GIS)
- Health technology
- Informatics
- Mobile health (mHealth)
- Multivoting
- Nominal group technique
- Organizational health literacy
- Personal health literacy
- Podcasts
- Telehealth
- Vlogs

LEARNING OBJECTIVES

Upon mastery of this chapter, you should be able to:

1. Describe effective communication strategies and the use of information and communication technologies in the care of people, communities, and populations.
2. Summarize the key issues related to health literacy.
3. Recognize group dynamics and the value of working with interprofessional community partners.
4. Discuss the value of contracting to both clients and community/public health nurses.

5. Examine the use of health technology in the provision of care to people, communities, and populations.
6. Describe the unique features of big data and areas of public health where it is most helpful.
7. Explain the main trends in mobile health, remote, and telehealth.
8. Analyze the use of geographic information system (GIS) as it applies to public health.

INTRODUCTION

Although you have learned how to effectively communicate with your patients in acute care settings, communicating with community/public health nursing (C/PHN) clients entails additional skills and techniques. Communication, collaboration, and contracting are primary tools for community health nurses. They form the basis for effective relationships that contribute both to the prevention of illness and to the protection and promotion of population health. Additionally, digital technology is now prevalent in all aspects of health, with rapid innovations changing how C/PH nurses provide healthcare. Health literacy must also be considered as a concept that is important because of its relationship to health promotion and disease prevention and management. For the nurse accustomed to communicating one-on-one with clients, communicating as part of an interprofessional team and with community groups requires new skills for effective collaboration.

Health technology serves as a powerful equalizer for improving health education and access to care among vulnerable and underrepresented populations by reaching people where they are and in whatever environment they live. This chapter examines these tools and discusses their integration into C/PHN practice.

COMMUNICATION IN COMMUNITY/PUBLIC HEALTH NURSING

Effective communication is vital to all areas of nursing and is considered to be a fundamental core competency needed in C/PHN practice. The Council of Public Health Nurse Organizations (CPHNO) Competencies include communication skills as one of the eight competency domains (CPHNO, 2018).

Nurses working in C/PH must be skilled in effective communication to be able to maintain relationships with individual clients, families, the community, members of the healthcare team, and community partners (Harmon et al., 2020). The lack of effective communication can lead to misunderstanding, poor performance, interpersonal conflict, ineffective program development, and medical mistakes, all resulting in poorer health outcomes. Ineffective communication is one of the major causes of preventable adverse events in acute care settings; effective communication skills and lessons learned through COVID-19 include transparency and collaboration between healthcare teams, clients, and the larger community (Agency for Healthcare Research and Quality [AHRQ], 2021, para 11).

- Include all interdisciplinary team members and apply innovative approaches to care.
- Provide transparent decision making and continuous communication; use all communication modalities available and assess health literacy.
- Employ distance communication for seamless integration of everyday rounding and communication with the interdisciplinary team, client, and family.
- Expand the use of telemedicine for real-time communication and diagnosing.
- Employ community learning and messaging through social media platforms with consideration for health literacy.

Successful nurses must use both sound clinical skills and good communication skills (Arnold & Boggs, 2020). Necessary communication skills include soliciting input from others and listening to others in a nonjudgmental way.

Communication provides a two-way flow of information that nourishes nurse–client and nurse–professional relationships. For communication to take place, client and professional messages are sent and received. As participants in the communication process, C/PH nurses play both roles: sender and receiver. The nurse must be able to elicit ideas as well as contribute to the planning process by speaking and acting in ways that promote information sharing.

The Communication Process

Communication, in its simplest form, is the sending and receiving of a message, a process by which one assigns and conveys meaning to create shared understanding. This process incorporates the conventional aspects of communication: sender, receiver, message, channel (e.g., verbal, nonverbal, social networking), encoding, decoding, and feedback (e.g., checking the message meaning, revising for clarity) (Salik & Ashurst, 2023). This process forms a communication loop, which is shown in Figure 10-1.

Strategies to Overcome Communication Barriers

Community/public health nurses should be aware of the barriers that block effective communication (Box 10-1). Overcoming barriers to effective communication requires the development of sound communication skills, including sending, receiving, and interpersonal skills.

Establish Trust and Rapport

Nurses are considered knowledgeable professionals who have a standing within the community. Those working for public health agencies have power and authority as government agency representatives. Clients may feel apprehensive about C/PHNs entering their homes.

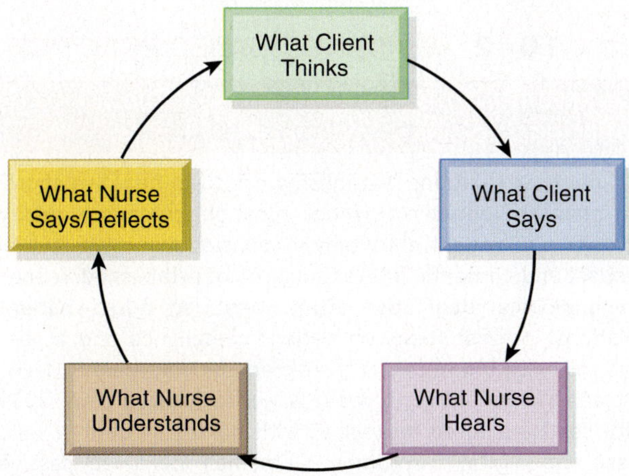

FIGURE 10-1 The communication process.

Therefore, the nurse needs to demonstrate respect for the client, especially for those clients who lack self-respect. Having an appreciation for the dignity and worth of all people, being nonjudgmental, and demonstrating empathy (acceptance and acknowledgment of the client's situation and feelings) are prerequisites for successful communication with clients in the community setting (Bryne et al., 2020). To establish trust and rapport with clients and to incorporate a patient-centered care mindset, a nurse must:

- Recognize client uniqueness: Recognize the uniqueness of each person where care is tailored to the client.
- Create partnership: Develop and maintain trust by being consistently trustworthy, reliable, sincere, and truthful with clients.
- Demonstrate professional practice: Partner with the client through a professional relationship with concern for the client's life and challenges. The nurse must demonstrate professional attributes such as respect, compassion, and nonjudgmental behaviors; professional competence; recognize the client's competence and their ability to decide; and meet the physical and emotional needs of the client. Additionally, the nurse must be flexible in offering choices while creating opportunities for engagement while freely giving information and listening with engagement.

BOX 10-1 Barriers to Effective Communication in Community/Public Health Nursing

Selective Perception

People interpret a message through their own perceptions, which are influenced by their own experience, interests, values, motivations, and expectations. This perceptual screen leads to possible distortion or misinterpretation of the meaning from the sender's original intent. Nurses can overcome this barrier by using the **feedback loop** to ask clients to voice their understanding of the message they just received from the nurse. This enhances clarification and correction of misunderstandings, which is an essential step in the communication process.

Filtering

Filtering is described as manipulation of information by the sender in order to make it seem more favorable to the receiver. Clients sometimes use filtering during the assessment process, giving only partial or distorted information because they think this is what health professionals want to hear. Filtering can also affect community/public health nurses. Cole (1990), in a classic work, noted that we have "filters" through which we view others—often influenced by culture, ethnicity, and socioeconomic class or even gender—and these can lead to miscommunication. Cole's (1990) premise is that people from different backgrounds actually view the world differently, thus confounding communication and leading to prejudice and stereotyping. Community/public health nurses should consider their communication style and those of the people with whom they come in contact.

Emotional Influence

How a person feels at the time a message is sent or received influences the meaning. Emotions can interfere with rational and objective reasoning, thus blocking communication. Nurses need to be aware of their own emotions and the emotional status of clients or health professionals with whom they are communicating. For example, it is important for community/public health nurses to remain calm and unruffled when dealing with families in crisis. Family communication may be angry, blaming, and confrontational because of a child's serious health crisis, for instance. A calm, firm, reassuring presence can go far in diffusing the situation and promoting clearer and more constructive communication. You may say, "I sense that you are feeling upset about Joey's diagnosis. Are there any questions I can answer for you? How can I be of help to you?"

Language Barriers

People interpret the meaning of words differently, depending on many variables, such as age, education, cultural background, and primary spoken language. For example, an adolescent might understand the term "lit" to mean that something is good or exciting, whereas an 80-year-old person might understand the word refers to lighting. In the community, nurses work with a wide range of clients and professionals whose disparate ages, education levels, and cultural backgrounds lead to different communication patterns.

Language of Nursing

The context of healthcare provides nurses with a unique vocabulary that may not be understood by clients, family, and community members. The use of scientific terminology or jargon by some health professionals can be confusing to clients. Communication techniques would be different when educating a new parent on proper breastfeeding techniques than when discussing community health needs with the director of a public health department.

Source: Cain et al. (2018); Cole (1990).

- Foster autonomy: Allow clients to make decisions about their care, to foster autonomy and participation. Balance the power between provider and receiver; allow for the sharing of knowledge (Bryne et al., 2020).

Many factors that are shaped by clients' cultural background and upbringing influence trust and rapport. For many, the societal norm is to agree with someone in a position of authority, such as a C/PHN, even if they do not fully understand what that person is communicating. This can lead to mistrust and poor client outcomes. Establishing a trusting relationship can empower clients to accomplish important lifestyle changes (Box 10-2). However, it is important to keep in mind that although nurses have a good deal of knowledge and education, to be effective they must appreciate the knowledge clients have gained through life experiences and the environments in which they live (Pratt et al., 2020) while appreciating the knowledge that each one possesses.

Showing respect is a fundamental behavior that conveys the attitude that clients and others have knowledge, importance, dignity, and worth (Kossenniemi et al., 2019). C/PHNs can work with clients in many ways to change their lives for the better. But just like acute care nurses need to "know the patient" in the hospital setting in order to pick up subtle cues that may indicate serious problems, we must begin with what is important to the client rather than our own agenda (Johansson & Martensson, 2019, p. 120). A new nurse making a home visit to a parent who has missed several immunization clinic appointments for their infant may think that the patient only needs information on why immunizations are important for their baby. However, the patient may be dealing with an abusive partner who has substance misuse issues. If the nurse begins the visit with a reminder about the missed appointments and the potential consequences involved, it may end abruptly. It is best to begin by asking about the client's concerns so the nurse can gain a deeper understanding of the client's experiences, fears, and perspectives while communicating a demeanor of understanding and the intention to help (Serin & Tuluce, 2021).

BOX 10-2 EVIDENCE-BASED PRACTICE

Community/Public Health Nurse—Client Relationship

The nurse—patient relationship can have negative short-term and long-term effects on patient outcomes, quality of care, and patient autonomy in decision making if mutual respect and authentic interaction are not established. A phenomenological qualitative study identified nurse—patient relationships that focus on patient compliance and a passive role with the nurse as the expert (Molina-Mula & Gallo-Estrada, 2020). Nursing records were reviewed from 2019 with semistructured interviews with nurses through a field diary and digital recordings. Outcomes identified passive patient responses such as following instructions, accepting the illness, and collaborating with the health team tied to nurse empathy, support, care, and a positive nurse—patient relationship. Complicit actions by the patient were more likely to be associated with a "good" patient.

The outcomes of the study identified that the nurse—patient relationship is viewed on the merits of the patient's obedience, thereby influencing quality, outcomes, and patient decision making. While good intentions come with a maternalistic perspective, patients cannot gain trust or honest communication if a reciprocal relationship is not established. Equal distribution of power allows patients autonomy in the decision-making process and respect of patient values and beliefs.

Source: Molina-Mula and Gallo-Estrada (2020).

Actively Listen

An essential skill is active listening, also referred to as reflective listening. **Active listening** is the skill of assuming responsibility for and striving to understand the feelings and thoughts in a sender's message, thus giving importance to the person speaking (Center for Creative Leadership [CCL], 2022). See Figure 10-2 for skills that promote active listening.

Active listening with nonjudgmental empathy (see Fig. 10-3) helps to communicate acceptance and increase trust. It also allows for an accurate understanding of another person's viewpoint and helps to bring issues and concerns into the open, where they can be more easily resolved (CCL, 2022). However, our own personal beliefs and values may confuse the message. A critical response to the client's message by

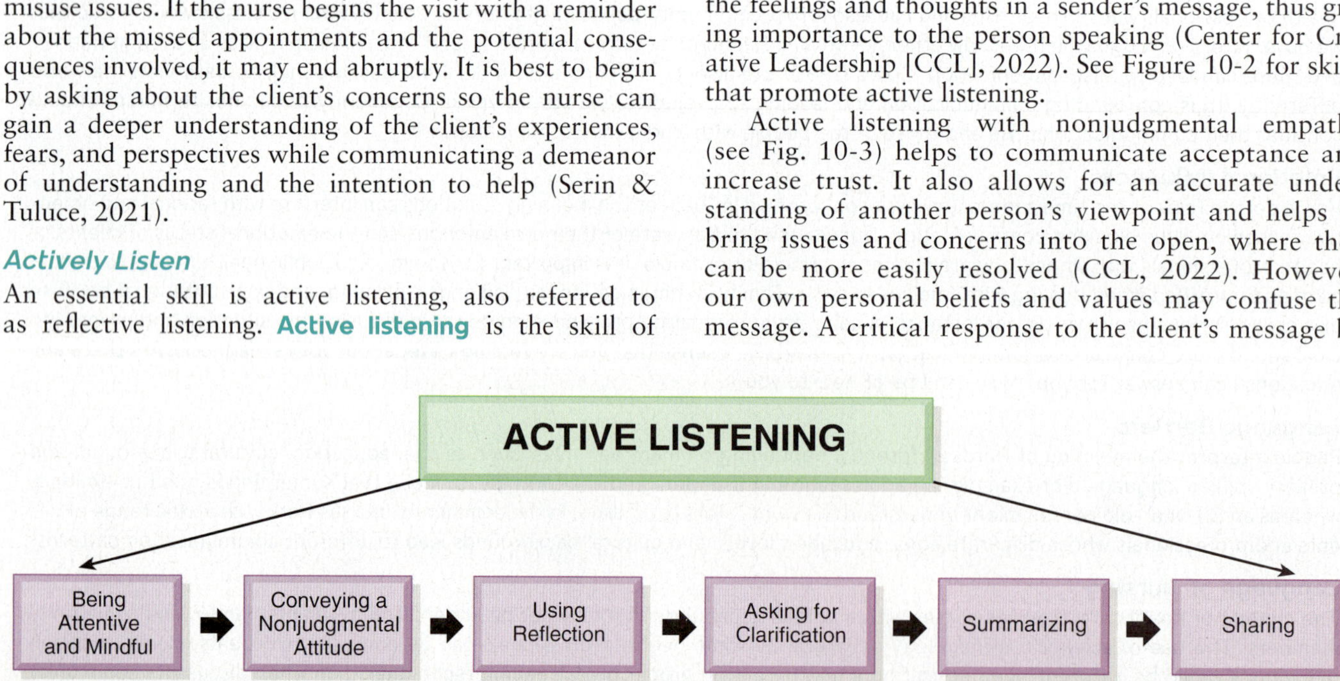

FIGURE 10-2 Six key skills for active listening. (Source: Center for Creative Leadership. (2019). Active listening: Improve your ability to listen and lead. Greensboro, NC: Author.)

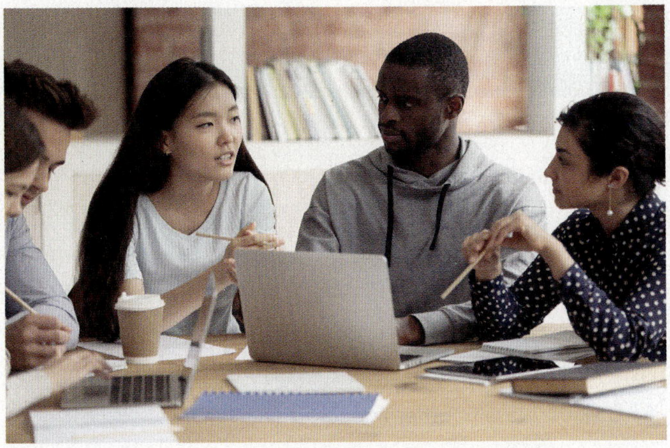

FIGURE 10-3 An example of active listening.

BOX 10-3 Motivational Interviewing: Key Principles

1. Express empathy: Listen carefully and convey that feelings, beliefs, and experiences are understood.
2. Support self-efficacy: Support the client's belief that they can change.
3. Roll with resistance: Avoid argumentative or defensive behavior if meeting with resistance. Help the client identify the problem and solution for themselves.
4. Develop discrepancy: Help the client identify discrepancies between their current situation and their future goals.

Source: Psychology Today. (2023).

the nurse can cut off communication and cause the client to disengage; therefore, a nonjudgmental approach better supports a therapeutic relationship (CCL, 2022). Students interested in learning more about active listening skills can listen to a podcast developed by the CCL (2022), which may be found at https://www.ccl.org/multimedia/podcast/the-big-6-an-active-listening-skill-set/.

Communicate Clearly

The Centers for Disease Control and Prevention (CDC) hosts a site that provides valuable resources to augment clear communication, including a clear communication index use guide, index widget, example material, and everyday words for public health communication found at https://www.cdc.gov/ccindex/. The basic rules for effective verbal or written communication can be summarized in this manner:

1. Write a clear and concise main message, including well-organized content with visual cues.
2. Use active voice.
3. Use everyday words.
4. Include evidence from subject-matter experts.
5. Provide a recommendation, a call to action, or a clarifying message (CDC, 2023a).

Promoting Effective Communication and Change: Motivational Interviewing and OARS

Many techniques promote effective communication. One of the most successful is using motivational interviewing (MI) to support clients in changing their behaviors. MI was first developed as a method of counseling to break through ambivalence and motivate clients to change problem behaviors such as excessive drinking (Miller & Rollnick, 2013). It involves "coming alongside the person and helping them to say why and how they might change for themselves" (Psychology Today, 2023, para 2). This technique can be used in conjunction with the Transtheoretical or Stages of Change Model to determine the client's stage from their statements (see Chapter 11). Listen carefully to what the client says about the issue (e.g., smoking, hypertension, dietary changes), and determine if the client is amenable to making changes (see Box 10-3).

OARS is an acronym encompassing the skills needed in MI:

- Open-ended questions: Rather than closed-ended questions that often result in only Yes or No answers, these questions open up conversation and help clients talk about thoughts and feelings, as well as behaviors and motivations for change. An example follows:
  Nurse: "What are your concerns for your baby (Rose)?"
- Affirmations of client strengths: These are genuine and congruent statements about clients' positive behaviors, skills, and accomplishments. An example follows:
  Nurse: "You were very caring in comforting Rose while she was getting her shots."
- Reflective listening: Similar to active listening, discussed earlier. It helps discern what the client is saying and if the nurse is hearing and understanding the client's meaning. Reflective comments demonstrate empathy and understanding and can move conversations to deeper levels. An example follows:
  Nurse: "So it sounds like you would like some information on how to sign up for Womens, Infants, and Children (WIC)."
- Summaries: Statements used to move the conversation into different areas or to review final highlights of a conversation; can also be helpful in adding information about resources or future planning. Two examples follow:
  Nurse: "Let me see if I understand what you said so far..."
  Nurse: "We talked about x, y, z; let me know if I understood you correctly or missed anything."

Through MI conversations, client statements may reflect indecision or motivation to change. If motivated to change, clients may discuss their desire, ability, or reasons for change along with importance and urgency. The nurse can help them mobilize these feelings by asking open-ended questions about their commitment to change, how they could begin to plan for change, and other steps they need to take to move toward their goal (Dobber et al., 2019; Haque & D'Souza, 2019; Psychology Today, 2023; Vowell, 2020).

Research demonstrates the effectiveness of MI and OARS delivered by counselors (including lay counselors), primary providers, nurses, and nurse practitioners working with a variety of clients:

- Physical activity, fruit and vegetable consumption, and hypertension (Mesters et al., 2022)
- Uncontrolled type 2 diabetes (Oz & Buyuksoy, 2022)
- Tobacco use among adults (Kumar et al., 2022)
- Coronary artery disease patients (promoting a healthy lifestyle; Dobber et al., 2019)
- Appalachian women supporting breastfeeding (Addicks & McNeil, 2019)

Cultivating Cultural Awareness

Effective communication is also strongly influenced by previous experiences and the culture of both the nurse and the client. For example, adolescents who are having difficulty with authority may hear the nurse's suggestion to "learn more about sexually transmitted diseases" as an authoritarian command or an effort to exert control. Differences in culture, ethnicity, and linguistics pose even greater challenges in establishing a helping relationship (Box 10-4). Consideration for basic principles of cultural awareness should be applied when working with clients (CDC, 2021; Table 10-1).

C/PH nurses often find themselves communicating cross-culturally and sometimes through an interpreter. This requires patience and constant effort to ensure accurate and inoffensive messages. Culture is dynamic, and C/PH nurses cannot make assumptions about a client's cultural background, but it has been shown that knowledge of someone's cultural background can aid in providing quality care within the cultural context of the client (AHRQ, 2019). See Chapter 5 for more information on culture within our communities.

TABLE 10-1 Principles of Cultural Competence

1. Define culture broadly.
2. Value clients' cultural beliefs.
3. Recognize complexity in language interpretation.
4. Facilitate learning between providers and communities.
5. Involve the community in defining and addressing service needs.
6. Collaborate with other agencies.
7. Professionalize staff hiring and training.
8. Institutionalize cultural competence (CDC, 2021, para 8).

Source: Centers for Disease Control and Prevention. (2021). *Cultural competence in health and human services.* Retrieved from https://npin.cdc.gov/pages/cultural-competence#what

Health Literacy and Health Outcomes

Personal health literacy refers to the degree to which a person can find, understand, and use information to make health-related decisions (Health Resources and Services Administration [HRSA], 2022). Essential elements of health literacy include the following:

- The ability to use information, not just understand it.
- The ability to use the information to make well-informed decisions.

BOX 10-4 PERSPECTIVES

Mr. Alverez Needs an Interpreter

I am a student in community/public health nursing now, but I work as an extern at our local county hospital in the emergency department (ED). A man came in one Saturday a month or so ago with a bad cut to his left foot; he is employed at the processing plant in town. The ED doctor asked him if he had received a tetanus shot recently, and he quickly nodded "yes." He spoke little English, and none of us spoke Spanish. The interpreter was not available. We cleaned his wound, closed it with stitches, bandaged it, and told him to keep it clean. He left the ED on crutches with the help of his son. He was given a prescription for an antibiotic medication, but a tetanus shot was not administered.

A short time later, Mr. Alverez was back in the hospital because his wound had gotten infected; he used a needle to drain the pus and developed tetanus. He ended up in the intensive care unit (ICU) on a ventilator. Mr. Alverez spent 30 agonizing days in the ICU because of miscommunication about the tetanus booster. We should have used an interpreter, and I truly understand the importance of a translator now. I have a few Spanish-speaking clients in my community/public health nursing rotation. Some of the nurses use the family to interpret, bit if the client does not understand English, I request that an interpreter accompany me on my home visits. I always remember Mr. Alverez and what can happen when you don't use an interpreter, and communication is not clearly understood.

Jessy, age 27

1. *What first comes to mind when you think of this scenario?*
2. *Can you imagine an incident like this occurring in your facility?*
3. *What barriers exist in using an interpreter? How can communication and understanding be validated in a situation where language is a barrier?*

- Organizations have a responsibility to provide health-literate information.
- Health literacy influences health equity (CDC, 2023b).

Health literacy is critical for understanding and evaluating health information. Arguably, the ability to comprehend and discern health information can have influence on one's ability to promote their own health and prevent disease or mitigate health issues. Health literacy is more than just readability, but encompasses technology, media, language, scientific completxity, and culture (Coughline et al., 2020). Vulnerable groups such as older adults, recent immigrants, migrants, ethnic underrepresented groups, and clients with low levels of education and dominant language proficiency are most affected by low health literacy. Low health literacy is associated with social determinants of health and has a direct influence on disease prevention (Coughlin et al., 2020). Low health literacy skills are associated with poorer health status, increased healthcare costs, and use of emergency care because patients with low health literacy levels may be less knowledgeable about their health conditions and are less likely to seek preventative care (Shahid et al., 2022). For more on health literacy, see Chapter 11.

Adequate health literacy among the nursing population is imperative in addressing the problem. Erunal et al. (2019) revealed that nursing students fail to demonstrate adequate health literacy skill levels. Hence, it is vital that nursing students (and nurses) improve their health literacy skills to communicate effectively with clients and fellow healthcare personnel (Erunal et al., 2019). The C/PH nurse has a role in addressing health literacy as low health literacy influences patient outcomes (Shahid et al., 2022).

The benefits of health outcomes include the following:

- Increase use of preventative health
- Lower unneeded emergency room visits
- Lower preventable stays in the hospital and readmission
- Lower dosing errors
- Better management of chronic conditions
- Improved health outcomes
- Increased patient satisfaction
- Increase in the six aims of quality improvement for safe, effective, patient-centered, timely, efficient, and equitable care (AHRQ, 2019)

Organizational health literacy "is the degree to which organizations equitably enable people to find, understand, and use information and services to inform health-related decisions and actions for themselves and others" (HRSA, 2022, para 1). The federal government has set standards to encourage health professionals and health organizations to consider clients' health literacy when communicating with them. Table 10-2 details the most relevant acts, guidelines, and standards addressing our nation's health literacy goal.

The U.S. Department of Health and Human Services (USDHHS) developed the National Action Plan to Improve Health Literacy based on the vision and principles that "(1) everyone has the right to health information that helps them make informed decisions and (2) health services are delivered in ways that are understandable and beneficial to health, longevity, and quality of life" (USDHHS, 2021, para 1). Online health literacy suggestions are found in Box 10-5.

To be sure that these goals are being met, the improvement of health literacy and health communication for our population continues to be a priority in the *Healthy People 2030* goals (Box 10-6).

Health communication includes health literacy, but it also incorporates health messages and campaigns targeted to populations. Population health promotion is best achieved by health communication that uses multiple communication channels to reach stakeholders, including television, radio, newspapers, websites, social media, smartphones/applications, text messaging, educational pamphlets, and nutrition and medication labels. To manage disease and promote health, we must make sure that our patients can understand the health information they see, hear, and read from multiple sources (CDC, 2023b). More information on these topics can be found in Chapter 11.

TABLE 10-2 Acts, Guidelines, and Standards on Health Literacy

Resource	Website Link
National Standards for Culturally and Linguistically Appropriate Services	https://minorityhealth.hhs.gov/omh/browse.aspx?lvl=2&lvlid=53
National Action Plan to Improve Health Literacy	https://health.gov/communication/initiatives/health-literacy-action-plan.asp
National Health Education Standards 2023	https://www.cdc.gov/healthyschools/sher/standards/index.htm
Federal Plan Language Guidelines	https://www.plainlanguage.gov/
Federal Plan Writing Act	https://www.plainlanguage.gov/law/
Health Literacy Training Agency for Healthcare Research and Quality	https://www.cdc.gov/healthliteracy/gettraining.html https://www.ahrq.gov/health-literacy/professional-training/index.html

BOX 10-5 Health Literacy Online Strategies Checklist

- Develop and disseminate health and safety information that is accurate, accessible, and actionable.
- Promote changes in the healthcare system that improve health information, communication, informed decision making, and access to health services.
- Incorporate accurate, standards-based, and developmentally appropriate health and science information and curricula in childcare and education through the university level.
- Support and expand local efforts to provide adult education, English language instruction, and culturally and linguistically appropriate health information services in the community.
- Build partnerships, develop guidance, and change policies.
- Increase basic research and the development, implementation, and evaluation of practices and interventions to improve health literacy.
- Increase the dissemination and use of evidence-based health literacy practices and interventions (USDHHS, 2021, para 1).

Source: U.S. Department of Health and Human Services: Office of Disease Prevention & Promotion (2021).

WORKING WITH INTERDISCIPLINARY TEAMS

An important aspect of communication in C/PHN involves working with interdisciplinary teams. C/PHNs are regularly involved in committees, task forces, support groups, and other work-related groups both inter and intradisciplinary (Fig. 10-4). Group communication patterns can be complex, and interaction requires skill on the nurse's part to elicit feedback from all members to generate a common understanding and a collaborative process. C/PHNs need to understand how to work with groups and how groups function and develop over time as well as techniques for facilitating group support and decision making. Failure to effectively communicate between team members can have a negative impact on patient outcomes (Verwijs et al., 2020; Whittington et al., 2020).

Group Development

In 1977, Tuckman and Jenson identified five stages of group development; this process continues to be used to identify the formation and functionality of groups (West Chester University [WCU], 2022; Box 10-7).

Techniques for Enhancing Group Decision Making

As a member of many decision-making groups in the community, the C/PH nurse can facilitate the process

BOX 10-6 *HEALTHY PEOPLE 2030*

Selected Objectives Related to Health Literacy or Health Communication

Core Objectives	
HC/HIT-01	Increase the proportion of adults whose healthcare provider checked their understanding
HC/HIT-02	Decrease the proportion of adults who report poor communication with their healthcare provider
HC/HIT-03	Increase the proportion of adults whose healthcare providers always involved them in decisions about their healthcare as much as they wanted
HC/HIT-04	Increase the proportion of adults who talk to friends or family about their health
HC/HIT-05	Increase the proportion of adults with broadband internet
HC/HIT-06	Increase the proportion of adults offered online access to their medical record
HC/HIT-07	Increase the proportion of adults who use IT to track healthcare data or communicate with providers
Developmental Objectives	
HC/HIT-D01	Increase the number of state health departments that use social marketing in health promotion programs
HC/HIT-D02	Increase the proportion of emergency messages in news stories that give complete information
HC/HIT-D07	Increase the proportion of doctors with electronic access to information they need
HC/HIT-D08	Increase the proportion of doctors who exchange and use outside electronic health information
HC/HIT-D09	Increase the proportion of people who can view, download, and send their electronic health information
HC/HIT-D-11	Increase the proportion of adults with limited English proficiency who say their providers explain things clearly

Reprinted from U.S. Department of Health and Human Services (USDHHS). (2020a). *Browse 2030 objectives.* Retrieved from https://health.gov/healthypeople/objectives-and-data/browse-objectives

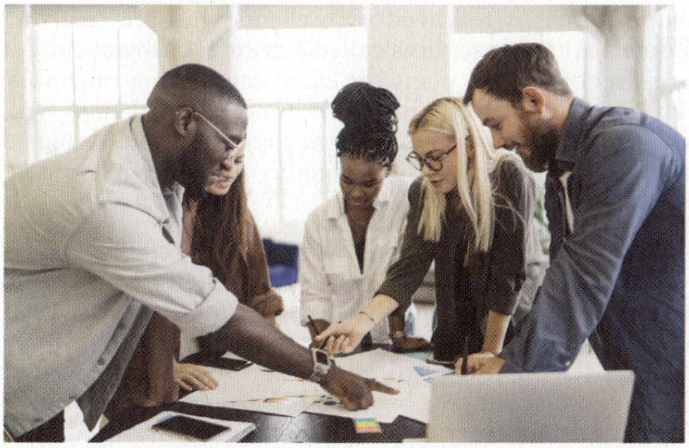

FIGURE 10-4 An example of a functioning group.

through certain techniques such as brainstorming, multivoting, and nominal group technique.

- **Brainstorming** is an idea-generating process that encourages group members to freely offer suggestions. Group members are asked to present creative ideas without criticism or discussion. This technique is helpful for generating creative possibilities and is most useful in the early stages of decision making. Research has shown that brainstorming is the most widely used method of generating creative ideas (Wilson, 2022).
- **Multivoting** is a decision-making tool that enables members to prioritize a long list of ideas, with minimal discussion and difficulty. Multivoting often follows brainstorming to narrow the list to a few items worthy of immediate attention. All the ideas are listed on a flip chart, and members are allowed to vote on one third of the total number of items (Minnesota Department of Health, 2022a).
- **Nominal group technique** is a group decision-making method in which group members are asked not to speak to each other but instead are asked to write down their ideas, along with the advantages and disadvantages of the issue being addressed. After everyone has completed the task, the members' ideas are presented to the group, and discussion takes place so that the information can be categorized and prioritized (American Society for Quality, 2023).

Advances in technology have resulted in the availability of a number of online tools and apps that can help facilitate group decision making, whether the groups are sitting together in a room or working virtually. A website that provides links to 14 free online applications that support various forms of group decision making can be found at https://tallyfy.com/brainstorming-tools/.

Other group communication settings might include the following:

- Group-teaching methods to change behaviors (see Chapter 11 for more on health teaching). Group teaching can be an effective tool for many healthcare challenges, such as diabetes education (Wang et al., 2022; Zeydeni et al., 2021).
- Community/public health nurses are also called on to share best practices and research findings. Public speaking is an important C/PH nurse skill. This involves developing public speaking and presentation skills that engage and draw in audiences, ultimately influencing improvements in health outcomes for people and populations.

BOX 10-7 Tuckman's Stages of Group Development

Forming

- **Members:** Feel awkward and hesitant and depend on the group leader to help them develop mutual trust and give them structure and guidance
- **Group leader:** Helps members become oriented to each other and to the work
  - Selects icebreaker activities at the first group meeting
  - Sets ground rules (e.g., confidentiality)
  - Defines scope of work and timeline for completion

Storming

- Group begins to work together
- Conflict and competition over different agendas, ideas, and approaches
- **Group leader:** Guides group in problem solving and setting goals, models maintenance roles (e.g., encouraging all to participate), and summarizes group feelings

Norming

- Group shows signs of cohesiveness, trust, openness, shared sense of "belonging"
- Work begins to progress
- Creativity and shared ideas and opinions
- **Group leader:** Continues to role model good maintenance behaviors

Performing

- May not occur with all groups
- **Members:** Can work as a total group, in subgroups, or independently
- Most productive stage, as group members are motivated and able to handle the decision-making process in a competent and autonomous manner
- High level of team satisfaction

Adjourning

- Emphasis is on wrapping up the project
- Withdrawal from both task and relationship or maintenance activities
- **Members:** Often feel happy to have accomplished goal but are sad about the loss or disbanding of the group

Source: West Chester University (WCU). (2022).

CONTRACTING IN COMMUNITY/PUBLIC HEALTH NURSING

Contracting means negotiating a working agreement between two or more parties in which they come to a shared understanding and mutually consent to the purposes and terms of the transaction. Contracts are common and include legal and nonbinding agreements. Contracts in community/public health nursing can be either verbal or written, and clients can make them with themselves, family members, healthcare practitioners, or other members of the healthcare team. Such contracts commit clients to a set of behaviors, with the goal of improving adherence to a health promotion program or plan.

Box 10-8 shows a contract used by C/PHNs when counseling clients who desire to stop smoking. Contracts in a collaborative relationship or a nurse–client alliance are flexible and changing and are based on mutual understanding and trust, making this a valuable tool for community/public health nurses (Ackley et al., 2020). The same format is followed with clients who are receiving home healthcare services called a **critical pathway**, and it consists of written plans for client care with a timetable. This is a more formal type of contracting that is typically a fiscally driven and agency-required tool designed to document standards and quality of care while reducing costs.

Value of Contracting

Community/public health nursing has used the concept of **contracting** for many years, developing partnerships with clients to address issues such as weight loss, exercise, and substance misuse. Without always labeling it contracting, these techniques are used with clients who want to lose weight, for instance. In this case, the contract involves mutual agreement on certain exercise and eating patterns for clients and teaching and support responsibilities for the nurse. Contracts set time limits (e.g., 6 months) within which to achieve the intended goal (e.g., weight loss). Nurses can help

BOX 10-8 Client Service Plan With Contract

Madera County Public Health Department
Public Health Nursing: Client Individual Service Plan

Client Name: Tilly Lopez-Davis Client's Signature: ____________

RN Case Manager: J. Silva, PHN Start Date: 3/1/2025

Date: 3/1/2025	Client Goal:	Case Manager: Teaching/Counseling/Referral Case Manager will:	Follow-up/ Reassessment Date: 6/2025
Strengths Identified: Tilly desires to improve the length and quality of life to be healthier to spend time with grandchildren Problems/Risks: Has smoked 1–2 packs per day for 20 years	Tilly will decrease to fewer than 10 cigarettes per day within the next 2 months. Contract agreement: Tilly will avoid temptations or situations associated with pleasurable aspects of smoking by the following: ■ Instead of smoking after meals, brush teeth or take a walk. ■ Limit social activities to where smoking is prohibited. ■ Find new activities that make smoking difficult such as swimming or bicycle riding. ■ Identify a new activity to spend time on during work breaks (reading, crosswords, etc.). ■ Avoid alcoholic drinks. ■ Keep oral substitutes such as carrots, pickles, and sugarless gum handy. ■ Take a yoga class to learn relaxation techniques. Tilly will explore community resources: ■ American Lung Association Program: Freedom from Smoking ■ California Smokers' Helpline: 1-800-NO-BUTTS	■ Promote positive expectations for success; encourage self-efficacy. ■ Prepare Tilly for relapse. ■ Assist in developing time frame with goal ultimately to be that Tilly will stop smoking completely. ■ Partner with Tilly for evaluation, feedback, and revision of health plan as needed. ■ Provide resources for Freedom from Smoking and California Smoker's Helpline.	Outcome/Evaluation Tilly will smoke fewer than 10 cigarettes (1/2 pack) per day by 6/2025.

Source: Gulanik & Myers (2022).

take a complex behavior and break it into manageable steps, such as by contracting to walk at a moderate pace for 30 minutes three times a week, which may seem more feasible than beginning by jogging 2 miles a day. Success in meeting the contract may encourage future efforts to increase exercise activities. Nurses and clients are, in effect, contracting even though they may see it simply as setting goals with clients (Ackley et al., 2020).

Contracting may be used when implementing health promotion programs or when planning to stop or reduce substance use, change eating habits, or increase physical activity. Contracting can also be done with groups or agencies (e.g., schools, businesses), such as when a school district may want to contract with a public health agency to provide C/PHNs and health educators to address pregnancy prevention. The nurse may informally contract with the students about sharing aggregate information gleaned in the small-group teaching exercises with their parents to encourage adolescent–parent communication.

Common benefits of contracting include the following:

- Involves client in promoting their own health
- Motivates client to perform necessary tasks
- Focuses on clients' unique needs, regardless of aggregate size
- Increases the possibility of achieving the health goals identified by collaborating with team members
- Enhances all team members' problem-solving skills
- Fosters client participation in the decision-making process
- Promotes clients' autonomy and self-esteem as they learn self-efficacy
- Promotes efficient and cost-effective health services (Gallagher et al., 2022)

Characteristics of Contracting

The concept of contracting, as used in the collaborative relationship, incorporates four distinctive characteristics: partnership and mutuality, commitment, format, and negotiation. Box 10-9 displays the concept and process of contracting.

Partnership and Mutuality

All aspects of contracting involve shared participation and agreement between team members; they become partners in the relationship (Minnesota Department of Health, 2022b). In a mutual partnership, the nurse and partner come to an agreement on what the partner needs and what the nurse can provide. Together, they develop goals, outline methods to meet those goals, explore resources to help achieve them, define the time limits for the contract, and outline their separate responsibilities (Fig. 10-5). The contract involves reciprocal negotiation and shared evaluation.

Commitment

Second, every contract implies a commitment. The parties involved make a decision that binds them to fulfilling the purpose of the contract (Minnesota Department of Health, 2022b). In community/public health collaboration, there is a pledge of trust and dedication to see the contract through to completion. All parties feel responsible for keeping promises; all want to achieve the intended outcomes. When the nurse and the partners identify their tasks, they commit to success.

Format

Format, the third distinctive feature of contracting, involves outlining the specific terms of the relationship. Clients and professionals gain a clear idea of the purpose of the relationship, their respective responsibilities,

BOX 10-9 Concept and Process of Contracting

Contracting is based on four distinctive features, shown here as spokes of a wheel, that form the basis of a nurse–client collaboration. This relationship is a dynamic process that moves through phases, represented here as the outer rim of the wheel, and is focused on meeting client needs and aiding in the achievement of their goals.

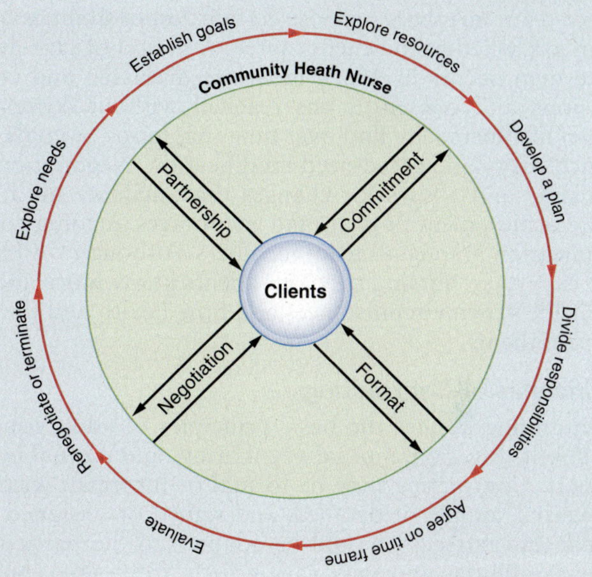

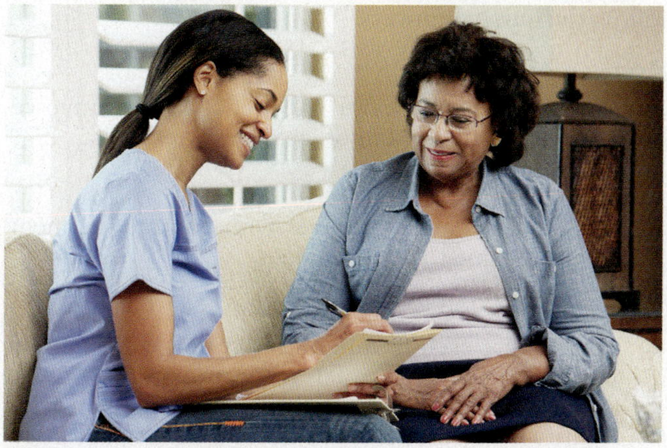

FIGURE 10-5 Contracting is an important aspect of client care.

and the specific limits of their work. Expectations are clarified for all parties involved. The format of contracting provides the framework for collaboration to clearly articulate the logistics, avoid the difficulty of terminating long-term relationships, and shift healthcare responsibilities from the professionals to the client.

Negotiation

Finally, contracting always involves negotiation (Minnesota Department of Health, 2022b). The nurse and other team members propose certain responsibilities and then ask whether the clients agree. A period of give-and-take then occurs in which ideas are discussed and conclusions and consensus are reached without coercion. Team members may find over time that terms or goals on which they had agreed need modification. Negotiation is dynamic and allows for changes that facilitate the ultimate achievement of goals and encourages ongoing communication among all team members. Although C/PHNs are experts in nursing care, our clients know more about their life's own circumstances and how health and illness impact them.

Principles of Contracting

Contracting applies the basic principles of adult education: self-direction, mutual negotiation, and mutual evaluation. Contracting may be formal or informal, written or verbal, simple or detailed, and signed or unsigned by client and nurse. It should be adapted to the particular client's abilities and may vary greatly from situation to situation. The nurse should date initial interventions as well as follow-up and plan for reassessment visits. Like all nursing tools, contracting enhances a client's health only if it is adapted to each particular client.

The Nursing Process and Contracting

Contracting follows a sequence of steps that are aligned with the nursing process. As a working agreement, it depends on knowing what clients want, agreeing on goals, identifying methods to achieve these goals, knowing the resources that collaborating members bring to the relationship, using appropriate outside resources, setting limits, deciding on responsibilities, and providing for periodic reviews. The tasks are incorporated into the contracting process and can be described in eight phases that follow the nursing process.

Assessment

- Assess the clients' health and needs, with the involvement of the clients and other relevant persons.

Nursing Diagnosis/Goal Setting

- Discuss goals and objectives with contracting members and come to an agreement.

Plan/Intervention

- Define what each member has to offer (clarifying the C/PHN role, client's role) and can expect from the others; identify appropriate resources and agencies.
- Identify methods, activities, and a timeline for achieving the stated goals.
- Negotiate the activities for which each member will be responsible.
- Set limits for the contract in terms of length of time or number of meetings.

Evaluation

- Conduct formative and summative assessments of progress toward goals at agreed-on intervals.
- Agree to modify, renegotiate, or terminate the contract.

As C/PH nurses use this process to negotiate a contract, they must adapt it to each situation. Nevertheless, the basic elements remain important considerations for successful contracting.

COLLABORATION AND PARTNERSHIPS IN COMMUNITY/PUBLIC HEALTH NURSING

Effective interdisciplinary and interprofessional collaboration is essential in the healthcare system to achieve quality healthcare and assure successful outcomes (Davidson et al., 2022). Collaboration is a purposeful interaction among nurses, clients, other professionals, and community members to develop strategies for improving the health of people, families, and communities (Minnesota Department of Health, 2022b).

Two examples of community collaboration are the **asset-based community development (ABCD)** approach and **community-based participatory research (CBPR)**.

- The *ABCD* approach is a methodology that starts with identifying community assets and strengths, including local persons, community associations and networks, natural resources, and institutions, as a means of working with residents to create sustainable communities. Rather than a needs-focused approach, ABCD starts with identifying the types of skills and resources already available in the community and then involves consulting with the community members on improvements they would like to make (Reddy & Barbalat, 2021). If you are interested in learning more about how to apply the ABCD methodology, you can access a free, easy-to-complete training at https://www.nurturedevelopment.org/. You will learn more about community assessment in Chapter 15.
- *CBPR* involves community members in the entire research process, from identifying a topic of importance to the community to implementing the research and disseminating the results (National Institute of Health, 2018). See more on CBPR in Chapter 4. Involving stakeholders in planning and implementing programs and research increases their buy-in and the likelihood of success as well as the quality of research findings (Symanski et al., 2023).

To meet the needs of clients, C/PHN practice draws on the expertise and assistance of numerous people. The list of team members can include many different interdisciplinary healthcare professionals, as well as the population being reached. All partners should be encouraged and allowed to use their skills and knowledge to optimize outcomes (Symanski et al., 2023).

Depending on the need to be addressed, C/PHNs may work with many people on a single project or on multiple endeavors. Remember to involve the most important team players, members of the client population, which facilitates addressing potential barriers.

Characteristics of Collaborative Partnerships in Community/Public Health Nursing

To explore the meaning of collaboration in the context of C/PHN, this section examines six characteristics that distinguish collaboration from other types of interaction: shared goals, partnering, partnership development, formalize the partnership, maintain and sustain the partnership, and end the partnership (Minnesota Department of Health, 2022b).

Shared Goals

First, collaboration in C/PHN is goal directed. The nurse, clients, and others involved in the collaborative effort or partnership recognize specific reasons for entering into the relationship.

Partnering

What potential resources, skills, and knowledge are needed by the partners? The collaborative partnership is designed to draw on the expertise of those who are most knowledgeable and in the best positions to influence a favorable outcome.

Partnership Development

Establish a common understanding of perspectives and contributions. How will the designated parties work together to meet the goals? Trust and rapport are built at this stage.

Formalize the Partnership

A formal agreement guides the relationship and action. The collaborating team members work in partnership and assume clearly defined responsibilities. Each member in the partnership plays a specific role with related tasks. Each member of the team develops an understanding of individual responsibilities based on realistic and honest expectations.

Maintain and Sustain the Partnership

Collaboration in community/public health practice has set boundaries, with a beginning and an end, that fall within the goals of the partnership. Communicate regularly and find a feedback process. Determine end results and termination. Once the purpose for the collaboration has been accomplished, the group as a formal entity can be terminated.

End the Partnership (or Not)

In some settings, the partnership may desire to continue to work on other, mutually agreed-on activities. Some partnerships are ongoing. For example, a university department of nursing might use a neighborhood community center for clinical experiences for their students. When people collaborate and work together in partnership, many possibilities exist (Minnesota Department of Health, 2022b).

Levels of Prevention

The levels of prevention are used to provide a framework for the collaborative process in C/PHN (see Box 10-10). One objective in Healthy People 2030 is the Environmental Health objective EH-04: Reduce blood lead levels in children aged 1 to 5 years (USDHHS, 2020a). To achieve this objective, community/public health nurses need to be able to collaborate effectively with community partners in the design and implementation of health programs that address this very significant issue.

The importance of effective collaboration to address lead contamination (Fig. 10-6) was highlighted when the United States witnessed the tragic contamination of publicly supplied drinking water in Flint, Michigan. The contamination occurred in 2014 when the community's water source was switched to the Flint River as a cost-saving measure (Gomez et al., 2019). Signs and symptoms of lead poisoning are primarily neurologic, especially in children, and include seizures, stupor, delirium, behavioral changes, and headaches (CDC, 2022a). Good communication between agencies is a necessity for good community health outcomes as noted during the Ohio derailment and community exposure to airborne toxic chemicals (Environmental Factor, 2024). For more information on environmental health and disasters, see Chapters 9 and 17.

Nurses played a major role in the public health response to the contamination in Flint, including assessing clients for lead exposure and offering health education aimed at primary, secondary, and tertiary prevention. Nurses also offered emotional support, particularly to those most vulnerable and underrepresented (Ruckart et al., 2019). This modern-day example of a major public health response involved nurses working in collaboration with the U.S. Public Health Service; the Centers for Disease Control and Prevention; the U.S. Surgeon General; county and state health departments; the Environmental Protection Agency; federally qualified health centers; the Red Cross; free medical clinics; local, state, and national political leaders; and a wide array of other community agencies.

Effective public health responses are possible only when interdisciplinary, cross-sectoral bodies collaborate efficiently and effectively. The Public Health Leadership Forum (2020) and the Health Care Transformation Task Force developed a framework aimed to support and improve collaboration between healthcare and public health bodies. Five primary elements of collaboration include establishing a governance structure, creating a financing plan, utilizing cross-sector prevention models, developing a data-sharing strategy, and ensuring that performance is measured and evaluated.

Fostering Client Participation

- This chapter has stressed that communication and collaboration are based on mutual participation. The extent of clients' participation varies, however, depending on their readiness and ability to participate (Minnesota Department of Health, 2022b). The client's level of wellness at the time of the initial nurse–client encounter directly influences participation.

BOX 10-10 LEVELS OF PREVENTION PYRAMID

Children's Health and the Environment

SITUATION: High lead blood levels were identified in a community
GOAL: Using the three levels of prevention:

- Develop programs and policies to prevent childhood lead poisoning.
- Screen children for elevated blood levels.
- Ensure that lead-poisoned infants and children receive appropriate medical care and environmental follow-up.

Tertiary Prevention*

Prevent Death and Further Disability	*Interventions*
▪ Restore child to healthful state. ▪ Restore the environment to a healthful state.	▪ Medical treatment as indicated ▪ Removal of child from environment ▪ Aggressive environmental remediation

Secondary Prevention*

Early Diagnosis	*Prompt Treatment*
▪ Surveillance and screening activities for early detection, treatment, and referral for management of lead exposure	▪ Identification of children with elevated blood lead levels ▪ Routine maintenance and repair of homes in high-risk communities

Primary Prevention*

Health Promotion and Education	*Health Protection*
▪ Identify populations at high risk for housing-based lead exposure. ▪ Develop strategies to ensure lead-safe housing. ▪ Collaborative partnerships to provide educational programs increasing knowledge of lead safety. ▪ Evaluate and redesign current prevention programs to achieve primary prevention.	▪ Identify high-risk geographic areas using surveillance data. ▪ Identify high-risk families who could benefit from immediate assessment. ▪ Educate community partners on the cost of inaction; highlight risk disparities. ▪ Incorporate lead hazard screening into home visits by community health nurses.

*The goal of primary prevention is to remove lead hazards from the environment before a child is exposed. The goal of secondary prevention (for those already exposed to lead) have blood lead testing, follow up care, and referrals. The goal of tertiary prevention is to prevent morbidity and mortality by preventing lead exposure.
Source: Centers for Disease Control and Prevention (CDC). (2022a).

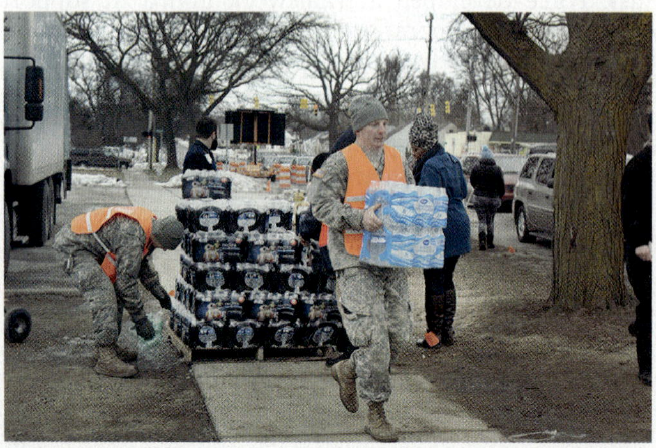

FIGURE 10-6 Emergency water distribution following the discovery of lead contamination of water supply in Flint, Michigan.

- Engaging clients in a collaborative process may be difficult at times. Clients with low literacy, with low income, or from different cultural backgrounds may need extensive encouragement to actively participate in a collaborative relationship. Sometimes, a client's previous experience with health personnel limits participation in collaboration (Bryne et al., 2020).
- The nurse's own view of collaboration also influences the degree of client participation. Nurses who see their position as more informed and the client's position as one of complete ignorance and need may find that a paternalistic relationship develops. All clients have resources on which to build, and the C/PH nurse should help clients to discover these resources and empower clients to enhance collaboration and attain health goals.

Barriers to Effective Collaboration

Communication barriers and miscommunication can inhibit effective collaboration. This is sometimes caused by misconceptions on the part of team members regarding the professional knowledge and motives of other team members. Stereotypes and the perception of unequal power and authority can sabotage the effectiveness of communication and collaboration. Conflict is inevitable when dealing with groups of diverse people, but how potential anger, resentment, and mistrust are handled is the key to getting beyond conflict (Community Toolbox, 2023). Agreeing on how conflict will be handled prior to any incidents sets a positive stage for resolution. One strategy is to use conflict resolution skills. Key principles for conflict resolution are presented in Table 10-3.

HEALTH TECHNOLOGY

Health technology is a term used to describe a broad range of technologies and applications that include medical processes and devices, IT infrastructure, artificial intelligence (AI), data analytics, cloud and storage systems, databases, and the many technologies that support health organizations and people's health (Lyamu et al., 2021). **Informatics** is a field of science that uses information technology to organize and analyze health records and other health data and information; an example of this is electronic health records (EHRs) (Jen et al., 2022). **Digital health** refers to those technologies that use or leverage information and communication technologies to deliver healthcare services or products for better health or well-being such as wearable devices, telehealth/telemedicine, and mobile health (mHealth) (U.S. Food and Drug Administration, 2020). Nurses use information technology to support care delivery and improve the health status of all. Health data, information, wisdom, and knowledge can be collected, stored, processed, and communicated. Nurses and other health professionals, administrators, policy and decision makers, consumers, and clients or patients can use information technology, hardware, and software (Lyamu et al., 2021).

TABLE 10-3 Key Principles for Conflict Resolution

1. Understand the conflict.
2. Communicate with the opposition.
3. Brainstorm possible resolutions.
4. Choose the best resolution.
5. Use a third-party mediator.
6. Explore alternatives.
7. Cope with stressful situations and pressure tactics.

Source: Community Toolbox. (2023). Training for conflict resolution. https://ctb.ku.edu/en/table-of-contents/implement/provide-information-enhance-skills/conflict-resolution/main

Electronic Health Records

Electronic health records (EHRs) are digital (computerized) versions of patients' paper charts. This enables a healthcare provider to record patient progress, place prescription orders, receive decision-support alerts and reminders, order laboratory tests, receive and review results electronically, message patients or fellow providers, and perform a variety of other documentation and clinical tasks using a software package. It may contain lab, x-ray results, medications, and medical history, along with administrative and billing information (Office of the National Coordinator for Health Information Technology [ONC], 2023).

The use of EHRs in community/public health has followed a slower progression than in hospitals. Reporting (e.g., communicable diseases, immunizations) has moved from paper to unidirectional electronic reporting in many areas. In public health, EHRs have been shown to improve efficiency, productivity, quality of care, cost reduction, and data management, although drawbacks include missing data, complex technology, and the learning curve (Pyron & Carter-Templeton, 2019; Tsai et al., 2020). Agencies may find EHRs helpful in areas such as epidemiology, large-scale planning, budgets, and grant writing. For example, an agency may search for specific characteristics and target vulnerable populations to best determine more effective planning and targeted interventions (e.g., clients with specific chronic diseases, clients who smokes currently). People may also gain access to their own health information, and this is especially helpful in the case of immunization records (McGreevy et al., 2023).

Data and Analytics

Massive amounts of data are captured daily as we browse the internet, use our credit cards, visit a clinic for a flu vaccine, or use social media sites. Other sources include biologic or genomic data, geospatial analyses (statistical analysis of geographic mapping) data sets, readings from personal monitoring devices people wear (e.g., GPS, FitBit, Smart Watch), EHRs, and continual volume of data from computer searches, online records, cell phone accounts, and social media (Ngiam & Khor, 2019).

- **Big data** represent "large-scale data collections" from a wide variety of sources and includes the unique methods of data processing, analyses, and storage (e.g., cloud servers, distributed data warehouses) needed to accommodate massive data sets (Zhu et al., 2019, p. 229).
- The four V's of big data include the following:
  - Volume: Denotes the massive amount of data (2.3 trillion gigabytes of data every day)
  - Velocity: Refers to the speed of data generation, collection, analysis, and transmission
  - Variety: Means the different types of data (often unstructured) that are collected that require sophisticated technology to overcome data inconsistencies
  - Veracity: Refers to assuring accuracy and trustworthiness of massive data sets that may be used for secondary analysis, have missing items, or need statistical cleaning to assure validity (Analytics Insight, 2021; Zhu et al., 2019)

Nurses in all settings add to big data through sharable and comparable documentation in the EHR. The use of big data makes it easier to drill down (or view more detailed information), drill up (or see data in an aggregate view), as well as combine different data variables than when using more traditional forms of data collection and analysis; this is the analytic aspect of what can be done with data once generated (SAS, 2023).

The goal of EHR documentation is capturing health and nursing care data in structured ways to help build a foundation for accurate, reliable, clinically meaningful measurement across systems and settings of care (ONC, 2023). Data are the core of that documentation; however, the lack of standardized data and a common data structure become barriers for analysis making it difficult for nursing research to identify outcomes of nursing care linked to assigned patients. The consistent and reliable use of data elements will allow information to be collected once and reused for multiple purposes (Zhu et al., 2019). If EHR systems are not integrated (e.g., if they do not work together and talk to each other), the task is much more challenging.

- The National Patient-Centered Clinical Research Network (PCORnet) is a central source of data from EHRs and provider billing that is currently used for healthcare research. Providers can be linked to patients and nursing researchers (National Patient-Centered Clinical Research Network [PCORnet], n.d.).
- The Nursing Value Data Model is a framework to guide data use in nursing research, and the National Database for Nursing Quality Indicators provides a means of measuring structure, process, and outcomes. (Harolds & Miller, 2022). Because nursing is a process-oriented profession, to effectively demonstrate nursing interventions and patient outcomes, data specific to nursing must be collected (Hersh, 2019).

Precision medicine (Fig. 10-7), using genomics and other big data, can provide more individualized care and treatments, along with more personally tailored medication regimens as well as disease prediction and differential diagnosis (U.S. Department of Health and Human Services, 2023). In the future, precision oncology and pharmacogenetics may be used to tailor healthcare. Data are used in precision public health to promote population health through epidemiology, disease surveillance, risk prediction, research, and preventive care. Big data has also been used to identify treatment and intervention in public health research on childhood obesity and asthma, HIV, misuse of opioid medications, use of smokeless tobacco, and the Zika virus (Bilkey et al., 2019; Fig. 10-7). For more information on studies using precision medicine in public health, follow the work of the CDC: https://www.cdc.gov/genomics/blog/index.htm

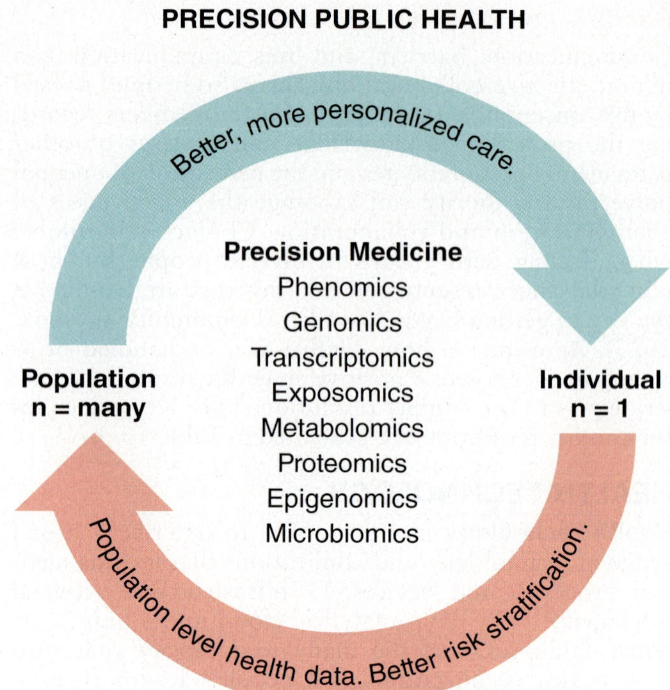

FIGURE 10-7 Precision public health infographic. (Reprinted from Bilkey, G., Burns, B., Coles, E., Mahede, T., Baynam, G. & Nowak, K. (2019). Optimizing precision medicine for public health. *Frontiers in Public Health*, 7(42). https://doi.org/10.3389/fpubh.2019.00042. This is an open-access article distributed under the term+l142s of the Creative Commons Attribution License (CC BY).

Mobile Health (mHealth)

Mobile technology provides an opportunity for nurses and other clinicians to improve health and healthcare through forms of interactive **mobile health (mHealth)**. mHealth includes the use of wireless technologies, such as smartphones, smartwatches, tablets, and notebooks for improving health. mHealth offers great opportunities for improving global health, safety, and preparedness. The potential of mobile technology's impact on sharing health information and collecting disease/health data is tremendous due to its portability, affordability, and availability; it also has the potential to save billions of dollars in healthcare costs (McCool et al., 2022). The potential of mHealth will be further established as patients' experiences with technology and clinical/psychosocial outcomes are evaluated (McCool et al., 2022).

Health apps allow clients to take control of their health; over 50% of current apps available are related to health and wellness (mHealth Intelligence, 2022). Four key features have become important for consumers:

- Health tracking and care support
- Usability
- Health data privacy
- Behavior-change techniques, such as reminders, prompts, and use of personal goals (mHealth Intelligence, 2022).

mHealth is extending healthcare to underserved and hard-to-reach areas. Technology puts healthcare providers in a position to change how healthcare is delivered, the quality of the patient's experience, and the cost of healthcare. Advantages include management of chronic disease, empowering older adults and expectant parents, reminding people to take medication, serving underserved areas, and improving health outcomes and medical system efficiency. However, there are big differences in the number of mobile devices that exist among nations.

In 2021, China and India (1.73 billion and 1.15 billion, respectively), followed by the United States (360 million), had the highest number of mobile devices, whereas several island nations (e.g., Falkland Islands, Marshall Islands, Cook Islands) had the lowest number—between 6000 and 17,000 (Central Intelligence Agency, 2021).

A report cited common uses for mHealth that include health monitoring, fitness and activity tracking, and smart and connected devices for in-home healthcare and remote monitoring, as well as continued access to call centers, reminders, and telemedicine (Mobile Health Technologies and Global Markets, 2022). Mobile wearable and integrated medical devices are projected to be growth areas for mHealth; sensor technology, interface of medical devices with wearable and integrated devices, and the use of AI for future wearable technology could change the landscape of health and healthcare (Mobile Health Technologies and Global Markets, 2022).

As an example of mHealth, medical apps are being used to augment patient information such as the medical information and procedure readiness for a colonoscopy procedure (Kernebeck et al., 2022):

- The COVID-19 pandemic saw a surge in mHealth usage for telemedicine consultation, remote interpreting of data, virtual education platforms, and virtual clinics.
- Ethical, legal, and privacy considerations must be considered for digital medical solutions (Kernebeck et al., 2022).
- The use of mobile phones for COVID-19 surveillance, contract tracing, and contact notification gives rise to the many applications and efficacies of this type of technology for public health (Mansouri & Darvishpour, 2023; Box 10-11).

Cellular Phones

Approximately 96% of Americans own a cell phone, and 85% of those are smartphones (Pew Research Center, 2021). Thirty percent of 18- to 29-year-olds in the United States rely on their cell phone for most online access as compared to all other age ranges (Pew Research Center, 2021).

Text messaging and the use of applications and other mHealth interventions can reduce geographic and economic barriers to health information and services. These interventions have the potential to reduce health disparities and leverage a profound effect on health, yet technologies are being designed without consideration of racial and ethnic populations (USDHHS, 2020b; Valdez & Rogers, 2022).

- A recent study found that there are racial and ethnic disparities in offer and access; Black and Hispanic patients were offered and accessed patient portals at a lower rate than White patients (Richwine et al., 2023). Optimizing websites for mobile devices could be helpful in reaching diverse populations and would enable a wide audience to test and review apps in development.
- In another study, non-White patients were apt to access their lab results if they had mobile access to their personal health information compared with only computer access (Graetz et al., 2019). Mobile phone technologies offer promising opportunities for nurses working in the community setting (Decker et al., 2022).

BOX 10-11 EVIDENCE-BASED PRACTICE

Using Mobile Phones as an Exposure Notification system During COVID-19

The COVID-19 pandemic was an unapparelled global event unleashing the infectious disease, SARS-CoV-2, in late 2019. Over 750 million cases were reported leading to more than 6.8 million deaths worldwide. Due to the rapid spread, morbidity, and mortality of this disease, there was interest in developing innovative tools for public health response. An exposure notification system was developed through an Apple—Google partnership, which provided app-based push alerts to anyone who was in close contact with another app user who tested positive for COVID-19. Users of the app could receive notifications and alert other users if they had tested positive. The system did not reveal personal information, such as names or phone numbers, to the app users. The apps could run on most Android and iPhones, allowing for real-time information. Twenty-six states adopted the exposure notification system over a 10-month period, with varying response and usage. Privacy was a common barrier to use, even though privacy and security were priorities in the design; this included privacy for those who downloaded the app, those notified on the app, and exposure notification to users on the app. Exposure notification technology may play a role in preventing the spread of disease through future use of exposure and notification systems.

1. *How could public health departments use mobile phone data to track communicable diseases in your area? Which data would be most critical?*
2. *In what other instances would knowledge of population mobile phone use in your area be helpful (e.g., disaster notification, health promotion, immunization reminders)? Are these being utilized in your area?*
3. *Find other research about digital technology in public health. Are the findings significant, valid, and helpful to your population?*

Source: U.S. Government Accountability Office (2021).

Text Messaging

Connected health offers the patient connectivity through just-in-time and "real-time" messaging opportunities that can be motivating, educational, and caring (Health Information and Management Systems Society, 2019). A disadvantage of cellular phones includes cellular access, dropped calls, and text message delays. Reminder and educational text messages can be disseminated widely and broadly, reaching a mass number of recipients quickly and inexpensively. Text messaging can overcome barriers of time and access to reach even high-risk populations; for many patients, it is now the expectation that they receive text messaging from healthcare providers (Tornetta, 2021).

Text message interventions can promote healthy lifestyle behaviors, have become widely integrated into routine daily life, and are simple, low cost, and nonlabor intensive. Use of text messaging to deliver information about more sensitive topics, such as sexual health and

BOX 10-12 Risks and Benefits of Health Text Messaging

Benefits

- Appointment reminders to reduce cancelations and absences
- Prescription reminders
- Support for the management of chronic conditions
- Ability to share health programs, education, initiatives, and campaigns
- Improved communication
- Enhanced patient engagement
- Cost savings

Risks

- Communication via text can be confusing due to brevity and its lack of verbal and nonverbal cuing that comes with in-person communication.
- Privacy issues (such as sending information to the wrong person) and lack of end-to-end encryption.
- To offset risks: Systems must include privacy, confidentiality, secure storage, and accurate content.
- Information related to diagnosis and treatment is part of personal health information and must be incorporated into the patient's chart.
- To avoid potential legal complications: Use HIPAA compliant platforms; information related to diagnosis and treatment is part of personal health information and must be incorporated into the patient's chart

Source: The HIPAA Journal (2023).

reducing risky behaviors, seems promising. Text messages may be used for simple reminders to have blood pressure checked, to notify people about an upcoming appointment, or to pick up prescriptions. Box 10-12 provides the risks and benefits related to provider-to-patient texting.

Nurses and other clinicians may use texting to assist patients and caregivers with management of chronic conditions and disease prevention. Text messaging provides a venue to deliver information to hard-to-reach populations and the opportunity to have a positive influence on health knowledge and behaviors, as evidenced by clinical outcomes in a recent study among college students (Arais, 2021). See Box 10-13 for considerations when texting patients.

BOX 10-13 Text Messaging Best Practices

1. Don't forget about HIPAA.
2. Understand your risks.
3. Be proactive on data security.
4. Get consent to communicate via text.
5. Think beyond patient health, including communication between healthcare personnel.
6. Manage who is authorized to access personal health information when communicating via text.

Source: Arais (2021).

Applications

An application, or app for short, may be defined as a self-contained software package to help the user perform specific tasks on a mobile or desktop device (Mills et al., 2021). Today's modern smartphones and smartwatches come with powerful processing capability, meaning nearly anything that can be done on a desktop computer can be done with smart technology. The portability of the app that allows the user to remain connected is very appealing to both nurses and clients. Many new mobile apps are targeted to assist people in their own health and wellness management. Other mobile apps are targeted to healthcare providers as tools to improve and facilitate the delivery of patient care and health information (Mills et al., 2021).

Following COVID-19, digital health is now considered a routine component of healthcare (Knowles et al., 2023). A national survey (Knowles et al., 2023) found that digital tool use through wearable devices is most popular with younger groups who have early adopter characteristics, college education, and higher income; conversely, wearable devices among older, lower educational attainment, and lower-income groups increased from 13% in 2019 to 21% in 2022 (Knowles et al., 2023). Those respondents who rated their health good or excellent were more likely to wear a digital device and were more likely to use wearables to track physical activity, heart rate, sleep, weight, blood pressure, diet, and calorie count (Fig. 10-8). Data security was important to participants with 70% reporting a willingness to share health data with their providers; respondents were less confident in the security of their data in the hands of health insurance companies, pharmacies, government organizations, and tech companies and were, therefore, less willing to share data with these entities (Knowles et al., 2023).

The Food and Drug Administration (FDA) is responsible for the protection of public health by assuring the safety, effectiveness, quality, and security of human and veterinary drugs, vaccines, and other biologic products, and medical devices (FDA, 2022). The FDA's mobile medical apps policy does not regulate the sale or general

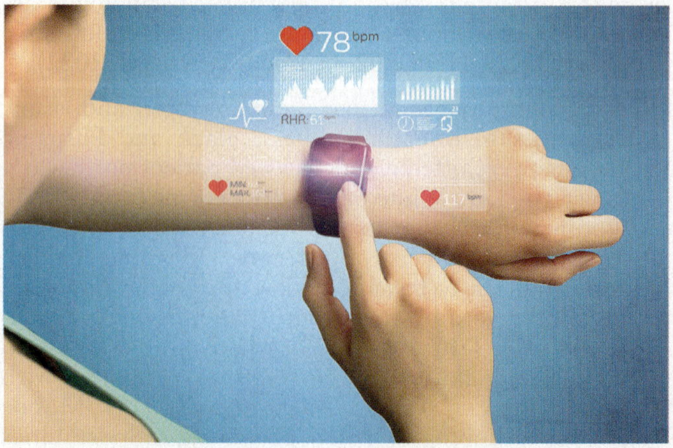

FIGURE 10-8 Social media and technology have the capacity to reach and influence the health behaviors of a wide audience.

consumer use of smartphones/watches and tablets and does not consider entities that distribute mobile apps or those that come from "app stores" to be medical device manufacturers (FDA, 2022, para 18).

Mobile Apps

Much research in public health has found that it is possible to use apps to help deliver health-related information and to aid people in disease management (e.g., diabetes) and make better health decisions such as smoking less and exercising more. During the COVID-19 pandemic, states and countries used texting to disseminate information including exposure notification. While the system had mixed reviews, the potential for mass communication, data sharing, racking, and dissemination of real-time information has set a new precedence (Colorado Department of Public Health and Environment, 2023).

Mobile apps are now available for free or purchase on most mobile device's "app stores." The integration of health and technology has allowed an explosion of interest by consumers. Convenience of access on a mobile device reinforces frequency and interest in use (see Box 10-14).

Social Networking Media

Social networking allows users to connect socially through digital formats such as websites, blogs, apps, vlogs, or other web-based broadcast posts. This digital social communication allows people to find and connect through the web in a way they may not have done in-person or geographically. Users access social media through computers, tablets, or smartphones, and it is generally composed of user-generated content.

Micro-messaging/microblogging

Micro-messaging/microblogging technology and an online social networking service enables users to send and read short 140-character messages called "tweets" or (with the rebranding of Twitter to X in 2022) "posts." Posts are delineated by a hashtag (#) symbol to organize topics (Yeung et al., 2021). Microblogging began with the advent of Twitter in 2006; it is a method of mass communication. "Followers" or users sign up to follow the microblog. Micro-messaging is in real time and designed for mobility. E-registered users can read and post tweets by computer or smartphone, and anyone on micro-messaging (not just followers) can see tweets on a public account. Micro-messaging can be used to provide important insight related to health and is a useful tool to promote healthy behaviors and engage patients (Yeung et al., 2021).

Nurses/clinicians and healthcare systems can use micro-messaging/microblogging to communicate timely information, both within the medical community and to patients as well as the general public. Short messages, or tweets/posts, are delivered to a group of recipients simultaneously, providing an easy and quick method to reach large groups in a limited time. There are obvious advantages to sharing time-critical information such as disaster alerts and drug safety warnings, tracking disease outbreaks, or disseminating healthcare information. Microblogging applications can deliver information about clinical trials, for example, or link brief news alerts from the CDC to reliable websites that provide more detailed information, as well as information related to public health surveillance (Masri et al., 2019).

Online Support Communities

Blogs or weblogs are web-based chronological journals (Sormunen et al., 2021). Blogs typically include date-stamped, multiple entries in chronological order and are updated frequently. Blogs usually focus on a particular subject or topic. One type of blog, referred to as a simple blog, is a form of online personal diary. Other blogs relate to group causes such as political or social concerns, and some may ask for contributions. Blogs may contain reflections, commentaries, comments, images, videos, and often hyperlinks to other information of interest to the blogger or that they feel will be of interest to their readers. The ability for readers to leave comments on a blog post depends on the settings that the blog administrator uses (Sormunen et al., 2021).

- Many journals, healthcare systems, nursing, and other professional organizations, healthcare provider networks, and educational institutions create blogs to provide the latest information and promote discussion (Sormunen et al., 2021).
- Many people create personal blogs when faced with an illness or are a family member/support for someone facing health challenges. Participating in the creation of health information through blogging and social networking contributions influences experiences and supports an person's understanding of their role in healthcare management and ability to copy with their disease process (Hu, 2019).
- Online blogs allow for contact and support that are available at any hour of the day or night via the internet. People who have joined an online support group benefit from venting their feelings and from the support they receive as well as feeling connected by helping and supporting others (Apperson et al., 2019).

Online supportive relationships generally provide a safe environment. Others' experiences can induce feelings of compassion, and one becomes less self-absorbed and may gain a better perspective (Wagner et al., 2020). Finding a safe place to share can be very empowering, and the value of first-person accounts, the appeal and memorability of stories, and the need to make contact with peers all strongly suggest that reading and hearing others'

BOX 10-14 Trends in Mobile Health Apps

- Personal health records (health diary)
- Medical equipment management
- Hospital management
- Medical bills
- Appointment booking
- Telehealth
- E-Prescriptions
- Medical research

Source: Interexy (2023).

accounts of their own experiences of health and illness will remain an important component of health management/care. For example, PatientsLikeMe (https://www.patientslikeme.com/) is a great example of a free internet-based tool for sharing and learning.

Another type of online support is **vlogs**. Vlogs are a type of blog where the content is in video format and typically centered around a topic or theme. Similar to a blog, creators develop a following connecting like-minded people to content that is educational entertaining, or inspiration (such as vlogging your cross-country trek) (The Arts Development Company, 2023).

Podcasts are digital audio files available for downloading on the web and listening to on mobile or desktop devices. The plethora of podcasts allows for most any subject, talk, or content to be recorded. If it can be audiotaped, it can be available as a podcast. Access to health material is limitless (Winn, 2023). The CDC offers healthcare downloadable podcasts on health and health promotion (https://www.cdc.gov/flu/resource-center/freeresources/video/media-podcasts.htm).

Video Games and Virtual Reality Games

As of 2019, 64% of American adults and 70% of American children play video games (TEConomy Partners, 2020). Public attitudes toward video games and the people who play them are complex and often mixed. Video games are typically thought of as entertainment. However, there is growing interest in video games to facilitate healthy behaviors. Exercise programs based on video game activities provide an alternative to motivate and increase adherence to activity and exercise (Suleiman-Martos et al., 2022).

Games can serve as a means to engage patients behaviorally in order to improve their health outcomes. Behaviors, often necessary to maintain and improve health, are reinforced.

- The use of an augmented reality (AR) game, Pokémon Go (Fig. 10-9), discovered that it provided opportunities for increased exercise levels suggesting an area for further research (Lee et al., 2021).
- A systematic review of virtual reality (VR) rehabilitation found some evidence of improvement in motor skills and balance for children with cerebral palsy and Down syndrome (Lopes et al., 2020).
- Researchers developed a game to help people with Parkinson disease improve coordination, gross and fine dexterity, and strength of upper limb muscle grip. Results showed significant improvement in the experimental group (Fernandez-Gonzalez et al., 2019).

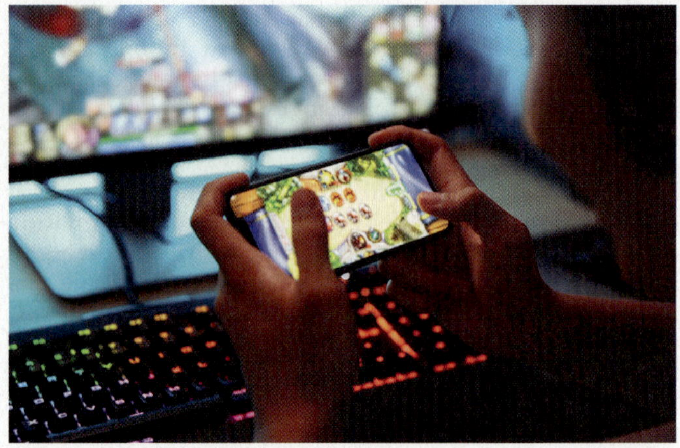

FIGURE 10-9 Person playing video game.

With game play, tension and fears are released in a safe setting, and aversive or shameful aspects of an illness may be managed. The focus of attention on an engaging distraction (the game) may explain how people manage aversive symptoms through video game play (see Box 10-15). An example of distractive use of a VR game is Virtual Meditative Walk (see Table 10-4 for description), which is used to distract patients during burn care.

BOX 10-15 POPULATION FOCUS

Use of Extended Reality Within Veteran Healthcare Facilities

Across the United States, veteran healthcare facilities are expanding the possibilities of treatment for several chronic conditions across the spectrum of acute and ambulatory care and behavioral health with innovative uses of Extended Reality (XR). XR is the inclusive term used to encompass AR and VR interventions that are nonpharmaceutical patient treatment modalities adjunct to traditional patient treatments for a wide variety of conditions. XR is utilized in many ways, such as fall risk assessment, neurologic assessment, pain management, anxiety, posttraumatic stress disorder, physical and occupational therapy, radiology phobias, and creative arts therapy (Rawlins et al., 2021). Veteran healthcare facilities most commonly use VR modalities as an adjunct or alternative for veterans with chronic pain, anxiety, stress, and posttraumatic stress, which is promising since veterans tend to experience pain and anxiety more frequently than non-veterans (Rawlins et al., 2021). For example, VR headsets reduce pain and improve mood (anxiety) and quality of life for outpatient and community living center patients by promoting relaxation and mindfulness. Further, a new program being introduced centers on veterans being assigned a VR headset with a written treatment plan over the course of numerous weeks and includes various levels of wellness experiences. Veterans may be provided a VR headset upon submission of a primary provider order. Concurrently, XR is also utilized to strengthen empathy and understanding among interprofessional healthcare staff by providing a "walk in my shoes" patient experience during the acute care discharge process. In conclusion, early research shows promising results with the integration of VR distraction as a nonpharmacologic modality to address chronic pain, anxiety, and stress. One study noted a decreased average pain intensity and correlating stress and anxiety with the use of VR distraction as an adjunct or alternative

BOX **10-15** POPULATION FOCUS (*Continued*)

within the veteran population for pain management (Rawlins et al., 2021). Evidence suggests that integration of nonpharmacologic VR immersion or distraction for pain management, stress, and anxiety is a beneficial treatment option (Rawlins et al., 2021). In another survey, a 72% decrease in opioid usage was found among veterans suffering from chronic pain (Rawlins et al., 2021) in addition to pain reduction. This is promising because of the potential decrease in negative effects of opioid treatments. Future study opportunities exist in the realm of long-term pain relief following the use of VR distraction as one progresses through daily activities (Rawlins et al., 2021).

Mona P. Tramont, DNP, RN, NE-BC

Definitions

Augmented Reality (AR) = the real world with a digital overlay; the real world is central, with a digital overlay enhancing the experience (e.g., work with patients with PTSD in which real-world scenarios/situations [e.g., war] are integrated into a controlled and safe environment) (Rawlins et al., 2021)

Virtual Reality (VR) = no interaction with the natural world (e.g., use of VR during stressful/anxiety-producing situations [e.g., chronic pain management]) (Rawlins et al., 2021)

References: Bailey, A., & Rawlins, C. (2021, February 1). *Veterans receive cutting edge virtual reality treatments.* VA News. Veterans receive cutting edge virtual reality treatments—VA News

Rawlins, C., Veigulis, Z., Hebert, C., Curtin, C., & Osborne, T. F. (2021). Effect of immersive virtual reality on pain and anxiety at a Veterans Affairs health care facility (2021). *Frontiers in Virtual Reality.* Retrieved July 18, 2023 Frontiers | Effect of Immersive Virtual Reality on Pain and Anxiety at a Veterans Affairs Health Care Facility (frontiersin.org)

Telehealth

Telehealth is the distribution of health-related information and services using technology for remote telecommunication (Association of State and Territorial Health Officials [ASTHO], 2023). A position statement from the Telehealth Special Interest Group of the American Telemedicine Association states: Telehealth is "remote healthcare . . . via electronic communications to improve patients' health status" using "different types of programs and services" (2019, p. 8). Telehealth gives the C/PH nurse an opportunity to see and speak with clients located at remote sites as well as to provide education and counseling. Telehealth consists of the delivery, management, and coordination of health services, integrating telecommunication and electronic technologies, to increase client access to healthcare and improve outcomes while lowering costs (ASTHO, 2023).

The boundaries of **telehealth** are limited only by the technology available, and new applications are being developed and tested every day. Telehealth provides access to care and the ability to export clinical expertise to people who require care (Donelan et al., 2019). During the COVID-19 pandemic, the Corona Aid, Relief, and Economic Security (CARES) Act expanded the use of telehealth and waived some restrictions and requirements

TABLE **10-4** Selected Health-Related Video Games and Virtual Reality Games

Name of Game if Specifically Named	Medical Condition Targeted	Game Description
Snow World	Burn pain	This game was created to minimize body motion during wound débridement by gameplay through the use of a joystick.
Mindscape Commons	Schizophrenia	360-degree VR immersion of what it might be like to experience psychotic episodes for an unmedicated person with schizophrenia
Packy and Marlon (Super Nintendo system)	Diabetes for children	The game was designed to better understand how to maintain stable glucose levels and manage their insulin.
Bronkie the Bronchiasaurus (Super Nintendo)	Asthma for children	Players help the characters keep their asthma in control by avoiding dust, smoke, and other triggers while on their quest.
Re-Mission 2	Cancer in adolescents and young adults	A collection of six games. The goal of the games is to improve treatment, with players controlling a nanobot named Roxxi, who flies through tumors with chemotherapy and radiation. Animations and direct interactions with environments provide information. Studies revealed greater knowledge, self-efficacy, and treatment compliance.
Virtual Meditative Walk	Pain therapy, phobias, fear, anxiety	A virtual meditative walk provides a peaceful, nondistracting, and safe environment. The VE uses a biofeedback loop and VR technologies for pain mitigation.

Source: Tao, G., Garrett, B., Taverner, T., Cordingley, E. & Sun, C. (2021). Immersion virtual reality health games: A narrative review of game design. *Journal of Neuro Engineering Rehabil, 18*(31). https://doi.org/1.1186/s12984-020-00801-3

(ASTHO, 2023). This allowed for billing Medicare and Medicaid-related services regardless of where the provider or patient was located, allowing for a broader range of providers for the duration of the public health emergency (ASTHO, 2023). Telehealth can be divided into two general types of applications: real-time or synchronous communication and store-and-forward or asynchronous communication.

- Real-time communication scenarios include a patient and clinician consulting with a specialist via a live audio/video link, a clinician and a patient in an examination room communicating through an interpreter connected by phone or webcam, or a patient at home communicating with a C/PHN via a live audio/video link (Fig. 10-10).
- Asynchronous telehealth applications (known as store-and-forward) do not require members to be present at the same time but share the same information at the time most convenient to each one. An example might be a follow-up where a picture of a skin wound is shared for later viewing (Siwicki, 2019).

In a survey of state health departments, ASTHO (Kearly & Oputa, 2019) found that over 51% used telehealth services to provide patient and professional health education. Other uses included behavioral health (42.4%), specialty care (40.2%), chronic disease (23.9%), and infectious disease (23.9%). Increased access was the greatest achievement (33.8%), whereas securing funding (22.4%) was the greatest challenge. Services are expanding; the U.S. Department of Health and Human Services provides an overview of telehealth services offered at https://telehealth.hhs.gov/patients/why-use-telehealth.

Telehealth shows great potential for advancing preventative medicine and the treatment of chronic conditions. Post COVID-19, there is an increase of 43% use in telehealth medicine (Call, 2022) and an upward trend in previously underserved groups:

- 73% of rural respondents use telemedicine (up from 63% in 2021)
- 50% of uninsured respondents use telemedicine (up from 37% in 2021)
- 76% of 55 years and older respondents use telemedicine (up from 64% in 2021)
- 82% of women use telemedicine (up from 73% in 2021)
- 82% of Hispanic respondents use telemedicine (up from 73% in 2021) (Knowles et al., 2023)

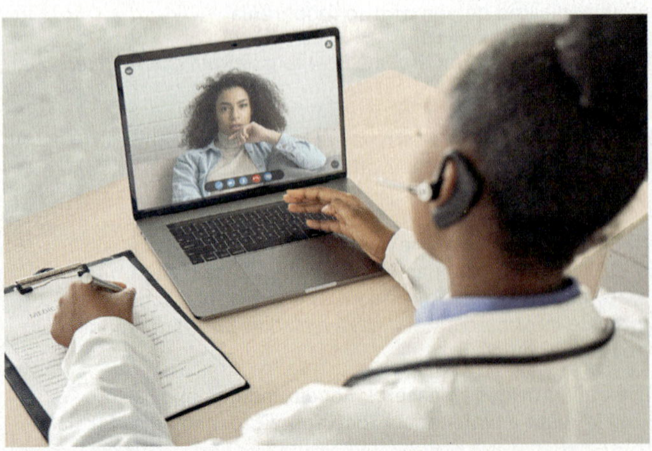

FIGURE 10-10. Telehealth gives the community/public health nurse an opportunity to see and speak with clients located at remote sites, as well as provide education and counseling.

Additionally, patients and providers view telemedicine positively with 80% satisfaction. Average visits were reduced by 45% with time and travel costs projected to save almost 90 billion annually (Call, 2022). The growth in telehealth services demonstrates continued demand for this service (FAIR Health, 2019).

There are nursing licensure barriers, as nurses working in telehealth must be licensed in the state where patients are located at the time services are provided. Licensure compact regulations provide for multistate nursing licenses through the Enhanced National Licensure Compact (eNLC), which requires criminal background checks and licenses within states and reporting between states participating in the compact (Mataxen, 2019). As of January 2020, there were 38 member states of eNLC, either enacted or pending (Gaines, 2023).

Geographic Information Systems

A **geographic information system (GIS)** is a special geographic system that creates, manages, analyzes, and maps geographic information to data (see Box 10-16). GIS allows the user to visualize, question, analyze, and interpret data to understand relationships, patterns, and trends. Spatial or mappable data are integrated with conventional data. Topographical maps on information such as watersheds, elevation, hydrography, transportation, land boundaries, and geographic features can be overlaid with additional data (United States Geological Service [SGS], n.d.). The use of GIS can provide information about demographic, epidemiologic, and logistical issues and emerging trends in relation to geographic areas and regions. The CDC interactive map can be used to view health trends in the United States using GIS data at https://www.cdc.gov/dhdsp/maps/atlas/sample_maps.htm.

GIS can provide the following:

- Better understanding of a current situation
- Planning/targeting of appropriate interventions
- Monitoring and revision of interventions as needed
- An opportunity for cooperation with other organizations and government departments through a culture of data sharing and working together

Sharing, comparing, and integrating GIS data will eliminate silos and result in better outcomes providing additional information to identify health disparities (CDC, 2020). There is great potential for GIS to inform C/PHN. Nurses can play an important role in demonstrating how various data sources come together to enable informed decisions for populations and people (DePriest et al., 2019). Understanding GIS may be considered an essential skill for the evolution of nursing practice (DePriest et al., 2019). GIS has tremendous potential to benefit healthcare delivery. Both public and private

BOX 10-16 STORIES FROM THE FIELD

Using GIS to Calculate Access to Providers for Patients Experiencing Heart Failure

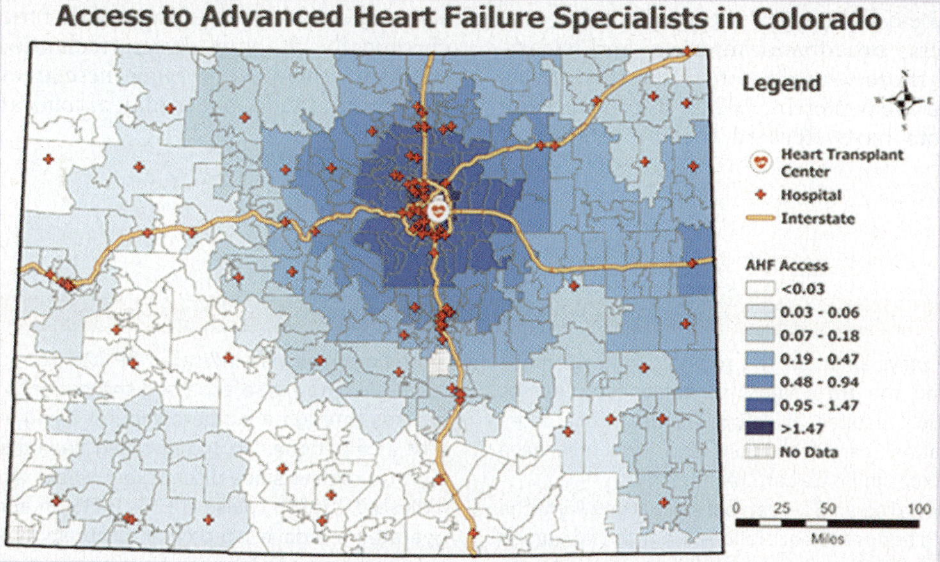

Researchers at The University of Colorado Anschutz Medical Campus are using geographic information systems (GIS) to calculate access to providers for patients experiencing heart failure (HF). Levels of care for these patients can be categorized into (1) primary care providers, (2) cardiologists, and (3) advanced heart failure (AHF) specialists. AHF specialists, which represent the highest level of specialty care for patients with HF, are more likely to be found in urban areas with hospitals specializing in heart care. These researchers are interested in how access to specialists varies by geography and whether better access is associated with better outcomes. In this work, GIS was used to calculate a measure of access to AHF specialists for each ZIP code using the Two-Step Floating Catchment Area method (Wang & Luo, 2005). ZIP code boundaries and population estimates were obtained from the U.S. Census, and provider billing ZIP codes were obtained for AHF specialists providing care to patients with HF in the Centers for Medicare & Medicaid Services database. In the first step of this method, a provider-to-population (P2P) ratio is calculated for every ZIP code using the providers and populations for every neighboring ZIP code within a 100-mile radius. In the second step, a measure of access is calculated by summing these P2P ratios and weighting them by distance. ZIP codes with the highest P2P ratios in their vicinity have the highest AHF Access index score (indicated by darker blue colors). Unsurprisingly, AHF specialist access was best in the Denver metro area where most of Colorado's population resides and where the state's only heart transplant center is located. Less expected was higher access for the rural plains of East Central Colorado. Researchers found that AHF specialists are spending part of their time in Western Kansas clinics to provide specialty services to patients with HF, which in turn increases access for Eastern Colorado. In addition to answering questions about access, GIS can be used to identify underserved areas that should be targeted by providers in the future. These maps can also be used to communicate research findings and resource locations to the public at large.

William B. Allshouse (Ben), PhD, BSPH
Instructor, Environmental & Occupational Health
Colorado School of Public Health, CU Anschutz Medical Campus

Reference: Wang, F., & Luo, W. (June, 2005). Assessing spatial and nonspatial factors for healthcare access: Towards an integrated approach to defining health professional shortage areas. *Health Place*, *11*(2), 131-146. https://doi.org/10.1016/j.healthplace.2004.02.003. PMID: 15629681

organizations are developing innovative ways to use GIS, from public health departments and public health policy and research organizations to hospitals, medical centers, and health insurance organizations. Public health uses of GIS include tracking child immunizations, evaluating the spread and clustering of diseases, conducting health policy research, and establishing service areas and districts (ArcUser Online, n.d.).

Electronic Health Literacy and the Digital Divide

The rapid development of communication technology affects every aspect of society as information is instantly available. Health communication and health information technology competencies are identified as vital skills of an informed consumer and essential for improving population health outcomes and healthcare quality. Electronic health literacy was first defined by Norman and Skinner (2006, para. 1) as the "ability to seek, find, understand, and appraise health information from electronic sources and apply the knowledge gained to addressing or solving a health problem."

Computer literacy and knowledge of the use of current technologies are part of health literacy. Increasingly, people must be able to use technology and navigate through a vast array of information, tools, and sources to acquire and critically analyze the information necessary to make appropriate and informed decisions (CDC, 2022b). The same is true for community/public health nurses, as noted in the Council of Public Health Nurse Organizations, C/PHN competencies (2018).

A digital divide exists between those who have easy access to computers, broadband internet, and smartphones/tablets and those who do not. Often this affects those living in rural areas (Perrin, 2021). Recent technological developments have elevated the importance of assessing how electronic health tools have empowered patients and improved health, especially among the most vulnerable populations. There is potential for electronic health technologies to aid in reducing communication inequalities and disparities in health. The need exists to educate at-risk and groups with functional needs (e.g., chronically ill) and design technology in a way that works for them. Addressing these areas may not diminish the digital divide, but it may ameliorate its consequences (Bevilacqua et al., 2021).

CASE STUDY **10 ESSENTIAL PUBLIC HEALTH SERVICES**

Home Care Technology

Today's technology plays an important role in caring for high-risk patients. During the early years of home care, nurses carried pagers, which resulted in delayed patient care coordination. Today, patient care transitions and outcomes have improved with advances in home care technology.

A nurse recently visited an 85-year-old discharged from the hospital with newly diagnosed heart failure. Prior to the nurse's visit, a home telehealth device was installed in the patient's home; it was programmed to provide heart failure information daily for 1 year. To use the device, the patient attaches a blood pressure cuff and O_2 oximeter and steps on a scale, and the device automatically records their blood pressure, pulse, O_2 saturation, and weight. The remote telehealth RN is able to review the patient's health data daily.

During the visit, the patient provided the nurse with health data from their telehealth log and asked questions about their diuretic therapy. The patient was concerned that they were constantly urinating during the day and multiple times at night and did not have time to always call someone to help them get up. The patient had a BMI of 20 prior to admission and had lost 5 pounds in the last few weeks. This telehealth records on the morning of the visit indicated BP 128/75, pulse 75, O_2 96% on room air. The nurse accessed the patient's clinic and hospital records through a laptop computer using a protected hotspot with a cell phone. No changes had been made to the patient's diuretic regime since discharge 6 weeks ago; hospital records indicated 150/85, pulse 82, O_2 94% on admission. The nurse operated a mobile lab device to obtain laboratory results and noted that no new labs had been obtained since discharge.

1. ***Recognize Cues:*** *Which findings require immediate follow-up, are unexpected, or are most concerning?*
2. ***Analyze Cues:*** *What information is noted or needed for interpreting findings?*
3. ***Prioritize Hypotheses:*** *Based on the information that you have, what is happening?*
4. ***Generate Solutions:*** *What intervention(s) will achieve the desired outcome?*
5. ***Take Action:*** *What actions should you take or do first?*
6. ***Evaluate Outcomes:*** *Were outcomes achieved? Why or why not?*
7. *Which Essential Public Health Services influence this situation? (See Box 2-2.)*

SUMMARY

- Information and communication technology is used to provide care, gather data, and inform decision making for people, communities, and populations.
- In community/public health, nurses will work with interdisciplinary teams; group communication and in-group decision making are necessary skills.
- Collaboration and partnership building are purposeful interactions among the nurse, clients, community members, and other professionals based on mutual participation and joint effort. It is characterized by shared goals, mutual participation, maximized use of resources, clear responsibilities, set boundaries, and collaborative relationships.
- Contracting is a helpful tool in promoting clients' participation, independence, and motivation. It is used at all levels of community/public health nursing to promote partnership in the collaborative process, to encourage commitment to health goals, and to ensure a format and a means for negotiation among the collaborating parties.
- Electronic health records (EHRs) are more prevalent in public health and are commonplace in hospital and outpatient settings.
- Big data include large and complex data sets that are analyzed to uncover trends, associations, and patterns. This is very helpful in public health agencies in the areas of disease surveillance, population health management, and immunization trends.
- mHealth involves the use of mobile devices (e.g., smartphones, tablets, notebooks) for communication between clients and community/public health nurses and can be useful in promoting health. Trends in mHealth include interactive (two-way communication), integrative (patient/provider and tracking systems), and multimedia uses (games/quizzes to promote health).

- Technology applications are used for computers, tablets, and smartphones, and more health-related apps are available every year. C/PHNs must be aware of reliable applications to assist in health promotion.
- Blogging and online support communities have proven to be helpful to those with chronic diseases or others needing emotional support.
- Video games and VR games, such as exercise programs, are being used for health applications, in addition to their usual entertainment value.
- Telehealth provides health information or healthcare to many people and groups who may otherwise not be able to access it, and its popularity is increasing.
- Electronic health literacy and the digital divide often prevent full use of technology among vulnerable and rural populations.

ACTIVE LEARNING EXERCISES

1. Pick a classmate and take turns practicing motivational interviewing (using OARS). Role play working with a client who has a problematic behavior (e.g., needs to eat healthier, exercise more). How will you approach them? Describe how you can demonstrate active listening and effective communication skills. How might you contract with the client to promote the achievement of client goals? (Objectives 1 and 4)
2. Think of a patient you have worked with who may have low health literacy. Give three examples of how to help them better communicate with their primary provider and other health professionals. Debate with a classmate if health literacy is important, not only for the patient as a person but for the community and society as a whole. Which of the 10 Essential Public Health Services (Box 2-2) is being utilized here? (Objective 2)
3. Discuss with a community/public health nurse or supervisor the importance of collaboration and collaborative skills. Ask about examples of types of collaborative projects or interventions. What facilitates effective collaboration in the community? What inhibits effective collaboration, and how can you overcome this? Describe how collaboration is essential in mobilizing community partnerships (see number 4 of the 10 Essential Public Health Services listed in Box 2-2). (Objective 3)
4. Search the literature for research examples of the use of big data in assessing public health problems and designing interventions. Were the findings significant and applicable to your community? From identified issues, what health technologies might be employed for people, communities, populations? Explain how these technologies will make a difference? How is this most useful in public health? (Objectives 5 and 6)
5. Consider the various types of technology available (e.g., mHealth, mobile health applications, video games, telehealth, GIS). Which would you find most effective as you design public health interventions for various age groups and populations (e.g., Spanish-speaking Latina people needing nutritional information; adolescents seeking information on STDs and sexual health; addressing an outbreak of foodborne illness in a large metropolitan area; 10- to 14-year-olds with asthma)? (Objectives 7 and 8)

CHAPTER 11

Health Promotion Through Education

"Of all forms of inequality, injustice in health is the most shocking and inhumane."

—Martin Luther King, Jr.

KEY TERMS

Affective domain	Health disparities	Planned change	Social determinants of health
Anticipatory guidance	Health literacy	Psychomotor domain	Stages of change
Cognitive domain	Health promotion	Revolutionary change	VARK
Evolutionary change	Learning theory		

LEARNING OBJECTIVES

Upon mastery of this chapter, you should be able to:

1. **Examine social determinants of health and how these determinants relate to health inequities and change through education.**
2. **Analyze the stages of change and associated change models/principles as they relate to health promotion with communities/populations.**
3. **Demonstrate the C/PHN role as an educator in promoting health and improving quality of life.**
4. **Link the domains of learning, learning theories, learning styles, and teaching models to educational activities that improve population health.**
5. **Develop teaching plans focusing on primary, secondary, and tertiary levels of prevention for clients of all ages and learning needs.**

INTRODUCTION

Think about one of your favorite teachers from nursing school, high school, or earlier. How did the teacher get and hold your interest? How can you apply that in your work with public health nursing clients? Teaching has played a critical role of the community/public health nurse (C/PHN) since the origins of the profession and is frequently a C/PHN's primary role or function. C/PHNs develop partnerships with clients to achieve behavior changes that promote, maintain, or restore health. This partnership focuses on self-care—the ability to effectively advocate and manage a person's own health. The rationale for health teaching is to equip people with the knowledge, attitudes, and practices that will allow them to live the fullest possible life for the greatest length of time.

This chapter begins by discussing the *Healthy People 2030* goals and objectives, as well as key concepts related to health promotion. It then covers the nature and stages of change and the process and principles of planned change. Next, we consider some foundational concepts related to learning and teaching, including the domains of learning, learning theories, health teaching models, and teaching at the three levels of prevention. Finally, the chapter concludes by providing guidance on effective client teaching, including some principles of learning and teaching, steps in the teaching process, teaching methods and materials, and teaching clients with special learning needs.

HEALTHY PEOPLE 2030 AND KEY CONCEPTS RELATED TO HEALTH PROMOTION

To understand the goals of health promotion and the C/PHN's role in meeting them, we must explore relevant aspects of the *Healthy People 2030* initiative and some key concepts, including the social determinants of health (SDOH), the socioeconomic gradient in health, health disparities, access to care, and quality of care.

Healthy People 2030

The vision of *Healthy People 2030* is for "a society in which all people can achieve their full potential for health and well-being of all people" (Office of Disease

Prevention and Health Promotion [ODPHP], n.d.-a, para. 4). The *Healthy People 2030* framework consists of a vision and mission with foundational principles that guide the overarching goals and objectives for the plan of action (Office of Disease Prevention and Health Promotion, n.d.-a). Attaining the full potential for health and well-being through the creation of social, physical, and economic environments is one of the five overarching goals of *Healthy People 2030* (CDC, 2023a). Furthermore, the *Healthy People 2030* objectives address SDOH, health equity, and health literacy (ODPHP, n.d.-b). *Healthy People 2030* objectives for Educational and Community-Based Programs are listed in Box 11-1 (ODPHP, n.d.-c). These objectives, when viewed in the broader context, can be used to identify client needs and align educational efforts that will advance this national initiative.

Social Determinants of Health

The World Health Organization (WHO) has defined the **social determinants of health** (SDOH) as "the conditions in which people are born, grow, live, work, and age and the wider set of forces and systems shaping the conditions of daily life" (WHO, n.d.-a, para. 1). These nonmedical conditions influence human beings across the life span and from their home to work and every place in between. The Centers for Disease Control and Prevention (CDC) have adopted the WHO definition and explain that economic systems and policies, societal norms and social policies, development agendas, politics, racism, and climate change impact SDOH (CDC, 2022a). The U.S. Department of Health and Human Services has identified five domains associated with SDOH. These domains include the following:

- Economic stability
- Access to quality education
- Access to quality healthcare
- Neighborhood and built environment
- Social and community context

The unequal distribution of these factors among certain groups contributes to health disparities that are persistent and pervasive. Between 2019 and 2021, the United States experienced a severe reduction of U.S. life expectancy. The biggest decline occurred among American Indian and Alaska Native (AIAN) populations with a decline of 6.6 years. Hispanic and Black populations experienced a decline in life expectancy of 4.2 and 4.0 years. In 2021, the average age of life expectancy was 65.2 for AIAN and 70.8 for Black populations compared to 76.4 years for White populations and 77.7 years for Hispanic populations (Kaiser Family Foundation, 2023a). The major contributing factor to this decline was related to COVID-19; however, SDOH can also be attributed to the decline. For example, AIAN populations under age 65 have the highest uninsured rate at 21%, followed by Hispanic populations under age 65 at 19%, Native Hawaiian and other Pacific Islander and Black populations at 10.9% compared to White populations at 7.2% (Kaiser Family Foundation, 2023b). *Healthy People 2030* provides an overview along with associated objectives, evidence-based resources, and actual community implementations, partnerships and related news updates (i.e., Healthy People in Action) associated with each domain (ODPHP, n.d.-a). See Box 11-2 for select objectives of *Healthy People 2030* social determinants of public health. Addressing these factors in a manner that has a positive impact on social, economic, and physical

BOX 11-1 *HEALTHY PEOPLE 2030*

Objectives for Educational and Community-Based Programs

Core Objectives

ECBP-01	Increase the proportion of adolescents who participate in daily school physical education
ECBP-02	Increase the proportion of schools that do not sell less healthy foods and drinks

Developmental Objectives

ECBP-D01	Increase the proportion of middle and high schools that provide case management for chronic conditions
ECBP-D03	Increase the proportion of worksites that offer employee health promotion program(s)
ECBP-D04	Increase the proportion of worksites that offer an employee physical activity program
ECBP-D05	Increase the proportion of worksites that offer an employee nutrition program
ECBP-D06	Increase the proportion of worksites with policies that ban indoor smoking
ECBP-D07	Increase the number of community organizations that provide prevention services
ECBP-D08	Increase the interprofessional prevention education in health professions training programs
ECBP-D09, D10, D11, D12, D13	Increase core clinical prevention and population health education in medical, nursing schools, dental, and pharmacy schools and primary provider assistant training programs

Reprinted from U.S. Department of Health and Human Services (USDHHS). (2020). *Educational and community-based programs objectives.* https://health.gov/healthypeople/search?query=ECBP

BOX 11-2 *HEALTHY PEOPLE 2030*

Key Factors for Social Determinants of Health (Selected Objectives)

Core Objectives

SDOH-01	Reduce the proportion of people living in poverty
SDOH-02	Increase employment in working-age people
SDOH-03	Increase the proportion of children aged 0–17 years living with at least one parent who works full time
SDOH-04	Reduce the proportion of families that spend more than 30% of income on housing
SDOH-05	Reduce the proportion of children with a parent who has served time in jail
SDOH-06	Increase the proportion of high school graduates in college the October after graduating

Research Objectives

SDOH-R01	Increase the proportion of federal data sources that collect country of birth as a variable

Reprinted from U.S. Department of Health and Human Services (USDHHS). (2020). *Browse objectives.* https://health.gov/healthypeople/search?query=social+determinants+of+health

conditions and supports positive health behavior change can improve the health of communities over time.

Health Disparities

Health disparities are preventable differences among populations in the quantity of disease, burden of disease, age and rate of mortality due to disease, health behaviors and outcomes, and other health conditions (CDC, 2023b; Duran & Pérez-Stable, 2019). Put another way, health disparities can be objectively viewed as a disproportionate burden of morbidity, disability, and mortality found in a specific portion of the population in contrast to another. When addressing health disparities, health equity must also be considered. Health equity is defined as "the attainment of the highest level of health equity for all people" (ODPHP, n.d.-d, para. 6). Health disparities impact populations of people that have experienced more systematic obstacles that are related to "racial or ethnic group; religion; socioeconomic status; gender; age; mental health; cognitive, sensory, or physical disability; sexual orientation or gender identity; geographic location; or other characteristics historically linked to discrimination or exclusion" (ODPHP, n.d.-d, para. 6). The *Healthy People 2030* framework provides guidance to address and reduce the health disparities and health inequities in the United States.

Reported disparities exist in the areas of quality of healthcare, access to care, levels and types of care, and care settings; they exist within subpopulations (e.g., older adults, people assigned female at birth, children, rural residents, those with disabilities) and across clinical conditions. Thus, to continue the work on eliminating health disparities, one overarching goal for *Healthy People 2030* is to "eliminate health disparities, achieve health equity, and attain health literacy to improve the health and well-being of all" (ODPHP, n.d.-c, n.d.-d, para. 1).

- Poor access to quality care and overt discrimination are examples of disparities.
- Discrimination can occur during service delivery if healthcare providers are biased against a specific group or hold stereotypical beliefs about that group.
- Providers may also not be confident about providing care for a racial or ethnic group with whom they are unfamiliar.
- Language barriers can be a problem, as can cultural values and norms that are unfamiliar to providers. Patients can also react to providers in a way that promotes disparities; patients may not trust the information given to them and may not follow it as explained, leading to inadequate care (Ndugga & Artiga, 2023).

Access to Healthcare

The Institute of Medicine's (2003) classic report *Unequal Treatment: Confronting Racial and Ethnic Disparities in Health Care* noted a large body of research highlighting the higher morbidity and mortality rates among all racial and ethnic underrepresented groups when compared with White populations. This report drew attention to an issue that continues today and remains relevant. Differences in healthcare access were also explained, be it in the form of inadequate or no health insurance, problems getting healthcare, the quality of care, fewer choices in where to go for care, or the lack of a regular healthcare provider.

- Residential segregation, although illegal, still exists and can play a role in health disparities.
- Historically, vulnerable populations, especially racial and ethnic underrepresented groups and populations with limited resources, have found access to healthcare difficult. Recent data shows rural areas experience reduced access to healthcare due to a healthcare provider shortage that results in longer travel times to care and lower healthcare coverage (Ndugga & Artiga, 2023).
- Other geographic factors can affect access to healthcare services. For example, the opioid epidemic has impacted all areas, but there are fewer substance use disorder treatment centers in certain geographic areas. A study found that people with substance use disorder living in a rural setting were over nine times more likely to lack a healthcare provider in their area

that was licensed to prescribe an essential medication-assisted treatment, buprenorphine (Rodriguez, 2023).

Quality of Healthcare

Quality of care is essential for positive health outcomes. The WHO explains that quality healthcare must be safe, effective, timely, efficient, equitable, people-centered, and integrated throughout the life span (n.d.-b). To receive quality care, people must be able to access it. In 2022, it was estimated that 112 million Americans (44%) struggled to cover healthcare costs and 93% felt that they did not receive adequate care for what they paid (West Health, 2022). Research confirms that underrepresented groups have more barriers to access healthcare when compared with White populations and use less care due to being under or uninsured. People of color are more at risk for being uninsured compared to White people (Tolbert et al., 2022). One factor contributing to the lower use of care could be the lack of diversity that exists in the U.S. healthcare system. It is reported that 64% of practicing primary providers were White; 20.6%, Asian; 6.9%, Hispanic; and 5.7%, Black or African American (AAMC, 2023). Research indicates that clients from ethnic and racial underrepresented groups feel more comfortable and satisfied with care from a healthcare provider who comes from the same racial and ethnic group (Fig. 11-1; Huerto & Lindo, 2020). Unfortunately, findings from the Robert Wood Johnson Foundation reveal that only 22% of Black adults reported being the same race as their healthcare providers compared to 73.8% of White adults and their healthcare providers (2023).

Lack of access to quality healthcare services is common among racial and ethnic underrepresented groups. Significant disparities in the quality of care can be attributed to healthcare staffing shortages. It is estimated that by 2034, the American healthcare system may experience a shortage in primary care providers, nurses, and healthcare technologists. In particular, these shortages will impact those areas already experiencing a healthcare shortage (i.e., rural areas). This then leads to additional barriers of transportation and work-related issues. Those populations experiencing a reduction of healthcare providers in their area must travel longer distances that require more of a time commitment (Wolters Kluwer, 2022). These barriers often lead to a reduction of participation in preventive healthcare and postponing care. It was reported that 42% of workers delayed care due to no available appointments (Mayer, 2023). Access to quality healthcare services is essential for positive patient outcomes. Solutions to overcome this problem include the use of telemedicine/virtual visits, after-hour services, and the use of remote patient monitoring systems (Wolters Kluwer, 2022).

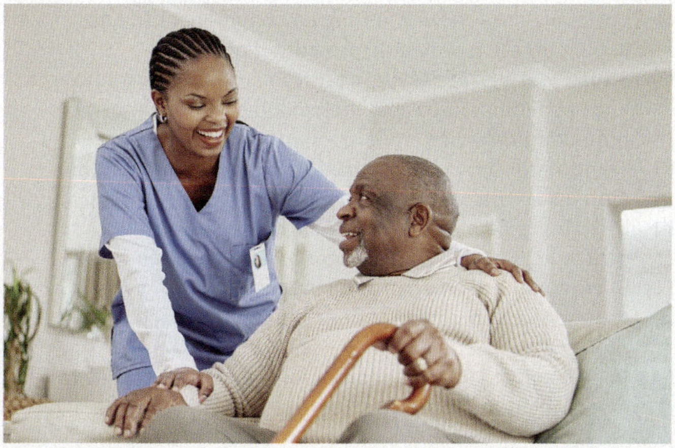

FIGURE 11-1 Clients from underrepresented groups often prefer healthcare providers from the same racial and ethnic background.

Health literacy is a key component related to positive healthcare outcomes. Underrepresented vulnerable populations are at a greater risk for experiencing communication problems in healthcare and have lower levels of health literacy. **Health literacy** consists of the information and services that people need to make educated health decisions. According to the Network of the National Library of Medicine (NNLM), "9 out of 10 adults struggle with health literacy" (para. 5). Health literacy involves more than the ability to read. Health literacy involves the ability to calculate the correct medication dosage and time for administration and the ability to understand medical jargon (i.e., fasting). There are several areas associated with health literacy:

- Personal health literacy refers to a person's ability to locate, understand, and use healthcare information to make decisions about healthcare for themselves or others. Examples of personal health literacy include understanding medication and health promotion instructions, healthcare forms, and the overall ability to understand the complex healthcare system (NNLM, n.d.).
- Organizational health literacy is the ability of the organization to provide people with equitable health information and services that are easy to find, understand, and use for making healthcare decisions for themselves or others. Examples of this include an easy-to-use appointment system, ensuring patient health education comprehension through the use of the Teach-Back method and providing communication using appropriate format, language, and reading level (NNLM, n.d.).
- Digital health literacy is the ability to access a computer or other electronic device and then search, understand, and ensure a reputable source for electronic information. Examples of digital health literacy include accessing personal electronic health records, using apps for health and wellness, using electronic communication for scheduling, bill payment, etc. (NNLM, n.d.).

Quantitative literacy, also known as numeracy, is defined as "a set of mathematical and advanced problem-solving skills that are necessary to succeed in a society increasingly driven by data" (National Association of Secondary School Principals, 2023, para. 1). Examples of numeracy include understanding insurance explanation of benefits, determining the best treatment option, and knowing what to do with a blood sugar or blood

BOX 11-3 Key Factors for Health Literacy (Selected Objectives)

Core Objectives

HC/HIT-D01	Increase the number of state health departments that use social marketing in health promotion programs
HC/HIT-01	Increase the proportion of adults whose healthcare provider checked their understanding
HC/HIT-02	Decrease the proportion of adults who report poor communication with their healthcare provider
HC/HIT-03	Increase the proportion of adults whose healthcare providers involved them in decisions as much as they wanted
HC/HIT-04	Increase the proportion of adults who talk to friends or family about their health

Reprinted from Office of Disease Prevention and Health Promotion. (n.d.-e). *Increase the health literacy of the population-HC-HIT-RO1.* https://health.gov/healthypeople/objectives-and-data/browse-objectives/health-communication/increase-health-literacy-population-hchit-r01

pressure result (NNLM, n.d.). Recommendations to improve health literacy are to ensure that healthcare providers are properly educated and trained regarding health literacy, develop clearinghouses of health literacy information for healthcare providers, ensure that health materials are in plain language and in different languages, and make health information accessible for everyone (NNLM, n.d.).

The C/PHN educator is essential in the improvement of health literacy. See Box 11-3 for select objectives related to health literacy in *Healthy People 2030*.

HEALTH PROMOTION THROUGH CHANGE

Health promotion has been defined as health behaviors that improve well-being and lead to a desire to meet one's human potential (Murdaugh et al., 2019). A term often confused with health promotion is *disease prevention* (or *health protection*), which is "focused on specific efforts aimed at reducing the development and severity of chronic diseases and other morbidities" (Rural Health Information Hub, 2023a, para. 3).

These two terms, so often used interchangeably, are clearly both important aspects of health education efforts, yet they imply a decidedly different motivation. For the C/PHN, both terms relate to practice at the primary level of prevention. Box 11-4 describes educational activities within both approaches in relation to primary prevention. For instance, a C/PHN may plan an educational program for community-dwelling older adults to learn about the need for a balanced diet, rich in fruits and vegetables. This would be an example of a health promotion focus, because there is no clear disease or condition at issue. As the nurse continues to work with these people, the nurse learns that several clients have had recent falls. Fortunately, none of the falls were serious, yet the nurse recognizes the need to discuss foods that will help reduce bone loss and promote healthy bone growth. To protect the client's health, the nurse provides information on a variety of foods rich in calcium and explains the need for adequate vitamin D, a safe home environment, weight-bearing exercise (Fig. 11-2), and medication review. This effort would be still primary prevention but with the purpose of health protection.

For the C/PHN, teaching is the primary means to influence health at all levels: primary, secondary, and tertiary. But consider the educational program just described: The C/PHN has provided a well-developed educational program that was well received by the participants. They

BOX 11-4 Theoretical Propositions of the Health Promotion Model

1. Inherited and acquired characteristics along with prior behavior influence beliefs, affect, and health-promoting behavior.
2. People engage in behaviors from which they anticipate deriving personally valued benefits.
3. Perceived barriers can constrain action to change behavior and the behavior itself.
4. Perceived self-efficacy to embrace a given behavior increases the likelihood to commit to action and implementing the behavior.
5. Greater perceived self-efficacy results in fewer perceived barriers.
6. Positive affect toward a behavior results in greater perceived self-efficacy, which can result in increased positive affect.
7. When positive affect is associated with a behavior, commitment and action are increased.
8. People are more likely to commit to and participate in health-promoting behaviors when significant others model the behavior, expect it, and provide assistance and support for the behavior.
9. Others—family members, peers, and healthcare providers—are important sources of influence that can positively or negatively influence commitment to and implementation of health-promoting behavior.
10. Situational influences can positively or negatively influence commitment to and implementation of health-promoting behavior.
11. The greater the commitment to a behavior change, the more likely the change will be maintained over time.
12. Distracting demands over which the person has little control may affect commitment to a behavior change.
13. Commitment to a behavior change is less likely to be maintained when other actions are more attractive and preferred.
14. People can modify the interpersonal and physical environments to create incentives for behavior changes.

Source: Murdaugh et al. (2019).

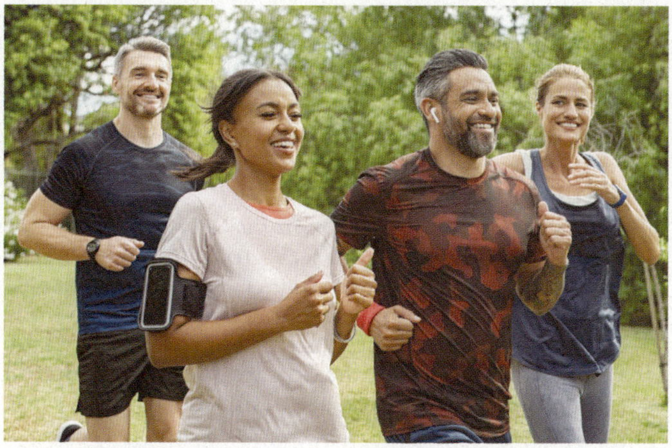

FIGURE 11-2 A goal of health promotion is to encourage clients to develop healthy behaviors.

listened attentively, took the nurse's well-prepared handouts home, and even promised to add more fruits, vegetables, and calcium-rich foods to their diet. A few weeks later, in another educational program, the nurse learns from the participants that they have not altered their dietary patterns in the slightest. This is an example of how understanding the principles of behavior change may provide guidance to this C/PHN in planning a more effective program, with a greater chance for success.

The Nature of Change

To be a C/PHN is to be a health educator with the goal of effecting change in people's behaviors. When nurses suggest that families adopt healthier communication patterns, they are asking them to change. Teaching parenting skills to teenagers is introducing a change. Promoting a community's self-determination in choosing a safer environment requires that the people involved must change. Therefore, it becomes imperative for C/PHNs to understand the nature of change, how people respond to it, and how to effect change for improved community health.

Definitions and Types of Change

Change is "any planned or unplanned alteration of the status quo in an organism, situation, or process," per Lippitt's (1973, p. 37) classic definition. This definition explains that change may occur either by design or by default. From a system's perspective, change means that things are out of balance or the system's equilibrium is upset (Roussel et al., 2020). For instance, when a community is ravaged by floodwaters, its normal functioning is thrown off balance. Adjustments are required; new patterns of behavior become necessary. The change process can also be described as sudden or drastic (revolutionary) or gradual over time (evolutionary).

Evolutionary change is gradual and requires adjustment on an incremental basis. It modifies rather than replaces the current way of operating. Some examples of evolutionary change include becoming parents, gradually cutting back on the number of cigarettes smoked each day, and losing weight by eliminating desserts and snacks. Gradual change may "ease the pain" that change brings to some people. Sometimes, this type of change may be viewed as *reform*.

Revolutionary change, in contrast, is a more rapid, drastic, and threatening type of change. It involves different goals and perhaps radically new patterns of behavior. Sudden unemployment, stopping smoking overnight, losing the town's football team in a plane accident, removing children from abusive parents, or rapidly replacing human workers with computers are examples of revolutionary changes. In each instance, the people affected have little or no advance warning and little or no time to prepare. High levels of emotional, mental, and sometimes physical energy and rapid behavior change are required to adapt to revolutionary change. If the demands are too great, some may experience defense mechanisms such as incapacitation, resistance, or denial of the new situation.

The impact of a proposed change on a system clearly depends on the degree of the change's evolutionary or revolutionary qualities, a factor to be considered in planning for change. Some situations lend themselves better to one kind of change than to another. A community in need of improved facilities for the handicapped (e.g., ramps, wider doors) can introduce this change on an evolutionary, incremental basis, whereas a community that is involved in an unsafe, intolerable, or life-threatening situation, such as a hurricane or pandemic, such as COVID-19, may require revolutionary change.

Examples of social and public health change occurred during the last decades of the 20th and 21st centuries. Dramatic decrease in tobacco consumption is an example of evolutionary change that occurred during that time. This change did not come about simply through education alone. Rather, state and federal legislative efforts were used along with social norming strategies bringing the problem to the attention of the American public. The combination of social influence and supportive legislation and policies changed health behavior (Comen, 2022).

Although cigarettes had been proclaimed a health risk in 1964, many people still smoked. It was not until smoking cessation research began to show promise and new over-the-counter treatments and medications became available that more people attempted to stop smoking. In 1992, secondhand smoke was declared to be a carcinogen. Mass media was used to educate the public on the risks of smoking and the benefits of quitting; this also began to change public opinion. At the same time, legislation to control the advertising of tobacco products and tighten sales to minors gained momentum. In 2009, federal excise taxes on tobacco increased with several states also increasing tobacco taxes. As of 2022, 28 states have laws banning smoking in public places, including workplaces, bars, and restaurants. These smoke-free policies and higher cigarette taxes made it more difficult for some to smoke. Research shows that adult smoking rates have declined from 23.5% in 1999 to 13.7% in 2018, with youth smoking rates decreasing from 26% to 8.8% (Comen, 2022).

Stages of Change

The phrase **stages of change** refers to the three sequential steps leading to change:

- Unfreezing (when desire for change develops)
- Changing (when new ideas are accepted and tried out)
- Refreezing (when the change is integrated and stabilized in practice)

Kurt Lewin first described these stages in the 1940s and early 1950s, and they have become a cornerstone for understanding the change process (Barrow et al., 2022; Lewin, 1947, 1951; Lippitt et al., 1958):

- Unfreezing: The first stage, unfreezing, occurs when a developing need for change causes disequilibrium in the system. A system in disequilibrium is more vulnerable to change. People are motivated to change either intrinsically or by some external force. The unfreezing stage involves initiating the change.
- Changing/moving: The second stage of the change process, changing or moving, occurs when people examine, accept, and try the innovation (Barrow et al., 2022). This is the period when participants in a prenatal class are learning exercises or when older clients in a center for older adults are discussing and trying ways to make their apartments safe from accidents. During the changing stage, people experience a series of attitude transformations, ranging from early questioning of the innovation's worth to full acceptance and commitment and then to accomplishing the change. The change agent's role during this moving stage is to help clients see the value of the change, encourage them to try it out, and assist them in adopting it.
- Refreezing: The third and final stage in the change process, refreezing, occurs when change is established as an accepted and permanent part of the system (Barrow et al., 2022). The rest of the system has adapted to it. People no longer feel resistant to it, because it is no longer viewed as disruptive, threatening, or new. As the change is integrated, the system becomes refrozen and stabilized. Refreezing involves integrating or internalizing the change into the system and then maintaining it.

Planned Change

Leaders in community health nursing have been change agents for decades. They have planned and managed change in a variety of systems. **Planned change** is a purposeful, designed effort to effect improvement in a system with the assistance of a change agent per Spradley's classic definition (1980). Planned change, also known as managed change, is crucial to the development of successful community health nursing programs, and various models of change have been proposed over the years (Table 11-1; Roussel et al., 2020). Regardless of the specific model used, the following characteristics of planned change are key to its success:

- *The change is purposeful and intentional:* There are specific reasons or goals prompting the change. These goals give the change effort a unifying focus and a specific target. Unplanned change occurs haphazardly, and its outcomes are unpredictable.
- *The change is by design, not by default:* Thorough systematic planning provides structure for the change process and a map to follow toward a planned destination.
- *Planned change in community health aims at improvement:* That is, it seeks to better the current situation, to promote a higher level of efficiency, safety, or health enhancement. Planned change aims to facilitate growth and positive improvements. Plans to provide shelter and healthcare for an unsheltered population, for example, are designed to improve this group's well-being.
- *Planned change is accomplished through an influencing agent:* The change agent is a catalyst in developing and carrying out the design; the change agent's role is a leadership role, often as an educator.

Planned Change Process

The planned change process involves a systematic sequence of activities that follows the nursing process. The eight basic steps lead to the successful management of change. These steps include (1) recognize symptoms, (2) diagnose need, (3) analyze alternative solutions, (4) select a change, (5) plan the change, (6) implement the change, (7) evaluate the change, and (8) stabilize the change (Table 11-1; Spradley, 1980).

Applying Planned Change to Larger Aggregates

C/PHNs use the change process when managing change at an organization, population group, community, and larger aggregate levels. For example, as a result of information gleaned from parents and other caregivers, C/PHNs, and other community health partners, as well as other data that track health outcomes, a nurse may suspect that there is a widespread lack of confidence among young parents (Fig. 11-3). This hypothesis could be tested through a social media survey to determine parenting needs among the entire community's population of young parents. If symptoms are present (step 1), the nurse, in collaboration with health department personnel or other appropriate professionals, could analyze the symptoms and reach a diagnosis (step 2) that many young parents in the community are lacking in confidence and knowledge of parenting skills. Several approaches to meeting this need could be considered, such as instituting a parenting center in the community with satellite clinics, organizing churches or clubs to sponsor parenting support groups, or working through the community college system to hold workshops and classes on parenting skills (step 3). The most feasible and useful alternative could be selected (step 4), and a parenting program for the community could be planned (step 5) and implemented (step 6). The nurse, with parents and other professionals involved, would then evaluate the outcomes (step 7) and make necessary adjustments in the parenting program before finally stabilizing it (step 8), making certain that this change, undertaken to meet a population group need, remains an established and effectively functioning service (Table 11-1).

TABLE 11-1 Change Models

Change Model	Steps in the Model	Example of Application
Six phases of planned change (Havelock & Havelock, 1973)	1. Develop the relationship 2. Diagnose the problem 3. Acquire resources for change 4. Select a pathway for the solution 5. Establish and accept change 6. Maintain the change (maintenance and separation)	A new family planning client is requesting birth control but is unsure of the method. Developing rapport and trust (relationship) is essential to allow the C/PHN to be able to identify the patient's needs (diagnose). Several birth control methods are discussed (resources), and the patient feels a long-acting birth control would be ideal (pathway). After education, a progesterone intrauterine device is inserted (maintenance).
Seven phases of planned change (Lippitt et al., 1958)	1. Diagnose the problem 2. Assess motivation and capacity for change 3. Assess the change agent's motivation and resources 4. Select progressive change objectives 5. Choose an appropriate change agent role 6. Maintain the change 7. Terminate the helping relationships	A patient's body mass index is 30 (diagnose). When the C/PHN asks if the patient has any health concerns, they report they are concerned with their weight (assess motivation). The patient is interested in working with the nurse to identify resources and a weight loss plan (assess change agent's motivation). A nutrition and physical activity plan is developed along with a return appointment (choose appropriate change agent). Upon the first return visit, the client has lost 4 lb in a 4-week period, and at the next visit in 4 weeks, the client has lost a total of 7 lb (maintain). Once weight loss goals have been accomplished, the visits end (terminate).
Innovation-decision process (Rogers, 2003)	1. Knowledge 2. Persuasion 3. Decision 4. Implementation 5. Confirmation	A client wants to stop tobacco use. She has tried several times but has been unsuccessful. The client seeks assistance from the C/PHN. The nurse provides information regarding the risks of tobacco use and tobacco cessation options (knowledge), and the need to set a stop date (persuasion). The client determines a stop date (decision), and with consultation of a primary care provider, a tobacco cessation medication is prescribed (implementation). A follow-up appointment is scheduled in 2 weeks, and the client is tobacco free. Additional follow-up is set up to track the client's progress (confirmation).
Kotter's 8-step model of change (Kotter, 2012)	1. Create a sense of urgency 2. Build a guiding coalition 3. Form a strategic vision and initiative 4. Enlist a volunteer army 5. Enable action by removing barriers 6. Generate short-term wins 7. Sustain acceleration 8. Institute change	Data reveal an increase in teen suicide (urgency). Several agencies, including the school system, the public health department, mental health providers, parents, caregivers, students, etc., schedule a meeting (coalition). The meeting consists of developing a vision to reduce teen suicide in the community (vision/initiative). Additional resources and support for the coalition are established (volunteer army). Focus groups with teens are conducted to determine concerns (remove barriers). Information from the focus groups is used to implement change (short-term wins). Interventions and evaluation continue (sustain acceleration and institute change).

Source: Havelock and Havelock (1973); Kotter (2012); Lippitt et al. (1958); Rogers (2003).

Change and Health Promotion Within Communities/Populations

Changes in behavior and health promotion can also be directed to even larger audiences—communities and larger populations. Similar approaches can be used but may be varied depending on age, most pertinent issues, and how to best reach targeted audiences. For instance, in an effort to increase physical activity in communities, the Office of Disease Prevention and Health Promotion partnered with 10 communities to implement Move Your Way. This campaign is designed to increase physical activity, thus increasing health and wellness. The program provides communities with resources to plan, implement, and evaluate community physical activity efforts (ODPHP, 2022). Preliminary research finds that exposure to Move Your Way increases the awareness of

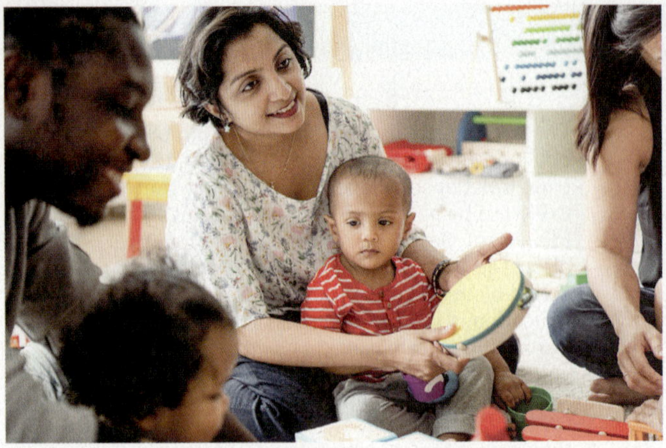

FIGURE 11-3 Parents and their young children in a playgroup.

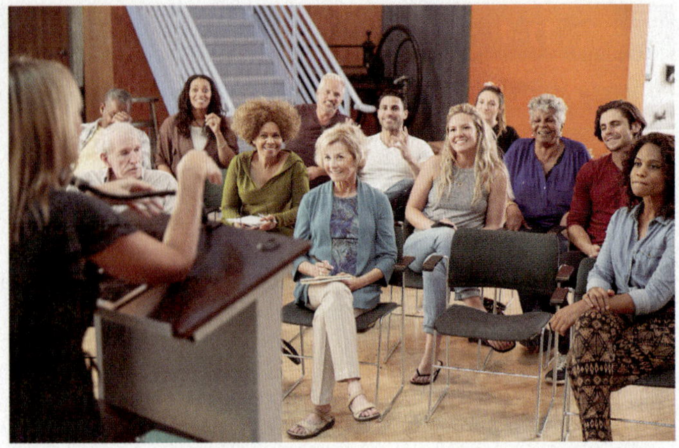

FIGURE 11-4 A group engaging in the planned change process.

the *Physical Activity Guidelines for Americans* and the aerobic and muscle-strengthening physical activity recommendations. Additionally, those aware of Move Your Way reported to meet the physical activity requirements (Olscamp et al., 2022).

Change and health promotion in communities begin with understanding the basics of health communication and social marketing. The CDC provides information regarding these six phases (CDC, 2022b):

1. Problem definition and description (e.g., health problem of concern, who this affects, how you can address it)
2. Problem analysis/market research (e.g., analyze data on the problem; target audience's values, behaviors, beliefs, attitudes, and barriers/facilitators to changing behavior)
3. Planning communication/market strategy (e.g., determine the target audience, what behaviors you wish to address, benefits offered [such as better health] with interventions to support change)
4. Program planning/interventions (e.g., methods you will use to influence change [for instance, a website to promote better nutrition/physical activity for adolescents], plan, objectives)
5. Implementation (e.g., plan for launching program, publicity, threats/opportunities)
6. Program evaluation (e.g., Was the program feasible, useful, accurate, ethical?)

This method has been used with many health problems and issues (e.g., arthritis, breastfeeding, drug misuse prevention, smoking cessation, HIV/AIDS, colorectal cancer screening, chronic fatigue syndrome, immunizations, influenza) and is a helpful means of reaching targeted populations (CDC, 2022b). See Chapters 10 and 12 for more on health promotion, communication, and use of technology in assessing communities and developing programs for health promotion.

Principles for Effecting Positive Change

C/PHNs introduce change every day that they practice. Every effort to solve a problem, prevent another problem from occurring, meet a potential community need, or promote people's optimal health requires change. For these changes to be truly successful, so that desired outcomes are reached, they must be well thought out and managed. There are several change models that define principles and guidelines for effecting positive change (Table 11-1).

Change is inevitable. Understanding the principles of planned change can assist the C/PHN in guiding people, families, and communities toward achieving the highest level of health (Fig. 11-4).

CHANGE THROUGH HEALTH EDUCATION

For the C/PHN, health education is a foundation of practice. Whether the nurse is providing one-on-one education to a new parent about the benefits of breastfeeding, briefing county officials on the need to maintain breastfeeding support centers, or working with community partners and grant funders to develop a web-based social marketing campaign to promote breastfeeding among adolescent parents, educational techniques are being used to promote health in the community. Knowledge of educational theories and teaching methods can assist the nurse in framing these "health messages" for the greatest impact and chance of success.

- *Teaching* is a specialized communication process in which desired behavior changes are achieved. The goal of all teaching is learning.
- *Learning* is a process of assimilating new information that promotes a permanent change in behavior. Learning is gaining knowledge, comprehension, or mastery.

After learning, clients are capable of doing something that they could not do before learning took place. Effective teaching is the cause; learning becomes the effect. To teach effectively, especially in the community where teaching is the focus of care, nurses need to understand the various domains of learning and related learning theories.

Domains of Learning

Learning occurs in several realms or domains: cognitive, affective, and psychomotor. Understanding the differences among these domains and the nurse's related roles provides the background necessary to teach effectively.

Cognitive Domain

The **cognitive domain** of learning involves the mind and thinking processes. When the meaning and relationship of a series of facts are grasped, cognitive learning has occurred. The cognitive domain deals with the recall or recognition of knowledge and the development of intellectual abilities and skills (Bloom, 1956), as follows:

- Remember
  - Recall basic facts
  - Example: A school nurse asks adolescents in a weight loss group to list foods high in fat
- Understand
  - Comprehend concepts when they are explained
  - Example: A school nurse asks adolescents in a weight loss group to identify ways to lose weight
- Apply
  - Transfer understanding into practice
  - Example: A school nurse asks adolescents in a weight loss group to keep a food and physical activity record for a week, draw up a diet, and share this plan with the group at the next meeting
- Analyze
  - Break down concepts into parts; establish the relationship among the parts
  - Example: A school nurse asks adolescents in a weight loss group to distinguish the fat content in a variety of packaged foods
- Evaluate
  - Validate information
  - Example: A school nurse asks adolescents in a weight loss group to select a menu that is low in fat
- Create
  - Produce new or original work
  - Example: A school nurse asks adolescents in a weight loss group to develop a menu that is low in fat

(Vanderbilt University Center for Teaching, 2019)

How to Measure Cognitive Learning. Cognitive learning at any of the levels described can be measured easily in terms of learner behaviors. Nurses know, for instance, that clients have achieved teaching objectives for the application of knowledge if their behavior demonstrates actual use of the information taught. Client roles in cognitive learning range from relatively passive (at the knowledge level) to a more active role (at the evaluation level). Conversely, as clients become more active, the nurse's role becomes less overtly directive. Not all clients need to be brought through all levels of cognitive learning, and not every client needs to reach the evaluation level for each aspect of care. For some clients and situations, comprehension is an adequate and effective level; for others, the nurse should focus on the application level. Table 11-2 illustrates client and nurse behaviors for each cognitive level (Iowa State University Center for Excellence in Learning and Theory, 2019).

TABLE **11-2** Domains of Learning

Level	Illustrative Client Behavior	Illustrative Nurse Behavior
A. Cognitive Learning: A Case Study in Controlling Diabetes		
Remember (recalls, knows)	States that insulin, if taken, will control own diabetes	Provides information
Understand (describes)	Describes insulin action and purpose	Explains information
Apply (uses learning)	Adjusts insulin dosage daily to maintain proper blood sugar level	Suggests how to use learning
Analyze (draws a connection)	Compares relationships between insulin, diet, activity, and diabetic control	Demonstrates and encourages analysis
Evaluate (judges according to a standard)	Selects a plan, incorporating above learning, for controlling own diabetes	Facilitates evaluation
Create (generates new ideas)	Designs a plan of diabetic control	Formulates own plan
B. Affective Learning: A Case Study in Family Planning		
Receptive (listens, pays attention)	Is attentive to family planning instruction	Directs client's attention
Responsive (participates, reacts)	Discusses pros and cons of various methods	Encourages client involvement
Valuing (accepts, appreciates, commits)	Selects a method for use	Respects client's right to decide
Internal consistency (organizes values to fit together)	Understands and accepts responsibility for planning for desired number of children	Brings client into contact with role models
Adoption (incorporates new values into lifestyle)	Consistently practices birth control	Positively reinforces healthy behaviors

Affective Domain

The **affective domain** involves learning that occurs through emotion, feeling, or *affect*. This kind of learning deals with changes in interest, attitudes, and values (Bloom, 1956; Miller et al., 2021). Here, nurses face the task of trying to influence what their clients may value and feel. Nurses want clients to develop an ability to accept ideas that promote healthier behaviors, even if those ideas conflict with the clients' values.

Attitudes and values are learned. They develop gradually, as family, peers, experiences, and culture influence the way a person feels and responds. These feelings and responses are the result of imitation and conditioning. In this way, clients acquire their health-related beliefs and practices. Because attitudes and values become part of the person, they are difficult to change unless the nurse is aware of how they develop.

Affective learning occurs on several levels as learners respond with varying degrees of involvement and commitment:

- At the first level, learners are simply receptive; they are willing to listen, to show awareness, and to be attentive. The nurse aims at acquiring and focusing learners' attention (Miller et al., 2021; Miller & Stoeckel, 2019). This limited goal may be all that clients can achieve during the early stages of the nurse–client relationship.
- At the second level, learners become active participants by responding to the information in some way. Examples are a willingness to read educational material, to participate in discussions, to complete assignments (e.g., keeping a diet record), or to voluntarily seek out more information (Miller et al., 2021; Miller & Stoeckel, 2019).
- At the third level, learners attach value to the information. Valuing ranges from simple acceptance through appreciation to commitment (Miller et al., 2021; Miller & Stoeckel, 2019).
- The final level of affective learning occurs when learners internalize an idea or value. The value system now controls learner behavior. Consistent practice is a crucial test at this level (Miller et al., 2021; Miller & Stoeckel, 2019).

Affective learning often is difficult to measure and is often attempted through self-report surveys or tools (Miller et al., 2021; Miller & Stoeckel, 2019). This elusiveness may influence C/PHNs to concentrate their efforts on cognitive learning goals instead. Yet, client attitudes and values have a major effect on the outcome of cognitive learning—which is desired behavioral changes.

Psychomotor Domain

The **psychomotor domain** includes visible, demonstrable performance skills that require some kind of neuromuscular coordination (Miller et al., 2021; Miller & Stoeckel, 2019). Clients in the community need to learn skills such as infant bathing, temperature taking, breast or testicular self-examination, prenatal breathing exercises, range-of-motion exercises, catheter irrigation, walking with crutches, changing dressings, and performing cardiopulmonary resuscitation (Fig. 11-5).

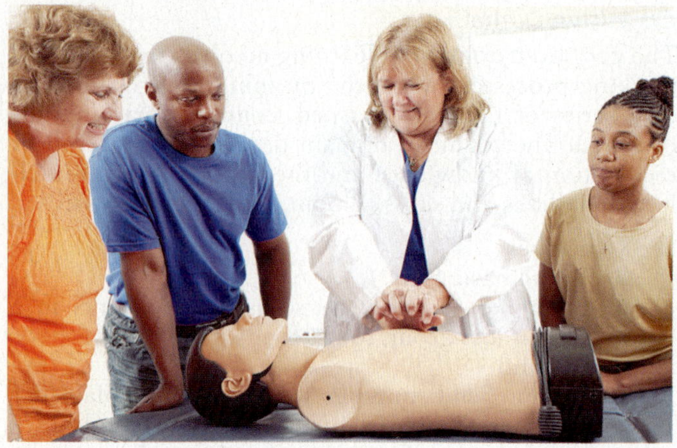

FIGURE 11-5 A C/PHN demonstrates cardiopulmonary resuscitation to clients before having them return the demonstration to show that they can put this learning into practice.

For psychomotor learning to take place, three conditions must be met: (1) learners must be capable of the skill; (2) learners must have a sensory image of how to perform the skill; and (3) learners must practice the skill.

- C/PHNs must be certain that the client is physically, intellectually, and emotionally capable of performing the skill. It may be difficult for an older person with diabetes who has trembling hands and fading vision to give their own insulin injections; it could frustrate and harm them. They may need some assistance or accommodations.
- Clients' intellectual and emotional capabilities also influence their capacity to learn motor skills. It may be inappropriate to expect people with significant developmental delays to learn complex skills. The degree of complexity should match the learners' level of functioning. However, educational level should not be equated with intelligence.
  - Developmental stage is another point to consider in determining whether it is appropriate to teach a particular skill. For example, most children can put on some article of clothing at 2 years of age but are not ready to learn to fasten buttons until they are past their third birthday.
- Learners also must have a sensory image of how to perform the skill through sight, hearing, touch, and sometimes taste or smell. This sensory image is gained by demonstration. To teach clients motor skills effectively, the C/PHN must provide them with an adequate sensory image. It is best to demonstrate and explain slowly, one point at a time, and sometimes repeatedly, until clients understand the proper sequence or combination of actions necessary to carry out the skill.
  - Another condition for psychomotor learning is practice. After acquiring a sensory image, clients can start to perform the skill. Mastery comes over time as clients repeat the task until it is smooth, coordinated, and unhesitating (Miller et al., 2021; Miller & Stoeckel, 2019). During this process, the C/PHN should be available to provide guidance and encouragement. In the early stages

of practice, you may need to use hands-on guidance to give clients a sense of how the performance should feel.

- When clients give return demonstrations, you can make suggestions, give encouragement, and thereby maximize the learning.
- For example, a C/PHN demonstrates passive range-of-motion exercises on a client's wife to show her how the exercises should feel (giving her a sensory image). The wife then learns to perform the exercises on her husband. During practice, feedback from the nurse enables the wife to know whether the skill is being performed correctly.
- At this guided response stage, objectives may include action verbs such as *fastens*, *manipulates*, *measures*, *organizes*, and *calibrates*.

The psychomotor domain, like the cognitive and affective domains, ranges from simple to complex levels of functioning. It is necessary to exercise judgment in assessing a client's ability to perform a skill. Even clients with limited ability often can move to higher levels once they have mastered simple skills. Nursing tasks that facilitate psychomotor learning in the client include the following:

- Determine the client's capability for learning by assessing the client's physical, intellectual, and emotional abilities.
- Physically demonstrate and explain the skill, providing the client with a sensory image.
- Encourage practice by providing guidance and positive reinforcement.

Learning Styles

It is important for the C/PHN to understand that learners have a learning style preference. These learning styles include the following: visual, aural/auditory, read/write, and kinesthetic (**VARK**).

- Visual learning style: These learners prefer diagrams, maps, flow charts, graphs, or other pictures that are used instead of words to convey the meaning of the information. It is important to note that visual preferences do not include PowerPoint, pictures, or videos. Instead, the visual preference incorporates symbols and other graphics that express an idea without using words (VARK Learn Limited, 2023).
- Aural/auditory learning style: Information that is heard or spoken is the preference of the aural/auditory learner. The content is best understood through lectures, podcasts, radio, and group discussions. Additionally, these learners prefer to speak the information and may talk to themselves as they interpret information. They may repeat something that has already been said or ask a question that was already answered (VARK Learn Limited, 2023).
- Read/write learning style: This style uses words through reading and writing as a way to interpret information. Activities such as reports, books, manuals, and essays are prime media for learning. These people thrive with PowerPoint, books, the internet, and other sources of words (VARK Learn Limited, 2023).
- Kinesthetic learning style: The learners with the kinesthetic preference learn best through experience and practice. Activities that allow the learner to actually do the skill or activity are the preferred method of learning. These learners value the personal experience rather than the experience of others. Real life experience, simulations, demonstrations, and case studies are examples of learning activities for this learning style (VARK Learn Limited, 2023).

Learning Theories

A **learning theory** is a systematic and integrated look into the nature of the process whereby people relate to their surroundings in such ways as to enhance their ability to use both themselves and their surroundings more effectively (Schunk, 2020). Each nurse has and uses a particular theory of learning, whether consciously or unconsciously, and that theory, in turn, dictates the way the C/PHN teaches clients. It is useful to discover what each nurse's learning theory is and how it affects the role of health educator. A brief examination of these learning theories can be viewed in Table 11-3.

Health Teaching Models

Theories on learning provide a general understanding of how people learn. In addition, various health teaching models specifically focus on explaining individual health experiences, behaviors, and actions. These models fit with the learning theories to give nurses a more accurate picture of the client and the client's learning needs. Four useful models are described here: the health belief model (HBM), Pender's health promotion model (revised) (HPM), the transtheoretical or stages of change model, and the PRECEDE and PROCEED models.

Health Belief Model

The HBM, which was developed by social psychologists and brought to the attention of healthcare professionals by Rosenstock (1966), is useful for explaining the behaviors and actions taken by people to prevent illness and injury. It postulates that readiness to act on behalf of a person's own health is predicated on the following (Rural Health Information Hub, 2023b):

- Perceived susceptibility to the condition in question
- Perceived seriousness of the condition in question
- Perceived benefits of taking action
- Barriers to taking action
- Cues to action, such as knowledge that someone else has the condition or attention from the media
- Self-efficacy—the ability to take action to achieve the desired outcome

Using the HBM, a study examined the perceptions of the severity and susceptibility of COVID-19 and the perceived efficacy of recommended health behaviors by age group. The study found that middle-aged and older adults were more concerned regarding hospitalization and death from COVID-19 compared to younger age groups. Additionally, the findings show that middle-aged and older adults felt they responded adequately to health recommendations compared to younger age groups (Bechard

TABLE 11-3 Learning Theories

Theory Type and Name	Theorists and Dates of Landmark Publications	Theory Description	Example of Theory in Practice
Behavioral			
Stimulus—response "bond" theory	Ivan Pavlov (1957)	With conditioning, certain causes (stimuli) evoke certain effects (responses).	C/PHN teaches a family client to take her birth control pill each morning after she brushes her teeth.
No-reinforcement approach	Edward Thorndike (1932, 1969)	The learner has an innate reflexive drive to accomplish the desired response after conditioning.	C/PHN repeatedly emphasizes to a group of pregnant patients that their prenatal classes promote a positive delivery experience and healthy newborns.
Conditioning through reinforcement	B. F. Skinner (1974, 1987)	Reinforcement through successive, systematic changes in the learner's environment enhances the probability of desired responses.	A school nurse gives rewards (e.g., stickers, activity books) to children who attend each class on safety.
Cognitive			
Theory of cognitive development	Jean Piaget (1966, 1970)	Each stage signifies a transformation from the previous one, and a child must move through each stage sequentially. Three abilities are used to make the transformation: 1. *Assimilation*: reacting to new situations by using skills already possessed 2. *Accommodation*: being sufficiently mature so that previously unsolved problems can now be solved 3. *Adaptation*: the ability to cope with the demands of the environment	The nurse uses puppets with 3-year-olds in a presentation on safety but group discussion with young teens with diabetes on the benefits and consequences of taking or not taking their insulin.
Insight theory		1. Learning is a process in which the learner develops new insights or changes old ones. 2. Learners intuitively and intelligently sense their way through problems. 3. However, the "insight" is useful only if the learner understands its significance.	The C/PHN provides a career planning class and Amy, who did not finish high school, realizes that she has limited job skills and that if she learned more computer skills, she could get a better job.
Goal-insight theory		The learner goes beyond intuitive hunches to tested insights.	Amy takes a beginning and then an advanced computer class and is offered a higher-paying job. The C/PHN discusses Amy's successes with her and asks Amy whether she ever thought about going to college. Amy begins to think about completing the requirements to go to community college, because if she had an associate degree she could be promoted to a supervisory position and make more money.
Cognitive field theory		The learner is purposive and problem centered.	Amy confers with the C/PHN about her choices and has changed her thinking about herself so much that she is planning to get an apartment in a neighborhood that is better for her child and she may continue taking classes.

TABLE **11-3** Learning Theories (*Continued*)

Theory Type and Name	Theorists and Dates of Landmark Publications	Theory Description	Example of Theory in Practice
Social Learning			
Overview of social learning theory	Bandura (1977, 1986)	1. Relationships often are dysfunctional and produce undesirable or inappropriate behavior. 2. The learner, influenced by role models, builds self-confidence, persuasion, and personal mastery. 3. Self-efficacy can lead to the desired behaviors and outcomes.	N/A
Coincidental association		Outcomes typically are preceded by numerous events, and the client selects the wrong events as predictors of an outcome.	Juanita had a negative experience with a person who wore a hearing aid. Afterward, all of her experiences with people who wore hearing aids were negative. Juanita may begin to separate her negative experiences with people from their hearing disabilities after attending a class on building self-esteem suggested by the C/PHN.
Inappropriate generalization		One negative experience provokes negative feelings for future experiences.	Three-year-old Ryan accidentally drank some spoiled milk. He generalized that milk tastes bad and now refuses to drink it. The nurse can suggest to Ryan's mother that she might have Ryan try chocolate milk. She then can slowly reintroduce plain milk.
Perceived self-inefficacy		"Persons who judge themselves as lacking coping capabilities, whether the self-appraisal is objectively warranted or not, will perceive all kinds of dangers in situations and exaggerate their potential harmfulness" (Bandura, 1986, p. 220).	An older client, William, tells the C/PHN about two missing Social Security checks but refuses to take a bus to the post office. He states that he does not know what to say to the postal clerk and has read about older adults getting mugged on buses. He refuses to follow-up on his lost income. The C/PHN introduces him to another gentleman in the apartment complex who feels confident in the neighborhood and improves William's self-confidence.
Humanistic			
Hierarchy of human needs	Abraham Maslow (1970)	A person's needs must be met in order of priority, with more basic needs having to be met before others. In order from most basic to least, needs are: 1. Physiologic (air, food, water) 2. Safety and security 3. Love and belonging 4. Self-esteem (positive feelings of self-worth) 5. Self-actualization	It would be difficult for a group of young parents to concentrate on learning about proper infant nutrition if they are worried about their babies crying in the next room. Their need to care for their children (need for love and belonging) would be greater than the need to learn about future health considerations (self-esteem and self-actualization).

(*Continued*)

TABLE 11-3 Learning Theories (*Continued*)

Theory Type and Name	Theorists and Dates of Landmark Publications	Theory Description	Example of Theory in Practice
Client-centered counseling approach	Carl Rogers (1969, 1989)	1. The learning environment is to be learner centered so that students become more self-directed and guide their own learning. 2. The learner is the person most capable of deciding how to find the solutions to problems. The client identifies the problem and, given time and space, can find a way through the problem to a solution. 3. The C/PHN acts as a facilitator in this learning process.	A 55-year-old person who wants to quit smoking after a prolonged upper respiratory tract infection that is aggravated by the habit comes to a stop-smoking class led by the C/PHN at the county health department.
Adult Learning			
Adult learning theory	Knowles (1984, 1989, 1990) Knowles et al. (2015)	Adult learners: 1. Are self-directed in their learning 2. Have a lifetime of experience to draw on when learning 3. Are more ready to learn when the learning is focused on helping them meet requirements for their personal and occupational roles 4. Have a problem-centered time perspective, in that they need to apply and try out their learning quickly	Susan, a 65-year-old retired librarian, was open to learning more about her type 2 diabetes after a recent discharge from the hospital. When the C/PHN arrived at her house, Susan was asked what she already knew about diabetes and included Susan in goal-setting regarding her health. Susan appreciated that the C/PHN provided information that built on her previous understanding of the disease and worked with Susan to find manageable solutions to improve her health.

Source: Bandura (1977, 1986); Knowles (1984, 1989, 1990); Knowles et al. (2015); Maslow (1970); Pavlov (1957); Piaget (1966, 1970); Rogers (1969, 1989); Skinner (1974, 1987); Thorndike (1932, 1969).

et al., 2021). C/PHNs may find the use of the HBM (and variations) to be helpful in assessing the health behaviors and beliefs of culturally diverse populations.

Pender's Health Promotion Model

First published in the 1980s by nurse Nola Pender, the Health Promotion Model (HPM) was envisioned as a framework for exploring health-related behaviors within a nursing and behavioral science context (Murdaugh et al., 2019). Reflecting the growing body of literature relevant to the HPM, Pender revised the model to reflect a number of major theoretical changes. The revised HPM includes three general areas of concern to health-promoting behavior: *Individual characteristics and experiences* are seen to interact with *behavior-specific cognitions and affect* to influence specific *behavioral outcomes* (Murdaugh et al., 2019). The revised HPM focuses on predicting behaviors that influence health promotion. In addition, the HPM includes the variable of interpersonal influence of others, including family and health professionals.

Being able to predict health promotion behaviors enhances the C/PHN's ability to work with clients. Awareness of their characteristics, experiences, comprehension of their health-related issues, perceived barriers, self-efficacy, support (or lack of it) from significant others, and commitment provides the nurse with a picture that clarifies the client–nurse role and gives direction for action taking. The HPM (Fig. 11-6) is based on the theoretical propositions found in Box 11-4.

Using these propositions, researchers examined the impact of the Pender health promotion model (HPM) on the health outcomes of pregnant people with cardiac disease. Findings revealed that after 12 weeks of education, the intervention group had increased health knowledge and lower rates of severe heart failure, cesarean delivery, preterm birth, and infants with low birth weight compared to the control group. The study concluded that the HPM can improve knowledge and reduce cardiac disease and improve infant outcomes (Zhang et al., 2022).

Transtheoretical or Stages of Change Model

The transtheoretical model (TTM) addresses change by anticipating relapses and recognizing those as opportunities to better plan for how to sustain the needed change in future attempts (Prochaska et al., 2007; Raihan & Cogburn, 2023). The model, sometimes called stages of change, is not linear but is depicted as a spiral, with

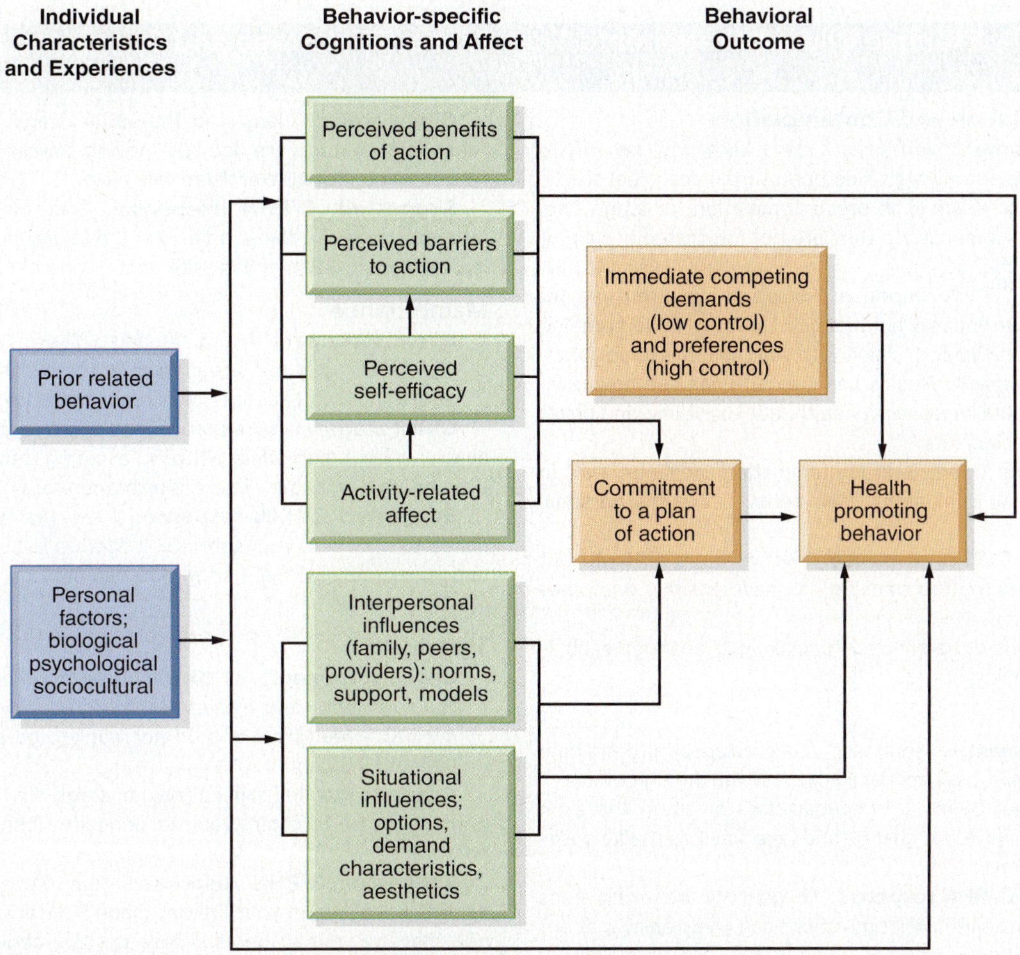

FIGURE 11-6 Health promotion model. (Reprinted with permission from Pender, N. L., Murdaugh, C. L., & Parsons, M. A. (2015). *Health promotion in nursing practice* (7th ed.). Prentice Hall. © 2015. Reprinted by permission of Pearson Education, Inc., New York, NY.)

plateaus, relapses, and false starts. It can be used with people, groups, and populations. The stages include the following (Prochaska et al., 2007, p. 39):

- Precontemplation—This is usually the normal state of denial or the problem may not be perceived (either the client doesn't know about it or doesn't want to acknowledge it). The client may say, "I don't really smoke that many cigarettes, so I don't have to worry about lung cancer or the other health problems."
- Contemplation—At this stage, the client is more realistic and may be more open to discussing the problem of smoking. However, the client may not be able to seriously consider behavior change or feel able to confront the issue. The client may say, "I know I should probably try to quit smoking, but I am really stressed right now and can't think about it."
- Preparation—During this stage, the client is moving away from contemplation toward action. The client may be trying to gather information and may be talking to others about how they quit smoking. They may be concerned that it may take more than one try in order to accomplish their goal. A client may talk to the primary provider about medications that are helpful, tell friends and family that they are planning to quit smoking, and may even begin to cut back on the number of cigarettes smoked each day.
- Action—This stage is the beginning of the behavioral change. The client sets a date to quit smoking, begins using a nicotine patch or medication, and finds replacement behaviors for smoking (e.g., using breath mints, exercising during usual smoking breaks). The client knows that this attempt may not be successful the first time and should be encouraged to acknowledge and plan for this.
- Maintenance—In this stage, the behavior has been changed. The smoker has stopped smoking but now needs to be vigilant in avoiding a relapse. The client needs a support system and rewards to encourage maintenance. If the client relapses, the C/PHN and others can help the client learn from this and begin their preparation and action stages again until longer periods of maintenance are achieved.
- Termination—This occurs when the former behavior is no longer appealing. The smoker no longer has an interest in cigarettes and does not have to exert the constant vigilance needed in the maintenance stage. Prochaska et al. (2007) note that not everyone can truly reach this stage, and therefore, it is not always included in health promotion programs or research.

BOX 11-5 Example Clients' Statements That Reveal TTM Stage and Suggested Nurse Responses

Precontemplation and Contemplation

Client statement: Jeff says: "I don't know why my wife is concerned about my high blood pressure. I don't feel sick."

Client stage: Client is in precontemplation, or stage one, in which clients demonstrate they are not interested in help or thinking about change.

Suggested C/PHN response: "Sometime symptoms are not always present, so you may not feel sick. However, understanding your diagnosis and what this means to your health is important."

Client statement: Jessica comments, "I can see how quitting smoking could improve my health, but I can't imagine never having another cigarette."

Client stage: Client is in contemplation, or stage two, in which clients may think about their behavior and the personal consequences of it.

Suggested C/PHN response: "I know this is difficult, but taking steps now to stop smoking can have positive outcomes for your health."

Neither client is committed to making a change; each is unaware or thinking of pros/cons.

Preparation

Client statement: Jamie states, "I feel good about setting a date to go into rehab, but I wonder if I can really go through with it."

Client stage: Client is in preparation, or stage three, in which clients think about change and take small steps like gathering information.

Suggested C/PHN response: "I'm glad you are taking steps to improve your health. What questions can I help answer about rehab?"

Action

Client statement: Kevin reports, "I have been on my low salt, low fat diet for a month now, and my blood pressure is better, but I'd really like to be able to eat fast food more often."

Client stage: Client is in the action stage, or stage four; those in this stage are actually moving toward their goal and feel more confident exercising willpower.

Suggested C/PHN response: "Incorporating change into your daily life takes time. You are taking positive steps to improve your health and modify your eating choices."

Maintenance

Client statement: Maria remarks, "These last few months of sobriety give me a feeling of accomplishment, but I still question if total abstinence is really mandatory."

Client stage: In maintenance, or stage five, people are successful with completing actions, avoiding temptations, and developing new habits. There is awareness of potential relapse.

Suggested C/PHN response: "I see that you are determined to stick with your sobriety. It is often too easy to slip into unhealthy choices, but I know you can stay on track with this lifestyle change."

Termination

Client statement: "I have modified my diet and exercise regularly now, and I have decreased my BMI and lowered my A1C. I feel great and do not want to go back to feeling unhealthy again."

Client stage: In termination, or stage six, people do not want to return to their previous unhealthy behaviors and will not relapse.

Suggested C/PHN response: "Your decision to include healthy behaviors in your life has made a difference in how you now manage your diabetes. These positive choices might also influence other family members."

Researchers have used this model with many topics related to health promotion and prevention (e.g., substance misuse, smoking cessation, weight loss, physical activity). A research study examined the effects of a TTM-based intervention combined with motivational interviewing on patients with depression and hospitalized with cardiac heart disease. The results found that the intervention was effective in reducing depressive symptoms in those patients hospitalized with cardiac heart disease (Li et al., 2020). Often, the nurse can determine the stage the client is in from the client's statements; see Box 11-5 for some example statements and suggested nurse responses.

The PRECEDE and PROCEED Models

First published by Green in 1974, the PRECEDE model was developed for educational diagnosis (Glanz et al., 2015). The acronym PRECEDE has been slightly revised from the original to stand for *p*redisposing, *r*einforcing, and *e*nabling *c*onstructs in *e*ducational/ecological *d*iagnosis and *e*valuation (Bartholomew et al., 2015; Green & Kreuter, 2005).

- The PROCEED model (Green et al., 2019, 2022) works in tandem with the PRECEDE model as the C/PHN proceeds to plan, implement, and evaluate health education programs.
- This acronym stands for *p*olicy, *r*egulatory, and *o*rganizational *c*onstructs for *e*ducational and *e*nvironmental *d*evelopment (Bartholomew et al., 2015). The entire PRECEDE–PROCEED model includes eight phases in the formulation and evaluation of health educational programs.
- The first five of these phases are included in the PRECEDE portion of the model and include (1) social, (2) epidemiologic, and (3) education/ecological assessments, followed by (4) administrative and policy assessment and intervention alignment, and (5) implementation.
- The PROCEED model is emphasized in the last three phases: (1) process evaluation, (2) impact evaluation, and (3) outcome evaluation.

A hallmark of the PRECEDE–PROCEED model is the emphasis on the desired outcome. The model both begins and ends with *quality of life*, which includes "subjectively defined problems and priorities of people and communities" (Green et al., 2019, 2022). The emphasis on what the person or community perceives as the problem, not what the professional believes it to be, is crucial. Outcome evaluation is logically linked back to that same person or community in assessing achievement of the desired change.

The steps in this model are similar to those of the nursing process. Because of this familiarity, the model has become a useful tool for nurses teaching in the community. The nurse builds on the assessment formulated from the PRECEDE model, determines the best interventions, and then proceeds to evaluate the outcome of those interventions. The emphasis on the perceived needs of the person or community as the starting point for all community efforts is consistent with public health nursing practice. The model reminds us of the importance of an organized approach to health educational programs, one that begins and ends with the "experts"—the people, families, and communities we hope to help through our efforts. The PRECEDE–PROCEED model is available at https://www.lgreen.net/precede-proceed-2022-edition.

This model has been used to address many public health problems. Over 1000 examples of published applications of PRECEDE–PROCEED may be found at www.lgreen.net, including studies on healthcare workers' hand hygiene behaviors, follow-up with multicultural people with atypical mammograms, implementation of church-based heart health promotion programs for older adults, developing a healthy-eating curriculum for schools, evaluation of a physical activity and nutrition program for older adults, and determining health promotion motivators in Asian populations. Other models used in community assessment and intervention may be found in Chapter 15.

Teaching at Three Levels of Prevention

C/PHNs should develop teaching programs that coincide with the level of prevention needed by the client. The three levels of primary, secondary, and tertiary prevention are demonstrated in the levels of prevention pyramid for nurses who teach clients, families, aggregates, or populations (Box 11-6).

Ideally, the C/PHN focuses on teaching at the primary level. If nurses reached more people at this level, it would help diminish years of morbidity and limit subsequent incapacity. Many people experience disabilities that could have been prevented if primary prevention behaviors had been incorporated into their daily activities.

BOX 11-6 LEVELS OF PREVENTION PYRAMID

Application to Client Teaching

SITUATION: Several examples of teaching at three levels of prevention.

GOAL: Using the three levels of prevention, avoid or promptly diagnose and treat negative health conditions, and restore the fullest possible potential.

Tertiary Prevention		
Rehabilitation	*Prevention*	
	Health Promotion and Education	**Health Protection**
▪ Restore function: a nurse teaches a stroke survivor about home safety, alternative housing options, physical therapy, and retraining opportunities	▪ Health teaching: a nurse teaches the stroke survivor about the importance of medication use, diet, rest, and exercise to prevent another CVA	▪ Maintenance: a nurse observes the stroke survivor's medication regime to ensure the client is taking medications properly

Secondary Prevention	
Early Diagnosis	*Prompt Treatment*
▪ Screening and case finding: a nurse takes blood pressure measurements from all family members at each home visit and teaches them the importance of maintaining a healthy blood pressure reading	▪ Treatment: a nurse teaches clients how to navigate through the complexities of the healthcare delivery system to receive prompt treatment

Primary Prevention	
Health Promotion and Education	*Health Protection*
▪ Health education: a nurse teaches a class on sensible weight control for teenagers	▪ Immunizations: a nurse teaches about the importance of pneumonia and flu vaccines for older adults, followed by an immunization clinic

Effective Teaching

Teaching is an art. It can be performed with such skill and grace that the client becomes part of a well-orchestrated event, with learning as the natural outcome. Instead of relying on prescribed teaching methods, the skillful C/PHN can make judgments based largely on client qualities, situations, and needs that guide the experience. The desired changes emerge during the interaction rather than at a level conceived before teaching. Before the C/PHN can reach this level of artistry, there is much to learn about being an effective teacher.

Client Readiness. The client's readiness to learn influences the C/PHN's teaching effectiveness. Four facets of client readiness have been identified (Kitchie, 2019):

1. Physical readiness, which deals with their ability, task complexity, environment, health status, and gender
2. Emotional readiness, which deals with the state of receptivity to learning (e.g., motivation, anxiety, developmental stage, risk-taking behavior)
3. Experiential readiness, which reflects the learner's past experiences with learning (cultural background, orientation, locus of control, coping mechanisms used)
4. Knowledge readiness, which encompasses the learner's knowledge and understanding (e.g., learning disabilities, learning style, current knowledge base)

For instance, one C/PHN found that a young primipara was not ready for prenatal teaching on fetal growth and development. She had strong fears that she would be unable to lose her baby weight and that this would make her sexually unattractive to her partner. Until these anxieties were addressed, the teaching would remain ineffective. Clients' needs, interests, motivation, stress, and concerns determine their readiness for learning.

Another factor that influences readiness is educational background. If a group of people who never completed grade school meet to learn how to care for a sick person in the home, material should be presented in a factual and easily accessible manner and in terms that they understand. To discuss complex concepts of health, illness, and scientific research would be above their level of readiness. However, you can begin to introduce more complex concepts as you work with them and assess their readiness for additional knowledge.

Maturational level also affects readiness. An adolescent parent who is still working on the normal developmental tasks of their age group, such as seeking independence or selecting a career path, may not be ready to learn parenting skills. Readiness of the client determines the amount of material presented in each teaching session. The pace or speed with which information is presented must be manageable. A small amount of anxiety often increases client receptivity to learning; however, high levels of anxiety can have the opposite effect.

Client Perceptions. Clients' perceptions also affect their learning, serving as a screening device or filter through which all new information must pass. Individual perceptions help people interpret and attach meaning to things.

Frequently, clients use selective perception. They screen out some statements and pay attention to those that fit their values or personal desires. For example, a C/PHN teaches a client about the various risk factors in coronary disease; the person screens out the need to quit smoking and lose weight, paying attention only to factors that would not require a drastic change in lifestyle. Nurses must know their clients, understand their backgrounds and values, and learn about their perceptions before health teaching can influence their behavior (Kitchie, 2019).

Educational Environment. The setting in which the educational experience takes place has a significant impact on learning (Kitchie, 2019). Students probably have had the experience of sitting in a cold room and trying to concentrate during a lecture or of being distracted by noise, heat, or uncomfortable seating. Physical conditions such as ventilation, lighting, room temperature, view of the speaker, and noise level should be controlled to provide a comfortable learning environment.

Equally important for learning is an atmosphere of mutual respect and trust. The nurse needs to convey this attitude both verbally and nonverbally. The way the C/PHN addresses clients, shows concern, and gives recognition makes a considerable difference in establishing clients' rapport and trust.

- Both the nurse and client need to be mutually helpful and considerate of one another's needs and interests.
- All participants in the educational experience should feel free to express ideas, should know that their views will be heard, and should feel accepted despite differences of opinion and perspective.
- According to the adult learning theorist Knowles, this requires that the nurse refrain from seeming judgmental or inducing competitiveness among learners. Knowles (1980, p. 58) adds that teachers should share their own feelings and knowledge "as a co-learner in the spirit of inquiry."

Client Participation. The degree of participation in the educational process directly influences the amount of learning (Stevanovic et al., 2022; Fig. 11-7). One nurse discovered this principle while working with a group of clients who were nearing retirement. After talking to them about the changes they would face and receiving little response, the nurse shifted to a different method of teaching. Handouts on Social Security benefits were distributed, and everyone was asked to read them during the week and come the next week with questions generated by the pamphlets. The C/PHN began the next session with a story about an older couple unprepared for retirement and the problems that they incurred. He then asked the group to share questions and concerns they had about retirement. This strategy prompted the group to slowly begin to participate in their own learning.

- Learning is facilitated when the student is engaged and fully participates in the learning process. C/PHNs should begin from the client's place of interest.
- When the client chooses their own directions, discovers their own learning resources, formulates their

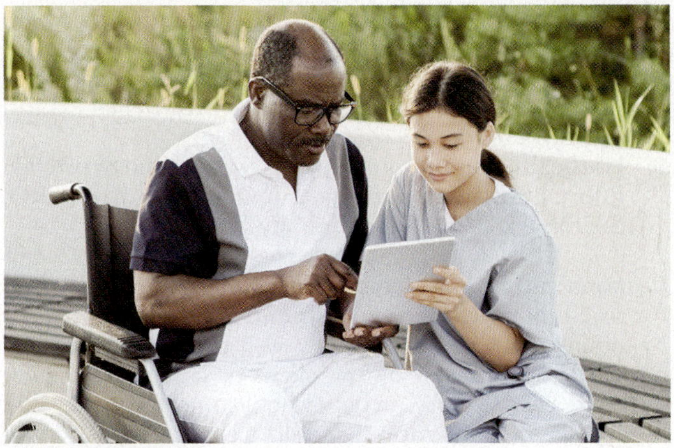

FIGURE 11-7 Client engagement is a key to successful health promotion programs.

own problems, decides their own course of action, and lives with the consequences of each of these choices, then the client has significantly maximized their learning.

- Contracting is a tool that allows the client to participate in the process as a partner to determine goals, content, and time for learning. This can contribute to client learning and active participation (see Chapter 10).

The amount of learning is directly proportional to the learner's involvement. In another example, a group of older adults attended a class on nutrition and aging yet made few changes in eating patterns. It was not until the members became actively involved in the class, encouraged by the nurse to present problems and solutions for food purchasing, understanding how to read nutrition labels, and preparing meals on limited budgets, that any significant behavioral changes occurred.

Subject Relevance. Subject matter relevant to the client is learned more readily and retained longer than information that is not meaningful. Learners gain the most from subject matter that is immediately useful to their own purposes. This is particularly true for adult learners, who have more life experiences that can be related to learning and who tend to see the immediate relevance of the material taught (Bastable et al., 2020; Knowles, 1980). When clients see the relevance in learning, they accomplish it more promptly. When the subject matter is relevant to the learner, more knowledge is retained.

Client Satisfaction. To maintain motivation and increase self-direction, clients must derive satisfaction from learning. Learners need to feel a sense of steady progress in the learning process. Realistic goals contribute to learner satisfaction. Objectives should be set within the learner's ability, thereby avoiding the frustration resulting from a task that is too difficult and the loss of interest resulting from one that is too easy. Once objectives are met, it is important to provide recognition or reward for the accomplishment. Setting objectives requires agreement on goals, periodic reviews, and revision of goals if they become too easy or too difficult (Bastable et al., 2020). Obstacles, frustrations, and failures along the way discourage and impede learning. Many clients who have had strokes and have potential for rehabilitation often give up trying to regain speech or move paralyzed limbs because they become frustrated and discouraged. On the other hand, clients who experience satisfaction and progress in their speech and muscle retraining maintain their motivation and may work on exercises without prompting. C/PHNs can promote client satisfaction through support and encouragement.

Client Application. Learning is reinforced through application (Bastable et al., 2020). Learners need as many opportunities as possible to apply the knowledge in daily life. If such opportunities arise during the teaching–learning process, clients can try out new knowledge and skills under supervision. Learners are given a chance to begin integrating learning into their daily lives when the teacher is there to help reinforce that pattern.

Teaching Process

The process of teaching in community health nursing follows steps similar to those of the nursing process:

1. *Interaction:* Establish basic communication patterns between clients and nurse.
2. *Assessment and diagnosis*: Determine client's present status and identify client's need for teaching through surveys, interviews, open forums, or task forces that include representative clients as members (keeping in mind that clients should determine their own needs).
3. *Setting goals and objectives*: Analyze needed changes, establish the goal (a broad statement of outcome), and prepare objectives that describe the desired learning outcomes. Objectives should be stated in measurable behavioral terms, using a grammatical structure that contains a subject, verb, condition/criterion, and time frame. That is, each objective should include a single idea that describes an outcome that can be measured within a certain time frame (see the example that follows these steps).
4. *Planning:* Design a plan for the learning experience that meets the mutually developed objectives; include content to be covered, sequence of topics, best conditions for learning (place, type of environment), methods, and materials (e.g., visual aids, exercises). A written plan is best; it may be part of the written nursing care plan.
5. *Teaching*: Implement the learning experience by carrying out the planned activities.
6. *Evaluation:* Determine whether learning objectives were met, and if not, why not. Evaluation measures progress toward goals, effectiveness of chosen teaching methods, or future learning needs.

Here is an example of a short-term goal, a long-term goal, and a set of objectives related to a specific client need:

Need: A group of smokers wish to end their dependency on nicotine.

Short-term goal: Within 1 month, all members of the group will reduce the number of cigarettes smoked.

Long-term goal: Ninety percent of group members will remain tobacco-free for 6 months.

Objectives: At the end of the program, all clients should be able to do the following:

- *List* three reasons why smoking is unhealthy.
- *Identify* at least two factors that influence their smoking habit.
- *Apply* a series of action steps leading to smoking cessation within 1 month.
- *Examine* the steps as they work to live tobacco-free in the first 3 months.
- *Design* a way to live a fulfilled, tobacco-free life.
- *Evaluate* successful strategies to remain tobacco free for 6 months.

Teaching Methods and Materials

Teaching occurs on many levels and incorporates various types of activities.

- It can be formal or informal, planned or unplanned. Formal presentations, such as group lectures, usually are planned and fairly structured.
- Lecturers tend to create a passive learning environment for the audience unless strategies are devised to involve the learners.
- Allowing time for questions and discussion after a lecture also actively involves learners. This method is best used with adults, but even they have a limited attention span, so breaks should be given every 30 to 60 minutes.
- Distributing printed material that highlights and summarizes, or supplements, the shared content also reinforces important points.

Some teaching is less formal but still planned and relatively structured, as in group discussions in which questions stimulate the exploration of ideas and guide thinking. Informal levels of teaching, such as counseling or **anticipatory guidance** (in which the client is assisted in preparing for a future role or developmental stage), require the teacher to be prepared, but there is no defined presentation plan. The C/PHN may use a handout or agency protocol steps as a guide. C/PHNs use one or a combination of methods, along with a variety of materials, to facilitate the teaching–learning process. Two-way communication is an important feature of the learning process. Learners need an opportunity to raise questions, make comments, reason out loud, and receive feedback to develop deeper understanding. When discussion is used in conjunction with other teaching methods, such as demonstration and role-playing, it improves their effectiveness.

Effective education also includes an understanding and awareness of health literacy and the need to evaluate patient understanding of medical information. Examples of how health professionals can mitigate low literacy may include the following:

- Assume all patients may have difficulty understanding medical information and implement health literacy universal precautions.
- Supplement instruction with appropriate materials.
- Ask open-ended questions (how and what) rather than closed-ended questions (yes and no).
- Have patients "teach back" or demonstrate a procedure.
- Teach so that age, culture, and ethnic diversity are considered.
- Provide information in the primary language for patients with limited English proficiency (LEP) (HRSA, 2019).
- Use health literacy tools (such as those found to provide information that patients can understand) (AHRQ, 2020a; CDC, 2019; Readability Formulas, 2020).

Demonstration. The demonstration method often is used for teaching psychomotor skills and is best accompanied by explanation and discussion, with time set aside for a return demonstration by the client or caregiver. It gives clients a clear sensory image of how to perform the skill. Because a demonstration should be within the visual and auditory range of learners, it is best to demonstrate in front of small groups or a single client. Use the same kind of equipment that clients will use, show exactly how the skill should be performed, and provide learners with ample opportunities to practice until the skill is perfected. The show-back method can be used to assess the level of understanding of the psychomotor skill that was demonstrated to the person. After the healthcare provider demonstrates the skill, the person/family will show the healthcare provider how to do a specific task or skill that was previously demonstrated. The show-back method is a great way for the C/PHN to evaluate the effectiveness of the health teaching and provides the opportunity to praise and provide feedback for improvement of the psychomotor skill (Agency for Healthcare Research and Quality [AHRQ], 2020a).

Role Playing. At times, having clients assume and act out roles maximizes learning. Members of a parenting group, for example, found it helpful to place themselves in the role of their children. In doing so, their feelings about various ways to respond became more apparent. Reversing roles can effectively teach conflicting couples better ways to communicate. To prevent role-playing from becoming a game with little learning, it should be planned with clear objectives in mind.

- What behavioral outcomes should be achieved?
- Define the context (the "stage") clearly, so that everyone shares in the situation. Then define each role ahead of time, making sure that participants understand their performance roles.
- Emphasize that no wrong or right performance exists and that participants should behave the way people behave in everyday life.
- Avoid having people play themselves, because it can embarrass them and make it difficult for them to achieve objectivity.
- After the role playing has concluded, begin the discussion with carefully prepared questions.

This technique can be used with staff, coworkers, young children, teenagers, and adults. However, it can be a risk-taking experience for some people, and they may be reluctant to participate. The nurse should use judgment, begin with volunteers, and avoid pushing this technique on unwilling or nonreceptive people. It is best to build up to full participation.

Teach-Back Method. The teach-back method is an evidence-based health literacy program that improves patient safety, adherence, and outcomes. This method is used to assess health education knowledge. The teach-back method requires the healthcare provider to ask the person/family to state in their own words what they need to know or do about their health. If the healthcare provider finds incorrect information provided, they can re-explain and check again. It is estimated that most people forget or don't understand 40% to 80% of health information provided to them (AHRQ, 2020a).

Here are effective components of the teach-back method:

- Ensure the tone of voice and attitude is caring.
- Provide appropriate eye contact and body language.
- Speak in plain language (avoid medical jargon/terms).
- Provide appropriate written or visual information to enhance the teaching when available.
- Use open-ended, nonjudgmental questions.
- Ask the person to explain the information that was provided in their own words.
- Explain to the person that this is not a quiz/test and the responsibility to provide clarity of information is on you as a healthcare provider.
- If the teach-back information is not correct or cannot be answered, provide the information again and re-check the person's answer.
- Document the teach-back method and individual response (AHRQ, 2020b).

Teaching Materials. Many kinds of teaching materials are available to the nurse (Fig. 11-8). They often are employed in combination and are useful during the teaching process.

- Visual images—such as PowerPoint presentations (using graphics, photos), pictures, posters, chalkboards, flannel boards, DVDs, online videos, bulletin boards, flash cards, pamphlets, flyers, charts, and gestures—can enhance most learning.
- Americans readily learn from television and the web, as there is visual and auditory appeal. Other tools, such as anatomic models and improvised or purchased equipment, provide clients with both visual and tactile learning experiences.
- Still others, such as interactive computer games or instruction, actively involve the learners.

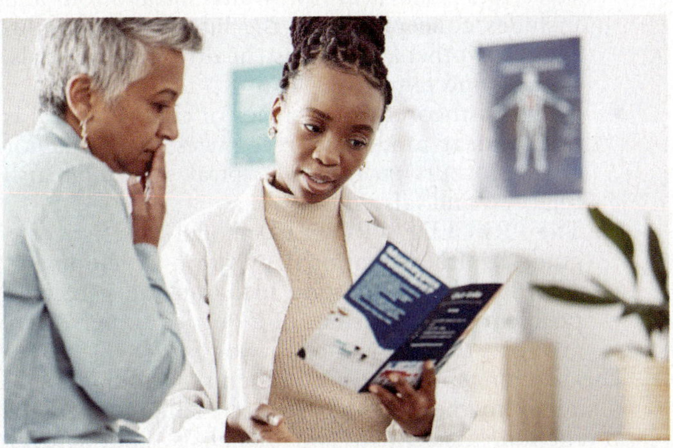

FIGURE 11-8 Teaching materials help to make your point.

The choice of teaching materials varies with the client's interests and abilities and the resources available. Teaching often occurs in casual conversations, spontaneously in situations when clients raise unexpected questions, or when a crisis arises. In these instances, C/PHNs draw on their background of knowledge and exercise professional judgment in their selection of content, methods, and materials.

Printed educational support materials are available, such as pamphlets, brochures, booklets, flyers, and informational sheets. Each should be evaluated for appropriateness and effectiveness with people, families, or groups. Many come from state and local public health sources. Nurses can create their own handouts, customizing them to the needs of individual clients. The nurse can get educational information from state, federal, and international health agencies.

- Examples include state health departments, the U.S. Food and Drug Administration, the CDC, the National Institutes of Health, and the WHO.
- Other materials come from nonprofit national agencies such as the American Diabetes Association, the March of Dimes, the American Association for Retired Persons (AARP), and the American Heart Association (AHA).

Factors to be considered with all educational literature include the material's content, complexity, and reading level. There are several ways to assess the readability of the printed word.

- One easy way is to use the Fry Readability Graph or the Gunning-Fog formula. These tools are a rough estimate to determine the years of schooling needed to understand printed material. It works by analyzing words and sentence length; the higher the number, the more difficult the reading level.
- A Gunning-Fog Index of 6 is a sixth-grade reading level, and a score of 11 is at the junior year in high school. Fortunately, most word processing programs now include a feature to allow assessment of the reading level in text.
- Another very common tool is the Flesch Reading Ease program, available in Microsoft Word grammar checker, which evaluates reading material. Like the Fry Graph, the Flesch-Kincaid Grade Level readability score rates the material in terms of typical grade level; however, it may not be as accurate, and you may need to adjust results downward (Medline Plus, 2019).
- The nurse should always consider the population when selecting a reading level, as many people cannot understand materials at even the sixth-grade level.
- Also, clients, including those speaking a language other than English, may not be able to read and write in their dominant language.

Culturally appropriate health education materials must be acquired or developed for the predominant cultural and linguistic underrepresented populations taught by the nurse. Developing printed materials is an important first step, but the development of video, audio, and public service announcements in community-appropriate languages is also necessary. It is important that materials are developed from a health equity lens using key principles and preferred terms from the select population (CDC, 2022c).

Finally, nurses teach by example. Actions speak louder than words. If a nurse teaches the importance of washing hands to reduce disease transmission and then begins a newborn assessment without hand washing, the message of observed actions carries more impact than the words. Nurses who exhibit healthy practices use themselves as teaching tools and serve as role models as well as health teachers.

Clients With Special Learning Needs

At times, the nurse experiences a challenging teaching situation with an individual, family, or group. These challenges may involve clients who have cultural or language differences, hearing loss, developmental delays, memory losses, visual perception distortions, and problems with fine or gross motor skills, distracting personality characteristics, or demonstrations of stress or emotions. Culture can play a role in communication because it influences belief systems, communication styles, and understanding and response to health information (NNLM, n.d.). The inability to see, hear, and understand health information can impact the health and health outcomes of those with disabilities. Regardless of the situation, C/PHNs will feel most comfortable and confident if they are prepared to deal with these situations before they are experienced.

Another difficulty that can arise is unexpected behavior from a client who disrupts the group process. The client may monopolize the discussion, answer questions asked of others, burst out with personal experiences that have no relevance to the topic, become irate at the comments of others, or sit silently and never speak. This can be unnerving to even the most experienced nurse. The C/PHN must tactfully diffuse any behavior that has the potential to distract the other learners. This is accomplished by considerately giving the recognition sought by the person while also setting limits.

SUMMARY

- *Healthy People 2030* objectives recognize the health and well-being of all people and communities through educational and community-based programs, SDOH, and health literacy.
- The purpose of health education is to effect change, which alters the equilibrium in a system.
- Change occurs in three stages: *unfreezing* when the system is ready for change, *changing* when the innovation is implemented, and *refreezing* when the change is stabilized.
- The cognitive domain refers to learning that takes place intellectually. It ranges in levels of learner functioning from simple recall to complex evaluation. As learners move up the scale of cognitive learning, they become more self-directed; the nurse then assumes a more facilitative role.
- Affective learning involves the changing of attitudes and values. Learners may experience several levels of affective involvement, from simple listening to adopting the new value. Again, as the client increases involvement, the nurse uses a less directive approach.
- Psychomotor learning involves the acquisition of motor skills. Clients who learn psychomotor skills must meet three conditions: they must be capable of the skill, they must develop a sensory image of the skill, and they must practice the skill.
- Learners have learning style preferences that include VARK. It is important for the C/PHN to assess the client's learning style preference.
- Learning theories can be grouped into four broad categories:
  - Behaviorist theories, which view learning as a behavioral change accomplished through stimulus–response or conditioning
  - Cognitive learning theories, which seek to influence learners' understanding of problems and situations through promoting their insights
  - Social learning theories, which explain dysfunctional behavior and facilitate learning
  - Humanistic theories assume that people have a natural tendency to learn and that learning flourishes in an encouraging environment. Knowles' adult learning theory provides a framework for understanding adult characteristics and appropriate teaching interventions.
- Health teaching models work together with the learning theories to give nurses a more accurate picture of the client and the client's learning needs.
  - The HBM is useful in explaining behaviors triggered by people interested in preventing diseases.
  - The health promotion model helps to predict behaviors that lead to health promotion and includes concepts about the interpersonal influence of others, such as health professionals, friends, and family.
  - The transtheoretical or stages of change model is not a linear model but recognizes that behavior change occurs more like a spiral, with plateaus, relapses, and false starts.
  - The PRECEDE–PROCEED model is designed to guide health educational program development. The model has a strong focus on the perceived problems and priorities of a particular person or group as they impact quality of life.
- The teaching process in community health nursing is similar to the nursing process, including steps of interaction, assessment and diagnosis, goal setting, planning, teaching, and evaluation.

- The teaching may be formal or informal, planned or unplanned, and methods may range from structured lecture presentations and discussions to demonstration and role-playing.

ACTIVE LEARNING EXERCISES

1. Using "Assess and Monitor Population Health" (1 of the 10 Essential Public Health Services; see Box 2-2), identify the leading cause of adult mortality in your community. Discuss the social determinants of health that may influence this mortality statistic. (Objective 1)
2. As a staff C/PHN, you have been asked to develop a sexual health educational program for group of students aged 14 to 16. Identify the process of change for this new program and how this relates to health promotion for the community. Explain your educational plan (include the domain of learning and the learning theory along with the need, goal, objectives, implementation, and evaluation methods). (Objectives 2 and 4)
3. Using behavioral objectives that match the learning level desired, develop a flyer or program for an educational presentation for clients. (Objective 3)
4. Go to https://www.cdc.gov/hepatitis/resources/patientedmaterials.htm and select a CDC patient educational handout. Determine the readability level of the handout and discuss the implications for a nurse using this handout in an educational program. Explain how it best meets the educational needs of your target population. (Objective 3)
5. Select a current research article that demonstrates the application of one of the health teaching models. How do the results compare with the constructs of the model? How did the author's approach change? What model was applied? (Objective 4)
6. Identify a population and a health issue. Develop a teaching plan focused on either primary, secondary, or tertiary levels of prevention. (Objective 5)

CHAPTER 12

Planning, Implementing, and Evaluating Community/Public Health Programs

"Community is a bunch of people looking after each other, seeing each other deeply, taking the time to really enter into a relationship with each other, to depend upon one another, to buttress each other's stories, and to buttress each other's behavior."

—David Brooks (2020), American commentator

KEY TERMS

Advisory groups
Authoritative knowledge
Benchmarking
Community action model
Community messaging
Enabling factors
Logic model
Population health
Predisposing factors
Quality indicators
Reinforcing factors

LEARNING OBJECTIVES

Upon mastery of this chapter, you should be able to:

1. Identify the knowledge, skills, attitudes, and resources a public health nurse must develop in order to plan, implement, and evaluate community and public health programs.
2. List sources of public health data and other information that can be used to identify group and community health problems.
3. Describe methods to gain input from target populations to define the scope of a health problem.
4. Explain the role and value of community partnerships in developing and promoting community/public health programs.
5. Identify change strategies that maximize cooperation of target populations.
6. Identify quality of care models that are useful in program evaluation.
7. Describe the role of community messaging in health promotion programs.
8. Locate appropriate grant funding sources for select health promotion programs.

INTRODUCTION

In the early 20th century, after suffering several personal tragedies, Mary Breckinridge committed herself to a cause: bringing effective healthcare to a resource-limited, remote region of the United States. A trained nurse and daughter of a politician, she used her skills and influence to establish a public health program, the Frontier Nursing Service (FNS) in rural Appalachia (Fig. 12-1). During the humble beginnings of the FNS, Breckinridge and her team of nurse-midwives rode through the hills of Leslie County, Kentucky, on horseback, providing primary care and midwifery services to the impoverished residents. Breckinridge dedicated her life to the effort, ultimately developing a network of clinics, a hospital, and a school to train midwives, and became an advocate for the region's economic development (Goan, 2015). Thanks to the FNS, the maternal mortality rate in Appalachia dropped from among the highest in the country to well below the national average. The school Breckinridge founded continues to operate today as Frontier Nursing University, which trains some of the nation's most influential nurse-midwives and nurse practitioners.

The COVID-19 pandemic underscored the value and importance of public health efforts. However, in the years before the pandemic, the public health workforce, including public health nurses (PHNs), had dwindled. There had been a 15% decline in the number of employees in local public health agencies between 2010 and 2020 (Castrucci & Lupi, 2020), and the proportion of nurses employed in public health had dropped from 3.2% of all nurses in

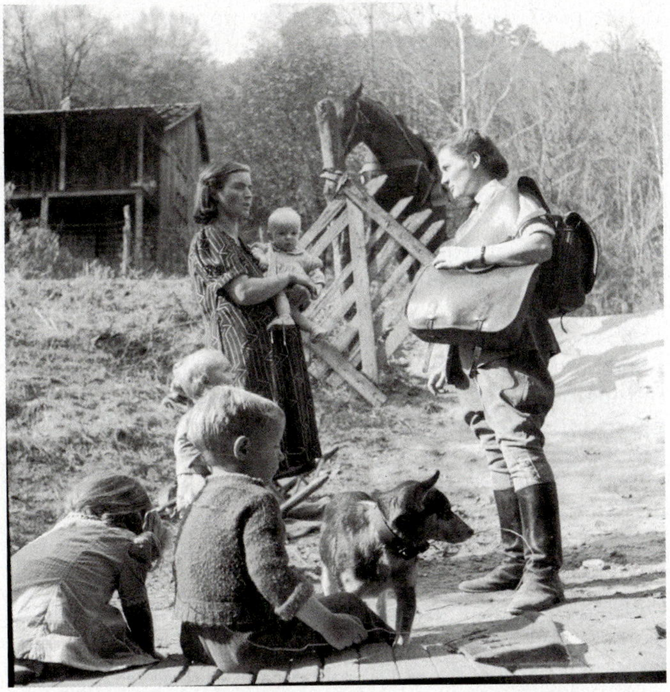

FIGURE 12-1 The Frontier Nursing Service used a public health program approach to improve the health of resource-limited families in rural Kentucky. (Photo Courtesy of Frontier Nursing University Archives. Used with permission. Retrieved from https://frontier.edu/about-frontier/history-of-fnu/)

2000 to 1.4% in 2018 (Pittman & Park, 2021). As part of the federal government's COVID-19 response efforts, the 2021 American Rescue Plan allocated approximately two billion dollars to assist state and local health departments in expanding the public health workforce. However, the demand for PHNs exceeds the supply.

The emerging role of the C/PHN offers nurses the opportunity to plan and implement programs that protect and enhance the health of entire communities. C/PHNs develop health promotion and educational programs for growing constituencies. In doing so, they address public health challenges that are just as significant in our generation as those faced by the FNS. C/PHNs collaborate with influential community leaders and organizations, write grant proposals, develop health programs through community partnership, create community messaging campaigns, evaluate the effects of health promotion programs, and are involved in many other activities that promote community health. Specific examples of these activities could include the following:

- Writing A Grant Proposal To Fund A Naloxone Distribution Program For A Community Struggling With Widespread Fentanyl Misuse And Overdose Deaths
- Collaborating with local school districts to assess students for mental health concerns and suicide risk
- Assisting a nongovernmental organization to create a social marketing campaign aimed at discouraging violence against people assigned female at birth in developing countries
- Gathering and interpreting data showing the impact of a home visitation program for people with dementia receiving in-home care from family members

This chapter builds on concepts discussed in other chapters and describes the knowledge, skills, actions, and resources that help C/PHNs become effective in planning, implementing, and evaluating community health programs.

PLANNING COMMUNITY HEALTH PROGRAMS: THE BASICS

Competent C/PHNs are able to apply the nursing process—assessment, diagnosis, outcomes/planning, implementation, and evaluation—at the community level (Fig. 12-2). The American Nurses Association (ANA) has established standards of practice for C/PHNs that include, in Standard 4, a list of competencies needed to plan effective community health strategies (ANA, 2022). Entry-level nurses may feel intimidated at the prospect of planning and implementing interventions for an entire community; however, robust baccalaureate nursing programs prepare them for this role. **Population health** is a domain of the American Association of Colleges of Nursing (AACN) essentials for baccalaureate nursing education. Population health includes the continuum of healthcare delivery settings, including hospitals, ambulatory care, and long-term care, and C/PHN. Nursing curricula should enable entry-level nurses to understand how C/PH interfaces with other healthcare settings and how to apply that knowledge in developing action plans to meet population health needs (AACN, 2021).

Although the responsibility of planning a health promotion program may seem overwhelming, the first part of this chapter is designed to take some of the mystery out of it.

In your nursing education program, you may have been assigned to develop a simple C/PHN intervention, work in an existing community health program, or simulate the health promotion process in a written assignment. The concepts you learned through those assignments are the same ones used in planning real-world community health programs. Successful community health programs take skill, time, patience, and, most of all, willingness to listen to the needs and opinions of the people who are the focus of your program—the target population.

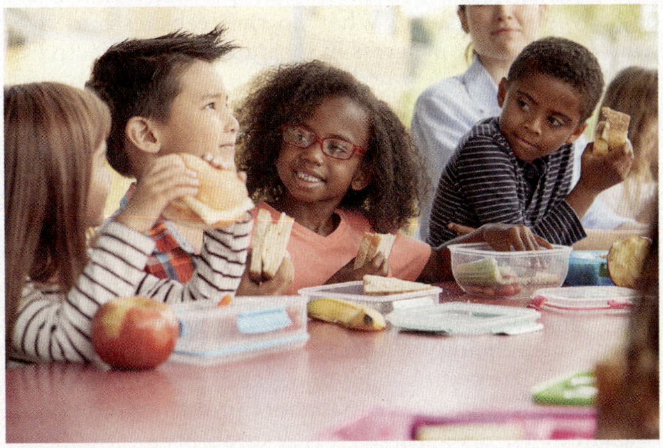

FIGURE 12-2 Contemporary public health nurses plan public health programs that improve the health of entire communities.

IDENTIFYING GROUP OR COMMUNITY HEALTH PROBLEMS

Nurses are educated in the care of people, families, *and* communities, yet nurses most often practice at the individual and family levels. When is it appropriate for a nurse to expand their practice to the community level? The most natural time may be when a nurse identifies a common, recurrent problem among a population at any point in the continuum of care. Examples of these problems may include an unusually high incidence of sexually transmitted infections among LGBTQ+ youth in a community-based clinic or overuse of the emergency department for pain medication prescriptions. Population health problems such as these should lead nurses to investigate the feasibility of community-based interventions. A key step in doing so is to look for and assess data about the problem. Data are available through federal, state, and local agencies and initiatives (see Chapter 4).

National and State Health Objectives and Initiatives

The U.S. Office of Disease Prevention and Health Promotion (ODPHP) establishes priorities for preventing disease and promoting health among Americans. In 1980, the ODPHP developed the Healthy People initiative—a set of national health-promotion objectives to be achieved by the end of the decade. At the beginning of each decade since then, a new set of priorities and objectives has been developed to address the most current public health trends and problems (ODPHP, 2022). There are many national- and state-level data sources that provide tools for identifying community health problems and potential solutions. State health department websites may provide links to data sets offering insights into state- and community-level health problems. Consider visiting the Healthy People 2030 website to view the most recent iteration of the initiative, as well as other resources that assist C/PHNs in identifying and addressing contemporary community health issues. As you explore, consider some of the following questions: What are the most significant areas of concern for health outcomes in the United States? What are the health promotion priorities of the state in which you live? What programs are being developed to meet the *Healthy People 2030* goals and objectives (Box 12-1)? What do the websites and data sources say about progress in meeting health objectives?

Local Health Priorities and Initiatives

Community agencies and organizations frequently network to establish community-wide goals, with state, county, or health departments spearheading the projects. The efforts may also be led or organized by community health or volunteer agencies. Examples of local community health goals could include decreasing the prevalence of community-acquired pneumonia among older populations or reducing the incidence of vaccine-preventable diseases. Nurses can collaborate and partner with key organizations and people to identify problems and potential solutions.

After a specific problem is identified, it is crucial to analyze the scope of the problem within the community. It is a poor use of resources to set up a program if the condition or situation is rare. For example, it would be a waste of resources to establish a program focusing on diabetes and pregnancy in a local homeless shelter that only serves 35 people assigned female at birth a year. Among those people, the percentage who are pregnant may be small, and considering that fewer than 10% of pregnancies are affected by gestational diabetes (Centers for Disease Control and Prevention [CDC], 2022), it may be years before an eligible client is found. A better target may be a community with a high proportion of people at risk for diabetes during pregnancy, such as non-Hispanic Asian individuals, among whom the prevalence of gestational diabetes is higher than it is for other racial/ethnic groups (Read et al., 2021). Another potential target group may be pregnant people aged 40 years or older, who are up to six times more likely to develop gestational diabetes as compared to younger groups (CDC, 2023a).

Using Data to Confirm Needs

Optimally, baccalaureate nursing students are trained to assess population health data and identify health patterns across populations (AACN, 2021). There are several ways a nurse can determine whether a problem affects enough of the population to warrant intervention. One way to start is by reviewing local, state, and national data available through government repositories. This can be done through online database searches, seeking help when needed from a university librarian, or by requesting specific data from local health and social service agencies, including police and judicial departments, and local school districts.

The National Center for Health Statistics (NCHS) offers public-use data through the CDC file server. The NCHS data collection systems include (1) population surveys, such as the National Health and Nutrition Examination Survey; (2) the National Survey of Family Growth; (3) vital records, such as the National Death Index; (4) provider surveys, such as the National Hospital Care Survey and other national healthcare surveys; and (5) historical surveys, which provide an overview of surveys and programs administered by the NCHS that have been completed (CDC, 2023b).

The U.S. Department of Health and Human Services (USDHHS) makes high-value health data accessible to the public via HealthData.gov. The data sets are collected from agencies within the USDHHS as well as its state partners. A feature of the HealthData.gov website is an abundance of data on COVID-19 and health equity. Health equity data are organized by themes such as access to care, cancer innovation, COVID-19 and long COVID, and others.

Target Groups and Neighborhoods

As PHNs and community groups narrow their focus to a community health intervention or program, they may be able to identify target groups and neighborhoods by using *geographic information system* (GIS) technology or studies. GIS uses digital mapping to link data to geographical locations (University of Kansas, n.d.-a). GIS can be used to identify target groups by race, age, and family status. GIS data are available through various federal

BOX **12-1** *HEALTHY PEOPLE 2030*

Recommended Leading Health Indicators and Objectives

Life Expectancy	■ Increase life expectancy (at birth)
Child Health	MICH-02 Reduce the rate of all infant deaths IVP-D03 Reduce the number of young adults who report three or more adverse childhood experiences
Self-Rated Health	■ Increase the mean healthy days (CDC-HRQOL-14 Healthy Days)
Well-Being	■ Increase proportion thriving on Cantril Self-Anchoring Striving scales
Disability	■ Reduce the percentage of adults ages 65 years and over with limitations in daily activities
Mental Disability	■ Reduce the rate of mental disability
Substance Use	SU-03 Reduce drug overdose deaths
Unintentional Injury Deaths	IVP-03 Reduce unintentional injury deaths
All Cancer Deaths	C-01 Reduce the overall cancer death rate
Suicide	MHMD-01 Reduce the suicide rate
Firearm-Related Mortality	IVP-12 Reduce firearm-related deaths
Mental Health	■ Reduce percentage of adults who reported their mental health was not good in 14 or more days in the past 30 days (i.e., frequent mental distress)
Oral Health Access	OH-08 Increase use of the oral health care system
Reproductive Health Care Services	FP-11 Increase the proportion of adolescent females[a] at risk for unintended pregnancy who use effective birth control
HIV Incidence	HIV-03 Reduce the number of new HIV diagnoses
Tobacco	TU-04 Reduce current tobacco use in adolescents
Obesity	NWS-04 Reduce the proportion of children and adolescents with obesity
Alcohol Use	SU-13 Reduce the proportion of people with alcohol use disorder in the past year
Immunization	■ Increase the proportion of children 19- to 35-month-old children up to date on DTaP, MMR, polio, Hib, HepB, varicella, and pneumococcal conjugate vaccines
Hypertension Rate	HDS-04 Reduce the proportion of adults with high blood pressure
Ambulatory Sensitive Conditions/ Avoidable Hospitalization	■ Reduce discharges for ambulatory care—sensitive conditions per 1000 Medicare enrollees (CMS-2[b])
Medical Insurance Coverage	AHS-01 Increase the proportion of people with medical insurance
Affordable Housing	SDOH-04 Reduce the proportion of families that spend more than 30% of income on housing
Environment	■ Improve the Environmental Quality Index ■ Lower the Heat Vulnerability Index
Education	AH-04 Increase the proportion of 4th graders with reading skills at or above the proficient level
Poverty	SDOH-03 Reduce the proportion of people living in poverty
Food Security	NWS-01 Reduce household food insecurity and hunger
Civic Engagement	■ Increase the proportion of voting eligible population who vote
Social Environment	■ Lower the Neighborhood Disinvestment Index ■ Reduce the level of residential segregation captured by the Index of Dissimilarity ■ Reduce the level of residential segregation captured by the Isolation Index

[a]In this box, "female" refers to a person assigned female at birth.
[b]CMS-2 is a chronic conditions composite measure developed by the Centers for Medicare & Medicaid Services.
Reprinted with permission from National Academies of Sciences, Engineering, and Medicine. (2020). *Leading health indicators 2030: Advancing health, equity, and well-being.* The National Academies Press. Retrieved from https://www.nap.edu/catalog/25682/leading-health-indicators-2030-advancing-health-equity-and-well-being

sources, including the CDC, the National Library of Medicine, the Environmental Protection Agency (EPA), and the NCHS. GIS mapping is useful in identifying priority health problems in neighborhoods and communities. This is illustrated in a study that utilized GIS to identify inequities in COVID-19 deaths in areas of social and economic vulnerability (Phillips et al., 2023) and in a study that used GIS to determine priority sites for colorectal cancer screening programs (Zhan et al., 2023). See Chapter 10 for more on GIS.

GIS offers significant potential for exploring the relationship between climate and health. The impact of climate on environmental and public health is felt in all populations, from the global community to small, targeted neighborhoods. Climate influences the seriousness and frequency of health problems (EPA, 2023). For example, the transmission of malaria occurs in tropical and subtropical areas because malarial parasites can only complete their growth cycle in hot, humid conditions (CDC, 2020). Changes in climate may contribute to new or unanticipated health problems among people or in places where they did not previously exist (EPA, 2023). GIS technology is increasingly playing a key role in measuring, analyzing, understanding, and managing the effects of climate on population health (Boulos & Wilson, 2023).

Collaborating With Other Healthcare Professionals

Collaborating with healthcare colleagues on population health issues is an essential competency for nurses (AACN, 2021). Discussing community health problems you have encountered with other nurses and healthcare professionals from other agencies may help you identify resources and solutions. Maintaining involvement in national professional organizations such as the Association of Public Health Nurses, or in state or county professional organizations such as school nurse collaboratives, provides other opportunities for sharing problems and ideas. Collaboration guides are available that promote relationships between state and local health departments, community agencies, and other health services. The National Association of County and City Health Officials (NACCHO, 2017) provides a toolkit for promoting collaboration between local health departments and community health centers; it includes tools for assessing opportunities, developing partnerships, and planning collaborative action.

A helpful source for evidence-based health promotion ideas is credible websites, such as The Community Preventive Services Task Force (CPSTF)—a federally sponsored collection of evidence-based community health resources. Its website, thecommunityguide.org, offers examples of successful community health interventions (CPSTF, 2023). The University of Kansas sponsors *The Community Tool Box* as a public service for people and agencies who are working to improve the health of communities. Some content is dated; however, The Community Tool Box offers classic resources in over 300 pages of free educational modules and other tools focusing on community assessment, planning, intervention, evaluation, and advocacy (University of Kansas, n.d.-b).

Engaging the Target Population

The next step, engaging the target population, may be the most important of all as it determines whether an intervention will succeed or fail. A key element in successful community engagement is understanding and respecting the views of the target population about an identified problem (Fig. 12-3). Nurses may have authoritative knowledge about health topics, such as first aid or vaccines and, therefore, conclude that their opinions on those subjects are superior to those of the target population. Nevertheless, the target population may hold just as strongly to their own beliefs.

Authoritative knowledge is knowledge that comes from sources or people who have power or authority in certain domains or areas. We learned from the COVID-19 pandemic that authoritative knowledge is not readily accepted when the target population is skeptical about the motives or credibility of the source. Walsh et al. (2022) evaluated the effectiveness of the coordinated efforts of government agencies and social media platforms to elevate authoritative content about the novel coronavirus. Many survey participants noticed the content online, but there was significant distrust of information shared by government and public health authorities. Similarly, Holroyd et al. (2021) tested a scale measuring public trust in public health authorities and identified two dimensions of trust: beneficence and competence. The authors found that trust in public health authorities was generally high, but a substantial proportion of study participants questioned their credibility. If nurses do not earn the trust and respect of the community, their success in planning and implementing effective health interventions will be limited.

Understanding the Target Population

When working with target groups, it is important to get as much information about the population as possible. Start by asking those you know, as colleagues and as patients/clients, about their local community. What are their thoughts about the problem of interest? What do they think about the quality of services currently available? What do they see as barriers to services? What barriers interfere with their adherence to treatment and other

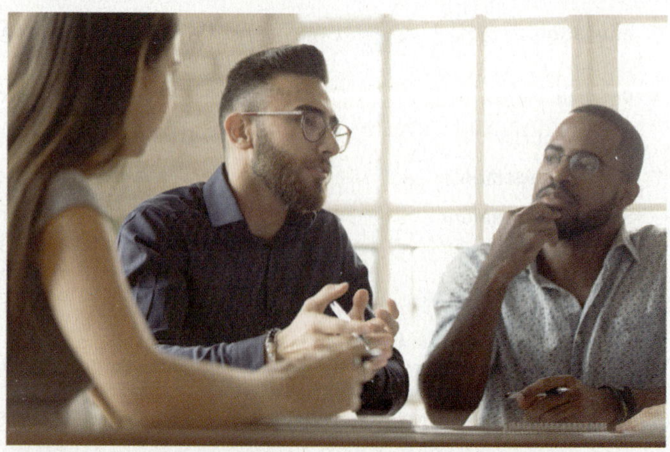

FIGURE 12-3 It is crucial to hear and respect the views of the target population.

recommendations? Who are their *formal* and *informal leaders*? The answers to these questions, and others, will provide insight into factors influencing health problems and help you understand how to work with the target population. Local knowledge affects community interest and buy-in, and it increases the effectiveness of community-based intervention.

Mobilizing Action through Planning and Partnerships (MAPP) is one of many tools that begin with community mobilization. The MAPP concept is that health must be viewed from the perspective of the community and that individual health cannot be fully achieved without the health of the community (University of Kansas, n.d.-c).

Using Evidence to Guide Interventions

Searching for evidence-based guidelines and interventions is important to program success. It is essential to review literature about health problems, factors influencing the outcomes of interventions, and the role of families and communities in adhering to interventions. The evidence prompts critical thinking about the problem and provides insights that may shape interactions with community members. Important questions to consider include how your target group compares to other populations in the literature and whether there is existing evidence about the problem you have identified. Nurses should be able to contemplate these factors and identify the best available evidence to support policy and program development (AACN, 2021).

Consider this situation: A C/PHN wanted to know why parents were using emergency departments for after-hours urgent care. A literature review identified studies focusing heavily on the "misuse" of emergency rooms by parents to treat urgent ambulatory care health problems, such as otitis media. Based on input from an emergency department nurse, the C/PHN decided to go directly to families in the community to ask what their doctors had told them to do if their child became ill at night. The families were told to take their children to the emergency room! None of the literature addressed what the families had been told to do for after-hours care. Seeking information from a variety of sources can promote understanding beyond what can be learned by relying solely on the literature.

Community Action Model

A participatory action research approach may be most effective in facilitating community change (Cusack et al., 2018; deChesnay, 2015). One such approach is the **community action model**, which aims to identify actions that are achievable and sustainable and propel change for the well-being of all. This model builds on concepts presented in the planned-change process, described in other chapters, and includes a cyclical five-step process (Fig. 12-4). The C/PHN can use this model to facilitate community participation and ownership of change that improves the community's health. An example of a successful application of the Community Action Model is the San Francisco Tobacco Free Project, which produced

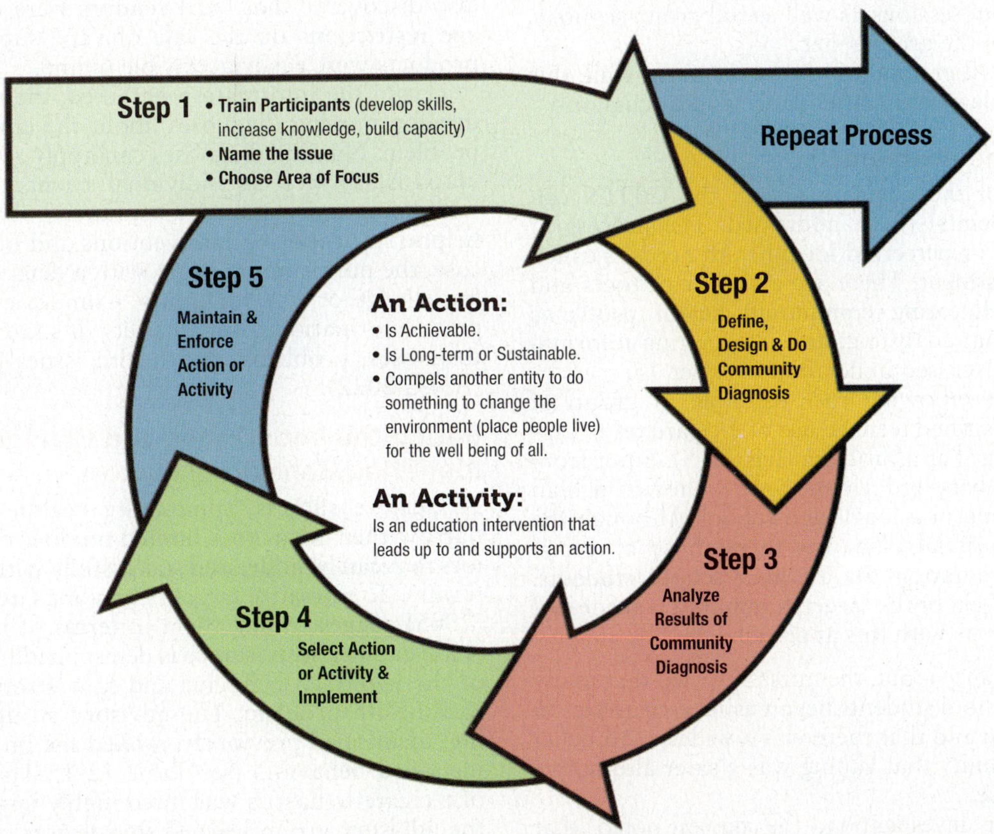

FIGURE 12-4 Community action model: Creating change by building community capacity. (Reprinted with permission from San Francisco Department of Public Health, Tobacco Free Project, and Bright Research Group. [September 2016]. *Community action in public health policy*. Retrieved from https://sanfranciscotobaccofreeproject.org/wp-content/uploads/CAM-Case-Study-Final-9.12.16-to-TFP.pdf)

tobacco control policies that have served as models for other communities (Conduent Healthy Communities Institute, 2023).

Advisory Groups

Competent C/PHNs work with a variety of community partners, healthcare colleagues, and other stakeholders in identifying factors contributing to local health problems and developing plans for improvement (ANA, 2022). In these collaborations, community members will begin to stand out because of their knowledge, networking capabilities, and interest in the subject. The C/PHN should consider engaging these members in **advisory groups**, such as community advisory boards, which provide the voice of the community on health promotion priorities and activities. Advisory group members should be as diverse as possible in race, ethnicity, age, gender, socioeconomic status, and other characteristics, to help the group understand the perspectives of a broad spectrum of local constituents. Inclusive advisory groups may help to promote health equity in the community. The advisory group's influence and responsibilities may range from serving in a strictly informative role with limited power, to serving as a board with decision-making abilities (Arnos et al., 2021). Successful advisory group meetings should have these features:

- Be well organized, punctual, and efficient.
- Focus on interpreting findings and community feedback and developing potential solutions.
- Include input from each member of the advisory group that should be sought and valued equally.
- Hold breakout sessions as well as full group sessions, depending on the group's size.
- Be documented in minutes to create a paper trail; this should include meeting attendance and discussions.

Delineating the Problem(s)

With the help of the advisory group, the C/PHN can define the problem(s) to be addressed. The process of determining real or perceived local health needs is called community assessment. There are a variety of tools and methods for delineating community health problems through collecting, analyzing, and interpreting information. These are discussed in detail in Chapter 15.

Consider the following case example. A group of school nurses identified teenage use of e-cigarettes ("vaping" or "JUULing") as a problem (Fig. 12-5). Input from community members and a data review showed a high rate of teen vaping in a local high school. Although the school nurses' original plan was to establish a special educational presentation for all high school students, input from members of the target communities suggested significant problems with this approach:

- From community input, the nurses learned that many of the high school students began using e-cigarettes in middle school and that there was a widespread belief in the community that vaping was a safer alternative to tobacco use.
- Upon further investigation, the nurses noted that e-cigarette users were predominantly people assigned male at birth, who did not understand the connection between gender and vaping.

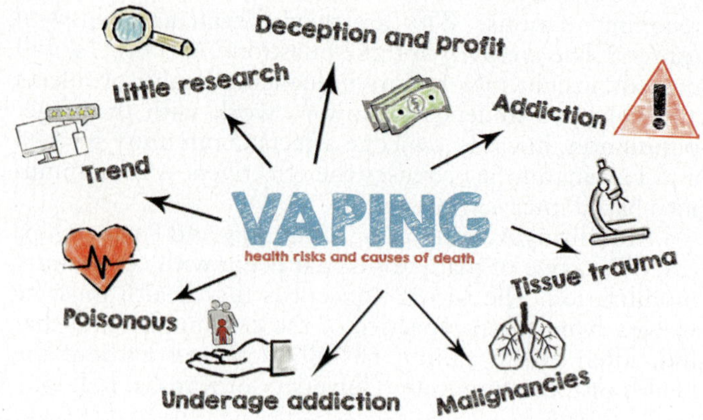

FIGURE 12-5 There are risks associated with e-cigarette use.

The advisory group helped the nurses identify the behavioral factors contributing to vaping in the target population. They informed the nurses that there was a high rate of tobacco use among adults in the community, and vaping was becoming increasingly popular. Teenagers in the target population were attracted to the flavors available with e-cigarettes, such as fruit, mint, and chocolate, and enjoyed vaping with their friends as an after-school activity. Additionally, many people assigned male at birth in the target group were high school athletes who used e-cigarettes to appear "cool" without realizing vaping involves risks. Through the advisory group, the nurses also discovered that local vendors were lax in enforcing age restrictions on the sale of vape supplies, and vape products were easily accessible online.

From the information gathered, the nurses began to develop nursing diagnoses about the community health problem. Nursing diagnoses can apply to aggregate populations, as well as individual clients. In conjunction with community assessments, nursing diagnoses may be helpful in proposing interventions and outcomes. In this case, the nurses might begin with a diagnosis of deficient knowledge or risk for injury. Competent C/PHNs integrate information from a variety of sources to determine diagnoses, problems, and health issues in communities (ANA, 2022).

Rating the Importance and Changeability of Identified Behavioral Factors

To achieve success, community health programs must narrow their focus to a limited number of health behaviors that can be addressed successfully within specific time frames. To prioritize target behaviors, Green and Kreuter (2005) suggest rating them in terms of importance and changeability. Importance is determined by the frequency of the identified behavior and how strongly it is linked to a health problem. The advisory group for teen vaping, mentioned previously, ranked the importance of the identified behaviors (see Table 12-1). The attractiveness of e-cigarette flavors was rated highly important because the advisory group learned that flavors are the primary reason youth begin using e-cigarettes (CDC, 2023c). The widespread use of tobacco among adults in the community, which modeled unhealthy practices for youth, was

TABLE **12-1** Importance Ratings of Behaviors Contributing to Teen Vaping at a Local High School

Behavior/Data	Basis for Rating
More Important Contributors	
A high proportion of high school students began vaping during middle school.	Long-established habits are more difficult to change than those which have been more recently adopted (Green & Kreuter, 2005).
Teenagers in the target population were attracted to the flavors available with e-cigarettes, such as fruit, mint, and chocolate.	Adolescents usually begin vaping with flavored e-cigarettes. Many teens are curious about the products, and flavors are the most common reason they begin using them (CDC, 2023c).
Although the legal age to purchase e-cigarettes was 18, local vendors were lax in enforcing the restrictions and vaping products were easily accessible online.	Unrestricted access to e-cigarettes supports widespread use and research showing early vaping is related to a greater chance of switching to cigarettes (Fairchild et al., 2019).
Teenagers in the target group indicated that they enjoyed vaping with their friends as an after-school activity.	Peer smoking behaviors are very influential and are more strongly associated with e-cigarette use during teenage years than smoking by adult family members (Wang et al., 2019).
Many people assigned male at birth in the target group were high school athletes who used e-cigarettes to appear "cool" without realizing vaping involves risks.	The perceived high status of the athletes may increase the influence of their conduct among fellow athletes as well as other students. There are significant risks associated with vaping, especially among children, teens, and young adults (CDC, 2023c).
Less Important Contributors	
There was a high rate of tobacco use among adults in the community.	Adult smoking is associated with uptake of smoking by young family members; nevertheless, sibling and peer smoking behavior more strongly influences teen vaping (Wang et al., 2019).

not rated highly important by the advisory group because the members felt the influence of peers was a much more important factor.

The advisory group was then asked to rate the changeability of the behaviors. Green and Kreuter (2005) indicate that the easiest behaviors to change are those that are still developing, have been adopted recently, do not have deep roots in culture or lifestyle, and have been attempted before with some success. In this round of assessments, the advisory group determined that it may be more effective to target middle school rather than, or in addition to, high school students, because they had not yet begun using e-cigarettes or the vaping habits were not yet deeply ingrained (Fig. 12-6).

After rating the identified problems by importance and changeability, the nurses and advisory group sought to narrow their focus to specific goals. Ranking the behaviors in a simple table, as seen in Table 12-2, is suggested (Green et al., 2014; Green & Kreuter, 2005). This effort yielded a table with the problems categorized in four groups: more important/more changeable, less important/more changeable, more important/less changeable, and less important/less changeable (Table 12-2). An issue seen as most important and changeable was the use of e-cigarettes among athletes assigned male at birth, who represented the subpopulation most likely to vape (high school students assigned male at birth) and who were influential among their peers. The change had support from coaches, so there was greater motivation to abandon unhealthy behaviors.

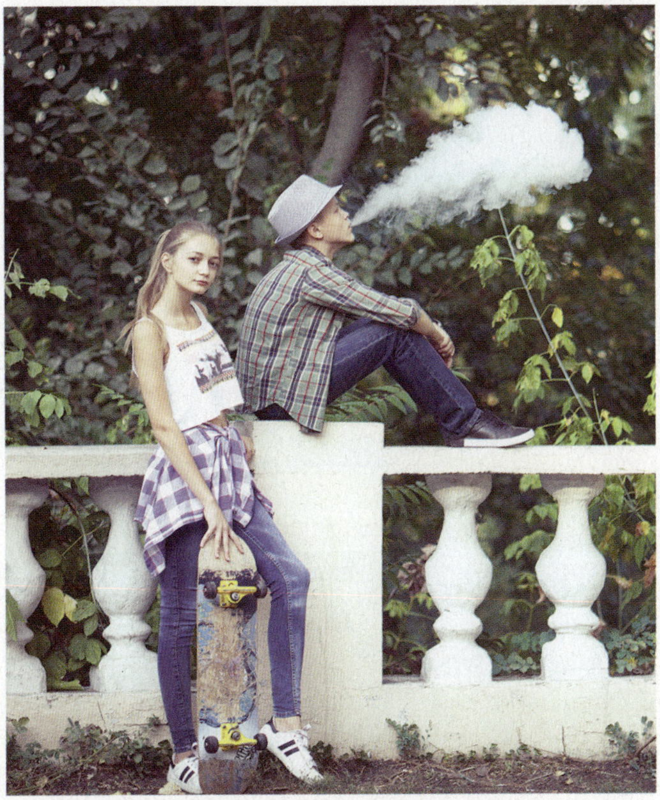

FIGURE 12-6 Vaping is increasingly popular among school-age children and is associated with significant health risks.

TABLE **12-2** Changeability Ratings of Behaviors Contributing to Teen Vaping at a Local High School

Changeability of Behavior	More Important Behaviors	Less Important Behaviors
More changeable	A high proportion of teenagers began vaping during middle school. Teenagers in the target group enjoyed vaping with friends. High school athletes assigned male at birth used e-cigarettes to appear "cool" without realizing vaping involves risks.	— — —
Less changeable	Teenagers in the target population liked the flavors available with e-cigarettes. Local vendors were lax in enforcing the restrictions, and vaping products were easily accessible online.	High rate of tobacco and e-cigarette use among adults in the community. —

Using this grid enabled the advisory group to focus on issues that were changeable and important. They determined behavioral objectives for each factor they hoped to change. These objectives identified *who* was targeted, *what* should change or what action should be taken, *how* the change would be measured, and what the *time frame* was for achieving the expected outcome. The following are their behavioral objectives:

- By the end of the fall semester, 90% of all high school athletes will sign a "no-vaping" contract as a condition of participation in high school sports.
- By the end of the school year, 90% of 6th through 12th grade students will attend a presentation aimed at preventing or discontinuing participation in vaping.

Factors That Influence Behavior Change: Predisposing, Reinforcing, and Enabling Factors

Three categories of factors affecting individual behavior can contribute or create barriers to successful behavioral change (Green et al., 2014; Green & Kreuter, 2005). These factors include **predisposing factors** providing the rationale or motivation for subsequent behavior, **reinforcing factors** providing motivation to repeat or persist in the behavior, and **enabling factors** promoting or facilitating the behavior (Fig. 12-7).

The advisory group used the PRECEDE–PROCEED model (see Chapter 11), which is one of several approaches to community health promotion, to organize their efforts. By following the model, they identified the predisposing,

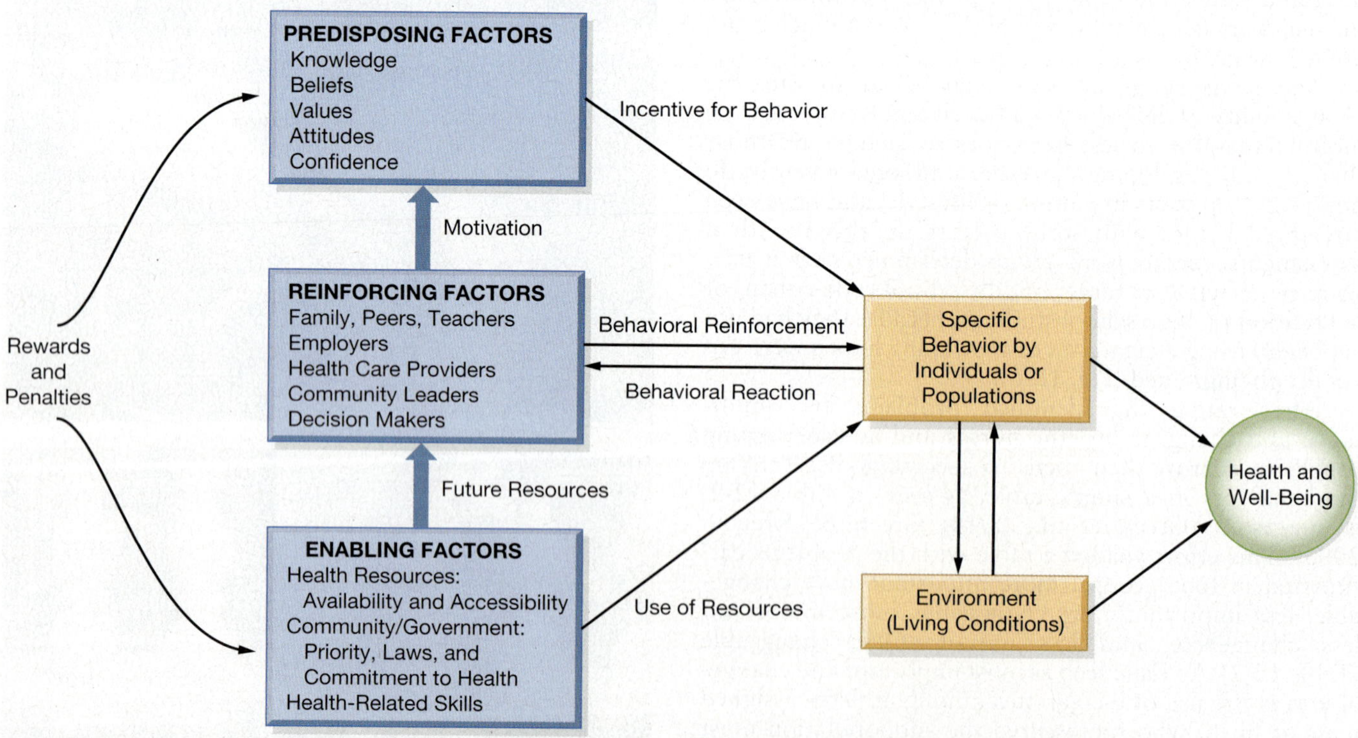

FIGURE 12-7 Predisposing, enabling, and reinforcing factors that categorize various behavioral influences. (Source: Hood, S., Linnan, L., Jolly, D., Muqueeth, S., Hall, M. B., Dixon, C., & Robinson, S. (2015). Using the PRECEDE planning approach to develop a physical activity intervention for African American men who visit barbershops: Results from the FITShop study. *American Journal of Men's Health, 9*(4), 262–273. https://doi.org/10.1177/1557988314539501.)

enabling, and reinforcing factors that affected each behavioral objective. For the behavioral objective, "By the end of the fall semester, 90% of high school athletes will sign a 'no-vaping' contract as a condition of participation in sports:"

- A *predisposing factor* was the athletes' belief that vaping would help them look "cool" among their peers.
- *Reinforcing factors* included the common use of tobacco and e-cigarettes among adults in the community, as well as the belief that e-cigarettes were a relatively safe alternative to tobacco.
- An *enabling factor* that promoted the change was the support of high school athletics coaches who agreed to monitor the conduct of the athletes while at school and enforce the no-vaping contract.

On the other hand, the apathy of local vendors in enforcing restrictions on the sale of vaping products to children under the age of 18 was seen as inhibiting change. In addition to the vaping education presentations, the advisory group decided to establish a peer-mentoring program, in which student leaders would work with the advisory group and provide mentoring and support to students who wanted to quit vaping (Fig. 12-8). Teachers were asked to nominate students for this intervention. The principal allowed the nominated students to attend educational classes conducted by the nurses to increase their knowledge about vaping cessation. The nurses worked collaboratively with the students to ensure that their mentoring and support approaches were effective. Student peer mentors suggested rewards that the students could work for that would encourage them to persist. One of the rewards that students felt should be offered was sports equipment for student use during recess and lunch periods. One local community-based organization offered to sponsor a fundraising event that would allow them to purchase sports equipment for the school.

Working with the advisory group, the nurses developed a program that outlined activities for each objective, as well as the individual responsible for the activity, the date by which the activities were to be accomplished, and how outcomes would be documented. This allowed the group to stay focused, share responsibilities, and monitor outcomes. For instance, student mentors were asked to meet with their assigned students to evaluate their progress and provide support at least once a week. The nurses were tasked with meeting each week with the student leaders to provide peer-mentoring training.

Working with the advisory group allowed the nurses to contextualize the problem of teen vaping within the target community. The advisory group ensured the nurses identified solutions that were culturally acceptable, appropriate, and effective. This process also helped them develop outcome measures consistent with the community's concerns. As nurses gathered data, they could interpret findings with input from the advisory group. This approach grounded the findings and ensured that interpretations were culturally consistent with the target population. Evaluation was facilitated by clearly defined goals that could be measured against actual results.

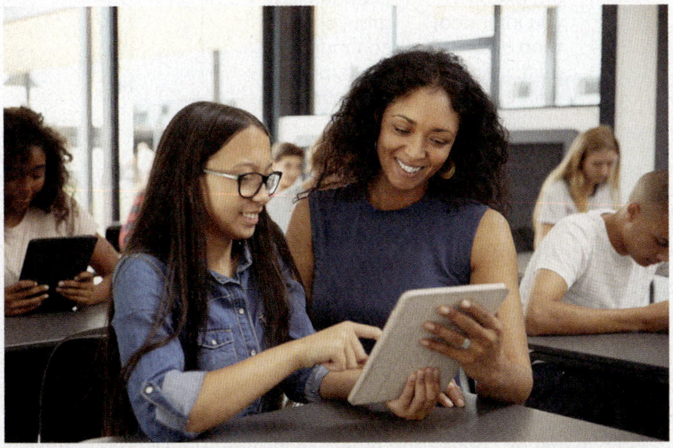

FIGURE 12-8 Peer mentoring can aid people in changing unhealthy behaviors.

EVALUATING OUTCOMES

The previous section of this chapter discussed the issues of program planning, implementation, and evaluation as they relate to a small health promotion program. This section focuses on programs and services provided by agencies. The CDC (2023d) proposes a framework and standards for program evaluation in public health, which includes six steps, usually taken in order (Fig. 12-9). There are several approaches and tools for evaluating healthcare agencies, programs, and outcomes, a few of which will be discussed in this section.

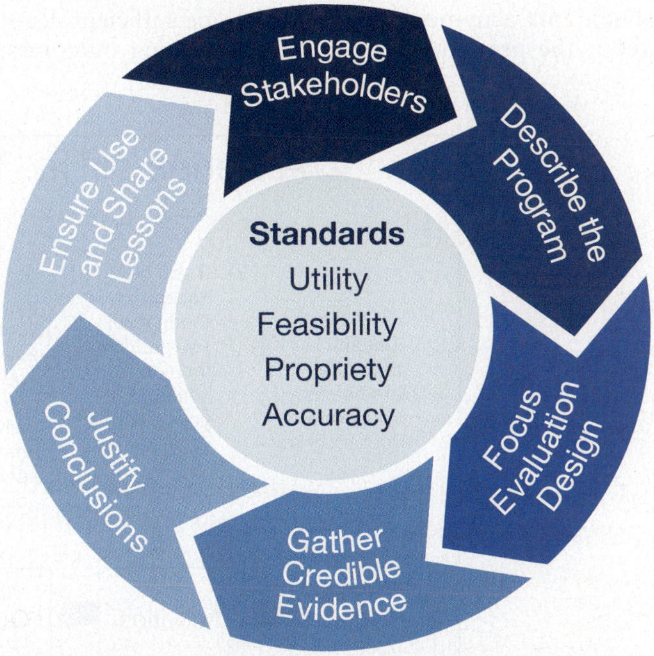
Engage Stakeholders
Describe the Program
Focus Evaluation Design
Gather Credible Evidence
Justify Conclusions
Ensure Use and Share Lessons
Standards
Utility
Feasibility
Propriety
Accuracy

FIGURE 12-9 The framework of the Centers for Disease Control and Prevention for program evaluation in public health. (Reprinted from Centers for Disease Control and Prevention. (1999). Framework for program evaluation in public health. *Morbidity and Mortality Weekly Report, 48*(RR-11), 4. Retrieved from https://www.cdc.gov/eval/framework/index.htm) Centers for Disease Control and Prevention (CDC) (2023). *Office of policy, performance, and evaluation.* https://www.cdc.gov/evaluation/)

Accreditation

Healthcare accreditation is a formal review process that allows healthcare organizations to demonstrate their ability to meet regulatory standards and requirements. The Public Health Accreditation Board (PHAB) is a nonprofit entity that is the sole independent accrediting body for public and community health agencies. The PHAB was launched in 2011 and, by September of 2023, had accredited or re-accredited a total of 366 U.S. health departments, including 41 state, 319 local, and 6 tribal agencies. Ninety percent of the U.S. population is now served by a PHAB-accredited health department (PHAB, 2023a). PHAB asserts that accreditation strengthens health departments by promoting a culture of quality and performance improvement, increasing capacity to respond to public health emergencies, and using equity as a lens to identify health priorities (PHAB, 2023b).

The National Association of County and City Health Officials (2023b) and PHAB assist health departments in assessing the feasibility of becoming accredited and offer tools to support a successful accreditation process. Several of the accreditation domains are particularly applicable to program development and outcome measurement.

Logic Models

A **logic model** is a diagram or image showing how an idea or initiative is supposed to work. It is a type of flow chart that shows the relationships between various parts of the plan. Effective logic models explain, visually and verbally, the activities involved in a health promotion program and what the results will be. To be effective, a logic model should link activities and effects, provide sufficient detail about the program and the forces affecting outcomes, and be visually appealing and thought-provoking (University of Kansas, n.d.-d). See Figures 12-10 and 12-11 for more on developing program logic models and evaluating program outcomes.

Setting Measurable Goals and Objectives

Using the logic model as a guide, planned programs should identify who the program should serve, what services should be provided, the length of time the services should be provided, and the needed resources. Measurable objectives can then be developed to describe the expected outcomes. Select verbs that indicate the expected level of achievement, such as "clients will be able to demonstrate safe administration of insulin after three home visits" or "parents will have their infants' recommended immunizations up to date by 24 months of age." Statements about measurable goals are then examined during the program evaluation. Without such statements, accurate evaluations cannot be conducted. Consider the overarching goal of the program, what you plan to accomplish, and why the program is important. The timeline and personnel resources must be considered, along with which actions must be taken to achieve the intended results.

The acronym, SMART, is frequently used in developing outcome measures. The consensus is that SMART stands for Specific, Measurable, Attainable or Achievable, Relevant, and Time Bound and may also include Evaluate and Reevaluate (SMARTER). Box 12-2 describes specific questions that must be asked and answered at each step of the SMART process.

In evaluating programs and services, outcomes must be measured against certain standards, which are guidelines for expected functioning. Standards can focus on the

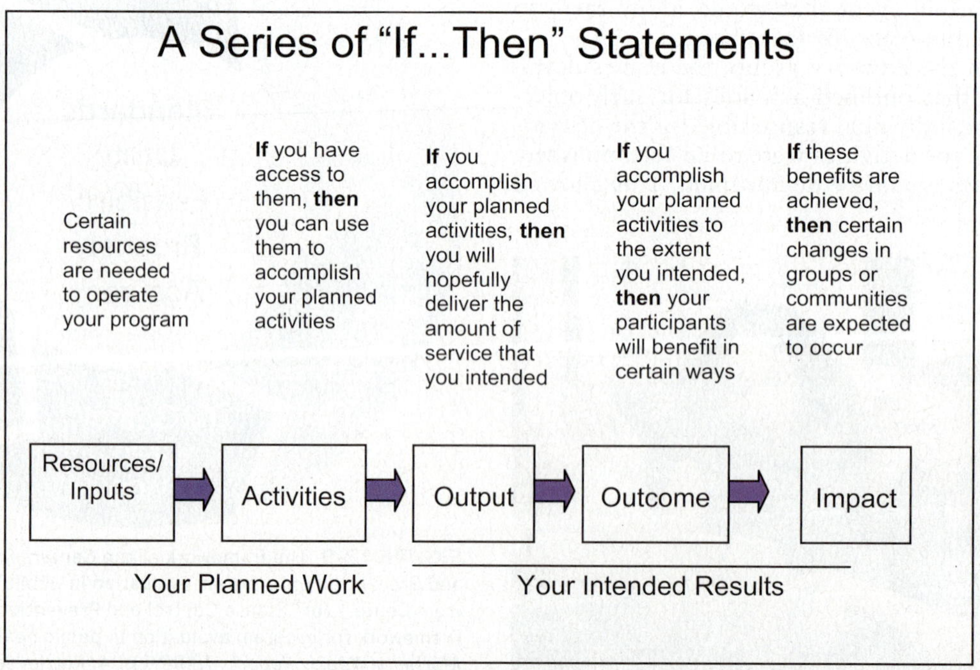

FIGURE 12-10 A series of "If...Then" statements to develop the program logic model by connecting inputs to interventions and outcomes to impacts. (From the Centers for Disease Control and Prevention, Division for Heart Disease and Stroke Prevention. [n.d.]. *Evaluation guide: Developing and using a logic model*. Retrieved from https://www.cdc.gov/cardiovascular-resources/media/pdfs/logic_model.pdf)

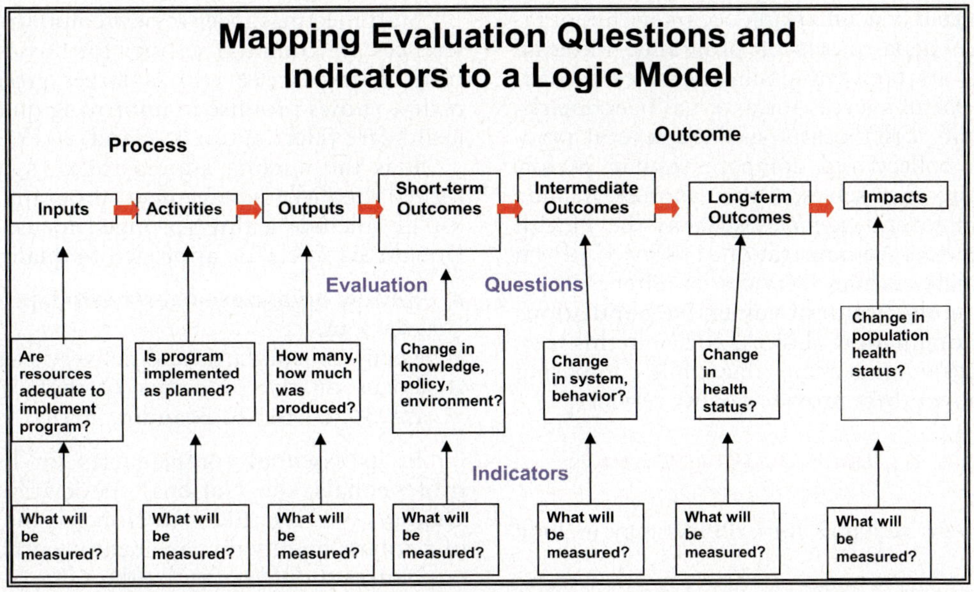

FIGURE 12-11 Mapping evaluation questions and indicators to a logic model to determine the effectiveness of a program. (From the Centers for Disease Control and Prevention, Division for Heart Disease and Stroke Prevention. [n.d.]. *Evaluation guide: Developing and using a logic model.* Retrieved from https://www.cdc.gov/dhdsp/docs/logic_model.pdf)

client, the caregiver, or the organization (e.g., finances). All care and services must also be measured against standards. The core standards of care, practice, and finance must be integrated and compatible if they are to ensure quality programs and services.

BOX 12-2 Developing SMART Objectives

Specific

- What: What do we want to accomplish?
- Why: Specific reasons, purpose, or benefits of accomplishing the goal.
- Who: Who is involved?
- Where: Identify a location.
- Which: Identify requirements and constraints.

Measurable

- How much?
- How many?
- How will we know when it is accomplished?

Attainable/Achievable

- Is the goal realistic?
- Are the needed resources available?
- How can the goal be accomplished?

Relevant

- Does this seem worthwhile?
- Is this the right time?
- Does this match our other efforts/needs?
- Are we the right group or agency?

Time-Bound or Timely

- When?
- What can we do 6 months from now?
- What can we do 6 weeks from now?
- What can we do today?

Source: Doran (1981).

Quality Indicators and Benchmarks

Quality indicators in healthcare are the measurable outcomes of a client's response to care. Optimally, the indicators are standardized and evidence based. Defining and quantifying client outcomes from quality indicators enables the nurse to evaluate the care provided. The goal of community healthcare is positive client outcomes. By starting with measurable indicators, successful outcomes can be quantified. When client care meets the standards set, client satisfaction—another quality outcome indicator—also tends to improve.

Quality indicators are part of broader quality management programs and are used to determine goal achievement. Accurate data are needed to determine whether quality indicators are being met; chart audits are a necessary and useful method of obtaining these data (AHRQ, 2022). For example, an agency may have a quality indicator such as "all infants younger than six months are weighed on each home visit." Every fifth chart of infants visited in March, June, September, and December during a designated year could be audited for documentation of the number of home visits and the number of infant weights recorded. A sample of charts is usually sufficient to evaluate the quality of care. It is generally accepted that a random selection of 10% of eligible cases provides useful information (Nock, 2016), with a minimum number of 20 cases. Nevertheless, statistical methods may be necessary to determine the appropriate sample size when the population is large, or the review is complex. Medicaid and Medicare regulations in some states mandate that a specific percentage of records be audited each year.

While striving for excellence and best practices, agencies may use the **benchmarking** process. Benchmarking compares the performance of an individual practice, department, or agency with an external standard. In quality improvement, a benchmark is considered achievable because it has already been achieved by another agency or institution. Internal benchmarking occurs within organizations, between departments or programs. External benchmarking occurs between similar agencies providing like services. Useful sources for external benchmarks include local quality collaboratives where several practices or agencies collect and compare similar performance data among themselves. Other sources include data reports from federal agencies such as the Health Resources and Services Administration (HRSA) Uniform Data System, which evaluate services or interventions aimed at improving the health of vulnerable populations and underserved communities (HRSA, 2023). In this way, an agency identifies what is achievable while comparing and contrasting how others provide quality services.

The Nurse's Role in Quality Assurance and Improvement

Quality improvement activities for C/PHNs may include the following:

- Daily prioritizing of care needs among a client caseload
- Seeking supervision or skills development for a difficult case
- Systematizing charting so that needed documentation is efficiently completed
- Proposing better ways to organize the care of chronically ill clients
- Establishing new agency procedures

Staff meetings, peer review committees, and case conferences are common settings for nurses to share lessons from their practice with a larger group. Nursing peer review shows promise in improving quality and safety in healthcare (Herrington & Hand, 2019).

It is the nursing administration's role to develop a formal quality management program. Such programs usually include a three-pronged focus, based on Avedis Donabedian's classic approach to quality management:

- Review organizational *structure*, personnel, and environment.
- Focus on standards and delivery methods (*process*).
- Focus on the *outcomes* of that care (Donabedian, 2003; Pelletier & Beaudin, 2018).

In its essential competencies for healthcare quality professionals, the National Association for Healthcare Quality (NAHQ, 2023) identifies eight key components of a robust quality management program (Fig. 12-12).

Nurses should recognize the value of quality improvement efforts and the importance of their role in ensuring that quality care is delivered. Direct service providers are the best judges of care problems and potential solutions. For this reason, quality assurance reviews and improvement activities should focus on issues relevant to staff and client concerns that can be accomplished quickly and with minimal effort. When these activities are clear, concise, and well-integrated into daily routines, they become

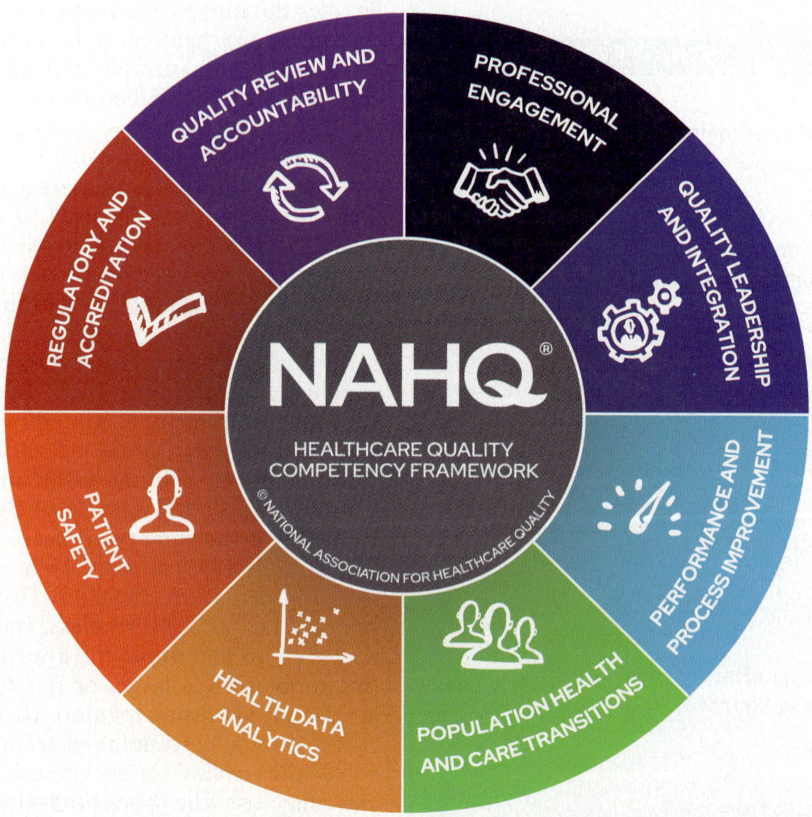

FIGURE 12-12 The National Association for Healthcare Quality (NAHQ, 2022) identifies eight key components of a robust quality management program. (Reprinted with permission from the National Association for Healthcare Quality. *NAHQ's Healthcare Quality Competency Framework*. Retrieved from https://nahq.org/wp-content/themes/yoko-nahq-child/includes/infographics/competency-framework/img/mobile-menu-wheel.svg)

less time-consuming, and staff members may view the positive client outcomes as rewards for their efforts.

Program Evaluation: Concepts and Tools

Whether small or large, healthcare agencies are complex organizations with many interrelated components. Assuring they provide services that protect or promote health can be an equally complex task. Donabedian's model not only offers a framework for quality management but also provides a foundation for the evaluation of healthcare quality initiatives. His concepts of structure, process, and outcomes offer a conceptual framework valuable in analyzing and evaluating quality of healthcare services.

Structure, Process, and Outcomes

The organizational *structure* should fulfill its mission statement or philosophy (Dunham-Taylor, 2015) and be client-focused with enough resources to maintain and develop more services, as needed. The organizational structure should operate efficiently and within budget, maintaining financial stability and promoting trust and confidence among stakeholders. There should also be a well-developed system for acquiring additional funding for new services through grants and contract expansion if needed. Finally, the organization should attract and retain clients and qualified, highly motivated staff.

The agency should develop and maintain *processes* that produce safe, effective, client-centered, timely, efficient, and equitable services (AHRQ, 2022). It should maintain standards that comply with or surpass those recommended by relevant accrediting bodies. Leaders should ensure that employee values and conduct are compatible with the organization's goals and that their knowledge and skills align with job requirements. The agency should foster a collaborative work environment in which quality of care is continuously monitored by using a variety of tools such as audit instruments, peer review, and incident reporting systems, and should encourage staff to contribute to the evaluation and revision of standards. Clients should also be invited to provide input and feedback, and the agency should act upon suggestions and opportunities for improvement. A supportive work environment in which leaders, staff, and clients have compatible relationships will help to minimize staff turnover, expand the client base, and create stability.

The agency should monitor client health *outcomes* that reflect the impact of services provided. However, outcomes are the result of numerous factors, including some that are beyond the agency's control. Reviewing client records will offer insights into preventable outcomes. For example, the charts of hospitalized clients may offer insights into teaching or care that could have prevented hospitalization. Clinic or home visit records of clients with poor outcomes may offer clues about teaching or care that could have prevented them. The agency's awareness of national, state, and local healthcare initiatives may help in identifying priority health indicators and outcomes. This awareness will help in developing SMART goals and aims (discussed earlier in this chapter) targeting the indicators and outcomes for the client population. In doing so, it is helpful to enlist people with healthcare analytics skills, within or outside the agency, to identify and analyze metrics that show whether or not goals for client outcomes are being met. Leaders can then modify and improve structure and processes as needed.

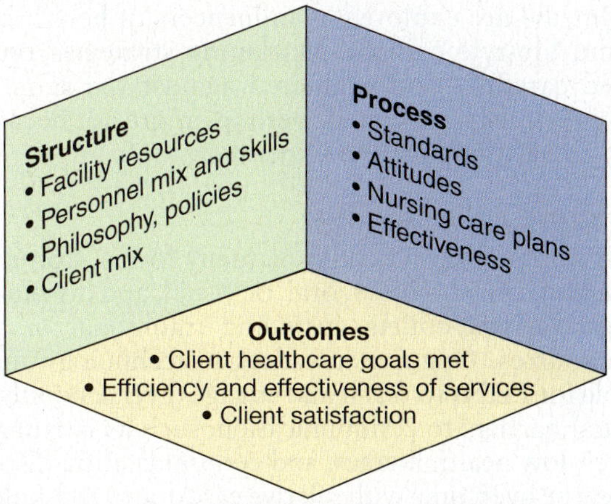

FIGURE 12-13 The Donabedian model uses the concepts of structure, process, and outcomes in evaluating quality of care.

Models Useful in Program Evaluation

Donabedian Model. As previously noted, Donabedian (2003) was the original proponent of using the concepts of structure, process, and outcomes in evaluating quality of care (Fig. 12-13). The Donabedian model is recognized as a basic model, linear in form, for measuring quality. Structure influences process which, in turn, produces outcomes. The Donabedian model is relevant to common domains of nursing and is widely used as a framework for more elaborate quality improvement models.

Omaha System. The Omaha System includes measurement approaches that make it a useful model for evaluating the quality of nursing care provided to people, families, *and* communities. Evaluation focuses on process indicators, client outcome measures, and satisfaction with care (Martin, 2005; The Omaha System, 2023). The model is currently used in "home care, public health, and school health practice settings, nurse-managed center staff, hospital-based and managed care case managers, educators and students, occupational health nurses, faith community staff, acute care and rehabilitation hospital/long-term care staff, researchers, members of various disciplines, and computer software vendors" (The Omaha System, 2023, para. 10). The evaluation components of the Omaha System include outcomes that are rated in terms of *knowledge* (what the client knows), *behavior* (what the client does), and *status* (how the client is). The outcomes are quantified on a range of severity, on a continuum toward or away from optimal health, and there is ongoing monitoring of the person, family, or community health outcomes to assess the quality of nursing interventions.

MARKETING AND COMMUNITY HEALTH PROGRAMS

Community health services are challenged to create health promotion programs that reach and engage their target populations. Communicating with the target community is essential in enlisting support and participation and in providing other relevant information about the program. In this section, the roles of community messaging and social media are explored as influencers of health behaviors and lifestyle choices. Marketing strategies must be selected carefully and evaluated against the same standards previously presented, perhaps more so, because of their potential impact and expense.

Community Messaging

Health communication comes in many forms. **Community messaging** can be written, oral, or visual, and disseminated through various outlets, including traditional or newer media sources. Ongoing advances in technology make it possible for PHNs to reach and engage diverse populations. Potential barriers to communication, such as language differences, low health literacy, and communication disorders, can now be overcome with relative ease due to technological advances. Most health communication, including community messaging, involves some or all of the steps identified in the National Prevention Information Network's Health Communication Strategies and Resources (2022, para. 3). These steps include the following:

1. Identifying the health problem and determining whether communication should be part of the intervention
2. Identifying the audience for the communication and the best ways to reach them
3. Developing and testing communication concepts, messages, and materials with the target audience
4. Implementing the health communication program based on testing results
5. Assessing the effectiveness of the messages and modifying them, as necessary

The 2021 "Vax-A-Nation" (United South and Eastern Tribes, Inc, n.d.) campaign illustrates the value of community health messaging. During the COVID-19 pandemic, underrepresented populations such as native American tribes were disproportionately affected. The COVID-19 vaccine was distributed among the tribes; however, there was low vaccination uptake among tribal nations in southern and eastern regions of the United States, leaving the recommended vaccination targets of 75% to 80% unmet. The Urban Indian Health Institute (2021) suggested that vaccine hesitancy among native Americans may be due to a long-established mistrust of government agencies. The Rescue Agency, a health communication company, was tasked with developing community messaging and a strategy to promote vaccination among tribal citizens.

After conducting research to understand perceptions and attitudes about vaccination among the target groups, the Rescue Agency determined key barriers and motivators in the communities. Perceived barriers were a lack of "proof" of the safety and effectiveness of the vaccine, and a threat to personal choice, while a significant motivator was protecting older and other vulnerable citizens. Based on the findings, the Rescue Agency developed a community messaging strategy that encouraged hesitant community members to consider the importance of protecting older people, families at risk, and community members. The messaging also addressed key concerns, such as the desire for autonomy (Seneres, 2023).

After developing the messaging, the Rescue Agency then developed a strategy for disseminating it among the target populations. It determined that tribal leaders were key in launching the Vax-A-Nation campaign, which included a toolkit that could be tailored to individual tribal community needs and preferences. The toolkit included posters, flyers, fact sheets, digital banners, social media graphics, and Facebook and Instagram messages focusing on four campaign areas (Fig. 12-14):

1. The duty of citizens to protect themselves and others from the threat of COVID-19
2. The relative safety of the vaccine as compared to the disease itself
3. The peace of mind coming from a personal decision to be vaccinated
4. The importance of seeking information from authoritative sources (United South and Eastern Tribes, Inc, n.d.)

Subsequent data showed that Native American and Alaskan Natives were vaccinated at higher rates than other racial and ethnic groups in 2021. This was attributed to the involvement of tribal leaders in vaccine prioritization and distribution efforts in their communities (Hill & Artiga, 2021). The Vax-A-Nation campaign highlights the importance of developing community messaging and dissemination strategies that are based on an understanding of the audience's distinct characteristics and values (Seneres, 2023).

Social Marketing of Community Health Programs

The term social marketing refers to marketing principles that change or maintain people's behavior related to products, services, or messaging. The National Social Marketing Centre (n.d.). The objective of social marketing in public health is to improve society's health by influencing changes in individual health behaviors (e.g., healthy eating) and implementing policies that improve the health behaviors of populations (e.g., seat belt laws). The integration of marketing with public health is seen to enhance the effectiveness of public health communication as noted through the CDC's *Let's Stop HIV Together* campaign (CDC, 2023e) (https://www.cdc.gov/stophivtogether/partnerships/social-marketing-toolkit.html).

Equity-Centered Public Health Communication

Public health communication must assure that the public understands, accepts, and acts on the information provided. As communication includes both context and language for communication messaging, communication must be respectful, inclusive, and nonstigmatizing (Calanan et al., 2023). Guiding principles to include in public health messaging:

- Use an equity lens (recognize and reflect the intended audience)
- Key principles (be clear, avoid blaming and stigmatizing, and use first-person language)
- Preferred terms (increase inclusiveness, engage community)
- Developing inclusive communication (intended audience)
- Inclusive images (how does it support community)
- Resources and references (follow best practice guidelines) (Calanan et al., 2023)

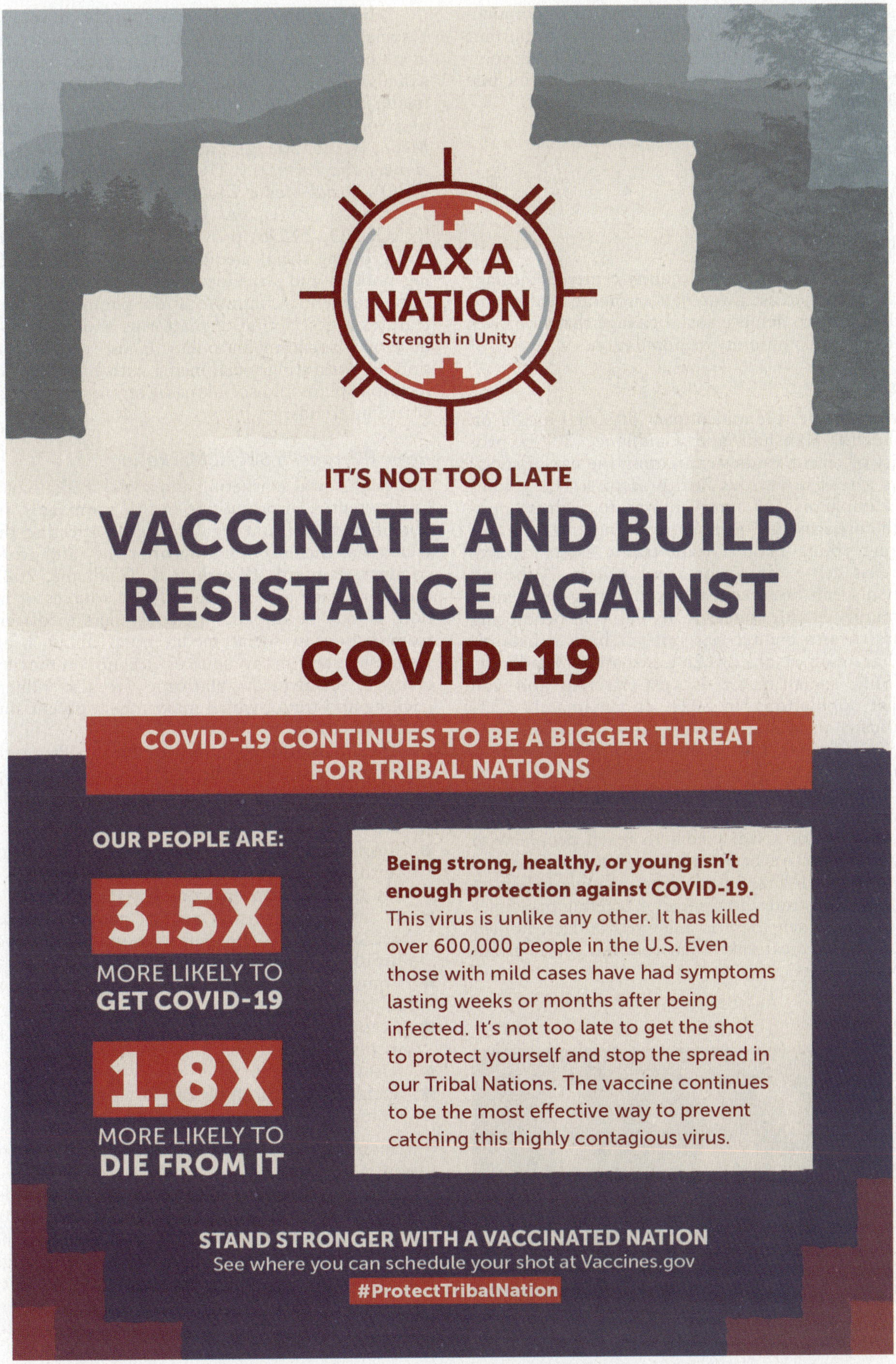

FIGURE 12-14 Vax-A-Nation campaign toolkit. (Reprinted with permission from United South and Eastern Tribes, Inc. *Vax-A-Nation Vaccine Campaign*. Retrieved from https://www.usetinc.org/vax-a-nation-vaccine-campaign/)

These guiding principles can be applied in conjunction with a social marketing plan connecting important messaging to the needs of the community. A social market plan brings awareness to the issue and should include the following:

- A problem description
- Market research
- Market strategy
- Interventions
- Implementation
- Evaluation (CDC, 2023e)

The use of marketing and equity-centered messaging is critical to increase awareness, promote health, and change behavior to achieve social change that improves the health of the community or population.

Social Media

In a review of the role and impact of social media on public health, Kanshan and Gaidhane (2023) provide a list of recent studies examining the use of social media as a tool in various health sectors. The studies include campaigns and interventions to address public health concerns such as risky drinking and cannabis use among young people, road traffic safety awareness, breast self-examination, and others. Although social media can be effective in promoting awareness of community health concerns, its value in promoting behavioral health change has not yet been substantiated (Gharamani et al., 2022; Kanshan & Gaidhane, 2023). Still, social media is cost-effective and can reach vast populations. In 2021, approximately 72% of Americans used social networking tools, such as Facebook, Snapchat, Instagram, X (formerly Twitter), and YouTube (Pew Research Center, 2021). By 2023, 60% of the world's population was using social media (Shewalte, 2023).

The capacity of social media to reach people with strategic and effective health messages is immense and must be harnessed (Fig. 12-15). The example below, in Box 12-3, demonstrates how social marketing principles can be utilized when there is a limited budget, limited time, and limited creativity. What role can social media play in these efforts?

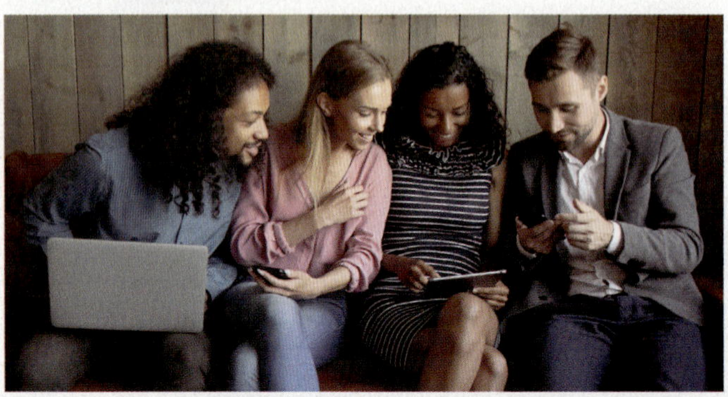

FIGURE 12-15 Social media and technology have the capacity to reach and influence the health behaviors of a wide audience.

When planning and beginning the development of a social marketing approach, there are many resources available to the PHN and other public health professionals. The CDC offers several webpages with social media information: *Gateway to Health Communications and Social Marketing* (CDC, 2023f), *Digital and Social Media* (CDC, 2023g), and *Social Media Tools for Consumers and Partners* (CDC, 2023h) among others. NACCHO's *Social Media Toolkit: A Primer for Local Health Department PIOs and Communications Professionals* (NACCHO, 2023b) provides information on initiating and growing social media programs, including developing policies and strategies, and integrating social media into emergency communication planning. This toolkit features a description of platforms and explains how to develop a social media policy. It also provides information on integrating social media with emergency communications plans and social media strategies, in addition to emerging trends.

Ethical Issues in Social Marketing

Although social marketing and social media have significant potential in promoting health campaigns, there are potential ethical and legal concerns affecting their use, which may include violations of privacy and professional conduct standards (Kanshan & Gaidhane, 2023). Furthermore, they are often unreliable sources of information. It may be difficult for consumers to discern truth from fiction in social media posts about health and wellness when many sources are not authoritative or credible. Social media platforms are also vulnerable to hacking and fraud, which makes them potent sources of misinformation.

The International Union for Health Promotion and Education (n.d.) is dedicated to promoting optimum health and well-being globally. Their values highlight the importance of ethics in health promotion:

- Respect—for the innate dignity of all people, for cultural identity, for cultural diversity, and for natural resources and the environment
- Inclusion and involvement of people in making the decisions that shape their lives and impact upon their health and well-being
- Equity in health, social, and economic outcomes for all people
- Accountability and transparency—within governments, organizations, and communities
- Sustainability
- Social justice for all people
- Compassion and empowerment

(International Union for Health Promotion and Education, n.d., para. 3)

Social marketing is not a panacea, but it does offer techniques that can support health education and promotion programs. The method can be expensive and elaborate or provide simple, straightforward messages. The point is that well-presented marketing can prompt behavior change. Media messages are not a replacement for a sound health promotion program, but they are a tool that can be used for profound impact.

BOX **12-3** STORIES FROM THE FIELD

Nursing Students and a Social Marketing Campaign

University campuses hold a wealth of often-untapped expertise. For nursing students working on a health promotion program, the health issue is often quite straightforward, but the presentation is more challenging. Many nursing schools are providing collaborative experiences for students, supporting partnerships with non-nursing students and faculty in addressing health education needs. The following is one example of how collaboration can be effective:

In conversation with an instructor, two nursing students learned that the university administration was concerned about a surge in measles cases statewide. The university recommended students be current on all standard immunizations prior to admission; nevertheless, it was not a requirement. After further discussion with their instructor, the nursing students sought input from several student organizations. From those discussions, they identified a low level of knowledge and concern about the issue among the students.

Recognizing that college students are not prone to worrying about measles, the nursing students sought help from the university's student health center. The health center administration agreed this was an important issue and collaborated with the public health department to offer free measles, mumps, and rubella (MMR) immunizations at the student health center. The student health center posted information about the free immunizations on its website, but there was little response from students.

The nursing students realized that they needed to spread the word about the importance of the issue and the availability of free immunizations. Based on input from the student groups, they decided to develop social media messaging that was informative, engaging, and brief. In conjunction with their instructor, they contacted the university's animation department and found an instructor who was willing to assign their students to develop an animated video promoting MMR vaccination. The nursing students provided information about the current measles outbreak, educational materials about the MMR vaccine, and details about its availability at the student health center. The graphic design students then developed brief animation videos, of which several outstanding videos were submitted.

The graphic design student's animation videos were posted on several of the university's social media outlets, including Facebook and Instagram. The campus newspaper also published an article about the MMR campaign and the collaborative efforts of the health center and students from different colleges. In response, there was a surge in students visiting the health center for free MMR vaccination. The campaign also reached parents who saw the videos on the web pages and social media. Many messages were sent to the university by the parents regarding the campaign, and the responses were handled by the nursing students.

The campaign was not expensive, it engaged the most skilled people for each task, and it provided much-needed information to the university students and their parents. Even though they had targeted the college students, the nursing students found that the parents were just as interested in the campaign.

1. *In what ways has social marketing influenced your actions or behaviors?*
2. *Can you think of an issue on your university campus that could benefit from social marketing?*
3. *Do you recognize any social marketing efforts sponsored by your university or your school of nursing?*

SECURING GRANTS TO FUND COMMUNITY HEALTH PROGRAMS

Public health departments and other community agencies often require outside funding to develop new health intervention programs. A customary practice is to seek grant funding. What is a grant? A grant is simply one individual or group providing another individual or group with support (i.e., money) for a specified purpose. It is important to note that grant support is often offered as funding to get programs started but not to facilitate long-term operations (Jaykus, 2017; Karsh & Fox, 2019). In health programs, grants offer a source of funding for program development or project support. These types of grants fall into certain categories: planning grants (i.e., initial project development), start-up grants (i.e., seed money), management or technical assistance grants (e.g., for fundraising or marketing), research grants, and facilities or equipment grants (National Institutes of Health, 2023).

Grants are not easy to locate, secure, or manage (once you have one), but they are vital in providing a wide range of programs and services to a community. Grants are available from government sources, private philanthropic sources, and corporations. Private organizations often have sections on their websites with information on available grant funding. Grant money is not typically paid back; however, it is a contractual agreement, and the terms and conditions are usually clearly delineated.

Federal Grants

Federal grants award government funds to implement projects that provide public service and stimulate the economy (Grants.gov, n.d.) and are available from 26 grant-making agencies. The funding categories most applicable to community health include the following: community development, disaster preparation and relief, food and nutrition, and health. Federal grants are available to a wide variety of groups, but typically, health-related grants are available to state or local agencies including public health departments, public housing organizations, educational organizations, and nonprofit organizations (Grants.gov, n.d.). Federal grants can be found on the website www.grants.gov or on individual federal agency websites.

The Grant Process

The grant process allows you to focus clearly on what you intend to accomplish, why it is needed, and what part you will play in the project's successful outcome. The first step is to select a funder that is a good match for your organization's mission, values, and goals and your program/project. For instance, applying to a faith-based organization that supports abstinence-only educational programs would not be a good fit for your program that seeks to provide contraceptive information in an after-school program for teens. It is wise to seek the help of an experienced mentor—someone who has been successful in grant writing—so they can guide you through the process of writing a proposal and offer suggestions prior to submission. In grant funding, experience counts! A proven record in securing grants and completing the requirements means you or your organization will have an easier time securing additional funding.

The Nurse's Role in Grant Applications and Management

Many health departments see grants as an integral part of their service delivery, even hiring grant writers and managers in some cases. For small nonprofit organizations seeking funding, an effective approach is to partner with a local university, which allows for more access to grant-locating programs, as well as to the expertise offered on the campuses (e.g., content area experts, experienced researchers, statisticians, business plan experts). For most health agencies, the task of locating grant funds, writing the grant application, and doing the work stipulated by the grant falls on the nurses and other professionals within those agencies. Grant proposal writing offers an opportunity for C/PHNs to explain to others what they can provide in terms of services and programs targeting the community's health.

SUMMARY

- The first step in developing effective community health programs is identifying the problem(s) to be addressed.
- National health objectives and initiatives, such as Healthy People 2030, and state and local priorities and programs offer ideas for community health aims.
- There are a variety of tools for identifying local health needs, including federal resources.
- Establishing partnerships with other healthcare professionals and community organizations, leaders, and members is a crucial element in planning community health programs.
- Nurses must integrate their own "authoritative knowledge" with the target population's "local knowledge" into the community health program.
- The Community Action Model is a form of participatory action research that identifies actions that are achievable and sustainable.
- A key factor in ensuring the success of an intervention is to appoint an advisory group, including representatives from the target community.
- The changeability and importance of healthy behaviors should be considered when developing community health programs.
- Successful community health programs require that the nurse listen to the target population and not determine the problem and solution without their assistance.
- Outcome measures should be consistent with the community's concerns, and evaluation can be facilitated by clearly defined goals measured against actual results.
- Accreditation is an evaluation process that promotes high-quality services among health departments.
- Quality indicators are measures of a client's response to care. The goal of community health programs is successful client outcomes.
- Benchmarking compares an individual entity's performance with an external standard. Local quality collaboratives are useful sources of external benchmarks.
- The concepts of structure, process, and outcomes offer the basis for Donabedian's and other related models of healthcare evaluation. The Omaha System provides standardized language for classifying problems, interventions, and outcomes.
- Effective community messaging and social marketing in public health can promote changes in individual health behaviors and policies that improve health behaviors of populations.
- Social media has immense potential for reaching people with public health messages; however, there is a lack of evidence confirming its effectiveness.
- Grants offer a source of funding for program development or project support. Nurses play a key role in grant writing and management.

ACTIVE LEARNING EXERCISES

1. With the information provided in the teen vaping example, work with a group of students to complete the planning of a viable program that meets the stated goals. List nursing diagnoses and develop measurable objectives (SMART objectives). Use Figure 12-7 as a guide to develop predisposing, reinforcing, and enabling factors related to teen vaping. Use the logic model diagrams in Figures 12-10 and 12-11, and other information on evaluation, to determine resources and activities, as well as available data that could be used to evaluate short-term and long-term outcomes. (Objectives 1 and 6)
2. Inquire about past and present public health programs targeted to specific populations in your area (or at the state level). How was the need discovered? What steps did they take to understand community concerns about this issue? Where was the data obtained? Was a model or framework used to develop an intervention (if so, which one)? How were the outcomes measured? Did program evaluation determine

if the intervention was effective? Describe how 4 of the 10 Essential Public Health Services (see Box 2-2) were used in this process. (Objectives 2 to 6)

3. Compare common quality improvement measures found in acute care (hospital) settings and potential areas for quality improvement in public health (e.g., CDC's continuous program improvement cycle or National Public Health Improvement Initiative). Is your local public health agency accredited? If so, ask an administrator how this has changed PHN practice and client outcomes. If not, ask for examples of public health quality improvement measures or benchmarks—how are community programs evaluated? (Objective 6)
4. Identify a health-related community messaging or social marketing campaign that you viewed recently on social media sites, in print, or on television. Alternatively, find a research article on the use of social marketing in public health. Who is the target audience? What is the main message it is sending? What is the target behavior or problem? Does it reach the target audience? What works? What doesn't seem to be effective? How could you improve on methods to reach the target audience? (Objective 7)
5. Talk with PHNs or PHN supervisors at your local or state public health department or other community health agency. How many and what types of grants do they have? What programs do they fund exclusively from grant writing? How are they involved in grant writing? How do they manage grant funding and data gathering to justify outcomes for grant funders? (Objective 8)

CHAPTER 13

Policy Making and Advocacy

"Never doubt that a small group of thoughtful citizens can change the world. Indeed, it is the only thing that ever has."

—Margaret Mead

KEY TERMS

Advocacy
Community empowerment
Health policy
Lobbying
Polarization
Policy
Policy analysis
Policy competence
Political action committees (PACs)
Politics
Power
Public policy
Special interest groups

LEARNING OBJECTIVES

Upon mastery of this chapter, you should be able to:

1. Describe the relationship between public policy and health outcomes.
2. Define health policy and explain how it is established.
3. Describe how a bill becomes a law on the federal level.
4. Discuss policy examples for legislation, regulation, and policy modification.
5. Contrast the rational framework with Kingdon's framework for policy analysis and identify when each would be most useful for public health nurses (PHNs).
6. Identify three ways a PHN can engage in policy activism.
7. Identify the difference between advocacy and lobbying, as well as the influence of both on policy.
8. Describe how the Patient Protection and Affordable Care Act impacts the health of the public.
9. Discuss the roles power and empowerment play in policy development.

INTRODUCTION

Public **health policy** consists of the legislation and funding that we, as members of the public, adopt to govern the provision, regulation, and research of healthcare for our fellow Americans. Because health policy outcomes are determined by the availability and quality of all health and social services, nurses must gain knowledge of health policy development and the political process. This allows nurses to advocate for and protect the people, families, and communities they serve and support their own nursing practice. Policy outcomes impact the communities in which we practice, our personal health, and the health of our neighborhoods and country. The community/public health nurse (C/PHN) needs to understand how to impact policy through advocacy and leadership.

In this chapter, we will discuss the current state of the health of people in the United States, how policy impacts health, the policy process, and how C/PHNs can be involved in health policy action.

HEALTH IN THESE UNITED STATES: HOW HEALTHY ARE WE?

The U.S. healthcare system is recognized worldwide for medical achievements such as the mapping of the human genome, advances in biomedical technologies, and pharmaceuticals that hold promise for the myriad of chronic and acute illnesses that affect the world's populations. The U.S. healthcare system is also known to be expensive. Current data indicate that the United States spends 18.3% of its gross domestic product on healthcare costs (U.S. Centers for Medicare & Medicaid Services [CMS], 2022a). This is twice as much as the average healthcare expenditures from countries with similar levels of economic development (Organization for Economic Co-operation and Development [OECD], 2023). High expenditures are not necessarily problematic if the nation can afford them and result in positive health outcomes. However, for the amount the United States spends on healthcare, are we achieving the results we desire (Box 13-1)?

BOX 13-1 WHAT DO *YOU* THINK?

Access to Healthcare

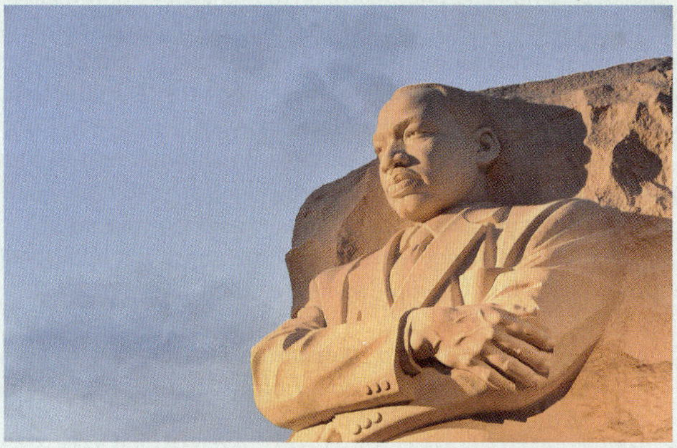

Martin Luther King, Jr. Memorial.

> "Of all the forms of inequality, injustice in health is the most shocking and the most inhuman because it often results in physical death."
>
> —Dr. Martin Luther King Jr.

Over time, the debate of whether access to healthcare in the United States was a right or a privilege has endured. What do you think? Should there be some basic rights regarding access to basic healthcare services as found in most other developed nations (e.g., a safety net)? Or is this a privilege that is accessed as a primary good for those who can afford to pay for it out of their personal resources? Should we ration healthcare based on social justice and provide it for those who need it the most? Should we ration healthcare based on market justice, making it accessible only to those who can pay?

The United States performs better than comparable countries in some areas and grossly underperforms in others. According to the OECD (2023), the United States performs worse than peer countries in these areas:

- Life expectancy and overall mortality
- Infant mortality and low birth weight
- Overweight and obesity
- COVID-19 deaths
- Traffic-related injuries
- HIV and AIDS
- Drug-related deaths (Box 13-2)
- Cardiovascular disease
- Chronic lung disease

The OECD (2023) also documents areas where the United States performs favorably when compared to peer countries, including the following:

- Cancer mortality
- Stroke mortality
- Overall avoidable mortality
- Tobacco consumption
- Survival of older adults
- Self-rated health
- Avoidable chronic obstructive pulmonary disease admissions
- Mammography screening
- Influenza vaccine (Gunja et al., 2023)

The areas in which the United States performs better than peer countries are, in part, a result of advances in early diagnosis and the development of new, more effective pharmaceutical treatments. Survival of older adults is also likely related to medication therapy and technological advances in old age. For those who live to age 75 years, their odds of living longer are greatly increased (Fig. 13-1). Self-rated health is high in the United States, possibly because our technological developments provide consumers with the perception of great medical advances from which it is logical to conclude that one's health outcomes are positive.

However, in general, people in the United States spend more money on healthcare and live shorter lives than those in peer countries (Arias et al., 2022). Among high-income countries, the United States has the lowest life expectancy and highest rates of preventable premature death (Gunja et al., 2023). The Peterson-Kaiser Health System Tracker (2023) shows that although mortality rates have fallen for all developed countries over the past decade, they remain higher in the United States than in similar countries.

Further, in the United States, there are significant health disparities that contribute to overall poor health outcomes. Since 2019, life expectancy for all racial and ethnic groups in the United States decreased. However, people of color are disproportionately impacted by this decrease. While the life expectancy for Black and Hispanic people decreased by over 4 years, life expectancy for White people decreased by only 2.4 years (Arias et al., 2022).

These outcomes are a result of problems within the U.S. healthcare system. Reasons for these health inequities are complex and include a lack of attention within the current healthcare system to the social determinants of health, challenges to access to healthcare, structural and systemic racism, and public policies that do not address the nonclinical causes of poor health.

This raises the question: What is health policy, and how is it relevant to community/public health nursing? If C/PHNs are to promote and protect the health of populations (American Public Health Association [APHA], PHN Section, 2013), they need to understand health policy as it relates to the health of the public. Policies affect our daily lives, regardless of whether they are related to health or work. Thus, C/PHNs need an understanding of health policy to better address the issues affecting the health of the communities they serve and improve health outcomes. Consider the following questions:

- How does health policy impact the health of the population?
- How is policy important in addressing both issues of access to care and of creating and supporting the social conditions that support health?

BOX **13-2** STORIES FROM THE FIELD

Opioids in America

Since 1999, more than 932,000 people died as a result of a drug overdose. In 2020, 75% of overdose-related deaths involved an opioid (including prescription and illegal opioids), making this eight times higher than in 1999 (CDC, 2023a). The causes of this epidemic are complex. One contributor was the increase in prescription of opioid medications, which lead to misuse before it was known that these medications are highly addictive (CDC, 2024). The number of opioid prescriptions tripled in the late 1990s and early 2000s. During that same timeframe, the number of opioid-related deaths also tripled (Positive Behavioral Interventions and Support, 2024). Misuse of prescription opioids often leads patients to seek nonprescription opioids. In some areas of the country, heroin is cheaper and easier to obtain than prescription opioids. Studies show that 80% of people who use heroin misused prescribed opioids first (National Institute on Drug Abuse, 2021). Further, the communities in which people live are influential factors in the opioid epidemic. Risk is compounded by overall poor health, poverty, lack of opportunity, and inadequate living and working conditions. The contributors to the opioid epidemic are public health policy issues.

Taylor is a 35-year-old who visits their primary care provider (PCP) for a chronic pain follow-up visit. During this visit, the PCP notes that the patient was prescribed an opioid for pain management 6 months ago. The patient has requested refills 4 to 7 days early each month. The patient reports limited pain relief and becomes agitated when the PCP offers alternative, nonopioid pain management options. By using motivational interviewing techniques, the PCP engages the patient in a discussion about their medication use. During this discussion, the patient shares that they have been misusing their opioid prescription for the past 5 months and has resorted to using nonprescription opioids when prescriptions run out. After much discussion, the patient acknowledges their misuse of opioids and asks for assistance in seeking treatment. Together, the PCP and patient develop a plan for next steps of care.

The healthcare system, in this case, functioned well in that Taylor had access to care and their provider practiced high-quality, evidence-based care to assist them in seeking treatment.

However, when Taylor leaves the clinic, there are additional resources necessary to help them reach their goals.

1. *Do they have access to transportation necessary to seek treatment? Such access could be related to where they live, or their income level.*
2. *Will Taylor's health insurance cover necessary follow-up and treatment options?*
3. *What community factors influence their opioid use? Does Taylor live in poverty, with limited opportunities for safe work and housing?*

The ability of Taylor to carry out a plan for treating their opioid misuse is related to policies that impact adequate housing, safe working conditions, social and economic stability, health insurance coverage, and access to illegal opioids.

1. *How does the healthcare system use its knowledge to influence such policies in ways that combat the opioid epidemic?*
2. *How can and should health professionals be involved in the development or implementation of policies to promote healthy lifestyles?*

Source: CDC (2023a); Dare and Bugen (2020).

- What is the relationship between politics and health policy?
- What do C/PHNs need to understand about health policy and its formation?
- How can nurses become involved in the political process and in promoting effective health policies?

In the remainder of the chapter, we will discuss policy, how it is formed, and how C/PHNs can gain policy competence to impact policy in their practice. We will also discuss the relationship between politics and health policy.

HEALTH POLICY ANALYSIS

What Is Policy?

Change in the healthcare system requires change in healthcare policies. What does that mean? Let's first define policy. While there is not a single clear definition of policy, at the most basic level, a **policy** is action that the government takes (or does not take) to address a problem or concern (Center for Civic Education, 2023). Key characteristics include the following:

- Policy is in response to an issue that requires attention.
- Policy is the course of action the government chooses to address the issue of concern.
- Policies may be laws or regulations.

Policy is made by the government on behalf of the public (Center for Civic Education, 2023). Policies lead to laws, regulations, or administrative rulings. When issued by national, state, or local governments, they are called public policies. Health policy refers to specific policies involving health and healthcare. There are different types of policies:

- *Substantive policy:* This is a policy that involves an action or activity, such as funding for a health program or health-related agency. One example would be federal funding for the Indian Health Service and its activities.
- *Procedural policy:* These involve the procedure by which an outcome is sought. An example of this is voting rights policies, which stipulate the process for voting eligibility.
- *Distributive policy:* These are policies that allocate services or benefits to specific groups of people. Medicare, for example, distributes resources to people who meet age and physical condition criteria.

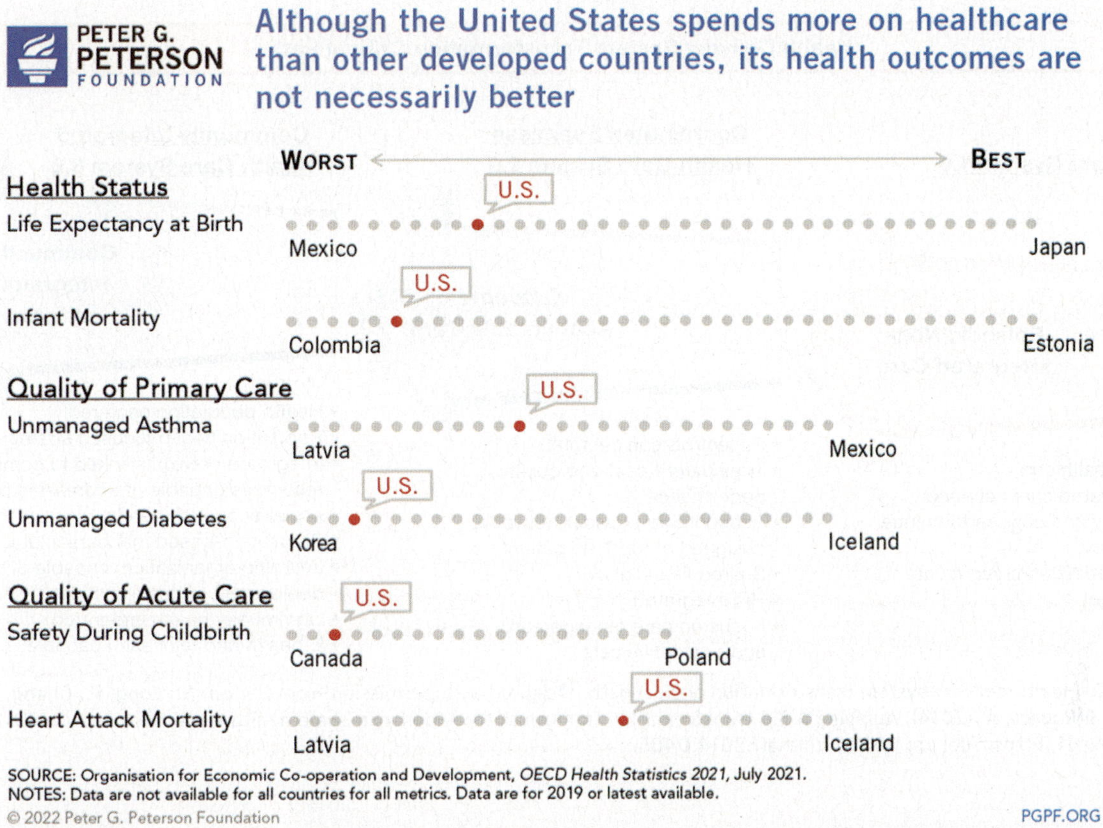

FIGURE 13-1 Global health outcomes rankings. (© 2022 Peterson G. Peterson Foundation. Used with permission. https://www.pgpf.org/blog/2022/01/us-healthcare-system-ranks-sixth-worldwide-innovative-but-fiscally-unsustainable)

- *Regulatory policy:* These policies limit the activities or behaviors of certain groups or people, such as age limits for the purchase of alcohol or health professional licensing regulations (Birkland, 2019).

Nancy Milio, a well-known C/PHN, wrote extensively on policy and public health nursing practice. In her classic work on health policy, Milio (1981) defined policy as option setting:

> "To bring about the largest improvement in health requires the development of policies that will change the options that organizations and individuals face today… It would provide new, easier opportunities, or reduce the cost of current options, in areas that now lack health-promoting resources." (p. 76)

Changes in the U.S. healthcare system are a result of changes in health policy priorities. Neal Halfon's 2014 illustration of how the U.S. healthcare system has evolved over time still holds true. Halfon showed that the healthcare system evolved in its policy options, moving from a focus on a short-term system of episodic nonintegrated care to a system of community integrated care—with an increased focus on population health strategies that address the social determinants of health (2014); see Figure 13-2.

What Is Politics?

While defining policy is important, understanding policy also requires knowledge about policy formation, implementation, and evaluation. An essential aspect of this is knowing the role politics plays in the policy process. **Politics** is defined as the process by which society determines who gets what, when they get it, and how they get it (Laswell, 1936). It is often discussed as the art of using influence to bring about change. This includes the efforts groups or people use to influence, gain power, or get their way. Politics includes discussions related to the values or ethics of a society, such as the conflict between individual needs and the needs of a community. Examples include the debate around assisted suicide or the continuing dispute regarding universal access to healthcare. The policy-making process may start with lofty goals, but the final product is usually the result of compromise often encouraged by special interest groups, coalition groups, political realities, or the current economic environment. This is politics.

Local, State, and National Level Policy

Government officials decide on **public policy** that impacts health and well-being at local, state, and national levels (Box 13-3). Because of this, it is essential to know whether the key decision makers are local, state, or national policymakers.

Local Policy

Many policies that impact healthcare are developed and implemented at the local level. Although local policies may also be subject to guidelines from other jurisdictions (e.g., state, federal), a hallmark of the U.S. governmental system has been to have robust local policy authority

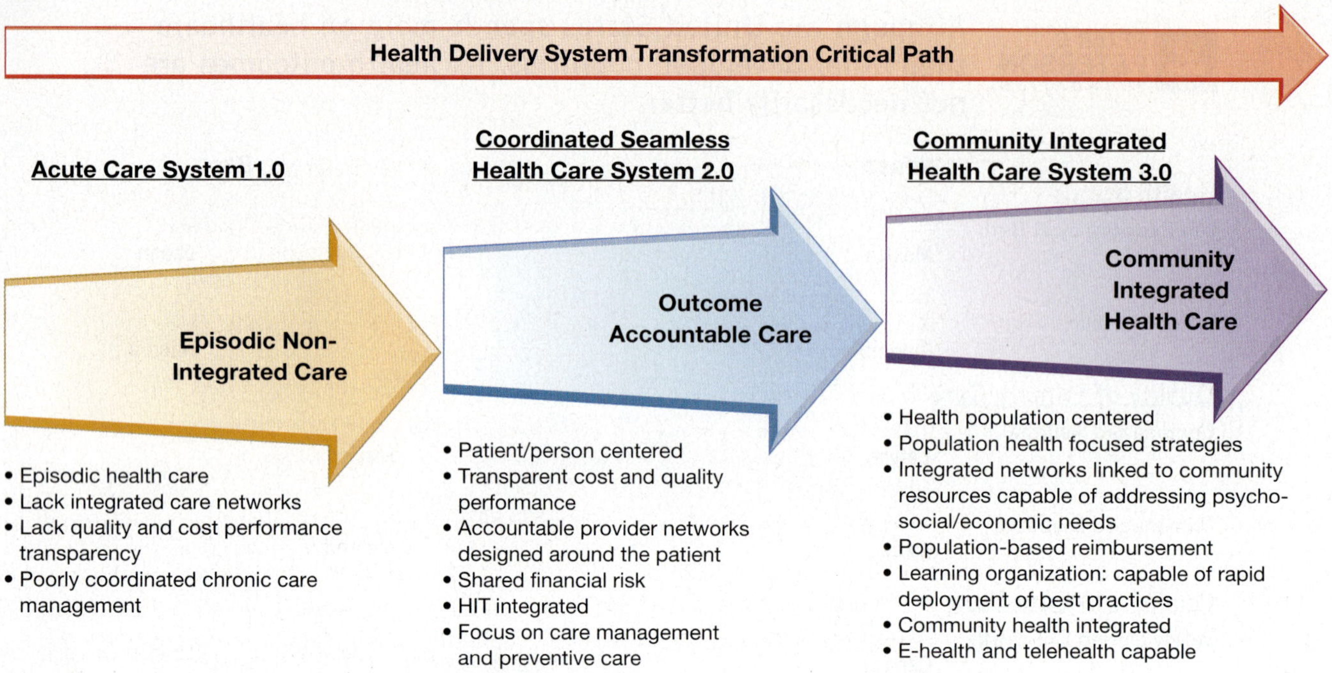

FIGURE 13-2 Health delivery system transformation critical path. (Adapted with permission from Halfon, N., Long, P., Chang, D. I., Hester, J., Inkelas, M., & Rogers, A. (2014). Applying A 3.0 transformation framework to guide large-scale health system reform. *Health Affairs, 33*(11), 2003–2011. https://doi.org/10.1377/hlthaff.2014.0485)

BOX 13-3 Policy Impacts at the Local, State, and National Levels

Local Policy

In 2016, the city of Chicago established the Tobacco Sales to Minors Program to prohibit the sale of tobacco products to anyone under the age of 21 years old (City of Chicago, 2023). This was 5 years before the federal policy that changed the minimum age from 18 to 21 years old. The local policy was changed as local leaders recognized the science that demonstrated that teenagers were the largest group of new smokers (Rhodes, 2016). This was a policy strategy to discourage local teens from using tobacco products.

State Policy

Since 2017, nine states have signed into law new regulations about prescription drug pricing (National Academy for State Health Policy, 2023). Maryland passed a law allowing the state's attorney general to sue generic drug manufacturers who engage in price gouging and return that money to consumers and others who pay for the drugs or make the drug available at its previous price. In 2023, the Maryland Prescription Drug Affordability Board was appropriated $1.4 million to investigate prescription drug pricing cases and explore the establishment of setting upper limits for prescription drug payment limits.

National Policy

Data indicate that climate change can have detrimental health effects on populations including increased respiratory and cardiovascular disease, injuries and premature deaths related to extreme weather events, changes in the prevalence and geographical distribution of food- and water-borne illnesses and other infectious diseases, and threats to mental health (National Institute of Environmental Health Sciences, 2023). National policy efforts, implemented by the Environmental Protection Agency (EPA), address climate change at the national level. In 2021, the EPA issued a final rule that will decrease the production and consumption of hydrofluorocarbons by 85% over the next 15 years. This is expected to decrease global warming predictions by up to 0.5°C (EPA, 2023).

Source: City of Chicago (2023); EPA (2023); National Academy for State Health Policy (2023); Rhodes (2016).

(National League of Cities, 2023). While the U.S. Constitution specifically details state authority, each state also gives powers to local governments. This means the policy-competent C/PHN needs to know what jurisdiction governs any relevant issue.

For example, public policies such as tobacco use in public places, requirements for gun ownership, or speed limits on public roads are often made by local-level governing bodies. At the local level, these policies are open to public involvement because the legislative and regulatory bodies are often easily accessed and composed of community residents. The C/PHN can use public health expertise to collect or interpret data that demonstrates the health impact of local policies. With this knowledge, the C/PHN can talk directly to decision makers about local policy concerns to influence decision making.

State Policy

There is a limit to municipal powers, and some policies are developed and regulated at the state level. Longest (2016) notes that the role of states in health policy includes being public health guardians (e.g., protect public health and welfare through laws and regulations), healthcare service purchasers (often in conjunction with the federal level; safety-net providers), and providers of education and public health laboratory services. Medicaid eligibility and services, health professional license regulation and scope of practice, and public health codes, including immunization regulations, are some of the functions that fall within state powers.

Policies vary widely from state to state and, therefore, have varied impacts across the country. For example, in states that have opted to expand Medicaid coverage in response to the passage of the affordable care act (ACA) in 2010, residents have increased access to health insurance and affordable care. This contrasts with states that have not opted to expand Medicaid, where many residents still lack access to healthcare (Kaiser Family Foundation, 2023).

National Policy

Public health policies are developed and implemented at the national level. Funding for Medicare, provisions in the ACA, parts of Medicaid, and health research are all national-level policies. This level of policy has the advantage of being broadly applicable across the country, with the potential for a significant impact on population health. However, it can be challenging to work at this level because there are many stakeholders and an enormous political bureaucracy for the creation, implementation, and evaluation of legislation.

Legislative Process at the National Level

The first step in becoming policy competent is to understand under which jurisdiction the issue falls (local, state, or federal). Next, one must know how policy is developed and regulated at that level. There are a wide variety of websites and descriptions of the legislative process, but the definitive version can be found on the House of Representatives website: http://www.house.gov/content/learn/legislative_process/. The federal model for how an idea becomes a bill and how a bill is passed into legislation is relevant across the country. States each have their own mechanisms that align with the federal process.

How a Bill Becomes a Law

This section will review the process for how a bill becomes a law at the federal level, but the process is very similar at the state level. See Figures 13-3 and 13-4 for federal and state examples.

Ideas for legislation originate from anywhere, including citizens like you. Once an idea is transformed into a bill, the bill is introduced in either the House of Representatives or the Senate by a legislator. When a bill is introduced to either side of Congress, it is assigned to a committee based upon the general area of focus (e.g., appropriations, agriculture). The committee structure is designed to allow members of each house to focus on a smaller number of issues in depth and then vote, as a whole, on issues that are deemed worthy of going before the whole legislature (i.e., going to the "floor") for a vote. Often, bills never leave the committee, stalling there because of a lack of interest from the majority party, whose members chair committees and thus set the committee's agenda in both houses. In fact, moving from a bill to a law is a complex process, with only a small fraction moving through the process successfully. It is estimated that 5% or less of bills introduced into any session of Congress become laws. In the first seven months of the 118th congressional session, less than one percent of bills were enacted into law (Civic Impulse, 2023).

Some bills have hearings, where experts are brought in to testify to facets of the bill and answer questions from the committee members. For bills where there is sufficient interest or political will, the bill will be discussed, amended as needed, and voted upon in the committee. If the bill passes in committee, it is sent to the full house for further discussion, possible amendments, and an ultimate vote (USAgov, 2023a).

If the bill passes the full house, it is sent to the other chamber of Congress, and the process begins again. Once more, the bill will be discussed, amended as needed, and voted upon in the committee. Similarly, if the bill passes in committee, it is sent to the full house for further discussion, possible amendments, and an ultimate vote. Sometimes, bills are introduced simultaneously to both houses, which can speed the process, as each committee and house reviews and votes on the bill during the same time period.

If the bill is passed in each house, but in a slightly different version, a conference committee that is composed of members of both houses is convened to discuss, amend, and vote on the bill.

- The bill can stall in the conference committee until the session of Congress ends, and then it would need to be reintroduced in the next session, as bills do not carry over from one session to the next.
- Alternatively, the bill may be passed by the conference committee and then be returned to each chamber for a final vote. At this point, amendments would not be added, or the bill would be stalled and have to go back through the process once again (U.S. House of Representatives, n.d.).

After both chambers of Congress pass the same version of a bill, it goes to the president for signature.

- The president can sign the bill, in which case it becomes law and is sent to the appropriate administrative agency for rulemaking.
- The president can actively or passively veto the legislation, in which case the bill needs to be sent back to each chamber for a 2/3 vote to override the president's veto, or the bill stalls again, and the process begins anew (U.S. House of Representatives, n.d.).

In summary, passing legislation is a complex process, designed for maximum debate and representation to avoid frivolous, dangerous, or unnecessary legislation (U.S. House of Representatives, n.d.).

HOW DOES A BILL BECOME A LAW?

1 EVERY LAW STARTS WITH AN IDEA

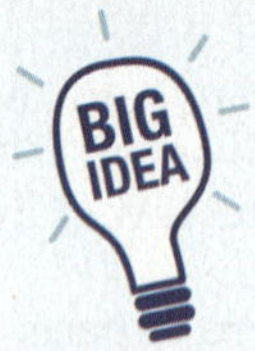

That idea can come from anyone, even you! Contact your elected officials to share your idea. If they want to try to make it a law, they will write a bill.

2 THE BILL IS INTRODUCED

A bill can start in either house of Congress when it's introduced by its primary sponsor, a Senator or a Representative. In the House of Representatives, bills are placed in a wooden box called "the hopper."

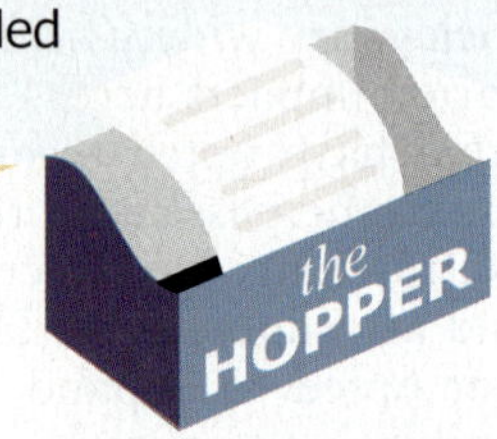

Here, the bill is assigned a legislative number before the Speaker of the House sends it to a committee.

3 THE BILL GOES TO COMMITTEE

Representatives or Senators meet in a small group to research, talk about, and make changes to the bill. They vote to accept or reject the bill and its changes before sending it to:

the House or Senate floor for debate or to a subcommittee for further research.

4 CONGRESS DEBATES AND VOTES

Members of the House or Senate can now debate the bill and propose changes or amendments before voting. If the majority vote for and pass the bill, it moves to the other house to go through a similar process of committees, debate, and voting. Both houses have to agree on the same version of the final bill before it goes to the President.

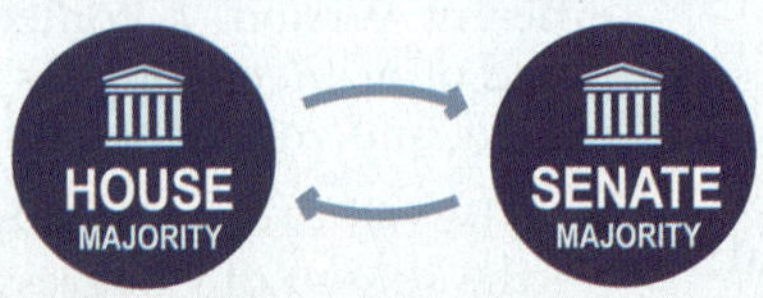

DID YOU KNOW?

The House uses an electronic voting system while the Senate typically votes by voice, saying "yay" or "nay."

5 PRESIDENTIAL ACTION

When the bill reaches the President, he or she can:

✓ APPROVE and PASS

The President signs and approves the bill. The bill is law.

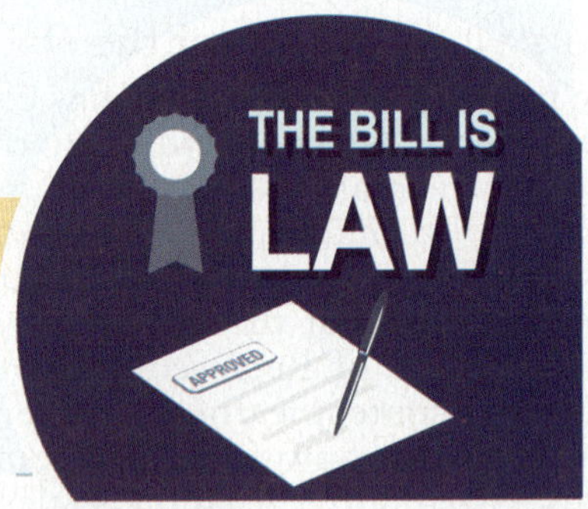

The President can also:

Veto

The President rejects the bill and returns it to Congress with the reasons for the veto. Congress can override the veto with 2/3 vote of those present in both the House and the Senate and the bill will become law.

Choose no action

The President can decide to do nothing. If Congress is in session, after 10 days of no answer from the President, the bill then automatically becomes law.

Pocket veto

If Congress adjourns (goes out of session) within the 10 day period after giving the President the bill, the President can choose not to sign it and the bill will not become law.

Kids.gov

Brought to you by usa gov

FIGURE 13-3 How does a bill become a law?—federal level. (Reprinted from *How laws are made and how to research them.* [2020]. https://www.usa.gov/how-laws-are-made)

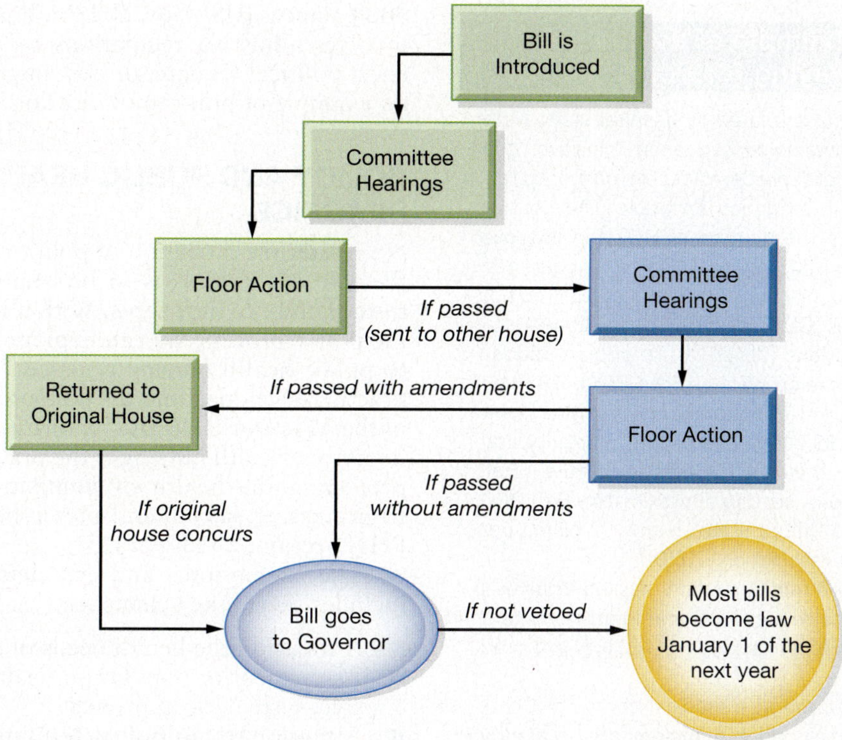

FIGURE 13-4 How a bill becomes a law—state process. The process may vary by state, but generally the schematic shows how the process unfolds. (Source: California Legislative Counsel.)

The C/PHN needs to be aware of other important aspects of the legislative process, including rulemaking, implementation, evaluation, and judicial action.

Rulemaking and Implementation

After a bill is passed and signed into law, it is sent to the appropriate administrative agency to develop rules, which are also referred to as regulations. This process is called rulemaking. Rulemaking is necessary to establish the process for policy implementation. Rules provide the "who, what, where, when, how, and why" of the law.

There are three different types of rules:

- Legislative rules: These types of rules are legally binding in a court of law.
- Nonlegislative rules: These rules do not have the force and effect of law; rather they are seen as guidance.
- Management and procedural rules: These rules concern administrative agency supervision, structure, and function (U.S. Department of Transportation, 2022).

After rules are developed by an administrative agency, they are published in the Federal Register with a designated time period for public comment. Comments are reviewed and used to revise and edit the rules as needed. This time of public comment presents an opportunity for C/PHNs to use their expertise to engage in the policy process. Once the period for public comment closes, the agency reviews comments and uses them to revise the rule. Once a final rule is established, it is published, along with an effective date for implementation. The final rule serves as guidance for policy implementation (Office of the Federal Register, n.d.).

Rulemaking is critical to the impact of legislation, as rules guide how the policy intent will be carried out (Office of the Federal Register, n.d.). Subtle changes to just one or two words can significantly alter the legislature's intent. For this reason, it is essential that C/PHNs understand the rulemaking process and their ability to have an impact.

Evaluation and Judicial Action

Policy evaluation is sometimes written into the law or sometimes requested as part of the rulemaking process as a step of implementation. Evaluation data can be used for policy modifications or for modifications of the rules for implementation. There are three types of policy evaluation.

- Policy content evaluation examines the policy content to determine if the policy will result in the intended change.
- Policy implementation evaluation examines implementation to determine if the policy was implemented as intended. This is essential to understand barriers and facilitators to implementation.
- Policy impact evaluation examines the outcomes to determine whether the policy has the intended short- and long-term impact (CDC, n.d.).

See Box 13-4 for an example of policy impact evaluation.

The judicial branch of government is designed to interpret laws and ensure they align with the Constitution. If a law is challenged, courts can void a law or require that it be changed to comply with the Constitution. If this

BOX 13-4 An Example of Evaluating Policy Changes: Paying for Performance

In the past, injury or illness related to hospital stays were often recognized as inevitable consequences. However, the Patient Protection and Affordable Care Act created a Hospital-Acquired Condition (HAC) Reduction Program. The goal of this program is to reduce the number of HAC and improve overall patient outcomes (CMS, 2022b). This is encouraged through reduced Medicaid payments for hospitals that do not meet benchmarks for HAC (CMS, 2022b). Central line–associated bloodstream infections (CLABSIs) are primary bloodstream infections that develop within 48 hours central line placement, with no apparent infection at another site (Joint Commission, 2023). CLABSIs increase patient mortality and healthcare costs. In fact, they are the most expensive of all hospital-acquired infections, costing approximately $45,000 per case, and costing the United States nearly $2 billion per year (Minnesota Hospital Association, 2020).

The promise of reduced reimbursement has led to several nurse-led interventions to reduce HAC and improve patient outcomes. A nurse-led effort to combat CLABSIs is explored below.

A nursing leadership team at a medical center in Charlotte, North Carolina, developed and implemented a quality improvement project to decrease CLABSI rates through a CLABSI-specific rounding team led by master's prepared clinical nurse specialists and clinical nurse leaders. Through use of an innovative infection prevention audit that was incorporated into standard nursing practice, the rounding team was able to provide real-time feedback and coaching to nurses to prevent CLABSIs while also easily tracking trends. Overall, this QI project resulted in CLABSI reduction. However, it should be noted that CLABSIs increase during two time periods when there was an increase in COVID-19 infection rates and subsequent decrease in infection prevention audits (Pate et al., 2022).

1. *Do you think nurses are generally aware of how legislation affects their workplace, practice, and patient outcomes? Why? Why not?*
2. *How could nurses become involved in the implementation of new laws/regulations and policy evaluation?*
3. *How might implementation or the impact of laws/regulations be affected by public health crisis such as a pandemic?*

Source: CMS (2022b); Joint Commission (2023); Minnesota Hospital Association (2020); Pate et al. (2022).

involves omitting part of the law, this can be done while implementation continues. However, if such a change negates the intent or desired outcome of the law, the legislative process would have to begin again to make any substantive changes.

This process of judicial action is designed to minimize the power of any branch of government: the legislators who wrote the law, the executive branch who administers the law, or the judicial branch who interprets the law. This is known as the American system of checks and balances (USAGov, 2023b). Policy modification often involves adjusting regulations to reflect changes in science, political climate, or cost impacts. See Box 13-5 for an example of policy modification.

POLICY AND PUBLIC HEALTH NURSING PRACTICE

No matter the definition of politics or the topic of debate, the role of C/PHNs is to be responsive to the needs of the community they serve. With a basic understanding of the policy process, we can explore how policy is relevant to public health nursing practice. The definition of PHN practice developed and disseminated by the PHN Section of the APHA in 1996 and reaffirmed in 2013 is as follows:

Public health nursing is the practice of promoting and protecting the health of populations using knowledge from nursing, social, and public health sciences (APHA, PHN Section, 2013, para. 5).

The definition, and its background statements, includes several key elements:

- A focus on the health needs of an entire population
- Assessment of population health using a comprehensive, systematic approach
- Attention to multiple determinants of health
- An emphasis on primary prevention
- Application of interventions at all levels—people, families, communities, and the systems that impact their health

Therefore C/PHNs, by definition, are interested in health policy broadly, including both healthcare services and policy as it relates to creating conditions in which people can be healthy by addressing the social, physiological, and behavioral determinants of health. Thus, C/PHN practice must address policy implications of health needs and conversely look at creating policies to promote and maintain health for communities and populations.

Recognizing that the public's health is not simply a result of healthcare systems but rather a result of the conditions in which people live, the APHA, CDC, and WHO all call for *Health in All Policies* (HiAP) (APHA, 2023; CDC, 2016; WHO, 2023). HiAP promotes collaboration between public agencies to create policies across sectors that promote healthy communities. By influencing policies in areas outside of healthcare such as education, housing, and transportation, we can promote health equity (WHO, 2023).

An example of how HiAP can impact the health of the public is suggested by the WHO (n.d.). Recognizing that air pollution is the cause of one in eight deaths across the globe, policies in every sector must be developed to ensure impact. Energy policies can decrease fossil fuel emissions and increase renewable power sources such as solar or wind. Transportation policies can prioritize the development of urban transit systems to decrease reliance on individual vehicle use. Urban planning policies can make cities more compact. Housing policies can promote energy efficiency through improved construction standards. Collectively, HiAP will result in greater impact than solely relying upon healthcare policies to impart change.

BOX 13-5 A History of Tobacco Legislation in the United States

The tobacco industry has been regulated through state and national legislation since the early 1900s, with several policies and policy modifications. Policies have been created and modified as a result of new scientific discoveries about the negative impact of tobacco use and in an effort to protect the health of the public. With the recent advent of electronic cigarettes, many tobacco policies have been created or modified to include new methods of tobacco use.

1906 The Food and Drugs Act of 1906 did not include mention of tobacco. However, a 1914 advisor groups recommended that tobacco be included in modified legislation but only when used to prevent or treat disease.

1914 The Federal Trade Commission (FTC) Act of 1914 empowers the FTC to take action preventing people or organizations from using "unfair or deceptive acts or practices in commerce." This is important legislation as it allowed the FTC to regulate advertising of tobacco products. The FTC completed seven formal cease-and-desist order proceedings for medical or health claims of cigarettes between 1945 and 1960.

1938 The 1906 legislation was superseded by the Federal Food, Drug, and Cosmetic Act (FFDCA) of 1938, which allowed the government to regulate tobacco products used to prevent or treat disease. For example, in 1959, the FDA asserted jurisdiction over Trim Reducing-Aid Cigarettes that claimed to aid in weight reduction due to the additive tartaric acid.

1965 Federal Cigarette Labeling and Advertising Act of 1965 required cigarette packages to include a warning label stating, "Caution: Cigarette Smoking May Be Hazardous to Your Health" but did not require this warning to be included on advertisements.

1969 The Public Health Cigarette Smoking Act of 1969 required the following to be placed on all cigarette packing and print advertising: "Warning: The Surgeon General Has Determined that Cigarette Smoking Is Dangerous to Your Health." This Act also prohibited radio and television advertising.

1984 The Comprehensive Smoking Education Act of 1984 requires four rotating warning labels on cigarettes about lung cancer, heart disease, pregnancy, and carbon monoxide. The Act also requires cigarette companies to provide a confidential list of ingredients to the government.

1986 The Comprehensive Smokeless Tobacco Health Education Act of 1986 required warning labels and prohibited radio and television advertising for smokeless tobacco products.

1987 Public Law 100—202 bans smoking on domestic airline flights 2 hours or less.

1992 The Synar Amendment to the Alcohol, Drug Abuse, and Mental Health Administration (ADAMHA) Reorganization Act of 1992 requires that all states adopt and enforce restrictions on the sale and distribution of tobacco to minors.

2009 The Family Smoking Prevention and Tobacco Control Act of 2009 gives the Food and Drug Administration (FDA) the authority to regulate cigarettes, smokeless, and roll-your-own tobacco.

2016 The "Deeming Rule": Tobacco Products Deemed to be Subject to the Federal Food, Drug, and Cosmetic Act extended the reach of the FDA to regulate "hookah, e-cigarettes, dissolvables, smokeless tobacco, cigarettes, all cigars, roll-your-own tobacco, pipe tobacco, and future tobacco products that meet the statutory definition of a tobacco product" (USFDA, 2016, para. 2).

2020 The Consolidated Appropriations Act amended the Federal Food, Drug and Cosmetic Act and the Public Health Act to prohibit the sale of tobacco products to people under the age of 21 years.

The history of tobacco legislation in the United States is an example of how policies are created and modified in response to science to protect the nation's health.

1. *Can you think of an example of a current policy that requires modification based on new or emerging science?*
2. *What modifications would you suggest?*

Source: Centers for Disease Control and Prevention (CDC) (2023b); Public Health Law Center (2019); U.S. Federal Drug Administration (FDA) (2016).

Public Health and Social Justice

The concept of social justice is seen as the very foundation of community/public health and community/public health nursing (deChesnay & Anderson, 2016). The American Association of Colleges of Nursing (2017) emphasizes that the guiding values of nursing include social justice at all levels of educational preparation, and the American Nurses Association (ANA) *Code of Ethics with Interpretive Statements* (2015) preface states that nurses should "act to change those aspects of society that detract from health and well-being." The ANA's *Public Health Nursing: Scope and Standards of Practice* document also highlights the basic value of social justice in community health nursing (2022). The many definitions of social justice depend on the discipline involved; for purposes of this chapter, social justice is focused on health equity, which is ensuring that people have an equal opportunity to maximize their health (deChesnay & Anderson, 2016). See Chapter 23 for more information on social justice.

As a C/PHN, you are expected to give voice to the health and social inequities found in the communities you serve (e.g., substandard housing, high rates of unemployment, death, and disability). These are disparities that often could be prevented or alleviated at early stages. In order to promote and protect the health of populations, your nursing interventions need to address not only health issues but also the educational, social, and economic issues that give rise to these disparities.

The nexus between social justice, advocacy, and policy is interrelated, complex, and one that will affect every aspect of your community health nursing career.

Power and Empowerment

Collaborating with underrepresented populations to elicit change can be a difficult task. Community participation is never particularly easy in communities excluded from political or economic resources. Community participation is often defined as getting people to participate—show up—for events, but a deeper perspective is that participation is on a continuum and numbers participating is one end moving all the way toward having communities define their own issues and be actively involved in setting advocacy and policy agendas (Narayan, 2023 and Health equity solutions, 2023).

Power can be defined as the ability to act or produce an effect, possession of control, or authority or influence over others. As public health professionals, nurses have a commitment to social justice and working with underrepresented communities. This means that nurses have a responsibility to ensure community participation in issues affecting them, and they must continually examine the relationship and position they hold within these communities. This is called **community empowerment** and is defined as the process of enabling communities to increase control over their lives (WHO, 2019). Community empowerment, therefore, is more than the involvement, participation, or engagement of communities (see Fig. 13-5). It implies community ownership and action that explicitly aims at social and political change. Community empowerment is a process of renegotiating power to gain more control over conditions impacting a community's life and health.

An empowered community is one in which members effectively use resources (human and fiscal) and collaborate to meet identified needs. People and organizations within empowered communities support each other, work together for conflict resolution, and increasingly facilitate social change, gaining power over the quality of life in their community. This demonstrates how the empowerment of communities is linked to empowerment at the individual and organizational levels.

How does the C/PHN ensure that preconceived ideas about certain communities are not forced on the community to meet the goals of the public health agency? In the past, community health promotion practices often only met one end of the community participation continuum, that of getting people to show up for events, while the professionals working with the community set the agenda. Health promotion and disease prevention may best be facilitated by using empowerment and assisting people and communities in articulating their problems and solutions. This suggests a change in the relationship between professionals and communities—a change from the customary hierarchical patient–provider relationship to one of a partnership. Community participation can be facilitated in a wide variety of ways, such as working with Community Health Workers, hiring staff from the community, engaging community members in sharing sessions, and training residents in specific useful skills to improve community health. Discovering what is most important to the community and providing access to that information while supporting leadership from within the community and encouraging them to overcome bureaucratic hurdles to action are important parts of community empowerment (Swider, 2023).

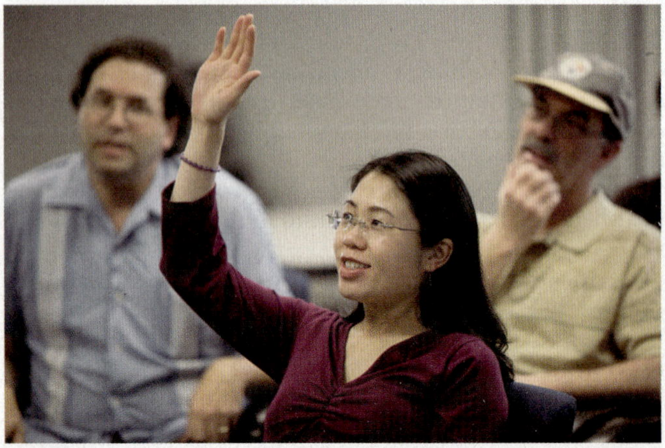

FIGURE 13-5 Town hall meetings promote community participation in public policy. (Photo courtesy of CDC Photo Image Library.)

POLICY ANALYSIS FOR THE C/PHN

Policy analysis is the technique of understanding a policy from a variety of perspectives. Such analysis can provide results for better understanding policy, finding ways to impact policy development, understanding the values behind policy, tracking the history of policy in specific areas, and other policy-relevant research and practice questions. C/PHNs can analyze the policy process to determine where they might become involved in creating "healthy public policy." Policy analysis can be done using a variety of approaches and methods.

Developing Policy Competence

For C/PHNs to be effective in the policy process, they need to be aware of policy implications on health planning and health-promoting interventions. Further, they must be prepared to provide data supporting policy recommendations that enhance health opportunities for a target group or community. This is called being *policy competent* (Longest, 2004). **Policy competence** means being able to do the following:

- Assess the impact of public policies on one's domain of interest/responsibility.
- Understand policy and the policy process sufficiently to be able to exert influence on the process and impact policy.
- Exert influence on the policymaking process.

For community/public health nursing practice, this means that C/PHNs can assess relevant policies and determine where the policy is in the policymaking process. The C/PHN must also be able to determine where action is needed to influence the policy process: data support, lobbying, development/testing of potential policy solutions, stakeholder convening, etc. The C/PHN might not be able to lobby due to their position (for instance, working for a government agency), but there are many other policy process activities that are relevant in planning and implementing health policy.

Exerting influence in the policy process can be done at a variety of levels. Because policy sets the context for much of C/PHN practice, policy competence is particularly important for C/PHNs, but all nurses should have some concept of how policy affects nurses, patients, and population health. For example, changes in Medicaid funding, at either the national or state level, might directly impact which clients the C/PHN can include in certain health promotion/disease prevention programs. Therefore, the C/PHN should understand this impact, the reasons for the Medicaid changes, and where useful input might be provided. This might be as straightforward as explaining to agency administrators what the impact of these changes will be on people in the community, or it may be more complicated and involve policy evaluation mechanisms or development of alternative policy solutions to meet the community's health goals.

Frameworks for Policy Analysis

For the purposes of policy competence in C/PHN practice, we will discuss two frameworks for policy analysis, the Rational Framework and John Kingdon's framework. These frameworks provide two interrelated mechanisms for looking at the policy process and are combined into a useful diagram by Longest (2016) (Fig. 13-6).

The Rational Framework

The rational framework is commonly found in policy texts as a straightforward way to comprehend the intent and effect of a policy. This logical analytic framework is very similar to the nursing process, in its structure and components, and as such is easily understood by C/PHNs.

- The first step of the framework involves defining the policy problem to be addressed. The clearer and more measurable this problem definition is, the more specific any policy response can be.
- The second step in this framework is to understand possible solutions to this policy problem and compare and contrast them to determine which is optimal in terms of being politically feasible, easily implemented, and likely to result in the desired outcome.
- The third step, based on comparing and contrasting the possible policy alternatives, is to select an alternative, implement it, and evaluate its effectiveness (Furlong & Kraft, 2020).

There are several challenges to using this framework. Much like the nursing process, it examines policy as a structured, linear process and that is often not the case. Challenges in defining the problem or in comparing viable solutions might often influence policy to be formed with insufficient data or based on the power and influence of specific stakeholders, meaning that all elements may not be considered carefully and in the order presented in the framework (Kraft & Furlong, 2020). Additionally, this framework does not assist the C/PHN in addressing the politics involved or in determining why one issue might be addressed when another—equally important to the community—might languish with no policy activity taking place.

Kingdon's Framework

A second policy analysis framework was developed by John Kingdon (2011) in his classic book, *Agendas, Alternatives and Public Policies* (Fig. 13-7). Kingdon set out in

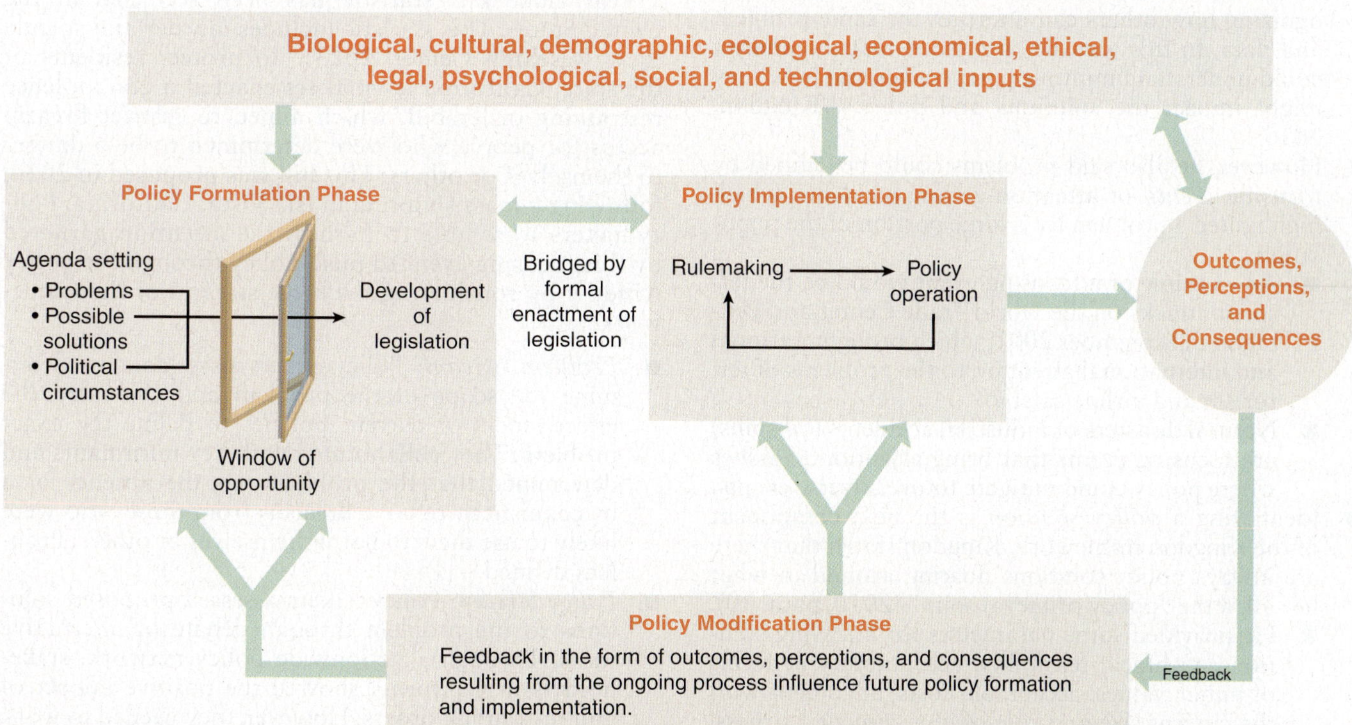

FIGURE 13-6 Longest's model. (Adapted with permission from Longest, B. B. (2016). *Health policymaking in the United States* (5th ed., p. 82). Health Administration Press.)

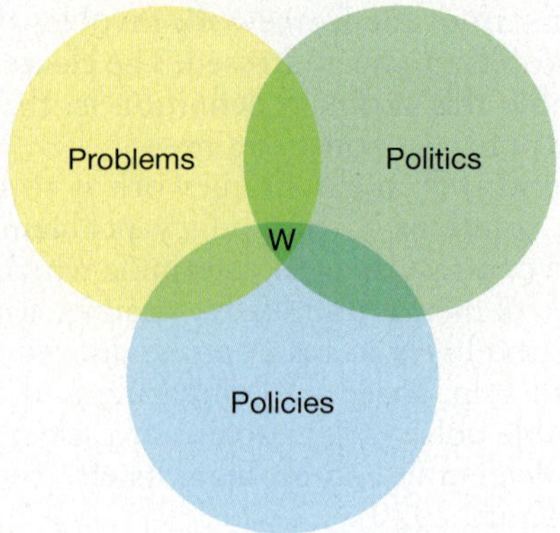

FIGURE 13-7 Kingdon's model of the policy process.

his research to address the question of why some issues came to the forefront of policy development and others did not.

Kingdon argued, based on his research results, that policy was enacted when a *window of opportunity* was opened. During this window, bills could be voted on and new legislation made. The window of opportunity opened when there was a confluence of a *policy problem*, a *viable solution* or solutions, and *political will* on this issue. This confluence opened a window of opportunity for the issue to be acted upon (however briefly).

Kingdon presented each component of the framework specifically.

- The *problem*, he contended, should be defined using *indicators*, that is, data to document its existence.
- Kingdon also argued that it was important to understand the problem from multiple perspectives, recognizing how others can interpret the same problem and data. In this way, he contended that the analyst could understand multiple perspectives and how they might impact the solutions and politics (Kingdon, 2010).
- However, he also said problems could be defined by *focusing events*, or attention-getting incidents, which highlighted a problem for a large portion of the population.
  - An example of a focusing event would be the terrorist attacks on the World Trade Center and Pentagon in September 2001, which brought national and international attention to the problems of terrorism and airline safety.
  - Natural disasters or industrial accidents (oil spills) are focusing events that bring attention to issues where policy could mitigate future adverse events.
- Identifying a *policy solution* is the next component of the Kingdon framework. Kingdon stated that there are always policy solutions floating around in what he called the "policy primeval soup" (2010, para. 10).
  - He provided some parameters for assessing solutions: technical feasibility, acceptability in terms of public values, acceptable costs, alignment with the current size and role of government, fairness, and equity. He used these parameters to compare solutions for those most likely to align with problems and politics (Kingdon, 2011).
- When analyzing the *politics* of an issue, Kingdon had several facets to consider, including the political climate and stakeholder perspectives.
  - For example, immediately after the 9/11 terrorist attacks, the U.S. political climate was focused almost entirely on safety and security, and very few other issues were being seriously addressed.
  - Kingdon (2010) also advised looking at stakeholders on both sides of an issue and assessing relative power and influence. This can be done by looking at the numbers of people they represent, resources available for lobbying, and political reputation and past achievements.

When a *window of opportunity* does open, Kingdon (2010, 2011) cautioned that it does not remain open forever. Sometimes, other issues take precedence. Sometimes, partial action is taken, and the public perceives the problem has been resolved, at least in the near term. Other times a window closes because the public loses interest in unresolved issues that have been around for a long time. In Kingdon's terms, policy activists should look for opportunities to open windows and, when windows are open, should act to capitalize on the opportunity.

Drawbacks to Kingdon's framework include the fact that it analyzes policy only to the point of passing a bill into law. It does not address implementation, evaluation, or policy modification.

An example of Kingdon's framework in practice:

Kingdon's Policy framework was used by researchers to analyze a gun violence protection policy in California (Tomsich et al., 2023). Gun violence is a public health concern in the United States. In 2021, 48,830 people died from gun-related injuries, the most in 1 year since this statistic has been recorded in the United States. This statistic includes murder and suicide (Pew Research Center, 2023). To protect residents of the state, California lawmakers enacted a gun violence restraining order bill, which aimed to restrict firearm access for people who were determined to be a danger to themselves or others. This bill was proposed in 2014, following a mass shooting in Isla Vista, California. Policymakers were able to harness the attention garnered by this focusing event to push policy through the policy window by considering the three streams of the framework.

- *Problem Stream:* Policymakers used data to determine the scope of the problem and evaluated the effectiveness of current policies to define the exact problem. They collaborated with key informants and determined that the problem was the absence of a mechanism to remove firearms from those who were likely to use them to harm themselves or others. Problem defined.
- *Policy Stream:* Policymakers assessed proposed solutions to the problem through debate of alternative ideas. Through a nationwide policy network, stakeholders in California showed the positive impact of gun restraining orders. However, they needed to work with and address those in opposition to this approach by showing economic and logistical feasibility. Policy developed.

- *Politics Stream*: Once the bill was proposed, policymakers engaged in bargaining with stakeholders to come to an agreement on a final solution. This included consideration of racial equity and misuse of the law. Ultimately, the bill was "softened" in order to gain enough momentum to push it through the policy window. Politics considered.

For the policy analyst, these frameworks present important components of understanding an issue. The rational framework allows the analyst to look post hoc at an issue and learn from the process as it unfolds. For policy activists, or C/PHNs who want to use policy effectively in practice (policy competence), the Kingdon framework allows you to examine a current issue in real time and determine if a window of opportunity exists or if one could be created. This helps the C/PHN, or a public health organization, to prioritize its time and resources and focus policy efforts where they can be most effective. Neither framework is perfect. Recognizing this, Longest (2016) combined the rational framework and Kingdon's framework into a figure encompassing all facets of policymaking.

Policy Analysis for Activism

Now, we will put this altogether to demonstrate how a C/PHN can use this information to be policy active in practice.

- The first step is to select a policy issue to address. Consider what health issue in your community has policy implications or is being impacted by current health policy or the lack thereof.
  - Perhaps there are water quality concerns in the community, or the most recent community assessment has identified an increase in STIs among adolescents and young adults. These are public policy issues; that is, they are issues that are impacted by public decisions about laws and regulations related to funding, services, or rights and behaviors.
- The second step, once the C/PHN has determined that the issue is indeed one of public policy, is to conduct a brief policy analysis using Kingdon's framework: What is the *problem*? Are there *policy solutions in place*, and are they adequate and appropriate? What are the *politics*—or who are the stakeholders and what is their level of influence?
  - This preliminary analysis will inform the C/PHN whether this is a new issue on the agenda or whether it is an issue of *implementation* or *evaluation* of existing legislation or regulations.

Given this analysis, the C/PHN can determine the next steps. Perhaps, the key concern is the problem; it may not be well defined, the definition may need to be expanded, or more data may be needed. The goal may be to get the issue on the policy agenda via outreach to policymakers. Action may be necessary to develop and test solutions based on practice standards and population needs. Perhaps the issue is the way a regulation is being implemented, and thus, change could be made by working with legislators to identify the problem and develop implementation modifications. The policy evaluation may lack clarity.

Once the C/PHN considers all factors, the necessary level of involvement can be determined. Given constraints on time, lobbying, access to data, and the priority of the issue, the level of engagement can be established. Several avenues for activism are available, based on the above criteria. Table 13-1 demonstrates how the analysis framework relates to concerns of the C/PHN and possible actions in response.

POLITICAL ACTION FOR C/PHNs

The definition of community/public health nursing practice describes efforts to promote and protect the public's health. When looking at *Healthy Public Policy*, community/public health nursing efforts to do so can take many forms, from active participation as an informed citizen to actions taken as part of community/public health nursing practice to promote *Healthy Public Policy*. To support this work, the Association of Public Health Nurses (APHN) put out a booklet for their community/public health nursing members to help them understand advocacy and policy in their practice (APHN, 2016).

The C/PHN as an informed citizen, who has valuable knowledge and experience in health and health promotion, can be involved at a basic level by being aware of health policy and using this awareness for informed voting in elections across levels of jurisdiction. Individual C/PHNs might choose to increase their involvement by serving in a campaign to support a legislator who espouses public policies promoting health and preventing disease. Additionally, the C/PHN might choose to share their expertise with others, to inform their voting and citizen involvement. The C/PHN could also choose to be involved in professional organizations or citizen organizations to advocate for *Healthy Public Policies* and the legislators who promote them.

C/PHN practice, looking broadly at health and the social determinants of health, can provide background that is valuable in a variety of settings.

- At the state level, the C/PHN can ensure that the state nursing organizations maintain a broad-based focus on the health of the public.
- Locally, C/PHNs can serve on health boards and can also provide valuable input into health and education by serving on school boards or parent–teacher organizations.
- C/PHN researchers can influence policy by focusing on research questions related to the social determinants of health or Health in all Policies and sharing results in a clear and persuasive manner with policymakers and legislators.
- C/PHNs can provide input by serving on policymaking bodies. A C/PHN serving on a hospital board could be critical in helping the hospital better understand population health and the role of the hospital in enhancing it. C/PHNs can serve on state or national advisory groups such as MedPAC (www.medpac.gov) or the Community Preventive Services Task Force (https://www.thecommunityguide.org/task-force/what-task-force).

TABLE 13-1 C/PHN Practice Mechanisms to Address Policy Issues

Component of Analysis Framework	Action Needed	Mechanisms of Action
Problem	Data to define	▪ Collect or analyze evaluation data; assessment data ▪ Collaborate with researchers on problem definition
	Expand definition	▪ Collaborate with researchers on problem definition
Policies/solutions	Develop/pilot possible solutions	▪ Develop and implement model projects
	Change context to increase solution viability	▪ Evaluate/collect outcome data on projects to evaluate process of implementation
Politics	Educate public or other stakeholders	▪ Letters, phone call, e-mails, office visits to key stakeholders ▪ Communicate via letters to the editor or social media ▪ Present program results or assessment results in public forum ▪ Disseminate reports on service outcomes or new conditions to key stakeholders
Implementation	Revise regulations to improve implementation	▪ Work with regulators to revise regulations and rules
	Expand implementation to others affected	▪ Work with legislators and regulators to expand eligible populations for interventions
Evaluation	Data needed to measure impact	▪ Evaluate services provided
	Disseminate evaluation results	▪ Present program results or assessment results in public forum ▪ Disseminate reports on service outcomes or new conditions to key stakeholders
	Policy modification needed (see Problem)	▪ Collaborate to collect data for problem definition

History of Public Health Nursing Advocacy

Nurses have a long history of advocacy, both for patients and in policy (Kalaitzidis & Jewell, 2020). **Advocacy** is defined as speaking for another on an individual or policy matter, to help them get what they need from a system to enhance their health. To advocate is to try to influence outcomes that affect people, communities, and systems. Advocacy is a process that includes identifying an issue, collecting information, identifying who can be influenced to make the required decision sought, building support, and acting. Advocacy also includes litigation and public education campaigns. Advocacy differs from lobbying in that **lobbying** involves advocacy on a specific legislative initiative (APHN, 2021).

The importance of early nurse advocates such as Lillian Wald, Sojourner Truth, Margaret Sanger, Clara Barton, Mary Seacole, Susie King Taylor, Mary Mahoney, and others is that they wielded influence even at a time when women were not allowed to vote (see Chapter 3). In fact, many women in the 1800s, regardless of socioeconomic status, did not attend school. Women during these times rarely, if ever, voiced their opinions about issues affecting their lives, the lives of their children, their families, or their communities; it was neither expected nor accepted. African American women in the early 20th century were legally forbidden to learn to read and write (Nickitas et al., 2016). For these women to influence policy during the 19th century is a tribute to their ability to take on the system in which they lived and to triumph over it.

The early pioneers are seen as feminists, and the entrance of these women into the political arena opened the way for others, such as Nancy Pelosi, the first-ever female Speaker of the U.S. House of Representatives, and the four current (and two previous) female Supreme Court justices. The numbers of women in elected office continues to grow, and after the 2022 midterm elections, 25% of members of the Senate and 28.5% of House members were female. In state legislatures, those numbers were 30% and 33.6%, respectively (Rutgers Center for American Women and Politics, 2023).

Advocacy and Lobbying

Nurses bring important expertise to the policy process. This is even more true for C/PHNs, whose work often involves the structural and social determinants of health most impacted by policy, including housing, food insecurity, and interpersonal and community violence. In order to advocate effectively for the communities within which they work, it is critical for C/PHNs to be policy competent. At the policy level, how can C/PHNs influence policies that affect the clients and communities they serve? How do we influence policymakers to hear these concerns and act on them?

Many professional organizations provide opportunities for advocacy and lobbying and can also guide nurses to participate individually. The APHN developed a toolkit as a resource for members: APHN Public Health Policy Advocacy Guidebook and Toolkit. The Toolkit provides guidance on effective lobbying and advocacy, and it outlines methods for contacting legislators and other policy stakeholders.

APHN (2021) discusses "inside" versus "outside" strategies for advocacy and lobbying, where "inside" means working with legislators and their staff and "outside" means public education campaigns. They also present samples of tactics for "inside" lobbying and advocacy methods:

- Letter writing
- Phone calls
- Testimony
- In-person visits

You can become more actively involved by communicating with legislators about the healthcare issues that impact the communities where you live and work. It is also vital to understand the importance of critically timing those communications. Effective communications with legislators should be tied to times when the issues are being heard in policy committee—thus, you must know when your issue is scheduled to be discussed in committee. For example, it is prudent to send letters on your issue—via e-mail or regular mail—close to the time of the committee hearing. Holding a press conference or getting other media coverage when the bill is introduced, or on the day it will be heard in committee, is quite effective in drawing attention to your issue. Writing letters to the editor of your local newspaper on health issues and writing articles for various publications are also effective methods of persuading others to back your issue.

Political Action Committees

Financial resources are essential to effective advocacy. **Political action committees (PACs)** are groups that exist to raise and spend money to influence political outcomes (Inouye, 2021). They raise money from those in concordance with their particular issue or candidate. They are governed by regulations from the Federal Elections Commission (FEC), which develops guidelines to enhance fairness and transparency in election processes (FEC, n.d.). Lobbyists may work for PACs or independently represent various special interests or groups. Professional organizations or other **special interest groups** (people who share a common interest and work politically to make their goals a reality) may retain paid lobbyists.

Lobbyists are professionals who know the rules governing the state or federal political process, have or develop relationships with policymakers, provide guidance for members of the organizations employing them on how to impact public policy decisions, and work behind the scenes to influence policy discussions and outcomes. States and the federal government have laws and regulations that determine the legal actions of lobbyists and the organizations that employ those (Inouye, 2021). Although the public perception of lobbyists is poor, they are an integral part of the process of establishing relationships with legislators to influence the political process (Gallup, 2022).

Volunteering and Voting

Money is *not* the only way to build a relationship with your legislator. Being involved in local and state elections can take many forms. Volunteering your time can be just as important (Box 13-6). Candidates develop position papers to tell their constituents where they stand on key campaign concerns. Nurses have the expertise to assist legislators in developing position papers and setting policy agendas for healthcare issues, including the structural and social determinants of health. Legislators and legislative candidates also need people to assist in everyday tasks such as phone banking, stuffing mailers, answering phones, putting up flyers and campaign posters, and walking door to door to spread support.

Voting is critical in policy development and in affecting public policy. RNs represent a substantial block of potential voters and yet vote at lower levels than other professionals (ANA, 2022).

BOX 13-6 PERSPECTIVES

A Volunteer's Viewpoint on Campaigning for an RN

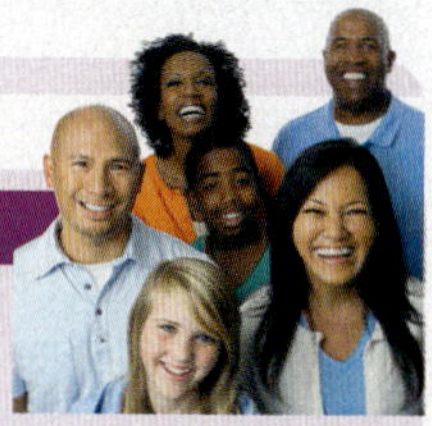

A registered nurse (RN) who had been through what I called the women's legislative career ladder—School Board, City Council, and the County Board of Supervisors—was now poised to run for the state legislature. Because we had had numerous contacts and I believed she would make a good state legislator and a voice for nursing and healthcare, I volunteered to work in her campaign office. I primarily answered the phones on the evenings I worked, but I met the office staff—many of them were much younger than me. And, even once, she came in while I was there. I talked with the staff about some of my experiences as a lobbyist, and they shared their experiences; many of them were fresh out of college.

She was successful in her run for office, and whenever I needed to meet with her or her staff, I was shown right in. I was also asked my opinion about the hiring of certain staff. Her staff knew me by name—many of them did not work on her campaign, but they were told about me by those campaign staff who were still around. After 3 years in office, she was appointed chairperson of a key committee, and I maintained access to her committee consultants and to her when necessary. We were able to work together quite successfully, and although we didn't always agree on every policy issue, I think the weeks I put in volunteering 3 years earlier really paid off for the clients and the issues I was representing.

Lydia, professional lobbyist

Professional Advocacy

One of the chief ways in which nurses have been successful in advocating is through membership in their professional organizations (Box 13-7). The late 19th century may be seen as the beginning of nurse activism. The Nurses Associated Alumnae of the United States and Canada and the American Society of Superintendents of Training Schools of the United States and Canada were formed in the 1890s (ANA, n.d.-a; National League for Nursing, 2016). Out of these groups came the ANA and the National League for Nursing (see Chapter 3). However, in the 1980s, with the stratification of nursing into various specialties and organizations, came the realization that the many nursing groups needed to coordinate efforts in order to be more successful, per a seminal article by Cohen et al. (1996). A significant outcome of this era was the development of *Nursing's Agenda for Health Care Reform* (ANA, 1994), which exemplified the maturing of nursing as a special interest group and demonstrated consensus building and collaboration among the more than 60 nursing and various healthcare provider organizations.

Throughout the next few decades, the nursing organizations realized, regardless of internal differences and competition, that to be politically successful, they must work together toward their common political goals. Over the past few decades, the formation of the following coalitions occurred:

- ***Council of Public Health Nursing Organizations***—a coalition of the leading public health nursing professional organizations including the Association of Community Health Nurse Educators, APHN, Alliance of Nurses for Healthy Environments, Rural Nurses Organization, National Association of School Nurses, and the Public Health Nursing section of APHA (formerly known as the Quad Council of PHN Organizations)
- ***Tri-Council for Nursing***—comprising the American Nurses Association (ANA), the American Association of Colleges of Nursing, the National League for Nursing, and the American Organization of Nurse Executives
- ***American Association of Nurse Practitioners (NPs)***—state and national NP groups initially met for a national forum and eventually to influence health policy
- ***Nursing Organizations Alliance (The Alliance)***—an alliance of National Federation for Specialty Nursing Organizations and Nursing Organizations Liaison Forum
- ***The Nursing Community Coalition***—a coalition of 63 nursing organizations across education and practice working to build consensus and advocate on a wide spectrum of policy issues

These and other coalitions permitted the organizations to lobby for common nursing issues, such as the maintenance of federal funding for nursing education and research, including the establishment of the National Institute of Nursing Research within the National Institutes of Health (NINR, n.d.). Many of the current state nurse practice acts and expanded responsibilities for NPs are the result of these new coalitions. But more

BOX 13-7 Expanding Practice Opportunities for Nurse Practitioners as a Result of Professional Advocacy

The Patient Protection and ACA is estimated to have decreased the number of uninsured in the United States from 10.2% in 2021 to 9.6% in 2022, with 46.5 million people uninsured in 2010 as compared to 25.6 million in 2022. Thus an estimated 20 million more Americans will have access to primary healthcare (Tolbert et al., 2023). The demand for nurse practitioners (NPs) or advanced practice nurses (APNs) is increasing; nationally, it is expected to reach an increase of 30% between 2016 and 2020 (Xue & Intrator, 2016). NPs are often thought by patients to provide quality care, excellent communication with patients, and clear education about self-management of chronic conditions (e.g., diabetes). Several provisions in the ACA promoted APN practice including the following:

- Five years of funds for demonstration projects to expand NP education programs.
- Increased funds for hiring NPs into the National Health Service Corps.
- Increased support for Federally Qualified Health Centers and Nurse-Managed Health Clinics, as safety-net providers, to hire APNs to care for their often vulnerable, high-risk clients.
- Medicare beneficiaries with functional limitations and chronic illnesses are able to receive home-based primary care from NPs through a 3-year project, Independence at Home Demonstration (Carthon et al., 2015).

In addition, COVID-19 led to reduced restrictions at the state level for APN practice (Kleinpell et al., 2023). Although these gains have been the hard-won result of consistent lobbying and advocacy efforts on the part of professional nursing organizations and people, the bright future on the horizon for APNs is at risk because of inconsistent scope of practice laws at the state level. In 2023, only 25 states and the District of Columbia had full autonomy rules for NPs (e.g., NPs could evaluate/treat patients, order/interpret diagnostic tests, and prescribe medications). That leaves 25 states with laws for NPs that restrict or reduce their scope of practice; often, this involves requiring primary provider oversight or collaboration (Kleinpell et al., 2023). Some states prohibit NPs from certifying home health or long-term care and limit their admitting privileges to hospitals. This restriction leads to barriers to NP practice and patient access to care. Although NPs are achieving success in the area of policymaking and expanded practice opportunities, it is still vitally important for them to advocate and politically support health policies that grant them full practice authority and benefit the clients they serve.

1. *What are the APN laws in your state?*
2. *How could allowing for APN full practice authority change how healthcare is provided in your community?*

significantly, the profession worked together to demonstrate that there is a difference between "self-interest" and "selfishness."

Despite nursing's early history of political activism and the fact that nurses are the largest group of healthcare providers in the United States, widespread political involvement has not been fully realized. The pursuit of personal agendas over the common good results in a piecemeal approach to problems and promotes polarization. **Polarization** is the process by which a group is severely split into two or more factions over a political issue. Polarization can be so intense that people perceive one another as good or bad, depending on their ideological opinions (Dimock & Wilke, 2020).

One of the primary goals of a professional nursing association is to build a collective voice for nurses. A strong professional association limits polarization by developing the political skills of its members and ensures that its structure and processes equitably meet the needs of its constituencies. This is the essence of politics: people must listen to each other, learn from others' viewpoints, and compromise to ensure the most positive outcomes from their endeavors.

In a review of the literature by Rasheed et al. (2020), they concluded that challenges to nurses' effective involvement in policy included power dynamics and marginalization of nurses in policymaking. Nurses were more often seen as the implementers of policy than its developers. When nurses were policy active, it was mostly around health promotion and healthy community initiatives and efforts to empower the professions.

Nurses are increasingly striving to become shapers of policy on both the local and federal levels due to their experience, perspective, and expertise in healthcare (Box 13-8). The realization that improving conditions for nursing also improves conditions for the communities we serve and the larger society in which we live, and work has enhanced our ability to organize. This increases our visibility, access to policymakers, and, more importantly, our capacity to influence the political process.

Nursing's Role in Healthcare Reform

Since the 1950s, the ANA has advocated for reforms in healthcare that will benefit both nurses and their patients. Their involvement in federal healthcare reform began in the 1960s with the passage of Medicaid and Medicare. In the 1970s, the ANA formed a PAC. PACs are organizations that raise money to contribute to political parties or candidates, with the understanding that those receiving financial and political support will be sympathetic toward issues of interest to members of the PAC.

In 1991, the ANA released Nursing's Agenda for Health Care Reform: A Call to Action—a plan so ambitious that Senator Edward Kennedy referenced this document when introducing his legislation on healthcare reform. The ANA continued to play a key role in the policy and political discussions on healthcare reform. As research and experience continued to show the need for healthcare reform, the ANA remained steadfast in its advocacy and updated the policy agenda on healthcare reform and progress toward a more balanced approach incorporating primary care, community-based care, and preventive services. Through these concentrated efforts and collaborations, healthcare reform became a reality in March 2010 (Lewenson, 2015).

Since the enactment of the ACA, ANA has worked to support implementation and to identify and disseminate the impact of any efforts to repeal the ACA (ANA, n.d.-b). The strongest efforts to repeal the ACA came at the end of 2016. The ANA carefully analyzed all proposals, compared them against the ANA's Principles for Health System Transformation (see https://www.nursingworld.org/practice-policy/health-policy/health-system-reform/), and made decisions regarding which proposals the organization would support. Due to these efforts, in 2017, the ANA was crucial in stopping the passage of legislation that would have repealed aspects of the ACA important to nursing practice and patient outcomes. Further, in May 2017, the ANA followed this same process

BOX 13-8 SPOTLIGHT ON ESSENTIAL NURSING COMPETENCIES

Safety through Legislative Involvement

Do not underestimate the power of nurses in action! On May 1, 2018, over 400 nurses from California visited the state capitol to push for important legislation that could impact them and the patients and populations they serve. They lobbied in support of A.B. 2874, which would require hospital systems to give the public 180-day notice before closing facilities or cutting specific services and would give the state attorney general the authority to approve or deny hospital closures. As a result, this bill was amended but became inactive. The nurses also advocated against A.B. 1795 and S.B. 944; these bills would allow paramedics to make clinical decisions about whether patients should be transported to emergency rooms or taken to other treatment sites, which the California Nurse Association worried could threaten patient safety and intrude on the RN scope of practice. Further, if passed, these policies could increase disparities in healthcare quality and access by providing a mechanism for vulnerable populations to be transported to subpar treatment facilities (National Nurses United, 2018). Both bills died in the Senate Assembly.

1. *Do you know about "lobby days at your local state capitol?" Do nurses participate?*
2. *Review legislation in your state. Analyze which legislation has an impact on patient safety or the potential to improve nursing care and patient outcomes.*

Source: National Nurses United (2018).

and was vocal in opposition to the American Health Care Act, which the organization believed would threaten the health of the public and compromise the quality of healthcare delivery in the United States.

Nurses represent the largest number of healthcare practitioners in America—almost 4 million—and are poised at the frontline in patient care to play a major role in the evolving healthcare system. However, to change the existing system, the barriers to competent, quality care (e.g., nursing shortages, faculty shortages, a lack of proper education and training) that prevent nursing from taking its rightful place among the cadre of providers must be addressed. To that end, the Robert Wood Johnson Foundation (RWJF) (2010), in collaboration with the Institute of Medicine (IOM), sponsored the report *The Future of Nursing: Leading Change, Advancing Health* (IOM, 2011). *The Future of Nursing* was a seminal document that addressed enhancing nurse preparation and practice environments to support the pivotal role of nurses in healthcare reform. Key recommendations addressed the need for nurses with baccalaureate preparation and for more nurses educated at the doctoral level, as well as implementing system changes to ensure that nurses are able to practice to the full scope of their license. RWJF supported the Center to Champion Nursing in America for over a decade to work on achieving progress in these recommendations (CCNA, n.d.).

In 2019, the National Academy of Medicine formed a workgroup to develop a report to build on this success (Wakefield et al., 2021). The resulting report focused on nurses' responsibilities for improving health equity in the nation. The recommendations from this report focused on enhancing nurses' knowledge and skills in assessing and addressing the structural and social determinants of health and working to enhance health equity (see Box 13-9).

These reports demonstrate that nurses are an important force in healthcare and should be at the table with other stakeholders when important decisions are being made. The National Academy of Medicine report clearly highlights the need for nurses, especially C/PHNs to take on a strong role in achieving health equity. "Nurses' regular, close proximity to patients and scientific understanding of care processes ... give them a unique ability to act as partners with other health professionals and to lead in the improvement and redesign of the healthcare system and its many practice environments..." (IOM, 2011, p. S-3). This is a mandate for C/PHNs to be actively involved in advocacy and influencing the future development of our healthcare system.

BOX 13-9 The Future of Nursing 2020–2030 Recommendations

- Address social determinants of health and health inequities.
- Address the nurse's role in advancing health equity.
- Address the healthcare needs of the nation: increase the number of nurses, increase the specialty distribution of nurses, assure a diverse nursing workforce, and remove barriers that affect workforce capacity.
- Eliminate restrictions on scope of practice for nurses and NPs.
- Design better payment models.
- Value C/PH nursing.
- Strengthen nursing education.
- Support nurse's health and well-being.
- Foster nurse's role as leaders and advocates.

Source: Adopted from Wakefield et al. (2021).

CURRENT U.S. HEALTH POLICY OPTIONS

What does the current healthcare system look like for C/PHNs? Earlier in this chapter, we discussed current health outcomes and the need for an increased focus on disease prevention and addressing the social determinants of health. The ACA has changed the policy options for healthcare on a national level; concerns persist regarding whether this is the best solution to ensuring access and controlling costs of care. However, in the past decade, policy and public health researchers examined the health outcomes as a result of the U.S. healthcare system as configured, with access to care largely through employer-based insurance and a focus on medical treatment. Although the system spawned innovations in pharmaceuticals and technological innovations, these services have often been effective for a small number of people in acute need and at a large cost. The healthcare system has been very successful in terms of education of healthcare professionals, pharmacologic treatments for many illnesses, surgical innovations, and diagnostic technologies. As discussed earlier, however, these achievements have not led to overall positive health outcomes for the population as a whole. The passage of the ACA (Kaiser Family Foundation, 2023) has led to policy changes designed to address these concerns (see Chapter 6 for more information on the ACA).

The ACA and C/PHN Practice

The ACA resulted in a dramatic change in U.S. policy options. Recognizing that the U.S. healthcare system was not addressing all the factors necessary to improve the health of the public and that it was costing U.S. taxpayers an ever-increasing and unsustainable proportion of the national budget, the Obama administration moved to pass healthcare reform legislation in 2010. The focus of the ACA, in the minds of the public, was to mandate health insurance coverage for all U.S. citizens. This would be done through a required employer minimal health insurance package, a mandate on employer provision of health insurance or employer contribution to a marketplace of insurance options for people to access, and government provision of subsidies for people who have a low income and are without employer insurance coverage. Indeed, data indicate that the ACA was initially successful at insuring those previously uninsured. The percentage of uninsured adults (ages 19 to 64) dropped from 20% in 2010 to 10.2% in 2018, but more people are underinsured (Collins et al., 2019; Corlette & Alker, 2023). This was aided by limitations on states' ability to restrict Medicaid enrollment implemented during the pandemic. These have now been lifted, and there is some concern that the rate of uninsured may rise again. Continued battles between political parties on the strength of the insurance provisions and eligibility continue to pose a threat to the ACA, depending on the outcome of upcoming elections.

Lesser known but equally critical aspects of the ACA include value-based purchasing and accountable care organizations, along with the expanded Internal Revenue Service requirement for nonprofit hospitals to conduct regular community health needs assessments and develop implementation plans based on these data for improving the health of their communities (Kacic & Castellucci, 2018).

The ACA began a movement away from the traditional fee-for-service care where health providers diagnose and treat people and are paid for each service provided (e.g., office visits, lab fees, prescriptions, follow-up visits) and that has been thought to have led to increasing healthcare costs (Kacic & Castellucci, 2018). This style of reimbursement for care has had the problem of indirectly encouraging additional care, as each service is reimbursed separately. National health policy has begun to reverse this by mandating no reimbursement for specific services required because of medical errors.

The ACA expands this with a move toward *value-based purchasing* or reimbursing a specific amount based on achieving the likely outcome for clients within specific diagnostic categories.

Instead of fees for office visits, lab fees, and prescriptions, the federal government is proposing paying for achievable health outcomes in a bundled manner based on the client's demographics and diagnosis. A person with diabetes would not have each service reimbursed, but rather a lump sum reimbursement would be provided upon the client achieving a level of stability in the disease (e.g., lab values for hemoglobin A1C within normal limits). This reimbursement would cover whatever services were required to achieve this outcome, which might be lab tests and medications, but might also include C/PHN-provided chronic disease self-management training or clinical nutrition counseling.

Such a change in reimbursement mechanisms would have a large impact on healthcare services, as clinical agencies would need to determine what services and providers were most effective at achieving the desired outcomes, with a focus on addressing the social determinants of health. This would provide an opportunity for C/PHNs to demonstrate the effectiveness of their practice interventions in improving health outcomes for people and populations (LaPointe, 2019).

Accountable Care Organizations are another feature of healthcare reform that is intended to emphasize quality over quantity. Primary providers and other healthcare and social service providers are forming groups, sometimes in conjunction with hospitals, and will be paid based on a patient's treatment outcomes (not the number of visits or tests). Early results of Medicare-funded demonstration projects of these models have shown promising results in terms of care coordination and outcomes for those with multiple social and health needs (Johnson et al., 2022). These models serve as ideal practice settings for PHNs.

Pandemic Preparedness, Public Policy, and PHN Practice

Discussion of the impact of health policy on health outcomes would be incomplete without looking at lessons learned from the recent COVID-19 pandemic. In many ways, the healthcare system performed remarkably, with rapid development of treatments and vaccines, and a Herculean effort to distribute those vaccines. On the other hand, there was great discord across all levels of society and political leadership about support for following the best available evidence on COVID-19 as it developed, leading to division and controversy at a time when local and national unity was needed most. Scholars and clinicians will review and write about the national response to COVID-19 over the upcoming decades. Early response from primary providers and nurses includes the following policy-relevant recommendations:

- Build a more resilient healthcare system, founded on equity, access, prevention, and addressing broadly the determinants of health and illness (Nash & Wohlforth, 2022; Williamson-Younce, 2023).
- Work to collaborate more effectively with all stakeholders, with a particular focus on those most often underrepresented, to build trust in public health efforts.
- Use technology to improve access and track progress before, during, and after emergent situations.
- Center the system on quality and safety for patients and employees.
- Build strong collaboration between public health and clinical care efforts.
- Realign financial incentives of the system to prioritize outcomes instead of services.
- Enact legislative and regulatory reform to enable rapid response capabilities in areas of healthcare license portability, access to telehealth, and quick access to personal protective equipment and other emergency supplies (Nash & Wohlforth, 2022; Williamson-Younce, 2023).

One thing agreed upon across sectors of society is that we will face future emergencies, including disease outbreaks. The time is ripe for nursing involvement in policy across all levels to help ensure that the healthcare system—and our communities—are better prepared to regain, maintain, and enhance the health of the public.

POLICY COMPETENCE AS AN INTEGRAL PART OF C/PHN PRACTICE

The U.S. healthcare system is undergoing significant changes to improve the health of the public and contain costs. These changes are impacting healthcare across the system but are particularly critical for those who work in communities with an increased emphasis on population health and disease prevention. The C/PHN can lead the way in addressing the social determinants of health and focusing efforts on prevention and long-term health promotion for families and communities. Along with other public health professionals, C/PHNs need to do this by understanding the policy process and then determining where their efforts would be most effective in improving overall population health. This is a critical time for nursing in general, and community/public health nursing specifically, as the healthcare system focuses attention on what has always been at the core of C/PHN concern—health where people live, work, play, and come together.

SUMMARY

This chapter briefly reviewed health outcomes in the United States.

- Health outcomes for Americans do not compare well with peer countries, particularly considering the high cost of the U.S. healthcare system; this is largely due to system issues and not addressing the social determinants of health.
- Health policy guides healthcare and governmental actions related to the social; C/PHNs can use policy in their practice to improve the health of the communities with which they work.
- Policy competence as it relates to local, state, and federal health policy—and how nurses are impacted by these policies—is an essential skill for C/PHNs.
- An understanding of how a bill becomes a law helps inform policy process, implementation, and evaluation.
- Frameworks such as the Rational and Kingdon provide guidance in health policy analysis.
- Policy analysis as a call for activism can be used to support social justice in public health, professional advocacy, and the C/PHN's role in healthcare reform, PACs, and volunteerism.
- Current U.S. health policy includes the ACA within community and public health practice, value-based purchasing, and accountable care organizations.

ACTIVE LEARNING EXERCISES

1. Using "Utilize Legal and Regulatory Actions" (1 of the 10 Essential Public Health Services; see Box 2-2) describe a legislative bill related to health at the state or federal level and identify where the bill is in the legislative process. Explain who is sponsoring the bill, who is opposing it, and why. Compare at least two populations to determine who will be affected most by the bill if it passes and in what ways they will be affected. Develop a political action plan to support or oppose the bill. (Objectives 1, 2, and 6)
2. Identify your state legislators. Examine one critical health issue in your state, and explain how your legislators responded to the issue. Select one state-level policy that impacts nursing practice and explain how your state legislators supported or challenged these efforts. Create a plan for how you might influence one of these policy issues. (Objectives 2 and 4)
3. Attend a meeting of a professional organization, board of directors, government agency, or council when a health policy or healthcare issue is on the agenda. Explain the purpose of the meeting and the important stakeholders present. For one policy issue discussed, compare the viewpoints of stakeholders. Defend the position of one stakeholder with your own evidence from the literature. (Objectives 4 and 6)
4. Identify the most important stakeholder groups for a particular health policy issue. Analyze the positions of the major interest groups involved. Critique the extent economics plays in the discussion. Defend who controls the discussion and why. (Objectives 2 and 9)
5. Develop a statement that explains whether nurses are the most qualified group to articulate national healthcare issues. Explain why or why not. (Objectives 6 and 7)
6. Apply either Kingdon's or Rationale's framework to a health issue or policy problem. Create a plan for how you would use frameworks to influence policy. Explain how you can use advocacy to make this issue a priority. (Objectives 3 and 5)
7. Explain a health issue that is important in your local community. Defend the need to address this issue through policy. Determine what stance your nursing professional organization has on this issue. (Objectives 6 and 7)
8. Compare two aspects of national health before and after the ACA. Explain the impact the ACA had on the health of the nation? (Objective 8)

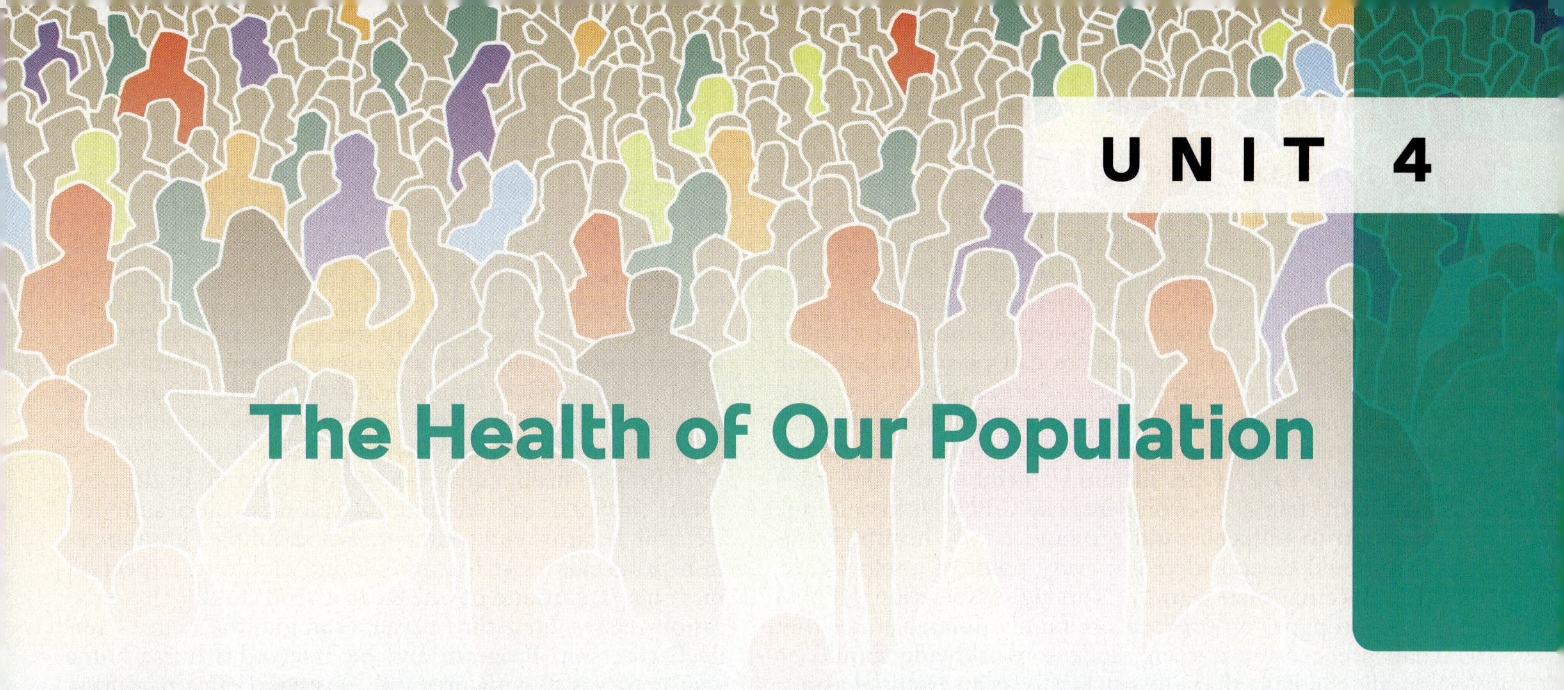

UNIT 4

The Health of Our Population

CHAPTER 14

Family as Client

"Healthy communities are comprised of healthy families. Hence, families as units of relationship are important components of communities, and undoubtedly, they are heavily affected by their community's state of health."

—Robinson, Padgett, & Smith (2022)

KEY TERMS

- Asset-based approach
- Conceptual framework
- Eco-map
- Family health
- Family health nursing
- Family life cycle
- Genogram
- Outcome evaluation
- Referral
- Resource directory

LEARNING OBJECTIVES

Upon mastery of this chapter, you should be able to:

1. Discuss characteristics all families have in common.
2. Identify the stages of the family life cycle and the developmental tasks of a family.
3. Discuss how a family's culture influences its values, behaviors, and roles.
4. Describe the functions of a family.
5. Analyze the role of the community/public health nurse in promoting the health of the family.
6. Describe the components of the nursing process as they apply to enhancing family health.
7. Describe safety measures the community/public health nurse should take when traveling to a home or making a home visit.

INTRODUCTION

Nurses interact with patients and families in everyday practice. The community/public health nurse (C/PHN) not only interacts with families but does so in the most intimate and natural settings where families gather.

The family plays a critical role in the health and influence of its members, and nurses can play a critical role in families. Health habits such as preventative care, diet, exercise, and physical activity are developed through your experiences in a family. Health beliefs, genetic influences, and care of the ill family member all take place within the family environment. The C/PHN is in a unique position to influence and promote family health. Families should be considered at every point of nursing care. The International Family Nursing Association (IFNA) position paper on prelicensure family nursing states that "all prelicensure nursing students worldwide should be taught curricula that identify family as an essential aspect of all person's lives" (IFNA, 2013, p. 2), and the position paper on generalist family nursing states "nurses have a commitment and moral obligation to support family and societal heath" (IFNA, 2015, p. 2).

Definitions of family according to discipline vary, here are some examples (Robinson et al., 2022):

- Legal—relationships through blood ties, adoption, guardianship, or marriage
- Biologic—genetic biologic networks among and between people
- Sociologic—groups of people living together with or without legal or biologic ties
- Psychological—groups with strong emotional ties

According to the Census Bureau, "[a] family is a group of two people or more (one of whom is the householder) related by birth, marriage, or adoption residing together; all such people (including related subfamily members) are considered as members of one family" (United States Census Bureau, 2021). Defining a family is not easy or all-encompassing because each family is unique and constantly changing. The legal definition is much more simplistic than is reflected in actual family groups found in the world today.

Today's C/PHN needs to be familiar with diverse families, each of which has unique health needs. For example, a young, single parent seeks help in caring for a toddler whom they do not believe is hitting developmental milestones. A 70-year-old provides care to their partner, who was recently discharged from the hospital after a stroke. A family from Egypt needs instruction on the purchase and preparation of food for the diabetic diet and medication one of its members has been given. The effectiveness of a C/PHN depends on understanding the diversity of families and considering policies that empower them.

This chapter draws from various theories to strengthen the student's understanding and appreciation of families as clients. This information will promote the effectiveness of interventions with families at the primary, secondary, and tertiary levels of prevention (Box 14-1).

The family is the basic element of a community and a population. The family's experience when accessing health services determines the health of the community and leads to a healthier population. Families have been impacted in recent years by the COVID-19 pandemic. With children being at home, much of the education fell on parents, which added to an already heavy burden of work, housework, and parenting (Pino-Gavidia et al., 2023). The changes in family dynamics and society during this time brought to the surface the importance of mental and physical family health. When the family faces challenges, they must work together to find a solution to the problem (Collier & Villareal, 2022).

Families need equal access to optimal healthcare, social services, and community resources in a supportive and healthy environment. For example, immunization programs exist for infants and children. Expectant birthing parents and partners can attend childbirth preparation classes. First-time parents can join the Nurse Family Partnership Program and be assigned a nurse home visitor to assist with prenatal, postnatal, and parenting support (Nurse Family Partnership [NFP], 2023). There are technological advances that allow older adults to visit with friends, family, and even primary providers remotely (Robinson et al., 2022). All these clients have one point in common: They are members of families. Regardless of stage of life, many families have access to resources and options within the community.

Within the family, the interactions are unique because a family member can knowingly or unknowingly influence another. The health of one family member can influence other members' perspective(s) about health or their social value system. The emotional state of a family member can be the deciding factor in another family member's choice for a career or the schools attended. Family members clearly influence each other and the entire family.

Just as each family is unique, so too are their homes. A public health nurse may feel more comfortable in some families' homes than others. A home is a structure or building where families live. Habitat for Humanity (2023) considers home "a place of refuge." It can be daunting for students to enter a home that is different from their idea of what a home should be. Each home brings its own set of unique challenges and strengths that can influence the way the public health nurse perceives and interacts with the community to promote health, prevent illnesses, and reduce risk.

Public health nurses rely on the nursing process when working with families, the "core unit of service," to promote health and wellness, prevent illness, and improve the overall health of the population. The delivery of care occurs in various community settings (i.e., homes, work settings, classrooms, clinics and outpatient departments, neighborhood centers, and shelters for people experiencing homelessness). Although caring for the family, as a unit of service, is an effective way to treat the population in the communities, practice does not always match a family nursing theory. The problem, in part, is that healthcare services are often tailored to a person and not to a family or a community. Third-party payer and reimbursement policies impose limits to the kinds of services funded. Public health agencies often organize services around people. The government requires that public health agencies structure disease statistics or service categories on a person instead of aggregated data on a family.

BOX 14-1 LEVELS OF PREVENTION PYRAMID

A Home Visit to an Older Adult During the COVID-19 Pandemic

SITUATION: A 75-year-old adult expresses fear of the COVID-19 virus. Their daughter takes them to the local health department clinic for their annual visit and shares this with the provider. A PHN is sent to his house for a follow-up home visit.
GOAL: Using the three levels of prevention, avoid negative health conditions, and promptly diagnose, treat, and restore the fullest possible potential.

Tertiary Prevention

Rehabilitation	*Health Promotion and Education*	*Health Protection*
▪ Patient and family are taught to monitor symptoms ▪ Work closely with the provider to ensure follow-up for concerns ▪ Be alert for any complication	▪ Patient and family are taught to recognize signs of inadequate oxygenation ▪ Patient and family are taught when to go to ED	▪ Support for long-lasting symptoms ▪ Continued family support ▪ Educate and follow-up regarding vaccines and boosters

Secondary Prevention

Early Diagnosis	*Prompt Treatment*
▪ Develops cold symptoms and fever ▪ Calls to inform doctor	▪ Testing ▪ Isolation and quarantine

Primary Prevention

Health Promotion and Education	*Health Protection*
▪ Discuss benefits of the vaccines and boosters ▪ Demonstrate thorough handwashing	▪ Review immunization schedule ▪ Stay home when sick and avoid others who are sick

When a C/PHN works with families, a family health assessment is an excellent way to get an accurate picture of family needs, concerns, and health. This creates a database from which a family diagnosis is generated, an essential step before planning, implementation, and evaluation of services.

The novice public health nurse must be able to practice within the nursing process. Moreover, when public health nurses address the health needs of the core unit of service, the family, the nurses are creating healthy communities and promoting the public's health (Association of Public Health Nurses [APHN], 2022). Public health nurses are the leaders in using accessible healthcare services to prevent illnesses and promote health in families (APHN, 2022). Family health is the cornerstone for community and population health, making the family the focus of healthcare and related services. Therefore, the health of the *family* is addressed through the nursing process that involves assessing, diagnosing, planning, implementing, and evaluating the family.

FAMILY HEALTH AND FAMILY HEALTH NURSING

Throughout history, the family has been the most basic unit. One of the first steps for nurses is to explore how a family influences the care that they provide and how they interact with the family. Most of nurses were raised in families and spent a good portion of their lives within families. Their first experiences with others were often influenced by their families of origin. People tend to think of family according to what they have personally experienced. So, nurses come to their nursing practice with unintentionally biased ideas about families.

- The U.S. Census Bureau (Census Bureau, 2021) views family as people living together and related by birth, adoption, or marriage.
- Robinson et al. (2022, p. 588) define family as "two or more individuals who depend on one another for emotional, physical, and economical support."
- Robinson et al. (2022, p. 6) define family health as a "dynamic changing state of wellbeing, which includes the biological, psychological, spiritual, sociological, and culture factors of individual members and the whole family system."

Family health is concerned with how well the family functions together as a unit. It involves not only the health of the members and how they relate to other members but also how well they relate to and cope with the community, outside the family. In fact, family health, like individual health, ranges along a continuum from wellness to illness. A family may be at one point on that continuum now and at a much different point 6 months from

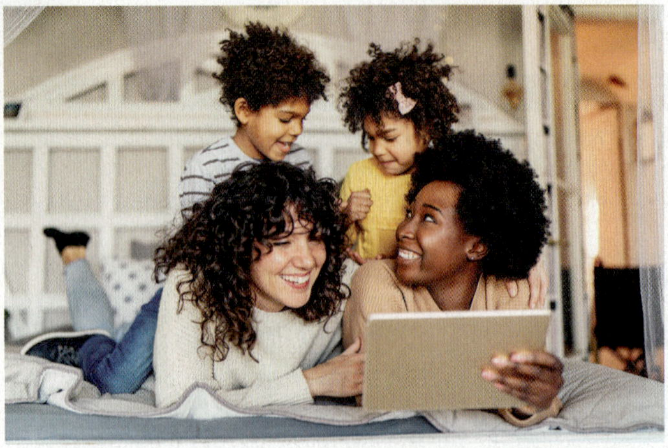

FIGURE 14-1 C/PHNs work with families and individual family members.

now. Family health refers to the health status of a given family at a given point in time (Robinson et al., 2022).

Family health nursing is how public health nurses care for people within the family or for the family as the client (family as context) or for the family as a system (Fig. 14-1). There are multiple ways that community health nurses can approach families. Some nurses view family nursing as part of other specialties such as public health nursing, maternal child nursing, or behavioral health nursing. However, some nurses view family nursing as its own distinct specialty, rich with its own body of literature and research. Each of these approaches with families has its own distinct set of beliefs.

Nurses work with people within families every day. Most often, that person is the recipient of care. While assessing the needs of the person, the nurse needs to include the family in the assessment, as the family is the pivotal provider of care. How does the family assist the individual family member or hinder their progress? What are their available resources (physically, emotionally, and spiritually)? What can the family share about the recipient of care that might improve health outcomes?

Nurses work with families as a system and view the family as part of a larger supersystem that includes many subsystems. The family becomes greater than the sum of all its parts. When one person in the family changes, the family system changes (Collier & Villareal, 2022).

When visualizing a family as a system, it may help to compare it to a mobile. Think of all the pieces suspended freely by a string. If you pull lightly on one piece, all the pieces move, just as a change in one member's health affects the entire family. Can you think of some examples of this in your own family?

FAMILY CHARACTERISTICS AND DYNAMICS

Several observations can be made about families. First, each family is unique, with its own distinct set of strengths and weaknesses. As a nurse, you want to focus first on the family's strengths. When you approach the door of a house to begin your visit, you do not want to begin with any assumptions about the family inside. You will have to gather information about the family to provide the best care possible. Starting with their strengths will ensure your success.

Families share universal characteristics with other families (Box 14-2). For instance, families in every culture throughout history have engaged in similar functions: They have produced children, physically cared for their members, protected their health, encouraged their education or training, given emotional support and acceptance, and provided supportive and nurturing care during illness. These characteristics provide an important key to understanding each family's uniqueness. No matter how many families a nurse may visit over the course of a year, each one will have universal features; it is important for C/PHNs to know each family's unique set of characteristics and their effects on family health.

Family Stage of Development

Many of the characteristics and defined developmental stages of individual growth also apply to families. For example, families change continuously. Families grow and develop as the people within them mature and adapt to changes. A family's composition, set of roles, and interpersonal relationships change with time. Families vary with each stage of the family life cycle. See Box 14-3 for some questions to ask yourself about your own family.

As Duvall and Miller (1985) first pointed out, no two children come from precisely the same family. Consider the following example of how families change over time. Destiny and Hassan, a young couple, begin their family after moving in together. Destiny has a 6-year-old child, Rose, who will be living with the couple. They are adjusting to their roles as a couple, Hassan is adjusting to a new role as a parental figure, and Rose is adjusting to all the

BOX 14-2 Universal Characteristics of Family Life

- Every family is a small social system.
  - Families are interdependent.
  - Families maintain boundaries.
  - Families exchange energy with their environments.
  - Families adapt.
  - Families are goal oriented (providing love, security, and a sense of belonging).
- Every family moves through stages in its life cycle.
- Every family has its own cultural values and rules.
- Family members share certain values that affect their behavior.
- Certain roles are defined for family members.
- A family's culture influences its distribution and use of power.
- Every family has certain basic functions:
  - Providing affection
  - Providing security
  - Instilling identity
  - Promoting affiliation
  - Providing socialization
  - Establishing controls
- Every family has structure.

Source: Duvall and Miller (1985).

BOX **14-3** WHAT DO *YOU* THINK?

Questions for Self-Evaluation

1. What are your first memories of family?
2. What is your definition of family?
3. How would you describe your own family?
4. Who do you include as family members?

changes. The couple marries after a year and have a new baby, Jackson. New roles are added to the family, and the dynamics change again.

Both family size and a reorganization of family occurred. The children entered school; Destiny went back to work, and soon, Rose is leaving for college. The family, like every family, is moving through a predictable and sequential pattern of stages known as the **family life cycle**.

C/PHNs who are knowledgeable about this cycle can provide anticipatory guidance to families. For instance, nurses can help prepare the family for parenting needs. The nurse can help the couple anticipate the responsibility and cost of raising their children. The nurse can assist the family in figuring out the monthly costs of childcare, breastfeeding versus formula, disposable versus cloth diapers, and clothing, equipment, and other medical costs.

To progress through the stages of the life cycle, a family must carry out its basic functions and the developmental tasks associated with those functions. Often, how we define family will determine how the family functions are filled. Unlike developmental tasks, which are specific to each age level, family developmental tasks are ongoing throughout the life cycle. The functions can change over time with generational differences (Collier & Villareal, 2022).

Some functions require greater emphasis at certain stages. Socialization, for example, consumes much of a family's time during the early years of child development. Duvall and Miller (1985) described these activities as "stage critical" family developmental tasks that must be completed before moving on to the next stage. Sample community health nursing actions with the family at different stages are presented in Table 14-1.

TABLE **14-1** Critical Family Developmental Tasks

Stage of the Family Life Cycle	Developmental Tasks	Role of the Community Health Nurse
Forming a partnership	Establishing a mutually satisfying relationship	Interact with family where they are at
Childbearing	Adjusting to pregnancy and the promise of parenthood Fitting into the kin network Having and adjusting to infants and encouraging their development Establishing a satisfying home for both parents and infant(s)	Assist them in developing strong relationships
Preschool-age children	Adapting to the critical needs and interests of preschool children in stimulating, growth-promoting ways Coping with energy depletion and lack of privacy as parents	Assist in preparing for family expansion through education and anticipatory guidance
School-age children	Fitting into the community of school-age families in constructive ways Encouraging children's educational achievement	Encourage time for each other as adults in a relationship separate from parenting role
Teenage children	Balancing freedom with responsibility as teenagers mature and emancipate themselves Establishing outside interests and careers as growing parents	Provide anticipatory guidance for the school-aged children as they grow into adulthood
Launching children	Releasing young adults into work, military service, college, marriage, etc., with appropriate rituals and assistance Maintaining a supportive home base	Provide anticipatory guidance for the contracting family as children leave home
Middle-aged parents	Rebuilding the relationship Maintaining kin ties with older and younger generations	Prepare adults for grandparenting role
Aging family members	Adjusting to retirement Coping with bereavement and living alone Closing the family home or adapting it to aging	Assist aging adults with emotional and financial security, as they approach retirement Prepare the aging adults with ways to cope with the losses of old age, including changes in space, work, health, status, and loss of friends and family members

Source: Duvall and Miller (1985).

Family Values and Their Effect on Behavior

Like most cultural values, many family values remain outside the conscious awareness of family members. These values, often not verbalized, become powerful determinants of what the family believes, feels, thinks, and does. Family values include those beliefs transmitted by previous generations, religious influences, immediate social pressures, and the larger society. Values become an integral part of a family's life and are difficult to change (Box 14-4; see Chapter 5).

Family Roles

Families distribute among their members all the responsibilities and tasks necessary to conduct daily family living. These roles can be based on culture, tradition, and the family's historical belief system. Each family determines what works for their family.

Family members may play several roles at the same time. A single parent often takes on the roles of two parents but may distribute responsibilities and tasks more widely. A grandmother or child may assume responsibility for chores and relieve some demands on the single parent. Among families, there is variation in expectations for each role and in the degree of flexibility in divisions of roles. An example may be how specific tasks are divided up between partners. For example, one partner may be responsible for childcare and cooking, whereas the other partner may be responsible for grocery shopping and yard tasks.

Many families enjoy the fellowship of organized religious or cultural groups. This fellowship can be a source of support or comfort and an additional role function for the family members. Family members can also participate in roles outside the family (e.g., local or regional politics, community improvement, volunteerism for nonprofit groups, or other groups that the community may offer). These diverse role relationships should enrich and energize the participants. The C/PHN may work with families to help them achieve a balance of activities that promote family health.

Power is the possession of control, authority, or influence over others—assuming patterns in each family. This power will look different depending on culture and family norms. In one family, it may be a parent, and in another, it may be a grandparent. The dominant family member holds most of the decision-making power, particularly over more important family matters such as employment, finances, and healthcare. It is critical the C/PHN knows who this is in the families they serve to get participation from the family. With changing societal influences, the present trend among American families is toward egalitarian power distribution.

BOX 14-4 Cultural Values

Cultural values such as the following shape most life decisions and choices:

- Education
- Gender roles
- Healthcare
- Courtship/marriage
- Lifestyle
- Childrearing
- Religion/spirituality

Family Social Class and Economic Status

As a C/PHN, it is important for your assessment to include the social class of families you are visiting. Social class has a powerful influence on health. How healthy we are and how long we live is often related to our social standing. The neighborhoods where families live and the schools their children attend are often determined by social class. This determinant of health has lifelong implications and shapes the history of families. See Chapter 23 for more on social determinants of health and the socioeconomic gradient.

Most people who experience homelessness are single adults. In 2022, 582,462 people were homeless (roughly 18 out of every 10,000 people):

- The vast majority were individual adults (72%).
- A notable share were people living in families with children (28%) (National Alliance to End Homelessness, 2023a).

Families that experience homelessness are not necessarily incomeless. They may include working parents who are not making enough money to pay for housing. Unsheltered families present the C/PHN with unique challenges. Primarily, the family is in crisis and often not able to provide for their most basic needs. When families cannot meet these needs, they cannot address other concerns such as medical appointments, healthy eating and exercise, and other preventative actions that nurses typically recommend. For those who are not working or have lost their job, homelessness causes problems with employment due to the inability to shower, access clean clothing, and provide an address when applying for or maintaining a job.

Children who experience homelessness have higher risks of emotional and behavioral problems, serious health problems, experience separations from families, school mobility, repeating a grade, and being expelled or dropping out of school and have lower academic performance (National Alliance to End Homelessness, 2023b).

Community health nurses should be aware of this and focus on first assisting the family in getting their essential needs met. They should also acknowledge that the behaviors seen in children may be the direct result of the situation that the family finds itself in. A C/PHN's knowledge of the resources available in the community is key in providing the family with the help to deal with the crisis and assisting in the provision of ongoing shelter, food, health, employment, and schooling needs. See Chapter 26 for more on unsheltered populations. You can check your state's rates at https://endhomelessness.org/homelessness-in-america/homelessness-statistics/state-of-homelessness/.

Family Composition

Family composition varies by demographic variables (Robinson et al., 2022). The meaning of family among the Hmong of northern Laos may include hundreds of people who make up a clan. In Mexico, families remain close, are large, and extend into multiple generations. In Germany and Japan, families are small and tend to the needs of their older adults at home.

In the United States, where families come from many cultural groups, many variations coexist within communities. Families come in many shapes and sizes (Fig. 14-2).

It is a privilege and honor to enter a family's home. This is a uniquely private space belonging to the family. The people who are members of this household interact, care for one another, and bond in ways that may never be fully understood by anyone outside the family. Therefore, being granted entrance into this system gives the community health nurse an opportunity to work with the family, which few other professionals experience. Each type of household requires recognition and acceptance by community health nurses, who must help families achieve optimal health.

Traditional Versus Modern Families

Both traditional families and modern families are the same in that they are both a constitutional construct. Traditional families are those that were the majority in history:

- The nuclear family—two parents and children living together in the same household. In nuclear families, the workload distribution between the two adults can vary. Both adults may work outside the home; one adult may work outside the home, whereas the other stays at home and assumes primary responsibilities for the household; or partners may alternate, constantly renegotiating work and domestic responsibilities.
- A nuclear dyad family consists of two adults living together who have no children or who have grown children living outside the home.
- A single adult family is one in which one adult is living alone by choice or because of separation from a spouse or children or both. Separation may be the result of divorce, death, or distance from children.

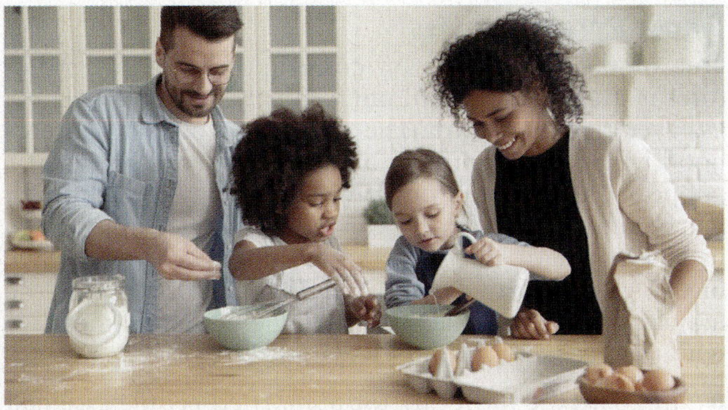

FIGURE 14-2 Families exist in many forms.

Today, in the United States, couples are putting off marriage as they start their careers. In the United States, as of 2021, 25% of 40-year-olds had never been married, which is a significant increase from 20% in 2010 (Fry, 2023). In the 1980s, just 6% of 40-year-olds had never been married, which indicates how much families are changing (Fry, 2023).

Sometimes, in close-knit ethnic communities, several nuclear families live in the same household or near one another and share goods and services. They may own and operate a family business, sharing work and childcare responsibilities, income and expenses, and even meals. Multigenerational living has grown in the United Stares for a variety of reasons, including rapid growth of the Asian and Hispanic populations who, along with Black Americans, are more likely to live with extended family, especially if they are immigrants. (Cohn et al., 2022). European Italian and Spanish families are also more likely to prioritize multigenerational support and entertainment than American families (Rodriguez-Gonzalez et al., 2020).

The number of young adults who continue to live with their parents is also on the rise. In 2022, 50% of adults ages 18 to 29 were living with one or both of their parents compared to 38% in 2000 (Fadeyi & Horowitz, 2022).

The number of children living with married parents has risen slightly since 2010. In 2020, 67% of children ages 0 to 17 lived with two married parents compared to 66% in 2010 (Childstats, 2021).

- The nuclear family has been a fundamental part of the cultural heritage shared by many Americans and reinforced by religion, education, and other influential social institutions. Historically, the nuclear family was envisioned as including a mother, father, and children; however, by thinking of this as the typical family, any variation was often treated as atypical, which could leave those who do not fit this description feeling isolated and alone.
- Families are changing for a variety of reasons; Americans are putting off previously expected milestones, families are getting smaller, and life expectancy is getting longer. There is an increase in single-parent adoptions; an increase in lesbian, gay, bisexual, transgender, or queer (LGBTQ+) couples and families; and high divorce and remarriage rates.
- The role of child-bearing partners in the family is changing; they are marrying at older ages, and children are being born outside of marriage.

Current media portray the family in various forms, showing that society is beginning to accept more contemporary definitions of family.

- Streaming sites allow families to pick the type of family shows they want to watch and the time they want to watch them. Series such as Blackish, Ginny & Georgia, and Fresh off the Boat are all examples of the ways families are portrayed in U.S. media. On the shows they watch, people want to see characters like themselves, going through similar experiences, with families that look like theirs.

- Social media impacts families in another way. It can have a positive or negative influence on the family and its members. People spend more time connecting with others online and less time in person. Because these activities are becoming more commonplace, the public health nurse should consider these factors when working with families (see Chapter 10).
- One of the positive aspects of social media is its use in promoting healthcare resources to families. Families often turn to online resources for many reasons and healthcare questions are no exception. Nurses can play a role in using social media to communicate and educate families with factual and evidence-based information.

Families Experiencing Divorce, Remarriage, and Blending

Divorce, remarriage, and blending of families can result in distinct emotional responses and developmental issues among family members.

Divorce. Divorce does not just affect the couple involved; it changes the entire family structure and each family member's life course. The Census Bureau reports that both marriage and divorce rates of U.S. people assigned female at birth aged 15 years and older declined from 2011 to 2021 but vary by state (Washington & Anderson, 2023). In 2000, there were 944,000 divorces in the United States, compared to 689,308 in 2021 (CDC.gov). This is a significant decline in divorce but continues to be a shift in family dynamics for nurses to consider.

Something new to consider today is the effect of social media on couples and relationships. It is easier than ever to form emotional relationships online. Through various online platforms, couples can reconnect with old friends and even make new ones. Social media boundaries are important for couples and families to discuss and agree on. The C/PHN should consider this when working on goals and interventions for the family.

Divorce affects all members of the family in a different way, since each is at a different stage in life. Each member is going through unique adjustments and transitions as they cope with their new normal.

- For children, it may require coping with a new geographic location and a new school, as well as adjusting to changes in the mental and physical health of family members.
- Children from divorced families may face an absent parent, interparental conflict, economic distress, parental adjustment, multiple life stressors, and short-term crises.
- New schools mean that children must find new friends and social groups, prove themselves, and try to gain acceptance in a completely new social setting. Their previous sense of security and comfort at home is forever changed. These adjustments take time, and C/PHN can provide support and resources for the children and families involved.
- Divorce and marriage are decreasing in the United States, with multigenerational living increasing. The C/PHN needs to consider this when planning interventions for families.

Remarriage and Blending. The U.S. Census Bureau uses the term "blended families" to describe families that bring nonbiologic children into a new family. In this structure, single parents marry and raise the children from each of the previous relationships together. If this arrangement is the result of divorce or death, this can be an especially painful transition.

- They may be custodial parents who have the children except during planned visits with the noncustodial parent, or they may share custody, so that the children live in the blended arrangement only part-time or possibly live in two separate blended homes.
- The family may include children from the couple, in addition to the children brought into the relationship. Not all divorced adults stay single; most remarry or cohabitate with another adult, who may or may not have children. This new couple may have children from their union, or adopt, creating an even more complex family.
- Merged or blended families require considerable adjustment and relearning of roles, tasks, communication patterns, and relationships.
- We all form new relationships with our own history. C/PHNs should consider the changing dynamics and complexity of the family in the above situations.

Because this emerging family pattern is becoming more prominent, it is probable that the C/PHN is familiar with this pattern or lives in such a family. The data on blended families can be challenging to track because the U.S. Census information is done only every 10 years. The American Community Survey done in 2021 found that 2,413,441 households included stepchildren (U.S. Census, 2021).

Nursing skills needed when working with divorced or blended families include the ability to listen, empathize, and address families genuinely. The nurse should meet the family where they are at and provide resources that the family may need. Resources may include support groups, reading materials, or interventions available in the community. Communication among all parents and family members should be encouraged. Peer support groups for children and adolescents and support from within the schools should be used, if available, or created if they do not exist. The school nurse is a supportive resource for families with school-aged children. The community health nurse can have a significant role in community-wide planning if services are needed but unavailable.

Single-Parent Families

One of the most common contemporary family structures is the single-parent family, mostly headed by people assigned female at birth. There are many paths to parenthood including intentional and unintentional pregnancy, adoption, assisted reproductive technology, and through marriage, and any of these can lead to single parenthood. In 1980, 18% of all people in the United States who gave birth were unmarried compared to 40% in 2021, and the majority of children living in single-parent homes live with their female parent (Childstats, 2021).

- In 2019, the birth rate for unmarried people assigned female at birth ages 15 to 44 was 40 births per 1000, with the highest birth rates for this group being ages 25 to 29 (Childstats, 2021).

- The rate for people assigned female at birth giving birth aged 15 to 17 years was at an all-time low; conversely, birth rates rose for those aged 30 to 44 years.

In part, the explanation of the data change is the result of more people assigned female at birth of childbearing age remaining unmarried than in the past (Childstats, 2021). The needs of the family will depend on their stage in the family cycle and experiences that brought them into the single-parent family.

Over time, the single-parent family has become more common in society. It is important for C/PHNs to view the strengths of single-parent families as they would any other family. Building on their current strengths can be most helpful in meeting the challenges they may face. These challenges will typically result from one parent being solely responsible for the financial income, caregiving, and support for the family. Single parents were hit especially hard during the COVID-19 pandemic. The workload of single parents specifically increased during the pandemic with children being home from school on top of the typical workload that was heavy prepandemic (Pino-Gavidia et al., 2023). This added significant strain on single-parent families. Nurses with their connections in the community can assist these families through advocacy and collaboration.

Families Headed by an Adolescent Parent or Parents

Statistics indicate that teenagers are increasingly the heads of single-parent families; some of these teen heads of households become pregnant in junior high or high school. The birth rate among teens 15 to 19 years old has continued a steady decline, but teen birth rates in the United States remain the highest among those in resource-abundant countries (Osterman et al., 2022).

- The birth rate for teens aged 15 to 19 years in the United States in 2020 was 15.4 births per 1000 teens, down 8% from 2019 (16.7).
- The number of births to teenagers aged 15 to 19 years was 158,043 in 2020, down 8% from 2019 (171,674).
- The 2016 birth rates for teenagers aged 15 to 17 years and 18 to 19 years were 6.3 and 28.9 births per 1000 teens, respectively, down 6% and 7% from 2019, record lows for both groups (CDC, 2021).

Teenagers are still developing physically, mentally, and emotionally and are not prepared to take on parenthood without help. Consideration should be given to helping the birthing parent on their life course as well as the baby. The adolescent parent needs support and structure to support the child. Home visitation programs such as the Nurse–Family Partnership can provide this stability for both parent and baby if available in the community.

Specific factors related to teen birth rates are low education and low-income levels of a teen's family, few opportunities in a teen's community for positive youth involvement, racial segregation, physical disorder, and neighborhood-level income inequality. Teens in child welfare systems are at increased risk for teen pregnancy and birth than other groups. For example, young people assigned female at birth living in foster care are more than twice as likely to become pregnant than those not in foster care (CDC, 2021). Also, teenagers may lack access to contraceptives and the education to use them properly. They may be afraid to ask for resources and fear judgment, which adds to risk of pregnancy and unsafe sex practices.

Partners of teen birthing parents can play an important role in the lives of teen birthing parent and newborns. Because teen parents are young and inexperienced, programs must be geared directly toward the parents and their specific needs. When programs meet the needs of the partners of teen birthing parents, they are more likely to participate (National Responsible Fatherhood Clearinghouse, n.d.). It has been established that partner involvement contributes positively to the outcomes in pregnancy (National Responsible Fatherhood Clearinghouse, n.d.; SmithBattle et al., 2019).

- A partner of the birthing parent who is emotionally supportive of their partner and actively helps raise the child and provides financial support, directly and indirectly, affects the well-being of the child.
- When the partner of the birthing parent is absent, children are at increased risk for behavioral difficulties and poor academic performance.
- When the teen partner of the birthing parent is involved in the preparation nad education of birth and early parenting, it benefits themselves, their partner, their babies, and the community (National Responsible Fatherhood Clearinghouse, n.d.).
- There are home visiting programs that include the partner of the birthing parent in the visits and activities (Nurse Family Partnership [NFP], 2023). This encourages a sense of inclusion and promotes healthy family relationships. Teens often feel misunderstood; this is even more true in the case of teen pregnancy. See Chapter 4 for research demonstrating the effectiveness of NFP.

The implications for the role of the C/PHN are greatest with the adolescent parent population. For example, nurses work with young teens through schools, clinics, or home visiting programs to ensure healthy pregnancies and teach parenting skills to the parents and grandparents.

- Nurses can ensure that the infant receives immunizations and primary care health services and reaches age-appropriate milestones. The nurse can also provide family planning information to the new parents.
- Teen birthing parents experience a profound disruption of life course development. C/PHNs can acknowledge this and recommend support groups and social events to provide a sense of normalcy.
- Teens may have trauma in their backgrounds that may not have been addressed. They may feel stigmatized, and this can prevent them from reaching out for help. C/PHNs can provide (and normalize) mental health resources and support that may disrupt the chain of trauma with the new baby.

- On a broader scale, C/PHNs should collaborate with other professionals to make sure that the community has resources for all levels of prevention, with a focus on primary prevention.

Families Headed by a Cohabitating Couple

Cohabitating couples' ages can range from young adults to older couples. The couples may be of any sexual orientation, and they may or may not share a sexual relationship. In some instances, these couples have their own biologic or adopted children. Cohabitation has become more common in America, especially among young adults. Roughly 9 million U.S. households were run by a cohabiting couple (Gryn et al., 2023). Fewer households led by a cohabiting couple had children in the home (3 million houses with children under 18) compared to couples with no children in the home (6 million) (Gryn et al., 2023). As young adults continue to put off marriage and parenthood, living with a partner creates a small family to enjoy life with.

Older couples may also choose to cohabitate after losing a spouse or experiencing loneliness but not wanting to go through a legal marriage. Like the other families mentioned in this chapter, cohabiting couples have become an accepted family structure in America.

LGBTQ+ Families

The Census Bureau included LGBTQ+ data for the second time in 2021, reporting roughly 1.2 million same-sex couples in the United States (Scherer, 2022). This family structure is increasing and, as any other family-type, requires health interventions aimed at their specific needs.

Healthy People 2030 addresses lesbian, gay, bisexual, and transgender health. The goal for the population is to improve the health, safety, and well-being of people in this group (HP, 2030). Specific *Healthy People 2030* objectives related to LGBTQ+ families are displayed in Box 14-5. The objectives speak to the importance of understanding the discrimination and oppression that LGBTQ+ families have faced. LGBTQ+ families have the same hopes regarding parenting that any family may have. In addition, they experience the stress that accompanies being stigmatized by much of society. It is critical that C/PHNs understand these challenges and care for families in a genuine and nonjudgmental way.

The nurse can become a valued resource for the family. Through education and anticipatory guidance, the nurse can help the family navigate the developmental stages of their children and the varied issues faced by families. The nurse can work with parents to anticipate what questions to expect from their children about their family.

Families With Older Adults

Aging is something that begins the day we are born; however, it is not focused on until a person turns 65 years or older or begins to experience declining health. It is often thought of as something negative rather than a process. Older adults are the fastest-growing segment of the population, and their value is often overlooked.

BOX 14-5 *HEALTHY PEOPLE 2030*

Objectives That Impact LGBTQ+ Families

Goal: Improve the health, safety, and well-being of lesbian, gay, bisexual, and transgender people.

Adolescents

LGBT-05	Reduce bullying of lesbian, gay, or bisexual high school students
LGBT-D01	Reduce bullying of transgender students

Drug and Alcohol Use

LGBT-07	Reduce the proportion of lesbian, gay, or bisexual high school students who have used illicit drugs
LGBT-D03	Reduce the proportion of transgender high school students who have used illicit drugs

Mental Health and Mental Disorders

LGBT-06	Reduce suicidal thoughts in lesbian, gay, or bisexual high school students
LGBT-D02	Reduce suicidal thoughts in transgender students

Public Health Infrastructure

LGBT-01	Increase the number of national surveys that collect data on lesbian, gay, and bisexual populations
LGBT-02	Increase the number of national surveys that collect data on transgender populations
LGBT-03	Increase the number of states, territories, and DC that include sexual orientation and gender identity questions in the Behavioral Risk Factor Surveillance System
LGBT-04	Increase the numbers of states, territories, and DC that use the standard module on sexual orientation and gender identity in the Behavioral Risk Factor Surveillance System

Reprinted from U.S. Department of Health & Human Services (USDHHS). (2020). *Healthy People 2030: Browse objectives.* Retrieved from https://health.gov/healthypeople/objectives-and-data/browse-objectives

Because Americans are getting older and families are getting smaller, there is an increase in older people and a decrease in adult children to care for them.

- In 2020, 56 million people in the United States were over the age of 65 years. This group is projected to increase to 73 million by 2030 (Agingstats, 2020).
- Many older adults live independently well into their 80s and maintain healthy contacts with family and friends.
- Others feel isolated because of chronic health problems that limit mobility, thereby reducing or eliminating the ability to interact or contribute meaningfully in society.
- The COVID-19 pandemic caused large periods of isolation and lack of relief for caregivers, with many community resources being shut down or limited.
- The way individual members of the family react to these factors will affect how the rest of the family copes. This is where the nurse can help.

The C/PHN needs to understand the complex dynamics of such situations and offer support and encouragement as family members work through chronic health problems. Adult children may become caregivers as their parents become older, which is a change in the family dynamic for nurses to keep in mind. Often, a nurse serves an entire community of older adults in an apartment complex in which residents are age 55 or older, an assisted living center, or a mobile home community, for whom maintaining wellness is the focus. Keeping physically active, eating healthy meals, receiving appropriate medical care and immunizations, and establishing and maintaining social contacts are some of the behaviors C/PHNs can encourage for the population to stay healthy well into old age. The community health nurse can intervene by advocating for the individual medical and social needs for older adults and involved caregivers.

Foster Families

Children removed from their families because of maltreatment due to abuse, violence, or neglect are often placed with foster families. In 2021, the number of children in foster care in the United States was down 11% from 2017, which is a 10-year low at 388,963 (Children's Defense Fund, 2023). This number was reached during the pandemic's isolation and could reflect that children were not in contact with as many mandated reporters.

- Foster families take a variety of forms, but all foster families have formal training to accept unrelated children into their homes temporarily, while the children's parents receive the help necessary to reunify the original family.
- Although this arrangement is not ideal, most foster families provide safe and loving homes for these children in transition.
- Black and American Indian/Alaska Native children are two to three times more likely to be in foster care as White children (Children's Defense Fund, 2023).
- Of every 1000 White children in the United States, 4.8% are in foster care compared with 9% of every 1000 Black children (Children's Defense Fund, 2023).
- Reunification with parents and foster placements was delayed during the pandemic due to court closures and related backlogs.

The pandemic led to isolation and less time spent in school and social environments. Even with the reduction in the number of children entering the foster care system, data regarding abuse and neglect were still astounding. In 2021, 583,476 children experienced abuse or neglect, which is roughly a child abused or neglected every 54 seconds in America (Children's Defense Fund, 2023). The C/PHN can assess families for feelings of overwhelm and frustration and offer opportunities for parenting education and self-care.

Implications of Family Composition Diversity for Community/Public Health Nurses

The variety of family structures raises three important issues for consideration:

- First, in order to be successful, C/PHNs must reassess their beliefs about what constitutes a family and must be prepared to work with and accept all types of families. Unless the C/PHN can accept the full array of family lifestyles and address the special needs of each, it is questionable whether they will be able to fully help the family and may even create additional challenges.
- Second, the structure of a person's family may change several times over a lifetime. For the person, each family form involves changes in roles, interaction patterns, socialization processes, and links with external resources. The C/PHN must learn to address clients' needs throughout these life changes, equipping people with the skills needed to deal with the inevitability of changing structures.
- Finally, each type of family structure creates different issues and problems that, in turn, influence a family's ability to perform basic functions. Nurses must identify and focus on strengths with families in planning nursing care (Robinson et al., 2022). This should be a community health nurse's starting point. What are the family strengths? How does the family see their strengths? All families have strengths, although sometimes these are not easily recognized. It is important for the nurse to identify these with the family's collaboration (Box 14-6).

The family is the basic unit of a community and a population. Maintaining the family's health transitions into the health of the community and population. Caring for family impacts the community's health, which in turn affects the population's health (APHN, 2022). This interdependence is evident even within the family because one

BOX 14-6 Questions the Nurse May Ask the Family

1. What are your strengths as a family?
2. If you had to tell me your three most favorite things about your family, what would they be?
3. Name one quality about a family member or caregiver that you really respect. Your partner? Your child?
4. What is your best memory of your family?

family member can positively or negatively impact other family members and the family unit itself. As a result, public health nurses must first understand what constitutes a "healthy family" so that they can use the nursing process with family-level problem-solving techniques for health prevention and promotion within the family and subsequently the community and the population.

Traits Associated With Healthy Family Functioning

A family is a health aggregate from the interrelationships of the family members. The health of the family is affected by each family member and all family members collectively. A healthy family promotes each family member's growth and resistance to illnesses so that the family's health can sustain members during times of crisis such as serious illness, emotional dilemmas, divorce, or death of a family member (Robinson et al., 2022). Conversely, a family with underdeveloped coping skills or a limited capacity for problem solving, self-management, or self-care is often unable to promote the potential of its members or assist them in times of need.

Adherence to cultural practices and family standards for family health can influence each member's health. In turn, these cultural norms dictate how family members will participate in their healthcare. This interlacing can either obstruct or facilitate the health of the family and the family members.

The description of a healthy family is challenging given the heterogeneity and subjectivity of the data related to family health. However, the following standards characterize a healthy family (Robinson et al., 2022):

- Communicates and listens
- Fosters table time and conversation
- Affirms and supports each member
- Teaches respect for others
- Develops a sense of trust
- Has a sense of play and humor
- Has a balance of interaction among members
- Maintains appropriate boundaries
- Spends quality time together
- Exhibits a sense of shared responsibility
- Teaches a sense of right and wrong
- Engages in rituals and traditions
- Shares a religious core
- Respects the privacy of each member
- Values service to others
- Admits to problems and seeks help
- Manages conflict and crisis when they occur
- Offers forgiveness, comfort, and support (Robinson et al., 2022, p. 6)

Healthy Communication Among Family Members

- Healthy families communicate in patterns that are regular, varied, and supportive (Fig. 14-3). Family communication impacts health and family functioning (Robinson et al., 2022).

Healthy families discuss problems, share ideas and concerns, and write or call each other when separated. They communicate through nonverbal means. This level of family communication sensitizes family members to one another. They watch for cues and verify messages to ensure understanding, which intensifies the family's recognition and dealing with conflict. Thus, a communicative family knows how to share and collaborate with each other.

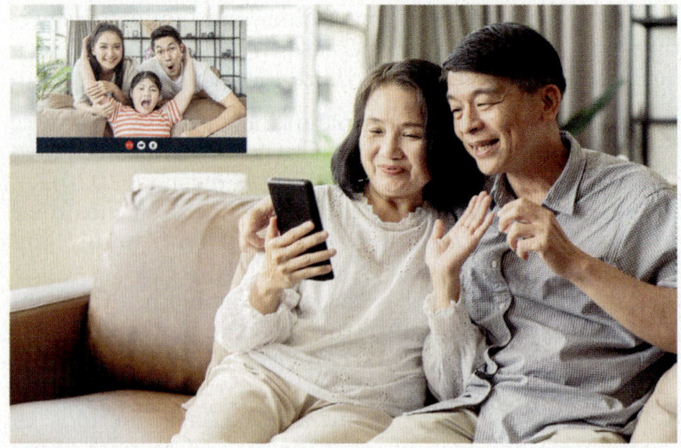

FIGURE 14-3 Good communication promotes healthy families.

Furthermore, family members use communication to demonstrate affection and acceptance, to promote identity and fellowship, and to guide behavior through socialization and social ethics. Importantly, effective communication patterns are associated with a family that promotes the health and development of each family member.

Enhancement of Family Members' Development

Healthy families respond to the needs of family members and provide the freedom and support necessary to promote each member's growth. A healthy family tolerates differences of opinion or lifestyle because each member has the right to be an individual, and the family respects this right. A healthy family encourages freedom and autonomy for each of its members, which contributes to the family's stability (Robinson et al., 2022).

Freedom and autonomy are supported even if the patterns of promoting family members' development vary from family to family. As a result, family members will experience increased competence, self-reliance, social skills, intellectual growth, and overall capacity for self-management among family members (Robinson et al., 2022).

Effective Structuring of Family Role Relationships

In healthy families, role relationships are structured to meet the family's changing needs over time (Robinson et al., 2022). In a stable society, families establish members' roles and tasks to maintain workable patterns throughout the life of the family. There is high role consistency because family members experience little to no external pressure or the need to change their role(s).

In a technologically advanced society, most families establish roles for the changing family needs that are created by external forces. The degree of role consistency is highly influenced by the permanency of the external forces on the family members' roles and expected tasks. Finally, changing life cycle stages require alterations in the structure of relationships. With each stage, family members change in their developmental needs so that the family must adapt their roles, tasks, and responsibilities in a healthy family (Robinson et al., 2022).

Active Coping Effort

Healthy families actively attempt to cope with life's problems and issues. When faced with a challenge, the family works together to meet the demands of the situation (Robinson et al., 2022).

Family members may pursue treatment opportunities for other family members to maintain the family's health. The collective support of family members may be essential for a family member to acquire any type of assistance outside the family. The healthy family recognizes the need for assistance, accepts help, and pursues opportunities to eliminate or decrease the challenges that affect it.

Even if most healthy families are dealing with less dramatic, day-to-day changes, healthy families remain receptive to innovation, new ideas, and creative and energetic ways to solve problems. Moreover, healthy families actively seek and use a variety of resources to solve problems, which may be internal or external within the family.

Healthy Environment and Lifestyle

Another sign of a healthy family is a healthy home environment and lifestyle. Healthy families maintain safe and hygienic living conditions for their members. Steps are taken to minimize the risk of injury or illness to any family member while maximizing the potential for health within the family.

A healthy family lifestyle encourages family members to find balance or harmony in their lives so that the family will have sufficient energy for daily living. A balanced and varied family diet is nutritious and appealing. Adequate physical activity helps to maintain a healthy weight while promoting cardiac health. Family members seek out and use health-care services and demonstrate adherence to recommended regimens. The emotional climate of a healthy family is positive and supportive of growth. Contributing to this healthy emotional climate is a strong sense of shared values, often combined with a strong moral–ethical orientation.

Regular Links With the Broader Community

Healthy families maintain dynamic ties with the broader community. They participate regularly in external groups and activities. They use external resources suited to family needs.

Healthy families also show an interest in current events and attempt to understand significant social, economic, and political issues. The families are exposed to a wider range of alternatives and a variety of contacts, which can increase options for finding resources and strengthen coping skills. Public health nurses need to assess and encourage a family's involvement within the broader community as it facilitates a relationship between the family and the community since healthy families make up healthy communities (Robinson et al., 2022).

FAMILY HEALTH NURSING: PREPARING FOR THE HOME VISIT

Because the nurse encounters most family members in their homes and neighborhoods, the focus of this section is on the home visit (Fig. 14-4). However, some nurses encounter families in other settings in the community, including on the streets, in shelters, and in the homes of relatives or friends. For more on family health nursing in nonhome community settings, see Box 14-7. Regardless of the family's location, the family is the client; the family is the unit of service in public health nursing (Robinson et al., 2022).

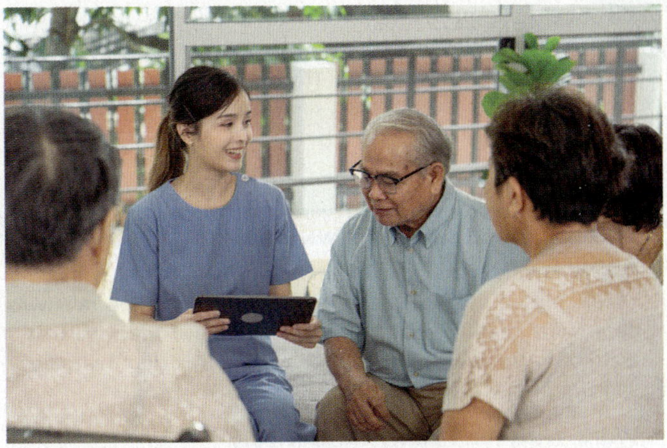

FIGURE 14-4 Family health assessments are foundational to the C/PHN's work with families.

In the unique setting of the patient's home, the nurse is permitted into the most intimate of spaces that human beings have. The key to this privilege is trust. Family members must have a certain amount of trust to let a stranger and representative of a governmental agency into their home. Family members believe that you are there to help enhance their ability to function as a healthy family with internal and external resources. In the same manner, the nurse must have a certain amount of trust to enter the family's home. Once the door closes, the nurse enters the client's world where they are the experts, and the nurse is the guest, a stranger. Nevertheless, you trust that the family welcomes your visit and is ready to work with you for healthier outcomes.

BOX 14-7 Working With Families in Nonhome Community Settings

There is a variety of nonhome settings or public places for visits to accommodate the family's schedules and routines provided the family member is comfortable with the nonhome setting. A visit may occur during a lunch break, after work/school, in a daycare or center for older adults, or public setting. Be mindful of maintaining a confidential atmosphere.

Visiting a family member in a public place can enhance the family assessment. It decreases the potential of issues in the home that impact the individual's response(s) to the questions. The nurse can assess a person's ability to function outside the home setting. The family member may feel comfortable talking about problems and issues related to the home environment away from other family members such as parents.

To be best prepared to enter a client's home, you must understand the skills of observation and communication, the components of the home visit, the various purposes for the home visit, and how to maintain your own personal safety while making the home visit. These topics are covered below. For general guidelines on public health nursing practice when the family is the client, see Box 14-8.

BOX 14-8 Public Health Nursing Practice Guidelines for Working With Families

The family is the unit of service in public health nursing (Robinson et al., 2022). The nurse assesses the family to determine what services are needed to move the family to a state of health, which can be determined by using five guidelines for practice.

Work With the Family Collectively

The family is a group of several people living together with a collective personality, collective interests, and a collective set of needs. The family functions collectively as a single entity with common attributes and activities so that all family members are involved in the nurse–client interactions (Robinson et al., 2022).

Start at the Family's Present Level of Functioning

The C/PHN begins by conducting a detailed family assessment to ascertain the needs and health level of each family member. The nurse can also recognize patterns of behaviors to determine collective interests, concerns, problems, risks, and priorities.

Adapt the Nursing Intervention to the Family's Stage of Development

Every family engages in the same basic functioning but not the same approaches to accomplish these functions within the family's development. A young family meets the family members' affiliation needs by establishing mutually satisfying relationships and meaningful communication patterns. The bonds of a family in the later stages of development change due to some family members becoming part of another family unit or family member(s) dying (Box 14-9). With this assessment, the nurse recognizes the family's appropriate level of functioning, determines the problems/risks, and implements the tailored interventions needed to move the family to a state of health (Robinson et al., 2022).

Recognize the Validity of Family Structure Variations

C/PHNs work with families from communities with varying family structures and individualized patterns of family functioning. The nurse must learn to understand and accept variations in family structure to address the needs of the families. Two principles guide this acceptance and understanding (Robinson et al., 2022):

1. Each family is unique in its combination of structures, composition, roles, and behaviors. This uniqueness is valid as long as the family functions effectively and demonstrates the characteristics of a healthy family.
2. Families are constantly changing throughout the life cycle, which leads to a family to adapt to its circumstances.

There may be a change in the family structure and the family members' roles due to internal and external environmental issues from the addition, loss, or alteration of persons related to the family. It is the C/PHN's responsibility to help the family to cope with these changes with a nonjudgmental and accepting manner about the family structure. As a professional, it is the nurse's responsibility to help promote the collective health of all families, despite any personal biases; all families are unique groups, each with its own set of needs that are best served through unbiased care.

Empower Families

Throughout the family visit, the public health nurse realizes that the ultimate goal is to assist the family in becoming independent of services (Robinson et al., 2022). This positive outcome is accomplished via the working nurse–family relationship, which can be guided by four suggestions:

- The current functioning of the family has worked for the family before meeting you.
- Before doing "something" for a family, consider who did this "something" before you.
- Find family strengths even in the most challenging and compromised family situation.
- Think about your ability to manage, cope, or function as well as the family members if you were in a similar situation.

With an **asset-based approach**, the nurse collaborates with the family to discern the family's strengths and positive potential embedded in weaknesses so that families feel empowered to handle challenges on their own. Regrettably, too often, C/PHNs perceive family weaknesses as *needs* or *problems*, which can undermine any hope of a therapeutic relationship between nurse and family as well as the use of an asset-based approach. It is the nurse's job to recognize the strengths in families and to help families recognize them and understand their potential for self-efficacy (Robinson et al., 2022). Focusing on a family's strengths sets the foundation for their future accomplishments. It also shows the family the genuineness of the nurse's wishes for the future of the family. This strengthens the relationships and connections between the nurse and family. C/PHNs must ensure that whatever assistance they offer/provide to a family will promote the family's independence and self-efficacy.

The C/PHN should be able to say, at the least, that the family is managing as best as possible so that the assessment can explore all aspects of family functioning, both positive and negative. It also emphasizes the positive outcomes, indicating to the family that they are important to the nurse—creating a collaborative relationship.

Through empowerment, the family can meet the needs of each family member and the demands made by systems outside the family unit. Of course, all behaviors must first be assessed in terms of promoting the family's functioning before being deemed a strength. Some behaviors that are considered as strengths are related to basic family functions, family developmental tasks, and characteristics of family health. Thus, it is the context in which the behavior exists that makes it a strength, not the behavior alone.

BOX 14-9 STORIES FROM THE FIELD

Factoring in the Ravina Family's Stage of Development

The Ravinas, a couple in their early 70s, recently moved to a retirement complex. They had received nursing visits after Mrs. Ravina's stroke 3 years earlier but requested service now because Mr. Ravina was feeling "poorly" all the time. He thought that perhaps his diet and lack of activity might be the cause and hoped the nurse might have some helpful suggestions. The couple had eagerly awaited Mr. Ravina's retirement from teaching, with plans to be lazy, travel, visit all their children, and do all those things they never had time to do when they were young. Now, neither of them seemed to have enough energy or the capacity to enjoy their new life. The move from their home of 28 years had been difficult: They were still trying to find space in the tiny apartment for their cherished books and mementos, although they had given many items away.

Ronald Bell, a C/PHN, recognized that the Ravinas were experiencing a situational crisis (leaving their home of 28 years) and a developmental crisis (aging and entering retirement) and may perhaps have some underlying health problems. Many of the Ravinas' expectations for this new life stage were unrealistic; they had not adequately prepared themselves for the adjustments that the loss of their home and retirement would demand. Through discussion, Ronald was able to help the Ravina family understand their situation and express their feelings. He completed physical assessments on the Ravinas and encouraged regular follow-up with their healthcare provider. He also helped them join a support group of retired people who were experiencing some of the same difficulties. Because this nurse was able to help the Ravina family through their crisis in a supportive and nonjudgmental manner, he found them receptive later to discussing preparation for the inevitable loss and bereavement that would occur when one of them died. He was adapting his nursing intervention to this family's stage of development.

1. *What concerns might the C/PHN have in this situation?*
2. *What strategies might the C/PHN employ for this situation?*

Skills Used During the Home Visit

Many skills are needed when assessing, diagnosing, planning, implementing, and evaluating families in their home at a variety of functional levels. Expert interviewing skills and effective communication techniques are essential for effective family intervention (see Chapter 10). Building rapport and a sense of comfort with a client is essential. A trusting relationship is the key to a productive home health visit and effective use of nursing skills (Healthy Families America, n.d.). Through home visits, nurses can assist families in promoting nurturing relationships leading to stronger family-centered healthy development (Healthy Families America, n.d.). The following paragraphs describe special skills required when making home visits.

Acute Observational Skills

You will be using your acute observational skills to assess both the family and the environment, which are equally important for a detailed assessment. This refers to the ability to take note of every detail (physical and nonphysical) that is directly and indirectly related to the family, the environment, the visit, and the entire process. Throughout the visit, the nurse focuses on the family members' concerns and the purpose of the visit, while being observant about the neighborhood, travel safety, home environmental conditions, number of household members, client demeanor, and body language, as well as other nonverbal cues. All this information contributes to understanding the family, identifying patterns, and recognizing how to navigate the neighborhood. Addresses on referrals may be incorrect, incomplete, or generally dubious. Confirm with the referring agency to identify any anomalies and environmental conditions in the neighborhood.

Observation of Home and Neighborhood Environmental Conditions. Conditions in the neighborhood and home environments reveal important information that can guide diagnosing, planning, and intervention with families. While traveling to and arriving at the family home, you have been gathering information about the neighborhood conditions and the physical appearance of the apartment or house. Observing the home environment conditions provides an assessment about the resources and barriers encountered by the family. The external environment may contradict the family's values, resources, and goals. They may have little control over the neighborhood or the building in which they live, especially if they are renting. Although these external factors may influence the behavior of the family, they may not define the behavior.

Observation of Body Language and Other Nonverbal Cues. You begin gathering data as soon as you knock on the door or ring the doorbell, greet the people in the doorway, and enter the home (Box 14-10). Observations of pre-visit nonverbal cues and body language contribute to your initial opinions and perceptions about the family. Also, *all* family members (present or absent) are doing the same with you (Box 14-11). Thus, you need to be aware of all family members; acknowledge and greet them. Inquire about those who are absent. Make this a habit on all visits. Each family member has opinions and healthcare needs, even if you only see certain members of the family on each visit.

Be observant of the family's nonverbal cues, such as body language and demeanor, because they provide information that must not be overlooked. Opening statements such as "You seem anxious today," or "Did I come at a bad time? You seem distracted," will encourage

BOX 14-10 STORIES FROM THE FIELD

A Home Visit to James Cutler and Brian Hoag

James Cutler and Brian Hoag have a 6-year monogamous relationship. A same-sex couple, they worked with an attorney to privately adopt a child. The arrangements were completed and their 2-week-old son, Adrian, arrived in their home last week. Helen Jeffers, a public health nurse, receives a referral from the county hospital where Adrian was born. The request is for an assessment of the home situation and parenting skills. At the hospital, the baby tested positive for cocaine with APGAR scores of 6 and 8 and had some initial difficulty sucking. Birth weight was 2900 g. Discharge weight, at 3 days, was 2850 g. At her first home visit, Helen finds a neat and orderly two-bedroom condominium that is well equipped with baby supplies. The infant has gained 200 g and is being well cared for by two fatigued parents whose previous contact with infants was limited. James and Brian have many questions and are anxious learners. Helen plans with the couple to make weekly home visits to assess infant growth and development, provide support, and answer questions. She suggests attending a neighborhood parenting class and finding a reliable babysitter. She also helps James and Brian develop an infant care work schedule. After 6 weeks of intervention, Adrian is thriving. Helen closes the case to home visits, feeling confident that the parents' goal of becoming knowledgeable and confident has been achieved.

1. *As the C/PHN, identify the family life cycle and developmental tasks of this family.*
2. *How can the C/PHN support this family in health promotion and education?*

family members to express what is on their minds, which otherwise might not be indicated or addressed. Through their facial expressions, hand gestures, subtle glances, eye movement, and body language, detailed information will be generated to address both direct and indirect concerns of the family. Overlooking body language makes it easy to continue with *your* agenda instead of the *family member's* agenda, although the family is distracted by another, more pressing issue.

Nonverbal Communication

It is equally important to be aware of your body language, which can tell the family a great deal about how you feel being in their home, dealing with the family members, and completing the home visit. Suggestive behaviors like fidgeting with car keys during the entire visit or appearing to be in a hurry or rushed can be perceived as nervousness, anxiety, or not wanting to be in the current situation. Minimal eye contact or continuously looking at your paperwork may be viewed as rudeness, unprofessionalism, and unknowledgeable about the family and the purpose of the visit. Your "fear" can be implied from the refusal to sit on any of the furniture or a shocked expression from a roach or mouse scampering across the floor. Your behavior impacts the family's trust in you, subsequent visits, and interventions.

Components of the Family Health Visit

The components of the family health visits align with the nursing process. Pre-visit preparation steps encompass assessment, diagnosing, and planning, which are necessary for implementation or completion of the actual family health visit. The documentation and planning for the next visit (or evaluation) terminates one visit and prepares the nurse for the next action needed.

Pre-Visit Preparation

Public health nurses identify preliminary family diagnoses and design a plan for the initial family health visit based on a referral to the agency. A **referral** is a request for service from another agency or person. They are the source of new cases and need timely responses. This request can be a form letter or the transferal of information from the originating agency to the receiving agency. Referrals may be formal (from primary providers or complementary agencies) or informal (verbal or telephone referrals from friends or relatives who believe that someone needs help). Some examples include the following:

- Labor and delivery hospital units request service for low birth weight babies and teen birthing parents.
- Social service agencies request a home assessment for a child being returned to parents after previous removal.

BOX 14-11 PERSPECTIVES

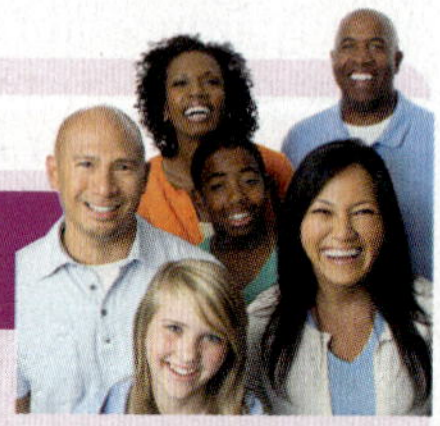

A C/PHN Nursing Instructor's Viewpoint on Home Visits—What Is Best for the Family Right Now

When making a home visit you usually have a goal. Your curriculum is planned, and you know the points you intend to make. However, when you enter the home, you can see that one member of the family is visibly upset. There is a baby crying in the crib and the other family members look exhausted. Would now be the time to pull out your carefully planned content and dive in?

Sometimes, our best laid plans are not appropriate. We need to engage the family and take time to really listen. Should we perhaps stop and ask the family what struggle they are facing? Will our teaching be effective if our topic of the day was to assist the family with healthy meal ideas, when they are dealing with a baby who is sick and kept them up all night? We can come back to our planned content later in the visit or at the next visit. When the C/PHN shows such consideration and compassion, the family is much more likely to keep their home visitation appointments. At every visit you should ask yourself, "What is best for the family right now."

Alice K., PHN

- A local health department may want a follow-up visit for an older adult who was seen for heat exhaustion.
- A shelter for people experiencing homelessness might be seeking services for people who are unsheltered or people in transitional housing showing signs of uncontrolled diabetes.
- A shelter for people experiencing intimate partner violence needs services to treat the emotional issues of both the person running from an abusive partner and their children.
- A person in a city 500 miles away requests that a nurse check on an older relative who lives alone in the community and has recently exhibited slurred speech or has been homebound.

Follow-up visits are based on the family's needs and agency protocol. Public health nurses must be equipped with the appropriate tools to establish a physical place to work:

- Access to a telephone, the internet, and other necessary resources
  - Educational material (pamphlets, brochures, and related web information)
  - Charting tools
  - Any other supplies required for home visits
- **Resource directory**, which is a list of resources for the broader community, or a nurse-made directory of resources created over years of working with people in the community
- A nursing bag or carryall tote (issued by an agency or devised by the nurse) for medical supplies
  - Specialized supplies depending on the visit (a tote for each type of visit)
  - Supplies to treat basic needs of a new parent and their infant or an older adult with hypertension

Once the nurse is prepared, the family is contacted to schedule a visit. The referral ideally contains a correct telephone number for the family, a relative, or a neighbor. The nurse needs to extract as much information as possible from the referral so that the preparation can be exact and specific for the health visit. This sets the stage for a thorough family assessment, appropriate family diagnosing, and family-oriented health promotion interventions (Robinson et al., 2022). If the referral does not contain this information, an unannounced visit is scheduled. During this visit, it is important to get a contact number for the family. When calling for the first time, you, the C/PHN, will do the following:

1. Introduce yourself.
2. Explain the reason for the call.
3. Give the reason why the family was referred.
4. Indicate what the visit will consist of.
5. Determine when a visit would be convenient for the family and you.
6. Get explicit directions to where the family is staying (the referral may have a different address, or the family did not mention that they are staying elsewhere).
7. Repeat the date and time of the scheduled visit.

The nurse's intention(s) may be questioned, with some people becoming defensive or suspicious. A new young parent may wonder, "Why is this nurse visiting me so close to my time in the hospital? Did I say or do something wrong with my baby when I was in the hospital?" The C/PHN will explain the following:

- The visit is a follow-up one to see if the move from the hospital to home went okay.
- The visit is an opportunity for them to ask questions that they might have about the baby since the return home. It is also a chance to learn more about handling the baby in the home, if needed.
- The visit is a service provided by the agency to all birthing parents.
- The visit is paid for by taxes or donations or by the client's health maintenance organization (if applicable). There is no direct cost to them or the family.
- The purpose of the visit is not to take anything away from the client but to provide resources, education, and information.

Following logical steps in the pre-visit preparation enhances the nurse's confidence in their ability to intuitively recognize patterns and trends from the referral information for preliminary diagnoses to guide preliminary care planning.

Making the Visit

It is recommended to call the family to remind them of the scheduled meeting and your arrival time prior to the scheduled visit. Restate the purpose of the visit and the anticipated length of time needed. Once you arrive, the following guidelines for initial contact should be used (Robinson et al., 2022).

1. Engage the family to build a supportive and trusting relationship (Box 14-12).
   a. Introduce yourself to the family.
   b. Explain the value of the nursing services provided by the agency.
   c. Spend the first few minutes of the visit establishing cordiality and getting acquainted (a mutual discovery or "feeling out" time).
   d. Become acquainted with all family and household members if you are making a home visit.
   e. Encourage each person to speak for themself.
2. Use acute observational skills.
   a. Use your "sixth sense" or intuition as a guide regarding family responses, questions they ask, and your personal safety (trust your feelings).
   b. Be sensitive to verbal and nonverbal cues.
   c. Be accepting and listen carefully.
   d. Be cognizant of possible internal and external stressors and effects on the mental status of family.
   e. Be aware of your own personality—balance talking and listening—and be aware of your nonverbal behaviors.
3. Help the family focus on issues and move toward the desired goals.
   a. Be adaptable and flexible (you may be planning a prenatal visit, but the person delivered their baby the day after you made the appointment, and now there is a newborn).

BOX 14-12 Developing a Trusting Relationship With the Stevenson Family

The public health nurse, Christopher, made an initial home visit after a referral by an outpatient primary provider who was concerned about possible child abuse. The primary provider suspected abuse after seeing bruises on the arm of a baby (Deshawn) who was in the emergency room for treatment of a laceration on the forehead. Tandrea Stevenson, the mother, claimed that the laceration resulted from Deshawn falling off a table when she was changing him. She also explained that the bruise happened when Larry (Deshawn's older brother) was playing too rough.

Christopher began the visit by stating that he was simply following up on the emergency room visit and wanted to see how Deshawn was progressing. Christopher made no mention of child abuse. He simply observed Tandrea and the children closely to learn more about the family's background and used the strengthening technique to create a trusting relationship interaction. Due to Christopher's supportive demeanor, Tandrea agreed to further visits, and at one of the visits, Tandrea confessed that her ring cut Deshawn's forehead when she tripped with him after smoking too much. "I could not get him to stop crying, no matter what I did," she whimpered. "I decided to smoke to calm my nerves but must have smoked too much and got dizzy." She also confessed that the bruises happened when she, not Larry, grabbed Eugene roughly to stop him from pulling and touching things he should not. Christopher learned that Tandrea's husband abandoned her while she was still pregnant with Deshawn.

Christopher realized that Tandrea would be particularly vulnerable to any criticism, so he concentrated on her strengths such as managing the home, dressing the children, and reading to little Deshawn. During subsequent visits, Tandrea and Christopher were able to discuss her feelings frankly and work toward improving the health of the Stevenson family. Tandrea started counseling to help with stress and her smoking habit, and she attended a support group for single parents counseling.

   b. Be aware that most clients are not extremely ill and have higher levels of wellness than are generally seen in acute care settings.
   c. Be prepared to develop a sustained continuity of care by actively collaborating with the family in addressing their issues.
4. Near the end of the visit, review the important points and emphasize the family's strengths.
5. Plan with the family for the next visit.

The length of the visit varies depending on its purpose and can influence the C/PHN–family relationship.

Less than a 20-minute visit:

- Not enough time for an initial intake, but ideal for
  - Dropping off supplies
  - Therapeutic conversation
  - Relaying information such as a referral
  - Sharing information
  - Stopping by at the family's request, such as for questions/concerns

More than a 60-minute visit:

- Avoid; not a productive way to provide nursing services.
- Any lengthy assessments should be conducted over two visits.
- Disruptive to the family with the potential for unwanted outcomes.
  - Families have routines that are important to them.
  - The family may feel that nothing of value occurred during a visit.
  - The family may not continue to make themselves available for future visits. This becomes a balancing act for the family and the nurse, and you may want to work at picking up on nonverbal cues.
- May reflect the nurse's hesitation in trusting the family to understand and follow the instructions and feedback.
- Limits the family's ability to seek out community resources for community-based healthcare.

Remember, the outcome of better health for family members must be demonstrated to support and validate the value and justify the cost of public health nursing services.

Concluding and Documenting the Visit

The current home visit concludes after planning for the follow-up visit with the family. You will say goodbye and pack up any paperwork, materials, and supplies used for this visit in your car.

Documentation or charting of each home visit should be completed according to the specific agency's protocol. It is important to be prepared for each visit of the day.

Agencies use various forms that help the nurse document fully and succinctly. Some forms use a checklist format that contains code numbers, letters, or checkmarks on developmental or disease-specific care plans. A four-paged postpartum visit and newborn assessment may consist of two narrative forms to chart the expectations for the birthing parent and baby plus two forms for the head-to-toe assessment of the newborn. There is a place to document parent teaching within the expected parameters and for listing other professionals' involvement with the family. Other forms may focus on chronic illnesses common in the agency's clientele (e.g., alcohol use disorder, chronic obstructive pulmonary disease, communicable diseases, diabetes, HIV/AIDS, hypertension).

Focus of the Family Health Visit

The focus of family health visits depends on the agency's mission and resources or services and the needs of the families. Some agencies provide education, recreational activities, and support groups for families of people with Alzheimer disease, asthma, or diabetes. Other agencies provide support for new parents, mental health concerns, or public health follow-up. In general, family health visits are designed to educate, provide anticipatory guidance, and focus on health promotion or prevention (Robinson et al., 2022).

Family Education and Anticipatory Guidance

Local health departments distribute their services based on the broader community's needs. The health department may contract with healthcare providers to treat a community with a high rate of teen pregnancies by offering educational classes at the local high school. The intervention may involve teaching prenatal, postpartum, and newborn care and providing anticipatory guidance to promote regular healthcare provider visits for the infant, immunizations, and safety awareness. The health department may address the needs of another community experiencing a significant number of illnesses in a particular zip code with vaccine clinics or treatment options.

Family Promotion and Illness Prevention

Family members can be taught health promotion activities for healthy living even within the limitations of chronic illnesses. These activities may include screening for hypertension and elevated cholesterol, performing a physical assessment, teaching about nutrition and safety, and promoting immunization.

Immunizations protect the health of all people and the larger community. Although such services are not brought into the home, it remains the C/PHN's responsibility to provide information about immunizations, teach the importance of following an immunization schedule, and follow-up with the family during home visits. A focus on population health shifts care to the community's needs and strengthens it on aggregate health promotion strategies that optimize personal health (APHN, 2022). Adding social determinants of health also contributes to the ultimate goal of creating "social, physical, and economic environments that promote attaining the full potential for health and well-being for all" (USDHHS, 2020, para. 4; see Box 14-13).

BOX **14-13** *HEALTHY PEOPLE 2030*

Selected Goals and Objectives Related to Family Health

Family Planning

Core Objectives

FP-01	Reduce the proportion of unintended pregnancies
FP-02	Reduce the proportion of pregnancies conceived within 18 months of a previous birth
FP-03	Reduce pregnancies in adolescents
FP-04	Increase the proportion of adolescents who have never had sex
FP-05	Increase the proportion of adolescent females* who used effective birth control the last time they had sex
FP-06	Increase the proportion of adolescent males* who used a condom the last time they had sex
FP-07	Increase the proportion of adolescents who use birth control the first time they have sex
FP-08	Increase the proportion of adolescents who get formal sex education before age 18 years
FP-09	Increase the proportion of females* who get needed publicly funded birth control services and support
FP-10	Increase the proportion of females* at risk for unintended pregnancy who use effective birth control
FP-11	Increase the proportion of adolescent females* at risk for unintended pregnancy who use birth control

Developmental Objectives

FP-D01	Increase the proportion of publicly funded clinics that offer the full range of reversible birth control

Adolescent Health

Core Objectives

AH-01	Increase the proportion of adolescents who had a preventative healthcare visit in the past year
AH-02	Increase the proportion of adolescents who speak privately with a provider at a preventive medical visit
AH-03	Increase the proportion of adolescents who have an adult they can talk to about serious problems
AH-04	Increase the proportion of students participating in the School Breakfast Program
AH-05	Increase the proportion of 4th graders with reading skills at or above the proficient level
AD-06	Increase the proportion of 4th graders with math skills at or above the proficient level
AH-07	Reduce chronic school absence among early adolescent
AH-08	Increase the proportion of high school students who graduate in 4 years

(*Continued*)

BOX **14-13** *HEALTHY PEOPLE 2030 (Continued)*

Developmental Objectives

IVP-D03	Reduce the number of young adults who report 3 or more adverse childhood experiences
EH-D01	Increase the proportion of schools with policies and practices that promote health and safety

Maternal, Infant, and Child Health

Core Objectives

Morbidity and Mortality

MICH-01	Reduce the rate of fetal deaths at 20 or more weeks of gestation
MICH-02	Reduce the rate of infant deaths

Infant Care

MICH-14	Increase the proportion of infants who are put to sleep on their backs
MICH-15	Increase the proportion of infants who are breastfeed exclusively through age 6 months

Health Services

MICH-08	Increase the proportion of pregnant women* who receive early and adequate prenatal care
MICH-19	Increase the proportion of children and adolescents who receive care in a medical home
MICH-20	Increase the proportion of children and adolescents with special healthcare needs who have a system of care

Developmental Objectives

MICH-D01	Increase the proportion of women* who get screened for postpartum depression

*In this box, "male" refers to a person assigned male at birth, "female" refers to a person assigned female at birth, and "women" refers to people assigned female at birth. Reprinted from U.S. Department of Health & Human Services (USDHHS). (2020). *Healthy People 2030: Browse objectives.* Retrieved from https://health.gov/healthypeople/objectives-and-data/browse-objectives

C/PHNs provide health promotion services during a family health visit in any setting. During prenatal classes, the C/PHN teaches couples about the expected changes during pregnancy, signs of preterm labor, and provides anticipatory guidance for safe infant care and postpartum care (NFP, 2023). The C/PHN screens older adults for hypertension or elevated cholesterol at the center for older adults, educates family members attending Alcoholics Anonymous, or provides mental and health assessments for people in shelters.

Personal Safety During the Home Visit

Being streetwise is essential when interacting and traveling throughout communities. Continuation of personal safety must be considered while maintaining respect for the families, a trusting relationship, and professionalism.

Traveling to and in the Neighborhood

When leaving your "base of operation," make sure you have all the necessary supplies, materials, and paperwork for the scheduled home visits. To ensure safety and promote coordination with your agency, always inform your agency about your planned itinerary and all contact information. Most agencies will have specific information they would like on file for each home visit on your schedule. It is important that someone knows where you are throughout your workday.

Requirements of traveling in an agency or private car:

- A full gas tank
- Addresses for families you are visiting, city/county map, or GPS
- A cell phone

Requirements of using public transportation:

- Change/bus card or smartphone app for each bus trip
- A current bus schedule
- Knowledge of the exit at the bus stop closest to your family's home
- Knowledge of the bus stop for the return trip to agency or to the next home visit
- A cell phone

You should ***always*** call ahead to the family and give them an estimated time of your arrival. Be "streetwise" when walking in neighborhoods. A C/PHN understands the value of safety measures used by expert nurses, following these measures for personal safety, and not challenging them. Another focus of concern is the perceived risk to self when making a home visit. Feeling and being safe can relate to the nurse's perception of a situation, views on risk-taking, awareness of the traveling conditions (e.g., the time and the setting), and coping process. What one person sees as a risk, another sees as a challenge or an opportunity, and another may see nothing.

We each perceive risks differently based on knowledge, experience, and personality.

Arriving at the Home

Make sure you are at the right house. Do not go into the home until you are assured that the family you are intending to visit does live there and is home. You are scheduled to visit 16-year-old Fatema and her 5-day-old infant, Dajon. A 60-year-old man answers the door when you knock. Give your name and ask if Fatema can come to the door because you are here to see her. Do not enter the house even if he invites you in to wait for Fatema. Smile and let him know that you are comfortable waiting for Fatema at the door. Remain outside the house and go inside ***only after*** you talk to Fatema at the door. This precaution ensures that the family members you want to visit are in the house and that this is the right address.

Dealing With Challenging Situations

Due to the nature of the home setting, you may encounter unexpected and challenging situations, including family conflict, family members under the influence of a substance, and the presence of strangers.

Friction Between Family Members. During a home visit, two or more family members may begin to argue or physically fight. You should immediately terminate the visit and inform the family what will take place regarding the home visit. Follow these steps:

1. Inform the family that the visit is now terminated.
2. Calmly let the family know that such distraction takes away from the purpose of the visit.
3. Inform the family that you will return at another convenient time.
4. Calmly and quickly remove yourself from the home.

When two or more family members are physically fighting, never intervene, try to stop the fight, serve as a referee, or assist an adult family member. You may be the next victim. Once you are out of the house, call 911, if necessary, from your cell phone. Once you are safe, rely on your acute observation skills to recall the altercation. These data may provide significant information about the family's structure, process, and health. Depending on your assessment and processing of the information, it may be appropriate to discuss the altercation and the friction in the family at a later visit.

Family Members Under the Influence. If the focus of the visit is on two family members, but a third member's behavior suggests the use of drugs or alcohol, use your judgment as to the best action to take. It is important for you to assess the situation and proceed accordingly within the parameters of guidelines provided by your agency or your school. If the person who is under the influence goes to another room and remains quiet/calm, it might be appropriate to continue the visit. You might want to discuss your observations with the two family members. If the person who is under the influence remains in another room but interrupts the visit by being abusive or distractive, it is best to terminate the visit. Let the two family members know that you want to reschedule when the third family member is not under the influence or is not present. Never put yourself in the middle of a situation that could deteriorate rapidly and compromise your safety.

The Presence of Strangers. In some families, it is common to have extended family members, neighbors, and friends present in the home. This may be the norm for the family but not for the nurse because it may be a different setting from their experience. The nurse may have to weave their way past five teenagers sitting on the front stoop to enter the home and step over three adults sleeping on the living room floor in the small apartment of a teenage parent and their infant. Children may be riding their bikes inside the house during a teaching visit to two young parents, who do not seem fazed by the commotion. These situations may not be indicative of danger, but they can make you feel vulnerable and uncomfortable and distract you from the purpose of the visit. Always rely on your observation skills; inquire about the people you observe in the periphery of the home visit; ask about their relationship to the family and if they should be included in the visit. The family may suggest that you ignore these people or say they are family members in transitional housing. It may be important to learn who they are, if they have unmet healthcare needs, or if their presence influences the health of the family you are visiting.

APPLYING THE NURSING PROCESS TO FAMILY HEALTH

The nursing process (assessing, diagnosing, planning, implementing, and evaluating nursing care) includes steps used to deliver care to families and aggregates in community health settings. These steps are, interestingly, the same ones used to care for clients in acute care settings and in the extensive clinic system. The difference in implementing this process in family health nursing is the context (the home), the client focus (the family), and the consideration of external variables not typically encountered in other contexts. In C/PHN, addressing the health needs of the core unit of service (in this case, the family) should always transition to addressing the health needs of the community and the population. The context and application of each step are tailored to the needs of the population by focusing on the core unit of service (APHN, 2022).

The nursing process commences on the first visit when the public health nurse performs an initial assessment (Box 14-14). Subsequent visits entail the nurse and the family working collectively to reach the targeted goals.

Preliminary Considerations

Before implementing the nursing process, the nurse must establish (1) a conceptual framework, (2) a clearly defined set of data collection categories, and (3) a method of measuring a family's functional level.

Conceptual Frameworks

"Nursing is a scientific discipline; thus, nurses are concerned about the relationships between ideas and data" (Robinson et al., 2022). Nurses use theory to help explain

BOX 14-14 C/PHN USE OF THE NURSING PROCESS/CLINICAL JUDGMENT

Family Health

Assessment/Recognize Cues
According to the American Nurses Association (ANA), the Nursing Process is the common thread that unites all specialties of nurses (ANA, n.d.). When CPHNs enter a home, one of their first tasks is to conduct a family assessment. Much like in the hospital, the nurse will make observations, ask questions, and begin to build a picture of the health of the family unit. This is considered the family assessment.

Diagnosis/Analyze Cues and Prioritize Hypotheses
Once the C/PHN can identify themes (both positive and negative), the family's strengths and weaknesses come to light. Like a diagnosis, this provides direction for the nurse to apply the interventions.

Planning/Generate Solutions
The nurse creates a family plan with specific goals and interventions to help the family reach a higher level of health and functioning.

Implementation/Take Action
The family comes to an agreement with the C/PHN, and community resources and tools are used to effectively work toward agreed-upon goals.

Evaulation/Evaluate Outcomes
The C/PHN will follow up and continually evaluate the effectiveness of the interventions by speaking with the family and examining the outcomes achieved.

phenomena and in family health theories can help nurses determine effective interventions for families. According to Robinson et al. family social science theories are the best for use with families. These theories and models include family functions, the environment–family interchange, interactions and dynamics within the family, changes in the family over time, and the family's reaction to health and illness (Robinson et al., 2022).

Other theories used in family health are nursing models/theories and family therapy theories, but they are not as developed as family social science theories. Frameworks guide the nurse in family health nursing. There is no one theory that is perfect for working with families, and the nurse should base the choice of a theory that fits each family's needs.

Even though these frameworks reflect models used by C/PHNs, they are the foundation for various methods of family assessment. Their concepts come together to design family assessments, diagnosing process, and intervention models.

Data Collection Categories

The **conceptual framework** gives the nurse a format to group the data about the family into specific categories to organize the collected data. These data may be useful for assessing, diagnosing, care planning, and serving as a guide for subsequent visits in which to obtain additional information. Data collection should include both subjective and objective data.

Methods of Measuring a Family's Functioning

Family function includes the relationships, interactions, and structural properties within the family system in which communication, conflict, cohesion, adaptability, and organization are assessed. The C/PHN will evaluate the strengths, resources, and protective factors of a family including any underlying behaviors that might create unsafe conditions.

Family Health Assessment

A thorough family health assessment relies on the public health nurse's commitment to understanding the family, determining the value of the referred information, and processing any prior opinions about the family to promote family health. See Box 14-15 for guidelines that can help the C/PHN conduct a detailed family assessment and organize data. See Box 14-16 for an application-oriented exercise in conducting a family assessment.

Assessment Methods

Assessment methods generate information about selected aspects of family structure and function, while matching the purpose for assessment. An informal approach consists of the nurse's acute observational skills and occasional questioning to confirm the observations and determine the next direction to take. A formal approach entails the use of specific questions and assessment tools to assess each family member in terms of health data, family history, physical data, family development, or potential health problems not detected by family members.

The **genogram** (Fig. 14-5) diagrams the family's genealogy, relationships, and complex family patterns. This tool is helpful as the C/PHN examines the strengths and weaknesses of the family (Robinson et al., 2022). Completing the genogram with the family encourages family expression, which can reveal family behavior and problems. Knowing a family's health and social history can be useful in linking health outcomes to preventive strategies based on potential health risks and guiding clinical and public health interventions (Centers for Disease Control and Prevention [CDC], 2024).

The **eco-map** (Fig. 14-6) shows the connections between a family and the other systems in the ecologic environment. A central circle represents the family or family member with smaller peripheral circles indicative of people and systems significantly relating to the central circle. Connecting lines between the central circle and smaller ones depict the strength of relationships.

Public health nursing agencies usually develop their own tools to fit organizational needs (for examples of family assessment tools, visit https://www.cdc.gov/public-health-gateway/php/public-health-strategy/public-health-strategies-for-community-health-assessment-models-frameworks-tools.html). One type of family assessment tool uses questions based on characteristics of healthy families and follows a checklist format

BOX 14-15 STORIES FROM THE FIELD

Assessing the Beck Family's Nutritional Status

A public health nurse had initial contact with Mr. and Mrs. Beck and their youngest child at the well-baby clinic. The 9-month-old child was over the 95th percentile for weight and at the 40th percentile for height. The nurse also noted that both parents had obesity. The nurse asked about the family's eating patterns, the baby in particular, and suggested a home visit to determine whether the Becks were interested in family nursing. The nurse explained the purpose of home visits (to assess all family members, coping patterns, eating patterns, and food purchasing choices) and the importance of including all family members and asked for a time that would be good for the family as a whole. The nurse explained that each person should be involved and committed to the agreed-upon goals and that, like a team of oarsmen, the family has to pull together to accomplish the purpose of the visits. To help the Beck family improve its nutritional status, the nurse might suggest a session of brainstorming to uncover many causes of poor nutrition. More brainstorming might also lead to more solutions and plans for action. On each visit, the nurse views the Becks as a group, so group responses and actions would be expected. Evaluation of outcomes will be based on what the family did collectively. The Becks were interested, and a home visit date was made.

1. *What developmental stages appear to have been achieved?*
2. *What is your plan of action for this family over the next three visits?*
3. *What are the goals for this family (immediate, midrange, and long-term)?*

that is useful to observe family growth or decline over a span of time. The novice C/PHN can use this tool to gather data and to document how the nurse's rapport develops with the family and the PHN's comfort level.

Another type of family assessment tool has an open-ended format that allows the nurse to create an informative document while limiting subjective observations (https://www.cdc.gov/public-health-gateway/php/public-health-strategy/public-health-strategies-for-community-health-assessment-models-frameworks-tools.html). A self-care assessment guide examines a family member's ability to provide self-care by measuring the family's stressors and self-care practices. This tool is used adjunctively, especially with families from various cultural groups. Videotaping is a method used to assess family interactions for structured observations and analyses of life-changing events. Using it with other tools enhances the breadth of data collection.

BOX 14-16 STORIES FROM THE FIELD

A Family Assessment for Lorenzo

You are a C/PHN assigned to a small suburb in Chicago. Your new client is Lorenzo, a 103-year-old White American adult. He is being released from the geriatric ICU of Uptown Hospital after being treated for severe pneumonia, three episodes of delirium, and pressure injuries. He resides in his own house in the center of Othertrackside. The local hospital is the only medical facility with a geriatric unit in a 75-mile radius that will accept Medicare clients.

His respiratory complications started 4 weeks ago. He experienced shortness of breath and pain with breathing after working in his garden 3+ hours at 43°F temperature while it was raining. The frequency and severity of the respiratory problems resulted in Lorenzo significantly decreasing his activities while increasing his time in the bed. When he was rushed to the hospital, due to severe chest pains and arrhythmia, his neighbor Adam, a 97-year-old African American individual, expressed to the admitting nurse, "Please help Lorenzo feel better; he has not been himself. He will not even speak to his sister and brother when they make their occasional visit or any of the neighbors who stop by to check on us." The nurse later discovered that Lorenzo and Adam are in a 50+ year commited relationship.

Your job is to facilitate Lorenzo's return to his home from Uptown Hospital, assist him in regaining his prior level of activity, and address issues affecting his mental health. The teaching over your scheduled visits will include, but is not limited to, the following:

- Signs and symptoms warranting follow-up
- Medication and administration
- Nutrition and fluid consumption
- Bladder, bowel, skin, and mental healthcare
- Activities of daily living and instrumental activities of daily living
- Physical activity/endurance
- Safety/injury prevention
- Altered significant other/family/neighbor processes
- Community resources

Consider the following questions:

1. *How will you empower the family to avoid Lorenzo's isolation (self-imposed and socially constructed), risky behavior, and potential for nonadherence to his treatment?*
2. *How would you prioritize Lorenzo's issues, both medical and psychosocial?*
3. *As the public health nurse, what interventions can you utilize to achieve the indicated goals without offending, embarrassing, alienating, or "outing" the core family system?*

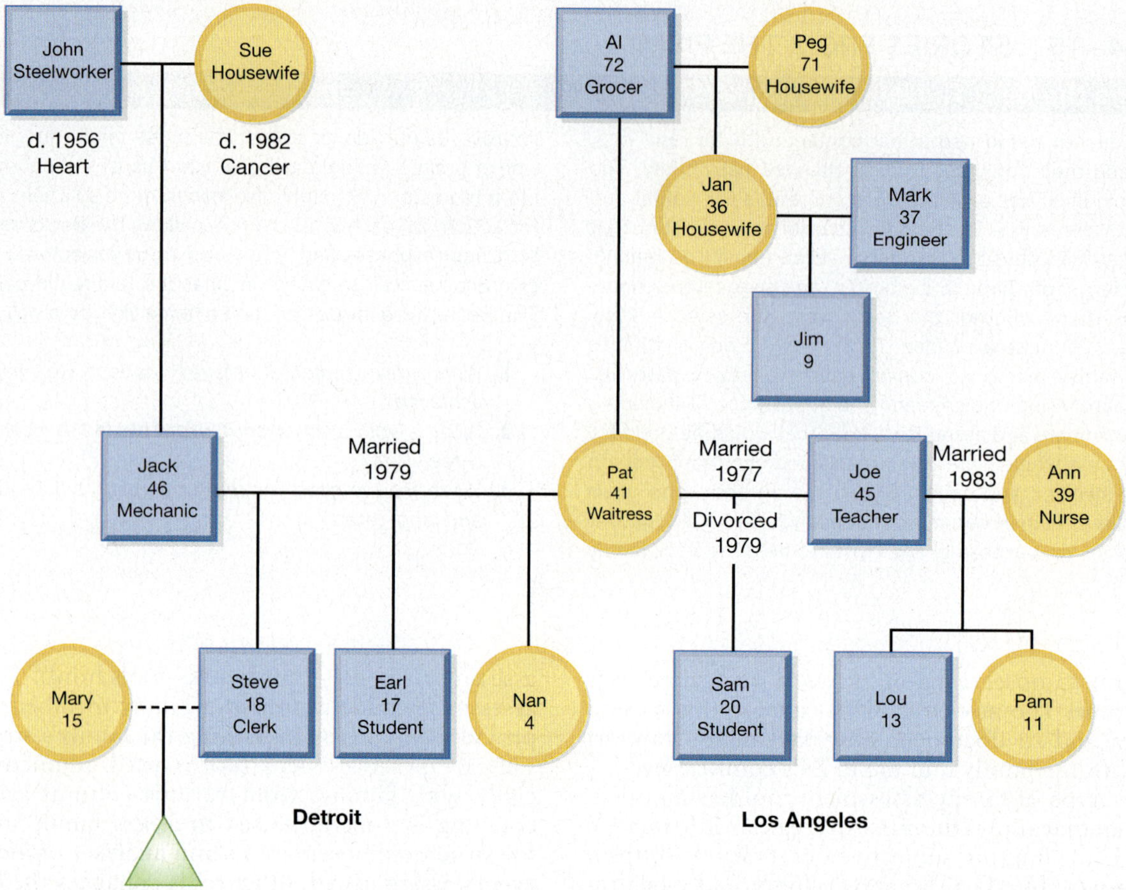

FIGURE 14-5 A genogram.

Guidelines for Family Health Assessment

Since a family health assessment results in a voluminous amount of data, there are five guidelines to use. These guidelines emphasize the family as the core service unit and will strengthen your ability to work collaboratively with the family—promoting a trusting relationship.

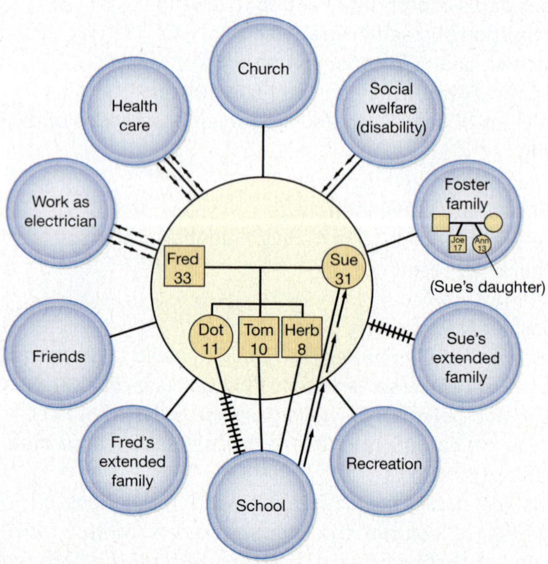

FIGURE 14-6 An eco-map of a family's relationship to its environment.

Focus on the Family as a Total Unit. The family is a single core service unit, and it is the family's aggregated behavior being assessed (APHN, 2022). The C/PHN ensures that the information is typical of the entire family.

Encouraging families to share their stories can be a health promotion tool by creating meaning for people and the family. The story can inform nurses what is important to the family and help develop interventions. Nurses can begin by asking the family "Who are you from?" rather than "Where are you from?"

When assessing the communication patterns of two family members, the nurse also considers how other family members communicate among themselves and with the two being assessed. After analyzing the data, the nurse may decide that the family communicates well and supportively even if one family member does not. The nurse documents this deviation and considers it in the care planning.

Ask Goal-Directed Questions. Nurses should be aware of their own communication style and how it may differ from the family's. The connections made in home visits depend upon successful and open communication between the family and the nurse. Goal-directed questions can help families share their perspectives while providing the nurse information for potential family goal setting.

Examples of goal-directed questions include the following (Robinson et al., 2022):

- How have you been talking about the situation you find yourselves in? Who has been involved?
- What sustains you in challenging times?
- Different family members have different talents or strengths: How do you most want to be involved?
- What have you found most helpful or useful to you as a family now?
- How are important decisions made in your family? How would you like important decision making to go now?

Thus, you watch everyone closely for signs of the family's response(s) to challenges and the ability to problem-solve any problems resulting from the challenge. Another more open-ended format or approach is to use assessment categories to stimulate questions to explore family support systems for a specific category.

Collect Data Over Time. Your approaches may include observations, interviews, identification of family strengths and weaknesses, and reflection after family visits (Robinson et al., 2022).

Timeliness also helps to develop a trusting and supportive relationship with the family since assessment can occur during any family activity such as mealtime. The family needs to feel comfortable with you, the observing nurse. Even if the C/PHN feels welcomed and comfortable at the initial home visit, it may take the family several visits to reciprocate that level of comfort.

Combine Quantitative With Qualitative Data. Both qualitative and quantitative data are collected when appraising a family's health and are used to create a database for planning care. Asking if family members engage in some type of behaviors is qualitative, and asking how often the family engages in the behaviors is quantitative.

One type of assessment tool evaluates a family's ability to enhance individuality by rating the family's behavior on a scale of 0 (never) to 4 (most of the time), which provides a way to compare the family's development over several home visits. The difference between the present and previous scores assists the C/PHN in executing the intervention(s). For this reason, it is useful to conduct periodic assessments when a case is reopened or every 3 to 6 months if it is kept open for an extended period.

Exercise Professional Judgment. The nurse may observe that a family makes good use of a community agency, but the decision that using this external resource contributes to the family's health results from a professional judgment. An assessment tool is only a tool, and its value should never be interpreted as an absolute and irrevocable statement about a family's health status.

As a professional, the C/PHN knows that the completion of an assessment tool should occur at the end of the home visit(s). The C/PHN may review the assessment tool before entering a family's home or keep it in a folder for easy reference or note during the visit. However, the assessment tool is not completed in the family's presence. Even with an eco-map or genogram, the C/PHN uses professional judgment to determine when the family is ready.

Family Health Diagnosis

The family diagnosing process moves the data from assessment to care planning, implementation, and evaluation. This process is an expected standard of practice for public health nurses (APHN, 2022). The C/PHN uses observational skills and clinical reasoning to understand the patterns in the data.

Specifically, the C/PHN identifies patterns of behavior, barriers preventing the family from being healthy, and internal relationships with the external environment (APHN, 2022). Next, the nurse prioritizes the information while taking the best action(s) for the desired outcome or goal (Robinson et al., 2022). The diagnosing process can occur as follows (Robinson et al., 2022):

1. Identify the family health problems.
   a. Determine what family members are directly and indirectly related to the problem.
   b. Determine what factors from the external environment are related to the problem.
   c. Describe the problem as it impacts the identified family members and external environment.
   d. Indicate the risks that are associated with the problem(s).
   e. Prioritize the problems along with their risks with an emphasis on the problems that are overlapping and have overlapping risks.
2. Indicate the factors from the family (family unit and family members) and the external environment associated with the health problems.
3. Determine the measurements (quantitative and qualitative data) that confirm or verify health problems.

The diagnosing process is an ongoing one with two major goals: improve the family health and give them the tools for health promotion. It should be completed several times, especially with a lot of assessment data so that the nurse can craft a plan of care to move the family toward a state of health.

Family Health Planning and Implementation

Planning, intervention, and evaluation for families should be viewed through the lens of health promotion and disease prevention. C/PHNs are familiar with health promotion frameworks and principles (Robinson et al., 2022). This approach allows family empowerment and reduces health inequities. The nurse will consider barriers to health and the social determinants of health.

Robinson et al. (2022) recommend using three frameworks to guide C/PHN intervention work with families and communities: the Alma Ata Declaration on Primary Health Care, the Ottawa Charter for Health Promotion, and The Health Promotion Model. Brief descriptions of each framework are provided below:

- The Alma Ata Declaration on Primary Health Care includes five main principles based on the social determinants of health. The principles include health promotion, accessibility, public participation, appropriate technology, and intersectoral collaboration.
- The Ottawa Charter for Health Promotion includes strategies to empower families to take control of their health. This framework uses five strategies: develop

personal skills, create supportive environments, build healthy public policy, strengthen community action, and reorient health services.

- The Health Promotion Model includes key assumptions to guide interventions. The key assumptions include recognition of determinants of health, the use of knowledge gained from research and practice, collaboration with families about the most appropriate action to care for them and building relationships with families based on mutual response and caring rather than on professional power (Robinson et al., 2022; see Chapter 11).

Health promotion and disease prevention frameworks provide the C/PHN guidance in planning, implementing, and evaluating interventions in an effective way.

Implementation includes making referrals and contacting appropriate resources.

Making Referrals

The nurse makes a referral so that the family can have access to services that might be beyond the agency's resources. The referral reflects the nurse's knowledge of resources within the community, which includes the eligibility requirements and availability of services, provided by official, voluntary, religious, and neighborhood organizations (Robinson et al., 2022). The nurse must also be aware of any updates or changes to the information about these organizations. Therefore, C/PHNs need to network with colleagues on a regular basis in order to remain up-to-date with community services for family referrals (APHN, 2022; Robinson et al., 2022).

Contacting Resources

Public health nurses know how to access key personnel in agencies, which can eliminate some of the red tape involved in obtaining services, while giving family members pointers on procuring needed services. When C/PHNs seek informal services for families, the nurse establishes a relationship with the agency's staff that can help nurses secure services for the family over time. This rapport can also be used to connect with other agencies, which increases the nurse's database of services.

Family Health Evaluation

Evaluation represents the final step in the nursing process and involves appraising the work with the family and preparing for the next visit. A formal evaluation concludes with the documenting of the outcomes, which facilitates the nurse in making appropriate referrals and contacting key resources to meet the needs of the family.

The components of the evaluation are the structure–process, the outcome, and the nurse's self-evaluation. Each one contributes to determining what made the visit a success and what made it less than successful by evaluating if the outcomes were achieved and if they can be advanced to the next level of family health. The nurse must be prepared to determine if a change is needed in the structure process, the nurse's level of preparedness, or the nurse's behavior to promote health in the family, the community, and eventually the population.

Structure—Process Evaluation

The structure–process evaluation should be completed first as it refers to the organization of the visit and how it proceeded. The nurse identifies where the organization or the flow of the assessment needs to be changed or modified to avoid distractions in the next visit.

Specifically, the nurse will analyze the available resources, number of persons present, timing of home visit(s), environmental factors, or materials/supplies used as well as the use of observational skills, people's attitudes, and reliance on standards of assessment and analysis. Every aspect must be used in the evaluation to effectively and thoroughly modify subsequent visits.

Outcome Evaluation

The **outcome evaluation** facilitates the nurse in deciding if the anticipated outcomes were achieved and what made them possible. This outcome evaluation, a formal appraisal process, happens with documentation of the home visits. The effectiveness of any achieved outcomes is determined with standards and agency-driven criteria.

The standards are the Nursing Outcomes Classification System, the Nursing Intervention Classification System, and the Omaha System (see Chapter 15). The agency-driven criteria may be the successful achievement of the indicated expectations for each client category or visit type. Evaluating the outcomes with the agency-driven criteria may be more exact if the effectiveness is demonstrated by small changes over time in the family dynamics as noted on a visit-by-visit basis instead of cumulatively as represented in the standards. Therefore, the nurse must use professional judgment to determine the success or failure of the family to achieve certain outcomes at the conclusion of agency services, with the family included in the decision process.

Self-Evaluation

The self-evaluation encompasses the nurse appraising the ability to facilitate the desired outcome during the home visit(s), the level of being prepared, the thoroughness in data collection, the degree of preparedness for subsequent home visits, and the pros and cons of completed home visits. In other words, this self-evaluation affords the community/public health nurse the opportunity to recognize their strengths and failings with internal measures to improve practice (Edelman & Kudzma, 2021).

In some agencies, routine peer evaluations are conducted to recognize strengths and weaknesses not indicated in a self-evaluation. The peer evaluation can be completed by an agency staff nurse who makes a family visit with the community/public health nurse and provides feedback based on their observations. This might be helpful when working with a family that has not made progress toward the desired outcomes. Another effective way for nurses to self-reflect is to have one-on-one meetings with program leaders (Harpin et al., 2022). These meetings provide the nurse with encouragement, empowerment, and a safe space to seek advice or guidance.

SUMMARY

- Because today the family is recognized as an important unit of service, an effective C/PHN must understand family theory and characteristics. Family health and individual health strongly influence each other, and family health affects community health.
- Although every family on the globe is unique in terms of its needs and strengths, each family is at the same time alike because of certain shared universal characteristics: every family is a small social system, has its own cultural values and rules, has structure, has certain basic functions, and moves through stages in its life cycle.
- The C/PHN needs to understand the different needs of various family patterns. Whereas the single adolescent parent needs the community health nurse's knowledge of family developmental theory, more complex interaction patterns and living arrangements are created by divorce, remarriage, the blending of families, and the unique relationships these arrangements create. LGBTQ+ families with children may also have specific needs, calling for a sensitive understanding of society's reaction to their family.
- The essential starting point in the community health nurse's work is to accept the family's definition of who their family is and listen to the family's ideas. The nurse and the family become partners in providing healthcare, with the nurse beginning the work by assessing the family's strengths, which will begin to build a positive relationship between the nurse and the family. The family unit remains the focus of service in public health nursing because each family member strongly influences the other, which affects the community's health.
- Healthy families demonstrate six important characteristics. These characteristics provide one assessment framework that public health nurses can use.
- Making family health visits is a unique role for nurses and is one of the activities common to most public health nurses.
- The nurse's preparation for the visit facilitates (1) an orderly and organized flow for the visit and (2) the nurse becoming acquainted with the family, which is indispensable for the comprehensive execution of the nursing process and development of a trusting relationship.
- For a comprehensive assessment, C/PHNs employ acute observational skills, good verbal and nonverbal communication, assessment skills, and intuition to guide them safely in the community and with the families they visit.
- The family is a total unit or single entity, and the nurse must consciously recall this point through the home visits and every stage of the nursing process, especially during assessment.
- To systematically assess a family's health, the nurse needs a conceptual framework, categories for data collection, and a measure of the family's level of functioning.
- The main broad categories of a family health visit are pre-visit preparation, the conduct of the visit, post-visit documentation, and preparation or planning for the next visit. Each step contributes to the success of the subsequent one.
- There are specific precautions for safety that a nurse must follow if using a personal or agency car or public transportation or walking to visit families. Safety must be considered in a family's home even if it means terminating the visit and rescheduling.
- The nurse empowers the family by establishing a verbal or written contract with the family so that the family members (1) understand their personal roles and responsibilities in the relationship and (2) feel confident in making independent decisions about their own health.
- The C/PHN makes referrals to other agencies on behalf of the family in order to provide all the services that a family needs; therefore, the C/PHN needs to know how and where to locate official and voluntary services within their community.

ACTIVE LEARNING EXERCISES

1. Listen to two to three stories on StoryCorps (https://storycorps.org/). What did you learn? Are there themes that you recognize among the stories? (Objective 1)
2. Analyze two families you know well (other than your own) and answer the following questions:
   a. If the financial providers were unable to work or lost their job(s), how would the family respond immediately and in the long term? (Objective 2)
   b. What are the strengths of the family?
   c. How could a nurse most effectively intervene in this situation (unable to work or loss of job)?
3. Talk with members of a family that is different from yours? Discuss the relationships with each member. What strengths can they identify in their family? How has this helped them adapt? (Objective 3)
4. Construct an eco-map of your family and ask a peer to do the same, which can be completed face-to-face or online (i.e., Google Docs). Compare the eco-maps. Assess the balance between your family and the resources in its environment. How does your eco-map compare with that of your peer? What changes are needed in each family system? Are you able to influence the changes that are needed? (Objectives 3 and 4)
5. Using "Build a Diverse and Skilled Workforce" (1 of the 10 Essential Public Health Services; see Box 2-2), watch one of the two YouTube videos, A Day in the Life of a Public Health Nurse (https://www.youtube.com/watch?v=n8FvhaMvcDQ) or A Day in the Life-Mary (Public Health Nursing) (https://www.youtube.com/watch?v=fGj5wncmuX0), with one or

two classmates. Evaluate the public health nurse in terms of structure–process and outcomes and a peer evaluation of the PHN. With your classmates, discuss the PHN's strengths and weaknesses, and identify what actions you would emulate, change, or leave as is. Identify five instances in the video that made you feel uncomfortable, discuss with your classmates why these occurrences affected you, and discuss ways to process these feelings. (Objectives 5, 6, and 7)

CHAPTER 15

Community as Client

"Of all the forms of inequality, injustice in health is the most shocking and inhumane."

—Martin Luther King Jr.

KEY TERMS

- Assets assessment
- Community as client
- Community development
- Community-oriented, population-focused care
- Community subsystem assessment
- Conceptual model
- Descriptive epidemiologic study
- Key informants
- Partnerships
- Priority setting
- Problem-oriented assessment
- Social determinants of health (SDOH)
- Windshield/familiarization surveys

LEARNING OBJECTIVES

Upon mastery of this chapter, you should be able to:

1. Assess a community utilizing the characteristics of the community from a population perspective.
2. Develop plan of care based on the prioritized needs of a community.
3. Conduct a windshield survey to gain knowledge of a community
4. Use the Minnesota Wheel to develop interventions that are focused on the person, the community, and the systems.
5. Participate with community partners/stakeholders to address community concerns.

INTRODUCTION

When you open the door of a center for older adults where you will be promoting cardiovascular fitness, advocating for exercise equipment, and suggesting changes in the on-site meal program, how might theories of public health nursing contribute to your success? When you approach your city council about the need to increase staffing for public health services, what models of public health nursing practice might support your argument? What are *theories, models, principles, and frameworks*, and what is their relevance to day-to-day public health nursing practice? These are the key issues explored in the first three sections of this chapter.

The remainder of the chapter explores the definition of a healthy community, the dimensions of the community as client, and the application of the nursing process to the community as client. Included in this discussion are the types of community needs assessment, methods of collecting and sources of community data, data analysis and diagnosis, and making, implementing, and evaluating plans for community health promotion.

WHEN THE CLIENT IS A COMMUNITY: CHARACTERISTICS OF COMMUNITY/PUBLIC HEALTH NURSING PRACTICE

Community and public health nurse (C/PHN) is a specialty in which the unit of care is a specific community or aggregate, and the nurse has a responsibility to promote group health. The goal of this specialty is health improvement of the community.

- Some of the skills required for excellence in public health nursing practice include epidemiology, research, teaching, and managing programs and influencing health outcomes.
- Public health nursing is characterized by community-oriented, population-focused care and is based on interpersonal relationships. In the following sections, each of these characteristics is examined in more depth.

A community is a collection of people interacting with one another because of geography, common interests, circumstances, characteristics, or goals/actions.

These interactions are facilitated through social institutions, such as schools, government agencies, and social services. The concept of **community as client** refers to a group or population of people as the focus of nursing service (Zeydani et al., 2023).

As described in Chapters 1 and 2, understanding the concept of the community as client is a prerequisite for effective service at every level of community nursing practice. Population-focused practice distinguishes C/PHN from other nursing specialties (American Nurses Association [ANA], 2022; American Public Health Association, Public Health Nursing Section, 2013).

Community orientation is a process that is actively shaped by the unique experiences, knowledge, concerns, values, beliefs, and culture of a given community. For example, when an outbreak of hepatitis occurs, the C/PHN does more than simply treat infection in people. The nurse also does the following:

- Uses disease investigation skills to locate possible sources of infection (see Chapter 7)
- Determines how the community's knowledge, values, beliefs, and prior experiences with infectious disease may influence its interpretation of the disease, response to the outbreak, acceptance of protective measures, and treatment preferences
- Works in collaboration with other health professionals and uses knowledge and suggestions gathered from the community to develop a community-specific program to prevent future outbreaks

A C/PHN who provides education about sexually transmitted diseases to a group of students at a Catholic university includes consideration of community values regarding sexual behavior. Similarly, a community-oriented nurse who provides nutritional counseling to a community of Hispanic older adults considers the meaning of food in their culture, the types of food most commonly consumed, and the cooking methods most commonly used.

A *population* refers to all people occupying an area, such as a city, county, or state. Parts of populations may be subpopulations or aggregates. Smokers and refugees are two examples of subpopulations. The nurse's place of employment commonly limits the population that the nurse serves. For example, a nurse who works for a county health department may be limited to caring for the residents within the geographical boundaries of that county.

A *population focus* requires that a nurse use population-based knowledge and skills such as epidemiology, community assessment, and community organizing as the basis for interventions. For example, a population-focused nurse employed by an autoworkers' union may study all cases of repetitive use injury occurring in the auto industry in the United States in the past 5 years, develop a program for reducing repetitive use injury, and lobby industry executives for adoption of the program.

Community-oriented, population-focused care is shaped by the characteristics and needs of a given aggregate, community, or population. For example, when C/PHNs count and interview people that are unsheltered and sleeping in a park and, based on these data, help develop a program to provide food, clothing, shelter, healthcare, and job training for this population.

THEORIES AND MODELS FOR COMMUNITY/PUBLIC HEALTH NURSING PRACTICE

As a nursing specialty, C/PHN is not only guided by theories and evidence that pertain to the nursing profession but also by theories and evidence that have been specifically developed and tested for the specialty. Borrowed and shared theories are also major parts of the practice of community and public health nursing. Examples of shared theories are health behavior, social cognitive theory, and diffusion of innovations.

A theory is based either explicitly or philosophically on a **conceptual model** (also referred to as a conceptual framework, a conceptual system, or a paradigm). These concepts are presented in a framework format used to explain the relationships among variables.

Betty Neuman's Systems Model provides a comprehensive holistic and system-based approach to nursing that contains an element of flexibility (Fig. 15-1). The theory focuses on the patient's response to actual or potential environmental stressors and the use of primary, secondary, and tertiary nursing prevention intervention for retention, attainment, and maintenance of patient system wellness. Table 15-1 shows an example of applying Neuman's model to the anxiety of older adults waiting for a colonoscopy.

Salmon's Construct for Public Health Nursing

Salmon proposed a model to specifically guide community health nursing practice. Salmon (1982, 1993) described public health as an organized societal effort to protect, promote, and restore the health of people and public health nursing as focused on achieving and maintaining public health.

The model describes three practice priorities:

- Prevention of disease and poor health
- Protection against disease and external agents
- Promotion of health

The three general categories of nursing intervention are as follows:

- Education that is directed toward voluntary change in the attitudes and behavior of the subjects
- Engineering that is directed at managing risk-related variables
- Enforcement that is directed at mandatory regulation to achieve better health

The scope of practice spans individual, family, community, and global care. Interventions target determinants in four categories: human/biologic, environmental, medical/technologic/organizational, and social.

Using Salmon's approach, a C/PHN attempting, for example, to reduce the transmission of COVID-19 would use education, engineering, and enforcement in working with the population of affected people and

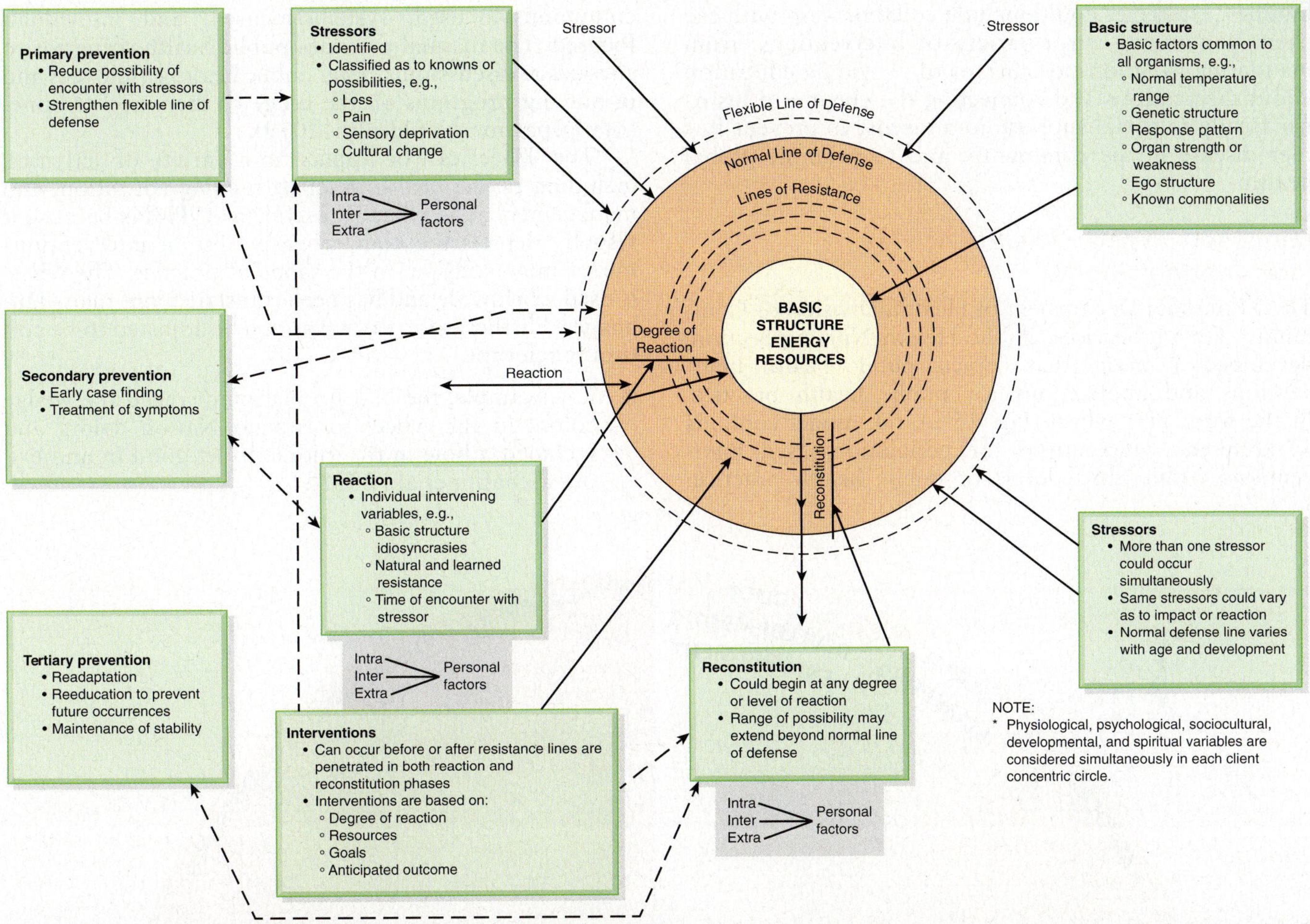

FIGURE 15-1 Neuman's healthcare systems model. (Adapted with permission from Neuman, B., & Fawcett, J. (2011). *The Neuman systems model* (5th ed., Fig. 1–3, p. 13). Pearson. Original diagram copyright © 1970 by Betty Neuman.)

TABLE 15-1 Applying Neuman's Model to Anxiety of Older Adults Waiting for Colonoscopy

Part of Model	Description	Application to anxiety related to colorectal cancer screening
Flexible line of defense	Buffer that expands and contracts to protect normal line of defense from stressors.	Primary prevention efforts include culturally competent education on risk factors for colon cancer and promoting health through regular exercise, healthy eating, limiting alcohol consumption, and not smoking.
Normal line of defense	Typical responses to stressors; changes over time. Behaviors strengthen or weaken this line in response to stressors.	Promotion of regular medical care, routine screenings, and maintaining a healthy weight.
Lines of resistance	These lines are final protection for the central core.	Providing culturally competent smoking cessation, healthy eating, and exercise programs. Encouraging referrals to nutritionist and medical specialists for continued follow-up of early signs/symptoms. Education on importance of continuing medications, diet, and exercise.
Central core	This component is the basic client system structure common to all people.	Colorectal cancer may be influenced by genetic factors as well as strengths and weaknesses of the system parts.
Stressors	These can originate in the external or internal environment.	Stressors include: ▪ Intrapersonal (within the self—e.g., how one deals with stress) ▪ Interpersonal (a result of how one copes with others/family/work) ▪ Extrapersonal (from outside the self—e.g., discrimination, financial crisis, no health insurance, limited healthcare providers)

Source: Larijani, F., Fotokian, Z., Jahanshahi, M., & Tabi, S. R. (2021). Application of Neuman's model on anxiety of older adults waiting for colonoscopy. *Nursing and Midwifery Studies, 10*(4), 236–242. https://doi.org10.4103/nms.nms_77_20

families. Strategies could include collaboration with the client community on a variety of interventions, from mandating isolation precautions to providing education about medications and connecting the client and his or her family to social support, in an effort to prevent further disease in the community and to promote global health.

Minnesota Wheel: The Public Health Interventions Model

The Minnesota Department of Health, Division of Community Health Services, Public Health Nursing Section, developed a model that depicts public health interventions and applications for public health practice. In the form of a wheel (Fig. 15-2), the model contains 17 different interventions for population-based interventions within three levels of public health practice: community-focused, systems-focused, and individual-focused. The manual provides public health scenarios to encourage discussion among public health employees and in nursing programs on the usage of the wheel (Minnesota Department of Health, 2019).

The Wheel can be applied in a variety of activities, including public health practice, nursing education, and management. The wheel is useful for C/PHNs because it visually depicts the comprehensive list of interventions nurses must consider in the scope of practice. The wheel is used worldwide and has been translated into many languages. Furthermore, the wheel can be adjusted to be culturally relevant.

- For example, the Navajo Nation changed the wedge colors in the wheel to Navajo Nation colors and included a hole in the middle to let good in and evil out (Schaffer et al., 2022).

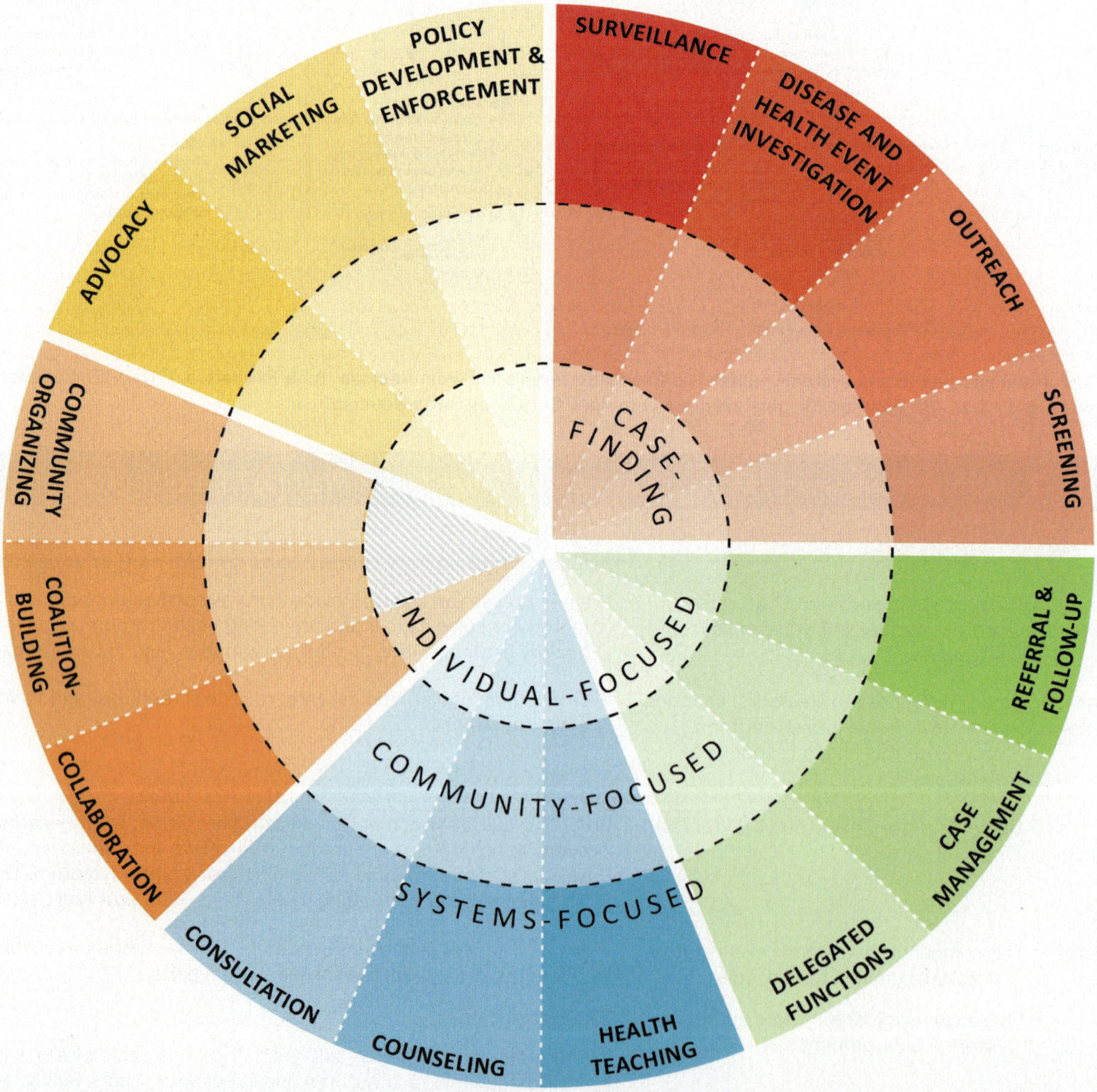

FIGURE 15-2 The Minnesota wheel. (Reprinted with permission from Minnesota Department of Health, Division of Community Health Services, Public Health Nursing Section. Retrieved from https://www.health.state.mn.us/communities/practice/research/phncouncil/docs/PHInterventions.pdf)

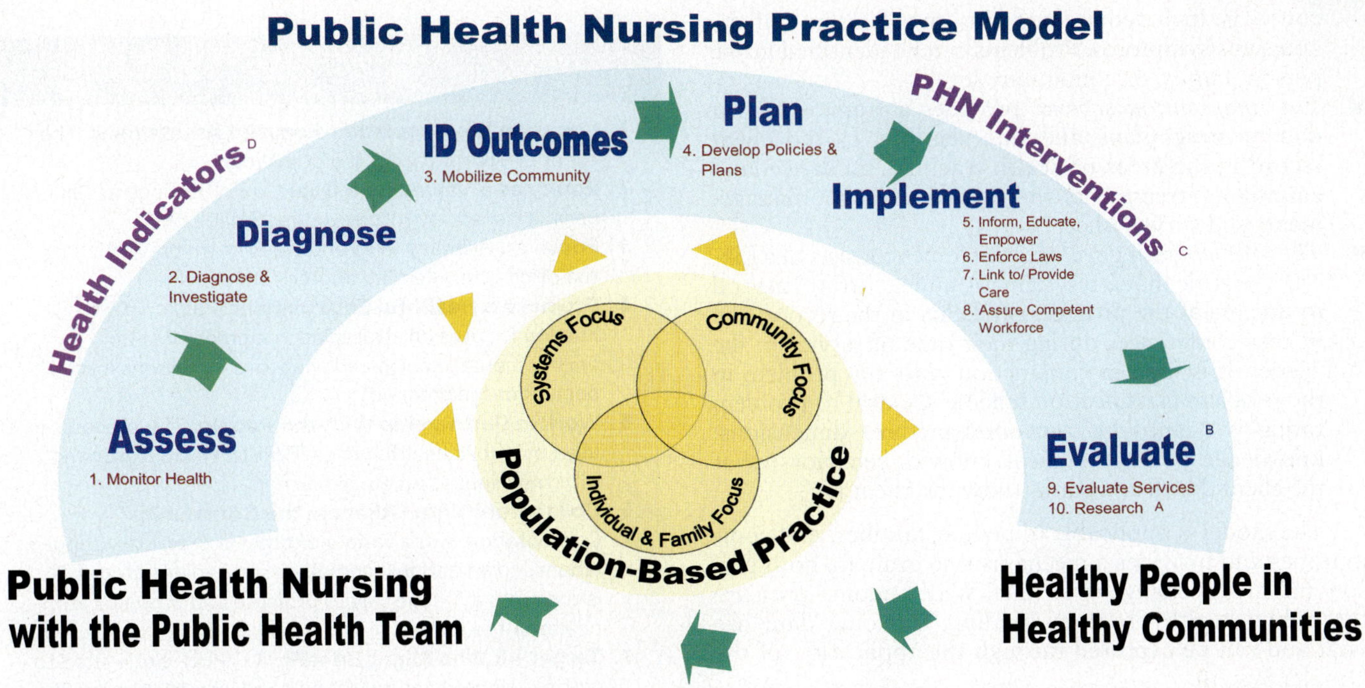

FIGURE 15-3 Public health nursing practice model. (Reprinted from the Los Angeles County Department of Public Health, Public Health Nursing. Retrieved from http://publichealth.lacounty.gov/phn/docs/PracticeModelFinal2.pdf)

Public Health Nursing Practice Model

The LAC PHN Practice Model (Los Angeles County Department of Health Services [LAC-DHS], 2013) integrates foundational nursing and public health guiding documents, including the Public Health Nursing Standards of Practice, the 10 Essential Public Health Services, the *Healthy People* health indicators, and the Public Health Nursing Practice Model (Fig. 15-3). The model has 10 criteria to consider:

- Concentrates on the entire population
- Focuses on the greater good rather than the individual or group good
- Designs conditions the people can grow in
- Utilizes population health statistics
- Considers determinants of health
- Applies the three levels of prevention, while emphasizing primary prevention
- Accounts for the three levels of focused practice
  - Individual, community, and systems focused
- Seeks out those who would benefit from services, rather than those who seek assistance
- Partners with other professions and organizations (LAC-DHS, 2013)

The principles of population-based practice are included in the LACDHS PHN Practice Model (LAC-DHS, 2013). C/PHNs integrate assessment, policy development, and assurance into their work. The three levels of population-based practice—people and families, community, and systems—are addressed, with the nursing process applied throughout the model. The 17 interventions, as first presented in the Minnesota Public Health Nursing Model described above, are also incorporated into the LAC-DHS PHN Practice Model.

Omaha System

The Omaha System (Fig. 15-4) is a multidisciplinary interface that incorporates documentation of assessment, care planning, and evaluation (Martin, 2005). This system consists of three relational components:

- *The problem classification scheme* is a holistic, comprehensive method for identifying clients' health-related

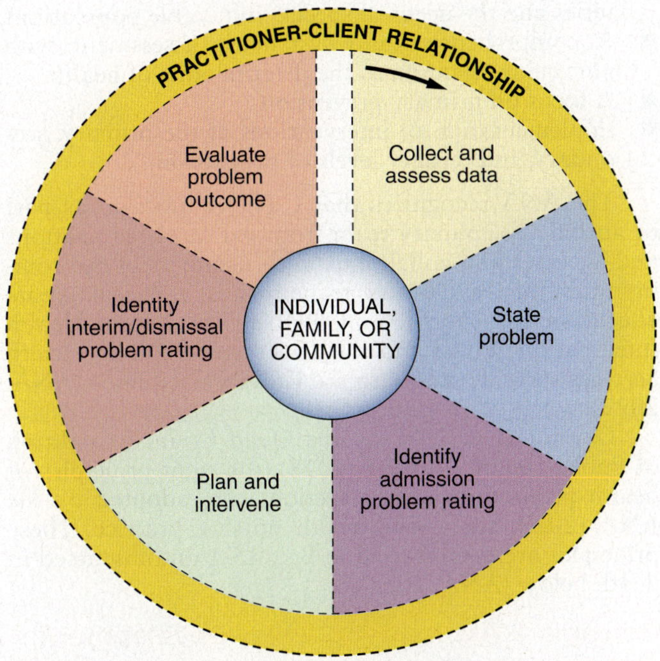

FIGURE 15-4 Omaha system model of the problem-solving process. (Reprinted with permission from Martin, K. S. (2005). *The Omaha System: A key to practice, documentation, and information management* (2nd ed.). Health Connections Press.)

concerns. Included are domains, problems, modifiers, and signs/symptoms. Problems can be identified at the person, family, or community level.

- *The intervention scheme* provides a framework for documenting plans and interventions in the client record in the areas of health teaching, guidance, and counseling; treatments and procedures; case management; and surveillance.
- *The problem rating scale* for outcomes consists of a Likert-type scale that is a systematic and recurring method to document the progress of clients in the record and in case conferences during their time of service in the agency. It is used in conjunction with any problem in the problem classification scheme. Central to problem rating is quantifying outcomes in three dimensions: knowledge (what the client knows), behavior (what the client does), and status (how the client is).

The model is applicable to people, families, and communities and provides a mechanism to evaluate both person and group change over time. With ongoing pressure for public health program funding, outcome data are vital and can be captured through the application of the Omaha System.

PRINCIPLES OF COMMUNITY/PUBLIC HEALTH NURSING

Public health nursing is "…the practice of promoting and protecting the health of populations using knowledge from nursing, social and public health sciences… [It] focuses on improving health outcomes by addressing social, physical, environmental, and other determinants of health…" (ANA, 2022, p. 2). The key elements of this practice include (ANA, 2022) the following:

- Population-level focus on issues including health inequities and the needs of special vulnerable populations
- A comprehensive and systematic assessment with particular attention to the determinants of health
- A focus on primary prevention
- Implementation of interventions at the primary, secondary, and tertiary levels of prevention

The ANA recognizes that C/PHNs function as part of an interdisciplinary team from various organizations and agencies and collaborate with members of the communities they serve and recommends a baccalaureate education for entry-level C/PHNs. The Public Health Intervention Wheel and the 10 Essential Public Health Services serve as guides to the C/PHN's activities (ANA, 2022).

Developed in 1997 by the Quad Council Coalition of Public Health Nursing (2018), the eight principles of health promotion and protection were adopted by the ANA (2022) for public health nursing practice. These principles are summarized in Box 15-1 and discussed in depth below (ANA, 2022).

BOX 15-1 Principles of Public Health Nursing

1. **Focus on the Population-Focused Assessment**. The client or unit of care is the population.
2. **Equity as a Value and a Goal**. Equity, defined as fairness, is necessary for the optimal health of all.
3. **Focus on Primary Prevention**. Primary prevention is the priority in selecting appropriate activities.
4. **Promote a Healthful Environment**. Public health nursing focuses on strategies that create healthy environmental, social, and economic conditions in which populations may thrive.
5. **Work in Partnership With the People**. The processes used by public health nurses (C/PHNs) include working with the client as an equal partner.
6. **Collaborate With Others in the Community**. Collaboration with a variety of other professions, populations, organizations, and other stakeholder groups is the most effective way to promote and protect the health of the people.
7. **Target All Who Might Benefit**. A C/PHN is obligated to actively identify and reach out to all who might benefit from a specific activity or service.
8. **Promote Optimum Allocation of Resources**. Optimal use of available resources to ensure the best overall improvement in the health of the population is a key element of the practice.

Adapted from American Nurses Association (2022, pp. 19–20).

Principle 1: Assessment, Policy Development, and Assurance

The primary focus of C/PH practice is on the core public health functions. Systematic and comprehensive population-focused assessment reminds us that the ultimate responsibility of public health nursing is to direct services to the population as a whole. Policy development and assurance activities are equally foundational in that they provide the basis for C/PHNs care for populations (CDC, 2022a). Even though PHNs may engage with families and groups, their primary responsibility is to the population as a whole (ANA, 2022).

Principle 2: Equity is a Core Public Health Value and a Goal

The second principle deals with the ethical obligation of the C/PHN to ensure optimal health and well-being for all members of the population. By collaborating with a diverse range of stakeholder groups, C/PHNs deliver the 10 essential services, which focus on achieving fairness for all (ANA, 2022) and give priority to the needs and preferences of the whole community over those of one person.

Principle 3: Focus on Primary Prevention

The third principle of public health nursing underscores the importance of primary prevention in promoting the health of people, as well as health protection. Public health nursing has an obligation to prevent health problems and injuries and to promote disease prevention strategies (ANA, 2022).

Principle 4: Strategies for Healthy Social, Environmental, and Economic Conditions

The fourth principle of public health nursing underscores the importance of addressing social determinants of health, including strategies developed through collaborative and participative problem-solving with affected community members. Advocacy and the impartation of advocacy skills are critical for addressing these issues (Dawes, 2020).

Principle 5: Partnerships Promote a Healthful Environment

The fifth principle requires the C/PHN to work in partnership with the community. The nurse and the community members (or groups) each bring their own values, beliefs, and expertise to the partnership (Yasmin et al., 2022). This includes being aware of "…perspectives, priorities, and values of the population when interpreting data, making policy and program decisions, and selecting appropriate strategies for action." (ANA, 2022)

Principle 6: Collaboration Across Organizations, Disciplines, and Stakeholder Groups

The sixth principle underscores the importance of collaboration with other nurses, healthcare providers, social workers, educators, spiritual leaders, business leaders, and government officials within the community. This interdisciplinary collaboration is essential to execute effective programs and improve health outcomes. Involvement of healthcare systems, legislative action, and social policy agendas can be leveraged to advance solutions for the populations served.

Principle 7: Target All Who Might Benefit

The seventh principle involves outreach strategies to meet the obligation to serve all people who might benefit from an intervention. This tenet requires that the nurse examine policies or programs to determine whether they are accessible and acceptable to the entire population in need and advocate for change if necessary (Ervin & Kulbok, 2018).

Principle 8: Optimal Use of Resources and Creation of New Evidence-Based Strategies

The last principle addresses resource allocation decisions. In most communities, the available resources are not sufficient to meet all needs of all people. The nurse must ensure that the community is using limited resources in ways that lead to the greatest improvement in health (Kavanagh et al., 2022).

- Know the latest research on the effectiveness of various programs in addressing needs
- Collect information about the short- and long-term costs of programs
- Evaluate existing programs and policies for ways to improve or discontinue them
- Communicate this information to community decision makers, so that they can make resource allocation decisions that are most likely to improve the community's health

C/PHNs should continue to work on all levels to promote greater funding for public health programs and more effective allocation of resources.

WHAT IS A HEALTHY COMMUNITY?

Just as health for a person is relative and will change, all communities exist in a relative state of health. A community's health can be viewed within the context of health being more than just the absence of disease and including things that promote the maintenance of a high quality of life and productivity. A key vision for healthy communities is presented in *Healthy People 2030*, the national agenda for health and well-being authored by the Office of Disease Prevention and Health Promotion (ODPHP) (n.d.) (see Chapter 1).

Healthy People 2030 objectives and targets provide guidelines for communities to follow to promote the health of their members. By encouraging collaboration across communities, empowering people to make better choices, and measuring progress toward set benchmarks, *Healthy People 2030* can be used as a road map for achieving longer and healthier lives for people living in the United States.

DIMENSIONS OF THE COMMUNITY AS CLIENT

The health of a community can be characterized through a number of perspectives. Donabedian's classic theory of structure, process, and outcomes provides unique insight into the health status of the community (Donabedian, 2005).

- *Status/people* is the most common measure of the health of a community. It typically comprises morbidity and mortality data identifying the physical, emotional, and social determinants of health.
- *Structure* of a community refers to its services and resources. Community associations, groups, and organizations provide a means for accessing needed services. Adequacy and appropriateness of health services can be determined by examining patterns of use, number and types of health and social services, and quality measures. These measures provide key information and correlate to health status.
- *Process* reflects the community's ability to function effectively. It includes processes within the community and between the community and the state or national levels to maintain health and improve outcomes.

These characteristics are discussed in more detail later in this chapter under the discussion on "Planning to Meet the Health Needs of the Community." See Chapter 1 for more information on healthy communities.

Addressing community health by examining the process, in addition to the structure and status dimensions, provides a broader view into the complexities of community health and community actions for change. It is key not only to examine health outcomes but also to consider how the interactions between process mechanisms and structures impact health outcomes (Public Health Accreditation Board, 2022).

Location

The health of a community is affected by location because placement of health services, geographic features, climate, plants, animals, and the human-made environment are intrinsic to geographic location. The location of a community places it in an environment that offers resources and also poses threats.

A healthy community is one that makes wise use of its resources and is prepared to meet threats and dangers. In assessing the health of any community, it is necessary to collect information not only about variables specific to a location but also about relationships between the community and its location. Do groups cooperate to identify threats? Do health agencies cooperate to prepare for an emergency such as a flood, tornado, or earthquake? Does the community make certain that its members are given available information about resources and dangers?

Table 15-2 describes the important community characteristics from a location perspective including the six location variables: community boundaries, location of health services, geographic features, climate, flora and fauna, and the human-made environment.

Community Boundaries

To talk about the community in any sense, one must first describe its boundaries. Measurement of health within a community must be preceded by the definition of geographic and informal boundaries around the target population.

- Nurses need to be clear, for example, that a target community of older adults includes a description of age and location (e.g., all people 65 years and older in a given city or county).
- Some communities are distinctly separate, such as an isolated rural town, whereas others are closely situated to one another, such as the suburbs of a large metropolis.
- Therefore, it is important for the nurse to know the nature of each location and clearly define its boundaries.

TABLE **15-2** Important Community Characteristics From a Location Perspective

Location Variables	Community Health Implications	Community Assessment Questions	Information Sources
Boundary of community	These serve as basis for measuring incidence of wellness and illness and for determining spread of disease.	Where is the community located? Is it a part of a larger community? Smaller communities included?	Google Maps State maps County maps City maps City directory Public library
Location of health services	Use of health services depends on availability and accessibility.	Where are the major health institutions located in the community? Outside the community?	www.Healthfinder.gov Chamber of commerce State health department County or local health departments Maps
Geographic features	Injury, death, and destruction may be caused by floods, earthquakes, volcanoes, or hurricanes. Recreational opportunities at lakes, seashore, and mountains promote health and fitness.	What major landforms are in or near the community? Which features pose possible threats? Which offer opportunities for healthful activities?	Atlas Chamber of commerce Maps State health department Public library www.NGMDB.USGS.gov
Climate	Extremes of heat and cold affect health and illness. Extremes of temperature and precipitation may tax community's coping ability.	What are the average temperature and precipitation? What climatic features affect health and fitness? Is the community prepared to cope with emergencies?	www.CLIMATE.gov Chamber of commerce State health department Maps Local government Weather bureau Public library
Flora and fauna	Poisonous plants and disease-carrying animals can affect community health. Plants and animals offer resources as well as dangers.	What plants and animals pose possible threats to health?	State health department Poison control center Police department Emergency rooms Encyclopedia Public library
Human-made environment	All human influences on environment (housing, dams, farming, type of industry, chemical waste) can influence levels of community wellness.	What are the major industries? Are there air, land, and water pollution concerns? What is the quality of housing?	Chamber of commerce Local government City directory State health department University research reports Public library

Location of Health Services

If the members of a town must travel 200 miles to the nearest clinic or dental office, the health of the community will be affected. When assessing a community, the community health nurse needs to identify the major health centers and know where they are located.

- For example, a treatment center for people with alcohol use disorder was located 30 miles outside of one city. This location presented transportation problems and profoundly affected the length of time clients remained at the center and their willingness to voluntarily seek treatment there.
- If a well-baby clinic is located on the edge of a high-crime district, parents may be deterred from using it. It is often helpful to plot the major health institutions, both inside and outside the community, on a map that shows their proximity and relationship to the community as a whole.

Geographic Features

Communities have been constructed in every conceivable physical environment, and environment certainly can affect the health of a community (see Chapter 9). A healthy community is one that takes into consideration the geography of its location, identifies possible problems and likely resources, and responds in an adaptive fashion. For example, Anchorage, Alaska, and San Francisco, California, are both located on a geologic fault line and are subject to major earthquakes. In such places, the health of the community is determined, in part, by its preparedness for an earthquake and its ability to cope and respond quickly when such a crisis occurs.

Climate

Winter weather patterns are expected to become more variable as average global temperatures continually increase. Research findings indicate that there is a relationship between temperature variability and health outcomes, including cardiovascular, respiratory, cerebrovascular events, and all-cause morbidity and mortality. Populations most vulnerable to global changes are older adults, residents of rural areas, children living in resource-limited countries, and those with preexisting medical conditions (World Health Organization [WHO], n.d., 2023).

Flora and Fauna

Plant and animal populations in a community are often determined by location. The way a community responds to these populations, whether wild or domesticated, can affect the health of the community.

Public health officials note chronic environmental factors as a possible cause for increased asthma cases: pollution from high-traffic areas, secondhand smoke in homes, and poor living conditions characterized by dust mites, mold, industrial air pollution, mouse and cockroach droppings, and animal dander.

C/PHNs need to know about the major sources of danger from plants and animals affecting the community under study.

- Are there community agencies that provide educational information about these dangers?
- Does the populace understand their significance?
- Are emergency services, such as a poison control center, available to community members?

The Built Environment

Every community is located in the midst of an environment created and transformed by human ingenuity. People build houses and factories, dump wastes into streams or vacant lots, fill the air with gases, and build dams to control streams. All of these human alterations of the environment have important implications for community health.

- A C/PHN might improve the health of a community by working with community members, legislators, and stakeholders to improve the design of the built environment, including universal design, to promote health and well-being.

Population Characteristics

When one considers the community as the client, examining the health status of the total population in a given community is a critical component. Table 15-3 presents the population perspective section of a community.

TABLE 15-3 Important Community Characteristics From a Population Perspective

Population Variables	Community Health Implications	Community Assessment Questions	Information Sources
Size	The number of people influences number and size of healthcare institutions.	What is the population? Is it an urban, suburban, or rural community?	State health department Census data Chamber of commerce
Density	High and low density often affects the availability of health services.	What is the density of the population per square mile?	Census data State health department
Composition	Composition of the population often determines types of health needs.	What are the population's demographic?	Census data State health department U.S. Department of Labor Statistics

(Continued)

TABLE 15-3 Important Community Characteristics From a Population Perspective (*Continued*)

Population Variables	Community Health Implications	Community Assessment Questions	Information Sources
Rate of growth or decline	Rapidly growing communities may place excessive demands on health services. Marked decline in population may signal a poorly functioning community.	How has population size changed over the past two decades? What are the health implications of this change?	Census data State health department
Cultural differences	Health needs vary among subcultural and ethnic populations. Utilization of health services varies with culture. Health practices and extent of knowledge are affected by culture.	What is the ethnic breakdown of population? What racial groups are represented? What subcultural populations exist? Are different ethnic and cultural groups included in health planning?	Census data State health department Social and cultural research reports City government Health planning boards
Mobility	Mobility of the population affects continuity of care. Mobility affects availability of service to highly mobile populations.	How frequently do members move into and out of the community? Are there any specific populations that are highly mobile? Is the community organized to meet the health needs of mobile groups?	State health department Census data Health agencies serving migrant workers Program serving people in transitional housing and people who are homeless
Income level	Economic disparities may lead to health disparities.	What percentage of the population is below federal poverty levels? How many children qualify for free or reduced cost school lunch?	Census data State data Local data (schools)
Education level	Education disparities may lead to health disparities.	What is the literacy rate?	State data Local data (schools)
Unemployment rate	Health insurance is often tied to employment. Lack of regular income can be a family stressor. Both can lead to health disparities.	What is the rate of unemployment? How variable is this rate?	U.S. Department of Labor State data Local data
Population by age	A high proportion of children and older adults can overburden healthcare and social systems.	What is the dependency ratio? Has this rate changed dramatically? What is the trend?	Census data State data Local data
Health status	Community members' status relative to the 10 Leading Health Indicators can impact overall community health.	What is the rate of obesity/people who are overweight? What are the rates of tobacco use and substance abuse? What is the immunization rate? What are rates of injury and violence? What are the STD and HIV/AIDS rates?	State data Local data Centers for Disease Control and Prevention (CDC) data Vital statistics—numbers of births, deaths, marriages, and infant mortality rate (Compare local to state data; state to national data)
Environmental health status	Poor environmental health (e.g., presence of coliform bacteria in well water, toxic chemicals, or poor air quality) can lead to increased incidence of communicable or chronic diseases.	What are rates of communicable or chronic diseases (e.g., *Escherichia coli* infections, asthma)?	CDC data State data Local data

Size

Knowing a community's size provides community health nurses with important information for planning. For example, when conducting emergency preparedness planning, knowledge of the population size will ensure that an adequate number of resources can be made available in the event of an emergency. See Chapter 27 for issues related to rural and urban population health.

Density

In some communities, thousands of people are crowded into high-rise apartment buildings. In others, such as farm communities, people live great distances from one another. Population density, or the number of people residing within a square mile area, is used to describe how many people live within a community.

- Studies suggest that high population density is associated with higher mortality rates for cardiovascular disease as well as increasing community members' exposure to pollution (Carnegie et al., 2022).
- A low-density community, however, may also pose problems. When people are spread out, provision of healthcare services can become difficult.

A healthy community takes into consideration the density of its population. It organizes to meet the differing needs created by its density levels (e.g., it recognizes differences in density between the city center and the suburbs and allocates services accordingly). See Chapter 27 for more on health risks specific to rural and urban areas.

Composition/Demographics

Communities differ in the types of people who live within their boundaries. Age, sex, educational level, occupation, and many other demographic variables affect health concerns (CDC, 2023). Understanding a community's composition is an important early step in determining its level of health. For example, when planning a cost-free vaccination program, knowledge of community demographics allows nurses to identify those who are eligible and those who would benefit most from the program.

Rate of Growth or Decline

Community populations change over time. Some change rapidly, as people leave to find new employment or weather climates and as political leanings change. Community morale may suffer, and community leadership may decline. Even a stable community can have problems (e.g., members may resist needed change because they notice little fluctuation in their population; commercial and residential properties may be abandoned or left vacant). This trend is widely observed across the country, as the United States has progressed from being a manufacturing society to a postindustrial and technologically focused one.

Cultural Characteristics

A healthy community is aware of the diversity and the needs of the cultural subgroups (ODPHP, n.d.). See Chapter 5 for more about transcultural nursing in the community.

Economic and Educational Level

Social determinants of health (SDOH) impact a wide range of health, functioning, and quality of life outcomes (Fig. 15-5; ODPHP, n.d.). They reflect social

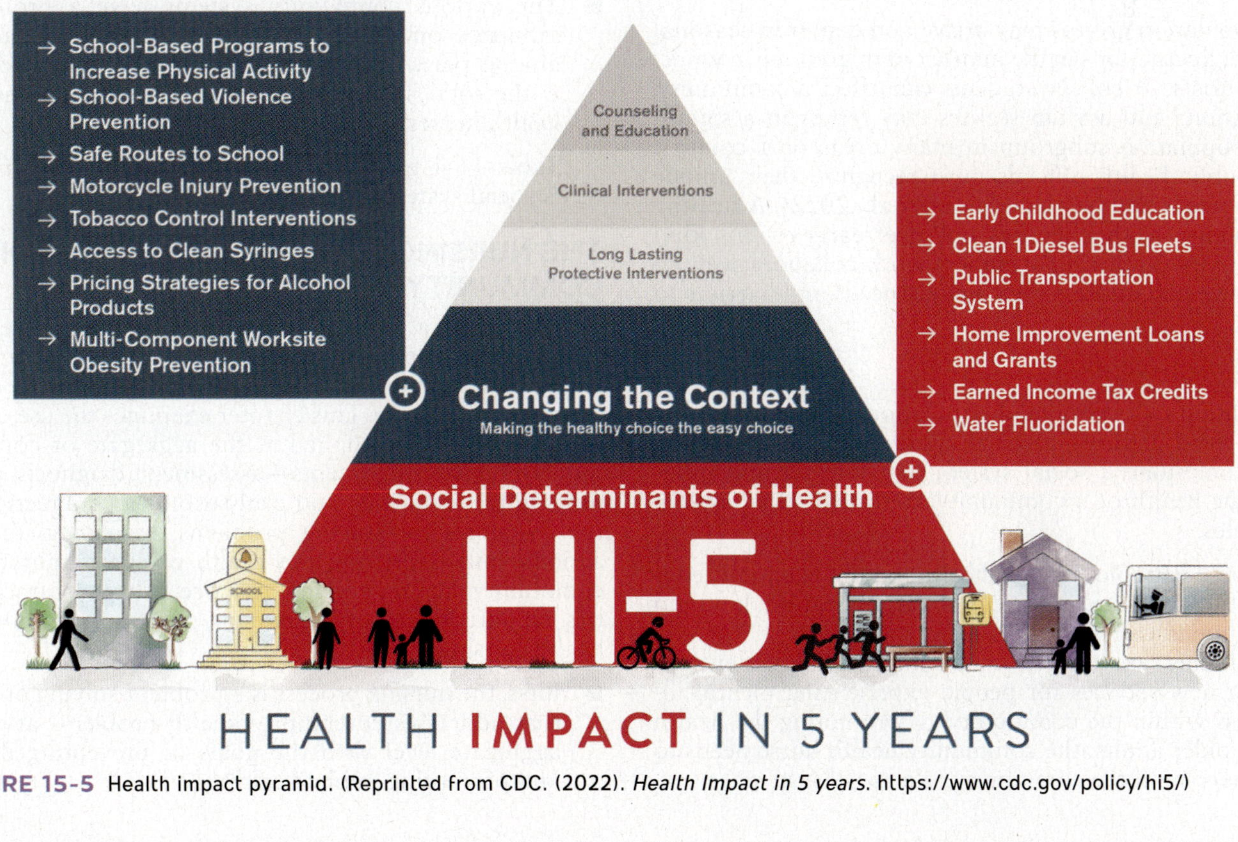

FIGURE 15-5 Health impact pyramid. (Reprinted from CDC. (2022). *Health Impact in 5 years.* https://www.cdc.gov/policy/hi5/)

factors and the physical conditions in the environment in which people are born, live, learn, play, work, and age. The SDOH affect our health more than genetics and healthcare access (CDC, 2022b). They are shaped by the distribution of money, power, and resources at global, national, and local levels and contribute to health inequities among different groups of people based on social and economic class, gender, and ethnicity. For these reasons, SDOH are an underlying cause of today's major societal health dilemmas and inequities (CDC, 2022b; see Chapter 23).

It is generally known that different groups have different health problems, as well as a variety of resources for coping with illness and diverse ways of using health services. A healthy community recognizes these differences and creates healthcare services to meet these varied needs.

Mobility

Americans are a mobile population. Outcomes from the 2023 American Community Survey estimate that approximately 20 million people moved annually within their region, 8 million moved to a different state, and nearly another 2 million were estimated to move to the United States from abroad that year.

- Oftentimes these fluctuations are linked to social and economic factors (U.S. Census Bureau, 2023).
- If the population turnover is extensive, continuity of services may suffer.
- Leadership for improving the health of the community may change so frequently that concerted action becomes difficult.
- High turnover may necessitate special attention to health education about local conditions.

Population groups may arrive and depart in seasonal swings; fluctuations in the number of migrant farm workers, tourists, or college students can affect a community. Immigrants and asylum seekers may represent a significant population subgroup in many areas of a country, and public health officials must recognize their unique health needs and barriers (Sherif et al., 2022). A healthy community neither ignores nor overreacts to this kind of mobility. Rather, its members work collaboratively to recognize and address their unique needs and barriers to health.

Social System

In addition to location and population, every community has a third feature—a social system. The various parts of a community's social system that interact and influence the health of a community are called social system variables.

- These variables include health, family, economy, education, religion, welfare, politics, recreation, law, and communication (Fig. 15-6).
- Whether assessing a community's health, developing new services for people experiencing mental illness within the community, or promoting the health of older adults, the community health nurse needs to understand the community as a social system.

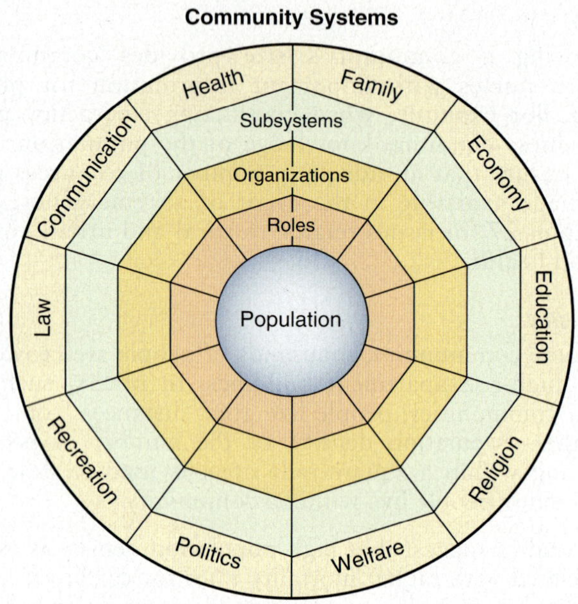

FIGURE 15-6 The community as a social system. Each of the 10 major systems of a community includes a number of subsystems that are made up of organizations. Members of the community occupy roles in these organizations.

- A community health nurse working in a tiny village in Alaska needs to understand and work with the social system of that village no less than a nurse practicing in New York City.
- When a group of organizations are linked and have similar functions, such as all those providing social services, they form a community system or subsystem.
- The various community systems have a profound influence on one another. Because this interaction among parts determines the health of the whole, it is the total social system that concerns community health nurses.

Table 15-4 guides the nurse in assessing a community's social system variables.

THE NURSING PROCESS APPLIED TO THE COMMUNITY AS CLIENT

Consisting of a systematic, purposeful set of interpersonal actions, the nursing process provides a structure for change that remains a viable tool employed by the community health nurse. This chapter examines the use of the nursing process as applied at the aggregate or community level. Five components—assessment, diagnosis, planning, implementation, and evaluation—give direction to the dynamics for solving problems, managing nursing actions, and improving the health of communities and community health nursing practice. Three characteristics support the use of the nursing process in community health nursing.

- First, the nursing process is a problem-solving process that addresses community health problems at every aggregate level with the goals of preventing illness and promoting public health.

TABLE 15-4 Important Community Characteristics From a Social System Perspective

Social System Variables	Community Health Implications	Community Assessment Questions	Information Sources
Health system Family system Economic system Educational system Religious system Welfare system Political system Recreational system Legal system Communication system	Each system must fulfill its functions for a healthy community. Collaboration among the systems to identify goals and problems affects health of community. Undue influence of one system on another may lower the health of the community. Agreement on the means to achieve community goals affects community health. Communication among organizations in each system affects community health.	What are the functions of each major system? What are the major subsystems of each system? What are the major organizations in each subsystem? How well do the various organizations function? Are the subsystems in each major system in conflict? Is there adequate communication among the major systems? Is there agreement on community goals? Are there mechanisms for resolving conflict? Do any parts of the total system dominate the others? What community needs are not being met?	Chamber of commerce Telephone book City directory Organizational literature Officials in organizations Community self-study Community survey Local library Key informants

- Second, it is a management process that requires situational analysis, decision making, planning, organization, direction, and control of services, as well as outcome evaluation. As a management tool, the nursing process addresses all aggregate levels.
- Third, it is a process for implementing changes that improve the function of various health-related systems and the ways that people behave within those systems.

The nursing process provides a framework or structure on which C/PHN actions are based (ANA, 2022). Application of the process varies with each situation, but the nature of the process remains the same. Certain characteristics of that process are important for community health nurses to emphasize in their practices. C/PHNs are expected to demonstrate competence, the expected level of performance, based on established professional standards of practice and must be familiar with their local laws and regulations which govern nursing practice (ANA, 2022).

Deliberative

The nursing process, like the research process in evidence-based practice, is deliberative—purposefully, rationally, and carefully thought out. It requires the use of sound judgment that is based on adequate information. C/PHNs often practice in situations that demand the ability to think independently and make difficult decisions. Furthermore, thoughtful, deliberative problem solving is a necessary skill for working with the community health team to address the needs and problems of aggregates in the community (ANA, 2022).

Adaptable

The dynamic nature of the nursing process enables the community health nurse to adapt it appropriately to each situation and apply it to meeting aggregate health needs. Furthermore, its flexibility is a reminder to the nurse that each client group and each community situation is unique. Based on assessment and sound planning, the nurse adapts services to meet the identified needs of each community client group.

Cyclical

The nursing process is cyclical and in constant progression. Steps are repeated over and over in the nurse–aggregate client relationship. The nurse engages in continual interaction, data collection, analysis, intervention, and evaluation. As interactions between nurse and client group continue, various steps in the process overlap with one another and are used simultaneously. The cyclic nature of the nursing process enables the nurse to engage in a constant information feedback loop: the information gathered and lessons learned at each step of the process promote greater understanding of the group being served, the most effective way to provide quality services, and the best methods of raising this group's level of health.

Client Focused

The nursing process is used for and with clients. Community health nurses use the nursing process for the express purpose of addressing the health of populations. They are helping aggregate clients, directly or indirectly, to achieve and maintain health. Clients as total systems—whether groups, populations, or communities—are the intended audience for the C/PHN's nursing process (ANA, 2022).

Interactive

The nurse and the community are engaged in a process of ongoing interpersonal communication. Giving and receiving accurate information is necessary to promote understanding between nurses and clients and to foster effective use of the nursing process. Furthermore, because of the movement toward informed use of healthcare, demands for clients' rights and the concept of self-care have gained emphasis. Client groups and community health nurses have increasingly joined forces to assume responsibility for promoting community health and effective partnerships, which are critical to the achievement of positive health outcomes for communities. The nurse–aggregate client relationship can and should be a partnership, a shared experience by professionals (nurses and others) and client groups (Duran et al., 2019).

Need Oriented

A long association with problem-solving has tended to limit the focus of the nursing process to the correction of existing problems. Although problem-solving is certainly an appropriate use of the nursing process, the community health nurse can also use the nursing process to anticipate the client's needs and prevent problems. The nurse should think of the nursing process as ranging from health problem identification to primary prevention and health promotion opportunities. This focus is needed if the goals of community health—to protect, promote, and restore the people's health—are to be realized.

Interacting With the Community

All steps of the nursing process depend on interaction, reciprocal exchange, and influence among people. Although nurse–client interaction is often an implied or assumed element in the process, it is an essential first consideration for community health nursing. This type of engagement was observed during the Flint water crisis, where C/PHNs established relationships with community members and were thereby able to identify and directly aid in addressing their needs. These relationships also facilitated communication between community members and service providers (see Chapter 10 for more details).

- Listening to a group of older people, teaching a class of expectant parents, lobbying in the legislature for people living below the poverty level, working with parents to set up a dental screening program for children—all of these involve relationships, and relationships require interaction.
- Mutual give and take between nurses, clients, and community stakeholders—whether a family, a group of parents on a Native American reservation, or representatives from resource agencies within the community—is an expected and much-needed skill that should be integrated throughout the nursing process.

Need For Communication

C/PHNs can serve as effective liaisons—facilitating communication between stakeholders and clients to ensure that health needs are both identified and adequately addressed.

Interaction and Effective Communication. Through open and honest sharing, the nurse (and others on the health team) can begin to develop trust and establish lines of effective communication.

- For instance, the nurse explains the nurse's role and purpose for being there.
- The nurse encourages the group members to talk about themselves.
- The nurse and group members together discuss their relationship and clarify the desired nature of that alliance.
  - Does the group want help to identify and work on its health needs?
  - Would its members like this nurse to continue regular contacts?
  - What will their respective roles be?

Effective communication, as a part of interaction, is essential to develop understanding and facilitate a free exchange of information between nurse and client.

Interaction Is Reciprocal. Sharing of information, ideas, feelings, concerns, and self goes both ways. The community health nurse (and other collaborating health professionals) represents one system, and the client group represents the other. Healthcare professionals tend to prioritize based on their own perspective and many times neglect to take the client's wishes into account.

- Whether the client is a parent group, people who are experiencing homelessness, or an entire community, this exchange involves a two-way sharing between the nurse and client group. The key elements of interaction are mutuality and cooperation.

Consider the following example:

- After several weeks of meeting with a community member focus group to discuss disease management and physical activity, a C/PHN noticed that community violence was a recurring theme during group discussions.
- Community residents described conditions in the neighborhood as unsafe and many indicted that they were afraid to adopt the nurse's recommendations to increase physical activity because of ongoing violence near their homes.
- The nurse initially felt unprepared to address this issue but, after consulting with other support agencies within the community, realized that resources were available.
- After meeting and coordinating with community members and support agencies, the nurse was able to develop a feasible and safe physical activity plan for residents.
- Engagement with community members and communication were the first step in reapplying the nursing process and allowed goals for the group to be accomplished.

Interaction Paves the Way for a Helping Relationship. As nurse and client interact, each learns about the other. For a female school nurse working with middle school students about health education and human sexuality, establishing interaction was more difficult at the time of the initial contact with the male students than with the female students. (Please note that in this paragraph, "female" refers to a person assigned female at birth, and "male" refers to a person assigned male at birth.) They had been reluctant to talk and felt embarrassed to discuss personal subjects with an adult they did not know. Nonetheless, their interests in bodybuilding and personal appearance were strong enough to bring them to these optional sessions. Interaction began with a friendly exchange on nonthreatening topics and gradually deepened, as the male students seemed ready to discuss personal subjects. Eventually, it was relatively simple to talk about a new "problem" (and start the nursing process over again), because a helping relationship had already been developed. The nurse had a track record. The male students trusted, respected, and liked the nurse, so they were happy to interact around a newly stated need.

Aggregate Application

As noted in earlier chapters, community health practice focuses largely on the health of population groups; therefore, interaction goes beyond the one-on-one with individual patients. The challenge that the community health nurse faces is a one-to-aggregate approach.

- A group of parents concerned about teenage alcohol misuse, people with physical disabilities needing access ramps, and a neighborhood's older adult population frightened by muggings and thefts are all aggregates or clients with different concerns and opinions.
- As defined in Chapter 1, an aggregate refers to a mass or grouping of distinct people who are considered as a whole and who are loosely associated with one another.
- Each person in an aggregate is influenced by the thoughts and behavior of other group members.
- Nursing interaction with an aggregate client demands an understanding of group behavior, group dynamics, and group-level decision making.
- It requires interpersonal communication skills applied at the group level. Interaction is more complex and challenging with an aggregate than with an person but also can be rewarding.
- Once community health nurses acquire an understanding of aggregate behavior, they can capitalize on the potential of group influence to make a far-reaching impact on the health of the total community.
- Chapter 10 more closely examines communication and interaction with groups.

Forming Partnerships and Building Coalitions

Community-level nursing practice also requires teamwork. The job of planning for the health of an entire community or a community subsystem requires that the nurse collaborate with other professionals. Usually, the nurse is part of an organized team, separate from the agency that employs the nurse. The team is brought together with the goal of improving the health of the community. Each group member brings expertise and a particular view of the problem. During times of crisis, collaboration across disciplines provides an opportunity for partners to facilitate sharing of best practices and address long-standing health and social inequities (Higgins & Cooper, 2021).

The need for and effectiveness of interdisciplinary collaboration in response to the COVID-19 pandemic is well documented. During the height of the pandemic, a group of faculty, students, and staff from Rush University Medical Center and homeless care service providers came together to develop a plan to protect the community of vulnerably housed people in Chicago, IL.

- These collaborators, which later became known as the West Side Homeless COVID-19 Response Group, were joined by more than 100 members of local hospitals, federally qualified health centers, advocates, and city officials to coordinate and deliver services to their community during the pandemic.
- Their efforts created additional housing and increased care access for high-risk groups while also creating housing for those who were healthy to protect them from frequent disease outbreaks (Michener et al., 2020).
- The group was later renamed the Chicago Homelessness and Health Response Group for Equity, and it boasts partnerships with several local academic centers, governmental agencies, and local public health service providers, working collectively to prevent disease and promote health for their community.

Partnerships are agreements between people (and agencies) that support a joint purpose. A partnership can be large (e.g., a multinational corporation and several high schools; a city government and the county jail system), or it can be a more modest endeavor (e.g., a group of older adult citizens and a preschool program; a Scouting America troop and a safe battery disposal program).

From 2009 to 2019 data from the Centers for Disease Control and Prevention's Youth Risk Behavior Survey (YRBS) reported a significant increase in adolescent suicide-related behaviors. It was determined that social isolation and loneliness resulting from the COVID-19 pandemic would further exacerbate this devastating trend and impact those with preexisting mental health conditions (Hertz & Barrios, 2021). To address this concerning trend, many state and local organizations collaborated to support their local communities.

- In New York, counselors, psychologists, and social workers from the South Oaks Hospital partnered with local school districts to develop a tailored approach to provide community education opportunities, professional development for staff and clinicians, newsletters, community events, workshops, and supporting students in need.
- The group worked collaboratively across local healthcare systems to increase access to care and ensure the availability of services to actively address at-risk populations and keep their communities healthy.
- This partnership paved the way for the creation of much-needed services and demonstrates the importance of community collaboration (South Oaks Hospital Northwell Health, 2023).

Community-wide partnerships require more planning and coordination than small partnerships.

- For example, because of increased student enrollment, a college may need two additional temporary and part-time faculty members who can teach the C/PHN course.
- The county public health department is interested in more new graduate nurses coming to work in the agency.
- The nursing program and the health department form a partnership and design a plan to solve both problems.
- The health department selects two staff nurses who have master's degrees and are qualified to teach undergraduate clinical courses in C/PHN one day a week for two semesters.
- The benefits for everyone are numerous.
  - The nursing program solves a temporary staffing problem.

- The nurses from the health department share their expertise with students, enhancing their practice and the students' learning experience.
- The health department successfully introduces a pool of students, who may be potential staff members, to the agency and the services that it provides for the community.

A coalition is an alliance of people or groups that work together to influence the outcomes of a specific problem. Coalitions are an effective means to achieve a collaborative and coordinated approach to solving community problems. Steps to coalition building include the following:

- Define a problem and how it affects the community.
- Identify key stakeholders.
- Arrange for stakeholders to meet as a group.
- Share viewpoints on the concerns.
- Discuss the current situation and what the ideal would be.
- Develop a vision for the community.
- Decide the next steps (U.S. Drug Enforcement Administration [USDEA], n.d.).

Staying in touch with the coalition members, running effective meetings, and keeping every participant involved are means of keeping the coalition active.

Sound public health practice depends on pooling resources—including people—in ways that will best serve the public. In planning for a community's health, the community (represented by appropriate people and agencies) must be involved. Community health nurses cannot lose sight of the need for client involvement at all levels and in all stages of community health practice (Box 15-2).

TYPES OF COMMUNITY HEALTH ASSESSMENT

Assessment is the key initial step of the nursing process; it involves collecting and evaluating information about a community's health status to discover existing or potential needs and assets as a basis for planning future action. Assessments are also a critical requirement for public health department accreditation (Public Health Accreditation Board, 2022).

Several models or frameworks can be used for assessment. Three such models follow:

- Mobilizing for Action through Planning and Partnerships
- Protocol for Assessing Community Excellence in Environmental Health
- State Health Improvement Planning

These models have been developed through partnership with the Centers for Disease Control and Prevention (CDC) to improve community assessment in relation to *Healthy People* goals (CDC, 2022a) and to assist communities in assessing health promotion and chronic disease prevention programs.

- The *Healthy People* website also provides planning tools and toolkits to assist local communities. These are all valuable resources that provide specific guidelines focusing on local-level strategies to improve the health of communities.

Assessment involves two major activities:

- Collection of pertinent data
- Analysis and interpretation of data

BOX 15-2 PERSPECTIVES

A Public Health Nurse's Viewpoint on Addressing Adolescent Depression

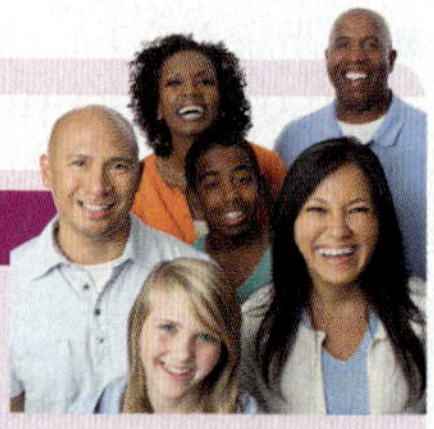

I am a public health nurse and my health department serves a community with a large proportion of adolescents and young adults aged 18 to 24 years. After reviewing data from a recent community health status assessment, members of our community council observed a significant increase in the number of high school students with depression after a recent natural disaster. We proceeded to convene a group of community stakeholders with the intention of partnering with them to identify and implement solutions to address these issues. Several meetings were held, and key members of the community were invited to participate, including a local church pastor, youth group leaders, school officials including nurses and teachers, parents, and administrators representing nonprofit organizations targeting this same issue. After further analysis of this issue, the group agreed to develop a plan to address depression among the age group and to also target resources toward secondary prevention in order to support those who had experienced depression within the past 6 months.

An assessment of community resources was conducted to identify available programs and resources. We searched the literature for best practices on this topic and collaborated with program planners to develop an implementation plan for our target population. The group engaged local leaders to request funding for areas where gaps in services were identified. After 2 months of planning, community resources were identified, and coordination was conducted to begin marketing and outreach efforts. Referral mechanisms in local clinics were used to link potential clients to our program, and we received several word-of-mouth recommendations for participants. The program consists of support help in schools, a mentor, counseling, participation in group informational sessions, and the assignment of a primary care manager in our community-based clinic. The program also provided support and counseling to the parents and siblings.

A 6- and 9-month outcome evaluation is planned to monitor the effect of our program. Anecdotal feedback has been resoundingly positive. The commitment of our partners is evident as our efforts have been embraced and supported by a wide range of leaders and community members. This commitment appears to have yielded a great response from program participants. Results have been positive as evidenced by a reduction in adolescent depression. Participants have remarked about the quality of services received, and many have commented on the quality of care they received in our program.

Joanna, public health nurse and school nurse

These actions overlap and are repeated constantly throughout the assessment phase of the nursing process. While assessing a community's ability to enhance its health, the nurse may simultaneously collect data on community lifestyle behaviors and interpret previously collected data on morbidity and mortality.

Community health assessment is the process of determining the real or perceived needs of a defined community. This can be accomplished by several means—through an extensive community study or through a cursory examination or windshield survey.

Windshield Surveys

Windshield/familiarization surveys are an activity often used by nursing students in public health courses and by new staff members in community health agencies. Nurses drive and walk around the community of interest; find health, social, and governmental services; obtain literature; introduce themselves and explain that they are working in the area; and generally become familiar with the community and its residents.

- This type of assessment is helpful for the C/PHN to become familiar with the community and is needed whenever the community health nurse works with families, groups, organizations, or populations.
- The windshield survey provides knowledge of the context in which these aggregates live and may enable the nurse to better connect clients with community resources (Box 15-3).

See an example in Box 15-4.

BOX 15-3 Community Familiarization (Windshield) Survey

A windshield survey is often done to help you become familiar with a new community or public health service area. Walking/driving around neighborhoods and interacting with community members can provide a context for further community assessment. You might begin at the local Chamber of Commerce or government building to determine history, current statistics, and demographics and to access maps and further resources for data you might use for a more formal community health assessment.

Physical

- Look at the age and conditions of the buildings, the density (apartments, houses on large lots) and materials used (bricks, plywood), and the zoning and maintenance of yards/empty lots. What clues does that give you about the community as a whole?
- How similar are the houses (are some neighborhoods resource-abundant, others resource-limited)? Are there abandoned vehicles, piles of excess trash, large numbers of stray animals/for sale signs, or vacant houses?
- Are there open spaces (parks, agricultural areas, public/private areas like golf courses) and are they being used? By whom?
- Are there boundaries separating the community (e.g., natural boundaries like rivers, economic boundaries, commercial/residential boundaries)?
- What about air/water quality, signs of pollution?

Economic

- Does the area look like it is a thriving community?
- Are there areas where people who are homeless gather? Soup kitchens?
- Is there adequate shopping (e.g., grocery stores, shopping centers)?
- Does it appear that food stamps are accepted/welcomed?
- Are there businesses, industries, manufacturing, and adequate places for employment? What is the unemployment rate?

Services

- Are there schools (how many, in what condition)? School nurses? What are the main concerns or problems with the educational system here (e.g., dropout rates)?
- Are there libraries? Do they provide additional services (e.g., internet)? Are they well used?
- Are there recreational facilities (e.g., gyms, playgrounds, soccer fields, baseball diamonds)? Are these being used and by whom?
- How many churches do you see? What denominations? What services do they provide to the community?
- Is there adequate healthcare? Does the community have a hospital? Are there adequate healthcare services (e.g., physicians, clinics, nurses, mental health/substance abuse facilities, PH department services, nursing homes, traditional healthcare providers)? Is it a medically underserved area or a health professions shortage area? Does the population need to travel outside the community for services?
- What types of social services are available (e.g., welfare/social workers, shelters, mental health counseling)? Do you see one main location for social services (e.g., government center) or are they dispersed around the community?
- What types of public/private transportation are available? Are highways and roads crowded with traffic? Accident rate? Are there bike paths/trails and adequate sidewalks? How is transportation access for people with disabilities?
- Does the community "feel" safe to you? Is there adequate fire and police protection? What is the crime rate? What are the most common types of crimes?
- Are there signs of political activity (e.g., posters, notices of meetings, predominant party affiliations)? Do people feel that they can be involved in decisions made by their local government?

Social

- Are there common "hangouts" (e.g., teen gathering spots, chess playing for older adults)? What about local newspapers, radio, and TV (e.g., satellite dishes)?
- Who do you see on the streets? Are there indications of homogeneity or diversity of ethnicities, languages spoken, SES (socioeconomic status), and occupations? How are people dressed?
- How do people feel about living in this community? What problems or concerns do they express? What strengths do they note? How "healthy" is their community?
- What are your impressions of this community?

Source: Anderson and McFarlane (2019).

BOX 15-4 STORIES FROM THE FIELD

Working With the Community on a Safety Assessment

Consider the following example: During a windshield survey a new C/PHN notices several churches, elementary schools, and parks that have limited use during certain days of the week. The nurse has been meeting with a community-member focus group to discuss obesity, nutrition, and physical activity, when he noticed that lack of community safety was a recurring theme during group discussions. Community residents described conditions in the neighborhood as unsafe, and many indicated that they were afraid to adopt the nurse's recommendations to increase physical activity due because of ongoing violence near their homes. The C/PHN initially felt unprepared to address this issue but after consulting with other support agencies within the community, he realized that resources were available. After meeting and coordinating with stakeholders, he was able to arrange for exercise and cooking classes in a church 3 days a week and at the schools on Saturdays. The program was a success, and, currently, there is a focus group to enlarge the program to different age groups. Engagement with community members and communication were the first step in reapplying the nursing process and allowed goals for the group to be accomplished.

1. *What should the C/PHN know about location, population, and social system to be better prepared to work with this group?*
2. *How can the C/PHN use the nursing process to direct the plan of care with this community?*

Problem-Oriented Assessment

A second type of community assessment, **problem-oriented assessment**, begins with a single problem and assesses the community in terms of that problem. Instead of working to gather information about the larger community, the nurse would identify resources, programs, and support networks of potential benefit to the family.

- Steps taken to complete this assessment would include collecting data on local prevalence and incidence, interviewing officials to obtain information on processes and policies, and identifying local programs and services.
- The problem-oriented assessment can be used when familiarization is not sufficient, and a comprehensive assessment is not feasible.
- This type of assessment is responsive to a particular need and should also seek to describe contextual issues associated with the need.
- The data collected can support community efforts to address specific problems.
- Data should address the magnitude of the problem to be studied (e.g., prevalence, incidence), the precursors of the problem, and information about population characteristics (e.g., community resources, strengths, and weaknesses), along with the attitudes and behaviors of the population being studied (Kirst-Ashman & Hull, 2018).

Community Subsystem Assessment

In **community subsystem assessment**, the C/PHN focuses on a single dimension of community life. For example, the nurse might decide to survey churches and religious organizations to discover their roles in the community. What kinds of needs do the leaders in these organizations believe exist? What services do these organizations offer? To what extent are services coordinated within the religious system and between it and other systems in the community?

In one situation, churches and other cultural leaders were instrumental in providing information to address the local public health department's concerns.

- A small county health department worked with the nearby university C/PHN clinical instructor and the instructor's students to determine why specific LGBTQ+ groups did not use free health clinics.
  - Students from the university conducted focus groups with local clergy and representatives from the groups to better understand the group's health-seeking behaviors.
    - Health department officials reviewed transcripts from the focus groups and discovered that most members of the groups were unaware of the services provided through the county health department.
    - The students then conducted additional interviews with community members and found that, as part of their cultural practice, members often avoid religious institutions for fear of ridicule and rejection.
    - They also learned that members of the group felt more comfortable with healthcare personnel from the community and that there was a provider meeting these criteria in a neighboring county.
    - As a result of these subsystem engagements, health department staff were able to tailor their service offerings to better meet the needs to these groups, and a partnership for health was established with local clinic administrators and group members.

Community subsystem assessment can be a useful way for a team to conduct a more thorough community assessment. If five members of a nursing agency divide up the 10 systems in the community and each person does an assessment of two systems, they could then share their findings to create a more comprehensive picture of the community and its needs.

Comprehensive Assessment

Comprehensive assessment seeks to discover all relevant community health information. It begins with a review of existing studies and all the data presently available on the community. A survey compiles all the demographic information on the population, such as its size, density, and composition.

Key informants are experts in one particular area of the community, or they may know the community as a whole. Key informants are interviewed in every major system—education, health, religious, economic, and others.

- Examples of key informants would be a school nurse, a religious leader, key cultural leaders, the local police chief or fire captain, a mail carrier, a school board member, public health officials, or a local city council person.
- Then, more detailed surveys and intensive interviews are performed to yield information on organizations and the various roles in each organization.

A comprehensive assessment describes the systems of a community and how power is distributed throughout the system, how decisions are made, and how change occurs (Anderson & McFarlane, 2019).

Because comprehensive assessment is an expensive, time-consuming process, it is not often undertaken. Performing a more focused study, based on prior knowledge of needs, is often a better and less costly strategy. Nevertheless, knowing how to conduct a comprehensive assessment is an important skill when designing smaller more focused assessments (Box 15-5).

Community Assets Assessment

Assets mapping focuses on the strengths and capacities of a community rather than its problems and evaluates variables such as the needs that exist, the goals to be achieved, and the resources available for carrying out the study (Ravaghi et al., 2023).

Although it is difficult to determine the type of assessment needed in advance, understanding the various types of community assessment in advance helps to facilitate your decision.

- Based on a classic model developed by McKnight and Kretzmann in the 1980s (Kretzman & McKnight, 1993), the assets assessment provides a framework for conducting a complete functional community assessment and serves as a guide to the community for the nurse, as well as the foundation for community development.

The previously mentioned methods are needs oriented and deficit based—in other words, they are *pathology* models, in which the assessment is performed in response to needs, barriers, weaknesses, problems, or perceived scarcity in the community. This may result in a fragmented approach to solutions for the community's problems rather than an approach focused on the community's possibilities, strengths, and assets. The **assets assessment** also provides the community the ability to know their strengths and a foundation on which to build on.

Assets assessment begins with what is present in the community (Ravaghi et al., 2023). The capacities and skills of community members are identified, with a focus on creating or rebuilding relationships among residents, associations, and institutions to multiply power and effectiveness. The nurse can then become a partner

BOX 15-5 PERSPECTIVES

A Public Health Nursing Student Viewpoint on Addressing the Health Needs of Migrant Workers and Farm Workers

After completing my Med-Surg courses, I was excited to begin my Community Health rotation. I looked forward to stepping outside of the clinical environment to engage community members, but I absolutely dreaded the thought of having to complete the perfunctory comprehensive community health assessment. To my delight, the assessment process had recently been revamped, so instead of repeating the task of collecting the same data that the previous classes had collected, my class was able to select from a list of community health projects for which data were needed. These projects were directly related to grants currently being written by staff and state-directed program evaluations that the department was working on. The fact that these were real-time projects made the assignment feel less like a task and more like a meaningful opportunity to contribute to the health of community members served by the department.

My class voted to collect data for a grant-funded project to address medical concerns of farm workers and migrant workers, and we set about creating our own survey tools, drawing from standardized assessment products. We were excited about our work and tackled the project like a bunch of detectives chasing down leads! We divided into subgroups, gathered data, problem-solved, and worked together to achieve our goals. We also worked with other agencies and NGOs and spoke with local healthcare providers and members of the community. Toward the end of our project, we collaborated with the public health department and the foreman for the workers to distribute questionnaires in Spanish to the workers so that we could gather information on their medical and emotional needs.

Due to the nature of the employment, we knew some of those who helped gather information may not be in the area for the duration of the process; therefore, building trust with the population was extremely important. It was imperative that the material was translated correctly and that we had interpreters to help with people who could not read or came from a region without a written language.

After speaking with healthcare providers and student nurse practitioners, we had a group interested in providing services in a clinic setting. Our next step was to apply for a grant to help buy a mobile clinic. Even though we were not able to see the finished product, we heard the following class was successful with the grant and has started equipping the mobile clinic!

Linsey, nursing student

in community intervention efforts, rather than merely a provider of services. Typically, seven categories are evaluated for this assessment:

1. Community demographic
2. Natural capitals
3. Economics
4. Infrastructure
5. Social and educational facilities
6. Health and social facilities
7. Social and cultural values and resources (Ravaghi et al., 2023).

The key, however, is linking these assets together to enhance the community from within. The community health nurse's role is to assist with those linkages.

METHODS FOR COLLECTING COMMUNITY HEALTH DATA

Various methods may be used to assess the community's health status. Regardless of the assessment method used, data must be collected.

Four important methods are discussed here: surveys, descriptive epidemiologic studies, community forums or town meetings, and focus groups.

Surveys

A survey is an assessment method in which a series of questions is used to collect data for analysis of a specific group or area. Surveys are commonly used to provide a broad range of data that will be helpful when used with other sources or if other sources are not available.

To plan and conduct community health surveys, the goal should be to determine the variables (selected environmental, socioeconomic, and behavioral conditions or needs) that affect a community's ability to control disease and promote wellness.

The nurse may choose to conduct a survey to determine such things as healthcare use patterns and needs, immunization levels, demographic characteristics, or health beliefs and practices.

The survey method involves self-report, or response to predetermined questions, and can include questionnaires, telephone, or in-person interviews (Polit & Beck, 2021).

Descriptive Epidemiologic Studies

A second assessment method is a **descriptive epidemiologic study**, which examines the amount and distribution of a disease or health condition in a population:

- By person (Who is affected?)
- By place (Where does the condition occur?)
- By time (When do the cases occur?)

In addition to their value in assessing the health status of a population, descriptive epidemiologic studies are useful for suggesting which people are at greatest risk and where and when the condition might occur. Their design and use are detailed in Chapter 7.

Geographic Information System Analysis

- In Chapter 10, the concept of Geographic Information System was introduced as health information technology. GIS technology is an integration of research methods and analytic techniques from both medical geography and spatial epidemiology. It has been well documented as a tool that can collect, organize, and display public health data, and it is widely used in assessment and research of health disparities, resource availability, and health-related behaviors (WHO, 2023). To help stop the spread of COVID-19, the WHO used GIS to help distribute COVID-19 vaccines to over 90 countries (WHO, 2021).

Harvard's T.H. Chan School of Public Health offers a website designated to the use of GIS in public health, including particular research studies.

- For instance, one line of research examines effects of air pollution on MI rates within the community of Worchester and spatial mapping of incidence and levels of pollution.
- Researchers are also working on developing a predictive model for pollution's effect on death rates in Eastern Massachusetts.
- A prospective study of normative aging began with data collected from a healthy cohort of 2500 people in the 1970s.
- GIS data on exposure are used to estimate cumulative exposure to pollution and its association with COPD, MI, and death (Harvard University, 2023).

Community Forums and Social Media

The community forum or town hall meeting is a qualitative assessment method designed to obtain community opinions. It takes place in the neighborhood of the people involved, perhaps in a school gymnasium or an auditorium. The participants are selected to participate by invitation from the group organizing the forum.

Members come from within the community and represent all segments of the community that are involved with the issue.

- For instance, if a community is contemplating building a pickleball court, the people invited to the community forum might include potential users of the court (residents of the community who do not have pools and special groups such older adults and citizens who are disabled), community planners, health and safety personnel, and other key people with vested interests.
  - They are asked to give their views on the court: Where should it be located? Who will use it? How will the cost of building and maintaining it be assumed? What are the drawbacks to having the court?
  - Any other pertinent issues the participants may raise are included.

This method is relatively inexpensive, and results are quickly obtained. A drawback of this method is that only the most vocal community members, or those with the greatest vested interests in the issue, may be heard. This format does not provide a representative voice to others in the community who also may be affected by the proposed decision.

Town halls are used to elicit public opinion on a variety of issues, including healthcare concerns, land usage and development, political views, and feelings about issues in the public eye, such as school safety.

Frequently, local news may stream important city government or school board meetings. Other methods of opinion gathering include e-mailing to support a particular view, web-based survey sites, and text messaging a Yes or No vote on an issue. Social media sites, like Facebook, Threads, and X (formerly known as Twitter), are also popular forums for opinion sharing. Digital media is often used to elicit grassroots opinions from local community members. See more ideas on the use of social media in Chapter 10.

Focus Groups

Focus groups are similar to the community forum or town hall meeting in that it is designed to obtain grassroots opinion with a small group of participants, usually 5 to 15 people. The members chosen for the group are homogeneous with respect to specific demographic variables.

- For example, a focus group may consist of community health nurses assigned female at birth, young people in their first pregnancy, or retired businesspeople.

Leadership and facilitation skills are used in conjunction with the small group process to promote a supportive atmosphere and to accomplish set goals. The interviewer guides the discussion according to a predetermined set of questions or topics. A focus group can be organized to be representative of an aggregate, to capture community interest groups, or to sample for diversity among different population groups. Whatever the purpose, however, some people may be uncomfortable expressing their views in a group situation.

The choice of assessment method varies depending on the reasons for data collection, the goals and objectives of the study, and the available resources. It also varies according to the theoretical framework or philosophical approach through which the nurse views the community.

- In other words, the community health nurse's theoretical basis for approaching community assessment influences the purposes for conducting the assessment and the selection of methodology. See Neuman's Model in Figure 15-1.

SOURCES OF COMMUNITY DATA

The community health nurse can look in many places for data to enhance and complete a community assessment. Data sources can be primary or secondary, and they can be from international, national, state, or local sources. Websites for many primary and secondary data sources are included in internet resources.

Primary and Secondary Sources

C/PHNs make use of many sources in data collection. Community members, including formal leaders, informal leaders, and community members, can frequently offer the most accurate insights and comprehensive information.

Information gathered by talking to people provides primary data, because the data are obtained directly from the community.

- Specific examples are health team members, client records, community health (vital) statistics, census bureau data, reference books, research reports, Healthcare Effectiveness Data and Information Set (HEDIS) measures, and community health nurses.

Secondary sources of data include people who know the community well and the records such people create in the performance of their jobs.

- Because secondary data may not totally describe the community and do not necessarily reflect community self-perceptions, they may need augmentation or further validation through focus groups, surveys, and other primary data collection methods.

International Sources

International data are collected by several agencies, including the World Health Organization (WHO) and its six regional offices and health organizations, such as the Pan-American Health Organization. The WHO publishes health statistics by country and information about specific diseases and health measures in their annual Global Health Observatory. Information from these official sources can give the nurse in the local community information about immigrant and refugee populations the nurse serves. More information on international health agencies can be found in Chapter 16.

National Sources

C/PHNs can access a wealth of official and nonofficial sources of national data (see Chapter 6 for more information). Official sources develop documents based on data compiled by the government. The following are the major official agencies:

USDHHS. This is the main agency from which data can be retrieved, and the National Center for Health Statistics at the Centers for Disease Control and Prevention (CDC) was specifically established under its auspices for the collection and dissemination of health-related data.

- This agency is the nation's principal health statistics agency, compiling data from many sources.
- These data provide information for many functions, including health status for various populations and subgroups, identification of disparities, monitoring trends, identifying health problems, and supporting research.

ODPHP, a part of the USDHHS, authored *Healthy People 2030* (ODPHP, n.d.), designed to focus America's attention on the major national health problems, including realistic goals for national, state, and local agencies to work toward over one decade. Other data sources are also available through the CDC (2022c).

U.S. Census Bureau. This agency undertakes a major survey of American families every 10 years, gathering data on health, socioeconomic, and environmental conditions. This information is available on the web or on a CD-ROM, allowing numerous variables to be viewed in combination, for easier development of a community profile (U.S. Census Bureau, 2023).

National Institutes of Health (NIH). This system focuses on improving the health of the nation. An emphasis is placed on discovery of new cures or treatments and preventing disease. Employees of these agencies prevent, diagnose, and treat diseases and conduct research and disseminate research findings (NIH, 2023).

Nongovernmental organizations (NGOs). Organizations have data sources generated from research they conduct that focuses on the population, disease, or condition they were developed to serve. Each agency collects data at the national level; however, the more accessible arm for services functions at the state, county, and local levels. Information from such national sources allows community health assessment teams to compare local data with national and state statistics and trends—a very valuable function.

- Examples of these agencies are as follows:
  - American Cancer Society.
  - American Heart Association.
  - American Association of Retired Persons.
  - Mothers Against Drunk Drivers.
  - Students Against Drunk Drivers.
- The Public Health Foundation (2020) offers information on many areas of interest to C/PHNs: team toolbox, critical thinking tools, population health driver diagrams, and other quality improvement tools for public health.
- The Kaiser Family Foundation and the RAND Corporation have a variety of fact sheets and compilations of data from various sources.
- The Gallup Poll provides national survey information on various topics, including health.
- The Robert Wood Johnson Foundation's (2024) County Health Rankings and Roadmaps is based on a model of population health that emphasizes the many factors that, if improved, can help make communities healthier places to live, learn, work, and play.
- Proprietary data sources include the American Hospital Association, the American Medical Association, or various health insurance companies.

See Chapter 6 for a list of data collection systems.

State and Local Sources

For nurses, the most significant state source of assessment data comes from the state health department. This official agency is responsible for collecting state vital statistics and morbidity data.

The Behavioral Risk Factor Surveillance System is the world's largest telephone health survey that monitors health risk at the state level (CDC, 2024). Supported by the CDC, the information is used at various levels to identify risk and prevent disease. As a resource to local health departments, the state health department provides invaluable support services, and it is the main source of health-related data on the state level.

Charitable hospitals are required by the Internal Revenue Service (IRS) to complete a community assessment every 3 years. Hospitals must comply with the specific criteria set forth by the IRS. These assessments are public information. For more information on the guidelines, hospitals must comply with go to https://www.irs.gov/charities-non-profits/community-health-needs-assessment-for-charitable-hospital-organizations-section-501r3

Nonofficial agencies have state chapters or headquarters and compile their information at the state level. Local nonofficial agency chapters have documents of compiled state and national data on the population, disease, or condition they address.

State and county budgets or public health agency websites may also provide helpful information. All states collect vital statistics (e.g., births, deaths), and many collect information on hospitalization and morbidities related to infectious diseases, cancer, or cardiovascular disease. State departments of education may have school-based data on immunizations and overall school health. Information on traffic accidents, mental health, and environmental hazards is often available at the state level. States may also organize their statistics by county level, making it easier to compare your county's data with others.

Many sources of information may be obtained at the local level. Some key sources are the local visitor's bureau, city chamber of commerce, city planner's office, health department, hospitals, social service agencies, county extension office, school districts, universities or colleges, libraries, clergy, business and service organizations, and community leaders and key informants. Some of these sources compile their own statistics, but all have views of the community particular to their discipline, interest, or knowledge base. Some agencies at the local level develop city or county directories.

- These are updated periodically and are valuable resources for community health assessment teams and community health nurses. More detailed information on national, state, and local health agencies, and information available from them, can be found in Chapter 6.

DATA ANALYSIS AND PLANNING

This stage of assessment requires analysis of the information gathered, so that inferences or conclusions may be made about its meaning. Such inferences must be validated to determine their accuracy, after which steps can be taken for collaborative prioritization of your findings.

The Analysis Process

First, the data must be validated: Are they accurate, complete, representative of the population, and current? Several validation procedures may be used (Northwest Center for Public Health Practice, n.d.):

- Data can be rechecked by the community assessment team.
- Data can be rechecked by others.
- Subjective and objective data can be compared.
- Community members can consider the findings and verify them.

Validated data are then separated into categories such as physical, social, and environmental data. In many instances, data spreadsheets are used to provide a structure for data organization. Next, each category is examined to determine its significance.

- At this point, there may be a need to search for additional information to clarify the meaning of the data. Then possible conclusions may be drawn.

Big data have increasingly become a go-to source for clinical and community health professionals seeking to learn more about communities' health status. Defined as large volumes of data that are amassed, managed, and analyzed from multiple sources, big data provide the level of detail necessary to predict and understand public health risks and to develop interventions for specific groups within a larger population.

- These data are used in disease surveillance, predicting health risk, targeting interventions, and understanding disease (Zhu et al., 2019).
- Big data can be found in clinical information systems (i.e., electronic health records), public payer data claims (i.e., Medicare), and research databases.
- Some computer programs are designed to analyze community assessment data. For large, complex, or ongoing community assessment plans, this may be the best method. For smaller, one-time assessments, the paper-and-pencil method may be sufficient and less unwieldy. Some communities may hire an outside professional assessment service. These teams often use the latest technology when analyzing data.
- Not all communities can afford such a service, and if key leaders become familiar with assessment, analysis, and diagnostic processes, an investment in a computer program may be worthwhile.
- Regardless of the analysis method used, data interpretation remains a critical phase of the process.

In data interpretation, the ever-present danger exists of making inaccurate assumptions and diagnoses. The importance of validation cannot be overemphasized. Before prioritizing findings, all assumptions must be validated: Are they sound? Community members should participate actively in validation efforts by clarifying perceptions, explaining the circumstances surrounding the situation, and acting as sounding boards for testing assumptions. Other resources, such as the healthcare team members and community leaders, are used to explore and confirm inferences. Data collection, data interpretation, and validation are sequential activities, with validation serving as the bridges between them. When performed thoroughly, these steps lead to accurate diagnoses.

COMMUNITY HEALTH IMPROVEMENT PLANNING

Planning is the logical decision-making process used to design an orderly, detailed series of actions for accomplishing specific goals and objectives. Planning for community health is based on an assessment of the community, but assessment alone does not prescribe the specific actions necessary to meet clients' needs. Actions must be based in evidence, focused on priorities, and have a clear and concise plan (Minnesota Department of Health, n.d.-a). See Chapter 12 for more on program planning.

Knowing that a group of children at the elementary school are at risk for obesity does not tell the C/PHN what preventions are needed. Further action is indicated, as the nurse must systematically develop an appropriate plan (Box 15-6). See Chapter 12 for more on planning, implementing, and evaluating community health.

The Health Improvement Planning Process

The improvement planning process is a four-stage system used to design new health-related programs or services in the community and includes the following:

- Priority setting
- Establishing goals and objectives
- Implementing health promotion plans
- Evaluating implemented programs

The process is often used by health educators when designing educational programs or by administrators in community health agencies when initiating new services. The nursing process is similar to the health planning process. Each model helps to promote service effectiveness in addition to maintaining standards of practice. Community health nurses familiar with both the health planning process and the nursing process should be able to work collaboratively with community health professionals using either model.

Planning Tools

- A wide variety of tools are available to enhance community health improvement planning; these include activity descriptions, templates, and models (Minnesota Department of Health, n.d.-a; National Association of County & City Health Officials, 2023).
- Such tools help prioritize health issues, develop goals and objectives, specify interventions, and anticipate client outcomes.
- Tools that assist with planning also enable the nurse to test ideas and adjust solutions before actual implementation. Finally, the use of standardized tools enhances the planning process and promotes the effectiveness of services, as well as professional standards of practice.

In addition to using tools, a systematic approach guides the community health nurse in the development of a feasible plan that adequately and appropriately addresses the needs of the community (National Academies of Sciences, Engineering, and Medicine; National Academy of Medicine; Committee on the Future of Nursing 2020–2030, 2021). As they do in the rest of the nursing process, community health nurses collaborate with clients and other appropriate professionals throughout each of these planning activities.

Setting Priorities

Priority setting involves assigning rank or importance to the identified needs to determine the order in which goals should be addressed.

There are numerous ways to set priorities in the planning process. Many have identified useful criteria that can guide ranking problems for order of action (National Association of County & City Health Officials, n.d.; Office of the Assistant Secretary for Planning and Evaluation, n.d.). A priority matrix may also be developed, but decisions must not be unilateral and should include input from all stakeholders, including community members. They are presented here as a combination of criteria:

1. Significance of the problem or the number of people affected in the community
2. Level of community awareness of the problem
3. Community motivation to act on the problem (Is this important to the community?)
4. Nurse and partnership's ability to reduce risk and/or influence the solution

BOX 15-6 LEVELS OF PREVENTION PYRAMID

The Problem of Childhood Obesity

SITUATION: Desire to reduce the prevalence of childhood obesity in a given community by 50% within 2 years.
GOAL: Using the three levels of prevention, avoid or promptly diagnose and treat negative health conditions, and maintain a healthy weight for the population of children residing in unnamed city.

Tertiary Prevention

Rehabilitation	***Prevention***	
	Health Promotion and Education	***Health Protection***
▪ Establish school programs for obese children, including nutritional training for parents and children, offer various physical activities and emotional support, and self-esteem building ▪ Rebuild the family unit if appropriate or possible	▪ Provide family education programs for families ▪ Develop resources to support health promotion programs	▪ Monitor children for harassment or bullying. Engage parents in program with family exercises and family outings.

Secondary Prevention

Early Diagnosis	***Prompt Treatment***
▪ Develop early detection programs through schools, clinics, and physicians' offices	▪ Establish programs to provide prompt treatment for children with obesity and their parents

Primary Prevention

Health Promotion and Education	***Health Protection***
▪ Assess factors contributing to childhood obesity ▪ Institute family life education programs through schools and community groups ▪ Develop community resources to support health protection programs ▪ Promote healthy eating	▪ Identify children in the community who are at greatest risk ▪ Develop community resources to support health promotion programs

- Cost of risk reduction in terms of financial, social, and ethical capital
- Ability to identify a specific target population for an intervention
- Availability of expertise to solve the problem within the partnership, coalition, or community
- Severity of the outcome if left unresolved or the consequences of inaction
- Speed with which the problem can be resolved

Establishing Goals and Objectives

Goals and objectives are crucial to planning and should be feasible, specific, and measurable.

- Goals are broad statements of desired outcomes.
- Objectives are specific statements of desired outcomes, phrased in behavioral terms that can be measured.

Target dates for the expected completion of each objective are also stated. Objectives are the stepping stones to help one reach the end results of the larger goal. For the group of older adults concerned about crime in the neighborhood, the need, the goal, and the objectives were defined as follows:

- *Need*: The group of older adults has altered coping ability related to their fear of crime.
- *Goal*: Within 6 months, this group of older adults will feel comfortable to walk the streets of their neighborhood without experiencing any incidents of criminal assault.
- *Objectives*:
  1. By the end of the 1st month, a safety committee (composed of older adults, nurses, police, and other appropriate community members) will be established to study the crime patterns in the neighborhood.
  2. The safety committee will develop strategies for crime reduction and older adult protection, which will be presented to the city council for approval by the end of the 3rd month.

3. Safety strategies, such as increased police surveillance, town watch patrols, and escort services, will be implemented by the end of the 5th month.
4. By the end of the 6th month, nursing assessment will determine that older adults feel free to walk about the neighborhood.
5. By the 6th month, there will be fewer reported incidents of criminal assault.

Development of objectives depends on a careful analysis of all the ways in which one could accomplish the larger goal. C/PHNs should first select the course of action that is best suited to meet the goal and then build objectives. For the group of older adults, other alternatives, such as staying indoors or always walking in pairs, were considered and rejected. The ultimate choice was to find a way to make their environment safe and enjoyable.

Some rules of thumb are helpful when writing objectives.

- First, each objective should state a single idea. When more than one idea is expressed—as in an objective to both obtain equipment and learn procedures—it is more difficult to measure the completion of the objective.
- Second, each objective should describe one specific behavior that can be measured. For instance, the fourth objective from the list states that the older adults will report feeling free to walk outdoors within 6 months. It describes a behavior that can be measured at some point in time. One can more readily evaluate objectives that include specifics—such as what will be done, who will do it, and when it will be accomplished. Then it is clear to everyone involved exactly what must be done and within what time frame.
- Writing measurable objectives makes a tremendous difference in the success of planning. See Chapter 11 for more information on writing behavioral objectives.

The acronym SMART is another useful guideline when writing objectives (Minnesota Department of Health, n.d.-b). SMART objectives have these features:

- **Specific:** Concrete, detailed, and well defined so that you know where you are going and what to expect when you arrive.
- **Measurable:** Numbers and quantities provide means of measurement and comparison.
- **Achievable:** Feasible and easy to put into action.
- **Realistic:** Considers constraints such as resources, personnel, cost, and time frame.
- **Time bound:** A time frame helps to set boundaries around the objective. Planning means thinking ahead. The nurse looks ahead toward the desired end and then decides what intermediate actions are necessary to meet that goal.

Sometimes, an objective itself describes the intermediate actions. At other times, an objective may be further broken down into several activities. For example, the second objective states that the safety committee will be charged with developing strategies, presenting them to the city council, and gaining their approval. Good planning requires this kind of detail.

Making decisions is an important part of planning. Decisions must be made during the process of establishing priorities. Decisions are necessary for selecting goals and for choosing the best course of action from many possible courses. Further decision making is involved in selecting objectives and taking action to accomplish the objectives.

- To facilitate planning and decision making, the community health nurse involves other people. Clients must be included at every step because they are the ones for whom the planning is being done. Without their insight and cooperation, the plan may not succeed. Additionally, the involvement of other nurses may be important.
- Team meetings, nurse–supervisor conferences, and nurse–expert consultant sessions are all useful resources for planning. In addition, it is essential that you confer with members of other health and professional disciplines (e.g., teachers, social workers, mental health professionals, hospital representatives, city planners, clergy). Interdisciplinary team conferences are valuable for gaining a broader perspective and enlisting wider support for the evolving plan.

IMPLEMENTING HEALTH PROMOTION PLANS FOR THE COMMUNITY

Implementation is putting the plan into action. The nurse, other professionals, or clients carry out the activities of the plan.

Implementation is often referred to as the action phase of the nursing process. In community health nursing, implementation includes not just nursing action or nursing intervention but collaboration with clients, stakeholders, and other professionals.

- Community Planning for Health Assessment: Frameworks & Tools provides a wealth of information on different health promotion plans (Public Health Professionals Gateway, n.d.).
- After community data are assessed and analyzed, the final step is to create an action plan by using SMART objectives. The action plan should include big-picture outcomes as well as incremental progress.

When bringing about change in a community organization, implementation involves the greatest commitment of time and planning. This often includes an implementation timetable, as well as funding or organizing physical/informational/staff/management resources, collaboration with outside agencies, finance resources, training staff and working with community volunteers as needed for program implementation, and putting into action those interventions created during the planning phase (New Mexico Department of Health, n.d.; Rural Health Information Hub, 2024).

Certainly, the nurse's professional expertise and judgment provide a necessary resource to the client group. The nurse is also a catalyst and facilitator in planning and activating the action plan. However, a primary goal in community health is to discover what the community needs from the community themselves and align these goals. To realize this goal, the nurse must constantly involve clients in the deliberative process and work in a partnership to achieve the goal. Other health team members, stakeholders, and community members also participate in carrying out the plan. All are partners in implementation.

Preparation

The actual course of implementation, outlined in the plan, should be fairly easy to follow if goals, expected outcomes, and planned actions have been designed carefully. Community members, stakeholders, and public health officials should have a clear idea of *who*, *what*, *why*, *when*, *where*, and *how*.

Do community members agree with and know what will be done to realize the outcomes?

- Who will be involved in carrying out the plan?
- What are each person's responsibilities?
- How will we know the interventions were successful in accomplishing the goal?
- Do team members know when and where activities will occur?

As implementation begins, all team members should review these questions for themselves as well as for clients. This is the time to clarify any doubtful areas, thereby facilitating a smooth implementation phase (Live Healthy South Carolina, 2019).

Even the best planning may require adjustments. For example, some nurses who planned a health fair for older adults discovered that the target group would not have transportation to the site because the volunteering bus company had withdrawn its offer. To smoothly implement the plan, the nurses arranged for volunteers from local churches to pick up the older adults, bring them to the health fair, and deliver them afterward to their homes. Implementation requires flexibility and adaptation to unanticipated events.

Activities or Actions

The process of implementation requires a series of nursing actions or activities:

- The nurse applies appropriate theories, such as systems theory or change theory, to the actions being performed.
- The nurse helps to facilitate an environment that is conducive to carrying out the plan (e.g., a quiet room in which to hold a group teaching session or solicitation of support from local officials for an environmental cleanup project).
- The nurse and other health team members prepare clients to receive services by assessing their knowledge, understanding, and attitudes and by carefully interpreting the plan to clients. This interaction nurtures open communication and trust between nurse and clients. Professionals and clients (or representatives if the aggregate is large) form a contractual agreement about the content of the plan and how it is to be carried out.
- The plan is carried out, or modified and then carried out, by professionals and clients. Modification requires constant observation and interchange during implementation because these actions determine the success of the plan and the nature of needed changes.
- The nurse and the team monitor and document the progress of the implementation phase by process evaluation, which measures the ongoing achievement of planned actions (Anderson & McFarlane, 2019).

EVALUATION OF IMPLEMENTED COMMUNITY HEALTH IMPROVEMENT PLANS

Evaluation is usually seen as the final step, but because the nursing process is cyclical in nature, the nurse is constantly evaluating throughout the entire process. For instance, in the assessment phase, the nurse must evaluate whether the collected data are sufficient and appropriate to beginning planning.

- Evaluation methods must be addressed during the planning phase as goals and objectives as well as interventions are identified (Rural Health Information Hub, n.d.).
- Evaluation refers to measuring and judging the effectiveness of goal or outcome attainment. Too often, emphasis is placed primarily on assessing client needs and on planning and implementing service. The nursing process is not complete until evaluation takes place.
- Ideally, the nursing process should be observed as cyclical instead of linear, and when this occurs, it is obvious that evaluation guides the next assessment.
- The Community Toolbox (n.d.) provides suggestions for participatory evaluation that includes examination of the process (e.g., how the assessment was conducted), implementation (e.g., how the program was designed and executed), and outcomes (e.g., if desired results were accomplished). Appropriate questions include the following:
  - Was all potential information assessed?
  - How effective was the service provided?
  - Were client needs truly met?
  - How has health status changed?
- Professional practitioners owe it to their clients, themselves, and other health service providers to fully and effectively evaluate a program (Box 15-7).

An example of evaluation to improve program plans includes the Health in Action Project (Nieves et al., 2020).

- In conjunction with the East Neighborhood Health Action Center, this project implemented a participatory grant-making process to fund projects that improved the community's health.

- The project engaged stakeholders in decision making by including local residents in the decision-making process for the allocation of grant funds.
- Evaluation findings showed that the inclusion of residents as part of the process for decision making was a strength of the project.
- Participants learned about the local organizations and services, and they felt included in a process that affected them and their neighborhood.
- Reciprocally, the funded organizations expanded their work and piloted new programs, forming new partnerships and building community networks (Nieves et al., 2020).

As stated earlier, evaluation is an act of appraisal in which one judges value in relation to a standard and a set of criteria. Evaluation requires a stated purpose, specific standards, and criteria by which to judge and judgment skills.

BOX 15-7 STORIES FROM THE FIELD

Community Assessment of a large county in a West Coast State

Our group completed a community assessment of a rural county in a west coast state. We found data from many sources (e.g., census, health department reports), including key informants and a community survey completed by community members. Many resources were available on the CDC website for Mobilizing for Action through Planning and Partnerships (https://www.naccho.org/programs/public-health-infrastructure/performance-improvement/community-health-assessment/mapp/phase-3-the-four-assessments) and from the community assessment conducted by the local charitable hospital (https://www.irs.gov/charities-non-profits/community-health-needs-assessment-for-charitable-hospital-organizations-section-501r3).

Windshield Survey

The windshield survey had the following findings.

Physical

In touring the area, it is noted that there are many older apartments in need of repair. Many do not have window screens, and balconies are cluttered with old furniture, children's toys, and trash. Some of the old apartments have been replaced with new high-end security apartment buildings and townhouses. Sidewalks are broken up, making them unsafe to walk on. No playgrounds are noted on this side of town. There is one motel advertising hourly rates. Several small ethnic grocery stores with window signs that say no cash on hand. Liquor stores are located on every corner with several people standing around smoking cigarettes. As the community begins to attempt gentrification, a large parking structure is torn down with rubble scattered among the vacant lot. Graffiti covers the rubble, and there are a few tents hidden among the concrete. Under the freeway overpasses are several homeless encampments. The elementary school children and their parents attempt to go around but find it difficult because of the busy street. The area has very few grass or tree areas. Children play in the parking lots of the apartment buildings.

Economic

There is only one major supermarket in the area, but it provides a wide variety of ethnic food that represents the community and is reasonably priced. In addition, there are several small neighborhood grocery stores that sell fruits/vegetables, meats, and baked goods. Convenience/liquor stores are found on every corner. The largest employer in the area is a large bagel bakery that has been in business for over 80 years, with generations of families having worked there. The bakery pays well and provides health insurance. The bagel business draws people from all over the city. The major streets are lined with small businesses and fast-food restaurants. Some small businesses have closed and/or are boarded up due to the poor economy in the area. Business owners are responsible for removing any graffiti on their buildings, which some do and others do not.

Services

Public bus transportation is extensive with most stops every 15 minutes during peak hours. One can see people running to catch the bus if the connecting bus runs late. Recently, a bus driver was stabbed and died as he took his break outside his bus. Medical transport services and cabs are available. Two major freeways run through both ends of the city. Many people drive their own cars, but bus ridership is the major source of transportation due to the high cost of maintaining a car. A community hospital is located in the middle of the city, and there are several small clinics scattered throughout. The city is located in a Health Professional Shortage Area (HPSA) for primary care, dental care, and mental health services. There is a county public health department with adult and pediatric services. Public health nurses operate out of the health department and make frequent home visits to different aggregates. Local churches provide food and overnight stays for those who need help. The community has several food banks that are open daily. Fire and police stations are located in the area. Federal and county courthouses are in the center of the city. City hall and a large library are located in the same area. There is one large high school with 2400 students that provides multiple services to students and their families. There are 10 elementary schools and three middle schools in the area. Each offer programs for adults and after-school programs for students. There is also a community college 5 miles away that many young adults attend. The nursing program is very difficult to get into.

Social

There is a local newspaper. Most people have access to TV/radio, and there are Spanish-language stations available. There are political bumper stickers on some cars and also billboards in populated areas. People can be seen smoking and occasionally vaping outside of stores or when walking downtown. People who are homeless gather in several areas of the county. High school students gather after school at local fast food restaurants. People shopping at grocery stores are overheard speaking English, Spanish, and Portuguese. After school is closed, one can see children and parents socializing outside.

BOX 15-7 STORIES FROM THE FIELD

Community Assessment of a large county in a West Coast State (*Continued*)

Data Collection

The data collected are shown in the following table.

	City	State
Population	200,467	39.5 million
Mortality Rates		
Average adjusted death rate	696.2 per 100,000	610.3 per 100,000
Diabetes death rate	30.3	20.4
Lung cancer death rate	38.4	27.5
Motor vehicle accidents death rate	15.5	9.5
Firearm death rate	10.5	7.9
Morbidity Rates		
Smoking (adults)	14.5%	11.3%
Hypertension on discharge	30.3%	28.4%
Adolescents who gave birth	30.4 per 1000 live births	15.7 per 1000 live births
Infant mortality rate	6.8	4.4
Prenatal care, 1st trimester	71.1	83.5
% Births late/no prenatal care	8%	2.9%
% Births ≤ 24 mo prior birth	16.8%	13.1%
Socioeconomic Data		
Ethnicity (majority)	53.5% Hispanic/Latino	39.3% Hispanic/Latino
Median household income	$25,742	$67,169
Children < poverty level	35.3%	22.8%
No high school diploma	30.1%	17.5%
Bachelor's degree or higher	10.2%	30.6%
Have health insurance	87.3%	91%
Unemployment	12%	5.3%
Of working population		
Worked 50–52 wk/y	40%	57%
Did not work/past year	32%	25%
Worked part of year/seasonal	28%	18%
Violent crime rate	4.6 per 1000	3.96 per 1000
Property crime rate	23.0	24.4

1. *List the assets and needs of this community.*
2. *Prioritize hypothesis.*
3. *What are some solutions that might be developed to address these issues? Identify one that your student group might be able to complete during this clinical experience.*
   a. Who would be involved (what partnerships would be needed)?
   b. What level of prevention (primary, secondary, tertiary) does the intervention represent?
   c. What outcomes could you measure to show improvement?
   d. How can your plan best be evaluated?

Types of Evaluations

To determine the success of their planning and intervention, community health nurses use two main types of evaluation: formative and summative evaluation.

The focus of *formative* evaluation is on process during the actual interventions. In formative evaluation, performance standards are developed and used to determine what is and is not working throughout the process. These could include the physical and organizational structure of the agency, as well as resources that provide a foundation for any interventions.

- Formative evaluation essentially looks at the step-by-step process of program implementation. Could I do anything better or different to increase my desired outcome?

- An example would occur when looking at the poor attendance at two sessions of an evening health promotion class for older adults.
  - The nurse identifies the reason for poor attendance as being older adults' reluctance to attend an evening class because they don't drive at night, have low vision at night, or fear coming out in the dark.
  - The class is rescheduled for midmorning, and the attendance dramatically increases.

Summative evaluation focuses on the outcome of the interventions: Did you meet your goals? Summative evaluation examines the outcomes of the interventions.

The *effect*, or degree to which an outcome objective has been met, informs the agency or program leader of the program's impact on clients' health.

- As an example, one manufacturing company had an 80% adherence rate for employees who were supposed to wear proper protective devices (goggles, safety shoes, and hard hats) in the plant.
- Noncompliance on the part of some workers was a concern to union representatives, the health and safety team, and the company management. They were concerned that 20% of their employees were at risk for injury that would cause pain, suffering, loss of work time, disruption to the manufacturing process, and reduced profitability.
- The occupational health nurse along with the safety officer began a month-long safety campaign that included safety mini-classes, posters, and incentives for departments with 100% safety equipment adherence.
- Three months after the program, 95% of the employees were adhering to the safety regulations.
- This 15% increase was attributed to the effect of the safety program.

The *impact* of a program determines how close it comes to attaining its goals. In the earlier example, the objective of the safety campaign was to increase safety equipment use, and use was significantly increased because of the program. However, if the goal of the program had been to decrease accidents and save the company money, the result could be determined only with additional information.

- Were there fewer injuries caused by accidents?
- Were there fewer days lost to injuries?
- Did the company save money as a direct result of employee safety adherence?
- What was the cost–benefit ratio?

Depending on the answers to these questions, the overall goal of the program may or may not have been met, even though the objective of the program was met. The full impact of the program cannot be determined without additional data. See Chapter 12 for more on program evaluation.

Community Development Theory

A **community development** perspective assumes that community members participate in all aspects of change—assessment, planning, development, delivery of services, and evaluation. With this approach, the focus is on healthful community changes generated from within the community, as a partnership between healthcare providers and inhabitants, rather than a commodity dispensed by healthcare providers.

- The outcomes are more positive when community members have a sense of ownership in the health programs and services that address their needs. This enhances empowerment among members of the community and enables them to more effectively control and participate in transforming their environment and their personal circumstances.
- This implies that healthcare agency infrastructures are appropriate additions to services that are planned and delivered in an acceptable manner to the community. This empowerment leads to greater resilience and ultimately, wellness (RAND Corporation, n.d.).
- Community members have mastered adaptation to the community, and they have firsthand knowledge of prevention methods and interventions that are appropriate to their lifestyles.
- Members of the community are engaged as leaders, and time is spent building trust and developing collaborative relationships with community members, stakeholders, and neighborhood healthcare providers.

The expertise of community members is valued and can be useful in designing recruitment strategies, as well as in data analysis. This experience can enrich the community, as well as the actual participants.

SUMMARY

- Public health nursing is a community-oriented, population-focused nursing specialty that is based on interpersonal relationships.
- The unit of care is the community or population rather than the person, and the goal is to promote healthy communities.
- Theories and models of community/public health nursing practice aid the nurse in understanding the rationale behind community-oriented care.
- Salmon's construct for public health nursing prescribes education, engineering, and enforcement with people, families, communities, and nations.
- Betty Neuman's System Model provides a comprehensive holistic and system-based approach to nursing. The focus is on a client's response to environmental stressors.
- Models used in public health nursing practice, the Minnesota Intervention "Wheel," the LAC-DPH

PHN Practice Model, and the Omaha System Model of the Problem-Solving Process provide guidance for C/PHNs to assess, plan, intervene, and evaluate the care they provide to communities.

- The eight principles of public health nursing provide a framework within which the nurse works to promote and protect the health of populations.
- Characteristics of healthy communities include those elements that enable people to maintain a high quality of life and productivity by increasing health and decreasing disease and disparities in health and healthcare delivery. The effectiveness of community health nursing practice depends on how well the nursing process is used as a tool to enhance aggregate or population health. The nursing process involves the appropriate application of a systematic series of actions with the goal of helping clients achieve their optimal level of health. The components of this process are assessment, diagnosis, planning, implementation, and evaluation.
- As noted previously, the concept of community as client refers to a group or population of people as the focus of nursing service. The community's health is reflected in its status (e.g., morbidity and mortality rates, crime rates, educational and economic levels), structure (availability, use, and quality of services and resources), and processes (how well it functions in regard to its strengths and limitations). The dimensions of a community's health may be seen in regard to its location (e.g., climate, vegetation, boundaries), population (e.g., diversity or homogeneity, old, young, pregnant, people with a substance use disorder, or academic members), and social systems (e.g., schools, businesses, communications, healthcare, and religious organizations, among others).
- Assessment for community health nurses means collecting and evaluating information about a community's health status to discover existing or potential needs and assets as a basis for planning future action. Assessment involves two major activities. The first is the collection of pertinent data, and the second is the analysis and interpretation of that data.
- Community health nurses may use various assessment methods to determine a community's needs. They include windshield and walking surveys; problem-oriented assessment, which focuses on a single problem and looks at the community in terms of that problem; *community subsystem assessment*, by which the community health nurse focuses on a single dimension of community life; a complicated and often time-consuming *comprehensive assessment*, to discover *all* relevant community health information; or an *assets assessment* that focuses on the strengths of a community as opposed to its deficits. Combinations may also prove useful (e.g., problem-oriented and assets assessments).
- Community data may be provided by many means—surveys, descriptive epidemiologic studies, community forums, and town meetings. Focus groups as well as primary and secondary sources (e.g., people who are familiar with the community and its character and history) are also common sources of data, along with websites, and government departments and agencies that compile statistics (e.g., U.S. Census Bureau, state, or county health departments). Sources can include national, international, state, county, and local agencies, as well as business and social organizations.
- Using the nursing process in the community would not be complete without looking at the role of the C/PHN as a catalyst for community health improvement. Community development theory is the foundation that supports citizen empowerment and use of key players in the community to plan for the health and safety of that community.

ACTIVE LEARNING EXERCISES

1. Using the characteristics of the community from a population perspective (Table 15-3), assess the 12 population variables of your own community. What did you learn about your community that you didn't know before? Which variables are assets to the community and how could they help your community? Which variables are a hindrance to the community? (Objective 1)
2. Based on your assessment, prioritize the needs of the community and develop a plan of care, taking into consideration the nursing process as outlined in the text. (Objective 2)
3. With a classmate, conduct a windshield survey (see Box 15-3) in a community unknown to either of you. Assess all the points under physical, economic, services, and social. What did you learn? Compare your windshield survey with other classmates. How were they similar and different? (Objective 3)
4. Choose one of the 17 interventions in the Minnesota Wheel that pertain to your windshield survey findings and develop interventions that are individual-, community-, and systems-focused. Are the interventions feasible with resources within the community? What community assets could help with the interventions? Which of the 10 Essential Public Health Services does this intervention address? See Box 2.2. (Objective 4)
5. Partnerships in the community are extremely important in community/public health nursing. Which community members could you partner with to develop your plan of care? Remember to have a member of the community as a partner as well. Ask your professors, church leaders, and community advocates if they belong to any partnerships and ask to attend. How do the members interact with each other? Is there an agenda for the meeting? Where do the members come from and how did they get involved? (Objective 5)

CHAPTER 16

Global Health Nursing

"When it comes to global health, there is no 'them'... only 'us'."

—Global Health Council (2010)

KEY TERMS

- Brain Drain Brain Gain
- Community health workers
- Demographic transitions
- Disability-adjusted life year
- Era of Chronic, Long-Term Health Conditions
- Era of Infectious Diseases
- Era of Social Health Conditions
- Global health
- Global burden of disease
- Primary healthcare
- 17 Sustainable Developmental Goals
- Years lived with disability
- Years of life lost
- World Health Organization (WHO)

LEARNING OBJECTIVES

Upon mastery of this chapter, you should be able to:

1. Compare and contrast global benchmarks, such as the global burden of disease, to identify health patterns across populations.
2. Recognize the impact of policies on population health outcomes.
3. Describe the role of the environment and climate change on population health and identify prevention measures that improve the population's health.
4. Identify global organizations and their role in the management of global disease during epidemics and pandemics.
5. Describe the concept of "Brain Drain Brain Gain" as it relates to global health ethics and the protection of population health.

INTRODUCTION

The world has come to us. We encounter the world every day where we live. In the Los Angeles Unified School District, the second largest K–12 district in the nation, students speak 98 languages other than English at home (Los Angeles Almanac, 2023). Even Montana, a sparsely populated state, has identified 21 world languages spoken in their homes (City-Data, 2023). Local health has become **global health**.

What do you think of when you hear the phrase "global health"? Would you first think about the survival rates of people during childbirth? Or basic nutrition as a foundation for health worldwide? More likely, you might think about the news of respiratory pandemics spreading from one country to another. What would you do if an international traveler from a pandemic-afflicted area is admitted to your unit for care?

- Knowledge about global health could guide you to find targeted resources when you write a nursing care plan for your traveler patient. These questions all point to the importance of understanding the concept of global health, or the "world as client," which is the focus of this chapter.
- How can the whole world be our client as the recipient of nursing care? Even if you think you will never practice nursing overseas, it is important to realize that global events affect nursing actions locally and the health of others globally.

This chapter describes the intersection of global health and C/PHN. It introduces basic global health concepts and how global events can impact the health and healthcare of a community, country, region, or the world.

- We begin with a quick review of the context for global health and some key events over the years that show the evolution of global health. Global health includes health within the borders of each nation, within population groups with unique cultures and languages, and across international borders and cultures.

- We briefly examine selected global health trends and examine the influence of global political initiatives. Usually when we think of global health trends, we think of data describing epidemiology and contagious diseases.
- One important trend since the COVID-19 pandemic is how trust in health institutions has been impacted by sociopolitical responses including the use of social media.
- Other trends are equally important, such as management of noncommunicable diseases and increased access to **primary healthcare**.
- One important initiative, *Health in All Policies*, aims to address the health impact of every program or initiative.
- We also consider how these trends influence global health goals. We know health promotion and disease prevention are important goals, but do some strategies work better than others?
- Smaller nations with emerging economies have figured out how to deliver quality healthcare despite limited resources and challenging infrastructure. Sometimes they partner with a nongovernmental agency, which is a nonprofit or voluntary citizens' group formed to address a social issue.

This chapter ends with a brief discussion of global health ethics. You are already familiar with the primary ethical concept in nursing of nonmaleficence, "first do no harm" (see Chapter 4). This is also a key principle in global health ethics. Someday you might have the opportunity to participate in an overseas internship or perhaps volunteer as a nurse following a disaster in another country. Being aware of the special ethical concerns unique to global health will help you be successful wherever you practice nursing. Ultimately, we want the nursing care we provide to be ethical and positive with lasting benefits, whether we care for patients down the street or across the world.

THE CONTEXT FOR GLOBAL HEALTH: INTERNATIONAL COOPERATION

The overarching perspective of global health nursing is one planet of interdependent nations. What happens in one country affects others in important ways. For example, air travel can transport health problems from any remote village halfway around the world to any major city within 36 hours. Detecting infectious diseases quickly has become more urgent for everyone's health. Other global issues with an impact on population health include ongoing efforts to eradicate old diseases such as TB or malaria along with newer ones such as HIV, all while maintaining efforts to improve basic healthcare services. As countries rush to help families and children affected by wars in their country, the world stands helpless. Yet, organizations, such as UNICEF, provide care as best they can. Many C/PHNs travel overseas to provide medical and prevention care (see Box 16-1). Measles and cholera outbreaks, the lack of safe drinking water, children not feeling safe, and upheaval of daily routines are a common occurrence for children in war-torn countries.

- Explore the stories of children found on the UNICEF website https://www.unicef.org/stories.
  - What are some common threads all these children experience?
  - Which of the 10 Essential Public Health Services are pertinent in these situations to help children?
  - Chapter 15 discusses community assessments. If one was to conduct a problem-oriented assessment what are some topics a C/PHN might focus on?

BOX 16-1 PERSPECTIVES

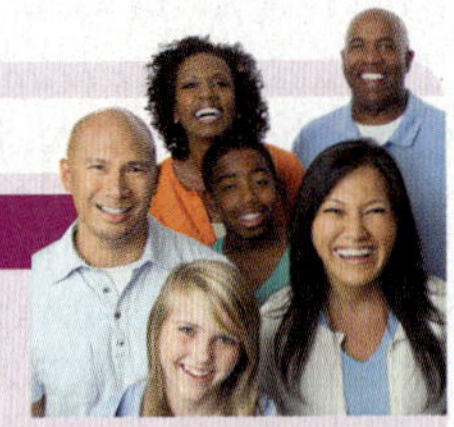

A Student Nurse's Experience in the Peace Corps

My experience in global health began as a Peace Corps Volunteer in the Dominican Republic from 2014 to 2016. Assigned to live in Río Limpio, a mountainous agricultural community bordering Haiti, my primary role involved working in a local elementary school. Through the time I spent working with the teachers, students, and families, I came to see how many children relied on government-provided meals. It became increasingly clear to me that for these children, learning couldn't flourish if their basic needs weren't met.

In a community of just over 2000 residents, the realities of life and death intertwined seamlessly into daily existence. Despite having a small clinic staffed by one dedicated community nurse, the absence of sufficient resources (e.g., reliable electricity, basic medications, etc.), as well as a primary provider, posed significant challenges. The nearest hospital, located 2 hours away in Loma De Cabrera, faced its own struggles due to limited resources, making it difficult to meet the needs of patients. Infrequent transportation compounded the issue, with families often bearing the financial burden of fuel costs for the government-provided ambulance, leaving essential healthcare out of reach for many.

Toward the end of my service, I translated for a medical mission that came to the community. The lengthy queues were filled with many unfamiliar faces from the more remote mountainous regions, spotlighting the urgent need for essential resources in underrepresented communities. Witnessing their journey to access healthcare services, such as tooth extractions, illuminated the profound challenges faced by all rural communities.

My time in Río Limpio serves as a constant reminder of the imperative to prioritize resource allocation and community empowerment in global health initiatives.

Andria De Filippi, BS in Political Science, International Relations, Senior BSN student (graduated May '24)

One Health: Healthy Environment, Healthy Animals, Healthy Humans

The One Health initiative involves all sectors of society from local, regional, national to global levels—an important approach that is especially crucial for countries with emerging economies. Because it is particularly important to prevent, predict, detect, and respond to global health threats, the World Health Organization formed the One Health initiative as a coordinated approach to addressing the root causes, recognizing the increasing interconnectedness between humans, animals, and our shared physical environment (CDC, 2023a).

- The operational definitions of One Health include communication, coordination of effort, and collaboration on activities at the animal–human–environment interface (CDC, 2023a).
- The United Nations Food and Agricultural Organization (2023) uses a One Health interconnected monitoring approach with an established early warning monitoring system. This allows for rapid notification of changes in zoonotic diseases, food and water safety, and agricultural production.
- In the United States, the CDC uses One Health to gain an understanding of how diseases spread among people, animals, and the environment. While we think of the CDC as a U.S. government agency, the CDC also has a global focus participating in global health security and coordinating outbreak investigations.
- Review the One Health in Action at https://www.cdc.gov/one-health/php/stories/?CDC_AAref_Val=https://www.cdc.gov/onehealth/in-action/index.html. Select one site for story links. Identify which partnerships were involved across locations and agencies, which animals were involved, and what was the environmental impact.
- What resolution for health was achieved? What was the role of cross-agency cooperation?

Sustainable Development Goals

At the 2016 United Nations (UN) Sustainable Development Summit, the **17 Sustainable Development Goals** were adopted by world leaders as the global development framework to be achieved by 2030 (UN, n.d.-a). Also known as Global Goals, the Sustainable Development Goals are not legally binding; however, governments are expected to address a range of social needs for their populations while tackling climate change (see Fig. 16-1).

- The Sustainable Development Goals are a collection of 17 global goals and "are a call for action by all countries—poor, rich, and middle-income—to promote prosperity while protecting the planet" (UN, n.d.-a, para. 1).

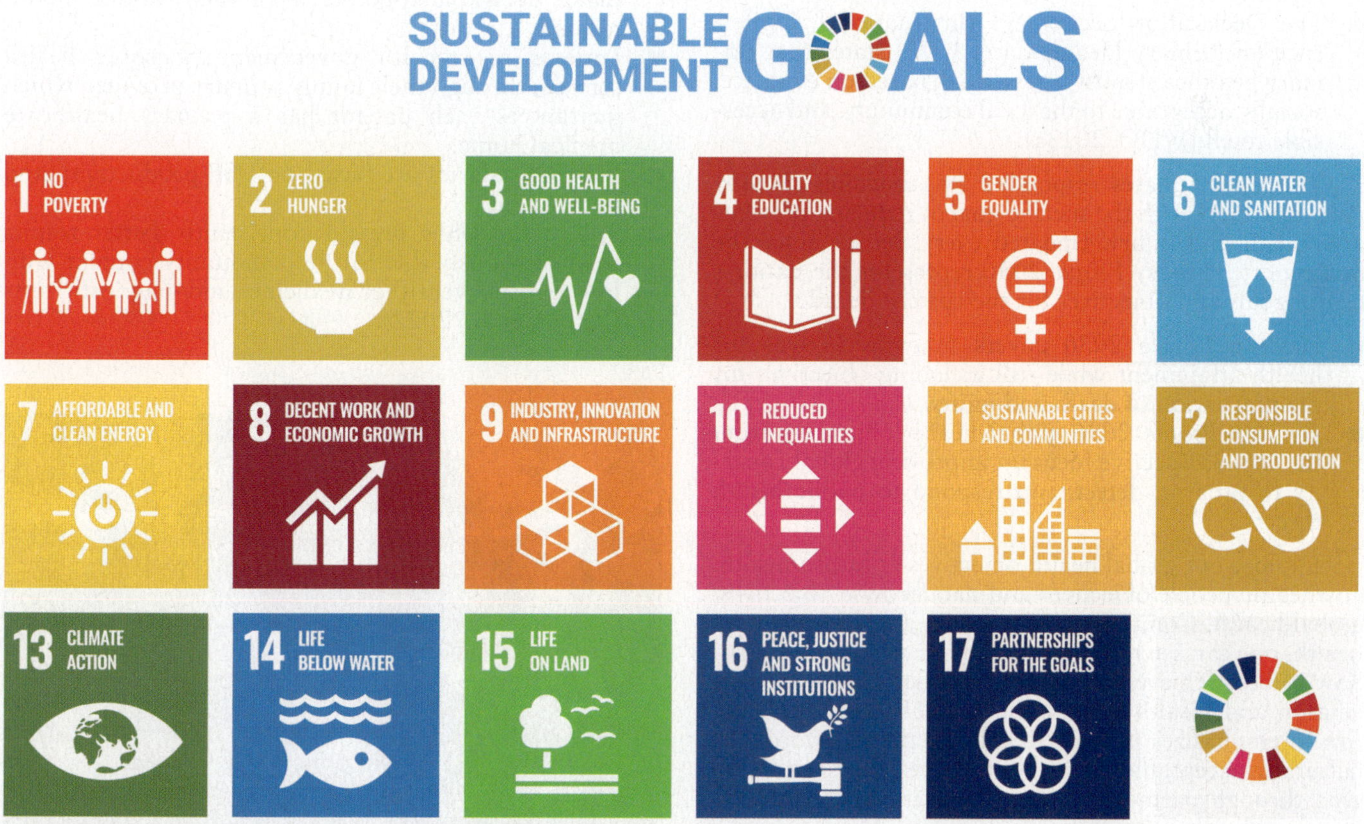
SUSTAINABLE DEVELOPMENT GOALS
1 NO POVERTY
2 ZERO HUNGER
3 GOOD HEALTH AND WELL-BEING
4 QUALITY EDUCATION
5 GENDER EQUALITY
6 CLEAN WATER AND SANITATION
7 AFFORDABLE AND CLEAN ENERGY
8 DECENT WORK AND ECONOMIC GROWTH
9 INDUSTRY, INNOVATION AND INFRASTRUCTURE
10 REDUCED INEQUALITIES
11 SUSTAINABLE CITIES AND COMMUNITIES
12 RESPONSIBLE CONSUMPTION AND PRODUCTION
13 CLIMATE ACTION
14 LIFE BELOW WATER
15 LIFE ON LAND
16 PEACE, JUSTICE AND STRONG INSTITUTIONS
17 PARTNERSHIPS FOR THE GOALS

FIGURE 16-1 Sustainable development goals. (Reprinted with permission from United Nations Sustainable Development Goals. https://www.un.org/sustainabledevelopment. The content of this publication has not been approved by the United Nations and does not reflect the views of the United Nations or its officials or Member States.)

- Interestingly, only Goal 3, Good Health and Well-Being, is specifically devoted to health and wellness. However, because the goals are all interconnected social determinants of health (SDOH), each goal reflects an important contribution to health.
- For an update on the progress of these goals refer to The Sustainable Development Guide Report 2023 at https://unstats.un.org/sdgs/report/2023/The-Sustainable-Development-Goals-Report-2023.pdf.

Together, these goals pledge to end conditions such as poverty, hunger, AIDS, and discrimination against people assigned female at birth and to "leave no one behind" (UN Development Programme, 2023, para. 3).

Health for All: A Primary Healthcare Initiative

The focus of the WHO in the years after World War II was on building hospitals and costly health establishments throughout the world. The thinking was that hospitals brought health to a region. However, many countries could not afford to build healthcare centers, nor could they afford to train large numbers of health professionals. Because of those emerging trends and a belief that a major change in thinking and practice was needed, many health leaders from throughout the world met in 1978 in Alma-Ata, Kazakhstan, at the International Conference on Primary Health Care.

- A sweeping set of recommendations emphasizing the importance of primary healthcare became the *Declaration of Alma-Ata* (see Chapter 1) or *Health for All*.
- The Declaration Section VI (International Conference on Primary Health Care, 1978) states that primary healthcare must be essential, based on evidence, socially acceptable to the local community, and accessible to all (WHO, 2023a).

The United States responded by launching *Healthy People* in 1979 with the specific goal of reducing preventable death and injury. Updated every decade since the first report, *Healthy People 2030* represents the nation's health goals and objectives for the current decade.

- *Healthy People 2030* covers many objectives for health attainment while still including objectives for the prevention of death and injury.
- *Healthy People 2030* global health objectives from the U.S. perspective focus on improving global capacity to prevent, detect, and respond to public health threats.

Explore our global health objectives at https://health.gov/healthypeople/objectives-and-data/browse-objectives/global-health. Compared to the initial goals for primary health, one can see the evolution in our understanding of how to best achieve health for all (Office of Disease Prevention and Health Promotion [ODPHP], n.d.). *Health for All* emphasizes primary healthcare that is affordable, culturally acceptable, appropriate, accessible, and delivered through partnerships between national health services and local communities.

- Communities assumed responsibility for identifying their own priority health concerns, with planning and implementing primary healthcare services to match their unique needs.
  - Common services include health promotion, disease prevention, treatment, and rehabilitative care provided by healthcare workers who live in the same community (Fig. 16-2; WHO, 2023b).

Health in All Policies

In 2006, *Health for All* was expanded to *Health in All Policies* as an essential component of primary healthcare. The idea of Health in All Policies is that good health requires policies across all sectors of society to actively support health. This expanded approach requires policymakers to consider the health impact of policies for transportation, housing, employment, nutrition, water and sanitation, and education. By acknowledging the impact that any policy has on health, optimal health is maintained for the community's benefit (World Health Organization [WHO], 2024a). See Chapter 13 on policymaking and advocacy.

Achievements of Primary Healthcare

One example of the achievement of primary healthcare is in Portugal, where comprehensive services have been expanded to the full population through Family Health Units ("USFs"—Unidades de Saúde Familiar) across the country.

- USFs are self-managed and self-selected groups of primary providers, nurses, and staff who work to provide care to local patients and families and make decisions together with them about health needs.
- Patients register for government-sponsored health services through their family primary provider, which guarantees each patient has a primary healthcare medical home.
- MD/RN salaries are based on USF productivity and performance.
- Today, the USFs present consistently better results than previously due to the community context with lower costs overall for medicines and diagnostic tests (Pereira et al., 2022).

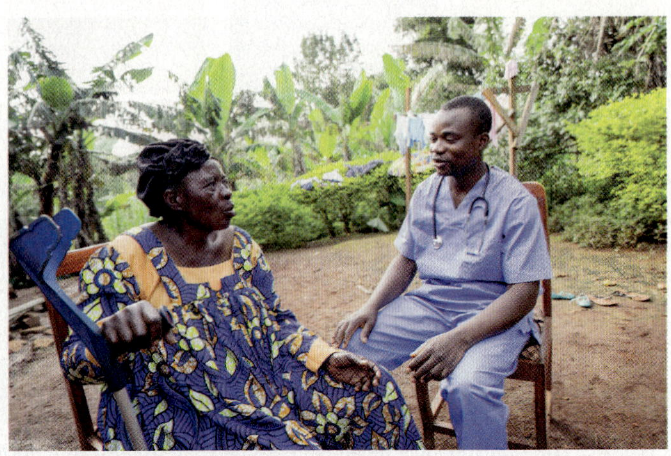

FIGURE 16-2 Community member waiting for free medical outreach care in an African village.

Many other nations are working toward *Health for All* by making healthcare a right for all citizens and expanding services to meet the needs of rural populations and high-risk groups.

- Future action regarding primary healthcare calls for strengthened collaboration among governmental agencies and NGOs in public and private sectors.
- Only when primary healthcare is accessible to all people will the world have a realistic chance of achieving all the goals set out in the Declaration of Alma-Ata (WHO, n.d.).

United Nations and World Health Organization

In 1945, at the end of World War II, the United Nations (UN) Charter was signed and ratified by 50 countries. As an international organization, the UN was to facilitate peace and security and to prevent threats to that peace; respect equal rights and the right to self-determine; promote international cooperation in solving problems and the protection of human rights and freedom; and be the hub for the coordinated actions (UN, n.d.-b). Listen to a reading of the Preamble (https://www.youtube.com/watch?v=GHrqzaFT0kw).

The UN today supports and manages several international funds, programs, and specialized agencies that focus on health.

Some of these existed 150 years ago under a different title (United Nations Global Market Place, 2024), and some, such as the Joint UN Programme on HIV/AIDS where 11 UN organizations came together to fight AIDS, were established more recently to meet emerging needs (UNAIDS, 2024).

The **World Health Organization (WHO)** is one of the specialized agencies under the UN. The Constitution of the WHO names principles of "happiness, harmonious relations, and security of all peoples" (WHO, 2020, p.1) with the main objective for "the attainment by all peoples of the highest possible level of health" (p. 2). As of 2024, there are 194 member states in the WHO divided into 6 geographical regions for the purposes of reporting, analysis, and administration (WHO, 2023c).

Other organizations also participate with the UN in promoting international health but are not necessarily sponsored by governments. Nongovernment organizations and civil society organizations are often philanthropic and some are for profit. See Table 16-1 for a list of selected global health organizations and their areas of focus.

TABLE 16-1 Global Health Organizations

Organization	Type	Funding Source	Purpose/Audience
World Health Organization (WHO)	Intergovernmental agency related to UN	Dues of member countries Donations (governments, private)	Directing, coordinating authority on international health Improves global health
United Nations International Children's Emergency Fund (UNICEF)	UN agency	Voluntary contributions of governments (70%) and private sources (30%): NGOs, foundations, corporations, and individuals	Promotes maternal and child health and welfare across the globe
United Nations Educational, Scientific, & Cultural Organization	UN agency	Voluntary contributions of governments, NGOs, foundations, corporations, and individuals	Assists people in forming peaceful and inclusive societies Preserves the heritage of countries (World Heritage Centre)
The World Bank	Intergovernmental agency related to the UN	Primarily financed by selling AAA-rated bonds in the world's financial markets, from reserves paid in by 188-member country shareholders	Not a bank in the ordinary sense but a unique partnership of five institutions to reduce poverty and support development with financial and technical assistance to resource-limited countries
Pan American Health Organization (PAHO)	Intergovernmental agency	Member country (52) assessments Funds from WHO, UN, private donations	Coordinating agency for public health in Western hemisphere Provides technical and epidemiologic assistance
U.S. Agency for International Development	Independent, bilateral agency of the U.S. executive branch, under the Secretary of State	Congressional justifications, annual appropriations bill, budget for the State Department	Strategic global health priorities for resource-limited countries: (1) preventing child and maternal deaths; (2) controlling the HIV/AIDS epidemic; and (3) combating infectious diseases Advances U.S. foreign policy

(Continued)

TABLE **16-1** Global Health Organizations (*Continued*)

Organization	Type	Funding Source	Purpose/Audience
Centers for Disease Control and Prevention (CDC; including the Center for Global Health)	U.S. federal agency within the U.S. Department of Health and Human Services	Congressional justifications, annual appropriations bill	Works 24/7 to protect America from health, safety, and security threats, both foreign and domestic
Partners in Health	501(c)(3) nonprofit corporation	Corporate and government donations, academic and public sector partners	To provide a preferential option for resource-limited people in healthcare, strives to achieve two overarching goals: to bring the benefits of modern medical science to those most in need of them and to serve as an antidote to despair
Médecins Sans Frontières (Doctors Without Borders)	NGO	International agencies and governments, along with private donors	International, neutral organization sending emergency medical assistance in times of war, epidemics, disasters, or denial of care
Bill and Melinda Gates Foundation	Private foundation	Endowment fund from the Bill and Melinda Gates Foundation Trust	Provides grants to U.S. tax-exempt organizations that are independently identified for partnership on global health, development, growth and opportunity, policy and advocacy, and U.S. educational improvement
International Council of Nurses	Professional federation	Membership dues, limited to one nursing organization per nation (The American Nurses Association is the organization representing U.S. nurses)	Represents the global interests and concerns of the nursing profession. Maintains the role of nursing in healthcare through its global voice Includes nursing organizations from 130 countries, representing 20 million nurses

NGO, nongovernmental organization; UN, United Nations.
Source: Bill and Melinda Gates Foundation (n.d.); Doctors Without Borders USA (n.d.); International Council of Nurses (2020); Kaiser Family Foundation (January 24, 2019); Partners in Health (n.d.); PAHO (n.d.); UNICEF (n.d.); World Bank Group (n.d.).

The Centers for Disease Control and Prevention

The Centers for Disease Control and Prevention (CDC) is the nation's leading science-based, data-driven, service organization that protects the public's health (CDC, 2022a).

- In addition to providing a home for health information and data on the people of the United States, the CDC's mission also includes supporting global health security and disease outbreak investigation throughout the world. CDC scientists work collaboratively through the Global Disease Detection Operations Center and partner with the U.S. Department of Health and Human Services Office of Global Affairs.

The CDC plays a leading role in global health security when outbreaks occur anywhere. CDC disease experts join with stakeholders to strengthen critical public health services globally in six areas:

- Surveillance, workforce development, laboratories, emergency preparedness and response, partnerships, and science monitoring, evaluation, and applied (evidence-based) research.
- The CDC also maintains an emergency surge staff of responders ready to be deployed as needed.
- Partners in the CDC response effort include the WHO and other international organizations, foreign governments and ministries of health, other U.S. government agencies, nongovernmental organizations, foundations, academic institutions, businesses and other private organizations, and faith-based organizations.

The 2022–2027 CDC Strategic Plan advances science and health equity and affirms the agency's commitment to one unified vision—equitably protecting health, safety, and security. The plan has five core capabilities:

- To maintain a diverse workforce
- World-class data and analytics
- State-of-the-art laboratories
- Rapid response to outbreaks at their source
- A strong global capacity with domestic preparedness (CDC, 2022b)

In 2023, the CDC made several structural changes to modernize efforts as part of their Moving Forward initiative. Core areas include sharing scientific findings and data faster, translating science into practice, easy to understand policy, prioritizing public health communications, developing a diverse workforce, promoting results-based partnerships, enhancing laboratory science and quality, integrating health equity, and modernizing data (CDC, 2023b).

Ultimately, these organizations share ideas and best practices for how we can all work together to deliver quality care to everyone, everywhere, at all times. The WHO Universal Health Coverage agenda coordinates efforts with the WHO and the World Bank, an agency that is the largest funder of global health within the UN system. To learn more about the current thinking on Universal Health Coverage and improving the quality of care, explore the free articles at https://www.bmj.com/qualityofcare, hosted by BMJ.

The C/PHN may participate with One Health principles anywhere and everywhere. The C/PHN's response during an infectious disease epidemic or pandemic may include one or more areas of focus as described by the WHO (2023b, 2023d):

Focus 1. Provide community education in support of a person's response to a local disease, such as wearing masks in public, handwashing, and physical distancing.

Focus 2. Explain evolving risk with communication to support lifesaving actions using local data indicators.

Focus 3. Facilitate access to timely treatment for people who display symptoms and ensure protection of the healthcare workforce.

View https://www.cdc.gov/globalhealth/stories/ for stories on creative global health partnerships with the CDC. Choose at least one country and one topic. What was the goal? What partners were involved? What was the outcome?

A FRAMEWORK FOR GLOBAL HEALTH NURSING ASSESSMENT

The slogan "think globally and act locally" captures the essence of caring for our interconnected world. When C/PHNs partner with the community client to assess health status, one useful guide is the universal imperatives of care.

- For instance, determining how many nurses a community needs depends in part on knowing the characteristics of the community, the people within it, and the predominant state of people's health. These universal imperatives are reflected in the elements of the following community assessment framework:
  - Patterns of care
  - Demographic transitions
  - Epidemiologic transitions

The principles of a community assessment remain the same no matter where the assessment takes place. Refer to Chapter 15 for an in-depth look at community assessments.

Patterns of Care

Using the nursing process, our first task is to assess the client. When the client is an entire population, the assessment can be quite substantial. In this case, we can use a framework to guide our review and look for patterns that represent commonalities and differences within our population of interest. Certain social conditions of living are known to influence and even determine health among all populations. When these SDOH are reviewed together, we can discern characteristics of the client population and their knowledge, behavior, and values. We also assess the health infrastructure within their country or region. Data describing these patterns have proven to be good predictors of the overall health of a population. Patterns allow us to design culturally appropriate care solutions affecting health, wellness, and illness of populations, both within and between countries and communities. These patterns of demographics are recognizable and measured across populations. What other aspects can you think of to add to the categories shown in Box 16-2?

Demographic Transitions

The **demographic transitions** model considers several factors that play a role in population size: birth and death rate and industrial and economic growth (Agarwal, 2022). Migration contributes to demographics transitions as people move in and out of areas (Johnson & Sabo, 2022). The model has four stages that describe a country's or region's population size.

Stage 1: Population size is stable due to high birth and death rates. The high mortality is due to poor sanitation and high disease rates. Birth rates are high due, in part, to the shortened lifespan of children. Communities are rural and rely on agriculture.

Stage 2: Population size begins to shift slowly. In this stage, birth rates continue to increase, while death rates decrease. The population benefits from improvements in medicine and sanitation, allowing for longer lives.

Stage 3: Population size and demographics shift as changes in birth and death rates occur. Fewer children are born, while death rates continue to decline. Medical advancements allow adults to live longer and healthier lives.

Stage 4: Population size either decreases or remains unchanged. Both the birth and death rates remain low. Fewer children are born, as adults live longer. In this final stage, society experiences many advances in industrial and economic growth (Agarwal, 2022).

Epidemiologic Transitions

The third concept in our framework of population assessment is to evaluate epidemiologic transitions. These are grouped according to the predominant health outcomes, or levels of public health, experienced by a society. There are three eras of epidemiologic transitions of public health, named according to historical trends of health and health conditions as described in a classic article by Breslow (2006) and Omran (2005). In resource-abundant nations, these eras progressed sequentially. However, in our world today, some countries may experience two or all three eras in different regions of their nation at the same time.

- The **Era of Infectious Diseases**: Throughout most of history, populations died from infectious diseases such as the plague, tuberculosis, puerperal fever,

BOX 16-2 Patterns of Care

- Patterns of place or the lived environment
  - Rural
  - Urban
  - Climate influence
- Patterns of perceptions of healthcare
  - Influence of culture
  - Influence views and acceptance of healing treatments
  - Influence acceptance of nurses and other healthcare providers
  - Affected by attitudes toward people assigned female at birth
- Patterns of privilege or inequality
  - Living conditions, including access to nutritional food and clean water
  - Daily functioning including physical safety
  - Quantity and quality of education for children, especially all ages of people assigned female at birth
  - Level of health literacy
  - Preference of learning style
  - Access to employment
  - Access to affordable healthcare resources
  - Informed healthcare decisions, including who lives or dies
- Patterns of population health differences (demographics)
  - Birth rates (fertility)
  - Infant and child survival rates
  - Life expectancy rates
  - Rates of infectious and communicable diseases
  - Rates of noncommunicable diseases and chronic illnesses (morbidity)
  - Death rates (mortality)
- Patterns of providers
  - Traditional healers
  - **Community health workers** who are trusted members with an understanding of the community and serve as a liaison between the community and services
  - Community health nurses
  - Midwives and primary provider extenders
  - Primary providers
  - Differing education levels and requirements for licensure
- Patterns of procedures and interventions
  - Sustainable and culturally appropriate
  - Primary care
  - Health promotion
  - Primary prevention
- Patterns of partnerships
  - Peripheral health unit and health station
  - District hospitals
  - Public health and governmental healthcare agencies
  - Nonprofit and nongovernmental organizations (NGOs)
  - Universities
- Patterns of politics and policies
  - Universal healthcare
  - Access to treatment and pharmaceuticals
  - Payment to providers
  - Local healthcare policies
  - Municipal governments
  - National governments
  - International collaboration
  - Cooperation versus conflict or violence
- Patterns of personal insight of healthcare workers
  - Personal health and physical well-being
  - Personal values and cultural beliefs, including religious beliefs and attitudes
  - Personal knowledge of community health nursing theory and practice

measles, and others. The death rate was high, and life expectancy was not very long.
  - During this era, the birth rate was also high. Families had many children because they knew that most children would die before adulthood and yet as adults aged, they depended on their children for care.
- The **Era of Chronic, Long-term Health Conditions**: With the advent of antibiotics, people survived common infections and started to live longer.
  - Because children survived into adulthood, the birth rate dropped.
  - As people survived infections and aged, they developed chronic, long-term illnesses such as heart disease, cancer, and arthritis.
- The **Era of Social Health Conditions**: More recently, new arrays of health conditions are affecting world populations. These new problems are anchored in social issues, as reflected in the observation that the places of our lives affect the quality of our health (Agency for Toxic Substances and Disease Registry, 2023a).
  - The wealth or poverty of your neighborhood reflects whether the streets are safe, housing is adequate, healthy food options are available, and schools and municipal services are adequate.
  - Personal lifestyle behaviors contribute to social health conditions, such as substance use disorders and obesity, while social behaviors contribute to others, such as gang membership, prostitution, sexual abuse, and deviant behavior.
  - The Geospatial Research, Analysis, and Services Program within the CDC Agency for Toxic Substances and Disease Registry works at the intersection of place and health to promote health and prevent disease (see Chapter 10).
  - Geospatial Research, Analysis, and Services Program provides expertise using geospatial science and geographic information systems to gain a better understanding and response to geographic determinants of health.
  - Interactive online maps showing the range of needs in a community are now available for online use with a special focus on the Social Vulnerability Index and the Environmental Justice Index (Agency for Toxic Substances and Disease Registry, 2023b).

- The goals of Geospatial Research, Analysis, and Services Program will be achieved when "everyone enjoys the same degree of protection from environmental and health hazards, and equal access to the decision-making process to live, learn, and work in a healthy environment" (Agency for Toxic Substances and Disease Registry, 2023c, para. 1).

Telehealth

Based on the WHO Global Strategy for Digital Health 2020-2025 (2021) including guidance from the WHO Consolidated Telemedicine Implementation Guide (WHO, 2022a), a telehealth services framework has been proposed that any country or healthcare system could adopt. The world experienced a shift during the COVID-19 pandemic toward greater acceptance and use of telehealth technologies for patient care, especially in rural or remote areas or even to avoid crowded urban hospitals.

- Prakash et al. (2023) observed that although several countries have established national telehealth plans, there are still hurdles to optimizing telehealth care.
  - They propose the six layers of TOASTS, an acronym that identifies different components of telehealth options, as follows: Technology type, Outcomes in health status, Application or purpose, Service provider who delivers the health service, Timing as real time or recorded, and in the Setting of hospital, home, or community.

Telehealth also serves to advance health equity and strengthens the opportunity to provide access to quality healthcare for all. Nonprofit organizations such as the World Telehealth Initiative (2023) are connecting healthcare workers everywhere through telehealth, providing a range of services from virtual care for refugees to building capacity where there are simply not enough primary providers or nurses.

- Read some of their many telehealth stories of impact at the World Telehealth Initiative website (https://www.worldtelehealthinitiative.org/blog). See Chapter 10 for more on technology and telehealth.

Bringing Together the Framework Components

Review each component in the community assessment framework. What examples from your own experience explain longevity in your community? Consider together the patterns of care, the demographic transition theory, and the epidemiology transition theory. How does the impact of communicable diseases and noncommunicable diseases potentially change the outcomes? See Figure 16-3.

Test your own worldview online by selecting one of the global demographic categories on the Gapminder website (https://www.gapminder.org/).

GLOBAL HEALTH METRICS

Key global health metrics include the **global burden of disease GBD**, **Disability-Adjusted Life Years**, **Years of Life Lost**, and **Years Lived with Disability**.

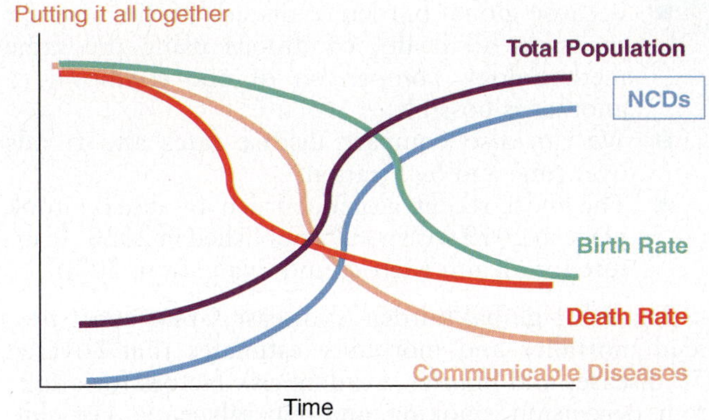

FIGURE 16-3 Demographic and epidemiologic transition theories combined. NCDs, noncommunicable diseases. (Reprinted with permission from Seymour, B., & Colburn, C. (2018). Module 1: global trends. In: B. Seymour, J. Cho, & J. Barrow (Eds.), *Toward competency-based best practices for global health in dental education: A global health starter kit* (p. 18). A project of the Consortium of Universities for Global Health Global Oral Health Interest Group. https://hsdm.harvard.edu/global-health-starter-kit; Data from: Omran, A. R. (2005). The epidemiologic transition: a theory of the epidemiology of population change. *Milbank Q, 83*(4), 731–757.)

Global Burden of Disease

Data collection and data analysis are an important part of the C/PHN toolkit. In addition to morbidity and mortality rates, one data tool used in global health helps measure what it costs society when not everyone is healthy and helps answer the following questions:

- If a member of your family dies, what is the impact on your family?
- What does it cost you and your family, your employer, and society, if you miss a month of work or school because of an illness?
- What does it cost a country where adults have high rates of diabetes or depression, or when the greatest cause of disability in children aged 5 to 14 years is from iron deficiency?

When populations or societies experience disadvantages socially, economically, or environmentally, these differences are called *health disparities*. The calculation of health disparities is the goal of a series of studies known as the *global burden of disease*.

- The first global burden of disease study was commissioned by the World Bank in 1990. This 1990 study found over half of the global burden of disease was due to communicable diseases and neonatal, maternal, and nutritional diseases. However, prior to COVID-19, the world experienced higher noncommunicable diseases, for instance cardiovascular disease and metabolic and behavioral risk factors (Institute for Health Metrics and Evaluation, 2020).
- Also in 1990, the WHO assumed responsibility for the global burden of disease study, which emphasized the impact of disability (morbidity) and death (mortality) rates.
- The Institute for Health Metrics and Evaluation now repeats the study and publishes the data at regular intervals.

- Because global burden of disease studies attempt to assess all health conditions using the same methodology, comparison of one condition to another is possible.
- We can also compare disease rates and trends over time and by location.
- The most recent global burden of disease took place in 2019 with results published in 2020 (Institute for Health Metrics and Evaluation, 2020).

The 2021 global burden of disease GBD report provided mortality and morbidity estimates that covered 359 diseases and injuries. Leading risk factors for adults are hypertension, smoking, and hyperglycemia. For children risk factors include low birth weight, short gestation period, and being underweight. Thousands of data points from a variety of sources were added (Institute for Health Metrics and Evaluation, 2024). This GBD data are also used to generate projections of health into the future through predictive analytics.

- Review disease, injury, and risk factsheets and other global burden of disease resource at the Institute for Health Metrics and Evaluation website (https://www.healthdata.org/research-analysis/diseases-injuries/factsheets). Global burden of disease is the measure for an entire population based on the disability-adjusted life years metric.
- Note that disability-adjusted life years is an equation that adds the total years of life lost due to diseases and premature mortality to the years lived with disability (Institute for Health Metrics and Evaluation, n.d.).
- The impact of public health interventions is calculated the same way but by using presumed years saved.

The basic metrics to know follow (Institute for Health Metrics and Evaluation, n.d.):

- **Years of Life Lost = Standard life expectancy – Age at death.** Years of Life Lost measures the impact counted in number of years of life lost due to deaths occurring earlier than the standard life expectancy.
  - For example, if a person's life expectancy is 80 years, and a person dies at the age of 50, the Years of Life Lost would be 30 years (80 – 50).
- **Years Lived with Disability = Prevalence of the condition × Disability weight × Duration of the condition.** Years Lived with Disability measures the nonfatal health impact of chronic diseases and injuries and quantifies the years of a healthy life lost due to living with that disability.
  - For example, if a person lives with a disability that has a disability weight of 0.5 (on a scale from 0 to 1, where 0 is perfect health and 1 is equivalent to death), and the duration of the disability is 20 years, the Years Lived with Disability would be 10 (0.5 × 20).
- **Disability-Adjusted Life Years = Years of Life Lost + Years Lived with Disability.** Disability-Adjusted Life Years represents the overall disease burden combining the impact of both mortality (Years of Life Lost) and morbidity (Years Lived with Disability).
  - For example, if the person's Years of Life Lost is 30 years and their Years Lived with Disability is 10 years, the total Disability-Adjusted Life Years for them would be 40 (30 Years of Life Lost + 10 Years Lived with Disability.

Let's use the Global Burden of Disease and Disability-Adjusted Life Years to assess one community's experience with measles and the impact of vaccinations. For several years, one community had a high rate of death from measles for children under 5 years of age, but after a measles vaccine campaign the next year, there were no deaths from measles.

- When the Disability-Adjusted Life Years are calculated for the year with measles, the C/PHNs are able to demonstrate the burden of measles on that community related to the lost lifetime productivity of the children who died.
- Comparing Disability-Adjusted Life Years to the year without measles demonstrates the impact of the vaccine.
- Children who might have died did not die, and they are now counted among those in the community who are healthy.
- Children who received the vaccine can become productive adults.
- The Global Burden of Disease on the community is lessened with the vaccine.

The information obtained from calculating the Global Burden of Disease informs decisions related to investments in health, research, human resource development, and physical infrastructure.

- Assessment of global and regional information on diseases and injuries can be reviewed directly online at http://www.healthdata.org/data-visualization/gbd-compare, using the *Global Burden of Disease Compare* interactive tool.

Compare the global disease trends by Disability-Adjusted Life Years for 1990 and 2019 in Figure 16-4. Notice that the 1990 chart shows a greater area for the burden of communicable diseases. By 2019, there was a noticeable shift, showing a greater burden of noncommunicable diseases. How might changing demographics account for that? Population data usually take a year or two to be collected and published. What changes might we expect to see with Global Burden of Disease and Disability-Adjusted Life Years for the years of the COVID-19 pandemic?

GLOBAL HEALTH TRENDS

Managing Global Diseases During Epidemics and Pandemics

An example of the interdependency of all nations is the cooperation needed when epidemics or pandemics occur. The WHO has led the way by developing an approach to respond to, coordinate, and assist all nations during such outbreaks via the Global Outbreak Alert and Response Network. This global network of technical institutions and other networks aim to deliver support in the prevention and control of infectious disease outbreaks and public health emergencies (Global Outbreak Alert and Response Network, 2023). The new strategy for

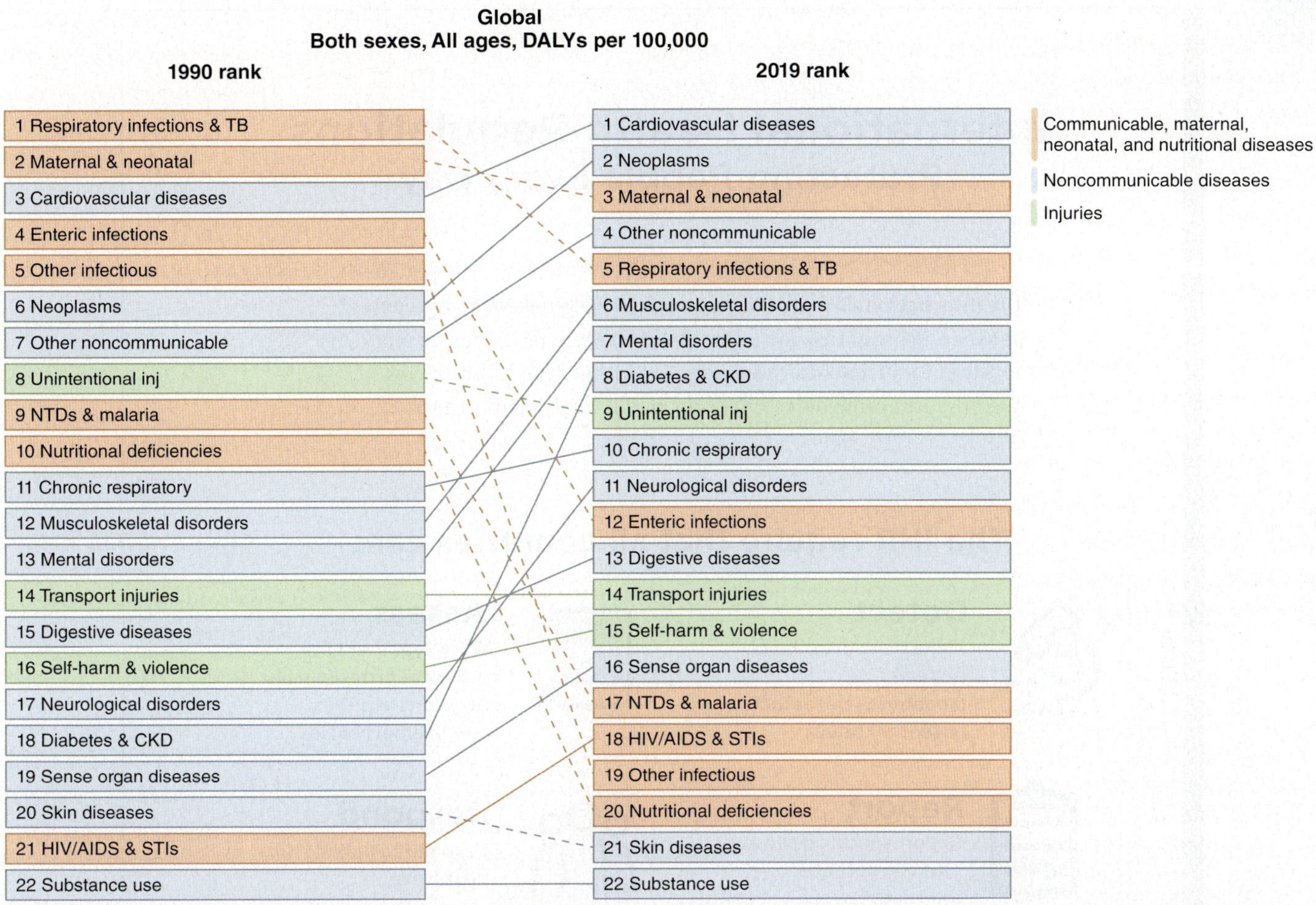

FIGURE 16-4 Global disease trends in DALYs by cause, 1990 and 2019. (From the Institute for Health Metrics and Evaluation. GBD Compare DALYs [global, by cause, all ages, both sexes]. https://vizhub.healthdata.org/gbd-compare/. Used with permission. All rights reserved.)

2022–2026 focuses on four strategic areas of response (Division of Global Health Protection, 2022):

- A community-centered approach
- Renewing commitment to the global public health emergency workforce
- Creating solutions for a better response
- Promoting collaborative response

The WHO Health Emergency Dashboard (https://extranet.who.int/publicemergency) is an interactive web-based platform, refreshed every 15 minutes, that shares real-time information about global public health events and emergencies. What current public health emergencies are listed on the WHO public emergency dashboard?

International Health Regulations

First adopted in 1969 to cover only six diseases, the International Health Regulations have been revised several times to cover many more. In 2005, the International Health Regulations was accepted as a legally binding, international treaty between all 196 WHO member states. Because the COVID-19 pandemic revealed gaps and shortcomings in the regulations, in 2022 at the 75th World Health Assembly (WHA75), an amendment was accepted to improve the global response to health emergencies (US DHHS, 2022).

The International Health Regulations require all countries to independently perform the following (Fig. 16-5):

- Detect: Make sure surveillance systems and laboratories can detect potential threats.
- Assess: Work together with other countries to make decisions in public health emergencies.
- Report: Report specific diseases, plus any potential international public health emergencies.
- Respond: Respond to public health events (CDC, 2022c).

Each nation has committed to meeting these four obligations within their own borders and to develop an internal public health strategy with an implementation plan for addressing domestic public health emergencies.

The International Health Regulations provides guidance before public health events happen by directing the WHO to provide tools, guidance, and training in support of any country. During public health events, the WHO offers decision support to affected areas for rapid assessment, critical information, and communications. Also, Global Outbreak Alert and Response Network coordinates sending teams with technical expertise upon request from a country as needed.

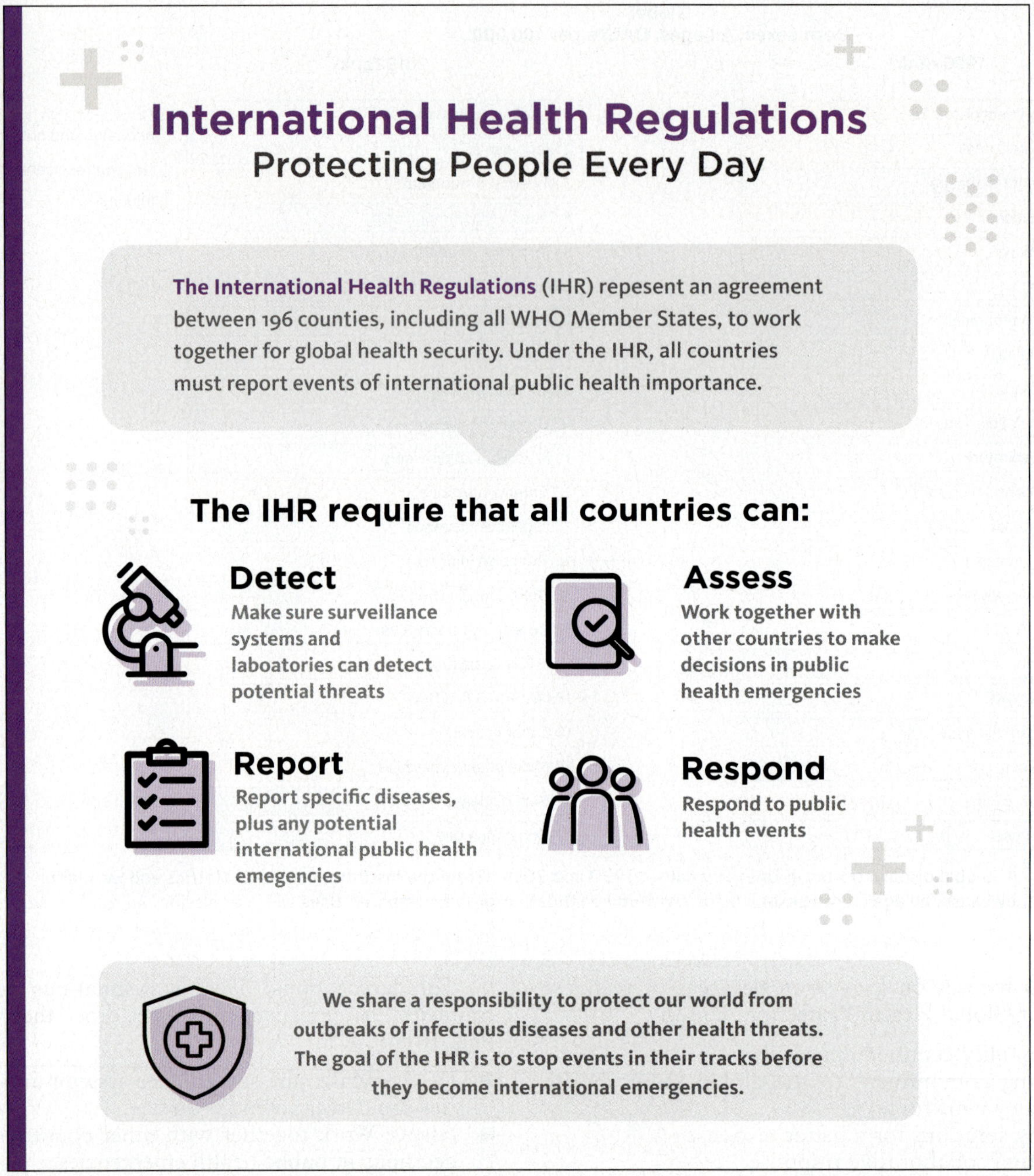
International Health Regulations
Protecting People Every Day
The International Health Regulations (IHR) repesent an agreement between 196 counties, including all WHO Member States, to work together for global health security. Under the IHR, all countries must report events of international public health importance.
The IHR require that all countries can:
Detect
Make sure surveillance systems and laboratories can detect potential threats
Assess
Work together with other countries to make decisions in public health emergencies
Report
Report specific diseases, plus any potential international public health emegencies
Respond
Respond to public health events
We share a responsibility to protect our world from outbreaks of infectious diseases and other health threats. The goal of the IHR is to stop events in their tracks before they become international emergencies.

FIGURE 16-5 International health regulations. (Reprinted from CDC. (2022). *International Health Regulations (IHR)*. Protecting people every day. https://www.cdc.gov/globalhealth/healthprotection/ghs/ihr/ihr-infographic.html)

According to the International Health Regulations reporting protocols, when a country detects a potential public health emergency of international concern, the affected nation first assesses the public health risk within 48 hours. If the event meets International Health Regulations reporting criteria, the country notifies the WHO within 24 hours. The WHO will assess the event using the Emergency Response Framework.

The framework provides guidance for the level of response that is indicated. There are four response levels, from Ungraded (requiring no response or monitoring only) to Grade 3 (requiring a major response across regions; see Table 16-2). The emergency response framework is based on risk, as follows:

- Very low or low-risk event: The WHO team may simply monitor the event. Mitigation, preparedness, and readiness may be part of the low-risk response.
- High or very high-risk event: The Incident Management System may be activated with an appropriately scaled response.

TABLE 16-2 WHO Emergency Response Framework Levels for Graded Emergencies

Level	Definition/WHO Response	Additional Information
Ungraded	A public health event or emergency Monitoring only ▪ **No** operational response	▪ Does not require a WHO operational response.
Grade 1	▪ Single-country emergency ▪ Requires **limited** response	▪ Exceeds the usual country-level cooperation that the WHO Country Once (WCO) has with the Member State. ▪ Most WHO responses can be managed with in-country assets. ▪ Organizational and external support required by the WCO is limited. ▪ Provision of support to the WCO is coordinated by an Emergency Coordinator in the Regional Office.
Grade 2	▪ Single-country or multiple-country emergency ▪ Requires **moderate** response	▪ The level of response required by WHO always exceeds the capacity of the WCO. ▪ Organizational and external support required by the WCO is moderate. ▪ Provision of support to the WCO is coordinated by an Emergency Coordinator in the Regional Office. ▪ An Emergency Officer is appointed at WHO headquarters to assist with the coordination of organization-wide support.
Grade 3	▪ Single-country or multiple-country emergency ▪ Requires **major or maximal** response	▪ Organizational and external support required by the WCO is major. ▪ Requires the mobilization of organization-wide assets. ▪ Provision of support to the WCO is coordinated by an Emergency Coordinator in the Regional Office(s). ▪ An Emergency Officer is appointed at WHO headquarters to assist with the coordination of organization-wide inputs. ▪ On occasion, the World Health Emergencies Programme WHE Executive Director and the Regional Director may agree to have the Emergency Coordinator based in headquarters. ▪ For events or emergencies involving multiple regions, an Incident Management Support Team at headquarters will coordinate the response across the regions.

Source: World Health Organization (WHO). (2024). *Emergency response framework (ERF), Edition 2.1* https://iris.who.int/bitstream/handle/10665/375964/9789240058064-eng.pdf?sequence=1 .

Public Health Emergencies of International Concern

Once Public Health Emergencies of International Concern are declared, the WHO coordinates an active response with the reporting country and with other countries as indicated. Since the implementation of the Public Health Emergencies of International Concern in 2005, the WHO has only declared it seven times (Wenham & Stout, 2024).

- The response may include controlling borders as well as containing the source of the public health threat.
  - Brazil followed these steps in 2016 with the Zika virus outbreak and in 2019 with the novel SARS-CoV-2 outbreak in Wuhan, China (Wenham & Stout, 2024).
- To see this process in action, review https://www.who.int/news/item/29-06-2020-covidtimeline for listings of the WHO's response to COVID-19.

Most epidemics or emergencies do not fulfill the criteria to be considered Public Health Emergencies of International Concern. For example, WHO Emergency Committees were not convened for the cholera outbreak in Haiti after the 2010 earthquake, for the use of chemical weapons in Syria in 2013, or following the 2011 Fukushima nuclear disaster in Japan.

- Four critical diseases will always be considered extraordinary and require mandatory notification: smallpox, poliomyelitis due to wild-type poliovirus, human influenza due to a new subtype, and severe acute respiratory syndrome (SARS).
- Other conditions are potentially notifiable events according to International Health Regulations criteria, whether infectious disease, biologic, radiologic, or chemical events (Division of Global Health Protection, 2022).
- Review https://www.cdc.gov/globalhealth/healthprotection/ghs/ihr/index.html for the International Health Regulations reporting requirements.

Global Influenza Surveillance Network

The Global Influenza Surveillance and Response System is a cooperative network of international laboratories established in 1952 by the WHO. This system has emerged as a critical player, coordinating worldwide efforts for surveillance and control of influenza. Functions of Global Influenza Surveillance and Response System include the following (WHO, 2022b):

- Maintaining physical presence in 148 National Influenza Centres, 7 WHO Collaborating Centres, 4 Essential Regulatory Laboratories, and 13 WHO H5 reference laboratories
- Recommending the composition of twice yearly seasonal influenza vaccine and aiding in its development
- Posting on an open-access platform the specific gene sequence of an influenza virus (reference viruses)
- Providing open access to confirmed lab protocols for testing and disease confirmation
- Developing test kits for shipping to requesting countries free of charge (Association of Public Health Labs, 2022)

Diseases With Global Impact

Coronavirus Disease 2019 (COVID-19)

COVID-19 is the disease caused by the SARS-CoV-2 coronavirus. It usually spreads between people in close contact. Within the first 3 years, 772 million cases and nearly 7 million deaths were recorded worldwide since December 2019, but the actual number is thought to be higher.

- After initially declaring COVID-19 a Public Health Emergency of International Concern in early 2020, then a global pandemic, the WHO announced the end of the emergency phase in May 2023.

The WHO continues to coordinate the global response in the endemic phase including the administration of 13.5 billion vaccine doses as of late 2023 (WHO, 2023e).

Ebola Virus

Ebola virus is an infectious disease caused by one of four viruses that has repeatedly caused outbreaks, mostly in Africa. Although the virus was first identified in 1976 in an outbreak near the Ebola River in the Democratic Republic of Congo, epidemiologic data suggest it has been around much longer.

- Population growth, deforestation, and cultural food habits (eating exotic animals or "bushmeat") are thought to have contributed to the frequency of Ebola virus outbreaks in our world today (CDC, 2023c).
- Vaccines used to protect against some types of Ebola virus have been used to control the spread of outbreaks, and other vaccines are in development.
- The initial outbreak in West Africa in 2014 became a global Public Health Emergency of International Concern, crossing international borders within months.

Numerous emergency responders from a variety of disciplines, including nursing, rushed to help as teams tried to contain the spread of the deadly virus. They met challenges with ingenuity as they struggled without adequate supplies initially. Two vaccines were ultimately developed and continue to be administered to vulnerable populations (CDC, 2023c).

Tuberculosis

Tuberculosis (TB) is an infectious disease caused by the tubercle bacillus (see Chapter 8). TB has been known for hundreds of years and was commonly referred to as *consumption*. Over time, the causative organism has become resistant to the medications used to treat it. Multidrug-resistant TB (MDR-TB) remains a public health crisis and a global health security threat. The WHO continues to classify TB as a worldwide chronic endemic disease with a Sustainable Development Goal to end TB by 2030 (WHO, 2023f).

- The WHO's previous Stop TB campaign realized a milestone in 2018 when 7 million people were diagnosed and treated. Because of that success, Stop TB has been replaced by the new End TB campaign (WHO, 2022c).
- End TB calls on governments to adapt and implement a strategy consisting of three pillars with interventions:
  1. Provide integrated patient-centered TB care and prevention
  2. Develop bold policies and supportive systems from governments, communities, and private stakeholders
  3. Intensify research and innovation.

Malaria

Malaria is an acute febrile illness caused by the parasite *Plasmodium falciparum* or *Plasmodium vivax*. Malaria is a vector-borne disease spread by bites of the female *Anopheles* mosquito, primarily in tropical and subtropical countries. The threat is highest in sub-Saharan Africa.

- Even though it is a serious disease, illness and death from malaria can usually be prevented with appropriate interventions such as sleeping under bed nets (Fig. 16-6) and complying with medical treatment.

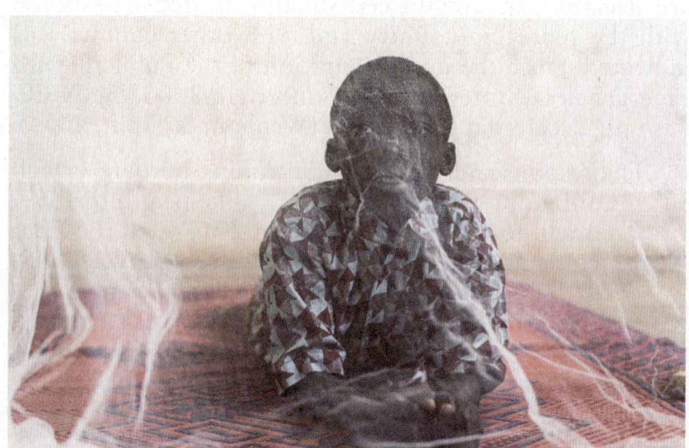

FIGURE 16-6 Little boy with mosquito net for protection against malaria.

- Malaria disproportionately affects people living in poverty, especially impacting people of working age with damaging effects on emerging economies.
- In 1998, half the world was at risk for malaria. The Roll Back Malaria (RBM) Partnership to End Malaria (2022), an ambitious international campaign, was launched with the goal of reducing the global burden of malaria. Between 2004 and 2020, two billion insecticide-treated mosquito nets were distributed worldwide, decreasing malaria by 70% in parts of the world. But more needed to be done. In 2022, there were 249 million cases of malaria, an increase of 5 million from 2021 (WHO, 2023g). Then, three interventions were developed in rapid order that gave the world hope that malaria could be entirely eliminated.
    - Insecticide-treated mosquito nets
    - Rapid diagnostic lab tests
    - Artemisinin-based combination therapy, an oral drug therapy (WHO, 2023g).

The first WHO-recommended malaria vaccine, RTS,S/AS01, has experienced success in a phased roll-out in three African countries with a substantial reduction in severe malaria and a 13% drop in early childhood deaths. A second safe and effective malaria vaccine, R21/Matrix-M, became available in late 2023 (WHO, 2023g). Additionally, the RBM Partnership to End Malaria Strategic Plan 2021–2025 (2020) can be found at https://endmalaria.org/sites/default/files/RBM%20Partnership%20Strategic%20Plan%20for%202021-2025_0.pdf, detailing objectives and interventions to control and eliminate malaria.

The WHO is currently concerned about a mosquito species mainly found in urban and human-made environments. In 2022, the WHO issued a vector alert on the *Anopheles stephensi* mosquito species. Until 2011, the vector was confined to a few countries; however, since 2012, it has expanded to seven countries on the African continent. The vector is resistant to many commonly used insecticides. Unlike other species, this species survives in hot, dry weather (WHO, 2022d).

- Countries were advised to do the following:
    - Increase surveillance and control.
    - Manage larval sites by removing them, provide sealed lids for water containers, and filling in or capping unused wells.
    - Enforce water container by-laws.
    - Dual-ingredient insecticide-treated nets and insulation of window screens.
    - For further information on the alert and advisement, see https://iris.who.int/bitstream/handle/10665/365710/9789240067714-eng.pdf?sequence=1&isAllowed=y.

The challenge remains in countries with emerging economies where there are large populations without sewer systems and clean water sources. Because people prefer to build their homes close to sources of water, mosquitoes that carry malaria are attracted to the standing water in those communities (Fig. 16-7; Box 16-3).

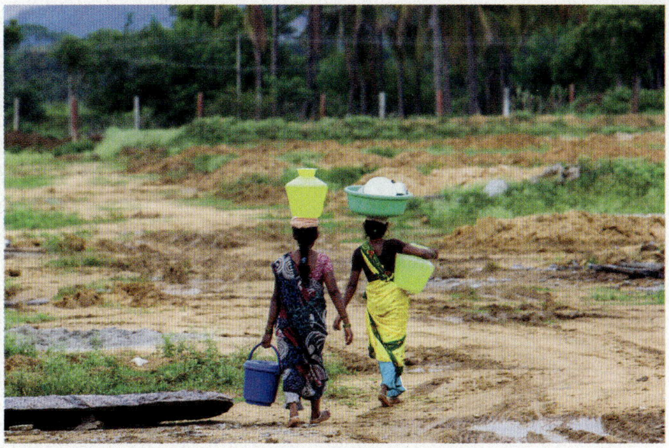

FIGURE 16-7 People carrying water buckets.

The primary role of the global health nurse in ending malaria is as a community educator. The topics of client education would cover simple measures:

- Proper placement and use of insecticide netting around a bed during the night.
- Educate on the risk of pools of standing water around the home.
- Intermittent preventive medication during their clinic visits.
- Partnership to End Malaria—https://endmalaria.org/. Visit the Malaria Vaccine Initiative website to explore the challenges of making a vaccine (https://www.malariavaccine.org/malaria-vaccines-biologics).

Global HIV/AIDS Response

HIV (human immunodeficiency virus) is a virus that attacks the body's immune system. If HIV is not treated, it can lead to AIDS (acquired immunodeficiency syndrome).

- Although there remains no cure for HIV infection, effective treatment controls the virus so people live productive lives. Treatment also helps prevent transmission. Current trends in HIV care focus on prevention, early testing, and treatment (WHO, 2023h).
    - Of the estimated 39 million people living with HIV in 2022, roughly 80% receive antiretroviral treatment (WHO, 2023i).

With surveillance testing, people can know their status and take measures to either remain HIV negative or start treatment, thus preventing transmission to others (see Chapter 8).

Role of the C/PHN for HIV/AIDS:

- Use the WHO Mortality Database at https://platform.who.int/mortality to explore how the causes of death worldwide have changed over time.
- Explore the WHO interactive webpage, Sexual and Reproductive Health and Rights and HIV linkages toolkit at https://toolkit.srhhivlinkages.org to learn more about recent, relevant, and important resources.

BOX 16-3 LEVELS OF PREVENTION PYRAMID

Malaria

SITUATION: Malaria, an infectious disease, occurs when a person is bit by a mosquito carrying the Plasmodium parasite. Malaria kills over 600,000 people yearly with the highest mortality rate among children under the age of 5 years. In 2022, there were 250,000 new cases.

GOAL: Reduce malaria cases, reduce mortality rates, and eliminate malaria. Using the three levels of prevention, partner with communities and families to avoid risk factors, to promptly diagnose and treat negative health conditions, to restore health to the fullest possible potential, and to prevent a resurgence of malaria in all countries that are malaria-free.

Tertiary Prevention

Rehabilitation	*Health Promotion and Education*	*Health Protection*
▪ Share resources across communities for rehabilitation from malaria ▪ Work together on providing community-based social support for people and families affected by malaria	▪ Disseminate new knowledge gained through research ▪ Participate in development of international networks for sharing expertise in management of malaria ▪ Coordinate efforts to ensure antimalarial drugs ▪ Collaborate on delivery of effective treatment protocols	▪ Continue research in vector control and new treatments ▪ Educate for prevention of recurrence and spread of disease ▪ Promote practices that prevent spread of disease

Secondary Prevention

Early Diagnosis	*Prompt Treatment*
Presence of the parasites by microscopic examination of blood smears and rapid diagnostic tests	▪ Provide artemisinin-based combination medication to only those who test positive to malaria to lessen risk of MDR ▪ Treat within 24 hours to decrease severe illness and death

Primary Prevention

Health Promotion and Education	*Health Protection*
▪ Educate population on risks of standing water where they reside ▪ Educate on proper placement of dual-ingredient insecticide nets around bed at night ▪ Educate parents of infants and of children under 5 years, pregnant people, and people with HIV/AIDs the risk of serious illness ▪ Collaborate on international public health campaigns to raise awareness regarding TB, HIV/AIDS, malaria	▪ Removal of larval sites ▪ Remove standing water ▪ Cap unused wells ▪ Provide lids for water containers ▪ Install window screens ▪ Provide WHO-approved dual-ingredient insecticide nets ▪ Indoor residual spray ▪ Immunization of children residing in moderate- and high-risk areas with RTS,S/AS01 or R21/Matrix-M ▪ Travelers to high-risk areas should consider chemoprophylaxis ▪ Chemopreventive therapies for high-risk populations

GLOBAL HEALTH SECURITY AGENDA

In 2014, the United States helped launch the Global Health Security Agenda, an independent group of more than 70 countries, international organizations, nongovernmental organizations, and private sector companies that also have as their vision a world that is safe and secure from infectious diseases. Today's global travel increases the risk of dissemination of infectious diseases. A disease threat anywhere is a disease threat everywhere.

The Global Health Security Agenda 2024 targets working directly with partner countries to strengthen public health systems and reduce the risk of infectious disease outbreaks. Each country has agreed to develop the leadership, technical knowledge, and collaborative foundation to sustain health security in the long term and reduce the risk of infectious disease outbreaks (Global Health Security Agenda, 2023).

The COVID-19 pandemic called attention to the shortcomings in how countries respond to infectious diseases (Global Health Security Agenda, 2023). The Stories of Impact provides evidence of how these issues were addressed. Review https://globalhealthsecurityagenda.org/stories-of-impact/ to learn more. See Figure 16-8.

KEY ACHIEVEMENTS OF GHSA FROM 2014—PRESENT

	Laboratory Systems	Surveillance Systems	Workforce Development	Emergency Management and Response
HIGHLIGHTS	18 countries can conduct lab tests to detect national priority pathogens that can cause disease, outbreaks, or death	18 countries have indicator and event-based surveillance at the central and intermediate levels	All 19 countries established or expanded their program to train disease detectives	All 19 countries have a Public Health Emergency Operations Center (PHEOC), and most of the countries have sent personnel to be trained at CDC's Public Health Emergency Management (PHEM) Fellowship course
WHY IT MATTERS	Confirming a diagnosis with laboratory results allows health workers to respond rapidly with the most effective treatment and prevention methods, reducing spread of disease and deaths	Effective disease surveillance along with rapid laboratory diagnosis enables countries to quickly detect and stop outbreaks and continuously respond to potential risks	To maintain global health security capabilities, countries need a disease detective workforce that can quickly investigate potential outbreaks and take swift action	PHEOCs bring together experts and stakeholders to efficiently and effectively coordinate response to an emergency or public health threat

FIGURE 16-8 Key achievements of the Global Health Security Agenda from 2014 to present. (Reprinted from Centers for Disease Control and Prevention. (2022). https://www.cdc.gov/globalhealth/resources/factsheets/5-years-of-ghsa.html)

Interdependence of Nations During Migration

When hardships come, people would rather try to adapt and stay where they are, but if there is limited assistance from their government to remain or the area becomes too hazardous to stay, then people will leave. Populations may relocate within their own countries or move across borders or oceans to find safety after natural or human-caused disasters. Climate change in today's world, causing more frequent and severe wildfires (Fig. 16-9; see Chapter 9) and rising oceans (from melting glacial ice), can result in population migration.

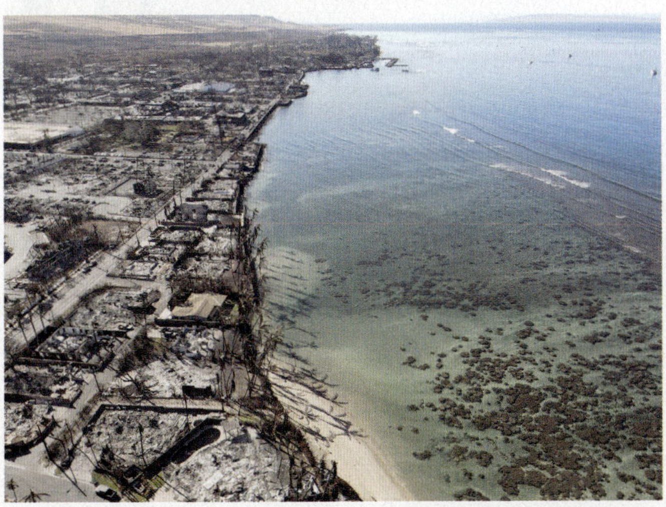

FIGURE 16-9 Views of Lahaina after the wildfires in Maui.

Population movement may also be in response to the following:

- Economic opportunities for workers and their families
- A nation's need to invite immigrants to offset low birthrates
- Large migrations of people fleeing violence or armed conflict (Fig. 16-10), or
- Food insecurity (UN, n.d.-d)

In each case, the challenge is to ensure that human rights are met first, followed by maintaining environmental law and refugee or migration law. In 2023, the UN (n.d.-d) expanded the Global Compact for Migration as a framework for international cooperation for orderly migration.

- Unfortunately, the actual migration process has become quite political.
- In 2023, the Rabat Declaration global agreement was the first to support present migration humanitarian crises or the impact on environmental rights breaches. The aim is to promote the inclusion of climate immigrants in national health systems (WHO, 2023i).
  - View the UN University video *How-to Guide for Environmental Refugees* at https://ourworld.unu.edu/en/how-to-guide-for-environmental-refugees for a description of the migration events of Carteret Islanders in Papua New Guinea.
  - Explore https://www.iom.int/wmr/ for information about the UN International Organization for Migration.

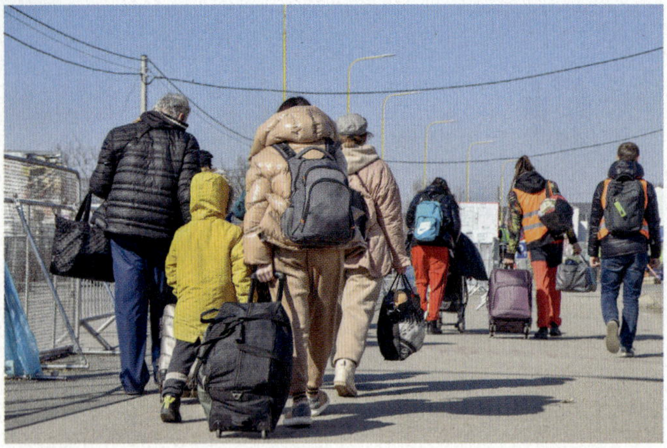

FIGURE 16-10 Refugees from Ukraine on the border with Slovakia.

Armed Conflict, Uprisings, Wars, and Humanitarian Emergencies

The UN Office of Genocide Prevention and the Responsibility to Protect has the overall objective of "advancing national and international efforts to protect populations from genocide, war crimes, ethnic cleansing and crimes against humanity, including their incitement" (UN, n.d.-c).

- Within this objective, the main priorities are to identify situations at risk (of genocide, war crimes, ethnic cleansing, and crimes against humanity; atrocity crimes); take early action to prevent them, and improve the protection of populations; and implementation of the Responsibility to Protect principle by Member States, regional organizations, and civil society.
- According to the UN (2023a), there are more violent conflicts taking place today than during WWII, affecting over two billion people living in violent conflict countries.
- Armed conflicts and uprisings initially cause governments and agencies to place a high priority on injuries, but the ability to sustain routine healthcare is reduced as time goes on.
- The health infrastructure itself becomes vulnerable during conflicts and uprisings as a consequence of political instability. Often, opposing factions raid hospitals and clinics.

During national conflicts, health services become disorganized with decreased resources from disrupted supply chains. Such actions have been repeated over the years as conflicts have emerged (see Box 16-4).

C/PHNs need to become aware of who is involved in an immediate local conflict and who is influencing the situation from abroad. Outside help is needed in these instances, and often, international help is available. Funding and sustaining health projects may depend ultimately on a variety of factors, not the least of which is providing care when the safety and survival of patients and nurses may also be threatened.

The CDC describes complex humanitarian emergencies as situations that affect civilian populations and distinguishes them from factors related to war or civil strife; shortage of necessities such as food, water, electricity, or fuel; and the displacement of local populations.

- During wars and other human-made disasters, infrastructures fail, and epidemics are almost inevitable.
- As conflict wears on, the healthcare needs of the combatants often take priority over the healthcare needs of civilians.
- As communities and families are relocated, thousands of children may be injured, orphaned, or become at risk for disease.
- Additionally, conflict disrupts food cultivation, harvest, and distribution, leaving populations at risk for malnutrition (Lin et al., 2022), which can lead to disease.

BOX 16-4 PERSPECTIVES

A World Health Organization Regional Advisor's Viewpoint on the Effect of War on International Cooperation

During the war in Yugoslavia, Bosnians and Serbs worked with the European Regional Office of the World Health Organization (WHO/EURO) in Copenhagen, Denmark, to develop interventions for women and children's health. WHO/EURO developed the training program to be held in Denmark but was not certain that the roads between Sarajevo and the coast would be open and safe for travel. Snipers had continued operating in the mountains surrounding Sarajevo and along the roads to the country's borders. Once the workshop started in Copenhagen, the nurses, primary providers, and midwives, both Bosnians and Serbs, collaborated professionally during breakout sessions. However, the facilitator had to ensure separate dining spaces, because casual communication was difficult and awkward while the conflict was ongoing.

Marie, WHO regional advisor

1. *What are some reasons people from the same area may be in conflict?*
2. *How does* The ICN Code of Ethics for Nurses *apply to this perspective? The Code can be found at https://www.icn.ch/sites/default/files/2023-06/ICN_Code-of-Ethics_EN_Web.pdf.*

BOX **16-5** WHAT DO *YOU* THINK?

Effects of Conflict on International Cooperation

In today's world, international cooperation could collapse due to changing national relationships, internal disruptions from natural disasters or violence, or political disagreements over policies such as withdrawal from the Paris Agreement on climate. Based on the material presented in this chapter and the current conflicts in the world, what would be some of the social, political, and economic consequences in terms of health if international cooperation were diminished?

- Countries in conflict are more likely to experience food insecurity and malnutrition than countries not in conflict. Countries affected by famine in 2022 were due to violence and war. Additionally, while starvation as a war technique is against international humanitarian law, we have seen it used as a method of war (UN, 2023b).
  - *Dangerously Hungry: The link between food insecurity and conflict* provides an in-depth look into the relationship between the two variables (https://www.wfpusa.org/wp-content/uploads/2023/04/Dangerously_Hungry_WFPUSA_Digital_Report.pdf) (see Box 16-5).

GLOBAL HEALTH ETHICS

Certain ethical considerations guide global health even as basic ethical principles guide the delivery of healthcare. Ethics of justice, equality, diversity, and inclusivity become even more important in an interconnected, multicultural world.

Brain Drain to Brain Gain

Brain Drain is defined as when someone who is highly trained and educated in one country migrates to another country for a variety of reasons, which is Brain Gain. In the healthcare arena, this exodus causes a lack of well-trained healthcare providers, including doctors and nurses. There are several important reasons for this:

- Physical and emotional abuse, largely experienced by people assigned female at birth
- The high nurse-to-patient ratios; other countries may not have ratio limits
- Lack of or poor continuing education and training
- Low pay
- Poor working conditions
- Lack of healthcare technology
- No respect for the nursing role in society (WHO, 2017)

Although this phenomenon is only considered to occur between countries, the exodus of nurses from rural communities in the United States to urban communities exists as well (WHO, 2017).

The WHO (2010) developed recruitment guidelines for countries to follow. The document states that countries should not recruit from resource-limited countries and countries in short supply of health professionals. This "push–pull" relates to wages, work conditions, and the country's characteristics (Adovor et al., 2021). When countries pull healthcare professionals over from another country, it is based on the need to fill a shortage of providers. Immigration policies and higher wages are used as a recruiting tool (Adovor et al., 2021). However, this **Brain Drain to Brain Gain** causes resource-limited countries to be short of healthcare professionals, as evidenced by the recruitment of nurses due to the COVID-19 pandemic.

Ethical Considerations

Global health volunteering dates back to the 17th and 18th centuries (Woldie & Yitbarek, 2021); while there is a long history of volunteering, ethical considerations still need to be considered. Prior to volunteering in global health, a C/PHN must be aware of ethical considerations. The desire to help others entails preparation and self-reflection. C/PHN volunteers should not presume that good intentions in providing free healthcare activities or work exempt them from ethical concerns. There are three words for the C/PHN to remember and reflect on before, during, and after volunteering: respect, humility, and trust (American Nurses Association [ANA], 2019). One important item to remember when inquiring about published guidelines on volunteering is that they may not be written by the host country (ANA, 2019). This may cause disillusionment in both parties and not provide what is needed or hoped for. C/PHNs need to be socially responsible and culturally humble, and the host country must be part of the planning (ANA, 2019).

C/PHNs should familiarize themselves with global health ethical considerations whether engaging with global communities to conduct research or deliver clinical care in the community. The ANA Position Statement on Ethical Considerations for Local and Global Volunteerism is a good starting point to learn more. See https://www.nursingworld.org/~4a346d/globalassets/practiceandpolicy/nursing-excellence/ana-position-statements/social-causes-and-health-care/ethical-considerations-for-local-and-global-volunteerism_final_nursingworld.pdf for the position statement.

Benefits and Consequences to the Volunteer and the Host Country

Benefits for the Volunteer and the Host Country

C/PHNs volunteer for several reasons including personal satisfaction and to help the community. Whatever the reason for volunteering, much can be gained from the experience.

- Increased knowledge and the role of SDOH
- Increased cultural and international awareness
- Increased awareness of public health

- Enlarged world outlook
- Lower depression rates (Woldie & Yitbarek, 2021; Ye et al., 2023)

Benefits to the host country require careful and purposeful planning between host and sending countries and mandates "do no harm."

- Exchange of knowledge
- Training and education of local providers, with goal that they train others
- Address health concerns as expressed by the host country (MacNiairn, 2019)

Consequences for Volunteers and for the Host Country

Volunteers in global health must be aware of possible consequences and risks.

- Lack of the healthcare infrastructure these nurses were accustomed to.
- Some healthcare professionals were unprepared for the violence and discrimination they faced due to COVID-19.
- Furthermore, some of the environments were unsafe leading to stress and mental health concerns (Downey et al., 2023; see Fig. 16-11).

Many times, C/PHN volunteers experience financial hardship due to loss of wages during their trip. Other times, nurses need to fundraise to cover the costs or pay out of their own pocket (Woldie & Yitbarek, 2021).

There are consequences for the host country as well:

- Host counties may feel a lack of respect for their culture and health interventions.
- Local care providers may not be included in decision making.
- Many times, collaboration between the two countries is lacking or superficial.
- There may be overlapping of services as one country leaves, and another arrives.
- Services are not culturally sensitive (Tracey et al., 2022).

Global volunteering can be very expensive and may not offer long-term health or financial benefits to the communities served; it may actually be burdensome (Woldie & Yitbarek, 2021; see Box 16-6).

Like transcultural nursing, described in Chapter 5, expanding one's horizons either in unfamiliar neighborhoods here or abroad can promote a broader understanding and provide richer experiences for the C/PHN. Many of our clients are not far removed from their countries of origin, and a global perspective provides C/PHNs with a more welcoming presence. The skills gained from global health experiences can help us better understand and work with all of our clients, wherever they may live.

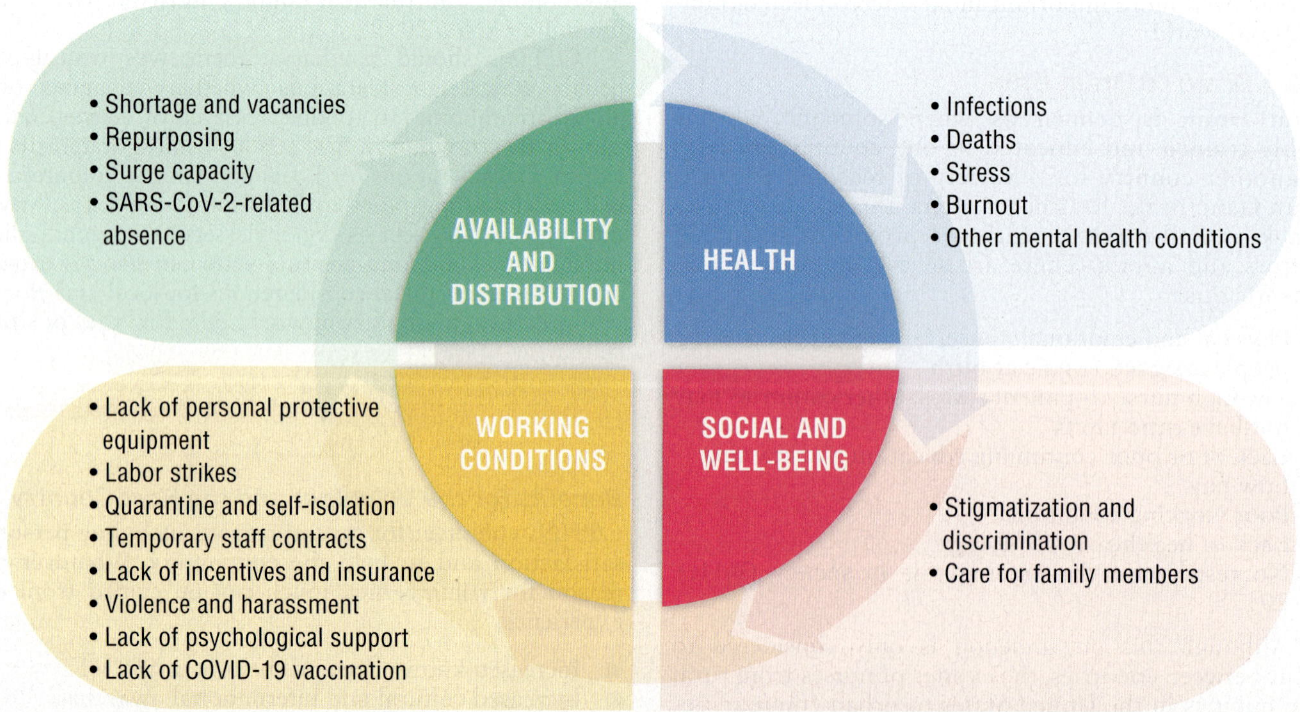

FIGURE 16-11 Multidimensional factors related to COVID-19 that affect Health Care Workers (HCWs). (Reprinted with permission from World Health Organization (WHO). Downey, E., Fokeladeh, H. S., & Catton, H. (2023). *What the COVID-19 pandemic has exposed: the findings of five global health workforce professions.* World Health Organization [Human Resources for Health Observer Series No. 28])

BOX 16-6 PERSPECTIVES

Volunteering as a Nurse-Midwife in Africa

Delivering babies in the United States is vastly different from the experiences I encountered while delivering babies for one year in remote areas near the Ethiopian border. I remember one case in particular. It was during the monsoon season, and I was called to help a young woman having her first baby. Because a hospital delivery was impossible due to a powerful rainstorm that made roads impassable, my aide and I walked for miles on very soggy dirt roads to reach the village.

When we arrived, people in the village said that the baby had died, and upon entering the house I rushed toward the limp baby girl. The mother had delivered the baby on the mat used to cover the dirt floor. I could still feel a very muffled heartbeat on the umbilical cord that was still attached to the young mother. I reached for my mask and bag and started resuscitation. I checked the heartbeat and continued bagging the baby.

Women in the small village had crowded into the house, which could be described as a hut; some had been crying and wailing. Now, they were quietly sitting or standing near the door, speaking to each other in hushed tones while watching me work. My aide checked the mom, who appeared to be stable and had only a little bleeding. I kept bagging the baby and asked the women to get me some warm water to help keep the baby's temperature stable. I alternated warm water with cold water to try to stimulate the baby to breathe on her own; she produced only an occasional breath. I removed excess air from the baby's stomach after inserting a nasogastric tube, and she pinked up. Within a short while, she began to breathe independently.

The mother was relieved, and I checked her to be sure that there had been no tearing. My aide and I remained there through the night to be sure that no further respiratory problems returned. Word of the baby's recovery spread quickly through the village. I felt that we had truly made a difference!

Robin, nurse-midwife

1. *What steps of the nursing process are demonstrated in this global health nursing story where the community is client?*
2. *Which of the 10 Essential Public Health Services are pertinent to this situation?*
3. *What follow-up might this family need?*
4. *What community interventions are needed to support this family? What challenges can the nurse expect?*
5. *How did this C/PHN demonstrate respect, humility, and trust with this family and community?*

SUMMARY

- Community/public health nursing services are critical to the ultimate health of a community, providing important primary, secondary, and tertiary levels of health promotion and prevention throughout the world.
- Community assessment includes a comprehensive review of the patterns of care, demographic transitions, and epidemiologic transitions.
- Major principles of global healthcare include the global burden of disease, Health in All Policies, Sustainable Development Goals, and One Health.
- The GBD is calculated in a population or country by adding Years of Life Lost to Years Lived with Disability to determine the Disability-Adjusted Life Year. The higher the DALY, the greater the GBD.
- The United Nations and the World Health Organization are the integrating agencies for health around the world. Additional international agencies also support global health efforts.
- The International Health Regulations guide the interdependence of nations at times of global epidemics or pandemics.
- The UN Global Health Security Agenda, UN Global Compact for Migration, and UN Office of Genocide Prevention and the Responsibility to Protect are initiatives that support national and international efforts to protect populations.
- Brain Drain Brain Gain is important in understanding the migration of healthcare professionals.
- Global service-based learning requires careful self-reflection of one's own personal motivation behind volunteer efforts.
- Global health volunteering has positive and negative consequences for the volunteer and the host country.

ACTIVE LEARNING EXERCISES

1. Use the GBD Compare interactive tool at https://www.healthdata.org/research-analysis/gbd to examine the most current population data for another country compared to the United States. Use all ages and all genders in your comparison (e.g., all-cause Disability-Adjusted Life Year per 100,000 map; Disability-Adjusted Life Year by causes treemap). How are the patterns different or similar? What factors could influence your findings? Compare the same two countries in 1990 and evaluate how the patterns of causes have changed for both. (Objective 1)
2. The idea of *Health in All Policies* is that good health in any society requires policies across all *sectors* that support health. Examine the achievements of a country found at https://www.who.int/activities/promoting-health-in-all-policies-and-intersectoral-action-capacities. What changes were noted in public health outcomes after *Health in All Policies* was

implemented? How do your findings compare with that of a classmate's? (Objective 2)

3. In 2022, the WHO Region of Africa saw roughly 464,000 deaths due to malaria in children under age 5. This accounted for 80% of deaths from malaria in that region (WHO, 2023c). What current efforts are being implemented to combat malaria? Over the last 25 years, what progress has been made in reducing the incidence, as well as morbidity and mortality for this disease? Why do children under age 5 have a higher mortality rate? List 3 of the 10 Essential Public Health Services as shown in Box 2-2 that have been utilized to combat these infectious diseases. (Objective 3)
4. This chapter discusses various global organizations and their role during epidemics and pandemics. As the global community reflects on prevention measures for future pandemics after the devastation caused by COVID-19, the organizations continue to strive for the health of populations. The Global Health Center Success Stories at https://www.cdc.gov/globalhealth/stories/topic-list.html highlight examples of how the CDC and partners throughout the world combated communicable diseases. Explore the link to learn more. What roles did the organizations discussed in this chapter play in combatting COVID-19 pandemic? (Objective 4)
5. Describe the concept of "Brain Drain Brain Gain." Why do healthcare providers such as registered nurses and medical providers leave their country of origin after training and migrate to a new country? What benefits are there for the new country and for the individual? How does this egression affect the country or community of origin population health? Investigate what some countries and global organizations are doing to slow this trend. Interview a healthcare provider who migrated to the United States from a resource-limited country to learn more about their reasons. (Objective 5)
6. Identify a country in which you would like to practice C/PHN. Before you begin a review of this country, write down your own knowledge, attitudes, and beliefs about the country, the people, and the culture. Examine your own motivations for wanting this experience. Identify how you might feel if you received services rather than provided services. (Objective 5)

CHAPTER 17

Disasters and Their Impact

"Current governance systems are built to prepare and respond to events with known frequency and manageable severity, but they are not fit for purpose to address worst-case scenarios, which are emerging, exponential, and global in scope."

—United Nations Office for Disasters Risk Reduction (UNDRR), 2023

KEY TERMS

Casualty
Directly impacted by disaster
Disaster
Disaster planning
Displaced people
Incident command system (ICS)
Intensity
Human-made disaster
Mass-casualty incident
Multiple-casualty incident
Natural disaster
Posttraumatic stress disorder (PTSD)
Resilience
Scope
Triage

LEARNING OBJECTIVES

Upon mastery of this chapter, you should be able to:

1. Describe a variety of disasters, including their causation, number of casualties, scope, and intensity.
2. Identify three factors contributing to a community's potential for experiencing a disaster.
3. Identify the phases of disaster management.
4. Describe the role of the community/public health nurse (C/PHN) in preventing, preparing for, responding to, and supporting recovery from disasters.

INTRODUCTION

In this millennium, we have witnessed multiple devastating natural disasters, such as Category 5 hurricanes, tsunamis, and earthquakes, and human-made destructive acts of terrorism (e.g., bombings) causing multiple fatalities, and increased gun violence and mass shootings. Natural and human-made disasters are ever-present possibilities regardless of where one lives or works; however, the increase in gun violence requires healthcare professionals to be skilled in disaster preparedness and response to mass casualties. This chapter will increase your understanding of the community/public health nurse's (C/PHN's) role in preparing for, responding to, and recovering from natural disasters, terrorism, and gun violence.

DISASTERS

A **disaster** is any natural or human-made event that causes a level of destruction or emotional trauma exceeding the abilities of those affected to recover without community assistance. Airplane crashes, mass shootings, and chemical explosions are all situations that are devastating to a community and, by definition, constitute disasters.

The geographic distribution and types of disasters vary around the world due to environmental, sociopolitical, and topographic factors. Throughout history, disasters have affected every section of the globe. However, technologic advances, such as satellite data, have improved disaster management worldwide (International Charter, n.d.).

Characteristics of Disasters

Disasters are often characterized by their causes.

- A **natural disaster** is caused by natural events, such as earthquakes and tsunamis.
- A **human-made disaster** is caused by human activity, such as mass shootings, the bombing of significant landmarks in major cities, or riots in major cities.

Other human-made disasters include nuclear reactor meltdowns, industrial accidents, oil spills, construction accidents, and air, train, bus, and subway crashes.

- A **casualty** is someone who has been injured or killed by, or as a direct result of, an accident or natural disaster.
- If casualties number more than two people but fewer than 100, the disaster is characterized as a **multiple-casualty incident**.
- Although multiple-casualty incidents may strain the healthcare systems of small or midsized communities, a **mass-casualty incident**—often involving many casualties—can completely overwhelm the healthcare resources of even large cities (County of San Luis Obispo Emergency Medical Services Agency, 2023).

Preparedness for mass-casualty incidents is essential for all communities. Community leaders should closely track and report through various media sources (e.g., weather models, shared databases) the path and anticipated time of full impact of an adverse weather pattern to inform residents in the target areas and support early evacuation of families and businesses if necessary. Communities can help minimize devastation from flooding and devastation from fires by supporting precautionary preventive measures and ensuring safety regulations are enforced.

Unfortunately, some disasters occur without warning. For example:

- Wildfires in California during 2021–2022, were uncharacteristically large and control was hindered by drought conditions, along with heat and high winds.
- The overwhelming number of mass shootings occurring without warning and most often committed by people with mental illness acting alone.

Some disasters, such as the natural gas leaks in some communities, are at first unknown to the public. Residents often begin noticing headaches, nosebleeds, respiratory problems, and other symptoms and then notify their healthcare providers and proper authorities. The **scope** of a disaster is the range of its effect, either geographically or in terms of the number of people impacted. The **intensity** of a disaster is the level of destruction and devastation it causes.

- For instance, an earthquake centered in a large metropolitan area and one centered in a desert may have the same numeric rating on the Richter scale yet have very different intensities in terms of the destruction they cause.
- As of May 2024, COVID-19, stemming from a novel coronavirus that started in Wuhan, China, in December 2019, had infected more than 775 million worldwide and caused over 7 million deaths (WHO, 2024).

The terrorist attacks on September 11, 2001, are the worst disaster in the U.S. history, as a total of 2996 people, including 19 terrorists, died in three attacks on U.S. soil. Every year on September 11th, the country remembers those who perished in the attacks and those living with and have died from 9/11-related illnesses due to exposure to the toxic materials in the aftermath of the disaster (Campinoti, 2023).

People Impacted by Disasters

Those who are **directly impacted by disaster** experience the event firsthand, whether fire, flooding, mass shooting, vehicular accident, or bombing. These survivors are likely to have adverse health effects from their experience, even if they are without physical injuries directly caused by the event. Some may be without shelter or food, and many experience serious psychological stress long after the event is over.

Depending on the cause and characteristics of the disaster, some direct survivors may become displaced people or refugees. **Displaced people** are forced to leave their homes to escape the effects of a disaster. Usually, displacement is a temporary condition and involves movement within the person's own country.

Those who are indirectly impacted by disaster are the relatives and friends of people directly impacted by the disaster survivors. These supporters often undergo extreme anguish while trying to locate loved ones or accommodate their emergency needs.

Agencies and Organizations for Disaster Management

In 1803, the United States first recognized the need to prepare for emergencies through law and dedicated organizations. The first law was written as a direct response to a major disaster, the Portsmouth, New Hampshire fire of 1803, which swept through the seaport town. The majority of subsequent legislation was in response to specific crises and created many different agencies to respond to those disasters. The one constant was that the response of the federal government to disasters remained more reactive than proactive and was ad hoc in nature, only becoming coordinated with the establishment of the Federal Emergency Management Agency (FEMA) in 1979 (FEMA, 2021a).

In the United States, FEMA, a part of the Department of Homeland Security (DHS), controls emergency management. Initially, the management of all disasters is at the local level through facility groups, police, fire, and EMS. Once local authorities become overwhelmed, disaster management transitions to the state level with FEMA acting as an assisting agency rather than an authoritative leader (FEMA, 2023a).

FEMA provides oversight of the National Incident Management System (NIMS), developed to allow responders from different jurisdictions and disciplines to work more cohesively and proactively in response to natural disasters, emergencies, and terrorist acts.

- NIMS defines operational systems that guide how personnel work together during incidents.
- NIMS is also designed to manage all types of incidents and incorporate standard command and management structures, emphasizing preparedness, mutual aid, and resource management.

- Nurses and other healthcare professionals must understand this system (Fig. 17-1) and are encouraged to take courses dealing with the **incident command system** ICS. These courses are available for free online at http://www.training.fema.gov/EMI/ from the FEMA Emergency Management Institute.

The most important courses for a nurse are as follows:

- IS-100 Introduction to the Incident Command System.
- IS-200.C Basic Incident Command System for Initial Response.
- IS-700 Introduction to the NIMS.
- IS-800.b Introduction to the National Response Framework.
- Students are encouraged to explore the FEMA distance learning platform at https://training.fema.gov/is/.

Public health has become recognized as a critical component of emergency planning, preparedness, and response. National public health response requires coordination with state and local authorities, including nongovernmental agencies (Centers for Disease Control and Prevention [CDC], 2024a). The CDC website https://emergency.cdc.gov/planning/index.asp#print has an assortment of educational materials such as videos, online modules, and statistics, to explore disaster preparation and response information.

Among disaster-relief organizations, perhaps none is as famous as the American Red Cross, founded in 1881 by Clara Barton and chartered by the U.S. Congress in 1905. The Red Cross was authorized to provide disaster assistance free of charge across the country through its more than half a million volunteers and staff. The duties assumed by the Red Cross in the event of a disaster are to provide shelter, food, basic health and mental health services, and distribution of emergency supplies (American Red Cross, n.d.).

After the attacks on America on September 11, 2001, President George W. Bush sought to consolidate the roles and responsibilities of agencies and organizations involved in disaster response into one large department and to align them with emergency support functions (ESFs; FEMA, 2021b).

- In November 2002, Congress passed the Homeland Security Act, which officially and formally created the DHS in March 2003, as a single, Cabinet-level department focused on coordination and unification of national homeland security efforts (Department of Homeland Security, 2023).

DHS is composed of 22 federal departments and agencies. Visit https://www.dhs.gov for a list of the DHS agencies and components.

Emergency Support Functions

ESFs (Table 17-1; FEMA, 2021b) provide the structure for coordinating federal interagency support for an incident. The necessary functions that provide federal support, either to states or other federal agencies, are grouped into Stafford Act-declared disasters and emergencies and non-Stafford Act incidents:

- **ESF #1:** Transportation
- **ESF #2:** Communications
- **ESF #3:** Public Works and Engineering

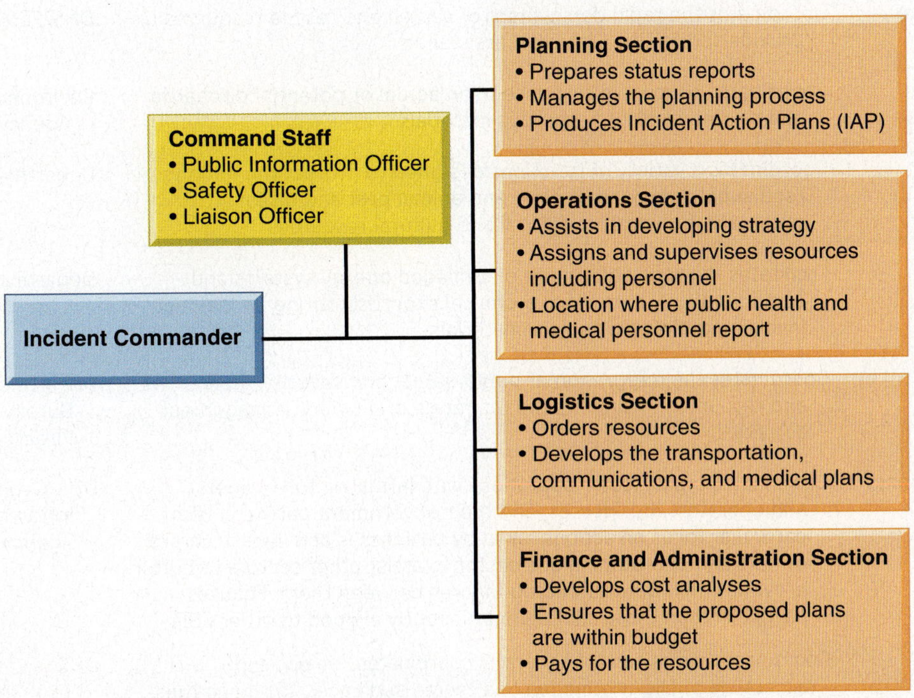

FIGURE 17-1 Incident command system. FEMA. *Incident Resource Center*. (Adapted from http://training.fema.gov/EMIWeb/IS/ICSResource/index.htm)

TABLE **17-1** Emergency Support Functions Responsibilities

ESF	Scope	Coordinating Agency
1. Transportation	Coordinates the support of management of transportation systems and infrastructure, the regulation of transportation, management of the nation's airspace, and ensuring the safety and security of the national transportation system	Department of Transportation
2. Communications	Coordinates government and industry efforts for the reestablishment and provision of critical communications infrastructure and services, facilitates the stabilization of systems and applications from malicious activity, and coordinates communications support to response efforts	DHS/Cybersecurity and Communications
3. Public works and engineering	Coordinates the capabilities and resources to facilitate the delivery of services, technical assistance, engineering expertise, construction management, and other support to prepare for, respond to, and recover from a disaster or an incident	Department of Defense—U.S. Army Corps of Engineers
4. Firefighting	Coordinates the support for the detection and suppression of fires. Functions include but are not limited to supporting wildland, rural, and urban firefighting operations	U.S. Department of Agriculture/U.S. Forest Service and DHS/FEMA/U.S. Fire Administration
5. Information and planning	Supports and facilitates multiagency planning and coordination for operations involving incidents requiring federal coordination	DHS/FEMA
6. Mass care, emergency assistance, temporary housing, and human services	Coordinates the delivery of mass care and emergency assistance	DHS/FEMA
7. Logistics	Coordinates comprehensive incident resource planning, management, and sustainment capability to meet the needs of disaster survivors and responders	General Services Administration and DHS/FEMA
8. Public health and medical services	Coordinates the mechanisms for assistance in response to an actual or potential public health and medical disaster or incident	Department of Health and Human Services
9. Search and rescue	Coordinates the rapid deployment of search and rescue resources to provide specialized lifesaving assistance	DHS/FEMA
10. Oil and hazardous materials response	Coordinates support in response to an actual or potential discharge and release of oil or hazardous materials	Environmental Protection Agency
11. Agriculture and natural services	Coordinates a variety of functions designed to protect the nation's food supply, respond to plant and animal pest and disease outbreaks, and protect natural and cultural resources	Department of Agriculture
12. Energy	Facilitates the reestablishment of damaged energy systems and components, and provides technical expertise during an incident involving radiologic/nuclear materials	Department of Energy
13. Public safety and security	Coordinates the integration of public safety and security capabilities and resources to support the full range of incident management activities	Department of Justice/Bureau of Alcohol, Tobacco, Firearms, and Explosives
14. Cross-sector business and infrastructure	Coordinates cross-sector operations with infrastructure owners and operators, businesses, and their government partners, with particular focus on actions taken by businesses and infrastructure owners and operators in one sector to assist other sectors to better prevent or mitigate cascading failures between them. Focuses particularly on those sectors not currently aligned to other ESFs	DHS/Cybersecurity and Infrastructure Security Agency
15. External affairs	Coordinates the release of accurate, coordinated, timely, and accessible public information to affected audiences, including the government, media, NGOs, and the private sector. Works closely with state and local officials to ensure outreach to the whole community	DHS

DHS, Department of Homeland Security; ESF, Emergency Support Functions; FEMA, Federal Emergency Management Agency; NGO, nongovernmental organization. Reprinted from The Department of Homeland Security. (2019). *National response framework* (4th ed., pp. 39–42). https://www.fema.gov/sites/default/files/2020-04/NRF_FINALApproved_2011028.pdf

- **ESF #4:** Firefighting
- **ESF #5:** Information and Planning
- **ESF #6:** Mass Care, Emergency Assistance, Temporary Housing, and Human Services
- **ESF #7:** Logistics
- **ESF #8:** Public Health and Medical Services
- **ESF #9:** Search and Rescue
- **ESF #10:** Oil and Hazardous Materials Response
- **ESF #11:** Agriculture and Natural Resources Annex
- **ESF #12:** Energy
- **ESF #13:** Public Safety and Security
- **ESF #14:** Cross-Sector Business and Infrastructure
- **ESF #15:** External Affairs

The Department of Health and Human Services is the lead federal agency for public health and medical services during a public health or medical disaster. Supplemental services are provided to state, local, and territorial governments and may include U.S. Public Health Service (USPHS) officers such as CDR Eduardo Cua (Fig. 17-2).

Governments often send their military personnel and equipment in response to international disasters. However, political agendas may prevent aid typically accepted by countries experiencing catastrophe to reach the impacted communities. The USPHS has also worked collaboratively with the U.S. Navy and Army to provide nursing and other medical care on combined humanitarian missions. The USPHS spent over 90 days in West Africa assisting with the management of the Ebola crisis (USPHS, n.d.).

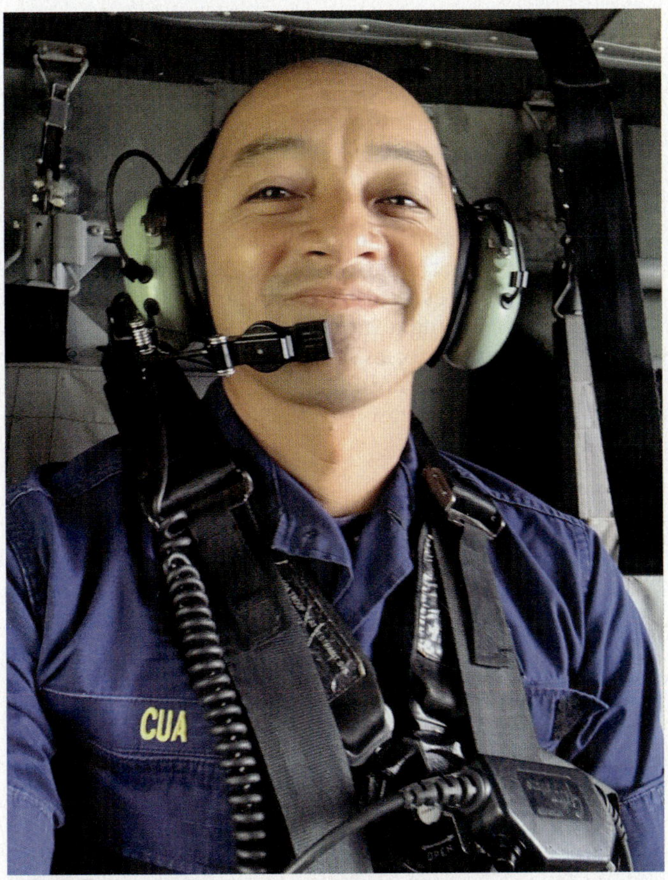
CUA

FIGURE 17-2 CDR Eduardo Cua of the United States Public Health Service. (Reprinted from USPHS February 2024 Officer Spotlight. https://www.usphs.gov/officer-spotlight/cdr-eduardo-cua/)

Phases of Disaster Management

To address the problem of disasters, it is important for the C/PHN to understand the phases of disaster management—prevention, mitigation, preparedness, response, and recovery—and become familiar with the language typically used in disaster preparedness (Fig. 17-3). Visit https://www.fema.gov/emergency-managers/nims for information on the NIMS stakeholder guidance for government, nongovernmental, and private sector disaster management strategies (FEMA, 2023b).

Prevention or Mitigation Phase

Activities during this phase are focused on preventing future emergencies or minimizing their effects. The shaping of public policies and plans that either modify the causes of disasters or mitigate their effects on people, property, and infrastructure are critical activities during this phase. Mitigation activities take place *before* and *after* disaster emergencies.

To reduce our vulnerability to disasters, the United States has strengthened its disaster management activities. The screening process at airports and shipping ports includes advanced imaging technology scanning and random hand-carried luggage or canine searches during the preboarding process.

- Nonpassengers are no longer allowed beyond the security entrance area, and photographic identification is required at two or more points before boarding.

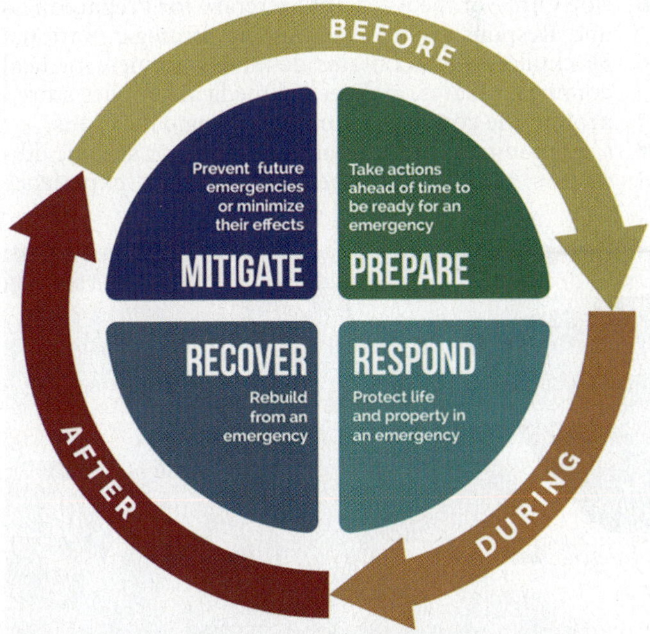
BEFORE
DURING
AFTER
Prevent future emergencies or minimize their effects
MITIGATE
Take actions ahead of time to be ready for an emergency
PREPARE
RECOVER
Rebuild from an emergency
RESPOND
Protect life and property in an emergency

FIGURE 17-3 Phases of disaster management. (Reprinted with permission from National Academies of Sciences, Engineering, and Medicine. 2024. Transportation for People with Disabilities and Older Adults During COVID-19: Lessons for Emergency Response. Washington, DC: The National Academies Press. https://doi.org/10.17226/27277. Figure 1).

Our global experience with the COVID-19 pandemic has fostered Global Health Security enhancements to help decrease the risk of pandemics. These steps include surveillance systems that detect possible threats, laboratories to identify the agent, a workforce for follow-up and containment, and emergency management systems to coordinate the activities (CDC, 2021). To prevent possible contamination by COVID-19, people are advised to stay current with COVID-19 vaccines, wear masks if known weakened immune systems, get tested if symptoms develop or with notification of exposure, if tested positive, stay home and away from others for at least 5 days (see Fig. 17-4). For additional prevention recommendations, visit https://www.cdc.gov/coronavirus/2019-ncov/prevent-getting-sick/prevention.html (CDC, 2024b).

Preparedness Phase

Disaster *preparedness* involves improving community and individual reaction and responses, so that the effects of a disaster are minimized. Disaster preparedness includes plans for communication, evacuation, rescue, victim care, and recovery. Pets are an important part of our society and for many an extension of their household and members of the family. Family disaster plans should include a plan for the pets in an emergency kit. Visit https://www.fema.gov/fact-sheet/are-you-petpared-disasters for recommendations (FEMA, 2023c).

- For instance, although plans may differ in states at higher risk of earthquakes from those in tornado alley, the preparedness plans apply to numerous disasters.
- Communities must ensure that warning systems are tested routinely to ensure appropriate notifications to residents of a tornado, hurricane, or any other potential threat.
- The Office of the Assistant Secretary for Preparedness and Response (n.d.) oversees the Strategic National Stockpile, which contains doses of vaccines, medical countermeasures, and needed medical supplies stored around the country in various strategic locations.
- Communities with increased diversity or specific ethnicities and limited access to resources experience inequities during disaster response and recovery. Data clearly show not only the need for systemic reinvestment in underrepresented racial and ethnic communities but also for disaster planners to prioritize these and other communities. Disasters affect everyone; however, the historical disparities and inequities experienced by people from underrepresented racial and ethnic groups, people with low incomes, and other communities with less power and access to resources are clearly revealed during these troubled times (Substance Abuse and Mental Health Services Administration [SAMHSA], 2024a).

Nurses have a significant role in disaster preparedness (Fig. 17-5). Preparedness activities take place *before* an emergency occurs. Nurses should also remember to prepare themselves and their families by having an individual and family plan and essential supplies (American Red Cross, 2023). Nurses are encouraged to enroll in disaster classes and register with a disaster agency such as the Red Cross (American Red Cross, 2024) to strengthen one's professional preparedness and to be a prepared responder during a disaster. Review "Nurses—the backbone of our nation's disaster response" from the Future of Nursing—Campaign for Action report, https://campaignforaction.org/ (2021).

Response Phase

The *response phase* begins immediately after the onset of the disastrous event and *during* the emergency. Response is putting your preparedness plans into action immediately, with the goals of saving lives and preventing further injury or damage to property.

- Activities during the response phase include rescue, triage, on-site stabilization, transportation of injured, and treatment at local hospitals and clinics.
- Disaster triage differs from triage done in the emergency departments. Simple Triage and Rapid Treatment (START), the most commonly used technique in the United States, consists of triaging people in 30 to 60 seconds during a mass casualty (Fig. 17-6).
  - The four categories consist of the walking wounded/minor (green tag), delayed (yellow), immediate (red), and deceased (black). These categories are

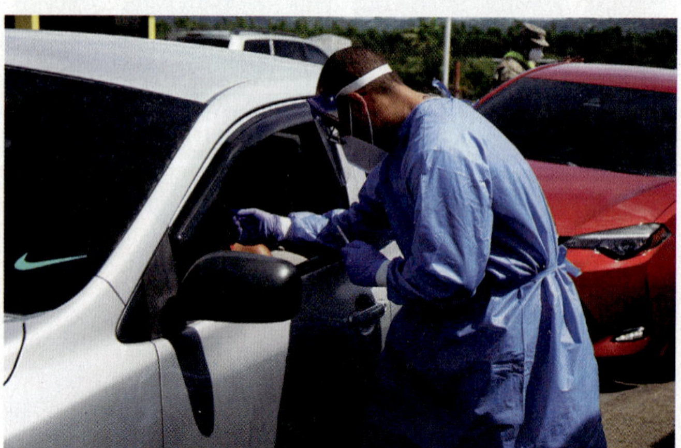

FIGURE 17-4 COVID-19 testing. (Reprinted from U.S. Department of Defense, photo by Army Sgt. José Ferrer, Puerto Rico Army National Guard. https://www.defense.gov/Multimedia/Photos/igphoto/2003016066/)

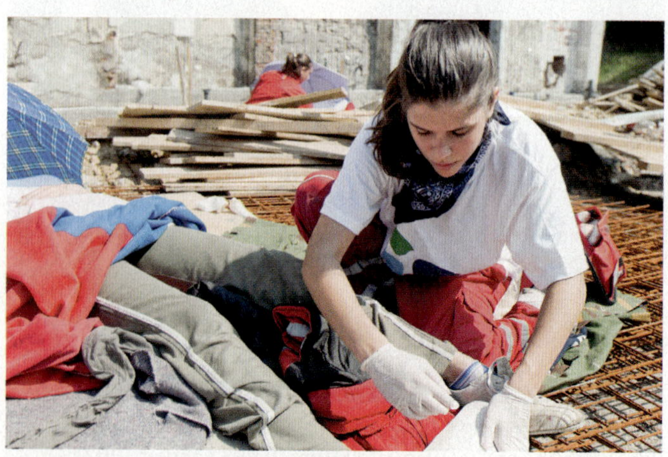

FIGURE 17-5 Disaster preparedness: simulated healthcare exercise.

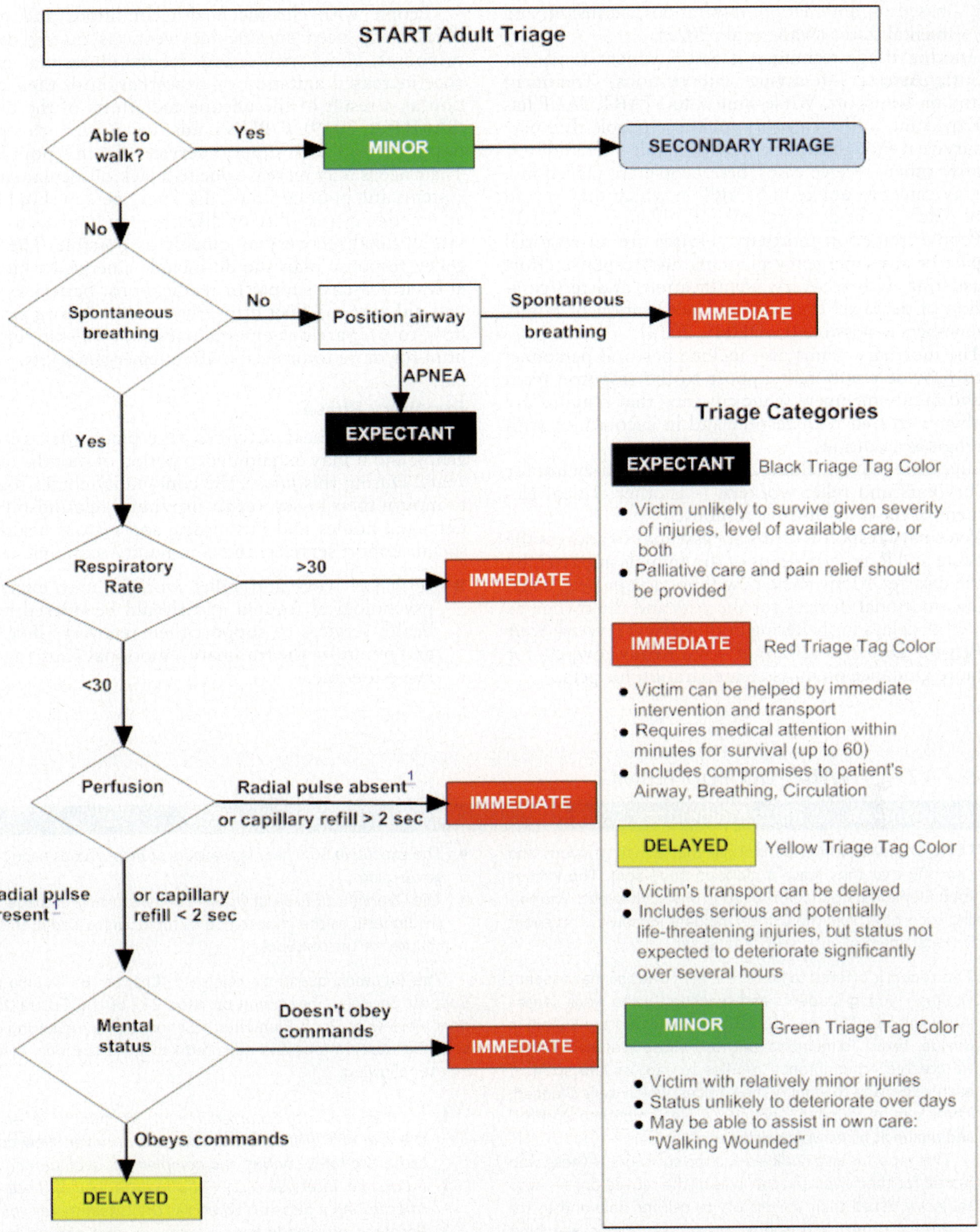

FIGURE 17-6 START Adult Triage Algorithm. (Reprinted from Chemical Hazards Emergency Medical Management, U.S. Department of Health and Human Services. https://chemm.hhs.gov/startadult.htm)

based on ambulation, respirations, perfusion, and mental status (Wang et al., 2022).

- Another triage technique is SALT, which stands for Sort, Assess, Life-saving interventions, Treatment and/or Transport. While similar to START, SALT has Expectant, a fifth category for those people that may survive if enough resources are available after and only after others receive care These people are placed in a gray category unlike in START in which they would be placed in the deceased category (Wang et al., 2022).
- People trained in mortuary services are an essential part of any emergency planning and response effort assisting with recovery, identification, and refrigeration of deceased remains until notification of family members is possible (USDHHS, 2024).
- The mortuary teams also include pastoral personnel to provide emotional support to the response team and family members while ensuring that remains are always treated with respect and in accordance with religious traditions.
- Supportive care, including food, water, and shelter for survivors and relief workers, is another critical element of the total disaster response.
- Veterinary response teams are essential to address the acute and long-term needs of the animals impacted by the disaster. Many shelters will not accept pets, causing emotional distress for the pets and the owner, as well as delays in sheltering both. Review *Prepare Your Pets for Disasters* (2023) at www.Ready.gov/pets for more guidance on disaster preparation for pets.

People with chronic health conditions and mental illness may need specific interventions during disaster responses. Those with serious mental illness may experience increased agitation or exacerbation of their condition as a result of the unexpected effects of the disaster (SAMHSA, 2019). C/PHNs must be aware of this potential effect and seek support services for this population. Their needs may increase due to a lack of regular support systems and poor coping skills. Every person should have an emergency response or disaster plan in place to facilitate optimal recovery as quickly as possible. The emergency response plan should include emergency kits with at least a 3-day supply of medications, batteries, water, first aid kits, etc. Visit https://www.redcross.org/get-help/how-to-prepare-for-emergencies/survival-kit-supplies.html for more information about emergency kits.

Recovery Phase

The recovery phase activities take place *after* an emergency, and it may extend over a period of months or even years. During this *phase*, the community comes together to mourn their losses, repair or rebuild relationships and damaged homes and businesses, and restore health and social support services, and community economic vitality.

- Both survivors and relief workers may experience psychological trauma and should be offered mental health services to support their recovery (Box 17-1) and minimize the traumatic emotional scars that may last a lifetime.

BOX **17-1** WHAT DO *YOU* THINK?

Active Shooter at Robb Elementary School

There are events in one's lifetime that are so grievous and horrific that they leave a mark on one's soul. The killings at Robb Elementary School in 2020 is one such event. The following excerpt is from the Critical Incident Review of this event (U.S. Department of Justice, 2024a, p. iv):

> This report is offered to honor the memories of the innocent victims—young students and teachers—who were senselessly killed on May 24, 2022, at Robb Elementary School in Uvalde, Texas. To memorialize those whose lives were taken, we created remembrance profiles to capture the spirit of each victim and to amplify their voices, which were silenced. These can be found in "Appendix A. Remembrance Profiles" and online at https://cops.usdoj.gov/uvalde.
>
> This report is also dedicated to the survivors—those who feared for their lives and the lives of their loved ones—who selflessly risked their own safety to call for help and to try to protect others and who witnessed the horror, watching in anguish as the event unfolded. To hundreds of survivors in this community, we know the negative impacts, including physical, mental, and emotional injuries, will not end and that your grief remains very heavy. Many of you continue to bear the scars and pain you suffered from the loss of your loved ones and the loss of your sense of safety in your own community.

- The Executive Summary is available at https://cops.usdoj.gov/uvalde
- The Overview of Factual Observations, starting on page xiv, underlines the importance of topics discussed in this chapter of the textbook.

The following questions relate to "Chapter 6: Trauma and Support Services," beginning on page 237 of the Critical Incident Review at Robb Elementary School. After reviewing the selected observations and selected recommendations, reflect on the following:

1. *If a mass casualty occurred in your community, reflect on the role of C/PHN and the role of a survivor. How could these two roles conflict and complement each other?*
2. *If possible, interview a C/PHN who experienced these two roles during a disaster. What was the takeaway for you?*
3. *Research policies in your community that pertain to the report's select recommendations. Is there more that needs to be done in your community?*
4. *Explore the plethora of training resources Chapter 6 of the report. Consider completing some in preparation for possible disasters.*
5. *What resources will the adults and children need in this community?*

- The Substance Abuse and Mental Health Services Administration (SAMHSA) offers guides, webinars, and podcasts to assist professionals and survivors with managing stress during and after a crisis. Visit https://www.samhsa.gov/resource/dbhis/guide-managing-stress-crisis-response-professions for resources for survivors and responders.

Role of the Community/Public Health Nurse

Understanding the phases of disaster, one should see the many ways the C/PHN can assist with implementing the disaster management plan.

Preventing Disasters

Disaster prevention may be considered on three levels: primary, secondary, and tertiary (Box 17-2).

Primary Prevention. Nurses play a central role in response efforts across all types of healthcare settings. They are able to provide education, community engagement, health promotion, and interventions to protect the public health status. They provide first aid, advanced clinical care, and lifesaving medications; assess and triage victims; allocate scarce resources; and monitor ongoing physical and mental health needs.

- Primary disaster prevention efforts should include awareness of a community's physical, psychosocial, cultural, economic, and spiritual stance. The C/PHN has the unique opportunity to educate people at home, at work, at school, or in a faith community, and the opportunity to be aware of the community perspective about safety and security focused on preventing a disaster.
- Primary prevention includes providing and participating in training sessions on the prevention of disaster risk factors, knowing high-risk groups through community assessments, and working with community partners (CDC, 2024a).

BOX 17-2 LEVELS OF PREVENTION PYRAMID

Responding to a Tornado

SITUATION: A natural disaster—Tornado

GOAL: Prepare, promptly diagnose, and treat and restore people, families, and communities to the fullest by using the three levels of prevention.

Tertiary Prevention

Rehabilitation	Prevention: Health Promotion and Education	Prevention: Health Protection
▪ Remain safe during the immediate recovery period. ▪ Accept help from others—friends, family, and community services. ▪ Rebuild family lives through counseling and other services to reestablish stable life physically, emotionally, spiritually, and financially.	▪ Educate community members about the need to enhance planning against damage from future natural disasters, based on experiences with the current disaster.	▪ Keep recommended immunizations current. ▪ Community physical structures need rebuilding, with infrastructure planning and supports that improve ability to withstand natural disasters.

Secondary Prevention

Early Diagnosis	Prompt Treatment
▪ Remain in your position of safety until a community all-clear warning signal is sounded or until rescued. ▪ Leave a damaged building cautiously, if able and not seriously injured, and do not return until it is declared safe.	▪ Rescue people promptly and get appropriate care for those injured as soon as possible. ▪ The infrastructure of the community becomes/remains intact, keeping community members safe from hazards such as live wires, broken gas lines, and fallen debris.

Primary Prevention

Health Promotion and Education	Health Protection
▪ Increase community awareness. ▪ Increase community preparation through education. ▪ Each person is as prepared as possible both physically and emotionally.	▪ Community members know what to do and where to go, whether at home, work, school, or elsewhere in the community. ▪ Get to safety before the impact—southwest corner of a home's basement or an interior room away from windows and under heavy furniture.

- Primary prevention of disasters is practiced in all settings—the workplace and home—with clearly defined processes to reduce safety hazards, to monitor risk factors, reduce pollution, and encourage nonviolent conflict resolution (CDC, 2024a).

The *Future of Nursing 2020–2030 Charting a Path to Achieve Health Equity* report recognizes the role nurses have with organizational logistics, operational response protocols, security measures, and statistical analysis of individual- and community-level data before, during, and after disasters (2021). The second aspect of primary disaster prevention is anticipatory guidance.

The C/PHN can assist community collaboration through planning, committee membership, organization of drills at the place of employment, or assisting with community-wide disaster drills on a regular basis.

Secondary Prevention. Secondary disaster prevention focuses on the earliest possible detection and treatment to yield an effective response. After a disaster, C/PHNs in the local health department work with the American Red Cross to coordinate and provide emergency assistance.

- Planned and organized early evacuation, identified shelters for patients with functional needs with adequate security outside the high-risk area, a well-designed volunteer cascading communication system, and pre-event evacuation drills have been proven to be most successful with response efforts.
- Many local communities have developed preparedness programs to inform, prepare, and ensure residents are ready for any type of human-made or natural disaster, such as the City of New Orleans's NOLA READY (for more details, visit https://ready.nola.gov/home/).
- The Emergency Prescription Assistance Program (Administration for Strategic Preparedness and Response, n.d.) provides medication, immunizations, and medical supplies and equipment for those without insurance in a federally identified disaster area.

Tertiary Prevention. Tertiary disaster prevention involves reducing the amount and degree of disability or damage resulting from a disaster. This level involves rehabilitative work and can help a community recover and reduce the risk of further disasters.

- The American Psychiatric Nurses Association provides many resources for nurses facing and managing traumatic events.
  - Visit https://www.apna.org/resources/trauma-informed-care-in-behavioral-health-services/ for a detailed list of resources for dealing with traumatic events.
  - Visit SAMHSA apps at https://store.samhsa.gov/product/samhsa-disaster for easy access when in the field.
- The Office of the Assistant Secretary for Preparedness and Response (2019) offers a three-module series at https://asprtracie.hhs.gov/technical-resources/resource/7216/disaster-behavioral-health-self-care-for-healthcare-workers-modules that covers compassion fatigue and secondary trauma for healthcare providers.

Preparing for Disasters

Disaster planning is essential for a community, business, and hospitals. Details of preparation and management by all involved, including community leaders, health and safety professionals, and lay people must be considered. Despite many disaster drills and numerous iterations of disaster plans before Hurricane Katrina, some hospitals in New Orleans were better prepared for terrorism events than for the hurricanes and flooding that were common to that geographic area. C/PHNs can be very instrumental in disaster preparedness (Association of Public Health Nurses [APHN], 2014), and they must ensure they have their own family disaster preparation plan in place. For information on nurses' personal preparation for disaster and online courses on disaster preparedness, see Box 17-3.

BOX 17-3 Nurses' Personal Preparation for Disasters and Available Training

American Nurses Association has educational opportunities for nurses on disaster preparedness. When we are a prepared profession, we can cope and help our communities recover from disasters better, faster, and stronger. See https://www.nursingworld.org/practice-policy/work-environment/health-safety/disaster-preparedness/ for the following documents from the American Nurses Association:

- Position Statement Background Information: Registered Nurses' Rights and Responsibilities Related to Work Release During a Disaster
- Position Statement Background Information: Work Release During a Disaster—Guidelines for Employers

Personal preparedness means that the nurse has read and understands workplace and community disaster plans and has developed a disaster plan for their own family (San Diego County Office of Emergency Services, n.d.). The prepared nurse should also have participated in disaster drills, have documented up-to-date vaccinations, be a certified basic life support provider, and be able to provide basic first aid. Nurses preparing to work in disaster areas as "spontaneous volunteers" should have copies of their nursing license and driver's license, durable clothing, and basic equipment, such as stethoscopes, flashlights, and cellular phones to facilitate appropriate task assignments during the disaster response.

To increase understanding of and the ability to work within an emergency situation, every nurse should become familiar with NIMS. NIMS is "a systematic, proactive approach to guide all levels of government, NGOs, and the private sector to work together to prevent, protect against, mitigate, respond to, and recover from the effects of incidents" (FEMA, 2023a). In essence, NIMS provides a framework for management of incidents in support of the national preparedness system. Free online courses are offered through FEMA at www.fema.gov.

Refer to *The Future of Nursing 2020–2030: Charting a Path to Achieve Health Equity*. Chapter 8. (2021). https://nam.edu/publications/the-future-of-nursing-2020-2030/

During disasters nurses respond by managing prehospital triage and treatment, providing onsite incident management, and designing and implementing community-based health education and training.

- Flexibility is essential because key authority figures may themselves be survivors of the disaster. It is critical to have a second-in-command with equal knowledge of the community's disaster plan who can step in without delay if needed.
- Reliable communication is often a point of breakdown for communities attempting to cope with major disasters. At times of heightened chaos and stress, as well as after physical damage to communication facilities and equipment, misinformation, and misinterpretation can cause delayed treatment and increased loss of life.
- Clarity and flexibility are the keywords for establishing efficient lines of communication.

The CDC sample, Single Overriding Communications Objective, is an effective template to disseminate information concisely and quickly to the media during a disaster (see Box 17-4).

Inefficient transportation routes can increase injury and loss of life. Disaster planners must consider what routes emergency vehicles will take when transporting disaster survivors to local and outlying hospitals or healthcare workers to the disaster site.

Responding to Disasters

- In many natural disasters, local weather service personnel, public works officials, police officers, or firefighters have the earliest information regarding any increasing potential for a disaster. They also advise the mayor's office or other community leaders of their recommendations for warning or evacuating the public and may recommend actions the community should take to mitigate damage and community panic or injury. Planners should never assume that all citizens can be reached by radio or television or that broadcast systems will be unaffected by the disaster. Broadcast media may indeed be a primary means of communicating warnings, but alternative strategies, such as social media or police and volunteers canvassing neighborhoods, should be considered (FEMA, 2024a).
- Social media options such as Facebook, X (formerly Twitter), and blogs are reliable methods used by news stations and public health agencies that must not be ignored. Over 20 million tweets were sent by utilities after Hurricane Sandy, and Google's web application, *Person Finder*, was especially helpful during the Boston Marathon bombings (SAMHSA, 2020).
- Messages should be broadcast in multiple languages according to the community cultural mixture.
- Information communicated should include the nature of the disaster, the exact geographic region affected, including street names if available, and the actions citizens should take to protect themselves and their property.
- A study on the use of GPS devices in a simulated mass casualty found the devices useful in tracking patient locations throughout the drill (Gross et al., 2019). Technology continues to improve tracking of people which can assist with managing injuries and fatalities in a timely manner.

An evacuation plan is an essential component of the total disaster plan (CDC, 2024a). The plan should include notification of the police, local military personnel, or voluntary citizens' groups as well as methods of notifying and transporting the evacuees. A coordinated response to rescue, triage, and treat disaster survivors is one of the first obligations of the response effort. A plan should also be made for responding to citizens who refuse to evacuate. For example, will police authorities forcibly remove an older adult citizen from their home to a shelter? Will evacuation plans include household pets? If farms or ranches are in the path of fires or floods, will animals be evacuated? How? Who will do this, and where will they be taken/sheltered?

BOX 17-4 The CDC Sample Single Overriding Communications Objective Template

- In one BRIEF paragraph, state the key point or objective you want to accomplish by doing the interview. This statement should reflect what you, the author or speaker, would like to see as the lead paragraph in a newspaper story or broadcast report about your topic.
- What are the three or four facts or statistics you would like the public to remember as a result of reading or hearing about this story?
- Who is the main audience or population segment you would like this message to reach?

Primary: general public   Secondary: policymakers (awareness)

- What is the ONE message you want the audience to take away from this interview/report?

Reprinted from CDC. (n.d.). *Sample single overriding communications objective (SOCO)*. https://www.cdc.gov/tb/publications/guidestoolkits/forge/docs/13_samplesingleoverridingcommunicationsobjective_soco_worksheet.doc

Responding to Disasters

At the disaster site, the job of rescue typically belongs to firefighters and urban search and rescue teams that have personnel with special training in search and rescue (Fig. 17-7). Depending on the disaster's character or type,

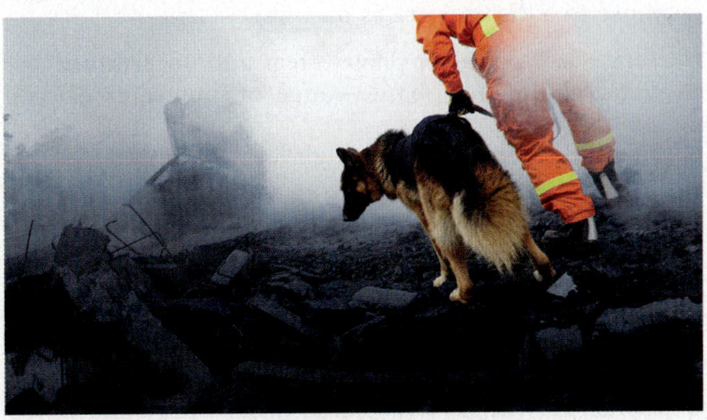

FIGURE 17-7 Search and rescue forces search through destroyed building with the help of rescue dogs.

protective gear, heavy equipment, and special vehicles may be needed, and recovery or mortuary teams including search dogs trained to locate bodies may be brought in (FEMA, 2021c). The C/PHN's population-based knowledge and awareness of community resources and particularly vulnerable people are needed throughout the response efforts.

Triage is the process of sorting multiple casualties in a major medical crisis or disaster when the number of casualties exceeds immediate treatment resources. The goal of triage is to effect the greatest amount of good for the greatest number of people. The most common method of triage used by first responders at a mass-casualty incident in the United States is the START process for adults and JumpSTART for pediatric patients.

- START and JumpSTART are forms of triage used to categorize victims into four categories (immediate, delayed, minor, or morgue/deceased) and are consistent with international triage system.

Prioritization of treatment may be very different in a mass-casualty event as opposed to an average day in a hospital emergency department. Under normal circumstances, a person presenting to a hospital emergency department with a myocardial infarction and showing no pulse or respirations would receive immediate treatment and have a chance of recovery. At a disaster site, a person without a pulse or respirations would most likely be placed in the nonsalvageable category.

- In mass-casualty occurrences, the broader community will need to become involved, including requests for rescue vehicles, firefighters, and police officers from neighboring towns, and the use of neighboring hospitals. Depending on the magnitude of the mass casualty, state and federal resources may also be needed.

Visit the SAMHSA website at https://www.samhsa.gov/dtac/disaster-survivors for information about disaster resource portal (SAMHSA, 2020).

Disasters impact not only the person but the community as well. There are six phases of a community's response to a disaster; each varies in length of time and with different emotions. It is important for C/PHN to be aware of the emotional impact on a community that follows a disaster and provide interventions to minimize emotional escalations. The six phases of a community's response to a disaster are as follows:

- Phase 1: Predisaster phase—fear and uncertainty
- Phase 2: Impact phase—range of intense emotional reactions
- Phase 3: Heroic phase—high level of activity with a low level of productivity
- Phase 4: Honeymoon phase—dramatic shift in emotion
- Phase 5: Disillusionment phase—realize the limits of disaster assistance
- Phase 6: Reconstruction phase—overall feeling of recovery
- Refer to https://www.samhsa.gov/sites/default/files/dtac/ccptoolkit/fema-ccp-guidance.pdf for a detailed look at these six phases and possible interventions.

Disaster nurses provide treatment on-site at emergency treatment stations, at mobile field hospitals, in shelters, and at local hospitals and clinics (Box 17-5). In addition to direct nursing care, on-site interventions might include arranging for transport once survivors are stabilized, and managing the procurement, distribution, and replenishment of all supplies, and food and beverages, including infant formulas and rehydration fluids. Safety responsibilities may include arranging for adequate, accessible, and safe sanitation facilities at the treatment location. The nurse very often may also recognize the need to arrange for psychological and spiritual care of survivors of disasters and responders.

C/PHNs must be aware of the covert physical and emotional injuries resulting from the disaster. Some survivors who seem physically uninjured may, in fact, be suffering from major injuries; however, they may be unable to relate their symptoms to a responder due to shock or anxiety.

BOX 17-5 New Nurse Practitioner Shares Community Hospital Disaster Response Experience

I had just come off of orientation in a new role as a nurse practitioner in an outpatient heart failure clinic that was located on the first floor of the affiliated hospital. A couple of the staff from my clinic were reassigned to different positions in the hospital to help meet patient needs, making us shorthanded in our clinic. We had to be creative in addressing the needs of our high-risk and complicated patient population. Patient management was further complicated as the patient population we serve is of a lower socio-economic status and thus has fewer resources available to them.

We always remained open as we needed to keep our patients stable and out of the ER, which was overwhelmed. We tried to shift appropriate patient appointments to virtual visits, and we mailed out scales and blood pressure cuffs to many of our patients. We also collaborated with homecare agencies, pharmacies with pill pack services, and our care management team to continue to deliver quality care to our patients, while trying to minimize the risk of them contracting COVID-19 by keeping them in their homes and not needing to travel to the hospital for their appointments.

As nurses, we are innovative and can adjust patients' care plans to meet their individual needs taking into consideration external factors that affect their health; the COVID-19 pandemic forced me to utilize that skill set in the setting of the many challenges that arose. This is not a skill set that is taught in a classroom or in a book, and it is a thought process obtained and strengthened while practicing as a nurse. I do not recall receiving any training from my hospital or schooling that could have even remotely prepared me for what we encountered during this pandemic, strategically or emotionally. The hospital did do a good job of quickly organizing a team of healthcare providers to write policies regarding management/visitation/masking and kept us abreast on how our hospital was being affected.

Jannae White, DNP, CRNP

Other survivors may be so emotionally traumatized by the disaster that they act out, disrupting efforts to assist them and other survivors and possibly engaging in dangerous activities. These survivors must be assessed for head trauma and internal injuries because their behavior may have a physiologic cause (SAMHSA, 2024b).

Identification and safe transport of the deceased to a morgue or holding facility is crucial, especially if contagion is feared, though this is rare in mass-casualty situations.

- Toe tags make documentation visible and accessible.
- Records of deaths must be accurately documented and maintained, and family members should be notified of their loved ones' deaths as quickly and compassionately as possible.
- If feasible, a representative from the area's faith community should be contacted to assist families awaiting news of missing loved ones.
- A family's recovery from loss is often delayed when notification of their relative is not possible because the recovered bodies are badly damaged or not found (USDHHS, 2024).

In addition to direct nursing care, on-site interventions might include arranging for transport once survivors are stabilized and managing the procurement, distribution, and replenishment of all supplies and food and beverages, including infant formulas and rehydration fluids. Safety responsibilities may include arranging for adequate, accessible, and safe sanitation facilities at the treatment location. The nurse very often may also recognize the need to arrange psychological and spiritual care for survivors of disasters and responders.

Recovery From Disasters

Disasters do not suddenly end when the rubble is cleared and the survivors' wounds are healed. Rather, recovery is a long, complex process often including long-term medical treatment, physical rehabilitation, financial restitution, case management, and psychological and spiritual support (FEMA, 2024b).

Long-Term Treatment. Long-term treatment may be required for many survivors of disasters, straining the local rehabilitative care facilities and resources.

- Challenges exist with a lack of adequate financial support for lifelong disabilities and medical care.
- Older citizens who have sustained serious injuries in the disaster might suddenly require relocation to a long-term care facility.
- Extensive property damage may cause some residents or businesses to relocate rather than rebuild on land they now deem to be disaster-prone.
- A disaster in a small community may alter the entire social fabric of that community permanently (SAMHSA, 2024b) causing an economic disparity.

Long-Term Support. Insurance settlements, FEMA funding, and private donations may assist in financing disaster survivors in need of funding to repair or rebuild their homes or to reopen businesses, such as stores, restaurants, childcare facilities, and other services needed by the community.

Psychological support is often required after a disaster, both for survivors and for relief workers (Fig. 17-8). Some people may experience **posttraumatic stress disorder (PTSD)**. Many survivors, especially older adults displaced from their homes, may quietly lose their will to live and drift into apathy, malaise, and depression. While some people may question their faith after a disaster, Sen et al. (2022) found religion and spirituality may assist with coping and coming to terms with the disaster. In assessing a community's citizens for counseling needs after a disaster, the PHN should not forget to include children. Often, children do not have words to express their feelings or fears and may act out in ways adults find difficult to understand, unless age-appropriate psychological intervention is provided. Medical responders to disasters are at risk of depression and PTSD; additional responses might also include decreased critical thinking skills, lower performance, and impaired decision-making skills (Alghamdi, 2022). Ritter et al. (2023) found that the U.S. Public Health Service first responders were at risk of moral injury due to the COVID-19 pandemic. Responders' moral values and codes of conduct were violated due to the overwhelming pandemic causing moral injury. Symptoms are similar to PTSD and include depression, guilt, and self-harm (Ritter et al., 2023).

Self-care, including stress education for all relief workers after a disaster, is a common practice and helps to reduce anxiety and put the situation into proper perspective. Critical incident stress debriefing (CISD) provides responders with professional debriefing. CISD is generally provided between 24 and 72 hours after the disaster event and typically produces positive outcomes, such as the following:

- Accelerated healing process
- Positive coping mechanisms
- Clarified misconceptions and misunderstandings
- Group cohesiveness
- A healthy, supportive work atmosphere
- Identifying people who require more extensive psychological assistance

Both relief workers and recent trauma victims can benefit from CISD, which seeks to limit secondary traumatic stress by promoting empowerment and collaboration, as well as providing safety and choices. Earlier

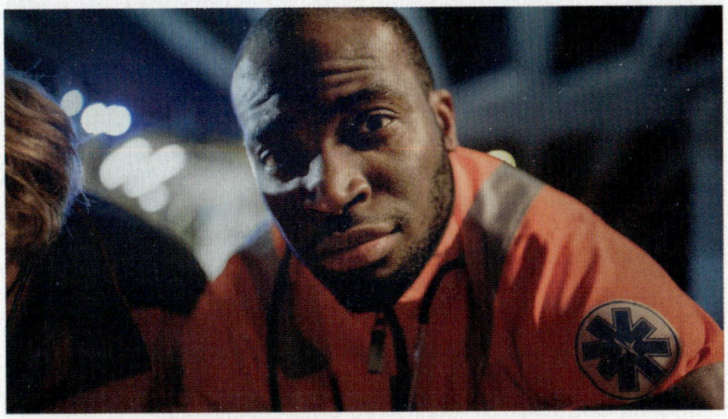

FIGURE 17-8 Paramedics provide medical help to an injured person on the street at night.

life experiences, such as abuse and neglect or systemic bias, may exacerbate experiences with traumatic events. Another helpful resource for survivors and responders is SAMHSA's (2024b) Disaster Technical Assistance Center at https://www.samhsa.gov/dtac. The website provides a host of information on the negative effects that stem from disasters as well as stress management tips.

More research is needed in the monitoring of long-term psychological effects and the evaluation of interventions following disasters (Généreux et al., 2019). Awareness of your perceptions and how your actions are viewed are essential in dealing with trauma victims.

- Literature indicates that healthcare professionals exhibit the same amount of implicit bias as the general public and that diagnosis and treatment may be affected.
- As health professionals, C/PHNs must be aware of their biases and prejudices (see https://implicit.harvard.edu/implicit/takeatest.html for a self-test for implicit bias).

In addition, trauma victims during a crisis may have previous unpleasant trauma experiences related to inequities, preventing them from seeking care or adhering to medical instructions and treatment.

The C/PHN and community mental health nurses, through education, screening, assessment, and referral, have an important role in the prevention of psychological disturbances due to a disaster.

Although a disaster, by its very nature, is often unforeseen, people's ability to cope with the disaster can be determined in part by the previous experiences and the resources available.

Health and Human Service (HHS) deployed public health workers to help Maui wildfire survivors in September 2023. The team of 25 officers from the U.S. Public Health Service Commissioned Corps included clinical psychiatrists, psychologists, social workers, and nurse practitioners (Fig. 17-9). "Public Health Services officers are trained and ready to respond to humanitarian missions and public health crises," said Admiral Rachel Levine, HHS Assistant Secretary for Health (U.S. Public Health Service, n.d.). The mission of the Commissioned Corp of the U.S. Public Health Service is to *protect, promote, and advance the health and safety of the nation*. The Corp, one of eight uniformed services, consists of public health officials who work across the nation. During national and global public health disasters or emergencies, such as assisting with the management of the Ebola crisis in West Africa and the COVID-19 pandemic, these public health officials are essential for the health of the nation and global communities (Box 17-6). Go to https://www.usphs.gov/about-us to learn more about the Commissioned Corp and the opportunities for C/PHNs.

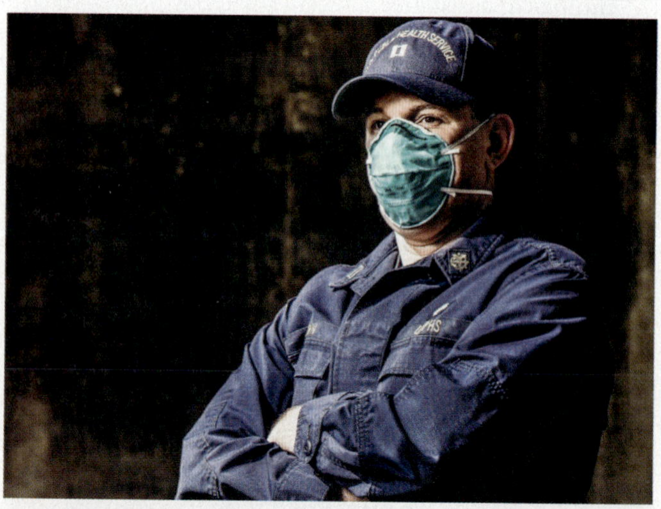

FIGURE 17-9 The Ready Reserve Corps is a group of Commissioned Corps that promote, protect, and advance the health and safety of the nation. (Reprinted from Commissioned Corps of the U.S. Public Health Service. https://www.usphs.gov/media/likbu44m/moaa2.jpg)

The American Psychological Association (APA) (2023) describes **resilience** as the process and outcome of successfully adapting to difficult or challenging life experiences, especially through mental, emotional, and behavioral flexibility and adjustment to external and internal demands.

- C/PHNs can contribute to primary prevention in the face of disaster by advocating for improving the social structure and economic conditions of the community, including housing, work, schools, childcare, and recreational areas.
- It is important for the C/PHN to advocate for the resources necessary for the community to meet both the physical and psychological challenges of a disaster by developing and participating in community disaster drills.
- One way to accomplish this is by supporting the Health in All Policies (HiAP) initiative, a collaborative approach that integrates and articulates health considerations into policymaking across sectors to improve the health of all communities and people.
- Initially outlined in the national prevention strategy and Healthy People 2020, HiAP is an approach to public policies that systematically takes into account the health implications of decisions, seeks synergies, and avoids harmful health impacts, in order to improve population health and health equity (Pan American Health Organization [PAHO], n.d.).
- Survivors of disasters often feel anxious and overwhelmed and may experience a *mental health crisis*, where their usual coping mechanisms are not effective.
- It is important for the C/PHN to be aware of the symptoms of stress-related disorders and make referrals to the available mental health professionals.

TERRORISM AND WARS

At the start of the 21st century, the world is a global community. This is particularly evident with the increased international communication and travel practices. The incidence and sophistication of terrorist threats and acts around the world highlight our vulnerability and dramatically emphasizes the need for increased preparedness within our communities for any type of biologic, chemical, or nuclear terror attacks. One only needs to turn on the news to learn of terror attacks throughout the world.

BOX 17-6 USPHS Nurse's Community Response to COVID-19 Pandemic

USPHS Nurse's Community Response to COVID-19 Pandemic

During the 2020 and 2021 COVID-19 (C-19) pandemic response, I was deployed four times across the country—each experience unique, challenging, and rewarding. In the early days of the pandemic, the world was clamoring for more knowledge about this virus and how to remain safe. I, as well as many other U.S. Public Health Service Commissioned Corps officers and healthcare professionals, worked to serve the public in a variety of capacities.

I was deployed for 23 days to the COVID-19 Community Based Testing Site in Katy, Texas, where my primary role was as the Quality Control Officer who provided oversight over the postcollection process of COVID-19 testing. I ensured the requisition form data points matched what was on the specimen tube, ensuring temperature control of the specimens prior to the shipment, counting, and packing specimens with a manifest for shipment and coordinating shipment to lab. However, I also supported training of clinical staff who were swabbers and check-in post assignees. Plus, I created an onsite Wellness Checklist due to extended hours of patient wait times in their vehicles, from Check-in to C-19 testing after a noted increase in heat-related incidences and other clinical episodes. As the Quality Control Officer, I provided 250+ specimens that were collected daily. In addition, I worked with the team lead, providing administrative support for data gathering and maintenance as well as serving as site liaison between federal components and state ensuring execution of federal guidelines.

I also served on the Centers for Medicare & Medicaid Services & Center for Disease Control Federal Task Force Strike Teams, in which I provided onsite technical assistance and education to three nursing homes in Pennsylvania experiencing outbreaks, to help reduce transmission and the risk of COVID-19 spread among residents. The Task Force Strike Teams were composed of clinicians and public health service officials from CMS, the CDC, and the Office of the Assistant Secretary for Health.

For 51 days, I was deployed at the Commissioned Corps Headquarters Command Cell as the Operations Section Chief. There I provided oversight and management of tactical operations and safety for augmentation and strike teams deployed within the fields across the United States. Oversight included the Chief Medical Officer, Chief Nurse Officer, and Chief Pharmacy Officer. In addition, I maintained close contact with the Incident Commander and Deputy Commander, subordinate Operations personnel, and other agency partners.

My last C-19 deployment was for 30 days at the Phoenix Indian Medical Center in Arizona, where I was a part of the Behavioral Health Team as a behavioral health nurse. In that capacity, I provided psychological first aid to the hospital employees, especially front-line staff. I compiled and provided resources for staff plus implemented wellness times for staff to come and talk about their experiences in which C-19 affected their families, tribal communities, and coworkers who had succumbed to the virus or were adversely affected long term.

Being deployed to different types of disaster or humanitarian responses requires knowledge and skills; however, it is equally important to be prepared. What has assisted me has been continuing education through training; completing Incident Command System courses, in order to be prepared for what to expect in a disaster situation; working collaboratively with state, federal, and nongovernmental organizations and stakeholders; and asking for assignments/tasks that I have not completed before in order to have working knowledge even if I am not an expert, which provides the opportunity to grow while deployed. Moreover, my nursing education and training has also prepared me to think critically while always using the nursing ADPIE (assessment, diagnosis, plannning, implementation, and evaluation) in many situations.

M. Baker-Bartlett, RN, CAPT USPHS

History of Terrorism

The U.S. Federal Bureau of Investigation (FBI, n.d.) categorizes terrorism in one of two ways—as international terrorism or domestic terrorism. International terrorism is committed by people or groups allied with foreign terrorist groups, whereas domestic terrorism is executed by people linked to U.S.-based extremist groups (FBI, n.d.). Generally, terrorism involves dangerous acts that are injurious to human life; it also involves a type of coercion or intimidation that affects government (U.S. Department of Justice, 2024b). Terrorism and terrorist acts are not new. The term *terrorism* can be traced to 1798, and the use of terrorist tactics precedes this date.

Bioterrorism and Nuclear and Chemical Warfare

Terrorists typically use biologic or chemical agents, explosives, or incendiary devices to deliver the agents to their targets.

A terrorist attack that involves nuclear weapons or aims at the destruction of a nuclear plant would cause multiple and prolonged deaths with extensive damage and negative effects for decades.

Bioterrorism is the intentional use of microorganisms to bring about ill effects or death to humans, livestock, or crops. The terrorist attacks on September 11, 2001 and the subsequent bioterrorist releases of anthrax led to an increased awareness of workplaces as possible terrorist targets. Chemical warfare involves the use of chemicals such as explosives, nerve agents, blister agents, choking agents, and incapacitating or riot-control agents to cause confusion, debilitation, death, and destruction (Organisation for the Prohibition of Chemical Weapons [OPCW], 2020).

Biologic warfare involves using biologic agents to cause multiple illnesses and deaths. Typical biologic agents (Table 17-2) are anthrax, botulinum, bubonic plague, Ebola, and smallpox and could be used to contaminate food, water, or air. Deliberate food and water contamination remains the easiest way to distribute biologic agents for the purpose of terrorism (Joint Counterterrorism Assessment Team, 2020).

TABLE **17-2** Categories of Biologic Agents

Category	Definition	Agents/Diseases
A	▪ Pose highest risk to national security/public health: ▪ Can be easily disseminated or transmitted from person to person ▪ Result in high mortality rates and have the potential for major public health impact ▪ Might cause public panic and social disruption ▪ Require special action for public health preparedness	▪ Anthrax (*Bacillus anthracis*) ▪ Botulism (*Clostridium botulinum* toxin) ▪ Plague (*Yersinia pestis*) ▪ Smallpox (variola major) and other pox viruses ▪ Tularemia (*Francisella tularensis*) ▪ Viral hemorrhagic fevers
B	▪ Second highest risk to national security: ▪ Are moderately easy to disseminate ▪ Result in moderate morbidity rates and low mortality rates ▪ Require specific enhancements of CDC's diagnostic capacity and enhanced disease surveillance	▪ Q fever (*Coxiella burnetii*) ▪ Brucellosis (*Brucella* species) ▪ Melioidosis (*Burkholderia pseudomallei*) ▪ Psittacosis (*Chlamydia psittaci*) ▪ Ricin toxin (*Ricinus communis*) ▪ Epsilon toxin of *Clostridium perfringens* ▪ *Staphylococcus* enterotoxin B (SEB) ▪ Typhus fever (*Rickettsia prowazekii*) ▪ Food- and waterborne pathogens
C	▪ Third highest priority agents include emerging pathogens that could be engineered for mass dissemination in the future because of: ▪ Availability ▪ Ease of production and dissemination ▪ Potential for high morbidity and mortality rates and major health impact	▪ Nipah and Hantaviruses

CDC, Centers for Disease Control and Prevention.
Reprinted from the CDC Emerging Preparedness and Response. (2018). *Bioterrorism agents/disease.* https://emergency.cdc.gov/agent/agentlist-category.asp#b

Trauma From the Warfront

Nurses, or people acting in that capacity, have provided comfort and care to soldiers long before Florence Nightingale arrived in Crimea during the mid-19th century (see Chapter 3). Nurses continued to help during the Civil War and both World Wars.

- Military nurses serving in modern-day wars provide care to those with serious injuries and multiple casualties often for extended periods of time.
- These nurses may experience disturbing long-term psychological effects when returning home including feeling disconnected from civilian lifestyles and levels of isolation.

It is critical that appropriate psychological and physical support and interventions are provided for these military nurses to facilitate their recovery, and C/PHNs should be aware of the needs of veterans and services available to them, especially during disasters and other traumatic events that may trigger memories of the traumatic past experiences. It is also important to ask patients if they have military experience during the initial assessment. This information may impact the planned interventions.

Factors Contributing to Terrorism

Political factors are the most common contributors to terrorism. Terrorist acts are committed against American military installations abroad, in airports, in airplanes, at American embassies, and even on American soil targeting civilian populations.

Within the United States, domestic terrorism involves extremist views of a social, environmental, racial, political, or religious nature (FBI, n.d.). According to the FBI (2023), a mass killing is defined as three or more deaths in one incident. In 2022, there were 13 mass killings at which 100 people were killed due to an active shooter; Robb Elementary School in Uvalde, Texas, had the highest number of fatalities (FBI and the Advanced Law Enforcement Rapid Response Training (ALERRT) Center at Texas State University, 2023; Fig. 17-10).

Role of the Community/Public Health Nurse

C/PHNs need to be prepared for the possibility of terrorist activity.

Primary Prevention

C/PHNs are in ideal situations within communities to participate in surveillance. They should stay alert by looking and listening within their communities for antigroup sentiments (e.g., antireligion, antigay, or antiethnic feelings) and appropriately report any untoward activities accordingly.

Although prevention of terrorist incidents is primarily the responsibility of the Department of Defense, the DHS, and public health and law enforcement agencies, C/PHNs must be ready to handle the secondary and tertiary effects of such attacks. Knowledge of the lethal and incapacitating chemical, biologic, and radiologic weapons potentially used by terrorists is important.

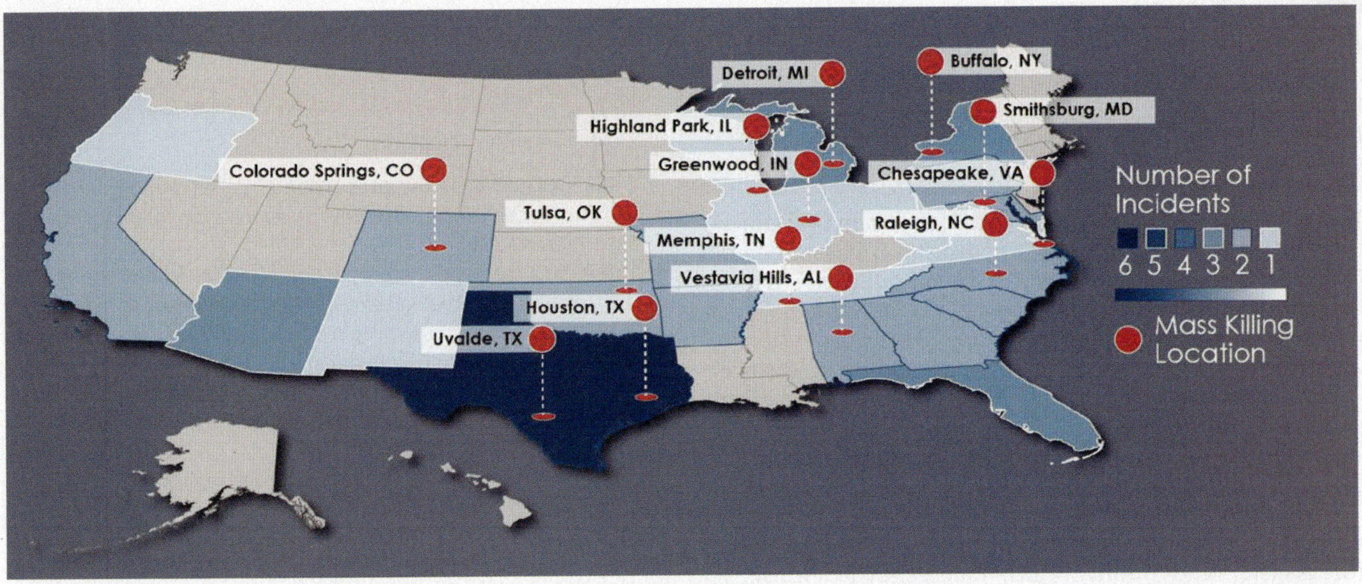

FIGURE 17-10 2022 active shooter incidents by location, including mass killings. (Reprinted from Federal Bureau of Investigation and the Advanced Law Enforcement Rapid Response Training (ALERRT) Center at Texas State University. (2023). https://www.fbi.gov/file-repository/active-shooter-incidents-in-the-us-2022-042623.pdf/view)

Realizing that terrorist attacks may result in large numbers of casualties, the C/PHN must be prepared to act quickly, safely, and competently, and to access information and effectively use resources rapidly. Formulating, updating, and following a disaster plan is one of the most effective community-based strategies to minimize injury and mortality from terrorism.

Most C/PHNs will not be on the front line of uncovering or immediately responding to terrorist activities; however, their skills will be needed with groups, families, or people who experience a terrorist-related event. C/PHNs provide direct care to survivors, help survivors with coping, or provide guidance to those who want to do something to help. After experiencing a traumatic event such as a terrorist attack, people do not know how to cope; they are warned to expect more attacks and to be vigilant. The terror C/PHNs must fight is often their own. This is a new experience for most people, and the C/PHN must have appropriate training and skills to help oneself and others cope effectively.

C/PHNs can make major differences in grassroots efforts to bring about change, on a day-to-day basis. For example, providing information on nonmedical treatment options such as support groups, hypnosis, and biofeedback is an example of how nurses can assist with coping mechanisms. Community resilience is the goal of the interventions.

Current and Future Opportunities

There are many ways in which nurses, especially nursing students, can prepare both personally and professionally for emergency events in their own communities. Various governmental and educational programs are available as free online training covering a broad range of topics. Many schools of nursing have now begun to include emergency preparedness plans in the curriculum and coordinate with local hospitals, public health departments, or faith institutions for collaborative training sessions. Nursing students should be aware of their role in the event of a local emergency, including discussing it with their faculty.

FEMA offers four particular courses within the incident command system (ICS 100, ICS 200, IS 700, and IS 800B), which are recommended for all healthcare personnel. Finally, make sure you have a family plan to reconnect with and care for children, spouses, parents, and pets.

During community exercises, nurses may be asked to participate in some community exercises as a "victim."

- Nursing students are encouraged to seek these opportunities, anticipating that the knowledge gained from the experience will improve their understanding of the response process and allow them to help identify gaps in services or areas in need of improvement.
- Volunteers may be asked to allow moulage to be applied to simulate injuries.
- The assigned health problem may be emotional or physical, allowing volunteers to demonstrate their understanding of behavioral health issues and crisis intervention.
- Just as immunizations help fight against infections, participating in an emergency preparedness drill can build competency for emergency response situations.

The American Red Cross (2024) and your local Medical Reserve Corps (Administration for Strategic Preparedness and Response, 2024) are two options to actively participate in emergency preparedness responses.

Disaster Preparedness and Public Health Emergency Response (National Academies of Sciences, Engineering, and Medicine, 2021) describes the role of nurses in disaster and public health emergencies before, during, and after disasters (https://www.ncbi.nlm.nih.gov/books/NBK573904/#top). Nurses must decide their personal level of involvement in the response effort and be aware of scopes of practice and licensure boundaries. Nurses are able to provide education, community engagement, and health promotion and implement interventions across boundaries for the greater good.

Objectives for *Healthy People 2030*

Healthy People 2030 includes four developmental objectives related to preparedness for disasters. These include (1) parents/guardians are aware of their children's school emergency and evacuation plans, (2) actions to take should a contagious disease occur, (3) adults who are aware of their transportation needs should a disaster occur and they need to evacuate, and (4) household emergency plan that includes at-risk persons (Office of Disease Prevention and Health Promotion [ODPHP], n.d.). See Box 17-7.

The Conclusions noted in Healthy People 2030 point out that the nation's nurses are not currently prepared for disaster and public health emergency response. A bold and expansive effort will be needed to fully support nurses in becoming prepared for disaster and public health emergency response. In advocating for population health, the gaps in nursing's disaster preparedness must be addressed across nursing education, practice, policy, and research.

BOX 17-7 *HEALTHY PEOPLE 2030*

Objectives Related to Disaster Preparedness

Developmental Objectives:

PREP-D01 Increase the proportion of parents and guardians who know the emergency or evacuation plan for their children's school

PREP-D02 Increase the proportion of adults who prepare for a disease outbreak after getting preparedness information

PREP-D03 Increase the proportion of adults who know how to evacuate in case of a hurricane, flood, or wildfire

PREP-D04 Increase the proportion of adults who have an emergency plan for disasters

Office of Disease Prevention and Health Promotion. (n.d.). *Emergency preparedness. Healthy People 2030.* U.S. Department of Health and Human Services. https://health.gov/healthypeople/objectives-and-data/browse-objectives/emergency preparedness

SUMMARY

- A disaster is any event that causes a level of destruction that exceeds the abilities of the affected community to respond without assistance. Disasters may be caused by natural or human-made/technologic events and may be classified as multiple-casualty incidents or mass-casualty incidents.
- In developing strategies to address the problem of disasters, it is helpful for the C/PHN to consider each of the four phases of disaster management: mitigation, preparedness, response, and recovery.
- An effective disaster plan establishes a clear chain of authority, develops lines of communication, and delineates routes and modes of transport. Plans for mobilizing, warning, and evacuating people are critical. At the disaster site, police, firefighters, nurses, and other relief workers develop a coordinated response to rescue survivors from further injury, triage survivors by the seriousness of injury, and treat survivors on-site and in local hospitals. Care and transport of the dead bodies and support for the loved ones of the injured, dead, or missing need to be included in the disaster plan as well.
- Survivors of disasters suffer physical injuries and psychological trauma that can affect them for life. The importance of prevention, early crisis intervention, and ongoing treatment for those in need is evident. The C/PHN plays a key role in assessing people for symptoms of psychological trauma and intervening to prevent long-term consequences. Self-care, including stress education for all relief workers after a disaster, helps to lower anxiety and put the situation into perspective.
- Terrorism is the unlawful use of force or violence against people or property to intimidate or coerce a government or civilian population in the furtherance of political or social objectives. Terrorism may be nuclear, biologic, or chemical and may involve the use of nerve agents and explosive devices. The C/PHN should be alert to signs of possible terrorist activity and prepared to address the secondary or tertiary effects of such attacks.
- Many opportunities are available for both student nurses and experienced C/PHNs to become involved in emergency preparedness and response efforts. Agencies such as the American Red Cross and the Medical Reserve Corps are options available to all nurses, including nursing students. *Healthy People 2030* includes recommendations to help nurses assist communities prepare for disasters and emergencies.

ACTIVE LEARNING EXERCISES

1. Choose one natural and one human-made disaster. The disasters could be from anywhere in the world. Make sure the disasters reflect something you want to learn more about. As you research, focus on the disasters' causation, number of casualties, scope, and intensity. Reflect on what you learned. Reflect on how you might use this knowledge in your future practice. Do you see yourself becoming more involved with disaster management? (Objective 1)
2. Conduct a focused community assessment on your local community and determine three factors that contribute to possible disasters. What can you do to lower the risk as a nursing student and as a resident

of the community? Which of the 10 Essential Public Health Services did you use to lower the risk of a disaster (Box 2-2)? (Objective 2)

3. The phases of disaster management are prevention, preparedness, response, and recovery. Talk with community members such as school nurses, C/PHNs, church leaders, community members, business owners, and families. Develop a community outreach to educate others about the four phases. (Objective 3)
4. Interview a C/PHN who was involved in a disaster. Topics to discuss with the C/PHN are how they prevented, prepared, responded, and supported recovery from the disaster on the community level and on a family/personal level. What changes would they recommend during a debriefing? What changes in your life and in your family's life would you make based on the discussion? (Objective 4)

CHAPTER 18

Violence and Abuse

"The constant incidents, the stories being broadcasted online and on television take a toll. The fear and trauma that is shared among everyone is real and something needs to be done, which is why I am happy that my classmates and colleagues are advocating and striving to stop this issue."

—Anonymous Older Adult Nursing Student

KEY TERMS

Abusive head trauma (AHT)
Child abuse
Child maltreatment
Compassion fatigue
Cycle of violence
Emotional abuse
Intimate partner violence (IPV)
Mandated reporters
Neglect
Older person abuse
Physical abuse
Protective factors
Risk factors
Secondary traumatic stress
Sexual abuse
Spectrum of prevention
Trauma-informed care
Vicarious trauma

LEARNING OBJECTIVES

Upon mastery of this chapter, you should be able to:

1. Apply the Social-Ecological Model to different types of violence.
2. Develop a plan of action to meet the needs of communities affected by violence.
3. Compare and contrast protective and risk factors associated with different forms of violence.
4. Advocate for community change as it relates to individual and population violence.
5. Identify the need for self-care when working with those affected by violence.

INTRODUCTION

Violence is a global public health issue. It is not limited by sociodemographic or geographic factors—anyone may experience violence or abuse at any point in one's lifetime. To learn about violence in our communities, one simply needs to turn on a television or look at the news on a smartphone. We all have our own experience, either personally or as a community, with violence. According to the FBI (2023), they investigated 2700 threats of domestic terrorism and 4000 threats of international terrorism since September 2023. Antisemitism and anti-Islamic sentiment are high, with domestic and international terrorism a constant threat (Center for Strategic and International Studies, 2024). Cybercriminals have targeted hospitals, educational institutions, and large corporations, in attempts to gain a ransom. At least 30 child pornography sites opened on the dark web within 1 month with one site gaining 200,000 new members within the first 3 weeks (FBI, 2023). Currently, there are 33,000 street gangs in the United States that include motorcycle, prison, and street gangs; these violent gangs are involved in human trafficking, drug sales, and murder (FBI, n.d.-a).

Acts of violence may occur once or multiple times. They may involve a single person conducting violence or a group. This person or persons may or may not be known to the person experiencing violence. Violence and abuse may occur in any setting—at home, in public, at work, or at school.

The World Health Organization (WHO, n.d., para. 2) defines violence as "the intentional use of physical force or power, threatened or actual, against oneself, another person, or a group or community, that either results in or has a high likelihood of resulting in injury, death, psychological harm, maldevelopment, or deprivation." Violence is a complex phenomenon affecting individuals, groups, communities, and all of society. There is no single risk factor that identifies who is more vulnerable to violence, nor is there one single intervention that prevents violence. Instead, there are a host of factors that must be addressed to identify and prevent violence. The Social-Ecological Model addresses four levels of prevention: individual, relationships, community, and societal (CDC, 2024a). Each level overlaps and must be addressed if violence is to be prevented before it occurs (CDC, 2024a).

Acts of violence can result in a crisis, which is a stressful and disruptive event (or series of events) that comes with or without warning and disturbs the equilibrium of the individual, family, community, or societal levels. A crisis can occur when usual problem-solving methods fail.

Regardless of their responses, people who are in crisis after experiencing violence need support, and C/PHNs have a unique opportunity and responsibility to provide support in a variety of situations and settings.

Primary and secondary prevention measures used by C/PHNs that help prevent crises include teaching families communication skills and coping strategies and connecting them with community resources. In addition to assessment and education, C/PHNs provide tertiary responses with direct assistance during times of crisis or in the immediate aftermath of experiencing violence. This chapter discusses the knowledge and skills C/PHNs use in their practice of violence prevention and intervention to promote improved health for individuals and communities who may be affected by senseless acts of violence.

Throughout this chapter, difficult topics are discussed that may bring up unwanted memories, feelings of anger related to abuse, assault, compassion fatigue, or secondary trauma. Those responding to a crisis or a traumatic violent act are at risk for compassion fatigue (Substance Abuse and Mental Health Service Administration [SAMHSA], 2023; Turgoose et al., 2021). **Compassion fatigue** is due to the combination of burnout and **secondary traumatic stress** (SAMHSA, 2023; Turgoose et al., 2022).

- Signs and symptoms of burnout:
  - Exhaustion, diminishment, or loss of empathy or caring
  - Thinking one is not doing enough to help
- Signs and symptoms of secondary traumatic stress:
  - Similar to posttraumatic stress disorder (PTSD) but the individual did not experience the event
  - Occurs from indirect exposure to the traumatic event
  - Feeling on edge all the time and avoiding similar areas or events
- Signs and symptoms of compassion fatigue:
  - Feeling overwhelmed, extreme exhaustion, confused, irritable, or frustrated
  - Shortness of breath, headaches, heart palpations, and insomnia

Healthcare providers that work in the field of violence need to be aware of **vicarious trauma**, which causes a shift in a person's worldview to positive, neutral, or negative (e.g., cynical or fearful) in response to working with trauma, people who have experienced trauma, and trauma services (Office of Victim Crime, n.d.).

DYNAMICS AND CHARACTERISTICS OF A CRISIS

Crises may be precipitated by a specific identifiable event that becomes too much for the problem-solving skills of those involved, may result from sudden unexpected or traumatic events, or may be related to a person's perception of an event.

When a community crisis occurs on a large scale or is so unexpected that it also involves people who are hundreds of miles away, it can affect distant friends and relatives. Examples include a fatal stabbing of a 15-year-old in a high school classroom; an arson at an apartment building that killed 12 people and injured dozens of others; 11 people being killed during a Lunar New Year celebration; the mass shooting at the Route 91 Harvest Music Festival in Las Vegas on October 1, 2017; and the terrorist attacks in New York City on September 11, 2001, which indirectly affected people hundreds of miles away. Medical centers are not immune to gun violence as evident in recent events that occurred in hospitals in cities in Oklahoma, Oregon, Georgia, and Texas (Boone, 2023). The list of community crisis events could fill a textbook, each one as important as the next to those who were present and to those who lost loved ones. Regrettably, by the time this textbook is published, new acts of violence will have occurred across the globe, replacing the examples above.

- A traumatic event or crisis is a stressful, unexpected, disruptive event arising from external circumstances that occur suddenly to a person, group, aggregate, or community. While some people can adjust to a crisis over time, for some, the external event requires behavioral changes and coping mechanisms beyond the abilities of the people involved (National Institute of Mental Health, 2024).
- The crisis occurs to people because of where they are in time and space. These events, which involve loss or the threat of loss, represent life hazards to those affected.
- C/PHNs may assist in various traumatic crises, including those arising from acts of violence. In each situation, people feel overwhelmed and need help to cope. Skilled intervention can make the difference between a healthy and an unhealthy response to the crisis.

OVERVIEW OF VIOLENCE ACROSS THE LIFE CYCLE

Violence affects people across the life cycle. It may involve chronic or long-term acts of abuse, neglect, maltreatment, or situational acts of violence that may be unexpected and sudden. C/PHNs encounter many different types of violence, including child abuse and neglect, youth violence, gang violence, bullying, intimate partner violence (IPV), dating violence, sexual violence, and abuse and maltreatment of older adults. Multiple types of violence can occur within a single household, community, or neighborhood, affecting people at different stages in life.

There is no single factor that can explain a specific act of violence. However, decades of research reveal that different types of violence are interconnected. For example:

- People who experience one form of violence are likely to experience other forms of violence.
- People who use violence in one context are likely to use violence in another context.
- Different types of violence share common short- and long-term biopsychosocial health effects that may contribute to chronic health conditions such as cancer, cardiovascular disease, lung disease, and diabetes.
- Different types of violence have shared risk factors and protective factors (CDC, 2024b).

Violence is a complex phenomenon. Understanding the neurobiologic effects, potential subsequent health effects, and overlapping causes of violence can help community health nurses enhance protective factors and reduce risk factors and can help inform violence intervention and prevention activities.

Neurobiology of Trauma

Over the past few decades, neuroscience research has clarified the neurobiologic response to trauma. Research on the effect of trauma on the brain is advancing. This body of research has provided professionals responding to acts of violence with a better understanding of human behavior and how people respond to trauma, has contributed to trauma-informed practices, and has enhanced the capacity of multidisciplinary responders to serve people who have experienced violence.

An expanded definition of trauma includes all the events and experiences that are subjectively traumatic to an individual, which are different from person to person. Just as the brain is complex, so are a person's potential reactions and behaviors in response to an experience. This complexity is further compounded by many potential extraneous factors, such as substance use, past trauma, underlying pathologies, and established neural patterns. Although there are common responses, there are no absolute responses for all people; this is a fundamental concept behind trauma-informed care. **Trauma-informed care** aids in accessing care, ensures treatment engagement, and provides a sense of safety to people that experienced trauma (Burns et al., 2023). Healthcare providers need to be culturally sensitive to those from underrepresented groups that experience health disparities and those who experience multiple traumas as a community, family, or individually (Burns et al., 2023). Nursing provides care to others in their most vulnerable state, many times related to trauma. Understanding and practicing trauma-informed care allows nurses to meet the needs of the client.

Protective Factors and Risk Factors

Many factors contribute to increasing or decreasing the occurrence of violence. **Risk factors** are factors known to increase the likelihood of experiencing violence. **Protective factors** are factors known to reduce the likelihood of experiencing violence or increase one's resilience when violence is experienced. Individual lived experiences and a person's own characteristics may also be risk factors or protective factors. For example, growing up in a high crime area and witnessing violence is a risk factor, whereas having communication and problem-solving skills that allow one to address conflict without using violence is a protective factor. The Social-Ecological Model addresses the interplay between the individual, relationships, community, and societal risk and protective factors (CDC, 2024b; Fig. 18-1). Preventive measures are discussed later in this chapter.

- *Societal level* includes the cultural norms of violence as either acceptable or discouraged; conflict resolution methods; equity of income, health, and education; and social policies and laws.
- *Community level* includes the backdrop of social relations that take place and seeks to address the characteristics of the setting that foster people to conduct violence.
- *Relationship level* encompasses our closest friends, family members, and partners who are instrumental in increasing or decreasing violence as a person conducting violence or as a person experiencing violence.
- *Individual level* addresses personal history such as income, education, history of substance misuse, and biologic components such as age (CDC, 2024a).

Community windshield surveys and other community-based learning opportunities often reveal community-level

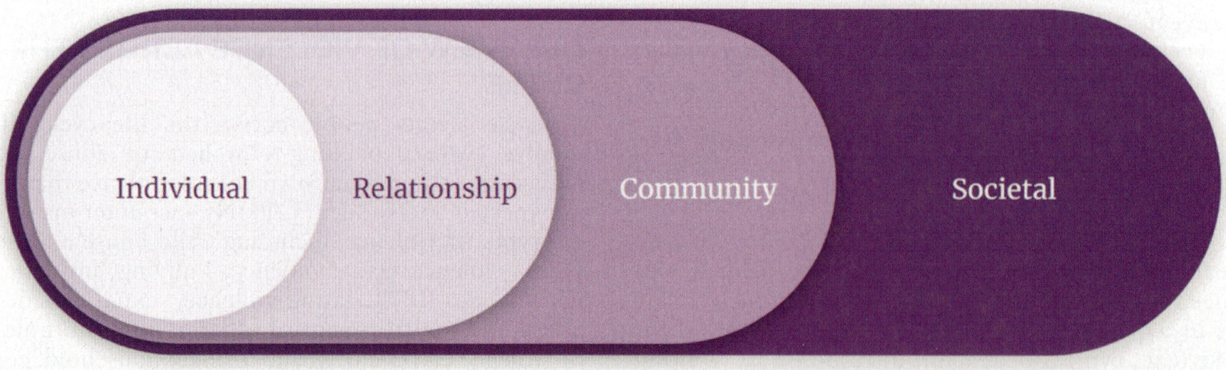

FIGURE 18-1 The Social-Ecological Model: a framework for prevention. (Reprinted from Centers for Disease Control and Prevention. (2024a). *About violence prevention.* https://www.cdc.gov/violence-prevention/about/?CDC_AAref_Val=https://www.cdc.gov/violenceprevention/about/social-ecologicalmodel.html)

risk factors and protective factors. For example, the level of safety described by residents can greatly vary from one neighborhood to the next. There are neighborhoods in all cities where residents describe feeling unsafe and witnessing crimes. In these communities, residents experience an overwhelming number of community risk factors compared with protective factors. In the 2014 landmark publication *Connecting the Dots*, the CDC (2024b) reveals the following:

- In neighborhoods where residents do not support or trust each other, residents are more likely to experience child maltreatment, IPV, and youth violence.
- People who are socially isolated and do not have supportive relationships with family, friends, or neighbors are at greater risk for using violence, including acts of child maltreatment, IPV, and abuse of older adults.
- A lack of economic and employment opportunities is associated with an increased risk for using violence, including acts of child maltreatment, IPV, self-directed violence (SDV), sexual violence, and youth violence.
- Communities in which societal norms support aggressive or coercive behaviors have an increased risk for violent acts such as physical assault of children, IPV, sexual violence, youth violence, and elder maltreatment.
- Witnessing community violence increases one's vulnerability to being bullied and the risk of using sexual violence against others.

To counteract community risk factors, residents need support to enhance their protective factors. For example, communities having coordinated resources and services among the different community agencies experience greater protective factors. Access to mental health and substance misuse services increases protective factors. Receiving community support and having connections within the community and with the family, prosocial peers, and school can also increase community protective factors and decrease individual vulnerability. What are some of the protective factors in your community?

HISTORY OF VIOLENCE AGAINST WOMEN AND CHILDREN

Violence against women and children is not new. For centuries, children were considered the property of their parents, and most countries had animal welfare laws long before child welfare laws were adopted.

- The first documented case of child abuse occurred in 1874, involving Mary Ellen Wilson. However, due to the lack of child abuse laws of the period, her case was filed under the Animal Welfare Agency.
- This 9-year-old was so badly beaten and neglected by her foster mother that the public was shocked during the trial in the New York Supreme Court. This case changed public opinion on society's role in the protection of children (Smithfield, 2016).
- In the early 1900s, leaders concerned with child welfare issues promoted the development of international agencies focused on factors affecting the health of children.
- In 1924, the League of Nations adopted the Declaration of the Rights of the Child, which later informed the United Nation's Declaration of the Rights of the Child in 1959 and the Convention on the Rights of the Child in 1989. This committee meets three times yearly to address global concerns related to children's rights, including violence against children (Office of the United Nations High Commissioner for Human Rights, 2020).

Historically, women were also treated as property and often experienced gender-based violence resulting in biopsychosocial injuries.

- Recent global prevalence figures indicate that 736 million women age 15 and older, or about 30% of this population worldwide, have experienced IPV or nonpartner physical or sexual violence, or both, in their lifetime (UNWomen, 2023).
- Research reveals that 640 million women are abused by intimate partners (UNWomen, 2023).
- During the COVID-19 pandemic, there was an increase in violence against women (WHO, 2022a).
    - The COVID-19 pandemic forced families to stay indoors and limited contact with the outside world. Furthermore, the pandemic caused women's resources to shut their doors, thus limiting help for women (WHO, 2022a).
    - A province in China saw a threefold increase in February 2020 when compared to the same period of the previous year (WHO, 2022a).
- The first global and regional estimates of violence against women were published in 2013, resulting in clinical and policy guidelines that have been widely disseminated. Working with many organizations, including the health sector, the WHO's goal is to end violence against women and children (Fig. 18-2) (WHO, 2022a).

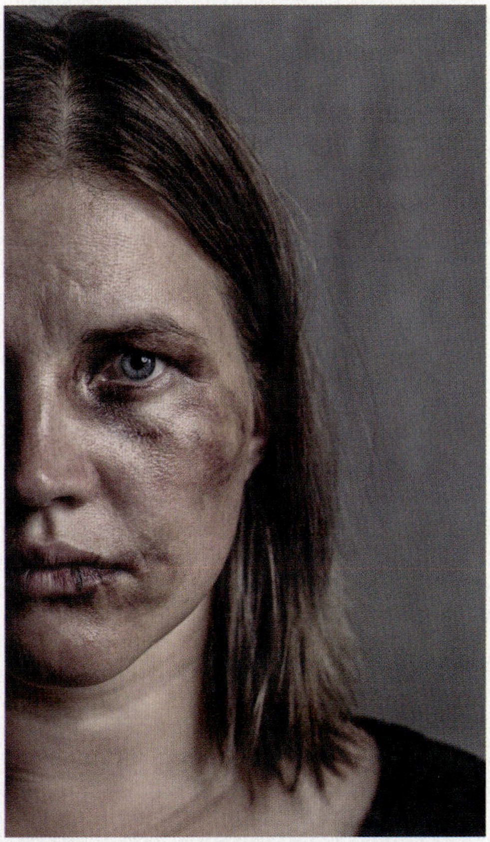

FIGURE 18-2 A person with bruises on their face as the result of abuse.

TABLE **18-1** Common Myths and Truths About Abuse in Families

Myth	Truth
Domestic abuse is only physical	Abuse can take all forms: physical, sexual, stalking, and psychological aggression.
Men are the only people conducting abuse	Domestic violence has no gender boundaries on the person conducting the abuse or the person being abused.
Domestic violence occurs most frequently among families with limited resources and education	Violence occurs across all incomes, educational levels, and across all racial, ethnic, and cultural groups.
The situation must be bearable if the person experiencing violence doesn't leave	People experiencing violence stay because of fear of the person conducting abuse, fear of deportation, lack of money, or concern for children, not because they are okay with the abuse.
People conducting the abuse cannot control their anger	Anger does not cause abuse. Abuse is a means to gain control.

Source: Arizona Law (n.d.); Paisner (2018).

Public Laws and Protection in the United States

In the 1960s, the Children's Bureau began to focus on child abuse and supported the development of a mandatory child abuse reporting law that could be used as a model for state laws. The law required health professionals and childcare workers to report suspected child abuse to appropriate officials. Since that period, laws have been refined and developed to protect children against abuse. The Administration on Aging supports similar programs including the National Center on Elder Abuse (n.d.-a) that works to educate and assist families, older adults, healthcare, and legal providers regarding the abuse of older adults.

Myths and Truths About Violence and Abuse

Many myths about violence and abuse need to be dispelled. Strongly held myths by members of society, including C/PHNs and other healthcare providers, may interfere with their ability to help people in crisis get the help they need. Table 18-1 displays some common myths and truths about violence and abuse.

VIOLENCE AGAINST CHILDREN

- **Child abuse** is defined by the federal CAPTA (42 USCA, 5106g) as "any recent act or failure to act on the part of a parent or caretaker which results in death, serious physical or emotional harm, sexual abuse or exploitation; or an act or failure to act which presents an imminent risk of serious harm" (USDHHS, 2023, para. 2).
- **Child maltreatment** is defined as abuse and neglect toward a child under age 18 including "physical and emotional ill-treatment, sexual abuse, neglect, negligence and commercial or other exploitation, which results in actual or potential harm to the child's health, survival, development or dignity in the context of a relationship of responsibility, trust or power" (WHO, 2022b, para. 2).

Identifying and gathering worldwide data about child abuse is difficult because many cases are not investigated, death reports may not be classified as a result of abuse or homicide, and definitions of maltreatment may vary. Despite, this, the following global statistics reveal a concerning reality:

- In 2021, Child Protective Services (CPS) investigated or had an alternative response for slightly over 2 million reports of child maltreatment, whereas 1.6 million reports were not investigated by CPS for a variety of reasons (U.S. Department of Health & Human Services, Administration for Children and Families, Administration on Children, Youth and Families, Children's Bureau, 2023). This number jumps to 3 million if a child experienced more than one instance of abuse and each report was counted as a separate offense.
- The younger the child, the higher rate of abuse.
- The highest level of abuse was neglect, followed by physical abuse, sexual abuse, and sex trafficking.
- Other maltreatment may include parental substance use disorder, lack of supervision, and threats of abuse or neglect.
- The highest percentage of people conducting abuse were parents.
- Across the United States, 1753 children died from abuse (USDHHS, 2023).

Nationally, measures have been taken to improve data gathering and information about violence toward children and outcomes for them. One of the largest investigations ever conducted to assess associations between childhood maltreatment and adult health and well-being is the Adverse Childhood Experiences Study. The seminal 1998 study conducted by Felitti et al. (1998) has led to new research on the long-term consequences of maltreatment in children.

Neglect

Neglect occurs when the physical, emotional, medical, or educational resources necessary for healthy growth and development are withheld or unavailable. Neglect is the highest form of maltreatment in children (Box 18-1).

C/PHNs need to assess if the neglect is due to a lack of knowledge of child development, lack of finances, or lack of healthcare. Providing services such as Women Infants and Children, education developed for health literacy level, and assisting parents to enroll children in a Child Health Insurance Program may provide the needed support for many families with children. Because of the invisibility of neglect, its prevalence is hard to estimate. Often, cases of neglect are brought to the attention of the proper authority only during the investigation of other forms of abuse or family issues. School nurses may be the first to suspect medical neglect when a parent does not provide the needed medication such as insulin after multiple attempts to contact and help the parent.

BOX 18-1 Signs and Symptoms of Neglect and Emotional Abuse

Signs and Symptoms of Neglect

Neglect may be suspected if one or more of the following conditions exist:

- Lacks adequate medical (including immunizations), vision, or dental care.
- Often sleepy or hungry.
- Consistently dirty, demonstrates poor personal hygiene, or is inadequately dressed for weather conditions.
- There is evidence of poor or inadequate supervision for the child's age.
- The conditions in the home are unsafe or unsanitary.
- Malnourished, failure to thrive, poor weight gain.
- Substance misuse.
- Parents may refuse to buy eyeglasses for a child who needs them or to access dental care for severely decayed teeth (medical neglect).
- An 8-year-old may get to school only 3 days a week, possibly without breakfast and no lunch money or packed lunch (educational neglect).
- A family with three children may live in a sparsely furnished apartment with very little food available and only intermittent heat and multiple people coming and going in the residence, while the children may appear at school unwashed and without coats in winter weather (general neglect).
- Emotional neglect may be seen when demands placed on a child are excessive or inappropriate for their development, or the caregiver berates or verbally humiliates a child frequently and without reason.

Signs and Symptoms of Emotional Abuse

Emotional abuse may be suspected if the child displays the following behavioral indicators:

- Shows extremes in behavior such as extremely demanding, passive, or compliant.
- Inappropriately takes on parent role or infantile in behavior.
- Physical or emotional development is delayed.
- Depression or suicidal thoughts.
- Unable to develop emotional bonds with others.

Source: Stanford Medicine (n.d.).

Physical Abuse

Physical abuse is intentional harm to a child by another person that results in pain, physical injury, or death. The abuse may include striking, biting, poking, burning, shaking, or throwing the child (Box 18-2). Some parents cannot control the degree of physical punishment they give their child (Child Welfare Information Gateway, 2022). A parent or caregiver may claim the injuries are the fault of the child, such as a 2-week-old rolling off the bed and hitting their head. C/PHNs need to know the stages of developmental growth to understand if a child can perform such a skill.

Sexual Abuse

- Sexual abuse of children includes acts of sexual assault or sexual exploitation of a minor and may consist of a single incident or many acts over a long period. Child sexual abuse (CSA) can be physical contact or nonphysical activities.
- CSA physical abuse includes intercourse, attempted intercourse, masturbation, oral-genital contact, and fondling (Lo Iacono et al., 2021).
- Noncontact abuse entails exposing children to pornography, prostitution, and sex trafficking (Lo Iacono et al., 2021).
- **Sexual abuse** is considered "The employment, use, persuasion, inducement, enticement, or coercion of any child to engage in, or assist any other person to engage in, any sexually explicit conduct or simulation of such conduct for the purpose of producing a visual depiction of such conduct" (Legal Information Institute, n.d., para. 1).
- Incest is sexual abuse among family members who are related by blood (e.g., parents, grandparents, older sibling). Intrafamilial sexual abuse refers to sexual activity involving family members who are not related by blood (e.g., stepparents, partner of a parent).
- Indicators of sexual abuse are expressed in various ways, and attention should be given to a history of sexual abuse, sexual behavior indicators, behavioral indicators in younger children and behavioral indicators of sexual abuse in older children and adolescents, and physical symptoms of sexual abuse (Box 18-3).
- As **mandated reporters**, C/PHNs should be aware that sexual abuse of a child may surface through a broad range of physical, behavioral, and social symptoms. Some of these indicators, taken separately, may not be symptomatic of sexual abuse and should be examined in the context of other behaviors or situational factors (Box 18-4).

Care for children who have been sexually abused varies, as the duration of the molestation, the age, and the symptoms of the child will influence their care measures. Long-term consequences of CSA have been well documented. Parents/guardians of such children may also need counseling and support following the investigation and proceedings.

Commercial Sexual Exploitation

- Commercial sexual exploitation of children (CSEC) is "a range of crimes and activities involving the sexual abuse or exploitation of a child for the financial benefit of any person or in exchange for anything of value (including monetary and nonmonetary benefits) given or received by any persons" (Office of Juvenile Justice and Delinquency Prevention [OJJDP], n.d., para. 1).
- Nonmonetary items may include food, shelter, clothing, drugs, transportation, or protection from another person.
- Forms of CSEC include child sex trafficking (prostitution of children), child sex tourism, production of child pornography, and transmission of live video of a child engaged in sexual acts in exchange for something of value.
- Internet-based marriage brokering, early-age marriages, and performing in sex-related venues are also forms of CSEC (OJJDP, n.d.).

BOX 18-2 Signs and Symptoms of Physical Abuse

Important Questions for the Nurse to Ask Themselves

- Does the child have frequent emergency department visits?
- Does the caregiver blame the child for the child's injuries?
- Was there a delay in seeking health/medical care or care, or does the child change providers frequently?
- Does the explanation of the injuries change, or does it not match the child's developmental ability, or does it contradict the injuries?

Signs of Physical Abuse

The most common systems affected are the integumentary, skeletal, and central nervous system signs of abuse may include:

- Unexplained injuries, explanation does not match the injury, or injuries are inconsistent with medical diagnosis such as.
- Injuries may include bruises, bite marks, abrasions, lacerations, head injuries, internal injuries, and fractures.
- Bruising from defensive injuries to forearms.
- Burns from cigarettes, ropes, or immersion into hot water or hot grid.
- Traumatic alopecia with possible hematoma area and is tender to touch.
- Trauma to ear.
- Appears depressed, withdrawn, anxious, or aggressive.
- Appears scared of parent and does not want to go home.

Healthcare providers including C/PHNs must consider language and cultural differences when interviewing a child and parent. Interviewing with a translator is important with these cases.

Behavioral Indicators of Physical Abuse

These behaviors are often exhibited by physically abused children:

- Attempts to hide injuries; child wears excessive layers of clothing, especially in hot weather.
- Frequently absent from school or misses physical education classes.
- Fearful, clingy, anxious, withdrawn, hypervigilant, or aggressive.
- The child is apprehensive when other children cry.
- Wary of physical contact with adults.
- Exhibits drastic behavioral changes in and out of parental/caregiver presence.
- The child suffers from seizures or vomiting.
- Exhibits depression, self-mutilation, suicide attempts, substance misuse, or sleeping and eating disorders.
- Fearful of going home.

Other indicators of physical abuse may include the following:

- A statement by the child that the injury was caused by abuse (chronically abused children may deny abuse).
- Knowledge that the child's injury is unusual for the child's specific age group (e.g., any fracture in an infant).
- Knowledge of the child's history of previous or recurrent injuries.
- Parent or caregiver shows little concern for the child or seeking or fails to seek medical care for the child's injury.

Source: Stanford Medicine (n.d.).

BOX 18-3 Indicators of Sexual Abuse

Physical Signs

- Sexually transmitted infections
- Trauma to the perineal area including bleeding, bruising, or pain; blood may be seen on sheets or undergarments
- Discharge from genitals or anus
- Pain during bowel movements or urination

Behavioral Signs

- Enuresis and fecal soiling in bed when behavior has been outgrown
- Inappropriate sexual behavior for age
- Not wanting to be left alone with certain people or fearful to leave parent or caregiver
- Refuses to remove clothing
- Has money, gifts, or toys unexpectedly
- Self-injury/suicide attempts
- Sexual promiscuity in teens
- Substance use

Emotional Signs

- Nightmares or fear of being left alone at night
- Extreme worry or fear
- Sexually explicit language or explicit knowledge about sexual topics beyond age of child
- Mood changes

Nursing students are encouraged to research the topic to learn more.

Source: RAINN (2023); Stop It Now! (2022).

Emotional or Psychological Abuse

- **Emotional abuse** of children involves psychological mistreatment or neglect, which impairs a child's self-worth and sense of security and being loved. Types of emotional abuse include humiliating, threatening, using sarcasm, ignoring needs, not showing love, or exposure to domestic violence (Child Welfare Information Gateway, 2022; NSPCC, n.d.).
- Emotional abuse is not defined or listed as a mandatory reporting law in all states. As a C/PHN, it is imperative to know state laws and definitions regarding all forms of child abuse (Child Welfare Information Gateway, 2022).

Specific Abusive Situations

The previous information addressed the major types of child abuse in families, yet other patterns of abuse against children need to be discussed. Abusive head trauma (AHT), factitious syndrome imposed on another (FDIA) (also known as Munchausen syndrome by proxy), and parental filicide are uncommon, but by the time the symptoms are recognized, it is often too late. Technology-facilitated crimes against children are an increasingly common fear of parents. Another area of growing concern for parents and communities is school violence (National Center of Education Statistics School Crime, 2023).

BOX 18-4 PERSPECTIVES

A School Nurse's Viewpoint on Child Sexual Abuse—Sandy's Secret

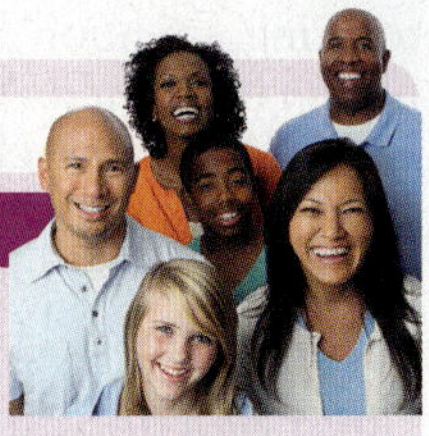

I am a school nurse at public elementary school in a metropolitan area. The majority of students do not speak English and come from families with incomes below the poverty level. I have a busy school nurse's office, but I try to be observant to subtle cues. Sadly, sometimes it's so busy that I worry I miss things. Sandy, a third grader, came to my office with stomachaches and vague complaints off and on for several months. Thinking back, this usually happened at the start of third period. When school is out, Sandy was to go to the after-school program on campus. The third-period teacher and a parent volunteer ran the after-school program. Each were well loved by staff and students. Sandy was a petite child, well behaved, very quiet, and usually only responded with a few words when I asked about her ailments.

One day, Sandy came in with another stomachache and wanted to lie down. When I asked what was going on, she shrugged her shoulders and didn't really respond. When the final bell rang, I told her if she didn't feel well enough to go to the after-school program, I could call her mother.

I had a feeling something was wrong. I remembered from a recent workshop on CSA that sometimes the hardest thing was to break through the guilt and shame for the child to open up. I told Sandy she could tell me anything, and I wouldn't think she was bad. She began talking. Well, it was more like "verbal vomiting"—the words just came spilling out. She told me the parent volunteer was "touching her" and showing her "bad" pictures and she "didn't want to go back there." She began crying as she told me the parent told her no one would believe her because her English "wasn't good enough." I told her we would call her mom and someone to talk with her about what happened. I also sent someone to get her second-grade teacher, a person she felt comfortable and safe with, who stayed with Sandy through the lengthy process.

Later, as I thought about the constant stream of children coming into my office every day, I wondered how many of those kids with subtle, vague complaints might have something going on that is as serious as Sandy's secret. Now I try to be even more vigilant and open to their concerns—whatever they may be.

—Jaime, school nurse

Abusive Head Trauma

- **Abusive head trauma (AHT)**, sometimes called shaken baby syndrome, is the intentional action of violently shaking a child, usually 2 years of age or younger; children 1 year of age and younger are at the greatest risk. AHT is the leading cause of death related to physical child abuse (CDC, 2024c).
- Injuries related to violent shaking of the body causing the brain to hit against the skull, blunt impact, or a combination of both may result in neurologic injury to the child. These types of injuries do not occur through play, as in minor falls or as a result of being tossed into the air (Fig. 18-3).

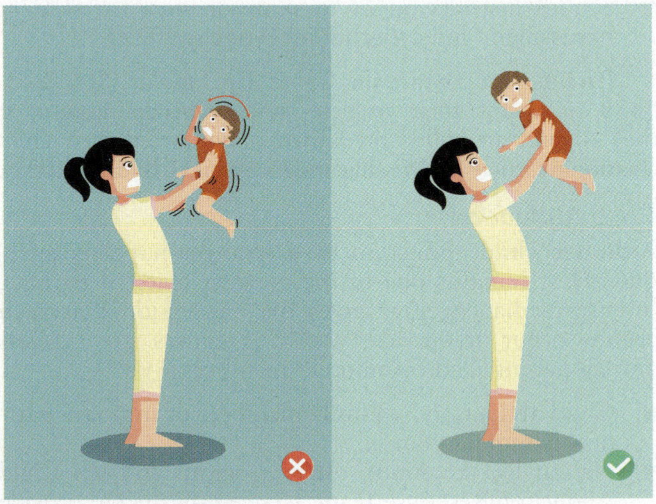

FIGURE 18-3 Never shake a baby. There are right and wrong ways to play with a baby.

- Symptoms of AHT may include bilateral retinal hemorrhage, subdural or subarachnoid hematomas, the absence of other external signs of abuse, breathing difficulties, seizures, dilated pupils, lethargy, and unconsciousness (American Association of Neurological Surgeons [AANS], 2023).

The National Center on Shaken Baby Syndrome at https://www.dontshake.org offers resources for parents and healthcare providers. Explanations for injuries are often vague such as stating the baby was "fine" and then suddenly went into respiratory arrest or began having seizures—both common symptoms of AHT—or they may attribute the injuries to falling out the crib or off of the sofa when the child is not developmentally able to roll or climb out of the crib (CDC, 2024c).

- In the United States, AHT is the leading cause of death in children under 5 years of age (CDC, 2024c).
- The caregiver becomes frustrated and violently shakes the child.
- AHT has a mortality rate of 10% to 30%.
- Risk factors include persistent, inconsolable crying and children under 1 year of age (CDC, 2024c; Yoon et al., 2022).

Children who survive AHT may require lifelong care. Children may develop learning, physical, visual, and speech disabilities; hearing impairment; cerebral palsy; cognitive impairment; and seizures (Yoon et al., 2022). Considering the person who causes the AHT is most often a parent or caregiver, C/PHNs can play a critical role in caregiver education and preventative mental health referrals.

Factitious Disorder Imposed on Another

FDIA, also known as Munchausen syndrome by proxy, is a mental illness in which the parent or caregiver attempts to bring attention to themselves by injuring or inducing illness in their child. About 85% to 98% of people who engage in FDIA are the child's birthing parent, who often forms close bonds with healthcare providers. Many of those who engage in FDIA have a mental health illness or were abused as a child (Abdurrachid & Gama Marques, 2022).

Child Murder by Parent

Filicide is a rare yet concerning type of child death, defined as child murder by a parent. Infanticide is defined as the murder of a child during the first year of life, whereas *neonaticide* is the murder of an infant within the first 24 hours of life.

- Measures for prevention and support to parents include parenting classes, emotional support, providing emergency numbers for support, as well as treating maternal substance misuse and postpartum depression.
- Safe haven laws are in place to prevent infant abandonment, leading to potential injury or death, by denoting safe places to relinquish a newborn infant, such as a fire or police station (Child Welfare Information Gateway, 2021).

Internet Crimes Against Children

Internet and technology-facilitated crimes are insidious because they come right into the home. Children may unintentionally or intentionally access a chat room or website developed or used by people who conduct abuse.

- The person who conducts abuse establishes contact, usually pretending to be a teenager or young man who has similar interests and is affectionate and understanding about the youth's "problems."
- After gaining the child's trust, the person who conducts abuse may engage in sexually explicit dialogue with the minor.
- If the minor meets the person who conducts abuse, the minor is at great risk for harm.

Technology-enabled child abuse has led to the U.S. Attorney General authorizing a national awareness and justice program focusing solely on technology-facilitated sexual exploitation and abuse against children, named *Project Safe Childhood* (USDOJ, n.d.-e) and the creation of Internet Crimes Against Children (ICAC) task forces. ICAC task forces assist federal, state, and local law enforcement agencies by enhancing their ability to investigate technology-facilitated crimes against children.

In one recent example of ICAC's work, 25 adults from several states were arrested for sexual exploitation of 19 children who were sexually abused, documented with videos sent over the internet (Saavedia, 2023). C/PHNs can assist families to prevent technology-facilitated crimes by the following:

- Encouraging parents to openly discuss with their children the dangers of online friendships that seek face-to-face meetings; downloading photos or uploading/posting photos to people they do not know; giving identifiable information about themselves (name, phone number, school they attend, home address); responding to e-mails or social media messages that are suggestive or harassing; and being aware of phishing and other forms of attempted identity theft.
- Establishing parent–child contracts for devices that can connect to web-based applications (e.g., computer, tablet, smartphone, gaming systems).
- Blocking or only permitting specific phone numbers for smartphone and web-based application calls and regularly checking for deleted phone calls and texts.
- Monitoring the amount of time that a child uses internet accessible devices and reviewing user history for applications used and websites visited.
- Placing computer and gaming consoles in a high-traffic area in the home, affording easy observation of usage by the child.
- Using available parental controls or blocking software on all devices with internet connectivity.
- Installing a firewall, antivirus, and malware/spyware programs that increase privacy and restrict usage.
- Discouraging downloading of apps, games, and other media that might contain hidden applications or programs that enable remote access by unauthorized users.
- Having access to their child's e-mail and other web-based accounts and randomly checking e-mails and text messages. Being aware of safeguards in place at their child's school, public areas the child frequents, and homes of their friends (Federal Bureau of Investigation [FBI], n.d.-b).

Cyberbullying and Cyberstalking

There is a constant stream of news around cyberbullying and cyberstalking incidents. Cyberstalking is "the use of electronic communication to harass or threaten someone with physical harm" (Merriam-Webster, 2020, para. 1). Nationwide, nearly half of all high school students have been cyberbullied with name calling and the spread of false rumors as the top two infractions. While a majority of high school students do not believe government officials or social media platforms are doing enough to stop it, they do think parents are actively involved in helping end internet bullying (Vogels, 2022). Teens also report that they think cyberbullies should be criminally charged.

- Cyberbullies should be banned from social media sites.
- Social media companies need to actively troll for cyberbullying.
- School districts ought to monitor sites for student harassment and cyberbullies (Vogels, 2022).

Parents can contact the Cyber Tip Line at (800) 843-5678 or access their website (www.cybertipline.com) if they suspect an online predator has contacted their child (National Center for Missing and Exploited Children, 2023).

Child Abduction

Although child abduction by a stranger happens infrequently, it remains one of the greatest fears of parents. Intense media coverage gives the impression that such crimes occur frequently, and this causes great stress among parents and community members.

- Child abduction by family members or intimate partners is more common.
- Nationally, the Amber Alert program and the Child Abduction Response Teams were established to provide an informed, prompt, and professional response to child abduction. Amber Alerts are sent through the radio,

television, road signs, and the Wireless Emergency Alerts system, which reaches millions of cellphone users.

- The goal of the Amber Alert is to provide instant collaboration and partnership in the community to assist in the search and safe recovery of the child and, as of January 2023, a total of 1127 children have been rescued (USDOJ, n.d.-a).

Prevention of child abduction is difficult, and at times, parents who think they have taught their children well may have a false sense of security. Kidpower (2021) recommends rephrasing the term "Stranger Danger" to "Stranger Safety" as most strangers are safe.

C/PHNs can help parents improve their child's safety by promoting close supervision of young children and practicing behaviors to promote anonymity, such as the following:

- Placing the child in the seat of a shopping cart and holding their hand when in malls or stores
- Keeping a young child in sight always when playing outside
- Sharing parental supervision with another parent when children play
- Not putting the child's name or initials in visible places on clothing or backpacks
- Teaching the child a "password," which only the parents and child know, to use when a different person is picking them up from an activity
- Teaching children to recognize when they feel unsafe and to go get help
- Involving children in making safety plans and having them practice getting help
- Helping children understand when it is okay to give personal information (e.g., at school, medical office, lost in a store) and when it is not (e.g., to a stranger they don't know)
- Practicing "think first" and "keep walking" activities with their children (Kidpower, 2021)

Older children and teens who go outside the home unattended by parents should be encouraged to use the following behaviors that promote safety: staying with groups of other children or teens, having a cellphone, leaving an itinerary with the parents, and not changing their plans without contacting parents.

Crimes Against Children by Babysitters

Abuse by caregivers is a fear of parents who work and leave their children with others. The C/PHN can help parents assess childcare settings by providing them descriptors for finding good childcare providers. The C/PHN ought to instruct parents to do the following:

- Obtain references and drop by the home or childcare setting at various times during the day.
- Assess their infants and follow-up on any bruises, rashes, burns, conditions, or behaviors they observe that are not normal for their child.
- Listen to their children and ask about their day and activities.
- Pay attention to signs, such as a child's fear of going to the babysitter or reports of spankings, being shouted at, or other inappropriate treatment.

Childcare centers and many home childcare programs are licensed by the state. When parent complaints have been filed with licensing agencies, those programs are monitored more closely, and the state is mandated to make changes or close the facility if necessary. Parents need to know that their child is safe and cared for when they leave them to pursue their employment or educational activities.

School Violence

Violence in the school setting is an area of growing concern for parents and communities. Violence in schools may range from bullying, slapping, or punching to weapon use (CDC, 2024d). Random shootings and hostage situations in schools over the past decades have fueled fears about the safety of students and promoted research on how to prevent this type of community violence from affecting children.

- Between 1999 and November 2023, there have been 389 school shootings.
- The majority of mass school shootings are committed by White students.
- Hispanic students are twice as likely to experience or witness school shootings.
- Black students are three times as likely to experience and witness school shootings.
- In 86% of the cases, the shooter used weapons from the homes of family, friends, or relatives.
- School violence dropped with the school closures due to the COVID-19 pandemic, but they have increased at a higher rate than in previous years once schools reopened (Cox et al., 2024).

Shootings have occurred at large universities, small community colleges, high schools, and elementary schools. They have taken place throughout the country, and no segment of the population is immune.

Bullying is defined as "any unwanted aggressive behavior(s) by another youth or group of youths, who are not siblings or current dating partners, involving an observed or perceived power imbalance and is repeated multiple times or is highly likely to be repeated" (APA, 2022a, p. 1).

- Bullying can be verbal, social, or physical or happen through electronic communication (cyberbullying).
- Middle school students experienced bullying at a higher rate than high school students (Schaeffer, 2023).
- Girls are bullied more often than boys (Schaeffer, 2023).
- Students from rural areas are bullied more than urban areas (Schaeffer, 2023).
- Youth who identify as LGBTQ+ were more likely than youth who identify as heterosexual to report high levels of bullying (CDC, 2024e).

The Youth Risk Behavior Survey collects information about health and prevention issues among adolescents. Included in the survey are questions about violence risks such as fighting, use of illegal drugs, carrying a weapon, and being threatened or injured with a weapon on school property. The Division of Adolescent and School Health highlights some 2021 survey results collected from a sample of youth in grades 9 to 12:

- Sexual assaults increased for the first time in 10 years.
- Among adolescents assigned female at birth, 60% felt persistent sadness, and 10% had attempted suicide.
- Among students who identify as LGBTQ+, 10% did not attend school because of safety concerns.

- Black students attempted suicide at a higher rate than other groups (Ethier, 2023).

Visit https://www.cdc.gov/healthyyouth/data/yrbs/results.htm to see the results of the 2021 Youth Risk Behavior Survey.

School violence has immediate and long-term effects on students that is demonstrated by an increase in depression, anxiety, psychological problems, difficulty in school, and fear (CDC, 2024d). See Chapter 20 for more on school-age children and adolescents.

The U.S. Department of Education, the Department of Health and Human Services, and the Department of Justice have collaborated to provide funding, programs, and training that improve school safety through the *Safe Schools Healthy Students Framework*. Five elements identified for attention in building safe school climates are as follows:

- Create a safe and violence-free school environment.
- Prevent behavioral health problems.
- Promote emotional, mental, and behavioral health.
- Provide early childhood psychosocial and emotional development programs.
- Connect communities, schools, and families (National Center for Healthy Safe Children, 2020).

Socioeconomics, peer groups, learning disabilities, individual temperament, level of parent involvement, discipline methods, and community involvement all have either a positive or negative effect on youth.

Youth development programs address these risk factors in schools and communities and promote activities to help students meet individual needs. Mentoring programs are beneficial for at-risk teens when the mentors are appropriately trained and supported. Social skills, conflict resolution, and programs supporting student sports, arts, and extracurricular interests decrease an individual's risk of being involved in violence. School and societal strategies include surveillance, maintenance of facilities, and consistent classroom management techniques, along with adequate student supervision (USDHHS, n.d.).

INTIMATE PARTNER VIOLENCE

Intimate partner violence is the abuse or aggression that occurs within close relationships that are either current or previous (Fig. 18-4). The four types of IPV are physical violence, sexual violence, stalking, and psychological aggression (CDC, 2024b).

According to the WHO (2024a), global prevalence figures indicate:

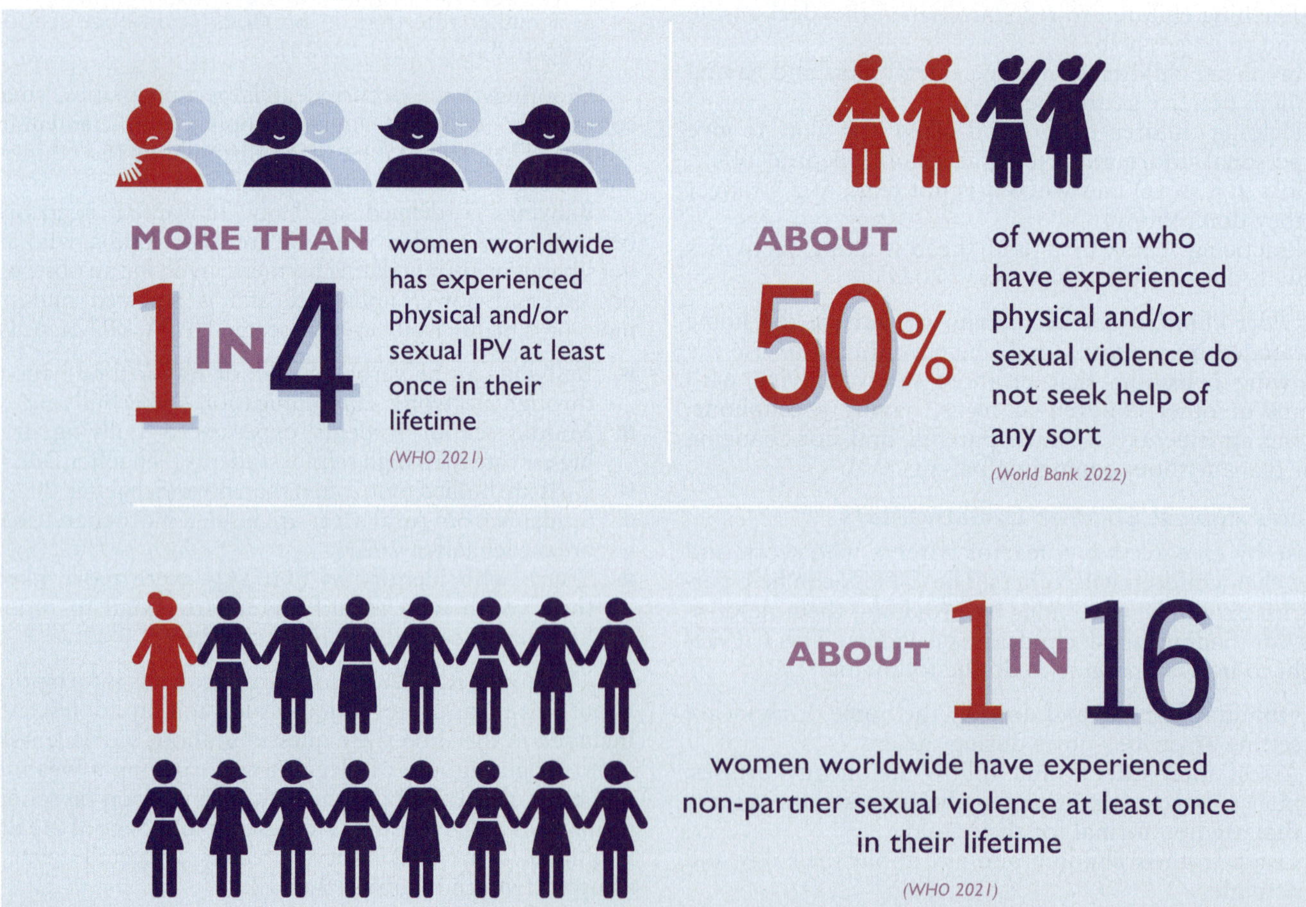
MORE THAN
1 IN 4
women worldwide has experienced physical and/or sexual IPV at least once in their lifetime
(WHO 2021)
ABOUT
50%
of women who have experienced physical and/or sexual violence do not seek help of any sort
(World Bank 2022)
ABOUT 1 IN 16
women worldwide have experienced non-partner sexual violence at least once in their lifetime
(WHO 2021)

FIGURE 18-4 Global statistics about intimate partner violence. (Reprinted from United States Agency for International Development. (2023). *Intimate partner violence and family planning*. https://www.usaid.gov/sites/default/files/2023-12/IPV-FP%20Infographic%20%282023%29.pdf)

- About 30% of women reported physical abuse by an intimate partner.
- About 30% of women reported sexual violence by an intimate partner or a nonpartner.
- Of all women murdered, 38% were killed by their intimate partner.

Among the LGBTQ+ community, 4.1 million have experienced IPV.

- Seeking formal support for IPV is hampered by stigma, lack of knowledge and understanding among certain therapists, and lack of formal support in the area.
- Seeking informal support from family and friends may be difficult; because some people may erroneously believe that only men conduct IPV and that therefore lesbian communities do not have IPV, those who expereince IPV in such communities may fear rejection, lack of support, and not being believed (Turner & Hammersjö, 2023).
- People conduct IPV equally in same-sex relationships, unlike in heterosexual relationships where the man is the main person who usually conducts IPV (Whirry & Holt, 2020).

Researchers often describe domestic violence, a form of IPV, as punching, grabbing, shoving, slapping, choking, kicking, biting, hitting with a fist or some other object, being beaten, or being threatened with a knife or gun by a spouse or cohabiting partner. The (USDOJ, n.d.-b, para. 2) defines domestic violence as "a pattern of abusive behavior in any relationship that is used by one partner to gain or maintain power and control over another intimate partner"; it may be emotional, economic, physical, psychological, or sexual in nature (Box 18-5).

Because of the nature of IPV, the problems are difficult to study and believed to be underreported. Much remains unknown about factors that increase or decrease the likelihood that one person will use violence against another person within an intimate relationship or while seeking that relationship. However, models have been developed to aid in the understanding of the repetitive cycles often seen in intimate partner and domestic violence.

Cycle of Violence

The **cycle of violence** is a repetitive, cyclic pattern of abuse seen in domestic violence situations (Box 18-6). Developed by Walker in 1979, the cycle is still in use today. The cycle includes the tension-building phase, the explosion (acute domestic violence incident), and the honeymoon phase. The relationship rarely starts in this cycle; rather, the person who conducts abuse romances the person experiencing the abuse in an attempt to gain control and power (Los Angeles Police Department [LAPD], n.d.).

- Tension-building phase
    - The person conducting the abuse attempts to control the person being abused.
    - Rules are set that are nearly unachievable to follow.
    - Consequences for not obeying rules: controlling money, limiting or denying family and friend contact, or telling the person where and when they can go somewhere.
- Explosion/acute domestic violence incident
    - Shortest phase of cycle
    - Most dangerous for person experiencing the abuse
    - Violence begins with slaps, hairpulling, and punching
    - Escalates to serious bodily harm or death
- Remorseful/honeymoon phase
    - Attempts to win forgiveness with gifts or promises to never repeat the violence.
    - Return to romantic behavior to gain control.
    - Blames person experiencing the abuse for the explosive phase because they did not follow the rules.
    - Cycle does not stop without professional help (LADP, n.d.).

The psychological dynamics of these three phases help explain why the person experiencing abuse feels guilty and ashamed of their partner's violence toward them and why they find it so difficult to leave, even when their lives are in danger.

Often, as the cycle of violence continues, the frequency of the cycle increases, with the tension-building phase and the acute domestic violence incident occurring more often, and with the diminishment or elimination

BOX 18-5 PERSPECTIVES

Viewpoint of a Person Who Experienced of Intimate Partner Violence

My parents were always shouting at each other. Although my parents didn't strike us or each other, many of our doors and walls had holes from my father hitting them. There was very little quiet time in our home growing up. The hitting wasn't nearly as bad as all the yelling. Now here I am in the same boat all over again—the yelling, the hitting, but now I've got this new baby to take care of. My partner was laid off, and money is very tight. I'm stressed, scared, and tired.

When the nurse showed up today to check on me and the baby, I swore to myself that I wouldn't mention last night. Then the nurse looked at me and asked if I felt safe, and that triggered me...I said "NO!" before I realized my mouth was even open. I told the nurse how he was yelling at me as I held the baby. I tried to walk away as he reached for the baby, but he got angry and pulled my hair to keep me near him. The nurse helped me look at my options. Because I was holding the baby when he pulled my hair, they said they were required to make a report of child abuse.

That was just awful news, and I started crying—but like the nurse said, I could have dropped my baby as he pulled my hair. I knew he'd be furious when he found out, and I really started to panic. Then the nurse told me about this place, a place downtown where I can stay with my baby, and helped me make arrangements. I'm so tired and scared, but I know now that I have to keep my baby safe. I hope he doesn't find out where I'm going—I know he'll get very angry when he finds out that I left with our baby.

—Angie

BOX 18-6 The Cycle of Violence

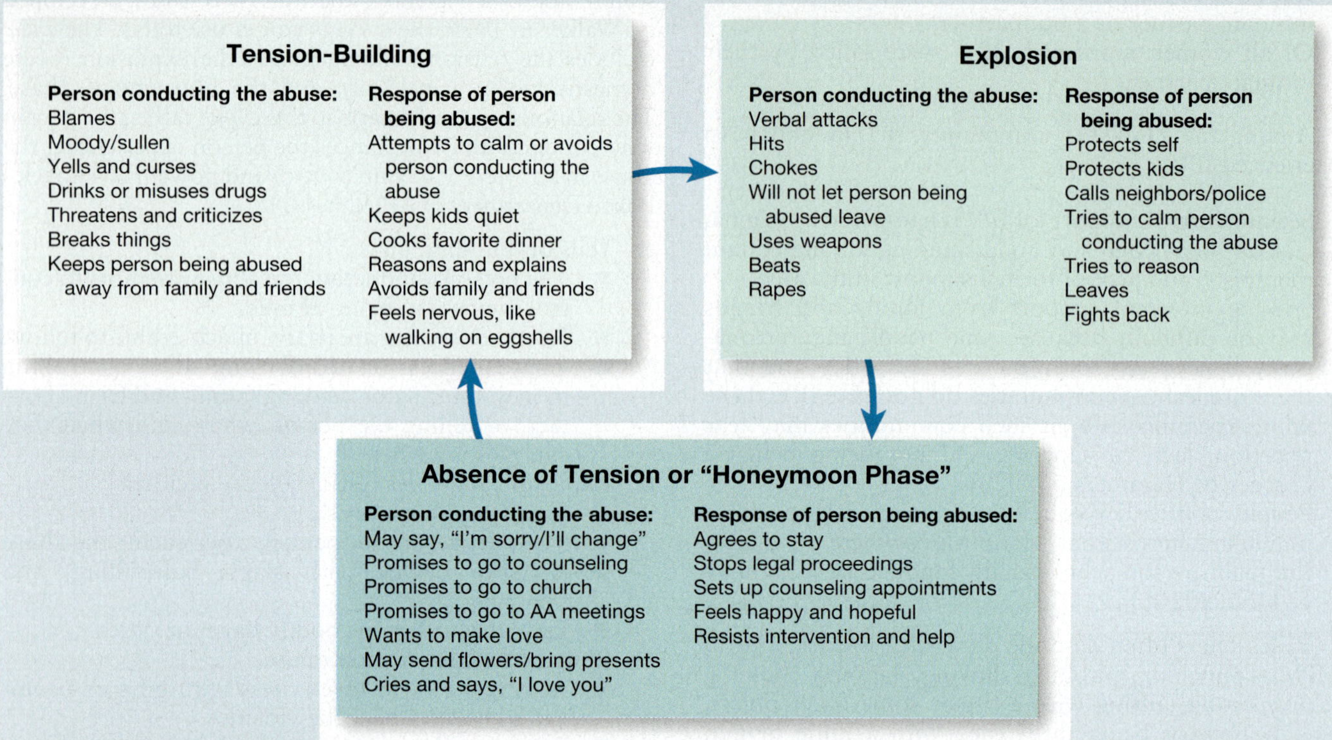

Tension-Building Phase

- Considered the longest of the phases—up to several weeks.
- Person experiencing abuse may feel like they are "walking on eggshells."
- Person conducting the abuse is edgy, negative mood, verbally abusive, and controlling.
- Minor augments occur.
- Person experiencing abuse attempts to appease partner in hopes of calming situation and to avoid the acute explosion phase.

Acute Explosion Phase

- Shortest phase usually lasting 1 to 2 days.
- Most violent phase as tension is released.
- Violence may take many forms such as sexual, physical, verbal, psychological, and emotional abuse.
- Phase is triggered by an external event or the state of mind of the person conducting the abuse.
- Person conducting the abuse may blame the abuse on the person experiencing the abuse.
- Person experiencing abuse may fight back, leave the person conducting the abuse, or try and placate the them.

Honeymoon Phase

- Person conducting the abuse may feel embarrassed and become withdrawn or attempt to justify actions.
- Person conducting the abuse expresses remorse and pledges it will not happen again.
- Person conducting the abuse promises to make behavioral changes such as work less, stop drinking, and be more attentive to person experiencing abuse.
- Person conducting the abuse is excessively romantic to person experiencing abuse, such as giving expensive gifts, flowers, candy.
- Person experiencing abuse forgives the person conducting the abuse.
- Intimacy may increase.
- Tension-building phase begins again.

Denial

- Common in each phase.
- Used to minimize seriousness of behavior.
- Creates a false sense of reality in person experiencing abuse.
- Family and friends use denial to lessen their responsibility.
- Person conducting the abuse uses denial to deny the abuse is their fault, that it was not abusive behavior, or that the behavior was deserved.

Source: White Ribbon Australia (2019); SexInfo Online (2017). Figure reprinted with permission from Hatfield, N. T., & Kincheloe, C. (2022). *Introductory maternity and pediatric nursing* (5th ed., Fig. 16-3). Wolters Kluwer.

of the loving reconciliation phase. Without intervention, this shorter, more violent cycle becomes increasingly risk filled for outcomes that may lead to incarceration or the injury, maiming, or death of a partner. Although early research focused on women who experience violence by men, men are not immune to abuse by women; according to the CDC (2024f), IPV occurs against men.

- One in three men have experienced sexual and physical violence and stalking.
- Of these men, 56% experienced IPV by age 25.

The Domestic Abuse Intervention Project in Duluth, Minnesota, developed a wheel of violence, identifying power and control at the center and citing eight categories

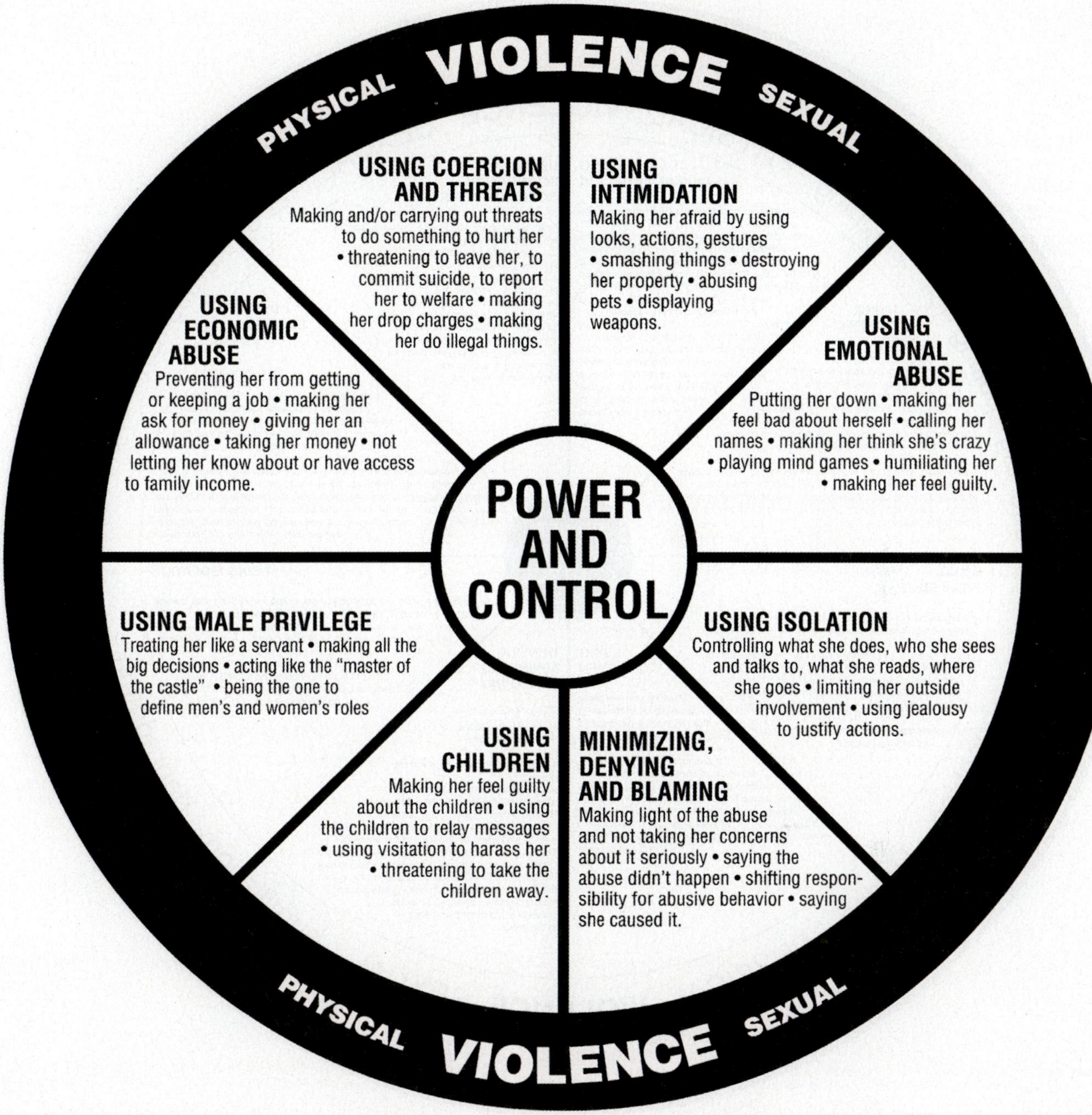

FIGURE 18-5 Wheel of power and control. Note that the language in this figure is not gender neutral because it is thes original model, which was based on women's experience of violence. (Reprinted with permission from Domestic Abuse Intervention Programs. https://www.theduluthmodel.org/wp-content/uploads/2017/03/PowerandControl.pdf)

of behaviors by people who conduct abuse (Fig. 18-5). This original model was based on women's experience of violence by men; hence, the language in it is not gender neutral. The examples given in the wheel are based on tactics to gain control and power that are used by men who conduct abuse (Domestic Abuse Intervention Programs, n.d.). Figure 18-6 highlights the power and control tactics often used within the LGBTQ+ community (Domestic Abuse Intervention Programs, n.d.). The wheels are used in therapy to help people experiencing abuse identify they are not alone, and people conducting abuse can see themselves in the pattern of abuse.

Reducing violence and its effects happens strategically at all three levels of prevention.

- Primary prevention efforts attempt to identify risk factors, reduce risks, enhance protective factors, and increase social support to prevent violence from occurring.
  - Examples include school or grade-based violence prevention classes or coping techniques.
- Secondary prevention effort involves screenings for people experiencing violence, holding classes and groups for people experiencing violence and those conducting violence, and developing an immediate response to violence that addresses the short-term consequences through emergency response and medical care.
- Tertiary prevention interventions work to address the long-term effect of trauma through counseling and rehabilitation for people experiencing violence and

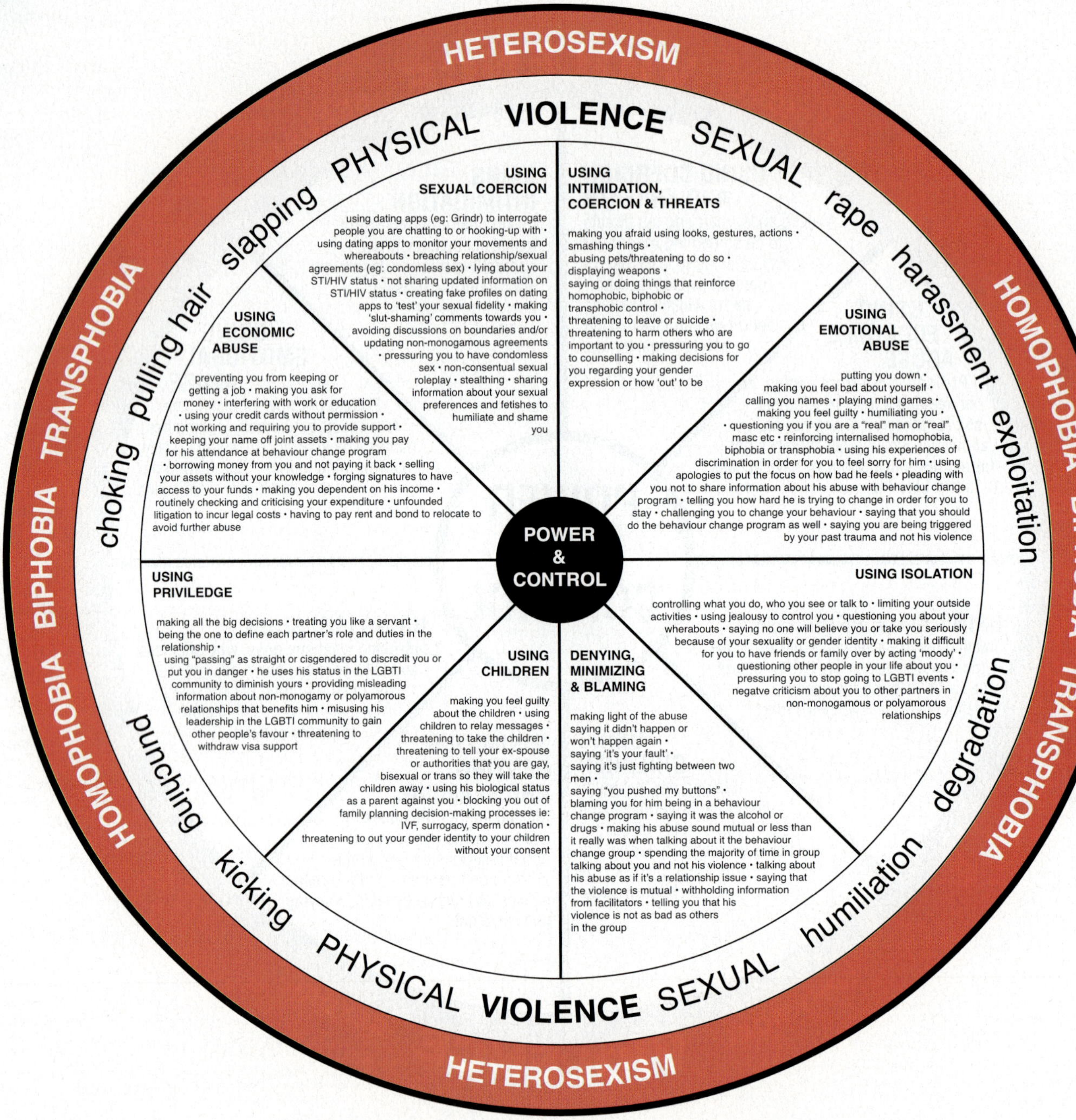

FIGURE 18-6 Wheel of power and control LGBTQ+. (Reprinted with permission from Domestic Abuse Intervention Programs. https://www.theduluthmodel.org/wp-content/uploads/2019/08/Power-and-Control-Thorne-Harbour-Health.pdf)

anger management for people conducting violence (CDC, n.d.-a).

Healthcare providers have a responsibility and opportunity to assess and initiate a safety plan when patients report experiencing violence. A compendium of assessment tools for IPV can be found on the CDC website.

Teen Dating Violence

Teen dating violence includes physical violence, sexual violence, psychological aggression, and stalking between teenagers who are or have been in a casual or serious dating relationship. It can be electronic or in person and might occur between an individual and a current or former partner (CDC, 2024g).

- The 2021 National Youth Risk Behavior Study indicated that slightly more than 8% of high school students reported physical dating violence and sexual dating violence in the past 12 months; furthermore, people who experience dating violence in adolescence are at higher risk for dating violence in college. Adolescents assigned female at birth and LGBTQ+ adolescents are at a greater risk of dating violence (CDC, 2024g).
- Documented risk factors include the following:
  - Childhood exposure to IPV by parents/caregivers, yelling or corporal punishment by parents, and teen delinquent behavior (Cheung & Huang, 2023).
  - If friend/peer groups condoned IPV, friends were more likely to be in IPV relationships, to be targeted

for violence by peers, to be sexually active prior to age 16, and to believe in gender inequality (Hunt et al., 2022).

Teens assigned female at birth experiencing dating violence are at risk for heavy binge drinking, depression, and smoking, whereas teens assigned male at birth experiencing dating violence are at risk for antisocial behavior and marijuana use. Both these populations experience suicidal ideation and PTSD (Cheung & Huang, 2023).

Programs through schools and communities, such as *Dating Matters: Strategies to Promote Healthy Teen Relationships* (https://www.cdc.gov/intimate-partner-violence/php/datingmatters/index.html), are part of a national effort to address harmful beliefs about dating violence and to promote healthy and respectful dating relationships (CDC, 2024g). Dating violence in adolescent relationships is a serious problem and because of its prevalence, community health nurses should include screening for dating violence in all encounters with teens.

Stalking

Stalking may occur by either partner in a relationship, demonstrated as a "pattern of repeated and unwanted attention, harassment, contact, or any other course of conduct directed at a specific person that would cause a reasonable person to feel fear" (USDOJ, n.d.-d, para. 2). The most recent statistics are from 2019:

- In the U.S. population, 3.4 million people age 16 and older were stalked, a decline from 2016.
- Because many believed stalking was not important enough to report, 81% did not report being stalked.
- The age group most often stalked was 20 to 24 years old, followed by people ages 25 to 34.
- Women are stalked twice as often as men.
- Stalking includes a person being followed, the person conducting the stalking showing up where they should not, harassment of family and friends for contact information, and sending unwanted items to the home or workplace of the person being stalked (Morgan & Truman, 2022).

Cyberstalking, a technology-based attack, can also take many forms that can involve harassment, embarrassment, and humiliation of the person experiencing the abuse.

In June 2022, President Biden established a task force to address online harassment and abuse consisting of researchers, law enforcement, people who had experienced abuse, parents/guardians, legal and medical professionals, and educators (The White House, 2023). This partnership is tasked with the development of a blueprint to stop online harassment.

Violence During Pregnancy

IPV during pregnancy increases the vulnerability of the birthing parent and the fetus. A systematic review conducted by Schrubbe et al. (2023) found social, physical, and economic demands of pregnancy may increase the risk of IPV.

- Prevalence rates of IPV during pregnancy vary, depending on where the data were collected, and the survey used.
  - Rates ranged between 2% and 13.5% and between 0.7% and 55%
- The following may increase the risk of IPV:
  - Low birth weight, miscarriages, preterm births
  - Inconsistent or lack of prenatal care
  - Insufficient weight gain of birthing parent during pregnancy
  - Depression and other forms of mental illness
  - Risk of birthing parent or neonatal death (Schrubbe et al., 2023).

Kah and colleagues found birthing parents were more likely to experience postpartum depression if verbal or physical abuse occurred and partner-related stress prior to and during pregnancy (Kah et al., 2022). See Chapter 19 for more on maternal–child health issues.

The prenatal care visit is one of the few times when providers have an important opportunity to identify patients who are abused and therefore at risk for homicide. It is imperative that C/PHNs conduct an assessment for danger and lethality so that the patient can be aware of their level of risk and take safety precautions as needed.

- A series of questions requiring a "yes" or "no" response and inquiries about occurrences of abuse, escalation of abuse, frequency, severity, weapons, drugs or alcohol use by the person conducting the abuse, and safety of other children in the home should be incorporated into prenatal home visit assessments.
- All healthcare providers, including C/PHNs, should have regular training on IPV.
- According to the American College of Obstetricians and Gynecologists (ACOG) (2022), when choosing a tool to assess for IPV, ensure it is culturally appropriate and avoid tools that include words such as "abuse," "rape," or "violence" because they may cause the person to feel stigmatized.
- Annual screenings for IPV and providing interventions and referrals are part of the Women's Preventive Services Guidelines (Health Resources Services Administration [HRSA], 2022). These are especially important for birthing parents who have not followed through with prenatal care, thereby not allowing healthcare professionals to monitor the progress of their pregnancies. C/PHNs are uniquely situated to screen for IPV during pregnancy, particularly through *Healthy Start* and *Nurse–Family Partnership programs.*

Characteristics of People Who Experience IPV

Increasing the abilities of the person who experiences IPV to manage and improve their behaviors and understanding of relationship patterns and abuse allows them to change their risk of being further victimized. Individual risk factors for IPV victims include the following:

- A prior history of IPV
- Being a person assigned female at birth
- Young age, especially if pregnant
- From resource-limited household
- Witnessing or experiencing violence as a child
- Lower education level
- Unemployment
- Being a single parent with children or being separated, divorced, or previously widowed
- For men, having a different ethnicity from their partner
- For women, having a greater education level than their partner
- For women, being American Indian/Alaska Native or African American

- For women, having a disability
- Experiencing childhood sexual and physical violence
- For women, having a verbally abusive, jealous, or possessive partner
- Being a veteran or active duty military (Pereira et al., 2020)

Effects of Violence on Children

Exposure to violence and abuse may hinder children's health and development and can have a lifelong impact, negatively affecting health and increasing the risks of experiencing further abuse and becoming a person who abuses others (WHO, 2022).

Literature reviews consistently suggest that a positive correlation exists between children witnessing IPV and some aspects of impaired child development. Young children are particularly vulnerable to violence, as they cannot understand the trauma. These children are likely to exhibit somatic complaints (e.g., headaches, eating or sleep problems) or behavior regression, such as clinging, whining, or becoming nonverbal (National Child Traumatic Stress Network, n.d.). Additional effects include the following:

- Are more likely to act out with delinquent behaviors or withdrawal
- Are at risk for depression, negative mental health effects, and consequences that last far into their adult lives
- Demonstrate behavioral (aggression and conduct problems), emotional (withdrawal, anxiousness, fearfulness), social, cognitive (learning disabilities), and physical
- Are less likely to be up to date on child immunizations
- Are seen more frequently in emergency rooms
- Have poor lung functioning
- Have a higher rate of obesity
- Experience deficient nutrition (Holmes et al., 2022)

Although, researchers have identified physical alterations in the child's brain when a child is exposed to IPV, much research is still needed. Holmes and colleagues (2022) completed a systemic review of published quantitative studies on the effects of IPV on children between 1975 and 2020. However, of the 381 empirical and systemic studies found, only 23 empirical studies and zero systemic reviews were found on the physiologic changes that occurred. There is agreement on the negative effects of witnessing IPV has on the autonomic nervous system, the hypothalamus–pituitary–adrenal axis, and increased levels of cortisol (Holmes et al., 2023).

- Mueller & Tronick's (2020) review of scientific findings identified the effects of IPV on brain maturation and socioemotional development as noted in the decrease of white and gray matter of sections of the temporal lobe in children between ages 3 and 13 who witnessed verbal abuse between intimate partners. A systematic review conducted by Doroudchi et al. (2023) found children who witnessed domestic violence were at a higher risk of poorer education performance, lower social skills, lower IQs, depression, PTSD, and aggression. These conditions ranged from moderate to severe and were either short or long term in duration.

Providers who work with children need to listen in a sincere, nonjudgmental manner and provide ongoing support when assisting the child and family with resources, such as counseling, education, or community violence prevention programs.

OLDER PERSON ABUSE AND MALTREATMENT OF OLDER ADULTS

Older person abuse, sometimes called elder abuse, is the "intentional act, or failure to act, by a caregiver or another person in a relationship involving an expectation of trust that causes or creates a risk of harm to an older adult" (CDC, 2024h, para. 1). Examples include physical (Fig. 18-7), sexual or abusive sexual contact, emotional or psychological abuse, neglect, financial or material exploitation, confinement, passive neglect, and willful deprivation (CDC, 2024h; National Council on Aging, n.d.). As with other types of abuses against vulnerable populations, the true incidence and prevalence of abuse of older adults are not known.

- It is estimated that 1 in 10 older adults experience some type of abuse (U.S. Department of Justice [USDOJ], 2023a). Worldwide estimates are as high as 1 in 6 adults over age 60 experience abuse (WHO, 2024b).
- Approximately two thirds of older adults who experience abuse are women (USDOJ, 2023a).
- About half of individuals have dementia (USDOJ, 2023a).
- Risk factors include low social support, dementia, poor physical health, and functional impairment (NCEA, n.d.-a).
- People conducting older abuse are often adult children or spouses, people assigned male at birth, and have a history of substance use disorders or mental health issues (NCEA, n.d.-a).
- The most reported abuse includes neglect, followed by financial exploitation and emotional abuse (USDOJ, 2023a).
- Over 88,000 adults age 60 and older experienced fraud, with a total loss of 3.1 billion dollars.
- The average loss per person was $35,000, but 5456 adults lost $100,000 (FBI, 2022).
- For more information on fraud and abuse of older adults refer to https://www.ic3.gov/Media/PDF/AnnualReport/2022_IC3ElderFraudReport.pdf

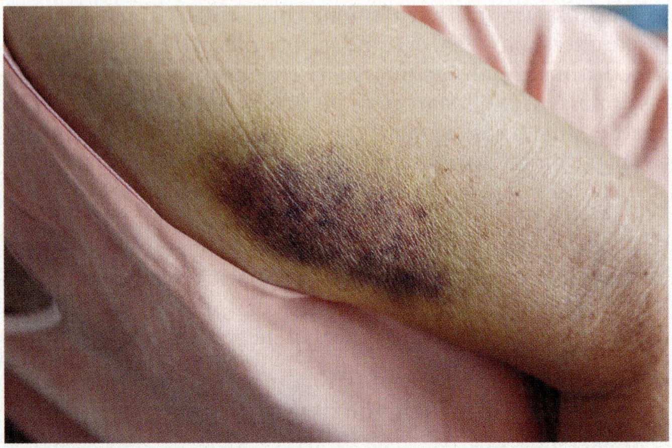

FIGURE 18-7 A bruise on the arm of an older adult who has been abused.

- Forms of physical abuse include rough handling during caregiving, pinching, hitting, and slapping.
- Emotional abuse, which can take many forms, includes being shouted at or threatened and having needed care withheld.
- Older adults may also be sexually assaulted or sexually abused.
- Some adults are neglected by those they depend on to meet their caregiving needs.
- Older adults with dementia and those requiring assistance for all activities of daily living are more vulnerable to maltreatment due to caregiver stress or burnout, factors known to increase the risk for maltreating older adults.
- A neglected older adult may appear unwashed and unkempt, be malnourished or dehydrated, or have pressure ulcers.
- Financial exploitation includes theft of Social Security or retirement money, savings or investments, and the use of these funds by the person conducting the abuse.
- Criminals often approach older adults with get-rich-quick schemes, sham investment opportunities, overpriced home repairs, or pose as collectors for illegitimate charities, thereby preying on the trusting nature of older adults (NCEA, n.d.-a; USDOJ, 2023a). See Chapter 22 for more on older adults.

Vulnerability Factors

Individual characteristics associated with vulnerability of abuse include poor health, increased age, and disability.

- Older adults who identify as lesbian, gay, bisexual, transgender, and queer/questioning (LGBTQ+) and those who are residents of an assisted living facility are also more vulnerable to experiencing maltreatment (NCEA, n.d.-b).
- The older LGBTQ+ community experiences discrimination due to age and sexual orientation, leading to social isolation.
- This population may experience discrimination from medical providers (Cassanova-Perez et al., 2022).

Dementia and newly diagnosed cognitive impairment correlate with occurrences of abuse. If violence or threats of violence by the older adult toward the caregiver accompany dementia, this contributes to the adult's risk for abuse.

Harmful effects of abuse for this vulnerable population include longer convalescence periods, permanent damage, premature death, depression, and anxiety (WHO, 2024b).

The *invisibility* of older in general, and abused adults specifically, increases an older adult's vulnerability to being abused. Reasons for invisibility among the older adults are multifaceted.

- Older adults may have less contact with the community because they are no longer in the workforce or in public regularly, which keeps their problems hidden longer.
- Older adults are reticent to admit to being abused or neglected.
  - Because the person conducting the abuse is often a family member, the older adult attempts to protect that person to avoid being entirely alone.
  - The older adult may fear reprisal from the person conducting the abuse for coming forward with a self-report of abuse or telling someone about the home situation.
- Cultural and societal values also contribute to keeping "family matters" private. A research study in New York City estimated abuse of older adults that was not reported was 24 times greater than the reported abuse. Researchers found shame, fear, and keeping the abuse private were contributing factors to the silence (New York City Department of the Aging et al., 2011).
- Older adults may be considered a vulnerable population for several reasons. Individuals may experience a diminished physical, cognitive, and psychological ability; death of family members and friends leading to lack of social support and isolation; stigmatization by the culture; discrimination by healthcare providers and not provided necessary care such as palliative treatments; and for economic reasons (Sanchini et al., 2022).
- Many older adults who are frail are dependent on others for some aspect of their day-to-day survival. The degree to which an older adult needs assistance is often kept hidden from others because the older adult fears being removed from their present living situation and being placed in a more restrictive environment.
- Additionally, vulnerability in older adults is increased when any of the following characteristics are present: (1) depression, (2) alcohol use disorder, (3) high dependency on others, (4) a decrease in health, (5) high stress levels with poor coping strategies, (6) shame and self-blame, (7) history of child physical abuse or/and neglect, and (8) poor relationship with caregiver (Storey, 2020).

Reporting and Prevention of Older Person Abuse

Awareness of abuse of older adults and education about the types of abuse via public and professional media campaigns has improved community recognition of the problem.

- C/PHNs need knowledge in screening procedures and risk factors for abuse and people who conduct abuse.
- Respite care can provide valuable relief to family members.
- Training for caregivers and for healthcare and social service providers focused on recognizing stress and initiating intervention measures has developed a new understanding of effective interventions.
- World Elder Abuse Awareness Day has been designated as an annual observance on June 15th to promote public awareness and prevention education regarding abuse of older adults (United Nations, n.d.).

Reporting laws differ among states. The Elder Abuse Guide for Law Enforcement website (https://eagle.usc.edu/state-specific-laws/) provides an interactive map with laws regarding abuse of older adults, mandated reporting laws, and where to report for each state. In addition, the website provides other resources including training videos, how to document pressure injuries, and photos of abuse in older adults.

OTHER FORMS OF VIOLENCE

Additional forms of violence include self-directed violence (SDV) (including suicide), homicide, sexual assault, and human trafficking.

Self-Directed Violence

Self-directed violence (SDV), an intentional act to cause injury to oneself, is a public health issue worldwide. SDV is considered a range of behaviors involving fatal and nonfatal self-harm. Examples of self-harm include cutting, head banging or hitting, self-scratching, self-biting, burning oneself, attempted suicide, and suicide. Suicidal ideation, although not a behavior, is often included due to an association with SDV (Banyard et al., 2021).

Suicide is taking action that causes one's own death. According to the CDC, suicide rates are rising in every state in the United States.

In 2021, 12.3 million people in the United States considered suicide, of those 3.5 million had a plan and 1.7 million attempted suicide (CDC, n.d.-b).

It is important to be aware of warning signs of potential suicide when working with people in crisis. Threats or comments that indicate a plan or giving personal items away are potential indicators of a person contemplating suicide. Isolation, sleeping too much, acting recklessly, and increased use of alcohol or drugs are high-risk behaviors for suicide. Moods that may reflect increased risk are depression, irritability, rage, humiliation, and anxiety. For more information on suicide, refer to your mental health textbook.

Gun Violence

- A Pew Research Center Survey discovered that 32% of Americans own a firearm and 40% live with someone who owns a firearm. Close to 50% of adults in rural areas own guns, followed by adults in suburbs, and then urban communities (Schaeffer, 2023).
- Most gun owners cite the Second Amendment to the Constitution as their right to own a firearm. Reasons for owning a firearm include protection (72%), followed by hunting, sport shooting, collecting, and requirement of job (Schaeffer, 2023).
- In 2021, 48,830 died from guns either by suicide (54%) or homicide (43%) in the United States. This is the highest number of homicides by guns since 1968 and the highest number of suicides by firearms since 2001 (Gramlich, 2023).
- Twice as many individuals have been injured by firearms than have died (American Public Health Association [APHA], 2023).
- Active shootings also saw an increase in 2021. In 2001, there were three mass shootings, whereas in 2019, there were 40. Regretfully, this number jumped to 61 in 2021 (Gramlich, 2023).
- Men have a much higher percentage of death by firearms and injury by firearms than women (CDC, 2024i).

In 2022, President Biden signed into law the Bipartisan Safer Communities Act. This law provides grants to states to improve gun control and decrease gun violence, more stringent background checks on buyers younger than 18 (Box 18-7), and monies to states for violence

BOX **18-7** STORIES FROM THE FIELD

The Younger Version of Me

When the topic of gun violence is discussed, I tend to look down and distract myself. This topic always makes me uncomfortable.

The younger version of me gets upset hearing the news or classmates discussing the topic of gun violence. The current version of me is more understanding. The constant incidents of violence, the stories being broadcasted online and on television take a toll. The fear and trauma that is shared among everyone is real and something needs to be done which is why I am happy that my classmates and colleagues are advocating and striving to stop this issue.

But what about the others? What about me? I know that sounds selfish but these questions linger in the back of my mind when the topic of gun violence is brought up. Younger me is yelling "No one cared when we were suffering?", "No one seemed to advocate or listen to us?" In my younger self's defense, these are valid questions. It is great that we are discussing gun violence, but we can't just focus on school shootings or movie theater shootings, not to imply that these are not important issues. But we must also advocate for urban communities, for Black, Brown, and Indigenous communities. These communities have been fighting for a long time, but no one seemed to listen and younger me wonders why. As I have gotten older, I understood that in this world the amount of money you have, your zip code, and the color of your skin are big determinants.

Some may read this and say that I need to get over it, that at least we are talking about it now, or that it wasn't a big problem before, and so on, but that's exactly what I mean. Others get the luxury to minimize and ignore what we, who have been dealing with the trauma in a different way, for a longer period, have been trying to get others to understand for a long time. Instead, we have had to sit here and watch nothing happen. We have had to sit here and be ignored. We have had to sit here and witness people finally care, but only once it started affecting those outside those communities I listed above.

So yeah, younger me is hurt because no one listened to her when she decided to speak up, so she is thinking, "Why speak up now?"

—*Anonymous Nursing Student*

Note: In class one day, this nursing student spoke about a police officer who was shot to death outside of the police station. The killing happened in her town and the community was saddened by the event. The person accused had a history of mental illness. As we talked more in the hallway, she described the community in which she grew up and how it differs from her current residence. She spoke about the constant gunshots she heard when growing up, the gang violence, and the murders that occurred. She learned to tell the difference between gunfire and fireworks by echo. As we spoke, she described her younger self. She graciously shared her account.

—*Dr. Charlene Niemi*

prevention programs (APA, 2022b). Finally, the act provided much-needed funds for mental health.

Homicide

Homicide is any non–war-related action taken to cause the death of another person. Globally, the number of homicides exceeded deaths due to terrorism and wars combined (UNODC, 2023).

In 2021, there were 458,000 deaths by homicide, of which 81% were men. Differences between the Americas and Europe are noted:

- In the Americas, most victims were between age 15 and 19, whereas in Europe victims ranged between 30 and 44 years.
- In the Americas, most deaths were due to firearms, whereas in Europe, deaths were due to sharp objects.
- In the Americas, most homicides were committed by organized crime and gangs, whereas in Europe, the majority of homicides were committed by intimate violence and family members (UNODC, 2023).

In 2021, there was a spike in global homicides due in part to the economic downturn with the ramifications and restrictions from the COVID-19 pandemic and a rise in gang and organized crime activity (UNODC, 2023). Hopefully, that trend will start to turn as evidenced by a decrease in homicides in 2022 when compared with the same time period in 2021 (UNODC, 2023).

Sexual Assault

Sexual assault is defined as "any nonconsensual sexual act proscribed by Federal, tribal, or State law, including when the victim lacks capacity to consent" (USDOJ, n.d.-c, para. 2). This definition includes threats of sexual violence, attempted rape, and rape. The person who conducts the assault can be of any gender.

Sexual assault is underreported and is the least reported crime to law enforcement due to the following:

- Fear of revenge by the person conducting the assault
- Fear assault would be made public
- Handled assault on own because did not want to involve the police
- Assault was viewed as a personal matter (Government of Canada, 2022)
- Shame

Groups at higher risk of sexual assault:

- People assigned female at birth
- Women with disabilities
- Young women and children (Government of Canada, 2022)

The person conducting the assault is most often known to the person experiencing the assault in one of the following ways:

- Acquaintance
- Friend
- Intimate partner
- Family member (Government of Canada, 2022)

Useful measures to prevent sexual assault must include the individual, relational, community, and societal levels for there to be change. In 2016, the CDC published *Sexual Violence Prevention Resource for Action* (Basile et al., 2016). This worthwhile publication provides a comprehensive, evidenced-based information and interventions to assist communities in eliminating sexual assault and violence. Refer to Figure 18-8 to learn more about strategies and approaches.

SART (Sexual Assault Response Team) consists of multidisciplinary members who are trained to understand the psychological and physical assessment needs of the person who experienced the assault as well as the legal requirements for an investigation and court proceeding (International Association of Forensic Nurses, n.d.). The CDC's Rape Prevention and Education program provides current tools, training, and support works (CDC, 2024j).

A common role in the SART is a sexual assault nurse examiner (SANE), who assists people who are affected by sexual violence, including people who experienced an assault, suspects, and the accused.

- For people who have experienced sexual assault, SANEs provide forensic medical examinations and appropriate follow-up referrals based on the patient's individual needs.
- SANEs may specialize in pediatrics, adolescents, adults, or a combination of all three.
- A SANE represents one subspecialty of forensic nursing practice; forensic nurses work in a variety of community settings and specialize in many different types of patient populations affected by violence including abuse of older adults, IPV, corrections, death investigations, and after a major disaster (International Association of Forensic Nurses, n.d.).
- To find more information on this specialty, explore the International Association of Forensic Nurses website at https://www.forensicnurses.org/page/WhatisFN/

Human Trafficking

The 13th Amendment to the U.S. Constitution, which bans slavery and involuntary servitude, provides the foundation of our current laws against human trafficking (USDOJ, 2023c). In 2022, over 27.6 million people were human trafficked (USAID, 2023).

The U.S. Department of Justice states, "Human trafficking, also known as trafficking in persons, is a crime that involves compelling or coercing a person to provide labor or services, or to engage in commercial sex acts. Coercion can be subtle or overt, physical or psychological. Exploitation of a minor for commercial sex is human trafficking, regardless of whether any form of force, fraud, or coercion was used" (USDOJ, 2023b).

Below is information about different types of organizations that fight human trafficking:

- U.S. Department of Homeland Security
  - Protect people who have experienced human trafficking
  - Intensify prevention efforts
  - Improve law enforcement operations
- DHS Center for Countering Human Trafficking (CCHT)
  - CCHT at Work
  - Annual report
  - Approach centered on the people who experienced human trafficking
  - Webinars
  - Resources

Strategies and Approaches to STOP SV

	Strategy	Approach
S	**Promote Social Norms that Protect Against Violence**	• Bystander approaches • Mobilizing men and boys as allies
T	**Teach Skills to Prevent Sexual Violence**	• Social-emotional learning • Teaching healthy, safe dating and intimate relationship skills to adolescents • Promoting healthy sexuality • Empowerment-based training
O	**Provide Opportunities to Empower and Support Girls and Women**	• Strengthening economic supports for women and families • Strengthening leadership and opportunities for girls
P	**Create Protective Environments**	• Improving safety and monitoring in schools • Establishing and consistently applying workplace policies • Addressing community-level risks through environmental approaches
SV	**Support Victims/Survivors to Lessen Harms**	• Victim-centered services • Treatment for victims of SV • Treatment for at-risk children and families to prevent problem behavior including sex offending

FIGURE 18-8 Strategies and approaches to stop sexual violence. SV, sexual violence. Note that the original gendered terms, which recognize that females are at higher risk for SV, have been retained in this figure. (Reprinted from Centers for Disease Control and Prevention. (2016). *Sexual violence prevention resource for action.* https://www.cdc.gov/violenceprevention/pdf/SV-Prevention-Resource_508.pdf)

  - https://www.dhs.gov/dhs-center-countering-human-trafficking
- International Trafficking Victims Protection Reauthorization Act of 2022
  - Holds counties accountable by withholding U.S. monies to countries that do not meet minimal standards of human protection
  - Protects domestic works of diplomatic officials
  - Enlarges international Megan laws
  - https://www.foreign.senate.gov/imo/media/doc/International%20Trafficking%20Victims%20Protection%20Reauthorization%20Act%20of%202022_Bill%20Summary.pdf
- U.S. Department of Justice (DOJ) (2023c) Human trafficking: Key Legislation provides a summary of various key legislation
  - https://www.justice.gov/humantrafficking/key-legislation

Despite the significant number of known cases, the actual prevalence of human trafficking is not known. This, combined with the well-established negative health consequences, has made this into a public health problem and one that is difficult to mitigate. However, people experiencing human trafficking most often do not mention this information during the healthcare encounter, and healthcare providers do not readily recognize individuals in this population (Hainaut et al., 2022). A review of human trafficking screening tools found that a great majority of the tools are not validated and are only given to individuals if a medical provider was concerned or noticed any red flags; the vast majority of tools focus on sex trafficking and not labor trafficking (Hainaut et al., 2022). Furthermore, tools did not highlight risk factors of the LGBTQ+ populations and people with developmental delays and intellectual disabilities even though both populations have an increased risk of trafficking (Hainaut et al., 2022). The limited education of healthcare providers and lack of validated tools in healthcare settings highlights the need for all of us to be educated about human trafficking and to conduct research on the tools used.

- A major response measure implemented by the USDHHS was the establishment of the National Human Trafficking Hotline (n.d.) at https://humantraffickinghotline.org/. The center is responsible for the 24-hour crisis line available in over 200 languages, plus additional texting (233733), live chat, and online resources to assist in the recognition and response to people experiencing human trafficking.

To learn about current human trafficking, one only needs to do an internet search and a host of examples can be found. The following examples are only two of many:

- Operation Blooming Onion took place across Georgia, Texas, Florida, and several Central American countries. This multilaw enforcement endeavor rescued more than 100 migrants who were forced to dig onions with their bare hands, paid 20 cents per basket of onions, threatened with violence, and retaliation against family members. Many were raped, kidnapped, or sold and traded to other farms. Living conditions were cramped and unsanitary with little to no water. What water was provided was untreated and not safe to drink (DOJ, 2021).
- In the deadliest human smuggling case in U.S. history, 53 migrants died from the Texas heat, and their cries for help went unanswered as they were locked in a tractor-trailer (Salinas et al., 2022).

Gang Violence

According to the FBI (n.d.-a), there are 33,000 violent gangs in the United States, consisting of street, motorcycle, and prison gangs (Fig. 18-9). Violent activities involve prostitution, human trafficking, drug sales, robberies, and gun trafficking.

Teens join gangs for several reasons:

- Identity or recognition
- Fellowship
- Intimidation
- Protection
- Criminal activity (Office of Justice Programs [OJP], n.d.)

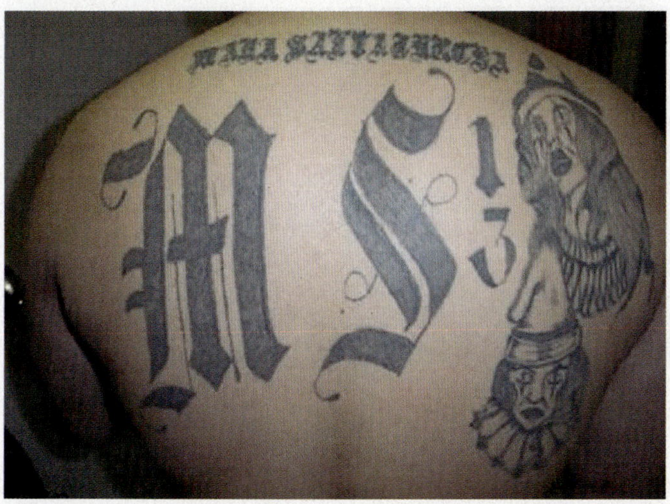

FIGURE 18-9 The tattooed back of a member of Mara Salvatrucha, also known as MS-13, which is one of the largest criminal street gangs in the United States. (Reprinted from U.S. Department of Justice Criminal Division. https://www.justice.gov/criminal/criminal-vcrs/gallery/criminal-street-gangs)

Teens involved in gangs are at higher risk of not graduating from high school, teen parenthood, and unemployment (OJP, n.d.).

For a list of gangs by state refer to World Population Review. (2023). *Gangs by state 2023*. https://worldpopulationreview.com/state-rankings/gangs-by-state

Workplace Violence

Workplace violence is defined as "any act or threat of physical violence, harassment, intimidation, or other threatening disruptive behavior that occurs at the work site" (Occupational Safety and Health Administration [OSHA], n.d., para. 2). Violence can take the form of threats, verbal abuse, physical assaults, or homicide (Fig. 18-10). According to the U.S. Department of Labor, those at greatest risk include healthcare providers, customer service workers, employees working in small groups or alone, public service employees, and law enforcement officers (OSHA, n.d.). See Box 18-8.

In hospitals, nurses working in emergency departments, intensive care units, and in-patient psychiatric units have the highest risk of injuries due to violence. Healthcare workers underreport workplace violence by patients because of unclear definitions of workplace violence, feeling that the patient was not responsible for actions due to mental status, or believing violence is part of the job (Joint Commission on Accreditation of Healthcare Organizations [JCAHO], 2021). The JCAHO standards and recommendations related to workplace violence are located at https://www.jointcommission.org/resources/patient-safety-topics/sentinel-event/sentinel-event-alert-newsletters/sentinel-event-alert-59-physical-and-verbal-violence-against-health-care-workers/.

Bullying or incivility among nurses is a common occurrence. It is estimated 50% of nurses and nursing students have been bullied within a healthcare setting (JCAHO, 2021).

Types of bullying:

- Verbal abuse
- Work interference, such as withholding patient information during shift change
- Intimidating, humiliating, threatening behavior

Risk factors:

- Inadequate staffing for census
- Heavy workload
- Poor management (JCAHO, 2021)

Fricke et al. (2023) found interventions should include the following:

- Emotional support after a violent act occurs
- Facilities must guarantee nurses' safety
- Offer training in violence prevention and de-escalation strategies
- Polices that protect nurses
- Guidance on management of role conflict between personal safety and professional role
- No single intervention is effective; multiple interventions must take place over time

While incivility is considered part of the job by some, it has a negative impact on healthcare. Horizontal and

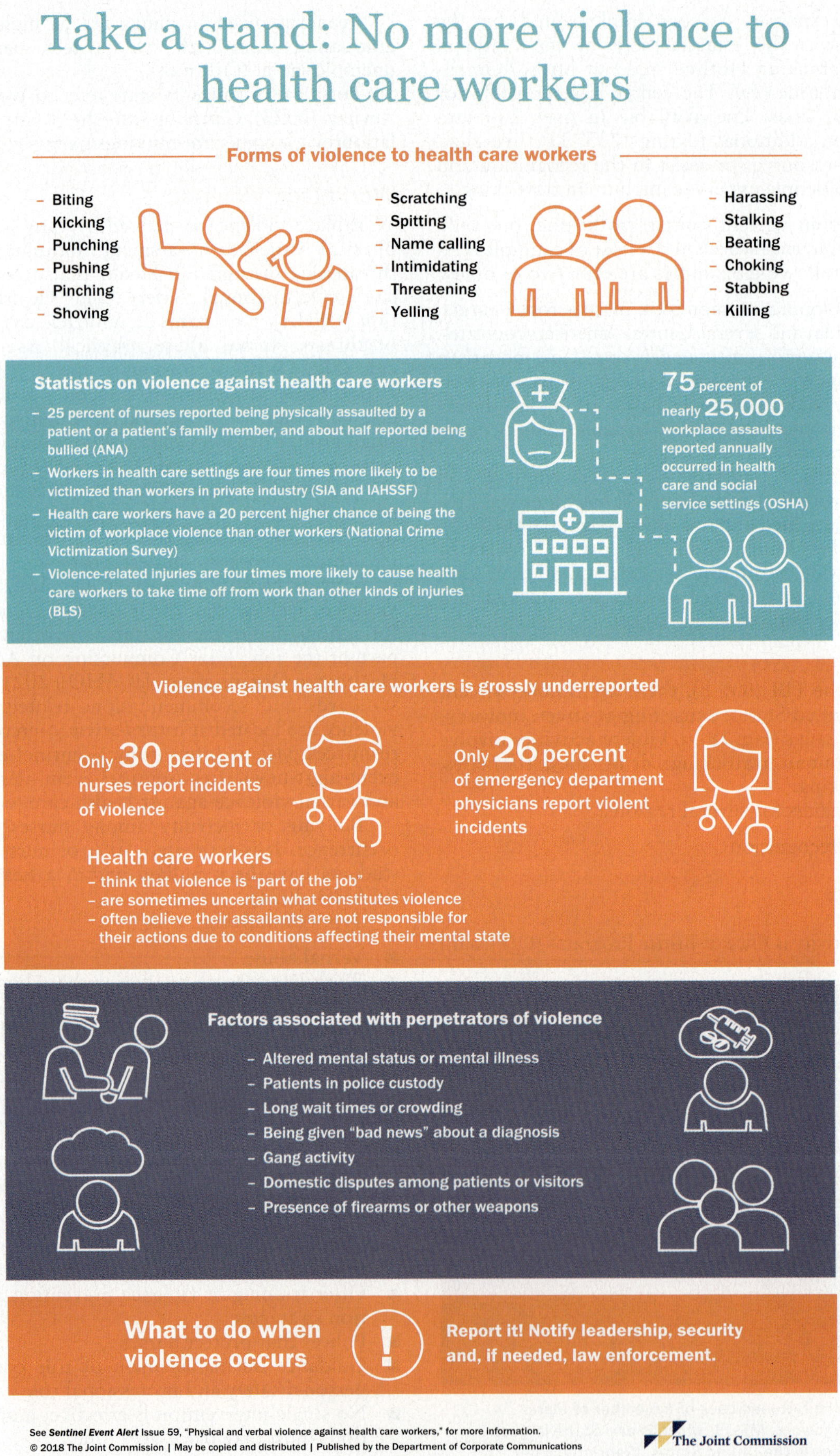

FIGURE 18-10 No more violence to healthcare workers. (Reprinted with permission from The Joint Commission. (2018). *Take a stand: No more violence to health care workers*. https://www.jointcommission.org/-/media/tjc/documents/resources/patient-safety-topics/sentinel-event/sea_59_wpv_infographic_3_30_18_finalpdf.pdf)

BOX **18-8** SPOTLIGHT ON ESSENTIAL NURSING COMPETENCIES

The Importance of Quality and Safety When Working in Correctional Health

Working in a correctional facility for a county, state, or federal institution is unlike working in any other setting. Prior to being incarcerated, many people may not have taken care of their health. Health problems for this population include infectious diseases such as HIV, STDs, hepatitis B and C, and tuberculosis. Mental illnesses are prevalent. When first arrested, individuals may experience drug or alcohol withdrawal (American Academy of Family Physicians, 2019). Chronic conditions such as hypertension, cancer, diabetes, asthma, and cirrhosis of the liver are seen in this population (USDOJ, 2016). Nurses need to be prepared to care for people experiencing diverse issues, such as a cerebrovascular accident, a drug overdose, or a myocardial infarction. Additionally, the stress and overcrowding of incarceration may exacerbate health concerns.

When assessing a person who is incarcerated, it is imperative to remember confidentiality; due to safety issues, custody is always with nurses when providing healthcare. Furthermore, nurses must remember not to self-disclose any part of their life outside of work. The three top reasons, in order, for federal prison incarceration include drug trafficking, offenses involving firearm violations, and sexual abuse (U.S. Sentencing Commission, 2024); to work in this field, the C/PHN must be able to put the crime for which the person was incarcerated aside to focus on providing safe and quality care while maintaining the safety of self and others.

1. *How might the nurse approach these issues?*
2. *Why would it be important to reflect on any implicit biases the C/PHN might have before working in correctional health?*

vertical bullying increases burnout, turnover rate, patient care errors, and costs (JCAHO, 2021).

C/PHN Self-care

While 2017 was the Year of the Healthy Nurse, these practices should become a part of our daily lives. Practicing health promotion themes throughout our careers places us in a better position to handle individual, family, community, and global violence. These topics should be a part of every C/PHN's daily routine. Some helpful practices to improve our self-care include the following:

Workplace

- Do not work more than three 12-hour shifts per week.
- Be consistent with shifts and do not rotate between nights and days.
- Prepare healthy meals for work.
- Have a place to retreat to for centering.

Home

- Engage in exercise/physical activity.
- Get adequate hours of sleep.
- Practice mindfulness (Williams et al., 2022).

HEALTHY PEOPLE 2030 AND VIOLENCE PREVENTION

The problem of violence is pervasive, affecting the people who experience violence directly and family members and society indirectly. Progress on select violence and abuse objectives for *Healthy People 2030* include the following (Office of Disease Prevention and Health Promotion [ODPHP], n.d.):

- Reduce homicides: In 2018, the baseline for homicides was 5.9/100,000. The target for 2030 is to decrease this to 5.5/100,000.
- Reduce emergency department visits for nonfatal self-harm injuries: Reduce these emergency department visits from 182.7/100,000 in 2017 to 144.7/1,000 for people 10 years and older.
- Reduce gun carrying among adolescents: In 2017, 4.8% of students in grades 9 through 12 carried a firearm at least 1 day within the past year. The target for 2030 is 3.7%.

See Box 18-9 for selected Healthy People 2030 violence-related objectives.

LEVELS OF PREVENTION: THE ECOLOGIC FRAMEWORK

The ecologic framework is made up of four levels: violence that affects the individual, family, community, and societal (see Fig. 18-11). This model can assist C/PHNs in implementing primary, secondary, and tertiary prevention.

BOX **18-9** *HEALTHY PEOPLE 2030*

Selected Violence-Related Objectives

Core Objectives

IVP-10	Reduce nonfatal physical assault injuries
IVP-13	Reduce firearm-related deaths
IVP-14	Reduce nonfatal firearm-related injuries
IVP-16	Reduce nonfatal child abuse and neglect
IVP-18	Reduce sexual or physical adolescent dating violence
OSH-05	Reduce work-related assaults

Developmental Objectives

IVP-D04	Reduce intimate partner violence
AH-D03	Reduce the proportion of public schools with a serious violent incident

Reprinted from Office of Disease Prevention and Health Promotion (ODPHP). (n.d.). *Healthy People 2030: Violence.* https://health.gov/healthypeople/search?query=violence

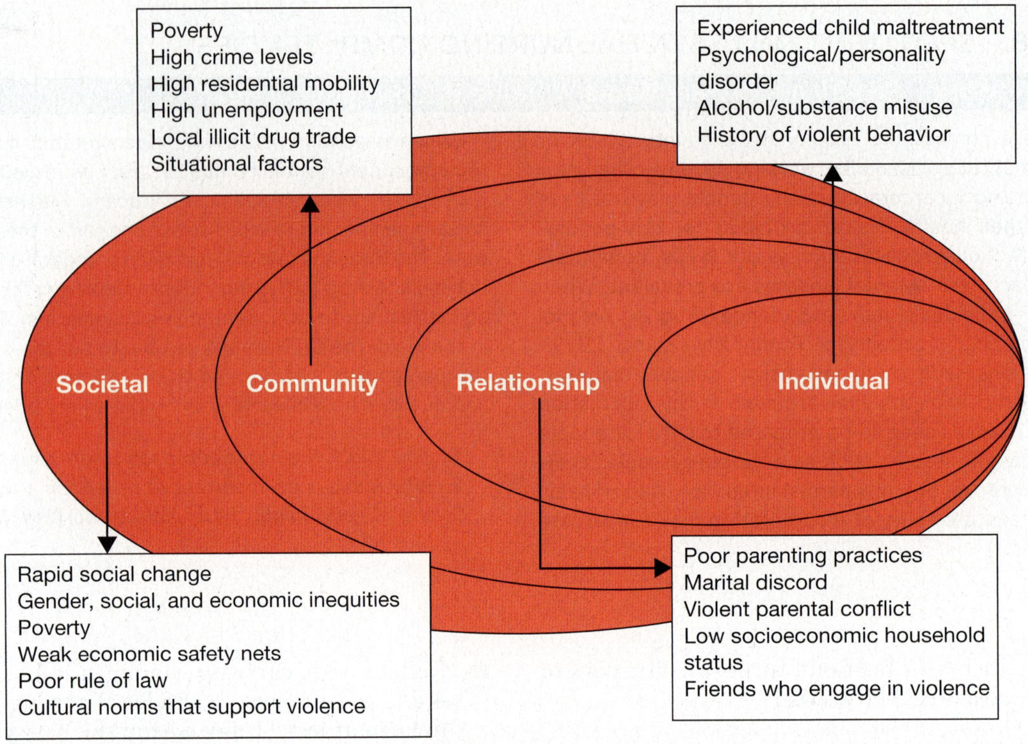

FIGURE 18-11 The ecologic framework: examples of risk factors at each level. (Adapted with permission from the World Health Organization. (n.d.). *The VPA approach.* https://www.who.int/groups/violence-prevention-alliance/approach)

All four levels must be addressed to make an everlasting change. By using the three levels of prevention in light of the ecologic framework, the C/PHN can advocate and make changes on all four levels of the framework.

Primary Prevention

Primary prevention is meant to prevent violence before it occurs. The **spectrum of prevention** offers a systematic framework for developing effective and sustainable primary prevention programs.

- Educate to all four levels.
- Change social norms on violence.
- Address environmental factors such as social determinates of health.
- Strengthen the social fiber of a community.
- Partner with community stakeholders including individuals, families, community, and society.
- Provide life skills and healthy relationship courses to adolescents.

Primary prevention is the most effective level of intervention in terms of promoting clients' health and containing costs. Primary prevention reflects a fundamental human concern for well-being and includes planned activities undertaken by the nurse to prevent an unwanted event from occurring, to protect current health and healthy functioning, and to promote improved states of health for all members of a community. For the C/PHN, any activity that fosters healthful practices will counteract unhealthful influences, thereby empowering an individual or family to avoid or better respond to a crisis. Health promotion considerations include the biopsychosocial and spiritual needs of the individual and family. The interrelatedness between families and communities cannot be overlooked or underestimated. Neighborhoods need to be enfranchised, developed, and attentive to the needs for the health and safety of all community members.

Secondary Prevention

Secondary prevention reaches out to individuals, families, communities, and societies most at risk.

- Screen at all four levels.
- Improve the living conditions of those at risk.
- Provide employment opportunities.
- Reduce the high density of liquor stores in communities.

Secondary-level prevention strategies focus on early diagnosis and prompt treatment of the effects of family crisis or violence. They seek to reduce the intensity and duration of a crisis and promote adaptive behavior. By creating a positive relationship with family members in their homes, the C/PHN can often uncover and intervene in a crisis or stop abusive situations.

People in crisis will seek and generally receive some kind of help, but the nature of that help may act in favor of or against a healthy outcome from which the participants can grow and evolve. A client's desire for assistance gives the helping professional a prime opportunity to intervene; this opportunity also presents a challenge to make the intervention as effective as possible.

One goal of crisis intervention should be to help the community, families, and individuals reestablish a sense of safety and security while allowing them to share their feelings and have those feelings validated. This process helps reestablish equilibrium at as healthy a level as possible and can result in growth.

Minimally, the goal is to resolve the immediate crisis and restore those affected to their precrisis level of functioning. Overall, intervention seeks to improve their functioning to a healthier, more mature level that will enable them to cope with and prevent future crises.

At times, the nurse may be responding to a referral regarding suspected abuse; at other times, an abusive or neglectful situation may be uncovered on a home visit made for another reason. In any case, the C/PHN has an important role in reporting suspected abuse and encouraging the child, partner/spouse, or older adult to go to the appropriate facility to seek care and to file required documentation about the abuse (Box 18-10).

Reporting Abuse

All states have reporting laws for suspected abuse, although states differ on aspects of the timeline for reporting, who to notify, and the sequence of events. The following steps represent one state's guidelines for reporting suspected child abuse (California Department of Education, 2020):

1. All mandated reporters must report known or suspected abuse or neglect.
2. Immediately, or as soon as practically possible, the designated agency such as the local child protective agency (police department after normal working hours) must be contacted by telephone and given a verbal report. During this verbal report, mandated reporters must give their name—which is kept confidential and may be revealed only in court or if the reporter waives confidentiality (others can give information anonymously)—the name and age of the child, the present location of the child, the nature and characteristics of the injury, and any other facts that led the reporter to suspect abuse or that would be helpful to the investigator.
3. The mandated reporter must notify the appropriate agency immediately or as soon as possible, followed by a written report within 36 hours. It is imperative that nurses know their state laws for reporting. If a mandated reporter fails to report known

BOX **18-10** STORIES FROM THE FIELD

Community/Public Health Nursing and a Potential Family in Crisis

You are a PHN employed at the Northville Health Department. You are following up on a referral from a community clinic's family planning clinic involving Susan, a pregnant teen who exhibited inappropriate behaviors with her 12-month-old during a clinic visit. Per the referral, staff observed the mother shouting at the child, accusing her of "being spoiled rotten." The mother also appeared quite anxious and seemed to have difficulty waiting the 15 minutes for her examination. Although the behaviors described were insufficient to warrant a report to social services, the staff felt that this young mother would benefit from intervention on the part of the nurse.

You discuss the case with family planning and immunization clinic staff, because the family receives services at both clinics. The staff are familiar with Susan and her boyfriend, Ryan. Their only interaction with Ryan was during a family planning clinic visit 2 months ago. They report Susan appeared anxious and rushed, stating, "I really need to hurry. Ryan is waiting in the car, and he gets impatient." Shortly after that, the staff tell you Ryan came running into the clinic shouting, "What the hell is taking you people so long?" He reportedly glared at Susan, and the two quickly exited the clinic.

Based on the family history you decide to make an unscheduled home visit to see how the family lives in the apartment. When you walk up to the apartment, you hear loud music coming from inside. Susan answers the door holding the baby on her hip. Ryan is in the small living room watching pornography on the TV. Susan recognizes you from the clinic and is glad to see you today. Once you introduce yourself to Ryan, you politely ask him to shut off the TV; he refuses to do so and tells you to mind your own business. You decide to meet with Susan in the kitchen. You explain that nurses often visit people who have given birth recently to assist them in finding resources. You add that as a PHN, you will be available to talk with her about her child's growth and development and the pregnancy. The client expresses interest in the visit and states, "I want you to show me some inexpensive foods to cook for my little one and my pregnancy. I need help figuring out what to do at night. Ryan is gone all night drinking with friends, leaving me to take care of the baby and clean up after dinner, and it's driving me crazy." You advise the client that you will be happy to discuss those issues with her and that you will bring information on your next visit to review together. As you leave, you inform Susan that pornography on the TV is not appropriate for small children. As you talk, Susan begins to cry and asks for advice. The nurse suggests that Susan take the little one to the park when Ryan is watching pornography or that she ask Ryan to watch it while the child is napping.

1. *Does this scenario provoke anxiety for you? If you were the nurse, how would you deal with your reaction?*
2. *How is this different from being in a hospital setting, where a supervisor is readily available?*
3. *Given this scenario, what actions would you take?*
4. *If you had been working in the family planning clinic on the day that Ryan came in, what, if anything, would you have done?*
5. *As young parents, Ryan and Susan are part of an aggregate that has unique risk factors for parenting. List as many of these risk factors as you can think of, and brainstorm about possible community/public health nursing interventions for each.*
6. *What methods would you suggest the clinic staff utilize to detect signs and symptoms of physical, sexual, or emotional abuse among this aggregate?*

or suspected instances of child abuse, they may be subject to criminal liability, punishable by up to 6 months in jail and a fine of $1000.

Similar steps are required for nurses when reporting abuse of older adults and other vulnerable adults. Such cases of suspected maltreatment are reported to a local area agency on aging, Adult Protective Services, or to the police, and a screening/documentation form is used to gather and record pertinent information. Guidelines for filing the report and agency notification are specific within each state. In cases of partner/spousal abuse, adults who are mentally competent cannot be removed involuntarily from the abusive situation. The C/PHN can communicate concern for the client's safety, emphasize the importance of being in a safe environment, and provide information regarding community resources, such as a shelter. If the adult has a life-threatening injury or illness, medical follow-up must be encouraged; however, the patient may still be reluctant to seek help.

Tools

Assessment of suspected abuse cannot be overemphasized. The C/PHN may be the only person entering the home of a family in crisis where abuse is occurring. Asking the right questions, being a careful observer, and following the correct reporting process and recording procedures may mean the difference between life and death for a person or family experiencing violence. Each state has their own forms for child and older adult abuse. A C/PHN must be aware of the forms appropriate for the state they practice in.

C/PHNs must be observant for hazards and personal safety. Follow agency policy if you ever feel a client is in harm's way. Some agencies assign nurses to go in pairs or with law enforcement to ensure safety. If the person who is violent is in the home, meet the patient in a public place and not in the home.

Tertiary Prevention

Tertiary prevention aids all four levels affected by violence and includes:

- Interventions to reduce recidivism.
- Ongoing assistance to those affected by violence—both those experiencing violence and those conducting it (CDC, 2022; Macassa et al., 2023).

Tertiary prevention focuses on the rehabilitation of the person, family, or community from the violence and crisis they have experienced. They may be alone, such as an adolescent who has experienced human trafficking and is estranged from their family. Or, they may never again have the same relationships because partners may separate—by choice, motivated by fear or hatred; by court order, if the person who conducted the abuse is incarcerated; or due to a death. Regardless of whether the people involved are an individual, a couple, a family, or a community, societal long-term intervention may be needed to establish a climate more conducive to normalcy.

Nurses may work at each level of the spectrum by educating individuals and high-risk target populations, working on coalitions to foster increased awareness and use of screening tools by healthcare providers, and working with multisector partnerships to foster change in workplace, organizational, and community policy.

VIOLENCE FROM OUTSIDE THE HOME

There has always been some degree of violence that affects people in their homes, such as burglaries, murder, or abduction (Fig. 18-5). Communities have developed resources such as the National Organization for Victim Assistance and crisis response teams, to assist individuals and groups experiencing a disaster or violent event (e.g., child murder or school shootings).

The *Global Study on Homicide 2023* provides an in-depth investigation into crime. Lethal violence can create a climate of fear and uncertainty. Intentional homicide victimizes individuals, families, and the community of the victim (United Nations Office on Drugs and Crime, 2023). Fear of violence can create psychological and physiologic stress reactions. These fears should not be ignored.

Nurses may work with extended family members of the victims or families.

THE CLINICAL JUDGMENT MODEL

Recognize and Analyze Cues and Prioritize Hypotheses

Initially, the nurse must assess the nature of the crisis and the client's or community's response to it in a focused community assessment. How severe is the problem, and what are the risks? Who is at risk? Assessment must be rapid but thorough and focused on specific areas.

- First, the nurse concentrates on the immediate problem during the assessment. Why have clients asked for help right now? What are the injuries? How do they define the problem? What precipitated the crisis? When did it occur?
- Next, the nurse focuses on the clients' perceptions of the event. What does the crisis mean to them, and how do they think it will affect their future? Are they viewing the situation realistically? When a crisis occurs in a family or group, some members see the situation differently from others.
- Determine who is available to offer support to the individual or family. Consider family, friends, clergy, other professionals, community members, and agencies. Who are the clients close to, and whom do they trust?
- Finally, the nurse assesses the clients' or community's coping abilities and resources. Have they had similar kinds of experiences in the past? What techniques have they tried in this situation, and if they did not work, why not? Clients should be encouraged to think of other stress-relieving techniques, perhaps ones they have used in the past, and to try them.

After the cues are analyzed, hypotheses are prioritized. Priorities should focus on Maslow's (1971) Hierarchy of Needs at the Physiological and Safety levels related to the act of violence. When the violence problem is more community centered, the Omaha System of documentation and information management may be useful as a nomenclature as it comprehensively includes the family and community as clients or modifiers. The system consists of three relational, reliable, and valid components used together: The Problem Classification Scheme, Intervention Scheme, and the Problem Rating Scale for Outcomes (Omaha System, 2019). The Problem Classification Scheme includes neighborhood/workplace safety in the environmental domain.

Generate Solutions

Several factors influence clients' reactions to crises. Nurses should try to determine what factors are affecting clients before making intervention plans. The nurse now also considers the clients' age, past experiences with similar types of situations, sociocultural and religious influences, general health status, and the actual assets and liabilities of the situation.

- This assessment helps clarify the situation and gives the nurse an opportunity to further encourage the clients' participation in the resolution process.
- If clients are defensive, resistant, and rigid, they are not processing clearly and can complete only simple tasks.
- It will take time before these clients can begin to solve problems related to the effects of the crisis on themselves and the loss they are experiencing, but the nurse will want to encourage them to reach this level.

A plan is based on multiple factors:

- The crisis
- The effect the crisis is having on clients' lives
- Where they are in coming to resolution of the crisis
- The ways in which significant others are affected and respond
- Their level of preparation for such a crisis
- The clients' strengths and available resources

Take Action

During implementation, the partnership between the nurse and clients is important. Discussions about what is happening, reviewing the family's plan and rationale for this approach, and making appropriate changes are necessary. Know the resources in the community so as to make referrals as needed. Referrals may include social workers, mental health practitioners, clergy, law enforcement, or support groups. The C/PHN needs to do the following:

- Demonstrate acceptance of clients.
- Use therapeutic communication.
- Assist clients in making and reaching achievable goals by using strengths.
- Communicate changes with clients prior to making them.
- Do not offer false reassurance.
- Discourage clients from blaming others.
- Help clients learn new coping skills by providing alternatives.
- Encourage clients to accept help from their social support system and spiritual resources as needed.

Evaluate Outcomes

In the final step, clients and the nurse evaluate, stabilize, and plan for the future. Evaluating the outcome of the intervention might address the following:

- Are the clients using effective coping skills and exhibiting appropriate behavior?
- Are adequate resources and support people available?
- Is the problem solved?
- Have the desired outcomes been met?
- Are modifications needed in the process?

SUMMARY

- Violence affects individuals, families, groups, communities, and all of society. Experiencing violence may result in a crisis, a temporary state of severe disequilibrium for people who face a threatening situation.
- Violence is a global public health issue. It is not limited by sociodemographic or geographic factors—anyone may experience violence or abuse at any point in their lifetime.
- Understanding the neurobiologic effects, potential subsequent health effects, and the overlapping causes of violence can help community nurses enhance protective factors, reduce risk factors, and inform violence intervention and prevention activities.
- Child abuse occurs among children of all ages, from infancy through the teen years, and may be physical, emotional, and sexual. Neglect and sexual exploitation are additional forms of child abuse.
- Community violence creates fear and uncertainty and impacts individuals and families that may live, work, play, and pray in close proximity.
- Maltreatment of older adults, often called older person abuse (or elder abuse), may involve physical, sexual, emotional, or psychological abuse; neglect; abandonment; financial or material exploitation; or self-neglect—or any combination of these mistreatments.
- C/PHN use three levels of prevention when working with families.
  - Primary prevention focuses on providing people with the skills and resources to prevent violent situations.
  - Secondary prevention involves immediate intervention at the time of the violent episode. Secondary-level prevention may include medical attention, emotional support, police, and social services involvement.
  - Tertiary prevention offers rebuilding services and helps establish equilibrium with a structure that may be different, but healthier. The spectrum of prevention offers a multidimensional approach to building community capacity to address issues of violence.
- Regardless of the method of intervention used by the C/PHN, the steps of the clinical judgment model provide an intervention framework. Assessing the assets

and liabilities, a person's willingness to change, and the nature of the violence helps the nurse form a nursing hypothesis. With this hypothesis, the nurse can begin to plan appropriate solutions to take action. Evaluation of the action plans provides the nurse with new data to assist with ongoing assessment of the progress and additional anticipatory guidance needs.

ACTIVE LEARNING EXERCISES

Some activities may be uncomfortable to participate in, please give yourself the freedom to decline any that cause undue stress.

1. The Social-Ecological Model (SEM) is a valuable framework when addressing violence. Violence affects every fabric of our being. Gather news stories that reflect all four levels of SEM. Review the risk factors highlighted in these events. How does the story narrate the event? Were you able to find news events that represent the various types of violence discussed in the chapter? Does your view of these events change after seeing them through the lens of SEM? Share your findings and reflections with your classmates and discuss your answers. (Objective 1)
2. Perhaps the "Younger Version of Me" in Box 18-7 reflects your experience. How would you respond to this student's experience and questions? Are we able, as a community and society, to answer these questions and address these concerns? Use a community's risk and protective factors to develop a plan of action for a community that has experienced gun violence. Provide all three levels of prevention. Every community has experienced some form of gun violence. Base this activity on a community you are familiar with and vested in. Return to the 10 Essential Public Health Services found in Box 2-2. Explain how equity played a factor in how you met these services. (Objective 2)
3. Explore CDC's Connect the Dots website at https://vetoviolence.cdc.gov/apps/connecting-the-dots/. Compare and contrast the risk factors for the different forms of violence. What risk factors are common among types of violence? Which types of violence have unique risk factors? What patterns do you notice? How might you use the listed protective factors to improve the risk factors? Examine your own community in which risk and protective factors are present? (Objective 3)
4. Figure 18-11 provides examples of risk factors at each level in the Social-Ecological Model. Under the societal level are risk factor examples. Choose either "gender, social, and economic inequities" or "cultural norms that support violence" and advocate for change. Identify stakeholders who can assist with changes. Who has the influence and desire to assist? Develop strategies such as social media campaigns and community forms to implement changes. (Objective 4)
5. Acts of violence affect the individual, the family, the community, and society. C/PHNs may practice or live in the area affected by the violence. As registered nurses, we must engage in self-care to care for our clients. What are some successful self-care methods you have practiced? Is there research that confirms your self-care practice? How might you use that research to help your clients? (Objective 5)

UNIT 5

Aggregate Populations

CHAPTER 19

Maternal–Child Health

"If you want to lift up humanity, empower women. It is the most comprehensive, pervasive, high-leverage investment you can make in human beings."

—Melinda Gates

KEY TERMS

- Abusive head trauma
- Alcohol-related birth defects
- Alcohol-related neurodevelopmental disorder
- Child abuse
- Fetal alcohol effects
- Fetal alcohol spectrum disorders (FASDs)
- Fetal alcohol syndrome (FAS)
- Gestational diabetes mellitus (GDM)
- Head Start
- High-risk families
- Infant
- Low birth weight (LBW)
- Preschooler
- Respiratory syncytial virus (RSV)
- Shaken baby syndrome
- Sudden infant death syndrome (SIDS)
- Toddler
- Very low birth weight (VLBW)

LEARNING OBJECTIVES

Upon mastery of this chapter, you should be able to:

1. Identify major health problems and concerns for childbearing people, infants, toddlers, and preschoolers in the United States and globally.
2. Examine the role of community partnerships and programs to improve health outcomes for childbearing families.
3. Examine the socioeconomic impact health promotion programs have on maternal–child populations.
4. Identify the role of the public and community/public health nurse (C/PHN) as a contributor to policy development, policy change, and improvements in disparities within the maternal–child population.
5. Recognize the role of the C/PHN as an advocate within the community they serve with the ability to engage in relationship-building and leadership to promote influence at a local, state, national, and global level.

INTRODUCTION

Maternal and child populations have always been priorities for public health and community and public health nurses (C/PHNs). These populations consist of childbearing people (including pregnant adolescents), infants, children, and adolescents. In this chapter, the focus is specifically on childbearing people (including adolescents) and children from birth through age 4 years. Often, more than half of the practice of C/PHNs in official public health agencies involves primary prevention work with birthing parents, such as family planning, preconception care, provision of prenatal care, and monitoring infant health. Why do maternal–infant populations require this amount of attention from C/PHNs? Despite advanced technology and availability of excellent perinatal services in the United States, it often has less than optimal birth outcomes—for instance, 311,932 low birth weight (LBW) and 383,979 preterm infants were born in 2021 (Centers for Disease Control and Prevention [CDC], 2023a). Also, certain segments of the maternal and infant populations, such as adolescent birthing parents, those with low incomes, and people of color, remain at high risk for disparities in regard to maternal deaths and complications and child risk and illness. Although some patients receive excellent prenatal care and benefit from diagnostic and technological resources, many others lack access to prenatal care.

This chapter addresses the following:

- The major areas of concern regarding population health for maternal–infant clients
- It also explores the global needs and related services available to the youngest and, thus, most vulnerable of society's members.
- Health services that are commonly available in the United States for pregnant and postpartum patients, as well as infants, toddlers, and preschoolers, and the role of the C/PHN in providing those services.

HEALTH STATUS AND NEEDS OF PREGNANT PEOPLE AND INFANTS

C/PHNs constitute a key group of health professionals involved in both program planning and the actual delivery of services to birthing parents and babies in the community. In the public health sector, these nurses are the largest group of professionals practicing public health. A solid understanding of vital statistics and other data is important to determine the appropriateness and effectiveness of programs and services. A review of the global and national vital statistics provides insight into the major issues that face the maternal and child populations.

Global Overview

In 2020, 287,000 birthing patients died in childbirth or shortly thereafter; 95% of those occurred in low and lower middle-income countries (World Health Organization [WHO], 2023a). While this is a stark decrease from numbers seen in the past, we are a far cry from reaching the sustainable development goal of 70 maternal deaths per 100,000 live births by 2030 (UNICEF, 2023). Programs such as Every Newborn Action Plan (WHO, 2024a) and groups such as Ending Preventable Maternal Mortality (WHO, 2024b) help C/PHNs globally ensure that the maternal mortality rate (MMR) continues to drop.

Maternal Mortality Rate

One of the major indicators of population health is maternal health, which is often measured by the MMR. The MMR is a measure of obstetric risk and is determined by dividing the number of maternal deaths by the number of live births per 100,000. The National Pregnancy-Related Mortality Surveillance, conducted by the CDC, helps our understanding of risk factors and the causes of maternal mortality (CDC, 2023b). Most maternal deaths are the result of direct causes (complications of pregnancy, labor, and delivery), hypertensive disorders, intervention omissions or incorrect treatment, the chain of events resulting from any one of these, and unsafe abortions. In resource-limited countries, the MMR is 430 per 100,000 live births, compared with resource-abundant countries, where the MMR is around 12 per 100,000 live births—a very wide disparity (WHO, 2023c). The U.S.'s MMR has risen from 20.1 per 100,000 live births in 2019 to 32.9 per 100,000 in 2021 (CDC, 2023p; Hoyert, 2023). More alarming is the significant disparity between Black patients' MMR of 69.9 per 100,000 and White patients' MMR of 26.6. According to Hill et al. (2022), MMR was higher in Black people at 41.4 and at 26.2 in Alaska Native (American Indian and Alaska Native [AIAN]) people when compared to White people at 13.7 per 100,000 births. Furthermore, pregnancy-related death increases with age and with lack of prenatal care for all races (Hoyert, 2023). The CDC has devolved multidisciplinary committees at the state and local levels in the majority of states and one territory to help move toward achieving the *Healthy People 2030* goal of reducing maternal deaths (2023d).

Primary causes of MMR include the following:

- Lack of or inadequate healthcare
- Limited or lack access to prenatal care
- Social and economic determinants of health
- Discrimination by healthcare providers
- Structural racism (Hill et al., 2022)

Infant and Child Mortality Rates

Another critical population health indicator are the infant and child mortality rates. Globally, 5 million children under 5 years of age died in 2020, which is a significant decrease from the 12.6 million who died in 1990 (WHO, 2022). More than half of the deaths of children under 5 years of age are preventable, and the interventions are affordable (WHO, 2022). In the United States, the infant mortality rate (number of deaths of children under 1 year) was 5.0 per 1000 live births in 2020 (CDC, 2021a). Although this is a decrease from years past, 19,582 infants still died in 2020 in the United States.

- Infant Mortality Rate (IMR) for Black populations was 10.4 per 1000 births, whereas for White populations, it was 4.4 per 1000 births.
- Similar to the White IMR, Hispanic IMR was 4.7 per 1000 births.
- AIAN and Native Hawaiian and Other Pacific Islander (NHOPI) differed slightly as well with rates at 7.7 and 7.2 (Hill et al., 2022).
- While IMR rates are highest in the southern states, 16 states meet the *Healthy People 2030* target of 5.0 per 1000 infant deaths (CDC, 2022a). See Figure 19-1 for U.S. IMR ethnic comparison data.

The causes of infant mortality include the following:

- Preterm birth
- Low birth weight
- Birth defects
- Sudden infant death syndrome
- Injuries to infant (Hill et al., 2022)

Black, American Indian, AIAN, and NHOPI people received less or no prenatal care and had higher rates of preterm births and LBW when compared to White people (Hill et al., 2022).

Another area of concern is that people of color either started prenatal care in the third trimester or did not start at all, placing the newborn at risk.

- NHOPI people were four times more likely to either start prenatal care in the third trimester or not at all when compared to White people at 19% versus 5%; for Black people, this discrepancy was 9% to 5% (Hill et al., 2022).

To learn more about MMR, IMR, and racial disparities, see Hill et al.'s 2022 research "Racial Disparities in Maternal and Infant Health: Current Status and Efforts to Address Them" (see References for further details).

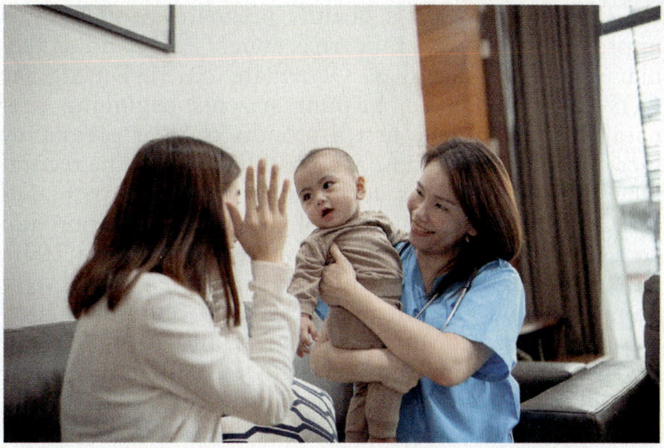

FIGURE 19-2 Support for birthing parents and children helps ensure healthier families.

National Overview

In the United States, birth rates continued to decrease from 13.5 live births per 1000 people assigned female at birth in 2009 to 11.4 live births per 1000 in 2019 (CDC, 2023e).

- The largest rate of decline was seen in those aged 15 to 29 years, with a slight increase in those aged 40 to 54.
- Birth rates declined for non-Hispanic White, Hispanic/Latina(x), and African American people.
- Just over 40% of births were to people who do not have a partner or spouse (Martin et al., 2019). When such individuals rely on a single income, financial resources are more limited, causing many of them to raise their children at poverty or near-poverty income levels, which impacts their health and their children's health over the life course of both (see Fig. 19-2).

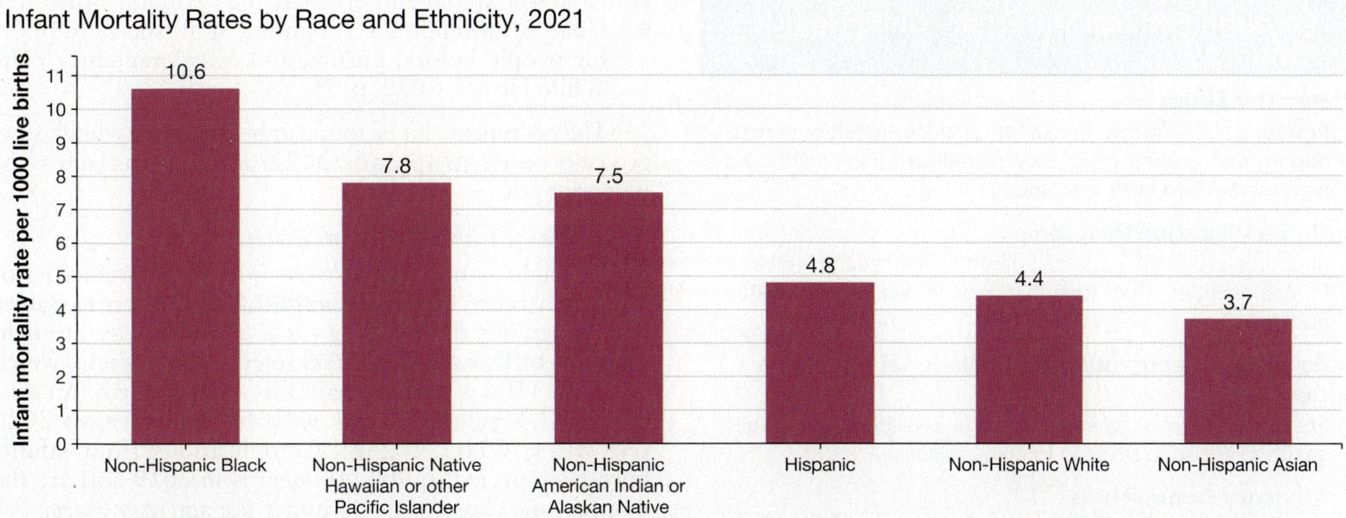

FIGURE 19-1 Infant mortality rates by race and ethnicity, 2021. (Reprinted from Centers for Disease Control and Prevention. (2023). https://www.cdc.gov/reproductivehealth/maternalinfanthealth/infantmortality.htm)

The likelihood of a healthy pregnancy and baby is improved when prenatal care is sought early and at regular intervals (Martin & Osterman, 2023). During the COVID-19 pandemic, birthing parents beginning prenatal care within the first 4 months of their pregnancy increased; however, those who had fewer than the recommended prenatal visits during their pregnancy increased by 22%. Overall, the number of patients with no prenatal care rose by 2.1% in 2021 compared to 2019. In 2020, 11.6% of childbearing people in the United States were uninsured, and 42% of the births that occurred in 2020 were covered by Medicaid (March of Dimes, 2020a). Seventy-two percent of those who were uninsured were least likely to receive adequate prenatal care. This correlates with health inequity characteristics such as race and ethnicity, poverty, and low maternal education levels (less than high school education).

Historically, the health of U.S. people assigned female at birth and children has largely fallen under the umbrella of Title V of the Social Security Act, enacted in 1935 (see Chapter 6). Title V is "the longest-standing public health legislation in American history" and came to fruition after other legislation established a National Birth Registry; provided *Infant Care*, the first educational pamphlet; established the Children's Bureau; and provided protection against child labor practices (i.e., the first Child Labor Law of 1916; MCHB, n.d.-a, para. 4). For an illustration of MCHB functions and programs, see Box 19-1.

Since the inception of Title V, many programs have been developed with the goal of improving the health of people of childbearing age, as well as infants and children.

- Research areas have included prenatal and pregnancy health, child development and parenting, and improving healthcare systems and delivery of care, as well as obesity, nutrition, medical homes, school services and outcomes, and behavioral health (MCHB, n.d.-a).

BOX 19-1 Types of Services Offered Through Federal Maternal—Child Health Funding

Healthy Start

Programs to improve health of birthing parents before, during, and beyond pregnancy to reduce infant death and increase positive birth outcomes

Home Visitation Programs

Supports pregnant patients, parents, and young children in communities that face barriers in achieving healthy outcomes

Adolescent and Young Adult National Resource Center

Specific programs to equip medical providers and public health agencies to respond to unique needs of youth

Advisory Committees

Committees on heritable disorders in newborns and children, infant and maternal mortality, innovation on maternal health community care, and innovation on maternal health

Source: https://mchb.hrsa.gov/programs-impact/programs (n.d.-b).

- Healthy Start grants were awarded in 1991 with the goal of reducing rates of infant mortality, LBW, premature births, and maternal deaths (MCHB, n.d.-b).
- Evaluation of Healthy Start programs reveals that almost all programs provide home visitation to prenatal clients, and most continued these visits to infants and toddlers.
- Health education, smoking cessation counseling, services for perinatal depression, and involvement of birthing parents' partners are hallmarks of most programs.

In 2021, $2.4 billion in expenditures was used under Title V to improve the health of birthing parents, infants, and children (MCHB, n.d.-c). Maternal, Infant, and Early Childhood Home Visiting Program (Home Visiting Program) accounted for $783 million of those expenditures. This program provides C/PHN visits, assistance from social workers, teaching from early childhood educators, and services from other professionals to expectant families (MCHB, n.d.-d). Early improvements in six benchmark areas were noted (MCHB, n.d.-e, p. 3):

- Maternal and newborn health
- Child injuries, child maltreatment, and emergency department visits
- School readiness and achievement
- Crime or domestic violence
- Family economic self-sufficiency
- Service coordination/referrals for other community resources/support

In 2022, the White House released White House Blueprint for Addressing the Maternal Health Crisis. The document addresses five goals to improve maternal health:

- Goal 1: Increase access to and coverage of comprehensive high-quality maternal health services, including behavioral health services
- Goal 2: Ensure those giving birth are heard and are decision-makers in accountable systems of care
- Goal 3: Advance data collection, standardization, transparency, research, and analysis
- Goal 4: Expand and diversify the perinatal workforce
- Goal 5: Strengthen economic and social support for people before, during, and after pregnancy (The White House, 2022, p. 2).

The document can be found at https://www.whitehouse.gov/wp-content/uploads/2022/06/Maternal-Health-Blueprint.pdf

Birth Weight and Preterm Birth

Birth weight is one of the most important predictors of infant mortality. **Low birth weight (LBW)** refers to babies who weigh less than 2500 g (or less than 5.5 lb) at birth; **very low birth weight (VLBW)** refers to babies who weigh less than 1500 g (or less than 3 lb 4 oz) at birth. An estimated 13.4 million infants were born preterm in 2020 (Fig. 19-3; WHO, 2023b). Complications from infants born preterm led to 900,000 deaths in 2019 and are the number-one cause of death under the age of 5 years.

Infant complications of preterm birth include a plethora of concerns:

- Hearing and vision problems; acute respiratory, gastrointestinal, and immunologic problems.

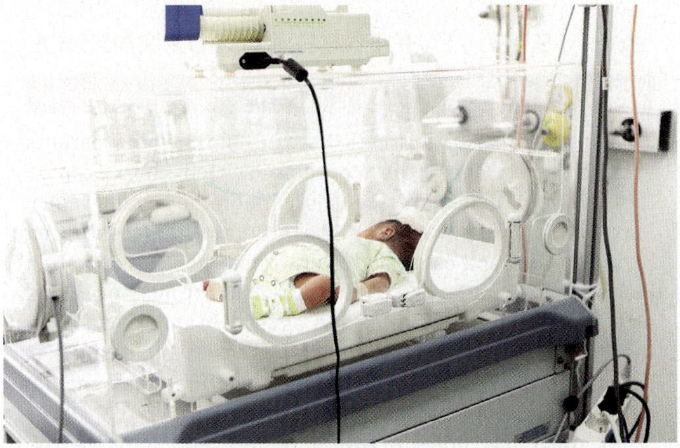

FIGURE 19-3 Infant in the neonatal intensive care unit.

- Central nervous system, motor, cognitive, behavioral, and socioemotional disorders.
- Growth concerns as well as acute and chronic health and developmental problems.
- Families of these infants are burdened with additional economic and emotional costs.
- Increased parental stress, poorer maternal mental health, or increased family stressors compared with those preterm infants who did not have feeding difficulties.

Maternal mortality, LBW, and VLBW are three areas requiring attention by healthcare providers and the public health system. Nurses can contribute to reducing these rates and societal costs through outreach, surveillance, health teaching, counseling, and referral (WHO, 2023b).

In addition to infant deaths and LBW, the effects of pregnancy and childbirth on birthing parents are other important indicators of health and reflect discrepancies in access to reproductive healthcare. The United States suffers from a lack of qualified maternity care providers, no guarantee of paid parental leave and provider home visits, as well as the highest MMR (Melillo, 2020).

One of the maternal–child objectives for *Healthy People 2030* is to improve the proportion of infants who are breastfed. Breastfeeding is beneficial to both birthing parent and infant, and recently, 83.2% of birthing parents reported ever breastfeeding, with only 24.9% continuing for the recommended 6-month period exclusively (U.S. Breastfeeding Committee (USBC), 2022). It is estimated that 3.6 billion dollars in medical costs could be saved if the exclusive 6-month breastfeeding rate was increased to the recommended level of 50% by the U.S. Surgeon General (Quesada et al., 2020). See Box 19-2 for a partial list *Healthy People 2030* maternal, infant, and child health objectives. A complete list of maternal, infant, and child health objectives is found at https://health.gov/healthypeople/search?query=maternal+child+health

Adolescent Birthing Parents

The teen birth rate (birthing parents aged 15 to 19) in 2020 was 15.4 per 1000 births, which is down 75% from a peak in 1991 of 61.8 per 1000 births (U.S. Department of Health and Human Services [USDHHS], n.d.). While the teen birth rate has continued to decline since 2009, the United States still has a higher teen birth rate than many other resource-abundant countries. Fifteen percent of the teen births in 2020 were not the first birth for these teens. See Chapter 20 for more on adolescent pregnancy.

BOX 19-2 *HEALTHY PEOPLE 2030*

Objectives for Maternal, Infant, and Child Health

Improve the health and safety of infants; prevent pregnancy complications and maternal deaths; improve patients' health before, during, and after pregnancy; and improve the health and well-being of children.

Core Objectives

MICH-02	Reduce the rate of all infant deaths
MICH-04	Reduce maternal deaths
MICH-05	Reduce severe maternal complications identified during delivery hospitalizations
MICH-06	Reduce cesarean births among low-risk women with no prior births
MICH-07	Reduce preterm births
MICH-08	Increase the proportion of pregnant women who receive early and adequate prenatal care
MICH-09	Increase abstinence from alcohol among pregnant women
MICH-10	Increase abstinence from cigarette smoking among pregnant women
MICH-11	Increase abstinence from illicit drugs among pregnant women
MICH-15	Increase the proportion of infants who are breastfed exclusively through age 6 months
MICH-17	Increase the proportion of children who receive a developmental screening

Developmental Objectives

MICH-D01	Increase the proportion of women who get screened for postpartum depression

Reprinted from Office of Disease Prevention and Health Promotion (ODPHP). (n.d.-a.). Pregnancy and Childbirth. *Healthy People 2030.* U.S. Department of Health and Human Services. https://www.healthypeople.gov/2020/topics-objectives/topic/maternal-infant-and-child-health/objectives and https://health.gov/healthypeople/objectives-and-data/browse-objectives/pregnancy-and-childbirth

Risk Factors for Pregnant People and Infants

Most pregnant people in the United States are healthy; they have normal pregnancies and produce healthy babies. Many factors contribute to the health problems of patients who figure in the statistics on infant mortality and LBW. The factors associated with LBW and infant mortality can be grouped into three categories (CDC, 2022b):

1. Lifestyle: smoking, secondhand smoke exposure, inadequate nutrition, alcohol consumption, substance misuse, late prenatal care, environmental toxins, stress, violence, and lack of social support
2. Sociodemographic: maternal age below 15 or above 35 years, low educational level, poverty, domestic violence, and unmarried status
3. Medical and gestational history: primiparity, multiple gestation, short interpregnancy intervals, premature rupture of the membranes, uterine anomaly, febrile illness during pregnancy, spontaneous abortion, genetic factors, gestation-induced hypertension, less-than-ideal weight gain during pregnancy, and diabetes

It is in the area of lifestyle choices that nurses can have the most significant impact on pregnancy outcomes such as LBW, preterm birth, and infant mortality. Programs that provide access to and funding for C/PHNs are available through federal, state, and local funding (Box 19-3).

Substance Use and Misuse

Another area of concern is substance use and misuse among the childbearing population. The adverse consequences associated with the use of tobacco, alcohol, and illicit drugs during pregnancy are wide ranging and include preterm birth, LBW, and fetal alcohol spectrum disorders (FASDs; described later in this chapter). This puts these patients and their fetuses in double jeopardy; not only are they at risk from the consequences of alcohol or drug use, but they also do not receive the preventive prenatal care that can eliminate or reduce other obstetric complications. This is most often related to the pregnant person's concerns about the legal ramifications of substance use while pregnant if they do seek care.

Substance misuse during pregnancy is a problem with staggering social and medical implications, such as preterm births, LBW, miscarriage, placental abruption, developmental delays, and child behavior and learning difficulties later in life (CDC, 2023f). A 2020 survey found that 20% of pregnant people had at least one drink containing alcohol in the past 30 days, and of these individuals, 40% had used other substances as well; also, 74% of pregnant people continued smoking cigarettes during pregnancy (CDC, 2023f).

Opioid use disorder diagnosed in pregnant people has nearly quadrupled in recent years (CDC, 2022c).

- Opioid use disorder causes serious health issues that range from low birth rate, stillbirths, maternal mortality, and neonatal abstinence syndrome (NAS) (CDC, 2022c).
- The United States has seen an increased incidence of NAS as a result of heroin or other opioid use in pregnancy, with a NAS diagnosis every 25 minutes (Anbalagan & Mendez, 2020).

BOX 19-3 EVIDENCE-BASED PRACTICE

Home Visiting

There are many ways C/PHNs can help birthing parents and babies. One of the programs in which a nurse can do this, in a very fundamental way, is through the Nurse–Family Partnership (NFP) program. The program was created by Dr. David Olds and came out of his experience working at an inner-city day care with preschoolers suffering the effects of the struggles of poverty and abuse. He quickly realized that to make an impact, he needed to reach families earlier in life with the help of trained nurses and first-time and at-risk birthing parents. Thus, the NFP was born.

Dr. Olds has done research to test and improve the program in Elmira, NY; Memphis, TN; and Denver, CO. The results have been consistent; NFP improves the lives of both birthing parents and babies through the tenacious work of a registered nurse (RN) and the relationship that is formed between the RN and the client. The client begins to see the nurse as part of the family, and someone that they can go to with any concern. The NFP nurse home visitor becomes a life coach, lifting the client up in what can be one of the most difficult parts of the life of a person assigned female at birth: pregnancy and the first 2 years of parenting a child.

NFP nurses offer praise and screen the baby to make sure milestones are being met. Parenting skills are taught, references are made, if needed, and encouragement is given. Clients can contact their NFP nurse with questions about their bodies, their babies, future plans, relationships, and so much more.

The program provides the kind of consistency and advocacy that many of the clients have never experienced. The NFP nurse is a true ally and fierce advocate for both birthing parent and baby in the critical early years. To date, the NFP has been funded by public and private sources and is now operating in forty U.S. states, the U.S. Virgin Islands, and many tribal communities.

Source: Nurse-Family Partnership (n.d.-a., n.d.-b).

- Between 1999 and 2014, there was a 333% increase in NAS (Anbalagan & Mendez, 2020).
- The states with the highest numbers of newborns hospitalized for NAS include West Virginia, Maine, Delaware, Kentucky, and South Dakota (U.S. Agency for Healthcare Research and Quality, 2019).

Yet, not all states mandate the reporting of NAS, and/or states may differ in the NAS definition, which causes problems in determining rates (Anbalagan & Mendez, 2020) NAS occurs because of the sudden discontinuation of fetal exposure to substances such as fentanyl, heroin, or opioids during pregnancy (CDC, 2022c). Withdrawal symptoms experienced by these infants include irritability, excessive or high-pitched crying, tremors, and gastrointestinal problems such as diarrhea. If nonpharmacologic care does not alleviate these symptoms, morphine is commonly used. The long-term effects of NAS are not fully known, but these children may have poor school performance, vision issues, cognitive disabilities, neurodevelopmental delays, and higher mortality rates (Anbalagan & Mendez, 2020). It is clear more research needs to be done on this vulnerable population.

Although substance use is uncommon during pregnancy, there are certain drug combinations to be aware of (CDC, 2023g):

- One or more alcoholic drinks and other substances
- Marijuana and tobacco use
- Illicit opioid use and alcohol
- Medically prescribed opioid use and tobacco

The primary, secondary, and tertiary prevention interventions of the C/PHN cannot be underestimated when drug use takes such a high toll on every aspect of the person, the family, and the community.

Alcohol Use

Another societal problem is the use of and dependency on alcohol. Among pregnant people, the alcohol use rate is 10.2%, with binge drinking at a rate of 3.1% (Dejong et al., 2019).

The conditions that can occur in a child due to maternal drinking of alcohol during pregnancy are collectively known as **fetal alcohol spectrum disorders (FASDs)**. The most severe type of FASD is **fetal alcohol syndrome (FAS)**, which can result in facial anomalies, delayed growth and development, neurologic congenital disorders, learning and sensory difficulties, and even death. What was once termed **fetal alcohol effects** is now separated into the more descriptive categories of **alcohol-related birth defects** (ARBD) and **alcohol-related neurodevelopmental disorder** (ARND) (CDC, 2023f). Whereas ARBD indicates difficulties with hearing, bones, heart, and kidneys, ARND indicates intellectual disabilities or behavior issues. Physical signs of FASDs are often much more subtle than in people who have FAS. However, those with FASD may have one or more of the following behaviors or characteristics (CDC, 2022d):

- Small size for gestational age or small stature in relation to peers
- Facial anomalies (e.g., smooth philtrum: the area between the upper lip and base of the nose is smooth and without ridges)
- Poor coordination
- Hyperactivity, attention issues, and learning disabilities
- Difficulties in school, especially with math
- Developmental disabilities (e.g., speech and language delays)
- Intellectual disability or low intelligence quotient
- Vision and hearing difficulties; issues with the heart, kidneys, and bones
- Poor reasoning and judgment skills
- Sleep and sucking disturbances in infancy

It is important to provide evidence-based primary prevention before pregnancy and to reach patients before drinking becomes such a large part of their lives that they are unable or unwilling to abstain during pregnancy. To learn more about the educational needs of this population, the CDC and state health departments collect population-based information on maternal preconception, prenatal, pregnancy, and postpartum behaviors and experiences through the Pregnancy Risk Assessment Monitoring System. By understanding these concerns, education can focus on primary prevention.

Working with people assigned female at birth of childbearing age to improve their general health behaviors and promote better preparation for pregnancy is essential. For people who use substances and are pregnant or have already had a child, maternal drug and alcohol treatment programs that focus on supportive parent–child attachment, enhancement of parenting and child-rearing capabilities, and encouragement of the use of support systems that can improve child health and cognitive development are needed. In-home family skills training and parenting education programs that are evidence based and promote C/PHN and client rapport can be effective methods of working with people with a substance use disorder and their children who are at risk; however, more studies are recommended. The NFP completed a study between 2014 and 2017 to see the program's impact on decreasing alcohol, cigarette, and drug use among patients. A decrease of 2.6% by 34 to 36 weeks was seen with patients enrolled in the NFP versus 1.9% of those with routine prenatal care (Catherine et al., 2021).

Tobacco Use

Roughly 10% of people assigned female at birth use tobacco products (Cornelius et al., 2023). The nicotine in tobacco is a major a substance that can induce dependency, and smoking is a dependency that many people find difficult to stop. Although the risk factors of smoking are well documented, some pregnant people continue to smoke. Smoking during pregnancy is one of the most studied risk factors in obstetric assessment. Pregnant people, who may have started smoking as adolescents, often continue to smoke in response to life stressors. From a population and C/PHN perspective, one study found that the higher the density of tobacco stores in a neighborhood, the higher the prevalence of smoking among pregnant people (Galiatsatos et al., 2020). The use of e-cigarettes, or vaping, is a health danger for pregnant people; this nicotine delivery system also poses threats to the developing fetus. Also, the exhaled aerosol that is advertised to be "water vapor" contains nicotine and other chemicals such as metals, nitrosamines, and volatile organic compounds (American Cancer Society, 2022). In a systematic review, Bell et al. (2023) found infants born to people who vaped during pregnancy were at risk for small-for-gestation age, preterm birth, and/or LBW. An initial health history of a pregnant person should always include the assessment of tobacco use, smoking status, and exposure to smoke in the personal environment. If a pregnant person lives with a smoker, both the person and their fetus can be negatively affected by the other person's smoking.

The C/PHN must not only advise clients to quit smoking but also offer supportive and empathetic approaches to stress reduction during smoking cessation, including methods or interventions that can help other symptom management that is associated with smoking cessation. For example, the C/PHN may do the following:

- Counsel clients individually.
- Refer for behavioral therapy.
- Provide self-help manuals.
- Recommend nicotine replacement therapy or medication.
- Encourage support groups.

Any permanent reduction in the number of cigarettes smoked, the amount of secondhand smoke inhaled, or the amount of smokeless tobacco products used is helpful in improving the health of both birthing parent and fetus.

Intimate Partner Violence

Intimate partner violence (IPV) is any sexual, physical, economic, and psychological abuse taken by someone against an intimate partner or ex-partner (Román-Gálvez et al., 2021). Pregnancy is a vulnerable period for pregnant people and can increase their risk for IPV. It is estimated that 15% to 40.5% of pregnant people experience IPV throughout the world (Román-Gálvez et al., 2021). Reasons for increased IPV during pregnancy can be an unintended pregnancy, increased stress related to supporting a child, and jealousy. People experiencing IPV may avoid prenatal care services for a variety of reasons such as injuries, control by their partners, and a lack of resources such as transportation or money for mass transit. Pregnant people who experience psychological IPV have a one-fold increase in the risk of suicidal ideation. IPV can also have effects on the newborn and infant (Román-Gálvez et al., 2021).

Sexually Transmitted Infections (STI) and Sexually Transmitted Diseases (STD)

Although STI and STD have been used interchangeably for some time, there are differences between the two terms. STIs refer to a person being infected but asymptotic, and STD is used when symptoms are present (Rudderown, 2019). The 2018 data from the CDC's STI surveillance program estimates that 1 in 5 people tested positive for an STI in a given day, which is about 26 million new cases, costing the healthcare system about $16 billion across the lifetime (CDC, 2022e). The CDC (2020a) has recommended STD screening of all pregnant people at the initial prenatal visit for *Chlamydia*, hepatitis B (and hepatitis C for high-risk patients), HIV, and syphilis. Further, they recommend screening high-risk pregnant people for gonorrhea.

STIs can pass from birthing parent to baby. Syphilis can cross the placenta and infect the fetus, as can HIV—which can also be passed to the infant through breastfeeding (CDC, 2022f). Congenital syphilis is on the rise at alarming rates. Between 2012 and 2017, the rate of congenital syphilis increased 750% in California (California Department of Public Health, 2019). This increase is seen across the United States, where there has been a 153% increase from 2013 to 2017 to 918 cases (Schmidt et al., 2019). Other STIs (e.g., gonorrhea, hepatitis B, *Chlamydia*, genital herpes) can infect the baby as it passes through the birth canal during delivery. LBW, stillbirth, conjunctivitis, blindness, deafness, neurologic damage, chronic liver disease, and cirrhosis, along with neonatal sepsis and pneumonia, are possible infant complications of maternal STIs. Birthing parents may have premature rupture of membranes and resultant infection or may have a premature onset of labor.

Pregnant people who discover they have an STI/STD often feel ashamed, betrayed, embarrassed, and angry. Those who are asymptomatic may not realize they are infected or deny the existence of the disease and fail to carry out the treatment plan after diagnosis. Although educating the pregnant client about the effects of STI/STD is critical, providing information alone is not enough. The C/PHN has a pivotal role in enhancing the empowerment of clients so they can act on the information they receive. The C/PHN engages with pregnant clients and helps them understand that they have control over their bodies. Usually, STI/STD are first discovered in pregnancy during routine prenatal screening, which places the clinic nurse and the nurse who may make home visits in the position to take an affirmative approach to treatment and follow-up.

HIV and AIDS

There were 39 million people living with human immunodeficiency virus (HIV) in 2022, and 46% of the new infections were in people assigned female at birth (HIV.gov, 2023). Most children with acquired immunodeficiency syndrome (AIDS) are children of birthing parents who are HIV positive (WHO, 2023c). Transmission of HIV from the birthiing parent to the child can be almost fully prevented with antiretroviral treatment for both (WHO, 2023a). To reduce this type of transmission, patients must seek prenatal care early enough in their pregnancies for the antiretroviral drug to be effective. The use of antiretrovirals has reduced the transmission of HIV in the United States and Europe to about 1% (HIVinfo.gov, 2023).

In the United States and other resource-abundant nations, patients with HIV infections are advised not to breastfeed their infants because there is a chance that the infants will become infected with HIV from breast milk (CDC, 2023h). The C/PHN focuses their teaching on providing a safe, available, and low-cost form of infant formula. In resource-limited countries, the lack of clean water makes formula feeding dangerous, and breastfeeding is usually recommended. The infection rate for HIV from breastfeeding and the mortality rate from formula made with impure water are about the same, resulting in a dilemma for patients and healthcare providers in such countries.

Poor Nutrition, Weight Gain, and Oral Health

Research has demonstrated a positive correlation between weight gain during pregnancy and normal birth weight in babies. In 2009, the Institute of Medicine (IOM) released new guidelines for weight gain during pregnancy based on body mass indices. The American College of Obstetricians and Gynecologists reaffirmed in 2023 that the 2009 Institute of Medicine gestational weight gain guidelines are important for clinicians to use. Weight gain recommendations are based on prepregnancy body mass indices of the patient (see Fig. 19-4), and clinicians should discuss weight gain, diet, and exercise goals initially and throughout the pregnancy to achieve these goals.

Studies have shown that about 48% of pregnant people in the United States gain more than the recommended amount of weight (CDC, 2022b). Gestational diabetes poses the greatest risk to pregnant people with obesity and increases the risk of preterm birth (CDC, 2022g). C/PHNs who work with pregnant people who have severe obesity can help them most by emphasizing good nutrition and by encouraging them to maintain their prepregnant weight without drastically reducing caloric

If before pregnancy, you were...	You should gain...
Underweight BMI less than 18.5	28–40 pounds
Normal Weight BMI 18.5–24.9	25–35 pounds
Overweight BMI 25.0–29.9	15–25 pounds
Obese BMI 30.0–39.9	11–20 pounds

FIGURE 19-4 Weight gain recommendation for people pregnant with one baby. (Adapted from Centers for Disease Control and Prevention. (2024). Retrived from https://www.cdc.gov/maternal-infant-health/pregnancy-weight/index.html)

intake. This can be accomplished primarily by a marked decrease in the consumption of "empty calories" from junk food and an increased intake of fruits, vegetables, and low-fat sources of calcium. Pregnancy is never a time for dieting. Nutritional counseling can have an additional benefit in that it may ultimately decrease the risk of obesity or eating disorders in the client's children. Exercise during pregnancy is essential; it can moderate maternal weight gain and improve overall fitness, which is desirable for the labor and delivery process.

After assessment, the C/PHN can determine whether any weight gain over the recommended amount is related to the consumption of additional calories, to limited activity, or to fluid retention. Each cause must be managed differently.

People who are lower weight have twice as many LBW babies as those whose weight is within the typical range. Nutritional teaching is part of the C/PHN's role when working with a pregnant person who has difficulty gaining the recommended weight during pregnancy. Finding ways to add calories to foods and increasing the person's desire to eat are effective methods to improve maternal weight gain. Insufficient caloric intake in pregnant adolescents (who themselves are still growing) is an additional concern for their future health and the health of the infant.

Periodontal infection may affect around 40% of people of childbearing age and is especially common among those who may not have adequate access to dental healthcare.

- Maternal periodontal disease has been linked to preterm birth, LBW, preeclampsia, and early fetal loss.
- Recent studies have not shown the reduction of preterm birth or LBW among those infants whose birthing parents received periodontal therapy in pregnancy.
- Not only is dental health important during pregnancy, but poor dental hygiene and disease have been linked to health conditions, such as cardiovascular disease and diabetes.
- High maternal levels of the bacteria that cause cavities have been associated with a greater chance of subsequent dental caries in the infant (American Dental Association, 2023).

C/PHNs should teach people of childbearing age the importance of regular dental health checkups and proper dental hygiene, along with making referrals for dental treatment when needed. Because there is frequently a shortage of dental providers to see low-income patients, the nurse sometimes must advocate for pregnant people who need oral health treatment, such as gingivitis or dental caries or infections. Dental health should be a part of general primary preventive education for all childbearing-age people and a major teaching and screening element of prenatal care.

Socioeconomic Status and Social Inequality

Poverty plays a role in pregnancy and birth outcomes. Social and economic disparities are factors in preterm birth in both resource-abundant and resource-limited nations and reflect some of the social determinants of health. These relationships may be indirect, as people with low income often lack health insurance, have less access to quality prenatal care services, have poorer nutrition, and are exposed to more situational and psychological stressors. In the United States, several factors contribute to early access to prenatal care: socioeconomic status, higher education, race, and where in the country the patient lives (National Conference of State Legislatures, 2021). Aside from rural areas being known for having lower median incomes and education levels, there are areas that have zero OB providers (OB/GYN or CNM) per 10,000 live births (see Fig. 19-5).

Social, economic, political, and cultural structures contribute to reproductive health issues. Practices that address inequalities are necessary for improving health outcomes while addressing national morbidity and mortality inequalities. Consider the following example. A C/PHN discovers during the interview that a pregnant patient with gestational diabetes has not been checking their blood sugar routinely. Rather than labeling the patient as nonadherent, the nurse asks the patient what challenges they have encountered that prevent them from completing this task and discovers that the patient lacks a stable living environment in which to keep their supplies. The C/PHN makes arrangements with social services to address the housing concerns (Whitman et al., 2022).

The C/PHN can play a role in reproductive healthcare and equity. Nurses can inquire regarding structural determinants such as access to food and safe water. Does the client have utility needs and is the home and community environment safe? Nurses can ensure access to social services and other services to support needs (Whitman et al., 2022).

Prenatal care is crucial to ensure good outcomes of pregnancy. Studies continue to reiterate the need for regular care visits, showing an association between regular and early care, fewer preterm deliveries, and higher infant birth weights. Significant disparities in prenatal care are present among Black, Hispanic, Pacific Islanders, non-Hispanic Native Hawaiian, and American Indian and Alaska Native people (HRSA, 2024). Access to obstetrical and gynecologic healthcare is difficult in many areas

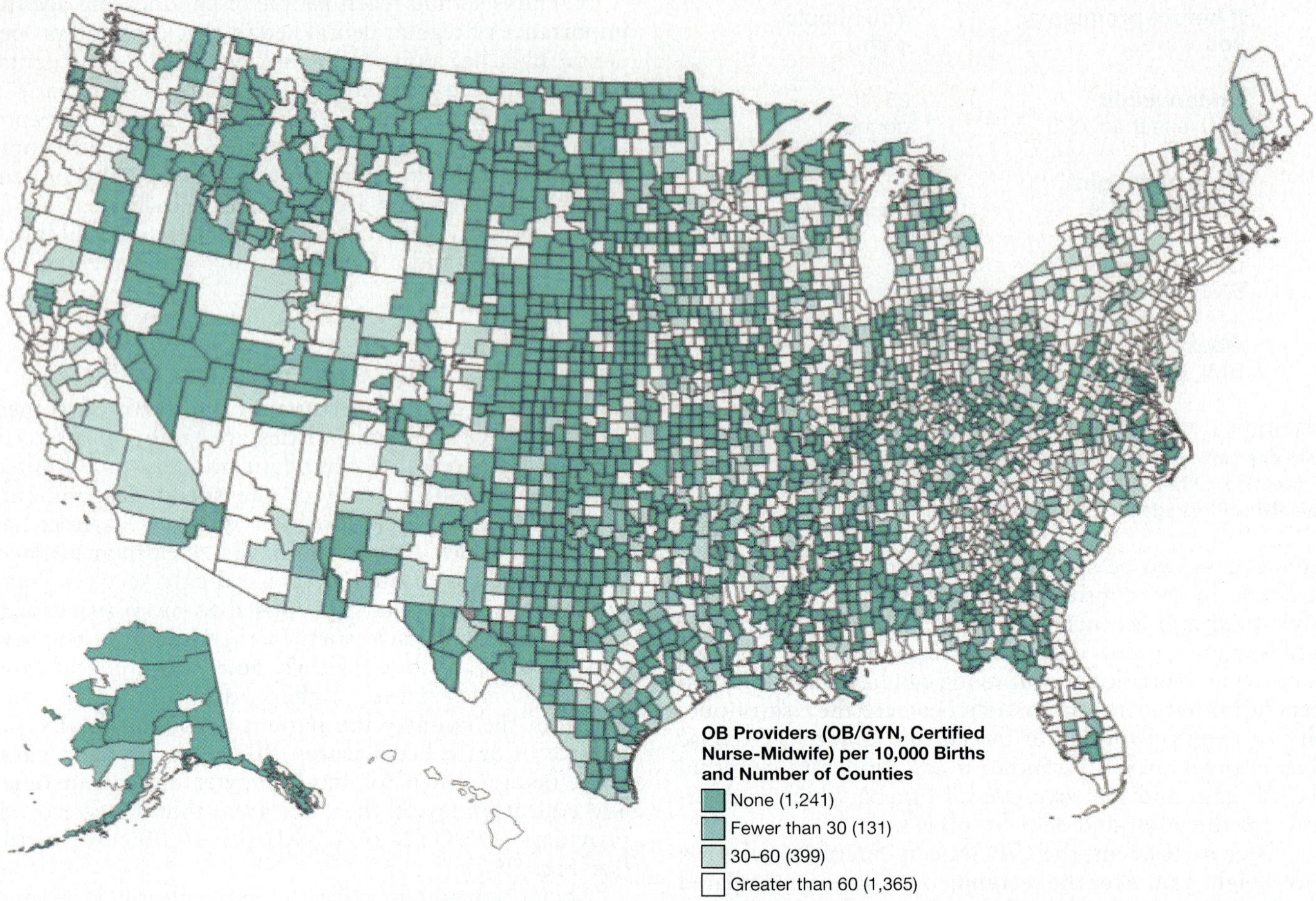

FIGURE 19-5 Distribution of obstetric providers by U.S. counties. (Reproduced with permission from National Conference of State Legislatures (NCSL). https://www.ncsl.org/health/state-approaches-to-ensuring-healthy-pregnancies-through-prenatal-care)

of the country. It is at crisis levels in some rural areas. Lack of adequate access to prenatal care leaves many pregnant people in danger (Box 19-4). Other factors, outlined in more detail in Chapter 25, may also affect the health of both birthing parents and babies.

Maternal Developmental Disability or Intellectual Disability

For couples that have developmental or intellectual disabilities, having a child puts increased stress on a system that is already burdened. Parenting requires attending to not

BOX **19-4** PERSPECTIVES

Racial and Ethnic Disparities in Maternal Health

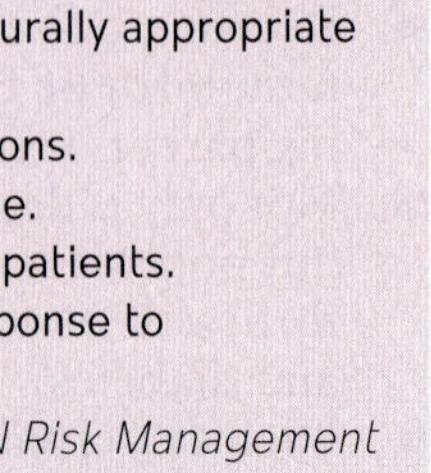

Pregnancy is an exciting time, a time to plan for the arrival of your expanding family, discuss your pregnancy plan, and ensure a healthy pregnancy. Prenatal care ensures you are taking good care of yourself and the fetus for a healthy pregnancy. While pregnancy rates are declining for 18- to 24-year-olds, they are increasing for 35- to 44-year-olds. Findings show more people are entering pregnancy as an older adult with preexisting conditions such as hypertension and diabetes, with Black and Hispanic individuals most at risk. Pregnancy and childbirth complications have increased especially for people of color, including disparities in maternal morbidity for that group from delivery through 6 weeks postpartum. Reducing maternal morbidity means knowing who is most at risk and designing tailored plans of care to support people of color.

- Be aware of implicit bias and provide culturally appropriate care to your patients.
- Prioritize management of chronic conditions.
- Make prenatal care accessible to everyone.
- Follow standards of care equitable for all patients.
- Standardize coordination of care and response to emergencies.

Lavita, RN Risk Management

Blue Cross Blue Shield. (2022). *Racial and ethnic disparities in maternal health.* https://www.bcbs.com/the-health-of-america/reports/racial-and-ethnic-disparities-maternal-health

Centers for Disease Control and Prevention (CDC). (2023). *Working together to reduce black maternal mortality.* https://www.cdc.gov/healthequity/features/maternal-mortality/index.html#:~:text=Black%20women%20are%20three%20times,structural%20racism%2C%20and%20implicit%20bias

only the child's physical care but also to socialization and developmental stimulation, well-child and illness healthcare, emotional nurturing, and age-appropriate supervision. Depending on the social support and coping skills of the parent with a developmental disability, the stress and need for emotional control and positive decision making can be monumental. Confounding variables included the environment of the home, parental affect, and child intelligence quotient. Even though there may not be strong evidence for these problems, children are still at risk for understimulation and environmental insecurity. Parent training/childcare skills programs, peer-to-peer support groups, community agencies, and careful home monitoring can reduce the risk of child abuse and neglect and promote more effective parenting (Connections for Families, 2023).

How does the C/PHN work with parents with developmental or intellectual disability effectively? Most importantly, nursing support must enhance the natural resilience of the family. The establishment of a trusting relationship between the nurse and the family is of foremost importance. Teaching by demonstration with many visual aids and prompts, along with games and creative approaches to engage and sustain attention, can challenge the nurse's creativity. Modeling of appropriate parenting behavior needs to occur on each visit. As part of the transition to other systems of care, C/PHNs often advocate for families with maternal developmental disability regarding the plan of care, interpreting it for other professionals and multiple disciplines. Many agencies employing nurses cannot provide the intensive follow-up that such a family requires. It is then necessary to make referrals to organizations that can provide support, such as The Arc or Exceptional Parents Unlimited. The nurse may stay involved as a consultant to the paraprofessionals or make periodic home visits at times of developmental or situational crisis.

Complications of Childbearing

Some maternal deaths are not preventable (e.g., amniotic fluid embolism). Morbidity is also a factor, and although some major risk factors among pregnant people and infants have been discussed, several common medical complications of childbearing bear mentioning. The effects of hypertensive disease in pregnancy, gestational diabetes, postpartum depression, and grief in families who have lost a child are important areas in which the C/PHN can intervene effectively. Following is a brief review of the complications of childbearing. For more detailed information, refer to your maternal/child textbook and lecture notes.

Hypertensive Disease in Pregnancy

Hypertension in pregnancy may be chronic or related specifically to pregnancy. Chronic is diagnosed prior to 20 weeks of gestation, and gestational (pregnancy related) is diagnosed after 20 weeks but goes away by 6 weeks postpartum. In 2019, chronic hypertension affected 2.3% of pregnancies, and gestational hypertension was seen in 13% (CDC, 2022i).

Preeclampsia occurs in about 3% to 7% of pregnancies, with 25% of cases developing in the postpartum period (Carson, 2022). Various methods are employed to attempt to prevent and control hypertension during pregnancy:

- Careful and constant monitoring of blood pressure
- Low-dose aspirin after 12 weeks of gestation
- Use of blood pressure medications if needed
- Frequent prenatal visits with monitoring of lab tests
- Diet rich in fresh fruits and vegetables
- Low-sodium food choices
- Adequate fluid intake and weight gain limitations
- Rest and regular exercise
- Intermittent fetal monitoring may be required

These remain the most common preventive suggestions that C/PHNs, in collaboration with the client's primary healthcare providers, can give to their pregnant clients. A calm environment, periods of rest, and the pregnant person either elevating their feet or reclining in a left-side lying position, are also recommended. Additional assessment data may guide the nurse to focus teaching on stress reduction techniques and modification or elimination of smoking. As care providers C/PHNs can provide frequent monitoring of blood pressure and other symptoms and encourage the client to be vigilant in keeping prenatal appointments. However, medication or even hospitalization may be necessary. The C/PHN can offer support and understanding while continuing to be a resource for the client as the pregnancy progresses and the infant is born.

Gestational Diabetes

For the patient with **gestational diabetes mellitus (GDM)**, there is a higher risk of hypertension, preeclampsia, urinary tract infections, cesarean section, and future risk of type 2 diabetes. Because growth and maturation of the fetus are closely associated with the delivery of maternal nutrients, particularly glucose, maintenance of appropriate glucose levels is essential to the health of the fetus. Daily self-monitoring of blood glucose levels is recommended. People should be encouraged to monitor blood glucose levels regularly 6 weeks postpartum and periodically throughout their life (CDC, 2022g).

The infant is at increased risk for fetal death because GDM has been associated with macrosomia, or large-for-gestational-age babies, birth injuries such as broken shoulders, breathing problems, and abnormally low blood sugars at birth (CDC, 2022g). The C/PHN can help in the control of GDM by encouraging the following:

- Early prenatal care
- Adequate nutrition
- Appropriate rest and exercise
- Adherence to the dietary recommendations
- Monitoring blood glucose regimen suggested by the patient's healthcare provider

Those C/PHNs working with pregnant people should provide education on early warning signs for GDM and the importance of regular prenatal care, including getting the glucose tolerance test around the 28th week of pregnancy, and follow-up.

Postpartum Depression

Prenatal stress is difficult to research because of the multiple variables that can affect prenatal stress. All areas of perceived stressors should be assessed (e.g., unintended pregnancy; nutrition; chronic stress and daily hassles; levels of social support; mental health issues, such as depression or anxiety, work stressors, racism, or discrimination; and any significant life events, such as death or other significant losses).

According to the CDC (2023i), one in eight people who give birth will experience postpartum depression. Risks for postpartum depression include a family history of psychiatric illness, previous history of depression, poor social support, stressful life events, pregnancy and birth complications, difficulty getting pregnant, preterm labor and delivery, pregnancy and birth complications, and being a teen parent (CDC, 2023i). Depression can affect anyone, even people without a history of prior depression. Perinatal depressive symptoms may not indicate major clinical depression. Nevertheless, symptoms may cause considerable psychological distress, such as irritability and restlessness; feeling hopeless, sad, and overwhelmed; having little energy or motivation and crying unexpectedly; sleeping and eating too little or too much; problems with cognition (memory, decision making, focus); loss of pleasure or interest in usually pleasant activities; and withdrawal from family and friends (Fig. 19-6).

There are several nonpharmacologic interventions the nurse can initiate in addition to the ones mentioned above. First, caffeine can lead to sleep disturbance, and alcohol is a depressant that has been implicated in depression. A simple yet helpful suggestion is to eliminate both. Additional nonpharmacologic considerations follow:

- Adequate sleep is important because sleep deprivation exacerbates psychiatric symptoms. Napping when the baby naps, resting throughout the day when possible, and going to bed early (albeit with the knowledge that sleep may be interrupted two or more times to feed the infant) will provide more hours of rest and sleep.
- Exercise is helpful and raises levels of endorphins. Anxiety symptoms often coexist with depression.
- Relaxation techniques that reduce anxiety can be helpful, including listening to relaxing music, doing yoga, or performing a simple exercise routine.
- Having a daily routine and setting realistic goals are also helpful (CDC, 2023i).

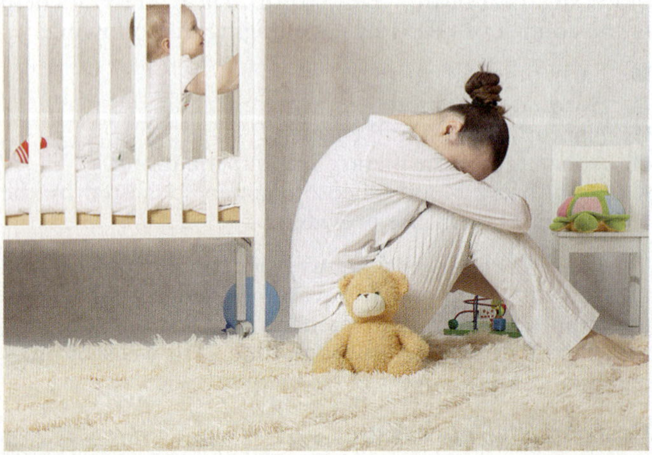

FIGURE 19-6 C/PHNs need to watch for signs of postpartum depression among their clients and offer assistance.

- Participation in a support group allows patients to identify with others who may be experiencing similar difficulties. Through discussion, participants provide each other with both emotional and practical support.

C/PHNs can intervene by initiating primary preventive mental health and coping measures that promote mental health throughout pregnancy and the postpartum period. Helping pregnant people to appreciate themselves and their strengths, embrace their new body changes, and positively anticipate their new role are primary preventive interventions for good mental health and the promotion of attachment to their infant. If patients are assessed to be at risk, mental health resources can be identified and then positive mental health outcomes may be fostered by supporting their self-esteem, optimizing the quality of their primary intimate relationships, providing anticipatory guidance on issues that may arise during pregnancy and the postpartum period, and reducing day-to-day stressors. At times, the nurse's efforts alone are not sufficient, and a referral to community mental health services for early detection and treatment is essential for the patients and their children.

Fetal or Infant Death

An infrequent role for nurses in maternal–child health is that of grief counselor, but this may be a role for the advanced practice nurse in certain settings or communities. A couple may experience a miscarriage or ectopic pregnancy, stillbirth, or the death of an infant from **sudden infant death syndrome (SIDS)**. The exact cause of SIDS is not certain, but it may be associated with brain stem control of heart and lung functions (Boston Children's Hospital, n.d.). It is more common in children assigned male at birth and most often occurs in infants between 1 and 4 months of age (Safe to Sleep, n.d.). Increased rates of SIDS are associated with side/stomach sleeping position, exposure to cigarette smoke, premature birth, co-sleeping, having a sibling who died of SIDS, and soft bedding in the crib. SIDS is the leading cause of death for infants from 1 to 12 months of age; about 2300 infants die annually from SIDS.

In each situation of loss, the C/PHN has an important supportive role. People respond to grief in a variety of ways: some express deep sadness, shock, or disbelief; some weep and are unable to talk; and others talk incessantly about regrets or guilt. Even if a miscarriage occurs early in a pregnancy, the bonding between the patient and fetus has begun, and expressions of grief may be as intense as with the loss of an infant or child. Patients often have feelings of abandonment, bereavement, and guilt, thinking that they did something wrong. When parents are unable to identify the exact cause of their fetal loss, they have a more difficult time letting go of grief and anxiety. Increased anxiety levels are also found, sometimes more frequently than depression. Psychological counseling has been associated with greater decreases over time in levels of worry, grief, and self-blame (March of Dimes, 2020b). For couples that have delivered a stillborn baby, the shock is compounded by the experience of carrying the pregnancy to full term, along with the anticipation of an imminent delivery and the expectation of an addition to the family. This is especially true if all signs before the birthing event itself were positive.

Patients who experience stillbirths recognize the need for spiritual and psychosocial support from professional caregivers. Families must acknowledge the death of the child and integrate the loss into their family lives. Home visitation and simply being there for the family and listening well are invaluable nursing interventions. Referral to mental health counseling or support groups specific to parents of stillborn children where they can share their feelings may be very helpful (March of Dimes, 2020b). Providing continuity and support to the family for months after the death of an infant gives the C/PHN an opportunity to assess the family for signs of unresolved grief. Grieving families may find comfort, support, and helpful information from support groups and resources such as Compassionate Friends or First Candle.

When a family experiences the loss of an infant after the baby has been brought home from the hospital, grief and guilt are compounded by the loss of an anticipated future and the disrupted continuity in family life. An infant may die of SIDS, a congenital anomaly, an infection, or an injury. There are constant reminders of the infant's presence in the home from memories, photos, videos, and accumulated possessions. This death disrupts family homeostasis and the psychological and physiologic equilibrium of the family. In many cases, the police are involved, and an autopsy is required, contributing to the anguish of the grieving family. This promotes both guilt and loss of self-esteem and can even threaten the relationship and marriage.

The *Healthy People 2030* (ODPHP, n.d.-a.) document encompasses specific goals and objectives for the maternal–child population, based on the previous achievements in the same or similar areas. After years of working toward improving maternal–child health, the United States has made limited progress. One objective, however, has been met: 70% of infants are now sleeping on their backs, up from a 35% baseline. The rate for SIDS has declined to 41% in 2020. This can be attributed to the national public health education campaign known as "Back to Sleep" (CDC, 2023j).

INFANTS, TODDLERS, AND PRESCHOOLERS

Healthy children are a vital resource to ensure the future well-being of nations. They are the parents, workers, citizens, leaders, and decision-makers of tomorrow, and their health and safety depend on today's decisions and actions. Their futures lie in the hands of those people responsible for their well-being, including the C/PHN, whose dominant responsibility is to the community and populations, such as dependent children.

The well-being of children has been a subject of great public health concern globally and in the United States. Its importance has been emphasized through the development of numerous laws and services, yet the needs of many children continue to go unmet. Young children (up to age 4 years) are totally dependent on their caregivers. This contributes to their vulnerability during these years. Too many young children often go to bed hungry; some infants and toddlers do not receive even the most basic immunizations before they reach school age. It is essential for C/PHNs to be aware of the factors associated with the leading causes of death among the very young.

Adverse childhood events (ACEs) are potentially traumatic events that occur in childhood (aged 0 to 17 years) such as experiencing violence or abuse, witnessing violence in the home or community, and having a family member attempt or die by suicide (CDC, 2023k). Any aspect of a child's environment that can undermine their sense of safety, stability, and bonding are linked to chronic health issues, mental illness, and substance misuse as an adult. According to the CDC (2023k), 64% of adults reported experiencing at least one type of ACE before the age of 18; one in six reported experiencing four or more types of ACEs. People assigned female at birth and underrepresented groups are at greater risk for experiencing four or more types of ACEs. The CDC-Kaiser Permanente ACEs study is the largest investigation of childhood neglect and abuse, showing the effects of violence exposure and later-life health and well-being (Felitti et al., 1998). This seminal study identified seven categories of ACEs that were correlated with multiple health risk factors later in life. ACEs can have lasting and negative effects on children, increasing the risk of injury, maternal and child health problems, teen pregnancy, sex trafficking, STIs, and a wide range of chronic diseases. It is estimated that the effects of ACEs can cost families, communities, and society billions of dollars each year (CDC, 2023k).

Home environment and safety are current areas of concern for many children and families. Children in families make up approximately 30% of the population who are homeless (National Alliance to End Homelessness, 2023). Children who are homeless have higher levels of emotional and behavioral difficulties and may have lower academic performance due to transience. Access to services and transition into permanent housing provides stability (National Alliance to End Homelessness, 2023).

Global History of Children's Healthcare

Only recently in the history of the world have children been considered valuable assets, even in countries where there are now well-developed programs of infant health promotion and protection, infant and child daycare services, and strict educational expectations for all children. In some countries today, however, infants and children assigned female at birth or those born with congenital anomalies are not valued. In some countries, selective abortions or infanticide depending on infants' sex assigned at birth may occur. In some countries, inequitable care for children exists depending on their sex assigned at birth. Cultural practices that are fostered by political forces prevent many countries from improving the health of infants and young children (Le & Nguyen, 2022). For these reasons, there are great differences globally in child healthcare systems. The health of children in one country can affect that of children in other countries, including the United States. Major natural disasters place whole populations at risk, especially the very young and the very old.

National Perspective on Infants, Toddlers, and Preschoolers

In the United States, the **infant** (birth to 1 year), **toddler** (aged 1 to 2 years), and **preschooler** populations (aged 3 to 4 years) are generally healthy years. Most U.S. children have a usual source of healthcare (96.8%), and their parents report them to be in excellent or very good health (CDC, 2023l). The growth and development of infants and young children should be monitored regularly. Pediatricians and C/PHNs often provide anticipatory guidance for parents so that they better understand what to expect as their child grows and can plan for safety issues that may arise. See the CDC online growth charts.

The mortality rate for children ages 5 to 14 years is 14.3 per 100,000. Major causes are unintentional injuries (motor vehicle crashes, falls, drowning, fires, and burns), cancer, homicide, and suicide (CDC, 2023l). Some variation in mortality rates continues among racial/ethnic groups.

Accidents and Injuries

Toddlers and preschoolers are at risk for many types of accidents and unintentional injuries, such as those caused by unsafe toys, falls, burns or scalding, drowning, motor vehicle crashes, and poisonings.

These unintentional injuries are the leading cause of mortality and morbidity for children from age birth to 19 years (CDC, 2023l, 2023m). Male children have higher rates of death from injuries than females, at almost twice the rate. Causes of injury deaths vary across age groups.

- For those children under age 1, about 80% are caused by suffocation
- Between ages 1 and 4, drowning is the leading cause
- In 5- to 19-year-olds, being a passenger in a motor vehicle crash was the most frequent cause of injury and death.

The loss of children's lives resulting from all injuries combined represents a staggering number of productive life years lost to society. Childhood unintentional injuries lead to approximately 7000 deaths annually (CDC, 2021b).

In an effort to reduce childhood inadvertent deaths, the *National Action Plan for Child Injury Prevention* was developed by the CDC in 2012 to address child safety and provide an agenda for injury prevention. This project provides partners with implementation tools through communication, education, and training on injury prevention. The program incorporates the levels of prevention to address the leading causes of infant, child, and adolescent mortality and morbidity. The program focuses on the prevention of injuries (e.g., safety latches on cabinets containing cleaning supplies or medications), minimization of injuries (e.g., child safety seats), and improving emergency response and care after an injury occurs (e.g., paramedic, trauma care). For instance, to prevent infant suffocation and SIDS, infants should go to sleep on their backs, in a crib or child-friendly bed without soft bedding or pillows, and parents should be cautioned about risk factors for SIDS and the potential dangers of sleeping with their babies. Information about the SIDS prevention campaign *Back to Sleep* should be provided to all parents of infants, and education should begin with hospital nurses and continue with C/PHNs in the community (ODPHP, n.d.-b). Although childhood mortality decreased 11% from 2010 to 2019, the current *Healthy People 2030* objective data shows an increase in those ages 1 to 19 at 29.5 per 100,000 population in 2021 compared to the baseline of 25.2 per 100,000 population. The *Healthy People 2030* target goal is 18.2 per 100,000 population (ODPHP, n.d.-c.). The *National Action Plan for Child Injury Prevention* continues to be an integral part of *Healthy People 2030* with resources available for C/PHNs.

Burn injuries can affect children of all ages. Bath water that is too hot can also cause serious scalding injuries. Cigarette lighters and matches are fascinating to young children. Toddlers or preschoolers may be able to start a flame, injuring or killing themselves or others. The sound of a smoke alarm may frighten young children, and it is important for C/PHNs to instruct parents not only to teach their young children about fire prevention but also to be aware of the sound of the alarm and know what actions to take when they hear it, such as the *Stop Drop and Roll* program taught in Head Start and other preschool programs (National Fire Protection Association, n.d.). The C/PHN should also take every opportunity on home visits and in other health education settings to ask or observe if parents have a functional smoke detector in their home. Several fire departments test and install smoke detectors at no cost. For instance:

- Illinois Fire Safety Alliance and the Office of the Illinois State Fire Marshal provide fire safety education and install smoke alarm to residents of Illinois (Illinois.gov, 2022).
- Residents in Loudoun County, Virginia, can request a smoke detector assessment and free replacement if needed (Loudoun County, Virginia, n.d.).
- Residents of Prince George's County, Maryland, are eligible to receive fire safety education and free smoke detectors and installation (Prince George's County, Maryland, 2023).

C/PHNs are encouraged to be aware of such programs in their areas and to be knowledgeable of state laws and regulations regarding smoke detectors. Another excellent resource is the American Red Cross *Sound the Alarm. Save a Life* (see https://www.redcross.org/sound-the-alarm.html). Preventing the sources of injury or death from burns may be accomplished by eliminating opportunity and source. Through child supervision, safe storage of matches and lighters, and keeping children away from stoves and electrical outlets, burns, and fires can be prevented.

Drowning is another category of unintentional injury in children. Brief lapses in supervision can have disastrous consequences. Young children are at risk for drowning wherever water occurs in depths exceeding a few inches—such as in toilet bowls, bathtubs, large buckets or cans filled with rainwater, puddles, ponds, spas, and swimming pools. Lakes, rivers, streams, and irrigation ditches or canals are other water hazards. Infants, toddlers, and preschool-aged children are especially vulnerable because they are not aware of water dangers, and they explore without fear. The C/PHN can work with community groups and recreation centers to promote swimming for children. Parents need to provide a drown-free environment. Guidelines include the following (CDC, 2022j):

- Bathe young children in shallow water.
- Never leave young children unattended during a bath.
- Keep toilet lids down and bathroom doors closed—preferably secured with childproof safety handles.
- Never leave full large buckets unattended.

- Eliminate water collection sites around the home by turning over or removing empty buckets, containers, flowerpots, and other items that can collect rainwater.
- Fence swimming pool areas and install childproof locks or alarm devices that sound when the water is disturbed.
- Promote water safety measures, including teaching young children to swim.
- Be aware of the dangers of open pool drains and suction outlets that can lead to drain entrapment and hair entanglement and ensure that drain covers and safety vacuum release systems are installed.
- Vigilant supervision of young children at play to prevent involvement with neighborhood water sources.

Supervising children in or around bathtubs, spas, pools, or other water receptacles is critical and requires close (arm's length) distances. Parents of young children should be encouraged to get cardiopulmonary resuscitation training, including Hands-Only CPR. Once certified to teach CPR and first aid, the C/PHN can teach CPR classes to a group of parents or child caregivers in the community. The real dangers of inadvertent drowning are related in the case study at the end of this chapter.

Injuries and deaths from motor vehicle crashes continue to be a major safety problem in the United States. Automobile accidents accounted for 607 deaths and more than 63,000 injuries among children 12 years of age and younger in 2020. Of children who were killed, 38% (211) were not wearing seat belts (CDC, 2022k). Although many families have car seats and use them regularly, it is estimated that 49% of those car seats are installed improperly, placing the child at as much risk as if there were no restraint (Davidson, 2023). The most current recommendations for safety seat use are categorized by age.

- For children birth up to age 2 to 4 years, a rear-facing seat should be used (placed in car's back seat); the child should continue in a rear-facing seat until they outgrow the rear-facing seat (reaching the height or weight limit of the seat).
- After outgrowing a rear-facing car seat, the child should use a forward-facing car seat (used in the back seat) until at least age 5 or until reaching the upper weight and height limit for the seat.
- After outgrowing a forward-facing car seat and until a seat belt fits properly, keep the child in the back seat with a seat belt–buckled booster seat until a seat belt fits properly (ages 9 to 12).
- Seat belts are properly fitted when the lap belt portion lays across the upper thighs (not the stomach area) and the seat belt lays across the chest and not the neck.
- Children age 12 and under should always be properly buckled in the back seat (CDC, 2022k).

There is much opportunity in this area for the C/PHN to educate the public and ensure that parents have the information and skills to secure their children properly when traveling by car. Safety seat clinics, where installations are checked and corrected, can help to promote the proper use of age-appropriate child restraints (Box 19-5).

BOX 19-5 EVIDENCE-BASED PRACTICE

Getting Families to Use Child Booster Seats

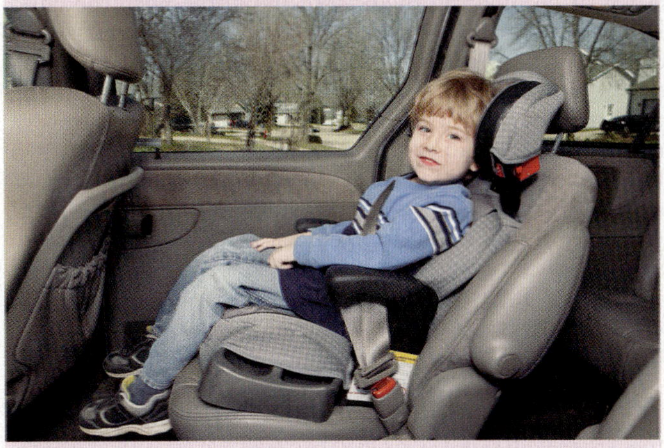

Many health departments, law enforcement, and social service agencies educate parents about the laws and benefits related to the use of child safety seats. Still, not every family consistently uses them. Education and awareness are essential to increase the use of child safety seats. One organization that provides a wealth of information related to car seat safety is the National Highway Traffic Safety Administration.

The National Highway Traffic Safety Administration has a mission to prevent injuries and death from motor vehicle accidents and to reduce the economic costs associated with these accidents. This organization works to accomplish this mission through the use of research, education, safety standards, and enforcement advocacy. Information regarding quality and safety ratings of car seats along with recall information can be found through this organization. Additionally, educational resources for parents include motor vehicle topics ranging from bike safety to teen driving to school bus safety.

Another activity this organization supports and promotes is "Child Passenger Safety" week and the "National Seat Check Saturday." These events occur each year in September with the focus on car seat safety education in communities across the United States. A series of public service announcements and promotional materials are available to be adapted for communities to use to promote this event. It is important for C/PHNs to use evidence and a variety of approaches to combat unintentional childhood death. For more information on selecting the proper car seat for children, visit: https://www.nhtsa.gov/equipment/car-seats-and-booster-seats

Source: National Highway Traffic Safety Administration (n.d.).

Poisoning is a constant safety concern for young children, and toddlers are most often at risk. Sources of poisoning include household plants, prescription medications, over-the-counter drugs, unintentional medication overdoses, household cleaning products, other chemicals stored within a child's reach, and lead. Parents should be provided with the number for the Poison Help Hotline (1-800-222-1222). Encourage parents to post the number next to each telephone and call immediately in the event of a suspected poisoning or overdose (American

Association of Poison Control Centers [AAPCC], n.d.-a). C/PHNs can also educate and demonstrate for parents how to childproof the home by eliminating major sources of poisoning. This includes keeping plants out of a child's reach or eliminating them from the home until the child is older, locking up household chemicals (e.g., toilet bowl cleaner, bleach, mouthwash, oven and drain cleaners, pesticides, gasoline, paint thinner, hair products) and storing them out of a child's sight and reach, using childproof medication containers, and storing all medicines in a locked box with a key that is kept out of reach (AAPCC, n.d.-a). Alcoholic beverages should also be kept out of reach, as should tobacco products. Outside hazards, such as wild mushrooms and poisonous plants, flowers, and berries, must also be considered (AAPCC, n.d.-a). It is also important to eliminate sources of lead in and around the home.

Lead Poisoning

Lead poisoning historically resulted in encephalopathy and death. Today, morbidity from lead poisoning is subtle and most often affects the child's central nervous system with long-term changes in behavior and cognitive ability. The CDC estimates that half a million children between the ages of 1 and 5 years have elevated blood lead levels or 3.5 μg of lead per deciliter of blood (CDC, 2023n).

- Lead in paint, dust, water, and soil can be inadvertently consumed, and lead also crosses the placental barrier.
- It can be transferred in breast milk and is also found in some infant formulas.
- Lead can be found in some toys, candies, cosmetics, traditional medicines, and eating utensils and drinking vessels imported from other countries. Many of these have been tested and revealed to have high levels of lead.
- There is no safe level of lead, and the elimination of elevated blood lead levels in children is a U.S. Health Goal.
- The primary sources of lead exposure in preschool-aged children continue to be lead-based paint and lead-contaminated soil and house dust.
- The critical age of exposure (or peak level) is thought to be between ages 18 and 36 months. Levels generally begin to decline after age 3 years.

Children who live in poverty and play in substandard housing areas remain at risk for direct exposure to significant sources of lead. Lead safety and housing code enforcement, along with periodic monitoring to detect new lead hazards, can help prevent future lead exposures (CDC, 2021c).

C/PHNs working together with environmental health sanitarians should promote opportunities for blood lead screening, especially if it is suspected that children in certain homes, apartments, or neighborhoods are at risk for lead poisoning.

Education and public awareness campaigns can help prevent this type of lead poisoning. The C/PHN can alert clients to the dangers of lead and its sources and work as an advocate for policies to reduce this danger for infants and children.

Child Maltreatment

Child maltreatment includes physical, emotional, and sexual abuse and neglect that occurs in anyone under 18 years old. Neglect is an act or acts of omission in which a child's basic needs are not met (e.g., withholding feeding or medical care). Children under age 4 years are at the greatest risk for severe abuse and neglect (CDC, 2022l).

Abusive head trauma (AHT) is often an overlooked form of abuse. In the United States, AHT, which includes **shaken baby syndrome**, is the leading cause of child maltreatment deaths for those under age 5 (CDC, 2022m). AHT can be suspected in infants or toddlers who exhibit traumatic brain injuries caused by violent shaking or impact. It is characterized by a triad of symptoms: retinal hemorrhage, subdural hematoma, and cerebral edema, with few signs of external trauma. The soft brain tissues are injured as they move violently against the rough cranial bones as the infant is shaken or thrown against a hard object (American Association of Neurological Surgeons, 2023). Nurses need to know the stages of development to help determine if the caregiver's explanation for the injury is developmentally possible. For an example, a 1-month-old baby cannot roll off a bed. The C/PHN has an important role in the prevention of AHT by providing parents with education regarding the triggers and intervention strategies. Educating parents that baby crying patterns are more severe in the first few months and progressively improve, along with teaching parents baby soothing techniques, is essential before and after delivery (CDC, 2022p).

Failure to thrive (FTT) is characterized by a slow growth rate in height and weight, as well as head circumference among infants and toddlers. If an infant's growth rate is consistently below 3rd to 5th percentiles, drops more than two percentiles, or is lower than the 80th percentile of median weight for height, a diagnosis of FTT may be made.

- Problems with growth may be due to food insecurities and many behavioral or physiologic etiologies for infants but can also be related to child neglect or abnormal maternal–infant bonding.
- Child neglect differs from **child abuse** in that the action of the parent or guardian is more one of omission rather than commission as in the case of an injury related to abuse.
- Risk factors that point to child neglect as the basis for FTT include those most often cited for abuse and neglect, along with specific concerns about parents intentionally withholding food, being resistant to recommended interventions, and having rigid beliefs about nutrition and health regimens that may jeopardize the infant.

The exact incidence of FTT is difficult to determine, and no accurate estimates are available. The C/PHN can take a careful nutritional history and determine the caregiver's knowledge of basic infant needs and, if possible, observe the caregiver feeding the infant. Other assessment information includes developmental milestone assessment, and a psychosocial history is also helpful (e.g., income/poverty level, cultural beliefs, social support networks, domestic abuse, substance misuse, mental health disorders), with careful attention to maternal/caregiver bonding and feeding practices. Growth problems in the first 2 months of life may result in cognitive, language/speech, and fine motor deficits in childhood, and early intervention programs that involve home visitation have been effective in attenuating the long-term effects of FTT (Smith & Badireddy, 2022).

C/PHNs play a role in the prevention and management of child abuse and maltreatment. Preventive strategies such as parent education should begin prenatally and continue throughout the life span. Parent training programs can help teach parents to cope, and child sexual abuse prevention programs may also be helpful. Home visiting programs that provide anticipatory guideline education will also help to prevent abuse and neglect. Early recognition and reporting of suspected abuse or neglect is a responsibility of C/PHNs. See Box 19-6.

Communicable Diseases

Infants, toddlers, and preschool-aged children experience a high frequency of acute illnesses, more so than any other age group. Acute conditions commonly seen from birth to age 5 include sore throat, ear pain, urinary tract infection, skin infection, and respiratory infections (including ear infections, colds, influenza). Communicable diseases are prevalent in these age groups, as very young children are building an immune system and are just beginning to come in contact with a greater number of people outside their families (Fig. 19-7) (American Academy of Pediatrics, 2023a).

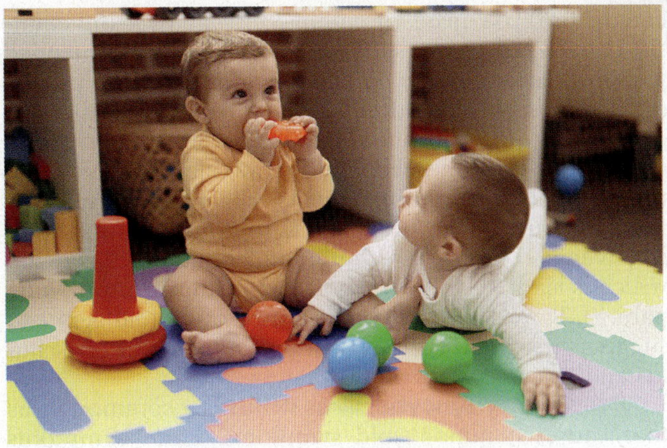

FIGURE 19-7 Infants, toddlers, and preschoolers are constantly putting things in their mouths and sharing items with others, contributing, in part, to the increased incidence of accidents and infections among them.

Acute upper respiratory infections are common in children under the age of 5 years. Most uncomplicated upper respiratory infections range in duration from 5 to 7 days with the common cold lasting approximately 10 days. Symptoms include nasal drainage, congestion, and

BOX 19-6 Reports of an Emergency Foster Home

The following are examples of the various situations from which abused and neglected children come, as reported by a couple who had an emergency foster home for the county Department of Social Services. The examples represent children placed with them over a 2-year period in which they cared for 256 children.

- A 2-week-old Jose was taken to their home because the parents (under the influence of drugs) were found swinging Jose upside down in circles in an infant carrier as they walked along a downtown street at 3 a.m. After being returned to his parents, he returned to foster care 1 month later after he was found abandoned in an infant carrier at the county fair.
- Andre, Otis, and Selma were siblings under the age of 8 years old. They went to the foster home when the social services agency discovered they had been living with their father in an abandoned car for 2 years. They stayed for 3 weeks while the social worker found suitable housing for this family and counseling for the father.
- Victoria, 5 years old, a loving and passive child, arrived wearing a diaper and appeared developmentally delayed. She had a history of being physically and sexually abused. Her family was very dysfunctional, and it took the social worker several weeks to sort out relatives and their intentions before placing Victoria in a long-term foster home.
- Ronald and Randall, 6-year-old twins who were sexually abused by their mother for several years, came to the emergency foster home before being placed with relatives while their mother underwent psychiatric treatment. The twins began counseling during their stay in the emergency foster home.
- A 7-year-old Antoinette had severe asthma and was very withdrawn. She came to the emergency foster home because her mother (and the mother's boyfriend) refused to care for her. The child came with every photograph of herself and personal mementos because the mother wanted no reminders of the child. The social worker located a grandmother who would be the child's guardian.
- A 13-year-old, Robert, came home from school one day and found his mother and all their furniture gone. After a few weeks of Robert living in the basement of the apartment building, someone alerted the social services agency, and he was placed in the emergency foster home for 2 months. His mother finally called social services after 6 weeks, saying Robert was too difficult for her to handle, but she may want to see him again someday. Robert was eventually placed in a group home.
- Quyn, a 17-year-old Laotian person, came into foster care after being referred by the school nurse because of wounds observed on her wrists and ankles. Quyn reported being strapped to a chair for 12 or more hours at a time by her father because she was not following the old ways and was shaming the family by being seen in public with a boy, and without a chaperone. Several meetings were held between the parents, a Southeast Asian community leader, and the social worker to resolve this situation so that Quyn could go home safely.

cough. C/PHNs need to emphasize that over-the-counter cough and cold medications are not recommended for children under age 6. The use of decongestants and antihistamines in children under 2 is contraindicated. Additionally, parents should be instructed to read labels carefully as even "homeopathic" cold and cough medications contain harmful ingredients. For example, some of these products have been found to contain "nux vomica, which contains strychnine and plumbum aceticum which is lead" (U.S. Food and Drug Administration, n.d., para 9). Parents need to be informed of the dangers and suggest safer interventions of supportive measures of fluids and rest.

Respiratory syncytial virus (RSV) is a common virus that causes common cold symptoms. Early symptoms include runny nose, diminished appetite, and coughing; however, in certain populations RSV may lead to the more severe symptoms of wheezing and difficulty breathing that are associated with bronchiolitis or pneumonia. It is a common cause of hospitalization in this age group with approximately 80,000 infants and children hospitalized each year. The majority of hospitalizations for bronchiolitis are for infants 6 months and younger. RSV is the cause in 70% of cases and can rise to 100% during winter epidemics. Although wheezing, tachypnea, and chest retractions can be frightening to parents, most healthy infants survive (95%). However, C/PHNs need to work with parents and pediatricians to ensure that infants receive monoclonal antibody products.

- Monoclonal antibody products include nirsevimab (Beyfortus) and palivizumab (Synagis) or RSV immunoglobulin.
- The CDC recommends that all infants under 8 months who are born during or entering RSV season (fall to spring) receive nirsevimab. One dose provides a 5-month window of protection.
- For those infants at a higher risk of RSV (i.e., premature and immunocompromised infants), a second dose of nirsevimab is recommended between 8 and 19 months of age when the second RSV season occurs.
- Palivizumab is available for infants and children under 2 years of age with health conditions that put them at a higher risk for severe RSV disease. Dosing is once a month during RSV season (CDC, 2023o).

Using these products combat RSV infection and prevent severe complications from the virus. Education regarding the prevention of RSV through good handwashing and avoiding those with cold symptoms is important for those caring for infants.

Vaccine-Preventable Diseases

Vaccines are one of the greatest achievements of public health. Since 1980, there has been a 99% or greater decrease in deaths because of the vaccine-preventable diseases of mumps, pertussis, tetanus, and diphtheria and 80% or greater decline in deaths associated with vaccines instituted since 1980: hepatitis A and B, *Haemophilus influenzae* type B, and varicella. Worldwide, vaccine coverage has increased because of effects of manufacturers and philanthropists (e.g., Bill & Melinda Gates Foundation). Smallpox has been eradicated worldwide, and the viruses for polio, rubella, and measles are no longer endemic in the United States. Newborns' immature immune systems and lack of exposure to antigens, along with somewhat porous physical barriers to microbes, put them at high risk of infection. By the age of 4 to 6 months, however, a brisker antibody response to vaccines becomes possible. Successful infant and childhood immunization programs have been responsible for high vaccine coverage and the subsequent decline in morbidity and mortality from these preventable diseases.

State-level immunization registries help track vaccine coverage at all age levels. Because daycare centers and schools require proof of immunization, vaccination rates have improved over the last two decades. The financing of immunizations for infants and children has significantly improved as a result of two major initiatives. The Vaccines for Children Program and the Child Health Insurance Program cover children on Medicaid, uninsured children, and American Indian/Alaska Native children. In addition, underinsured children who receive immunizations at federally qualified health centers and rural health clinics are covered. Additional state programs and funds help provide free or low-cost vaccines for children who are not covered by the other programs. There are several ways for C/PHNs to help all families obtain free or low-cost immunizations and contribute to maintaining adequate levels of community immunity to communicable diseases.

Even if financial barriers are removed, there are other barriers. Transportation is a significant problem for some parents, especially in rural areas, and for families in urban areas who have several children and need to take public transportation. A recent study found that rural families were less likely to have current vaccines due to parental vaccine hesitancy, negative experiences in healthcare clinics, primary care providers referring patients to other clinics for vaccines, and distance to receive the vaccines (Albers et al., 2022). Despite public health announcements in the media, some caregivers remain unaware of the disabling consequences of diseases such as pertussis and measles and do not realize the importance of fully vaccinating their children. Also, as more vaccines become available and the deadly diseases they prevent become a distant memory in the public's mind, more concerns about the safety of vaccines emerge. Some parents may believe that there is link between thimerosal, an ethyl mercury preservative used in vaccines, and autism (CDC, 2020d). However, thimerosal was removed from all childhood vaccines in the United States in 2001, while autism rates remained the same (CDC, 2020d). Numerous websites have emerged that advise against childhood immunization and provide graphic horror stories about the handful of severe reactions to vaccination. Media coverage and online websites about vaccine adverse events also contribute to decreased compliance on the part of parents in getting their children immunized. C/PHNs and other health professionals are encouraged to provide parents of very young children with meaningful stories of preventable deaths because of vaccines and to educate parents about scientifically based websites and resources rather than relying solely on dispassionate facts and figures.

Chronic Diseases

Infants and young children can be afflicted with chronic diseases that affect their quality of life.

Dental cavities are the most common unmet health need in the United States (CDC, 2021d). It is estimated that 45% of children have a cavity before age 19. Young children's diets, often unreasonably high in sugar, increase the incidence of dental caries in this population group.

- Allowing infants to feed from the bottle beyond 15 to 16 months, or to fall asleep with a bottle, can lead to *baby bottle tooth decay* or *nursing caries*.
- Baby bottle tooth decay occurs when giving toddlers and preschool-aged children milk, juice, sodas, or sugared drinks continually throughout the day (American Academy of Pediatrics, 2022).
- Frequent snacking and sippy cups filled with juice or sugary drinks can lead to cavities. It is recommended that sugary foods be avoided.
- Between ages 6 and 12 months, sippy cups are often used to wean infants from the breast or bottle, but between-meal drinks should be avoided. Between meals, drinks should only be fluoridated water (American Academy of Pediatrics, 2023a).
- Parents of infants older than 6 months who have several erupted teeth should be instructed to rub the infant's gums with a damp, clean cloth and to begin tooth brushing, using a soft pediatric toothbrush with a very small amount of fluoride toothpaste—about the size of a grain of rice.
- The first dental examination should be made within 6 months of the first tooth eruption.

Addressing parental misconceptions about dental health and understanding cultural beliefs and practices related to dental health and hygiene are important (American Academy of Pediatrics, 2022).

Dental caries is a preventable condition that can be addressed with proper nutrition and hygiene. The younger the age when dental caries first appear, the greater the risk for future tooth decay, which increases the risks of chronic health conditions due to the inflammatory response. Untreated dental caries can also lead to serious infections. Pain can interfere with learning at school. Many health departments are using fluoride varnishes as a means of preventing dental caries in young children. Dental hygienists and C/PHNs may be trained to apply the sealants and varnishes while making home visits, or children and families may visit clinics for treatment (American Academy of Pediatrics, 2022).

Asthma symptoms may begin in infants and toddlers. Approximately 4.7 million children ages 0 to 17 years have asthma (CDC, 2023p). Children from underrepresented groups and from resource-limited settings are disproportionately affected, and asthma hospitalizations are common. C/PHNs can assist families in finding appropriate healthcare providers and encourage the proper administration of asthma medications and treatments. They can also teach families to reduce the presence of asthma triggers in their homes.

Autism is a developmental spectrum disorder (ASD) that is often first noticed in toddlers. Parents become aware that the child's communication and interaction with others are different and that the child may also display obsessive and narrow interests. Autism spectrum disorder (ASD) is a complex developmental disorder, and the spectrum of ASD indicates that symptoms for each child varies and may range from mild to severe (CDC, 2023q). A child's communication skills and interaction with others are most often affected, along with obsessive behavior and narrowed interests. Behaviors associated with autism include:

- Language problems (no language, delay in language, repetitive use of language)
- Motor mannerisms (often repetitive rocking, hand flapping, object twirling)
- Fixation on objects (restricted interests)
- No spontaneous play or make-believe play (Fig. 19-8); no interest in peers (problems making friends)
- Little or no eye contact (may also resist hugging)

Children assigned male at birth are four times more likely than children assigned female at birth to develop autism. An estimated 27.6/1000 or 1 in 36 children were identified to have ASD in 2020 (CDC, 2023r). The causes of autism are unclear—some genetic links have been found, but environment may also be a factor. There is a higher risk of subsequent children having autism in a family with one autistic child or a parent with ASD (CDC, 2022n). It is often associated with other disorders (e.g., congenital rubella syndrome, Down syndrome, fragile X syndrome, tuberous sclerosis), being born to older parents, and birth complications, but the exact causes are not fully understood (CDC, 2022n). Families may need to be referred to early educational intervention programs and social service agencies for assistance. Treatment involves multiple modalities that include behavioral, developmental, educational, pharmacologic, social-relational, psychological, and other alternative therapies that are used in conjunction to manage ASD (Hyman et al., 2020). Parents need to make daycares and preschools aware of their child's environmental sensitivities. It is important for C/PHNs to educate parents that parenting practices are *not* a cause of autism and that multiple, large-scale research studies on childhood immunizations have shown that there is no relationship between immunizations and autism (CDC, 2021e).

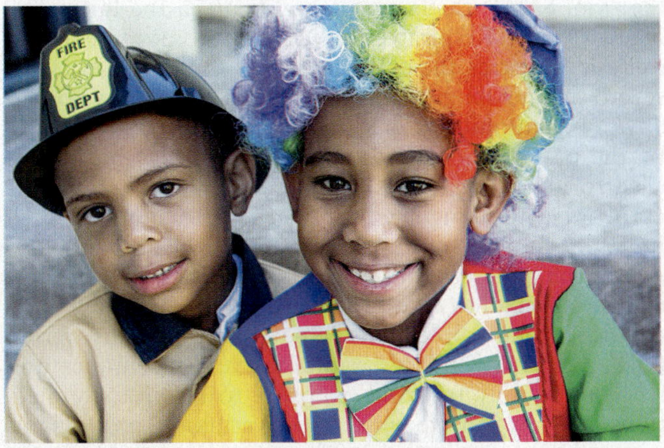

FIGURE 19-8 Dress-up and playtime are important for toddler and preschooler development.

Sickle cell disease, an inherited blood disorder, affects thousands of children in the United States, most often those of African or Hispanic Caribbean ancestry. The characteristic chronic and severe anemia is common in young children with this condition, and it can affect memory, learning, and behavior. Children can also exhibit jaundice, gallstones, and joint pain. When both parents have the genetic mutation, the newborn will be afflicted with the disease. Those with the sickle cell trait have no symptoms of the disease but can pass it on to their offspring. In many states, routine newborn screening for sickle cell anemia is offered. Because sickle cell anemia can lead to splenic sequestration (or pooling of blood in the spleen), many children either have nonfunctioning spleens or have had them surgically removed. The risk of infection is always a concern when this occurs before age 5 (CDC, 2023s). C/PHNs working with populations at risk for this disease can educate and refer families for diagnosis and treatment.

Food allergies are a growing problem in children. Approximately 8%, or 1 in 13, children in the United States have a food allergy (CDC, 2022o). Infants with close family members who have atopic diseases are at risk for the development of allergies. Prolonged breastfeeding for 1 year is recommended for these infants or the use of hypoallergenic infant formula. The American Academy of Pediatrics does not recommend a delay in the introduction of the most allergic foods (milk, eggs, and peanut products) for infants past the usual 4 to 6 months of age (in baby-safe soft presentation) as this will not prevent a child from developing an allergy (MacMillan, 2023). Fortunately, once allergies are diagnosed, they can be managed through dietary changes and by avoidance of allergy-triggering foods. Parents need to be educated so that they can consistently read food labels and alert family members to the young child's allergy so that inappropriate foods are avoided. Parents are encouraged to inform the school healthcare team of any allergies and emergency medication if needed.

Cystic fibrosis is a genetic disease that is screened for in infancy and affects about 35,000 people in the United States (CDC, 2022p). Cystic fibrosis is characterized by a persistent cough or wheeze, shortness of breath, poor weight gain despite a good appetite, and a salty taste to the skin. Sticky, thick mucus builds up in the lungs and digestive tract. Respiratory infections become increasingly more frequent as the child ages. It is the major cause of severe chronic lung disease in children. Chest physiotherapy to help mobilize secretions is performed daily, usually by the parents. Sometimes, a vibrating inflatable vest is used to loosen mucus. Aerosolized antibiotic treatments and mucus-thinning medications help to improve lung function and reduce respiratory infections. Mucus also affects the pancreas and prevents the release of digestive enzymes needed to digest food and absorb nutrients. Pancreatic enzyme supplements help with nutrient absorption (CDC, 2022p). C/PHNs reinforce these techniques and teach the family to avoid exposure to respiratory infections and to initiate prescribed antibiotic prophylaxis promptly. As much as feasible, the young child should be involved in his own care, offered valid choices, and encouraged to participate in decision making. The family needs genetic counseling and emotional support as members work through feelings of anticipatory grief.

Nutrition

Proper nutrition is foundational to well-being later in life. Exclusive breastfeeding is recommended for the first 6 months of life then gradually adding solid foods along with breastfeeding until 1 year of age (Patel & Rouster, 2022). Bonding between birthing parent and infant and overall maternal health are predictors of infant weight gain. Both nutrition and bonding can be accomplished by breastfeeding (Fig. 19-9). Along with convenience and no to low cost, there are other benefits of breastfeeding, which include the following (Patel & Rouster, 2022):

- *Nutrition*: Breast milk provides sugar, fat, and protein; the proteins are easily digested, and fats are well absorbed; it is the most complete form of nutrition for human infants.
- *Antiinfective and antiallergic properties*: Breast milk contains immunoglobulins, enzymes, and leukocytes that protect against pathogens, and it decreases the incidence of allergy by eliminating exposure to potential antigens. Babies exclusively breastfed for 6 or more months have fewer respiratory illnesses, ear infections, and cases of diarrhea. The chance of hospitalization for infants that are breastfed for more than 4 months is reduced.
- *Infant growth*: Breastfed babies usually gain weight at a more moderate rate and are leaner than bottle-fed babies; rapid weight gain in infancy has been associated with later chronic diseases.
- *Long-term health effects*: Breastfeeding exclusively for at least 6 months is associated with reduced risk of overweight in later life, and less change of developing atopic dermatitis, asthma, and leukemia and lymphoma. There has also been a 30% reduction in the risk of SIDS among breastfed babies and a decreased incidence of type 2 diabetes.
- *Benefits for breastfeeding parents*: Breastfeeding burns extra calories, helps to reduce postpartum bleeding, and delays ovulation and menstruation; it also lowers the risk of later ovarian and breast cancers. Studies

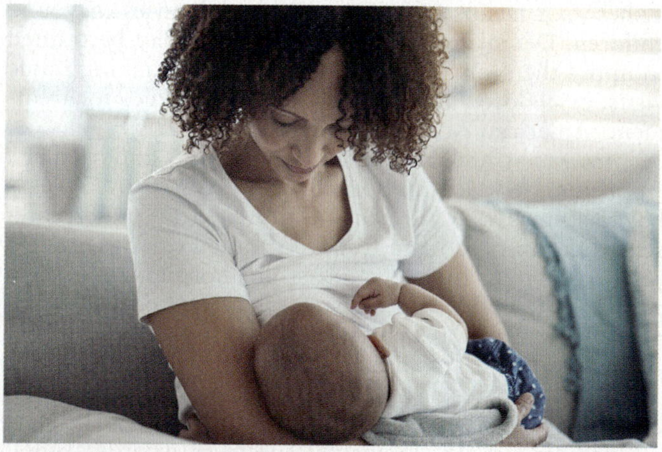

FIGURE 19-9 Breastfeeding has many benefits for both the infant and the breastfeeding parent.

show that the longer the period of lactation, the lower the chance of developing hyperlipidemia, hypertension, cardiovascular disease, and diabetes.

The C/PHN can encourage pregnant people to consider the benefits of breastfeeding their infants and provide education and interventions to assist them with the most common barriers: concern about an insufficient supply of breast milk, problems with the baby latching onto the breast, painful nipples, and scheduling problems. Patients often choose to breastfeed their babies when they fully understand the health effects for their infants and themselves and when they receive positive influence from family and friends. The C/PHN can join with labor and delivery nurses and lactation consultants in promoting breastfeeding among parents in the community.

Child and adolescent obesity prevalence in 2017 to 2020 was 19.7% (Stierman et al., 2021). In 2017 to 2020, there was a higher prevalence of obesity among Hispanic children and adolescents (26.2%) and non-Hispanic Blacks (24.8%) than among non-Hispanic Whites (16.6%) and non-Hispanic Asians (9%) (Stierman et al., 2021). The Orr et al. (2019) study identified food insecurities associated with childhood obesity as mediated through feeding practices and beliefs.

Overfeeding can lead to nutrition problems and poor infant growth. The pattern of growth may also be important, such as growth problems in infancy along with being overweight in later childhood. The most common sources of energy and nutrients for infants and toddlers are breast milk, formula, and milk. Fortified foods (e.g., grain-based foods with added vitamin A, folate, and iron) become increasingly more significant in toddler diets. In general, most nutrition recommendations include providing for a wide variety of foods for children. C/PHNs can encourage parents to continue to introduce new healthy foods to their toddlers and not give up or give in too soon.

HEALTH SERVICES FOR INFANTS, TODDLERS, AND PRESCHOOLERS

A variety of programs that directly or indirectly serve the health needs of very young children may be found in most communities. Nurses play a major and vital role in delivering these services especially for workers with low income and for vulnerable populations. In public and community health, programs fall into three categories, which approximate the three priorities of C/PHN practice: prevention, protection, and promotion.

Preventive Health Programs

Neighborhood community centers found in urban and rural settings provide families with parenting education, health and safety education, immunizations, various screening programs, and family planning services. In some areas, nurse-run clinics are established at local schools or community centers to assist in outreach services to the community. In collaboration with an interdisciplinary team, C/PHNs are often the primary care providers in these programs. The major goal is to keep communities healthy by focusing on primary and secondary prevention services. Three examples of preventive health programs for infants and young children are immunization programs, parent training programs, and quality daycare health services.

Immunization Programs

The Vaccines for Children Program (VFC) provides no-cost vaccines to qualifying children. The VFC program is provided through health departments, community clinics, and private healthcare providers to offer immunizations against the major childhood infectious diseases—measles, mumps, rubella, varicella, polio, diphtheria, tetanus, pertussis, hepatitis A and B, and Hib—some of which can cause permanent disability and even death. Pneumococcal, meningococcal, and influenza vaccines are also recommended, as is the vaccine for rotavirus, COVID-19, and RSV (CDC, 2022q). Many of these diseases no longer plague infants and children, and newer vaccines offer an even greater promise of health. The current immunization schedule can be found on the CDC (2023t) website: https://www.cdc.gov/vaccines/schedules/hcp/imz/child-adolescent.html

Although the threat of these diseases has been substantially reduced, vigilance is still essential. Low immunization levels in certain communities in the United States signal the need for constant surveillance, outreach programs, and innovative educational efforts. The C/PHN can help young families find low-cost vaccinations by using the VFC resources: (https://www.cdc.gov/vaccines/imz-managers/awardee-imz-websites.html) (CDC, 2020c). Whenever infants and young children come in contact with public health and other community clinics, it is always important to check immunizations and provide the necessary vaccines. C/PHNs are deeply involved in preventive activities that promote immunizations. One important intervention is to provide each parent with an immunization record so they can keep track of their children's immunizations. Immunization information systems are in place but vary from state to state; therefore, it is essential that parents maintain a record (CDC, 2020d).

Parent Training Programs

Parent education and training programs have been useful in providing parents with the tools needed to deal with the stresses and challenges of parenting effectively. These programs provide education regarding appropriate growth and developmental milestones, anticipatory guidance, positive discipline techniques, parenting skills, appropriate play, and parent–child interaction promotion (Child Welfare Information Gateway, n.d.-a). There are a variety of programs available for parents at local, state, and national levels, and resources are available at https://www.childwelfare.gov/topics/preventing/prevention-programs/parented/

Quality Daycare and Preschool Programs

It is estimated that 59% of children under the age of 5 spend time in nonparental care with 62% attending daycare, preschool, or a prekindergarten program (National Center for Education Statistics, 2021). Quality childcare centers improve school readiness, reduce family stress, and result in overall improvements in health and well-being for children and their families (The Children's Cabinet, 2020).

Although safe, affordable childcare is important, the long-term benefits of early childhood education are numerous. These benefits include higher rates of high school completion, college attendance, and full-time employment and lower rates of felony arrests, convictions, and incarcerations (The Urban Child Institute, 2023).

Head Start, a federally funded program that offers early childhood education to low-income children between ages 3 and 5, has consistently demonstrated significant improvements in preschoolers' social, emotional, and cognitive development.

- Children attending Head Start do better on several developmental and educational measures.
- Head Start children are also more likely to receive dental and health screenings and to have up-to-date immunization coverage.
- School attendance improves, and children are less likely to be held back in school.
- The benefits of Head Start extend to families because more Head Start parents read more frequently to their children than do parents of children not enrolled in the program (National Head Start Association, 2023).

However, the quality of daycare and preschool programs varies considerably; licensing laws can regulate only minimum safety and health standards. In addition, numerous childcare operations are too small to require licensing, leaving quality and compliance unevaluated. As educators, C/PHNs play a role in providing education and referrals. Also, nurses can influence and advocate for quality of daycare and preschool programs through active childcare consultation efforts that focus on health educational efforts for staff, monitoring of health and safety standards, and working to improve the state's or community's role in passing stronger licensing laws.

Health Protection Programs

Health protection programs for infants and young children are designed to protect them from illness and injury. Ultimately, these programs may even protect their lives.

Safety and Injury Protection

Accident and injury control programs serve a critical role in protecting the lives of children. Efforts to prevent motor vehicle crashes, a major cause of death, may include driver education programs, better highway construction, improved motor vehicle design and safety features, and continuing research into the causes of various types of crashes. Injury prevention and reduction have been addressed through strategies such as state laws requiring the use of safety restraints (e.g., seat belts, child safety seats), availability of front and side driver and passenger airbags, substitution of other modes of travel (air, rail, or bus), lower speed limits, stricter enforcement of drunk-driving laws, safer automobile design, and helmets for motorcyclists, bicycle riders, and skaters. It is essential that infants, toddlers, preschool-aged children, and children age 12 and under be properly restrained in an approved child restraint seat. C/PHNs collaborate with other community agencies, hospitals, law enforcement, and others to provide training, education, and child safety seat checks. Lead poisoning prevention programs can be found in most state and local health departments. The Lead Contamination Control Act of 1988 provided for CDC funding and programs to eliminate childhood lead poisoning (CDC, 2023n). The CDC provides technical assistance, training, and surveillance at a national level. Another role of the C/PHN is to help with targeted screening and case management and provide education to clients and communities about lead poisoning at the local level. They also work with environmental health personnel and epidemiologists to reach out to at-risk neighborhoods and communities for testing. See more on this in Chapter 9.

Protection From Child Abuse and Neglect

Services to protect children from abuse and neglect begin with a collaborative approach that includes social services, law enforcement, education, community health providers, and child advocacy. Protection begins with prevention efforts. Child abuse and maltreatment can be prevented by strengthening family economic and social support systems. Furthermore, C/PHNs must advocate for policies that support improved family economic and social systems (CDC, 2022r). There are several states that have implemented legislation to protect children from abuse and neglect. These programs include home visiting programs for pregnant people and their children, safe haven laws, shaken baby prevention programs, and prevention councils or task forces (Crane, 2020).

Additionally, social support systems and quality childcare and early education programs for children in communities are essential for the prevention of child abuse and maltreatment. Working alongside community leaders, C/PHNs strive to ensure that communities have adequate resources to support the healthy development of children (CDC, 2022s, 2022q). Protecting children from abuse and maltreatment also includes the importance of early recognition of the signs of abuse and reporting this to authorities. Nurses along with daycare providers, teachers, social workers, doctors, clergy, coaches, and all others who work with children and suspect child abuse or maltreatment are required by law to report it. In addition, animal humane workers and commercial photograph developers are mandated reporters. Child abuse or maltreatment must be reported to local child protective services or a law enforcement agency when it is suspected (Child Welfare Information Gateway, n.d.-b). Most states have hotline or toll-free numbers available for reporting (Child Welfare Information Gateway, 2019).

To promote safe and nurturing relationships and environments where children live and play free from abuse and violence, ACEs must be addressed in our communities. C/PHNs must recognize those at risk for ACEs and the history of ACEs in adults when referring clients and families to resources; ACEs are preventable. To combat ACEs in the community, Washington state has developed legislation that aims to reduce prevalence through primary prevention of child maltreatment and community engagement to improve the public's health. Secondary measures include policy enacted through Temporary Assistance for Needy Families to strengthen families dealing with ACEs through Head Start parenting programs.

Tertiary efforts include additional support for juvenile high-ACE offenders through functional family programs (CDC, 2023u).

Primary Prevention. Primary prevention measures include the use of social norming that promote positive parenting, family support groups, and public awareness campaigns about child maltreatment and how to report it, along with establishing community education to enhance the general well-being of children and their families. Educational-type services are designed to enrich the lives of families, to improve the skills of family functioning, and to prevent the stress and problems that might lead to dysfunction and abuse or neglect (CDC, 2023v).

Primary prevention also focuses on parent preparation during the prenatal period; practices that encourage parent–child bonding during labor, delivery, the postpartum period, and early infancy; and provision of information regarding support services for families with newborns. This is often the ultimate outcome sought by home visitation programs carried out or managed by C/PHNs. It is also helpful to provide parents of children of all ages with information regarding child-rearing strategies, anticipatory guidance for developmental milestones and tasks, and community resources. A helpful resource for parents is the CDC (2023w) Milestone Tracker app located at https://www.cdc.gov/ncbddd/actearly/milestones-app.html.

Secondary Prevention. Services are designed to identify and assist families who may have risk factors for impaired parenting to prevent abuse or neglect. **High-risk Families** are those families that exhibit the symptoms (risk factors) of potentially abusive or neglectful behavior or that are under the types of stress associated with abuse or neglect. These can include families living in poverty, those with substance misuse or mental health issues, parents who were abused when they were children, and parents or children with developmental disabilities. Early intervention with families at high risk can improve emotional and functional coping and help prevent further problems. High school parent education programs for pregnant adolescents, home visitation programs targeted to at-risk families, and respite care for families of children with disabilities are all examples of secondary prevention actions. Family resource centers in schools or community centers located in low-income neighborhoods can offer resource and referral services to families who may be dealing with multiple sources of stress. Evidence-based home visitation programs, such as the Nurse–Family Partnership, Early Head Start, and Healthy Families America, provide parental support and education and promote healthier family functioning, which have resulted in decreased rates of child abuse and neglect (Child Welfare Information Gateway, n.d.-c).

Tertiary Prevention. Intervention and treatment services are designed to assist a family in which abuse or neglect has already occurred, so that further abuse or neglect may be prevented and the consequences of abuse or neglect may be minimized. Often, families are referred to mental health counselors to improve family communication and functioning. Some families may require crisis respite when they feel they cannot manage the stresses of childcare. There are several evidence-based programs that have found parent mentoring or parent partner programs to be effective in reducing the reoccurrence of child abuse (Casey Family Programs, 2021).

The C/PHN and school nurse have major roles in all levels of prevention of child maltreatment. In addition, the nurse is in a unique position to detect early signs of neglect and abuse. The nurse must establish rapport with families and assist with appropriate interventions and referrals at the secondary and tertiary levels of prevention. The advanced practice nurse may also work with families of abused and neglected children as part of an interdisciplinary approach with teachers, the Department of Social Services, the judicial system, foster families, and other healthcare providers if needed. The effectiveness of local programs depends, in large measure, on the willingness of health professionals to increase their awareness and work as a team to detect, report, develop, and evaluate interventions for the perpetrators and victims of abuse and neglect. Ongoing education of healthcare providers is recommended to increase awareness of changing child abuse patterns, new reporting laws, and resources available to families.

Health Promotion Programs

Early childhood development and intervention programs are designed to have positive effects on the outcomes of children's cognitive and social development. Some health promotion programs have considered children's physical health, and others have focused on parent–child interaction and child social development. All are considered important health promotion programs from birth through preschool years.

Infant Brain Development Research and Parent—Child Interactions

Research into the normal brain development of infants and toddlers has revealed that brain maturation in the first few years of life is very rapid: the brain grows to 80% of adult size by age 3, and the myelination pattern of an 18- to 24-month-old child is similar to that of an adult (First Things First, 2023). The prefrontal cortex of 4-year-olds is already functional and becomes more organized throughout later adolescence. Early environment exerts a lasting influence on brain development, even in the womb. Appropriate early nutrition and stimulation promotes healthy development.

- Early in life, rapid myelination is taking place, and children need higher fat levels in their diet (50% of total calories should come from fat). Breast milk or formula will provide this fat during the first year of life, then breast milk or whole milk can be used after the first birthday. After age 2, children's fat consumption should be 30% of their calories, and 1% or 2% milk should be given instead of whole milk (Verduci et al., 2021).
- Meaningful parent–child interactions should be established early; they include holding, rocking, comforting, touching, talking, and singing. When parents talk to infants and read to young children, children

later demonstrate more advanced language and literacy skills. Providing a caring and supportive environment, with opportunities to learn and explore, is supportive of healthy brain development and promotes secure infant attachment (CDC, 2023x).

- Important parental behaviors that promote social development include gazing into an infant's eyes, paying attention to and interacting with toddlers, and listening to and answering preschoolers' questions.
- Providing infants and young children with secure, learning-rich environments where they can use their senses to discover new things helps them to maximize their potential.
- Emotional comfort and a secure environment ensure that young children will better deal with their feelings.

It is important for the C/PHN to provide information to parents on the most current research results about brain development as well as tangible suggestions such as low-cost brain-stimulating toys and community resources to encourage quality parent–child interactions that promote appropriate physical growth and cognitive and social development.

Developmental Screening

With an emphasis on infant and early childhood development, C/PHNs often routinely carry out developmental screenings (Fig. 19-10). The American Academy of Pediatrics recommends developmental screening surveillance for children at each health visit along with an evidence-based developmental screening tool used at 9, 18, and 30 months, or anytime there is a concern. Autism-specific screenings are recommended at 18 and 24 months, and social–emotional screenings should be conducted at regular intervals (CDC, 2023y). The CDC provides a free app with a variety of developmental screening resources available at https://www.cdc.gov/ncbddd/actearly/milestones-app.html (CDC, 2023t).

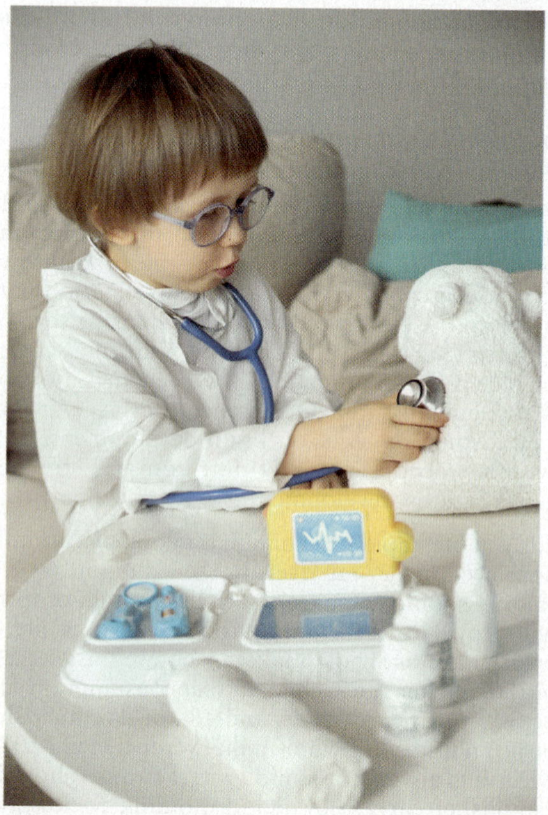

FIGURE 19-10 Allowing children to play with healthcare equipment can help alleviate fear and anxiety.

Developmental screening tools are also helpful in educating parents about normal child development and can provide a means of anticipatory guidance on developmental milestones and future safety issues. *Bright Futures*, an important resource for nurses and parents, provides tools to help families determine appropriate developmental milestones and expected behaviors, along with suggestions about when to seek help from professionals. A variety of screening tools available to nurses and other health professionals, ranging from parent report instruments to those that involve direct assessment of behaviors and skills, can examine overall physical and cognitive development or screen for such things as temperament, behavior, autism, and speech and language problems. It is important for the C/PHN to use tools that have reported validity and reliability. Early identification of problems can lead to interventions such as enrollment in early intervention programs and help children with school readiness. These early intervention programs are available in most communities or through the public school system (Bright Futures, 2022).

Programs for Children With Disabilities

Many children have special needs. They may have a congenital or acquired developmental disability, birth defect, or a chronic emotional, mental, or physical disease. Each year, about 1 in every 33 U.S. infants is born with a birth defect each year (CDC, 2023z). Some children suffer injuries after birth (Box 19-7). Autism and other mental or behavioral disorders develop after infancy and may require special services. Educational, health, and social or recreational services should be available for all children.

Federal law mandates early identification and intervention services for those with a variety of developmental disabilities. Developmental delays are characterized by slower development in one or more areas. The Individuals with Disabilities Education Act provides early intervention services, usually at home, for those from birth to age 2 who have developmental delays in physical, cognitive, communication, social/emotional, and adaptive development. Intervention services are also available to children with a mental or physical problem that is likely to result in a developmental delay. Newborns can receive infant stimulation services at home or in some schools specially designed to meet the needs of the very young. These programs are offered on a part-time basis for 1 to 2 hours, two to three times a week. Special education preschools are available for young children from ages 3 to 5. By preschool age, children may advance to half-day programs. Additional services can be provided to assist the families in getting children to the programs. Door-to-door bus service in specially equipped small buses or vans safely transports young children who arrive at school in wheelchairs or with other assistive devices (CDC, 2022t).

Most communities offer additional social and recreational programs for children who are disabled. For

BOX 19-7 STORIES FROM THE FIELD

A Case of Kernicterus

A young mother was hospitalized for the birth of her second daughter, a beautiful little girl born without incident. The infant had difficulty latching on for breastfeeding and was not an active feeder. The mother told her obstetrical nurse that the infant seemed very different from her first child. The infant was irritable, but the nurse reassured the mother that the baby was fine and "not all babies are alike." Still, the new mother was concerned.

By the second day, the mother noticed that the baby was not very alert and did not want to feed. She also noticed that the baby's color was "yellowish," and the mother notified the nurse. Again, the nurse reassured the mother that this was "normal" for infants of Asian descent. The baby still was not feeding well, and there was yellowish-orange color stool in the baby's diaper. The mother notified the nurse and asked the nurse to call the doctor. The nurse refused and told the mother that she was "overreacting." The nurse again reassured the mother that the baby was "fine" and no action was taken. The young mother was not satisfied with the nursing care and requested additional assistance. A referral was made to the breastfeeding specialist at the hospital to help the new mother feed her infant. There were no phone calls documented to the primary provider nor was there documentation of the "yellowish-orange" stool. (The young mother kept the diaper for further proof of her concerns, though.) There was no documentation of irritability, inability to breastfeed, lethargy, or jaundiced appearance of the skin. The primary provider discharging the infant did not receive any information regarding irritability, yellowish stool, and yellowish tone of lower extremities and abdomen. No blood work was done. No referrals were made to home health or public health for follow-up.

Within 48 hours of discharge, the young mother brought her lethargic baby to the hospital's emergency room. On day 4 of life, the infant's bilirubin was 46. The infant was severely neurologically damaged, and the brain damage that resulted was irreversible. She was diagnosed with severe cerebral palsy, secondary to kernicterus (excessive bilirubin). The child has normal intelligence but will never be able to walk or talk. She will be fed through a gastrostomy tube for the rest of her life. The family was devastated.

The primary provider and hospital (nurses) were sued. The nurses on duty could not defend their actions with their charting or lack thereof. The attorneys for the hospital, representing the primary provider and nurses, could not defend the actions of their clients. A multimillion-dollar settlement was granted, and the nurses were fired. Unfortunately, this is not an isolated case. The irreversible brain damage that occurs as a result of untreated hyperbilirubinemia should not occur in the 21st century. This was a no-win situation that could have been avoided with proper nursing intervention. Hyperbilirubinemia should always be in the forefront of newborn assessment during the first few days of life.

The nurses involved in this case were not acting as the patient's advocate. The primary provider should have been notified immediately when signs and symptoms were first noted. Incorrect assumptions were made because of the nationality of the patient, an indication of lack of cultural competence. Home health nursing or public and community health nursing care should have been arranged for infant follow-up after discharge.

Susan N., nurse consultant

1. *As a new C/PHN, what services do you think this family needs? Do you believe these services will change over time? If so, what type of anticipatory guidance should you provide the family and child?*
2. *How can you become culturally competent when working with a culture you are not familiar with?*
3. *You decide to develop some culturally competent care modules geared toward healthcare providers. Who are the stakeholders? What community members can you ask to help?*

example, American Lung Association affiliate offices sponsor camping programs for children with asthma or other lung diseases. Often, these are camps for school-aged children that may last up to 1 week and be located in mountain or beach areas, but they may also be day camps, with parents in attendance for preschoolers. Many of these camps have C/PHNs either working or volunteering. Nationwide programs, such as the Special Olympics, offer recreational competition for children in a variety of sports, such as bowling, track and field, skiing, and swimming. The C/PHN best serves families as a resource for such programs. Some parents are not aware of the rights or services available for their children with disabilities. Nurses can advocate for parents and help establish services in communities where needed services are lacking. For more information, refer to Chapter 24.

Nutritional Programs

Adequate nutrition must begin before birth. One of the most productive health promotion programs is the Special Supplemental Food Program for Women, Infants, and Children (WIC). In addition to supporting pregnant people and young children with nutritious foods and achieving the initial goals of decreasing the rates of preterm and LBW babies, increasing the length of pregnancy, and reducing the incidence of infant and child iron-deficiency anemia, WIC also improves pregnant people's nutritional status. WIC is not an entitlement program, but rather, Congress sets funding and eligibility requirements yearly (U.S. Department of Agriculture, n.d.).

WIC provides information to parents about eating healthfully and promoting healthy rates of growth. Parents become more aware of the need to reduce the consumption of saturated fat, salt, sugar, and over-processed foods. The C/PHN, through nutrition education, reinforcement of positive practices, and referral, plays a significant role in promoting the health of infants and young children (Box 19-8). For more information about WIC, see Chapter 20.

BOX 19-8 LEVELS OF PREVENTION PYRAMID

High Incidence of Low Birth Weight in Newborns

SITUATION: High Incidence of Low Birth Weight in Newborns Born Within a Community
GOAL: Improve birth weight in newborns within this community by using the three levels of prevention

Tertiary Prevention

Rehabilitation

- Establish rehabilitation programs for infants with LBW to lessen long-term effects
- Provide parents of LBW infants with resources and advocacy methods to improve their child's future

Health Promotion and Education

- Provide families with long-term education on the needs of their child, if possible
- Reevaluate education programs to determine if the incidence of LBW infants has decreased and modify programs as needed

Health Protection

- Continue monitoring and providing support to birthing parents who continue high-risk behavior
- Educate on prevention of LBW infants and risk factors
- Promote practices that decrease risk factors

Secondary Prevention

Early Diagnosis

- Screen at-risk people
- Conduct a community needs assessment
- Notify providers of the high incidence of LBW infants and ensure they screen clients at each visit
- Patient starts prenatal care early in the first trimester and continues care at regular intervals throughout the pregnancy

Prompt Treatment

- Establish programs to provide prompt treatment for birthing parents of infants at high risk for LBW
- Establish safe and private counseling for these patients

Primary Prevention

Health Promotion and Education

- Institute parent education programs through partnerships with community stakeholders and community members
- Install infographics for proper nutrition during pregnancy in supermarkets, transportation ports, and community gathering spots
- Increase community awareness of community resources such as WIC

Health Protection

- Identify people in the community who are at greatest risk of delivering a LBW infant
- Develop community resources that support health promotion (e.g., grants and community volunteers)

ROLE OF THE C/PHN

C/PHNs face the challenge of continually assessing each population's current health problems as well as determining available and needed services. Interventions are implemented for the maternal, infant, toddler, and preschool populations that focus on health promotion, health protection, and early intervention. Interventions may include work in family planning or high-risk clinics, telephone information services and hotlines, outreach interventions, childcare consultation, or home visitation programs. The nurse uses educational and health coaching interventions when teaching family planning, nutrition, safety precautions, and appropriate health-seeking or childcare skills. Such interventions involve providing information and encouraging client groups (parents and young children) to participate in their own healthcare. Other interventions include strategies in which the nurse uses a greater degree of persuasion or positive manipulation, such as conducting voluntary immunization programs, working in a lead screening program, encouraging smoking cessation during pregnancy, preventing communicable diseases, and encouraging appropriate use of child safety devices such as car seats. Finally, the nurse may use interventions that motivate people to adhere to laws that require certain immunizations or mandate reporting of suspected child abuse and environmental health standards violations, such as sanitation issues. Home visiting programs are effective in addressing the needs of high-risk and hard-to-reach families (Health Resources & Services Administration, 2023).

CASE STUDY **10 ESSENTIAL PUBLIC HEALTH SERVICES**

Bathtub Drowning

A Head Start nurse is assigned to a small rural community. The young mother that the nurse was working with had placed her 11-month-old infant in a bath seat and had walked away to retrieve her cell phone. She was gone no more than 5 minutes, but when she returned the bath seat had tipped over, and her child was unconscious and submerged in the tub's water. The child had likely reached for a toy and the seat tipped over, the suctions on the bottom are not a guarantee of seat stability. EMTs were unable to revive the baby, and despite hospital efforts, the baby did not survive.

Bathtub drownings can occur in less than 2 in of water. Bathtub rings and seats cannot prevent drownings. Never leave an infant or child unsupervised near water (Water Safety Council of Fresno County, n.d.).

1. ***Recognize Cues:*** *Which findings require immediate follow-up, are unexpected, or are most concerning?*
2. ***Analyze Cues:*** *What information is noted or needed for interpreting findings?*
3. ***Prioritize Hypotheses:*** *Based on the information that you have, what is happening?*
4. ***Generate Solutions:*** *What intervention(s) will achieve the desired outcome?*
5. ***Take Action:*** *What actions should you take or do first?*
6. ***Evaluate Outcomes:*** *Were outcomes achieved? Why or why not?*
7. *Which Essential Public Health Services influence this situation? (See Box 2-2.)*

Source: Water Safety Council of Fresno County. (n.d.). *Facts and stats.* https://www.watersafe.org/bathtubs-households

SUMMARY

- Maternal–child health clients are an important population group to C/PHNs because their physical and emotional health is vital to the future of society.
- The United States does not fare well in comparison to other resource-abundant nations on maternal–child health indicators.
- Problems of substance abuse, STIs, and teen pregnancy can lead to less-than-optimal outcomes for newborns.
- Complications of pregnancy and childbirth, such as hypertension, gestational diabetes, postpartum depression, and fetal or infant death, offer opportunities for C/PHNs to provide education, outreach, monitoring, and support.
- IMRs in the United States are higher than those in many other countries around the world. Toddler and young child mortality and morbidity are often related to unintentional injuries.
- Preventive services include immunization programs, along with quality daycare and preschool programs.
- Health protection services include accident and injury prevention and control, as well as services to protect children from child abuse and neglect.
- Health promotion services include infant development through effective parent–child interaction, developmental screening, and services to children with special needs.

ACTIVE LEARNING EXERCISES

1. Carefully examine the care needs for any one of the chronic diseases discussed in the Infants, Toddlers, and Preschooler section of this chapter. What are the mortality and morbidity statistics in the United States, in your state of residence, or globally? How do these statistics compare and contrast? (Objective 1)
2. Using the chronic disease chosen for Objective 1, what are the specific health issues and the *Healthy People 2030* goals directed toward those issues? Examine the resources available to these families within your state of residence. Are these resources enough to meet the needs of this population? Justify your answer. Which of the 10 Essential Public Health Services (Box 2-2) did you use in the activity? (Objective 2)
3. Adverse childhood experiences (ACEs) have a negative socioeconomic effect on people, communities, and society that costs billions of dollars. What health promotion programs are implemented in your community to help combat ACEs? Are these interventions effective and an efficient use of limited resources? Develop an infographic that describes these programs and their effectiveness. (Objective 3)
4. During a home visit regarding a child with a high lead level, you discover that the father works in a battery manufacturing plant. Furthermore, after speaking with other C/PHNs in the area, you discover an unusually high caseload of children with elevated blood lead levels. After speaking with the plant's management, you discover they do not have a policy regarding end-of-shift decontamination of the employees' clothing. Research current information on the decontamination of employees clothing when working with environmental hazards such as lead. The stakeholders in the policy development would include partners such as environmental health officials, union representatives, and plant management. Are there other groups that should be included? What role would a C/PHN take in the development of this policy? What is the downstream effect this contamination will have on maternal-child health? (Objective 4)

5. Interview a C/PHN who acts as an advocate for their community. How do they engage in relationship building and leadership to promote the overall health of their community? Interview a faculty member or a nurse leader on ways they advocate for birthing parents, infants, toddlers, and preschool-age children at the local, state, and national level. What leadership roles do they have to promote health in this population? List some advocacy measures you can take and complete one. (Objective 5)

CHAPTER 20

School-Age Children and Adolescents*

"Children are the world's most valuable resource and its best hope for the future."

—John F. Kennedy

KEY TERMS

Adverse childhood experiences (ACE)
Anorexia nervosa
Asthma action plan
Attention deficit hyperactivity disorder (ADHD)
Autism spectrum disorder (ASD)
Binge eating
Bulimia nervosa
Learning disorders
Obese
Overweight
Pediculosis
Social determinants of health

LEARNING OBJECTIVES

Upon mastery of this chapter, you should be able to:

1. Examine poverty as a significant social determinant of health in children and adolescents.
2. Identify major health problems and concerns for U.S. school-age children and adolescents.
3. Discuss the relationship of academic achievement to health status.
4. Analyze mortality and injury trends among school-age children and adolescents.
5. Evaluate Healthy People 2030 objectives affecting children and adolescents and the barriers involved in attaining them.
6. Appraise health promotion programs and services for school-age children and adolescent populations at the primary, secondary, and tertiary levels.

INTRODUCTION

According to Erik Erikson's developmental framework, the school-age and adolescent years are a time of task mastery and development of competence and self-identity. During these years, children grow physically as well as emotionally and socially. They move from being under the total control of parents and families during the infant and toddler years to being more and more influenced by those outside the home—classmates, teachers, peers, and other groups (Hockenberry et al., 2019).

Poverty, a significant social determinant of health, poses a challenge to the health of many school-age children and adolescents. Other challenges for this population include chronic diseases, behavioral and learning problems, emotional and mental health issues, disabilities, injuries, communicable diseases, developmental issues, school concerns, and the risk behaviors characteristic of the teenage years. The COVID-19 pandemic dramatically altered how children and adolescents experienced those years and the impact on their living, learning, and lives since the pandemic. This chapter explores the health needs of school-age children and adolescents and describes various services that address those needs, along with the community health nurse's role in assisting families with children.

SCHOOL: CHILD'S WORK

Children and adolescents spend most of their waking hours in school. The quality of their educational experiences (e.g., teacher–child interactions) can influence learning, and their academic success can predict future education, employment, life skills, and a livable income. Therefore, their future success as tomorrow's parents, workers, leaders, and decision makers depends in good measure on the achievement of their educational goals today.

*In this chapter, "male" refers to a person assigned male at birth, and "female" refers to a person assigned female at birth.

Child health has been linked to school success—healthy children are found to be more motivated and prepared to learn (CDC, 2022a)—and coordinated school health programs are linked to academic achievement (CDC, 2023a). This is well known to school nurses and community and public health nurses (C/PHNs) who work in schools.

In 2022, approximately 49.46 million school-age children and adolescents (5 to 18 years old) attended elementary and secondary schools in the United States. Of these students, approximately 48 million were educated in public schools, with 9% of the K–12 students being educated in private schools (National Center for Education Statistics [NCES], 2024a). In 2022, the U.S. population ages 0 to 17 years was 44% White/non-Hispanic, 15% Black/non-Hispanic, 5.5% Asian/non-Hispanic, 29% Hispanic, 9% American Indian/Alaska Native, and 5% identified with two or more races (NCES, 2024a).

POVERTY: A MAJOR SOCIAL DETERMINANT OF HEALTH IN SCHOOL-AGE CHILDREN AND ADOLESCENTS

Although the United States is making strides against poverty, around 14% of children still live below the poverty level ($20,050 for a family of four). In 2020, an additional 6.2 million children lived in extreme poverty. Moreover, this burden of poverty is not equally shared among racial and ethnic groups. In comparison with White children, children of color are almost three times as likely to live in a household with limited resources. One of every 10 White children live below the poverty line, and approximately one of every three Black, Hispanic, and Native American children live below the poverty line (National Center for Children in Poverty [NCCP], 2024).

As noted by the United Way (2022, para 9), "Child poverty can have a profound and lasting impact on a person's life. Growing up in poverty can lead to poorer health outcomes, lower educational attainment, and increased difficulty finding employment as an adult. Children who experience poverty are also more likely to experience food insecurity, poor housing, and limited access to healthcare. All of these factors can contribute to a cycle of poverty that is difficult to break."

Children living in poverty have poorer health overall and are more likely to experience the following:

- Chronic health conditions (e.g., asthma, anemia)
- Injuries and accidents
- Behavioral problems, including academic failure, alcohol use disorder, antisocial behavior, depression, substance misuse, and adolescent pregnancy
- Poor brain growth, neurodevelopment, and learning
- Developmental delays
- Stress
- Child maltreatment, trauma, and abuse
- Exposure to environmental toxins, inadequate nutrition, and decreased cognitive stimulation
- Increased susceptibility to illness (Ballard Brief, 2020; Children's Bureau, 2019; Child Trends, 2022)

Social determinants of health (SDOH) are the socioeconomic and environmental conditions that influence individuals' health outcomes and access to healthcare services (Chelak & Chakole, 2023). These determinants are powerful contributors to health disparities—irrespective of socioeconomic standing—as they encompass factors such as income, education, employment, housing, access to transportation systems, and social support networks. When examining the growth and development of children and adolescents in America through the lens of SDOH, it becomes evident that these factors play a pivotal role in shaping overall well-being (see Chapters 11 and 23).

In the United States, the impact of SDOH on the growth and development of children and adolescents is profound.

- Socioeconomic disparities significantly affect access to quality education, safe neighborhoods, and nutritious food.
- Children from families with low income may face barriers to educational attainment due to inadequate resources, which can hinder their cognitive and social development.
- Limited access to nutritious food, "food insecurity," can lead to malnutrition and hinder physical growth and cognitive development among young individuals.
- Something as simple as transportation resources can help a child get to an important health visit.

Furthermore, *housing instability* and overcrowded living conditions can expose children and adolescents to environmental hazards, contributing to health issues such as asthma and developmental delays.

The *availability of safe play* areas and recreational facilities also varies based on socioeconomic status, influencing opportunities for physical activity and social interaction, both crucial for healthy growth and lifelong habits (Fig. 20-1).

Access to healthcare is another critical aspect influenced by social determinants.

- Children and adolescents from underrepresented backgrounds may encounter *barriers to healthcare services* due to lack of insurance, transportation, or proximity to medical facilities.
- In the United States, this can affect rural and urban families in different ways. Preventive care and timely

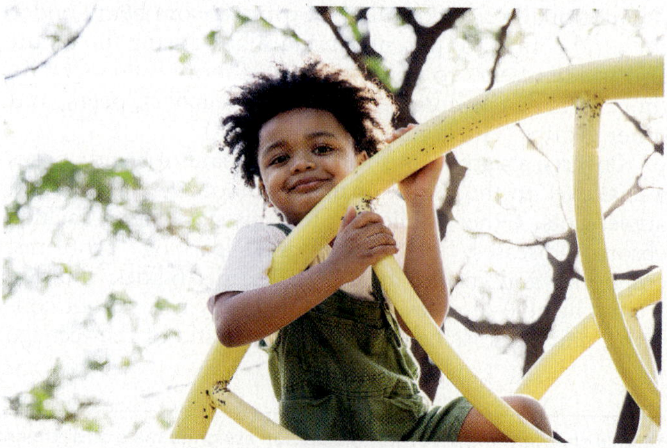

FIGURE 20-1 A child playing outdoors.

interventions are essential for monitoring growth, addressing developmental concerns, and preventing chronic illnesses.

Addressing SDOH is imperative for promoting equitable growth and development among children and adolescents. Policies and interventions that focus on improving socioeconomic conditions, ensuring affordable housing, and expanding access to quality education are crucial steps. Additionally, community-based programs that provide support to families, such as parenting resources and early childhood education initiatives, can mitigate the impact of adverse social determinants on children's development. By recognizing the role of factors such as income, education, housing, and healthcare access, society can work toward reducing health disparities and creating an environment that fosters the well-being of all young individuals. Efforts to address social determinants holistically are essential for ensuring that children and adolescents have equal opportunities to thrive, regardless of their socioeconomic backgrounds.

A classic longitudinal study, along with a series of preliminary studies, on the many stresses of childhood poverty (e.g., crowded homes/classrooms, inadequate childcare, low socioeconomic status, family/peer problems) found that levels of the stress hormone cortisol influenced results on school readiness testing and affected cognitive functioning (e.g., impulse/emotional control, planning, attention), which, in turn, affects school success (Blair, 2012). For children from more affluent backgrounds, other stressors (e.g., divorce, learning disabilities, harsh parenting) can affect stress levels and outcomes. Continuing periods of high stress can lead to either high levels of cortisol or levels that are immediately high but then drop very low, blunting children's responses to new challenges. Both those with blunted responses and those with very high cortisol responses were found to have lower executive function and more problems with writing, math, and reading, as well as poor self-control in class. The reverse was found for those with more characteristic patterns of cortisol response (elevated with a stressful event and then normalized afterward).

The children in this study were tested in Head Start and again in kindergarten. Parenting style was also examined, and parents with lower socioeconomic status were more prone to harsher forms of discipline that demanded obedience. Their children had lower executive functioning and either high or blunted cortisol levels. Parents using a more sensitive approach, who interacted with children during play and allowed more exploration, had children with better executive function and normal cortisol response. Researchers saw this as evidence that parenting style was an important part of child stress response. They noted that psychological stress in childhood "can substantially shape the course of their cognitive, social, and emotional development ... and impair specific learning abilities in children, potentially setting them back in many domains of life" (p. 67).

The negative impact of childhood poverty on learning and later income, along with health, continues to be well documented. Van Ryzin et al. (2018) indicate, "Researchers found that attaining economic security later in life did not completely attenuate this link between early poverty and health problems, suggesting that poverty and adverse social experiences early in life made the strongest contribution to negative long-term health effects" (p. 130).

Because the lifelong effects of poverty can be deeply rooted in children and adolescents, countering its effects requires a multilayered public health approach. Prevention programs that increase childhood nurturing have been shown to decrease behavioral, emotional, cognitive, and neurophysiological problem development and may be either family or school based.

Family-based prevention programs focus on teaching family management skills and improving family relationships. Change outcomes associated with these programs involve cultivating skills for monitoring and managing child behavior, negotiating conflicts, and improving overall family environment quality. Studies indicate that parenting programs can alter cortisol rhythms, improve stress regulation, and improve the standard of living over time. One of these programs, the Nurse–Family Partnership program, has directly led to decreased use of welfare and other governmental assistance, improved employment for birthing parents, and improved birth spacing (see Chapter 4).

School-based programs focus on child development and the need to remediate the effects of low-income and deficient home environments. Change outcomes involve social–emotional and character development, such as improving decision-making skills, improving the management of difficult situations, and establishing positive relationships. An example of a school-based program is Cooperative Learning, which focuses on instructional strategies and can be used in elementary, secondary, and postsecondary education settings. It involves group learning methods such as peer tutoring, reciprocal teaching, and collaborative reading. Teachers design their own small-group activities that focus on "positive interdependence." Members of the group are each responsible for achieving their goals and the success of the group. Such activities improve friendships, increase personal acceptance, and foster academic achievement (Van Ryzin et al., 2018).

Reaching families in need and disseminating programs to larger populations require policy initiatives and funding at the local, state, and national levels. Prevention programs can be implemented through improved access to healthcare systems. Using new technology strategies such as telehealth enables health service access and reduces provider-level barriers to healthcare. All of the strategies and programs discussed require ongoing evidence-based practice and community partnerships to educate the public and policymakers, with the goal of disrupting the intergenerational effect of poverty (Van Ryzin et al., 2018). For more on poverty, see Chapter 23.

Several government programs and legislative reforms have helped many move out of poverty. Legislation reforms enacted in 1996 (such as the Personal Responsibility and Work Opportunity Reconciliation Act) have been successful in moving many families from welfare to work. With a combination of welfare time limits, increasing work requirements/sanctions, and reducing financial disincentives for work, welfare reform, and work success programs were projected to lead to greater employment. After 22 years, however, many are questioning whether the resulting safety net of Temporary Assistance for Needy Families (TANF) is adequate. The number of families receiving cash assistance through TANF decreased since its implementation from 68 of every 100 families in poverty receiving cash assistance in 1996 to 21 of every 100 families in poverty receiving cash assistance in 2020 (Center on Budget and Policy Priorities [CBPP], 2022). COVID-19 has influenced economic instability and household poverty levels; TANF is not reaching families most in need. Eligibility requirements may differ between states, with Black and Hispanic children most at risk for not receiving services (CBPP, 2022). The Supplemental Nutrition Assistance Program (SNAP), formerly the Food Stamp Program, is one of the largest programs offered by federal Food and Nutrition Services. In 2023, 2 million households used SNAP benefits (Desilver, 2023). Positive health benefits for children are linked with SNAP (Carlson, 2022). However, the benefits fall short of meeting family food needs (Child Trends, 2024).

HEALTH PROBLEMS OF SCHOOL-AGE CHILDREN

The well-being of children is a concern both nationally and internationally. Many organizations have focused their resources on improving the health and well-being of children, including the World Health Organization (WHO), United Nations International Children's Education Fund, and U.S. governmental agencies, nonprofit groups, and charitable foundations. Unfortunately, the needs of millions of children in the United States and worldwide remain unmet. The *Healthy People 2030* framework for children is shown in Box 20-1.

Even in the wealthiest nations, many children face complex and often chronic health problems that cause them to miss school days or marginally participate in the classroom. Childhood is a critical period during which certain health behaviors or conditions can develop that can lead to more serious adult illnesses. The chronic health problems of children younger than 18 years are characterized by the duration and persistence of symptoms and their impact on social functioning. Examples of chronic conditions in school-age children include the following:

- Asthma
- Autism spectrum disorder (ASD)
- Diabetes
- Neuromuscular disorders
- Poor oral health
- Seizure disorders
- ADHD
- Nutritional problems—anemia or obesity/overweight
- Food allergies
- Mental illness (CDC, 2021a)

Chronic Diseases

Chronic health problems can affect a child's ability to learn and their physical and social development. Forty percent of all school-age children have a chronic condition requiring daily management and assessment for potential emergencies (CDC, 2021a). Serious conditions, such as asthma, diabetes, hypertension, seizure disorders, food allergies, and poor oral health, are common in the school setting and have effects on academic achievement and educational attainment, affect the entire family, and can lead to developmental and social issues for children, as well as missed school days and potentially school failure. Understanding the influence of chronic diseases in children and families is key for public health and school nurses as they assist children and families in managing health (National Association of School Nurses [NASN], 2021a).

With the number of children with chronic conditions increasing, more children with significant health problems are present in schools (NASN, 2021a). Some children require specialized physical healthcare procedures, such as catheterization, suctioning, or ventilator care while in the school setting, even though school nurses are not always present in each school building every day.

The Individuals with Disabilities Education Act (IDEA) and Section 504 of the Rehabilitation Act of 1973 mandate that services must be provided for children identified as *disabled*. Many conditions may be characterized as disabling under these two laws, including

BOX 20-1 *HEALTHY PEOPLE 2030*

Objectives to Improve the Health and Well-Being of Children

Core Objectives

EMC-01	Increase the proportion of children and adolescents who communicate positively with their parents
EMC-02	Increase the proportion of children whose parents read to them at least 4 days per week
EMC-03	Increase the proportion of children who get sufficient sleep
EMC-04	Increase the proportion of children with developmental delays who get intervention services by age 4 years

Research Objectives

EMC-R01	Increase the proportion of children with developmental delays who get intervention services by age 4 years

Developmental Objectives

EMC-D01	Increase the proportion of children who are developmentally ready for school
EMC-D02	Reduce the proportion of children and adolescents who are suspended or expelled

Reprinted from U.S. Department of Health & Human Services (USDHHS). (2020). *Healthy People 2030: Browse objectives.* https://health.gov/healthypeople/objectives-and-data/browse-objectives

autism, deafness or hearing impairment, blindness or vision impairment, emotional disturbances, intellectual disability, specific learning disabilities, speech or language impairments, or other health impairments (e.g., ADHD, asthma). Once identified as disabled, children may qualify for special education services. Children with chronic health conditions that can affect learning (e.g., diabetes, seizure disorders) may receive medications or other related services while in school to maintain health and promote their ability to learn (U.S. Department of Education, n.d.).

Many children with chronic health conditions take multiple medications at home and at school. This is a critical time for teens to develop schedules and optimal health behaviors. Medication adherence challenges can be particularly daunting for adolescents as they prepare to manage their health as adults. Common medication adherence barriers may include medication adverse effects, scheduling challenges, desire to appear "normal," and lack of family, social, or medical support. Working with the school nurses, families can coordinate care by creating individualized health plans that highlight the plan of care and communication between family, the student, and the school setting (CDC, 2022b). The use of mobile apps and technology may now be part of managing children's and adolescent's chronic health (Lee et al., 2023).

Asthma

Asthma is one of the most common chronic diseases of childhood. In 2022, it is estimated that 9.9% of children younger than 18 have asthma (National Center for Health Statistics, 2024). Asthma attacks in children have declined due to better recognition and diagnosis of the disease; however, overcrowded conditions and exposure to air pollution (indoor or outdoor), allergens, and irritants in the environment are probable culprits and may trigger asthma attacks (Asthma and Allergy Foundation of America [AAFA], 2024).

Recent research indicates that the pathogenesis of asthma can be influenced by many factors, including an inflammatory response to early life exposures or events such as infections and environmental exposures (air pollution, tobacco smoke). Additionally, obesity, genetics, early-life nutrition through breastfeeding, airway and gut microbiome, and preterm infants can influence the predisposition for asthma (Pignenburg et al., 2022).

Children and adolescents with asthma may have attacks triggered by infections, exposure to cigarette smoke, stress, strenuous exercise, or weather changes (e.g., cold, wind, rain). Asthma disproportionately affects underrepresented groups and families living below the poverty level (AAFA, 2024). Children with asthma incur greater healthcare costs associated with increased emergency department visits and hospitalizations. Treatment for chronic asthma usually includes:

- Quick-relief medicine (inhaled short-acting beta2-agonists [SABAs], oral corticosteroids, and short-acting anticholinergics)
- Long-term control (corticosteroids, biologic medicine, leukotriene modifiers, inhaled mast cell stabilizers, inhaled long-acting bronchodilators, and allergy shots) (National Heart, Lung, and Blood Institute, 2024).

Asthma education programs are central to effective disease control and management. The CDC's educational program EXHALE focuses on the following evidence-based strategies:

- E—Education on asthma self-management (AS-ME)
- X—X-tinguish smoking and secondhand smoke
- H—Home visits for trigger reduction and asthma self-management education
- A—Achievement of guidelines-based medical management
- L—Linkages and coordination of care across settings
- E—Environmental policies or best practices to reduce asthma triggers from indoor, outdoor, and occupational sources (CDC, 2024a)

School nurses and C/PHNs often work with students, families, and physicians to develop an **asthma action plan** to control, prevent, or minimize the untoward effects of acute asthma episodes. Asthma action plans to be used with children and in school settings can be found here:

- https://www.cdc.gov/asthma/action-plan/documents/asthma-action-plan-508.pdf
- https://www.nhlbi.nih.gov/resources/asthma-action-plan-2020

C/PHNs are in a unique position to implement many of the EXHALE strategies, especially education for children and their families. Education should include foundational asthma self-management (AS-ME) concepts, including medication use, asthma self-management techniques, symptom recognition and appropriate treatment, and asthma trigger reduction. Monitoring asthma medications and teaching proper methods of inhaler use are vital to school nursing or C/PHN functions.

Autism Spectrum Disorder

Autism spectrum disorder (ASD) is a complex developmental disorder frequently noticed within the first few years of life and typically lasts throughout a person's lifetime. The spectrum of ASD indicates that symptoms for each child vary and may range from mild to severe and from gifted to severely challenged (CDC, 2024b). A child's communication skills and interaction with others are most frequently affected, along with obsessive behavior and narrowed interests. Behaviors associated with autism include the following:

- Social communication and interaction skills
  - Does not respond to name by 9 months of age
  - Avoids eye contact
  - Does not play simple interactive games by 12 months
  - Does not show facial expressions by 9 months
  - Does not share interests with others by 15 months
- Restrictive or repetitive behaviors or interests
  - Repeats words/phrases over and over (echolalia)
  - Plays with toys the same way every time
  - Is focused on part of an object
  - Has obsessive interests
  - Must follow routines
  - Gets upset with minor changes
  - Has unusual reactions to how things smell, taste, feel, or look

- Other characteristics
  - Delayed language
  - Delayed movement
  - Delayed cognitive or learning skills
  - Unusual eating or sleeping behaviors
  - Unusual mood or emotional reaction (CDC, 2024b)

Autism has become an urgent public health concern, with prevalence estimated at 1 of every 36 children (CDC, 2024b). The disorder varies among racial/ethnic groups and communities, with greater prevalence among males than females. Current data identified an increase in populations with ASD (29.3% Black, 31.65 Hispanic, and 33.4% Asian/Pacific Islander) as compared to 24.3% of White children at 8 years of age (CDC, 2023b). The yearly expense for children with ASD is four times higher as compared with children without ASD. This estimate includes various costs including healthcare, special education, and indirect costs such as lost parental productivity (Matin et al., 2022). Risk factors for ASD include the following:

- A sibling with ASD
- Genetic or chromosomal conditions
- Complications at birth
- A child born to older parents (CDC, 2024b)

Through the CDC-sponsored multiyear Study to Explore Early Development (SEED), there are research findings on the growing knowledge of ASD:

- Forty percent of children with ASD on public insurance were not using community services as compared to those with private insurance; those on public insurance alone were also more likely to receive psychotropic medication and less likely to receive behavioral therapy. Increasing access and availability of evidence-based behavioral services may improve outcomes (Rubenstein et al., 2019).
- Research is on-going into the risk factors and causes of autism. But much more is needed. Recent research can be found at the National Institute of Environmental Health website https://www.niehs.nih.gov/health/topics/conditions/autism

C/PHNs may contact families dealing with autism through work in well-child or immunization clinics. It is important to assist families in accessing services for their children (early intervention is advantageous). It is also important to educate that parenting practices are *not* a cause of autism and that multiple, large-scale research studies on childhood immunizations do not indicate a relationship between immunization and autism (CDC, 2024c).

Diabetes

Although diabetes ranks lower as a prevalent childhood chronic illness, it is associated with significant complications and self-management challenges.

- Type 1 diabetes mellitus (T1DM) is usually diagnosed in early childhood and is the leading cause of diabetes in children and adolescents, with non-Hispanic White children having the greatest number of new cases.
- Type 2 diabetes mellitus (T2DM) is generally diagnosed later in life and associated with metabolic syndrome and being overweight. In the United States, it is more prevalent in underrepresented groups than in non-Hispanic White populations (CDC, 2024d).
- Both type 1 (T1DM) and type 2 diabetes (T2DM) are found in school-age children, with T2DM rising almost exponentially in this age group, leading some scientists to call this a major public health crisis. This epidemic is thought to stem from increasing rates of childhood obesity, sedentary lifestyle, and the predisposition of certain ethnic groups (e.g., African American, Native American/Alaska Native, Hispanic/Latino, Pacific Islander) to the disease. A family history of T2DM and having one or more conditions related to insulin resistance also plays a role (CDC, 2024d; Oranika et al., 2023).

Research continues on the pathophysiology of diabetes and prevention strategies (e.g., lifestyle changes, causes of autoimmunity), as well as refining methods of diagnosis and treatment (e.g., insulin pumps, continuous glucose monitoring [CGM], closed-loop systems).

- School-based interventions focusing on lifestyle modifications, weight loss, healthy eating, and exercise have effectively decreased T2DM risk factors short term. Additional research to determine long-term effects is recommended (Geria & Beitz, 2018).
- Social isolation, stigma, shame, anxiety, and a feeling of blame are barriers to medication adherence in adolescents. Additional expectations from family for the minor to manage their own care and the lack of family support hinder compliance. Other considerations include lack of provider support and SDOH (Bransteter et al., 2024).

Younger children with T1DM, especially those who use insulin pumps, may need careful monitoring, something that is not always possible for the school nurse assigned to several school sites. It is important for C/PHNs and school nurses working with children and youth who have diabetes to consider their psychosocial needs as well as their physical needs (Box 20-2). A multidisciplinary team approach coordinating family, school staff, and physician collaboration is optimal.

Children and adolescents with diabetes may be reluctant to comply with their medical regimen, but strict adherence has proved to reduce later microvascular complications. Intensive insulin regimens are recommended for T1DM and for some cases of T2DM. Automated insulin delivery systems should be considered, and glucose levels should be monitored multiple times each day. With the advancements in technology, people with diabetes now have choices in how they monitor their disease. These technologies include CGM systems, blood glucose meters, insulin pens, and insulin pumps that provide greater accuracy, reduce hypo and hyperglycemic swings, and are less invasive (American Diabetes Association, n.d.).

Research is ongoing regarding the long-term effects of diabetes and best management strategies. It is important for school nurses and C/PHNs to understand each child's unique needs and circumstances and keep in mind a child's developmental stages. In addition to meeting the obvious emergency health–related concerns for diabetic

BOX 20-2 C/PHN USE OF THE NURSING PROCESS/CLINICAL JUDGMENT

School Nursing Practice Framework

School Nursing Practice Framework™

Supporting Students to be Healthy, Safe and Ready to Learn

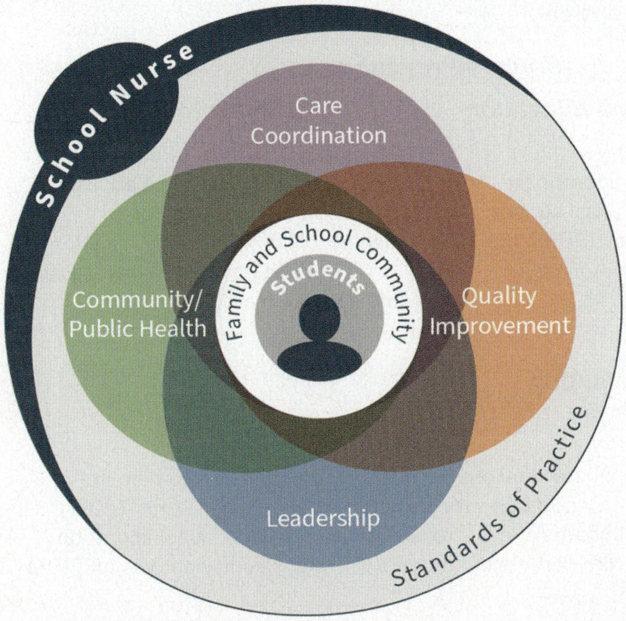

Care Coordination

- Provide direct care for emergent, episodic, and chronic mental and physical health needs.
- Connect student and family to available resources.
- Collaborate with families, school community, mental health team (including school counselors, social workers, and psychologists), and medical home.
- Develop and implement plans of care.
- Foster developmentally appropriate independence and self-advocacy.
- Provide evidence-based health counseling.
- Facilitate continuity of care with family during transitions.

Leadership

- Direct health services in school, district, or state.
- Interpret school health information and educate students, families, school staff, and policymakers.
- Advocate for district or state policies, procedures, programs, and services that promote health, reduce risk, improve equitable access, and support culturally appropriate care.
- Engage in and influence decision-making within education and health systems.
- Participate in development and coordinate implementation of school emergency or disaster plans.
- Champion health and academic equity.
- Share expertise through mentorship/ preceptorship.
- Practice and model self-care.

Quality Improvement

- Participate in data collection for local, state, and national standardized data sets and initiatives.
- Transform practice and make decisions using data, technology, and standardized documentation.
- Use data to identify individual and population level student needs, monitor student health and academic outcomes, and communicate outcomes.
- Engage in ongoing evaluation, performance appraisal, goal setting, and learning to professionalize practice.
- Identify questions in practice that may be resolved through research and evidence-based practice processes.

Community/Public Health

- Provide culturally sensitive, inclusive, holistic care.
- Conduct health screenings, surveillance, outreach, and immunization compliance activities.
- Collaborate with community partners to develop and implement plans that address the needs of school communities and diverse student populations.
- Teach health promotion, health literacy, and disease prevention.
- Provide health expertise in key roles in school, work, and community committees/ councils/coalitions.
- Assess school and community for social and environmental determinants of health.

Standards of Practice

- Ensure practice consistent with the scope and standards of school nursing practice, health and education laws (consider the Individuals with Disabilities Education Act, Section 504 of the Rehabilitation Act of 1973, Nurse Practice Act, state laws regarding school nursing practice and delegation), federal/state/local policies and regulations, and NASN position statements and code of ethics.
- Employ clinical judgment and critical thinking outlined in nursing process and prioritization.
- Integrate evidence and best/promising practices (consider multi-tiered systems of support, clinical practice guidelines).
- Safeguard privacy of students and data (consider Health Insurance Portability & Accountability Act, Family Educational Rights and Privacy Act).

NASN National Association of School Nurses

National Association of School Nurses. (2024). (Reprinted with permission from Tanner, A., Griffin, R., et al. (2024). A Contemporary Framework Update for Today's School Nursing Landscape: Introducing the School Nursing Practice Framework™. *NASN School Nurse, 39*(3), 140–147. https://doi.org/10.1177/1942602X241241092. https://higherlogicdownload.s3.amazonaws.com/NASN/8575d1b7-94ad-45ab-808e-d45019cc5c08/UploadedImages/PDFs/frameworkhorizontal_FINAL_4_3_24_V2.pdf)

children, it is imperative to teach children and families that proper diet, oral antidiabetic medications or insulin administration, physical activity, and blood glucose testing are vital strategies to keep blood glucose levels as close to normal as possible. This includes alerting teachers and school personnel to signs and symptoms (and treatment) of hypoglycemia. Alerting teachers to these concerns may help them better understand the academic complications of this disease and ensure their support (NASN, 2022).

The prevention of T2DM through education and improvement in exercise, nutrition, and lifestyle can be one of the most important areas of focus for health professionals who work with the school-age population—including C/PHNs who may come into contact with them during immunization or child health clinics (Box 20-3). Health education and health promotion to decrease childhood obesity and sedentary lifestyles may help stem the tide of T2DM in children and adolescents (CDC, 2023c).

Seizure Disorders

Epilepsy is a disorder of the brain in which neurons sometimes transmit abnormal signals, causing seizures. Epilepsy is considered one of the most common disabling neurologic conditions, and it is most common in the very young and in older adults (CDC, 2023d).

Approximately 470,000 children under the age of 14 have epilepsy. That's roughly 6 out of every 1000 students (Epilepsy Foundation, 2024). Those with seizure disorders may miss school, are more likely to use special education services, have difficulties in school, and are less likely to participate in sports (CDC, 2023d). Although there are some instances of intractable or drug-resistant epilepsy, many children diagnosed with seizure disorders/epilepsy can have their seizures controlled with antiepileptic medications.

Treatment is based upon many factors including the type of seizures, history, and physical status. Neurostimulation therapies, surgeries, and ketogenic diets are used in

BOX 20-3 LEVELS OF PREVENTION PYRAMID

Prevention of Type 2 Diabetes Mellitus in School-Age Children

SITUATION: The public health nurse and children with type 2 diabetes (T2DM)

GOAL: By using the three levels of prevention, avoid or promptly diagnose and treat negative health conditions and/or restore the fullest possible potential.

Tertiary Prevention

Rehabilitation	*Primary Prevention*	
	Health Promotion and Education	***Health Protection***
▪ Monitor the child's health ▪ Work closely with the child, family, physician, and teacher to ensure proper follow-up ▪ Be alert to monitor for any possible complications (e.g., medication side effects)	▪ Continue to promote a healthy lifestyle that includes appropriate food choices, daily physical activity within the limitations of T2DM, and medication adherence	▪ Educate teachers on safety precautions for children diagnosed with T2DM in their classroom ▪ Monitor children taking medications for T2DM (e.g., over- or underdosage and adverse reactions)

Secondary Prevention

Early Diagnosis	*Prompt Treatment*
▪ Teach older children to calculate their body mass index (BMI) ▪ Monitor BMI scores ▪ Yearly screenings for height and weight (calipers are useful) ▪ Complete health histories on at-risk children	▪ Initiate referrals for healthcare provider follow-up in collaboration with parents of students at risk for T2DM ▪ Initiate referrals to healthcare providers in collaboration with parents of students with signs and symptoms of T2DM

Primary Prevention

Health Promotion and Education	*Health Protection*
▪ Educate to promote good nutrition and a physically active lifestyle ▪ Provide classroom contact in the early primary grades to encourage children to make good food choices ▪ Limit passive activities and increase sports and physical activity ▪ Teach older children how to make better food choices at fast-food restaurants	▪ Advocate for policies that limit access to sugary beverages and snacks at school and programs that raise awareness and family involvement in better nutrition and promote physical activity for families ▪ Organize T2DM prevention programs, focusing on healthy nutrition and physical activity

some cases when other treatments have failed (Mayo Clinic, 2022). The causes of childhood seizures vary and may be a response to a fever, head injury, genetic, infection, or other brain disorder (Epilepsy Foundation, 2024). School nurses play a critical role in working with students and their families developing a health plan and training for school supporting staff (Epilepsy Foundation, n.d.). School nurses should be aware of emergency medication administration practices including state laws and school district policies: Rectal diazepam is commonly prescribed for younger children and those with developmental disabilities, yet nurses are not always available to make an appropriate nursing assessment of the child before the drug is given to stop a seizure. Often, school staff are trained to give emergency medication—highlighting the conflict between education laws and nurse practice acts (Lowe et al., 2021).

Parents may be reluctant to disclose a seizure diagnosis due to associated stigma. Children and adolescents with seizure disorders may feel embarrassed or be the victims of teasing or bullying. They may exhibit signs of school avoidance, or they may have problems learning. Seizure activity, along with the side effects of antiepileptic medications, may lead to memory and learning problems and changes in behavior. Moreover, seizures can affect short-term memory or language functions. Healthcare providers are in a position to educate and support families as they cope with the unique challenges of epilepsy (CDC, 2023d). It is important to monitor medication adherence and teach school staff about first-aid measures for seizure victims. When teachers are anxious about having a child with epilepsy in the classroom, educational programs for them and other school staff members can be provided. C/PHN or school nurses can help allay fears and promote appropriate and timely care.

Childhood Cancers

In 2024, it is estimated that over 9000 new cases of cancer will be diagnosed in children from 0 to 14 years. While cancer rates have declined by 70% from 1970 to 2020, cancer is still a leading cause of death in children. Leukemias, brain and other central nervous system tumors, lymphomas, malignant soft tissue sarcomas, malignant tumors, and bone tumors are the most common types of childhood cancers (National Cancer Institute [NCI], 2024). Five-year cancer survival rates for children have increased from 58% in the mid-70s to 85% due to major treatment advances (American Cancer Society, 2024a). More children are surviving childhood cancers, and concern has shifted to later complications of treatment rather than about cancer recurrence. Survivors are at greater risk of physical, emotional, or cognitive impairments affecting growth and development. Late effects may include changes to organs, tissues, or body functions, as well as emotional and psychological effects. Children who have been treated with chemotherapy and/or radiation may develop other long-term effects (NCI, 2021). The cause of most childhood cancers remains unknown with most cancers caused by (acquired vs. inherited) gene mutation leading to uncontrolled cell growth. Other factors such as radiation, Down syndrome, and other genetic syndromes (e.g., Beckwith-Wiedemann syndrome) have been linked to a higher risk for some childhood cancers. Parental smoking may be linked to increased cancer risk, but evidence for this is also inconclusive (American Cancer Society, 2024b).

Because many children return to school after initial hospitalization and treatment for cancer, school nurses or C/PHNs can help make this transition easier by educating classmates about cancer (e.g., it is not contagious), helping the children make necessary adjustments, and vigilantly protecting any immunocompromised students from communicable diseases (NASN, 2021b).

Behavioral and Learning Problems

Other childhood health problems, less easy to detect and measure but often just as debilitating, are those of physical, learning, language, or behavioral development. Disabilities can be caused by many factors including genetics, complications during birth, maternal or infant infections, exposure to smoking and alcohol in utero, and environmental toxins such as lead; however, the majority of the causes remain unknown (CDC, 2024e). Specific learning disabilities are prevalent in childhood. It is estimated that 2.3 million children, or 35% of those receiving special educational services in the United States, have learning issues. Students with learning disabilities are in every school across the United States, yet many remain unidentified and underserved (Learning Disabilities Association of America, n.d.).

Learning Disorders

Learning disorders (LDs), also known as learning disabilities, are often recognized as the child progresses in school, and special education services may be needed. Some LDs are apparent in early school years, whereas others do not present problems until early adolescence. Battles over homework, poor grades, acting out in school, or frequent child complaints about school, teachers, or schoolwork are often harbingers of LDs. Children with LDs are more likely to repeat a school grade, miss multiple school days, be suspended from school, and drop out (Learning Disabilities Association of America, n.d.). Early identification and intervention are key to the success of a child with LDs. Students must first be carefully identified through specialized testing; then, special education or resource teachers can build on the child or adolescent's strengths while working to compensate for weaknesses.

Learning disabilities range in severity and typically fall into these categories:

- Oral language (listening, speaking, understanding)
- Reading (phonics, decoding, fluency, recognition, comprehension) (Fig. 20-2)
- Written language (spelling, writing fluency, and written expression)
- Mathematics (number sense, computation, math fluency, problem-solving) (Learning Disabilities Association of America, n.d., para. 4).

If LDs are not dealt with in childhood and adolescence, they can lead to later, more serious, problems related to employment, relationships, and quality of life in adulthood (Learning Disabilities Association of America, n.d.). The C/PHN and school nurse can assist individuals and families in recognizing LDs and locating necessary resources. Some students with significant LDs may qualify for special education services, and school nurses can be helpful in facilitating this process along with teachers and learning specialists.

Attention Deficit Hyperactivity Disorder

Attention deficit hyperactivity disorder (ADHD), is a disorder that includes the inability to pay attention, stay focused, control behavior, and also includes hyperactivity (Learning Disabilities Association of America, n.d.). The behaviors occur in childhood and may continue in adolescence and adulthood. From 2020 to 2022, 11.3% of children 5 to 17 years were diagnosed with ADHD with males having higher prevalence than females (CDC, 2024f). White, non-Hispanic children were more likely to be diagnosed (13.4%) as compared with Black (10.8) and Hispanic (8.9%) children ages 5 to 17 years (CDC, 2024f).

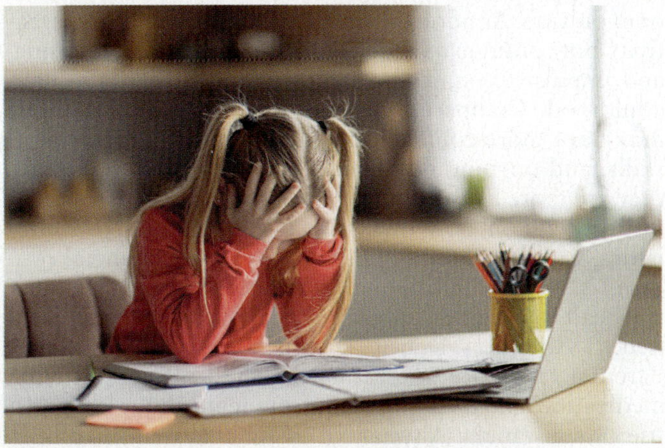

FIGURE 20-2 Reading is important to education and may be problematic for children with learning disabilities.

Treatment for ADHD can be managed using various methods including medications and behavioral management (CDC, 2024g). For children less than 6 years old, the American Pediatric Association recommends behavior management as the first line of treatment. For children 6 and older, medication and/or behavior management is recommended. Medications include both stimulants and nonstimulant pharmacologics. Behavior management can include therapy and intervention techniques to be used in the home and at school (CDC, 2024g). Diagnosis of ADHD involves a several-step process and should include reports from parents/guardians, teachers, and mental health providers if applicable. The primary care clinician generally makes the final diagnosis after considering all symptoms and reports and ruling out other possible symptom causes (CDC, 2024g).

Collaboration among the child's family, school, and physician is needed to diagnose ADHD and to plan appropriate interventions and educational accommodations. Although parents have a wealth of knowledge about the child, teacher confirmation of ADHD-related behaviors is very important. School nurses and C/PHNs can assist parents in recognizing the symptoms of ADHD and in obtaining appropriate treatment and follow-up. A multimodal treatment approach is recognized as the most effective. The main goals of medical treatment are to strengthen positive behaviors and decrease unwanted behaviors. Behavioral management techniques may include the following:

- Create routine
- Be organized
- Limit distractions
- Limit choices
- Give clear directions
- Break down tasks
- Make realistic goals
- Effective discipline
- Provide a healthy lifestyle (CDC, 2024g)

At each stage of development, those with ADHD are presented with distinct challenges. For example, children in elementary school may be involved in conflicts with peers and have problems organizing tasks. They may be more prone to accidents and may have more school-related problems, such as grade retention and suspension or expulsion. As adolescents, they may show less hyperactivity but continue to have restlessness, difficulty focusing, and impulsiveness. These symptoms often continue into adulthood. Compared with teens without ADHD, they may have more conflict with their parents, poorer social skills, and ongoing problems at school. As young adults, they are more likely to experience lower job performance, disorganization and time management issues, memory issues, haphazard focus, relationship issues, financial concerns, substance misuse and substance use disorder, mental health struggles, poor physical wellness, and legal issues (Attention Deficit Disorder Association, 2024). Parental resistance to treating the child may result from medication side effects or stem from fears about later misuse of substances. Alternative treatments that have been tried but not proven effective through research include yoga or meditation; special diets with decreased sugar and allergens such as wheat or milk, vitamin or herbal supplements, or increased omega-3 oils; and increased exercise (National Institute of Health, 2024). School nurses and C/PHNs can work closely with school staff, parents, and physicians in determining the efficacy of treatment regimens.

Behavioral and Emotional Problems

Monitoring and understanding children's mental health is an important public health issue and includes children's mental, emotional, and behavioral well-being (CDC, 2023e). Approximately 20% of U.S. children experience a mental health disorder each year. Forty percent of students 12 to 17 years have persistent feelings of sadness or hopelessness and 18.8% considered attempted suicide, 16% made a plan, and 8.9% attempting suicide (CDC, 2023f). Depression and anxiety have increased over time, as have depression and suicide; these behaviors were exacerbated over COVID-19 (Agency for Healthcare Research and Quality, 2022). The Youth Risk Behavioral Survey (CDC, 2023g) indicates students are struggling with their health and well-being. Female children are experiencing record-high levels of violence, mental health issues, and suicide risk, with 1 in 4 seriously considering suicide. LGBTQ+ students continue to face mental health challenges with more than half experiencing poor mental health in the previous month (CDC, 2023e).

The prevalence of any mental disorder among 13- to 18-year-olds is 49.5%, with anxiety in 32% and depression in 13% (United States Department of Health and Human Services [USDHHS], n.d.). An already tenuous health issue for children and adolescents was made much worse with the COVID-19 pandemic. School closures, disruptions, social isolation, family loss and illness, and financial hardships affected the well-being and mental health of America's youth with 1 in 3 high school students experiencing poor mental health with just under half the students feeling persistent sadness or hopelessness (CDC, 2022c). Living in an environment where children are not safe or that undermines their stability or ability to bond—such as households with mental health issues, substance misuse, or separation due to incarceration—can have lasting and negative effects on their health and well-being. **Adverse childhood experiences** (ACE) are traumatic events that occur in childhood (ages 0 to 17), such as violence, abuse, or having a family member attempt or die by suicide. ACE are linked to mental illness, substance misuse, and chronic health problems; they can also negatively impact employment opportunities and education (CDC, 2021b). Associated conditions related to ACE (such as food insecurities or living in under-resourced or racially segregated neighborhoods) compound an already stressful environment, leading to toxic stress. As children grow up, they may have difficulty forming healthy or stable relationships, with these effects being passed on to their children; this chain reaction can result in such individuals or their children being more likely to perpetrate or be the victims of acts of violence (CDC, 2021b). ACE are preventable through education, strong economic support for families, legislation that protects against violence, and community support for safe and nurturing environments for children.

Children are barometers of their environment. About 40% to 50% of couples in the United States divorce, and the second marriage rates of divorce are even higher. In 2016, 65% of children aged 0 to 17 years lived with two married parents, 22% of children lived only with their birthing parents, 5% lived only with the partner of their birthing parent, 5% lived with unmarried parents, and 4% did not live with either parent. Children of divorce are more likely to exhibit behavior problems; children who are products of highly contentious divorces are most at risk (Child Stats, 2023; Kids Health Alliance, 2020).

- Being aware of a child's family situation and living arrangements is helpful for understanding social, economic, and developmental well-being. C/PHNs can be alert to early symptoms and refer parents to marital counseling or suggest family therapists. Some schools also offer support groups for children of divorce.
- School refusal, where a child develops a pattern of refusing to go to school or remain in school for the entire school day, is common in school-age children and differs from truancy. Unlike truancy, school refusal is commonly associated with symptoms of emotional distress—usually anxiety or depression—but may also be associated with oppositional defiant disorder, ADHD, or other disruptive behavior disorders. Often, the children complain of headaches, stomachaches, or other physical ailments, but some are motivated to miss school to gain parental attention. School refusal is most found in children between ages 5 and 7 or ages 11 and 14. Transitional periods, such as school entry or moving to middle school or high school, are often the most difficult.
- Children usually present to the school nurse or C/PHN with headaches and/or abdominal pains. They may throw tantrums, cry, or show panic and fear to their parents to stay home from school. Sometimes, children are afraid of something in the school environment (e.g., bullies, teachers, test taking), or they may have separation anxiety. Family enmeshment, detachment, or high levels of family conflict may contribute to school refusal problems, as well as parental anxiety disorders like agoraphobia and panic disorder (Kids Health Alliance, 2020).
- The best interventions include an early return to school, with parental involvement in school, systematic desensitization (graded exposure to the classroom), relaxation training, emphasis on positive aspects of going to school, and counseling being the most effective (ADAA, n.d.). If symptoms persist, evaluation by a mental health provider is recommended. C/PHNs and school nurses can serve as liaisons with the child, family, school, and healthcare/mental healthcare providers to promote a positive outcome.

Disabilities

From 2021 to 2022, the number of children ages 3 to 21 years served under IDEA was approximately 7 million—accounting for 15% of the total school-age population. Specific learning disabilities and speech or language difficulties were the two most common disabilities reported, followed by other health impairments (asthma, chronic illnesses), and autism. Less common disabilities include developmental delays, intellectual disabilities, emotional disturbances, multiple disabilities, hearing and orthoperiodic impairment, visual impairment, traumatic brain injuries, and deaf-blindness. American Indian/Alaska Native children (19%) had the highest prevalence, followed by Black (17%), White (15%), Hispanic and Pacific Islander (both at 12%), and Asian (8%) (NCES, 2024b).

Many children with perceived disabilities or problems are referred for assessment and considered for placement in special education programs each year. School nurses often serve as liaisons between parents, physicians, and educators and are part of the team developing an individualized education plan (IEP) for children who qualify for special education services. Most children receive special services in a regular classroom because *full inclusion* or *mainstreaming* legislation mandates that fewer children be segregated into special classes or separate schools (see Chapter 24 for more on clients with disabilities).

Injuries

The loss of children's lives that results from all injuries combined suggests a staggering loss to society in the number of years of productive life lost. An injury is damage to the body, either unintentional or intentional, but the use of the word accident is considered incorrect, as injuries may be prevented through environmental, individual behavioral, legislative, and institutional policy changes.

- In the United States, unintentional injuries are the leading cause of death and disability for children between the ages of 1 and 19 years. Falls, bicycle-related accidents, drownings, airway obstruction (suffocation), and home injuries (fires and firearms) are the leading causes of injuries between 0 and 19 years (Stanford Medicine Children's Health, 2024). Injuries not resulting in death often cause permanent disabilities or emotional and physical consequences for children and their families. Although injury death rates have dropped over the past two decades, injuries are responsible for approximately 75% of deaths during adolescence.
- Unintentional firearm injury deaths from 0 to 17 were greatest for 11- to 15-year-olds (33%), followed by 0- to 5-year-olds (24%), 16- to 17-year-olds (24%), and 6- to 10-year-olds (14%) (CDC, 2023h).
- One-third of all accidents were related to motor vehicle accidents (MVAs). Children under 13 should be restrained in the backseat and infants and toddlers should remain rear-facing until at least 2 years (American Family Physician, 2020).
- Homicide rates have increased with a 27.7% rise in overall homicide rates for 0- to 17-year-olds from 2019 to 2020 affecting 27.1% Hispanic, 24.3% White, and 32.6% Black children (Office of Juvenile Justice and Delinquency Prevention, 2023).
- A public health concern contributing to child and adolescent motor vehicle crashes (MVCs) is alcohol use. A large-scale study examining the relationship between alcohol policies and fatal MVCs found that alcohol was a factor in more than 25% of cases of motor vehicle fatalities involving children,

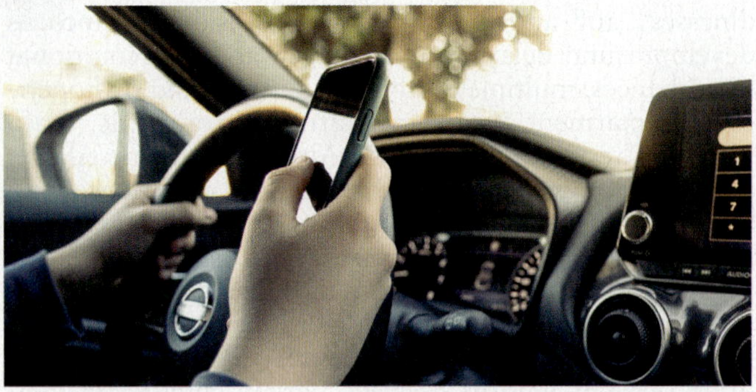

FIGURE 20-3 Cell phone use while driving—whether the driver is talking, texting, or using an app—is dangerous.

adolescents, and young adults less than 21 years of age. Research indicated that restrictive alcohol policies are associated with reduced alcohol-related MVC among youth (Koob, 2023).

- The use of cell phones while driving is another concern for adolescents (and the general population) (Fig. 20-3). Adolescent cell phone use while driving has been legislatively banned in many states and yet reports indicate continued cell phone use while driving. Research investigating self-reporting sending and responding to text messages indicates adolescents text even through they believe other drivers that do so are unsafe. Reasons for texting are social, importance, and entertainment. Reading versus sending is more commonly done. Teens that understand risk factors are less prone to texting. Increased education and intervention are recommended public health interventions for the adolescent population (Taylor & Blenner, 2021).

During the 2021–2022 school year, approximately 67% of public schools reported having at least one violent incident and 59% reported having at least one nonviolent incident. Sixty-one percent of schools reported at least one physical attack without a weapon; 4% of those attacks were with weapons. Three percent of schools reported a hate crime (approximately 3000 schools). Bullying was reported in 10% of elementary schools, 28% of middle schools, and 15% of high schools. Cyberbullying accounted for 6% of incidents in elementary school, 37% in middle school, and 25% in high schools (Bagley, 2024). C/PHNs can promote injury prevention and control through education, promotion of safety engineering and environmental protection strategies, and legislative advocacy.

- C/PHNs can advance the prevention of unintentional injuries and deaths by working with families to initiate the consistent use of seat belts and child safety seats in vehicles and the use of helmets and other protective gear for children riding bikes and skateboarding (Box 20-4).
- Where water is a natural hazard, wearing life jackets while boating and swimming can help decrease accidental drowning.
- Promotion of smoke and carbon monoxide detectors, poison prevention, and sudden infant death syndrome education can help to further decrease injury death rates.

BOX **20-4** STORIES FROM THE FIELD

Why Parents and Caregivers Are Inconsistent in Their Use of Car Restraints for Children

A leading cause of childhood injury and death continues to be MVCs. The use of restraints (seatbelts, infant car seats, child booster seats) has been shown to be an effective population-level intervention that reduces fatalities and serious injuries (CDC, 2024t).

I was part of a team of nurses, epidemiologists, and physicians from an Eastern Center for Injury Research and Prevention who studied factors about parent and caregiver use of booster seats. Our goal was to understand why parents and caregivers inconsistently use car restraint systems. Our group designed a cross-sectional online survey with a convenience sample of parents in the United States. Survey participants were greater than 18 years of age, spoke and read English, were the parent or caregiver of a child between 4 and 10 years of age, and had driven their child at least six times in the past 3 months. Participants answered questions about the situational use of car seats and booster seats with their child and carpooling children.

Our research found that parents and caregivers using booster seats did not fully restrain a child due to practical reasons more often than parents/caregivers using car seats did. Practical situations for not using a child restraint system included driving short distances, too many people in the car, and not having a CRS in the car.

Decreased use of child restraint systems puts children at a high risk of injury. It is imperative that healthcare providers continue to educate parents/caregivers and implement programs to promote CRS use.

—Catherine, RN

1. *As a C/PHN, what resources would you provide to a family with young children using a car seat?*
2. *What does the data in your community indicate regarding childhood morbidity and mortality for MVA? What strategies would work best for prevention in your community?*

Source: CDC (2024v).

- Teaching parents about presetting hot water heaters to lower than 130°F, recognizing the hazards of infant walkers, storing matches and lighters safely, and using pool fencing can help to prevent common unintentional injuries.
- Advocacy for stricter seat belt and child safety seat enforcement, as well as programs to provide child safety seats and bicycle helmets, has been shown to positively affect mortality and injury rates. Enforcement of seatbelt laws, graduated driver licensing programs, and adolescent education about MVC causes are also effective (CDC, 2024h). C/PHNs can work with their local health departments and community action groups to provide seats and helmets to families who cannot afford them, organize clinics to educate about proper installation and use, and encourage local law enforcement to enforce seat belt and safety seat laws.

Communicable Diseases

The mortality rates of school-age children 5 to 14 years old are comparatively low and have decreased substantially over the last century, a reduction that can be attributed to the effective prevention and control of the acute infectious diseases of childhood, a significant achievement in the last century. Although mortality rates are low in this country, worldwide mortality because of communicable diseases continues with lower respiratory infections being the deadliest. Globally, among children ages 5 to 14 years, the risk of dying from communicable disease has significantly decreased, whereas the prevalence of mortality related to injuries has increased and is the leading cause of death. COVID-19 represented 8% of the global cases and 0.1% of the deaths (WHO, 2022).

- It is estimated that immunizations save 33,000 lives, prevent 14 million causes of disease, and save approximately $40 billion. The U.S. public health efforts (Healthy People 2030) focus on reducing vaccine-related illnesses and diseases. School-age children must show proof of required vaccinations before they are allowed to enroll in school, although most states still allow exemptions for personal or religious beliefs (for information on which states allow religious and philosophical exemptions, visit http://www.ncsl.org/research/health/school-immunization-exemption-state-laws.aspx). Vaccine hesitancy by parents has been linked to outbreaks such as measles (Marcus, 2020). As early as 2006, 75% of pediatricians encountered vaccine hesitancy (9.1 % refusal). By 2013 that figure has increased to 87% (16.7% refusal). Interestingly, as many as 1 in 5 people still believe there is a link between vaccines and autism (Marcus, 2020).
- Results from a 2018 national immunization survey revealed that around 90% of children between ages 19 and 35 months received vaccinations for polio, MMR, varicella, and hepatitis B (CDC, 2023j).
- Black and Hispanic children were less likely to receive the full immunization series than non-Hispanic White children. Children in poverty, those covered by Medicaid, and children without insurance were also less likely to receive the full immunization series (CDC, 2023j) (see CDC for childhood immunization schedule, available at https://www.cdc.gov/vaccines/schedules/easy-to-read/child.html).

The National Immunization Survey–Teen (NIS-Teen) indicates that adolescent vaccination coverage in the United States has gradually increased. However, disparities continue with teens living in nonmetropolitan statistical areas being under vaccinated. Over the past several decades, the incidence of vaccine-preventable deaths has decreased; however, infectious diseases continue as a major cause of childhood illnesses, disability, and death. Vaccines are one of the most cost-effective health promotion services. Strong campaigns have been taken by health departments to get children immunized.

- Strategies shown to improve vaccination rates include the Vaccine for Children (VFC) Program, cost reduction, home visits, and linking vaccination opportunities with WIC visits.
- Public health professionals should continue to focus on eliminating socioeconomic barriers, strengthening school-entry requirements, and addressing vaccine misinformation.
- A Cochrane review by Jacobson Vann et al. (2018) indicates that vaccination increases are seen in all age groups when reminders by telephone or text message, letter, or postcard are used. Combinations of reminders were also effective; however, reminding people over the phone are the most effective.
- Cancer prevention for preteens and adolescents through HPV vaccinations is effective. While HPV immunization rates have increased 5% from 2020 to 2021 with 76.9% of adolescents receiving the first dose to start the vaccine series, and 61.7% of adolescents completing all vaccinations in the series, there is still room for improvement. Parental resistance and a focus on vaccinating only female children can inhibit successful immunizations efforts in communities (CDC, 2022d).

Community-acquired methicillin-resistant *Staphylococcus aureus* is another communicable illness seen in the school-age children population. C/PHNs and school nurses must be alert when skin infections or other conditions do not resolve quickly in children and adolescents. Sports teams, for instance, may spread this infection as team members come into close contact or use common-use facilities such as swimming pools. Referral to an infectious disease specialist may need to be considered (CDC, 2024i).

Pediculosis (head lice), another highly communicable disease, is a frustrating and common problem for many preschool and school-age children, and the incidence has been increasing with approximately 6 to 12 million 3- to 11-year-olds infected annually.

- Preschoolers and elementary-age children and their caregivers and family members are at the highest risk for head lice.
- Close crowded conditions can also be a risk factor. Although lice are wingless, because children frequently play close to each other, they easily move from child to child.

Head lice may be white, gray, or brown in color—about the size of a sesame seed. They attach to the scalp and lay eggs (nits) in the hair. Nits typically hatch within 8 to 9 days. They reach adulthood during the next 9 to 12 days and live about 30 days. Without treatment, the cycle repeats every 3 weeks. Complete eradication generally requires that all viable nits be removed along with lice; family and close contacts should be checked for head lice and, if found, treated at the same time. Treatment typically involves over-the-counter insecticide shampoos (or pediculicides).

School nurses and C/PHNs also need to educate families about reducing reinfestations by carefully applying pediculicides, retreating in 2 weeks if necessary, and cleaning any fomites (e.g., combs, hats, towels, sheets, clothing, and upholstered furniture), and removing any viable nits. Drying sheets, blankets, and towels on high heat and washing all hats and clothing are effective measures. It is not necessary to use fumigant sprays, as they can be toxic.

Other Health Problems

Other health problems found in this age group include nutritional problems (primarily overeating and inappropriate food choices) and poor dental health. Obesity often begins in childhood and is a risk factor for cardiovascular disease, diabetes, cancer, stroke, and osteoarthritis later in life. The percentage of children and adolescents with obesity has more than tripled in the last 40 years. Risk factors contributing to childhood obesity include genetics, metabolism, short sleep duration, eating and physical activity behaviors, and community environment (CDC, 2024j).

Food allergies can also play a role in poor nutritional status, especially in school-age children and adolescents. Researchers estimate that about 5.6 million children have food allergies, with teens and young adults being at greatest risk of anaphylactic reactions (Food, Allergy, Research, and Education [FARE], n.d.). Food allergies can be especially problematic in the school setting as strict avoidance of the food is the only way to prevent a reaction. It is recommended that parents and adolescents carefully read labels at the time of each use and that education systems have a plan to prevent allergic reactions and a response plan if an emergency should arise (FARE, n.d.).

Dental caries is another common problem among school-age children. Approximately 18.6% of U.S. schoolchildren (5 to 19 years) have untreated cavities. In 2015, 84.7% of children aged 2 to 17 visited a dentist during the year (CDC, 2023k).

Childhood Obesity

- About one in five U.S. children are obese, making childhood obesity a national concern. The CDC uses the term **overweight** for children and youth with weight at or above the 85th percentile and less than the 95th percentile for youth the same age and gender. Children with a BMI greater than the 95th percentile are defined as **obese** (see Box 20-5 for an explanation and examples).
- Children with obesity are more likely to become adults with obesity and are at increased risk of chronic health diseases such as asthma, sleep apnea, bone and joint problems, metabolic syndrome, type 2 diabetes, cancer, and heart disease. They are also more likely to be teased, bullied, and suffer from social isolation, depression, and poor self-esteem (CDC, 2024j).
- Preventive measures and early management of cardiovascular risk factors are now considered more effective forms of treatment than just clinical treatment of the disease complications after the fact.
- Multiple factors influence childhood obesity including genetics, decreased physical activity, increased

BOX 20-5 LEVELS OF PREVENTION PYRAMID

Obesity in a School Setting

HEALTH ISSUE: Obesity in a school setting

Tertiary Prevention

Rehabilitation Move to	*Health Promotion and Education*	*Health Protection*
■ Work closely with the child, family, physician, and teacher to decrease body mass index (BMI)	■ Continue to promote healthy lifestyle choices and daily physical activity	

Secondary Prevention

Early Diagnosis	*Prompt Treatment*
■ Conduct yearly screening of students' heights and weights to calculate BMI ■ Complete health histories on at-risk children	■ Initiate referrals for healthcare provider follow-up in collaboration with parents of students at risk for obesity

Primary Prevention

Health Promotion and Education	*Health Protection*
■ Limit passive activities and increase sports and physical activity ■ Teach children how to make better food choices at fast-food restaurants ■ Educate children and teachers to promote good nutrition and a physically active lifestyle ■ Promote a change of policy to take junk food out of vending machines	

television time, familial weight, poor nutrition knowledge, food insecurity, parental smoking, not having family mealtime, perceived neighborhood safety, and low economic status.

- Early childhood may be the best time to modify preventable factors influencing obesity. Studies recommend a variety of factors such as healthy eating, exercise, lifestyle modifications, and behavioral therapy to reduce the risk of childhood obesity (Salam et al., 2020).

A legislative goal was to provide balanced nutrition for children and reduce childhood obesity. Ninety percent of schools now report that they meet updated national meal provision standards, school lunch revenues have increased, and children are being educated to choose healthier food options (CDC, 2022e). Practice applying the nursing process to the problem of childhood obesity is shown in Box 20-6.

The causes of childhood obesity are multifactorial, so healthcare providers should take a multiple health

BOX 20-6 C/PHN USE OF THE NURSING PROCESS/CLINICAL JUDGMENT

Addressing Childhood Obesity

James Lopez is entering third grade. His teacher comes to you, the school nurse, because she is concerned about his poor school performance. He frequently comes to school late, puts his head on his desk, and appears to be falling asleep. You notice that James gained a significant amount of weight over the summer. His face is much fuller now than in his second-grade class photo.

Assessment (Initial Visits)/Recognize Cues

You do the following:

- Call James' mother and make an appointment for a home visit.
- Complete a health history, noting family history of diabetes, current eating, activity, and sleeping patterns for James and the family, and determine whether he has a regular physician and insurance or Medicaid.
- Assess his vital signs, height and weight, hearing, and vision.
- Talk with James' teacher about his playground activity level and any signs of excessive thirst, hunger, or general fatigue.

Diagnosis/Analyze Cues and Prioritize Hypotheses

After a home visit, a meeting with James' teacher, and two observations and interviews with James, you decide a nursing diagnosis would look at:

- James' body requirements are more than what is required. James has a sedentary lifestyle and may be eating to cope.
- Changes in the family's home life. Mother is single and attending classes necessitating several days' absence at a time. James is cared for by a married teenage sister and her husband.

Planning and Implementation/Generate Solutions and Take Action

For the past 3 months, since his mother started her class, James has been eating large quantities of snack food and fast-food meals. He stopped participating in soccer and baseball because of lack of transportation. James' bicycle was recently stolen, and he now spends a lot of time playing video and computer games. James says that he misses his mother when she is away and that he "stays up late watching television" and "has trouble getting up for school" when he is at his sister's house.

You plan to work with the family to refer James to his physician to rule out diabetes. A family meeting is scheduled to provide health education on childhood obesity and inactivity. You discuss some possible interventions that the family can put into place:

- Decrease reliance on fast-food meals.
- Have a regular evening mealtime and encourage less snacking.
- Provide fresh fruit and vegetable snacks and decrease purchases of high-calorie, high-fat snack foods.
- Decrease sedentary activity (e.g., video and computer games, television viewing) and increase physical activity (e.g., team sports, walking, bicycling, active outdoor games).
- Establish a reasonable bedtime and consistently enforce it.
- Offer referral for family counseling so James can discuss his feelings in a safe environment.
- With the family's input, seek ways to improve contact between James and his mother and opportunities for his sister to improve understanding of good parenting practices.
- Meet with the teacher, family, and James to discuss ways to help with school performance.
- Continue to monitor James' progress with monthly height and weight checks, personal interviews, home visits, and teacher conferences.

Evaluation/Evaluate Outcomes

The physician reported that James does not have diabetes; however, if he continues to gain weight and remains inactive, he is at a higher risk for type 2 diabetes. Evaluation of the two nursing diagnoses includes the following goals:

- The family will report less reliance on fast food and more meals cooked at home.
- The family will report more purchases of fresh fruits and vegetables and fewer purchases of high-calorie, high-fat snacks.
- James will report more physical exercise (he will track this on a calendar) and fewer hours spent in sedentary activity (corroborated by family).
- James will exhibit less tardiness and fewer signs of sleep deprivation at school, and his school performance will improve.
- James and his family will complete sessions with a family counselor.
- As James' height increases over time, James' weight will remain stable or will decrease.

behavior approach. Parental support and influence are keys. Parents can help their younger children develop healthy eating habits by following these recommendations (CDC, 2022f):

- "Eat the Rainbow." Provide a variety of fruits and vegetables. Let children pick fruits and vegetables and have them help cook or prepare them.
- Choose lean meats, poultry, and beans for protein.
- Watch out for added sugars. Avoid/limit sugar-sweetened drinks.
- Help kids be physically active for at least 60 minutes each day (Fig. 20-4).
- Serve whole-grain/high-fiber cereals and breads.
- Serve low-fat and fat-free dairy products (two to three cups of milk daily).
- Read food nutrition labels—pick healthy nutritional foods.
- Be a role model—help your child develop healthy habits early (CDC, 2022f).

Inadequate Nutrition

Poor nutritional status of schoolchildren is a global issue but also a problem in this country. Undernutrition can also have serious consequences, including effects on the cognitive development and academic performance of children and chronic health. Irritability, lack of energy, and difficulty concentrating are only some of the problems that arise from skipped meals or consistently inadequate nutrition. Infection and illness that lead to loss of school days can affect academic progress and interfere with the acquisition of basic skills, such as reading and mathematics. Food insecurity has been associated with child development problems, psychological and social issues, and poor general health:

- In the United States, 13 million children face hunger daily.
- At least 1 in 5 children do not know where they will get their next meal.
- Families with children experience economic burdens affecting food choices and affordability of food; families of color are disproportionally affected.
- Approximately 33% of households headed by single birthing parents experience food insecurity (Feeding America, 2024).

A national study suggests that there is an association between food insecurity and obesity in adolescent children (Fleming et al., 2021). A study by Ortiz-Morron et al. (2022) provides additional validation that there is a significant relationship between food insecurity and a lower quality diet, obesity, and longer screen time in households that experience food insecurity.

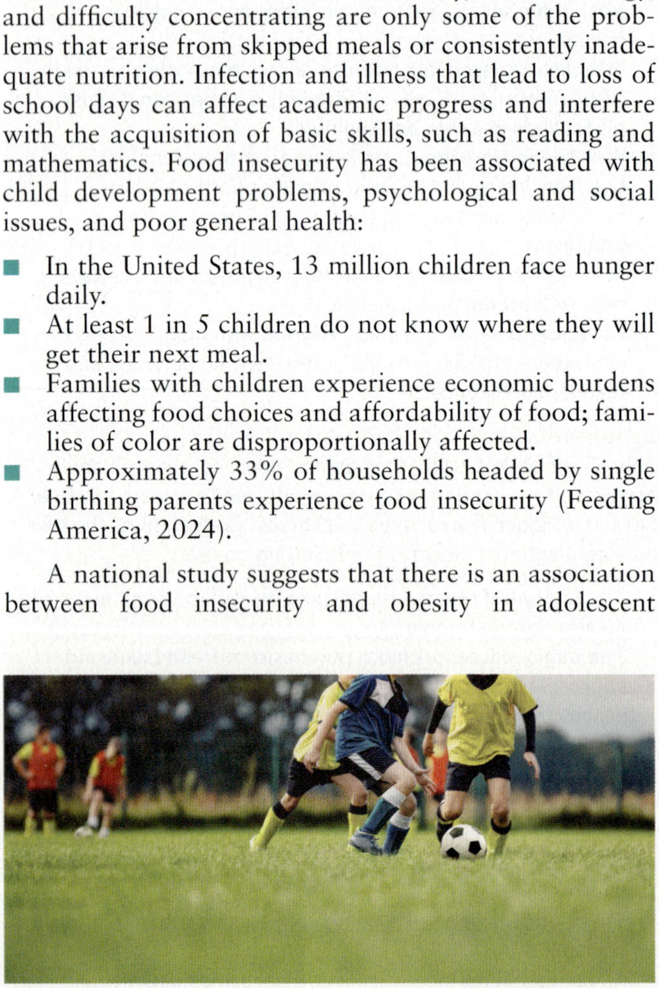

FIGURE 20-4 Physical activity is important for health and in childhood obesity prevention.

Undernutrition is frequently associated with poverty and hunger, but social pressure to be thin can also spark purposeful undernutrition. Because prepubertal children often exhibit a period of adiposity before a growth spurt, they are at risk for developing eating disorders. Along with childhood obesity, prevention of eating disorders is also a high priority in this age group.

A systematic review found an association between youth with T2DM and elevated scores on the Diabetes Eating Problem Survey-revised (Mateo et al., 2024). Ravi and Khan (2020) indicated an association with ADHD and obesity and eating disorders. Research also indicates that youth with a history of obesity are at a higher risk of disordered eating. Signs of disordered eating include food rituals, refusal to eat foods once enjoyed, avoiding meals, overexercising, secret eating, preoccupation with food, calorie counting, fear of becoming fat, binge eating, and food phobias. Other concerning behaviors include depression, irritability, sudden mood changes, and anxiety around food and eating. Parents and healthcare providers alike should be aware of symptoms and seek evaluation of the child or adolescent (Chaves et al., 2023).

- School nurses and C/PHNs should be aware of signs and symptoms of this disorder, noting that children with T1DM may be at higher risk, and watch for unexplained weight loss, stunting of normal growth patterns, concerns about body image, delayed puberty, and abnormal or restrictive eating.
- They can provide families with the necessary information to promote healthful eating and exercise, as well as provide guidance and support (Chaves et al., 2023). Some school districts include BMI screening programs as part of healthy lifestyle promotion.
- The CDC recommends that schools have a series of safeguards in place before launching a BMI measurement program. This includes fostering a safe and supportive environment for all students and a comprehensive program to prevent and reduce obesity (CDC, 2022g).

Inactivity

An association between poor eating habits and physical inactivity has been found in numerous research studies. More television watching, fewer family meals eaten together at home, and living in an unsafe neighborhood were shown to be associated with being overweight (D'Souza et al., 2020).

- In the 2021 Youth Risk Behavioral Survey, 19% of students attended physical education classes and 24% were active 60 minutes a day (American Academy of Pediatrics, 2023).
- High-impact obesity prevention standards recommend screen time limits for children, with no viewing during snack or meals (CDC, 2024k).
- Youth 6 to 17 should have 60 minutes of moderate to vigorous physical activity a day (CDC, 2022h).

School nurses and C/PHNs can work with families to increase their levels of physical activity and encourage limited television viewing for school-age children. They can also advocate for increased physical education in the school setting and for increased safe recreational opportunities in all neighborhoods.

Dental Caries

Dental caries is thought to be the most prevalent chronic childhood infectious disease.

- Thirteen percent of children 5 to 19 years old have untreated dental caries.
- Approximately 87% of children 2 to 17 years old had a dental visit (CDC, 2024l).
- Hispanic children have the highest rates of decay and non-Hispanic Black youth have the highest prevalence of untreated caries (The Children's Partnership, 2022).

The prevalence of dental caries in school-age children has decreased significantly since the early 1970s because of community fluoridation projects and the use of fluoride toothpaste. Fluoridated drinking water, the availability of school-provided fluoride rinse or gel, and dental sealant programs are cost-effective, proven methods of reducing dental caries in school-age children (Nassar & Brizuela, 2023). The peak incidence of dental caries is found among school-age children and adolescents, although the effects of decay are observed in adulthood as caries activity recurs or various restorations fracture or wear out and must be replaced.

- Approximately 5 million children are on Medicaid and have a difficult time locating dental professionals who accept this insurance.
- Of the children enrolled in Medicaid, 56% do not receive dental care.
- Of the children on Medicaid, 34% had one dental visit and 29% received preventative oral services (The Children's Partnership, 2022).

Yet, access to dental care is still problematic as many families live in areas with dental health professional shortages. Barriers to dental care are more prevalent among children from families with low incomes and children of color. Financial barriers, lack of education, and limited numbers of dentists accepting Medicaid lead to poor dental health values and adversely affect the appropriate use of early dental services and conscientious personal oral healthcare (CDC, 2024m).

The Division of Oral Health (CDC, 2024m) recommends integrating medical and oral health services to reduce barriers to care. Integrating oral health into primary care addresses access to care, timely interventions, and continuity of care improving patient outcomes (Adeghe, 2024). C/PHNs and other community health nurses working with school-age children and families can promote good dental health through education and advocacy, as well as through collaboration to provide adequate dental services to uninsured children and promotion of fluoridation and sealant programs.

ADOLESCENT HEALTH

Adolescence is a time of self-discovery, movement toward self-reliance, increasing opportunities, and pivotal choices that can affect the remainder of an individual's life.

- Adolescence generally begins with puberty and encompasses the ages between 10 and 24; it consists of early adolescence (aged 10 to 14), middle adolescence (15 to 17), and late adolescence (18 to mid-20s).
- Adult society largely segregates adolescents and often has ambiguous expectations for them. Adolescents are part of a subculture, one with its own language, dress, social mores, and values.
- The tasks of adolescence remain fairly constant: Adolescents must become autonomous, come to grips with their emerging sexuality, and acquire skills and education that can prepare them for adult roles, all while resolving identity issues and developing values and beliefs (National Academies of Sciences, Engineering, and Medicine, 2019).
- The search for and expression of developing identity, along with the strong drive for social acceptance, are evident in the personal home pages and blogs of adolescents on social networking internet sites such as X (formerly called Twitter) and Facebook (Office of Population Affairs, n.d.-a).

Identity formation for adolescents is an iterative process where they question values, beliefs, and meaning. As part of their identity formation, adolescents also develop sexual identity. How an adolescent defines themself as a member of society and how they feel sexually can possibly be confusing and difficult as a youth may struggle with societal, family, and religious norms and practices. The most recent Youth Risk Behavioral Survey (CDC, 2023l) shows that 24% of adolescents identify as something other than heterosexual. There are 42 million adolescents and young adults between 10 and 19 in the United States. Adolescents are generally healthy, but multiple health-related behaviors and social problems begin during this stage of development. Examples include mental health disorders, substance misuse, tobacco use, nutrition-related disorders, sexually transmitted diseases, unintended pregnancy, homelessness, homicide, suicide, and MVCs (Office of Population Affairs, n.d.-a).

The leading causes of morbidity and mortality for U.S. youth are related to risk-taking behaviors. Six health-related adolescent and young adult behaviors are monitored by the Youth Risk Behavior Surveillance System (YRBSS). These include behaviors contributing to unintentional injuries and violence; tobacco use, alcohol use, and substance use; sexual behaviors including unintended pregnancy and sexually transmitted diseases; dietary behaviors; and physical activity.

During the period that generally encompasses the teen years, adolescents encounter many complex changes physically, emotionally, cognitively, and socially. Rapid and major developmental adjustments create various stresses with concomitant problems impacting health and risk-taking.

- Because the amygdala influences adolescent brains more than the frontal cortex, teens base their decisions more on emotion—solving problems differently than adults. As a result, it is important to guide adolescents through the decision-making process before they engage in risky behaviors.

- The U.S. Office of Adolescent Health (Office of Population Affairs, n.d.-a) explains that in stressful situations, adolescents are more likely to:
  - Think one way but act or feel differently
  - Misinterpret social cues
  - Participate in risky behaviors

For 2022, the death rate for adolescents 15 to 19 was 59 per 100, 000 with Alaska (111), Montana (108), and Louisiana (100), having the highest rates. Accidents or unintentional injuries (including MVAs, poisonings, and overdoses) are 22 per 100,000, homicides are 13 per 100,000, and suicides are 10 per 100,000 (Ann E. Casey Foundation, 2024a).

- Unintentional deaths have shifted from a decrease in deaths associated with MVAs to drug overdoses and poisonings. Poisoning and overdoses make up 31% of unintentional deaths, an increase of 7% since 2002. In this same time period, MVAs fell from 75% to 55%.
- Homicide rates are at their highest level with the rise driven by firearm deaths with males being four times as likely to die from homicide (Fig. 20-5). Gun violence (for any reason) has become a leading cause of death in youth and a leading cause of mortality for children 5 to 14 years.
- Half of teen suicides were by firearm with 49% caused by guns up from 42%.
- Inequities in adolescent death can be noted by race: Black (111 per 100,000), American Indian/Alaska Native (84 per 100,000), Hispanic (55 per 100,000), White (49 per 100,000), two or more races (39 per 100,000), and Asian/Pacific Islander (28 per 100,000) (Ann E. Casey Foundation, 2024a).

Public health interventions are key to reducing teen injuries. Safety mechanisms for firearms are essential. This might include "smart" gun safety technology, removal of guns from the home, and safer firearm storage. Other public health safety interventions include mental health screening using depression and suicide screening tools and counseling for those at risk for self-harm or harm to others. C/PHNs and other health team members must advocate for laws, training, and education that support communities and families regarding firearms and gun safety (Lee et al., 2022).

While death rates have gone down, MVAs in adolescents remain an issue. Male adolescents in the 16 to 19 age are most at risk and are three times more likely than youth in their 20s to have a fatality. The presence of other teens in the vehicle increases an adolescent's risk with a crash risk highest for those initially licensed. Of MVA deaths, 44% occurred between 9 p.m. and 6 a.m. increasing to 50% on weekends (CDC, 2024n). Education has played a key role in reducing MVAs in this age, continued education is necessary in the following areas:

- Wearing seat belts: 43.1% of adolescents do not wear a seat belt.
- Texting while driving: 39% of adolescent drivers texted while driving.
- Speeding: 35% of males and 18% of females speed.
- Driving and substance use: 29% of adolescents who had a fatal crash were drinking alcohol; 16.7% of adolescents have driven with someone who has been drinking alcohol; and 13% of adolescents drove after using marijuana (CDC, 2024n).

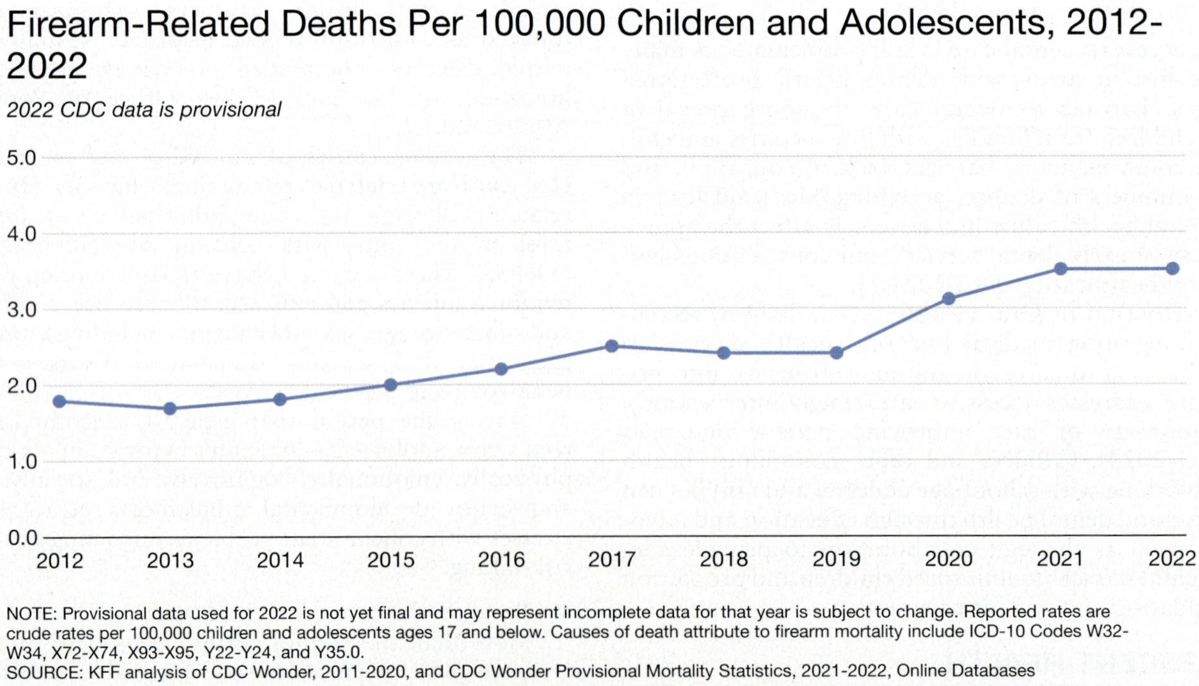

FIGURE 20-5 Firearm-related deaths in children and adolescents. (Reprinted with permission from Kaiser Family Foundation. (2024). *The impact of gun violence on children and adolescents.* https://www.kff.org/mental-health/issue-brief/the-impact-of-gun-violence-on-children-and-adolescents/)

Social stressors and strained relations with peers and parents/guardians are also linked to adolescent health complaints.

- Common complaints of adolescents include sleep deprivation, fatigue, chronic insomnia, acne, and concerns about weight and body image (Hockenberry et al., 2019). As children become adolescents, their sleep patterns change—they move from early risers/sleepers to staying up later and sleeping in later or catching up on sleep over weekends. This transition becomes more apparent through high school.
- Recent studies confirm the support for delaying adolescent school start times and indicate several health risks associated with sleep deprivation, including mental health issues and poor academic performance (Sliwa et al., 2023).

Adolescents have grown up with the internet and social media where digital technologies can provide information on an area of content from education, health, and entertainment. This cultural shift of access to any information day or night and across the globe exposes youth to both positive and negative interactions. Ninety-five percent of all adolescents have a smartphone with one in three reporting they are on social media constantly. The average 10th grader spends 3.5 hours per day on social platforms; adolescents who stay socially connected more than 3 hours a day are at twice the risk for experiencing poor mental health outcomes (Annie E Casey Foundation, 2024b; National Academies of Sciences, Engineering, and Medicine, 2024). The negative effects of social media use in adolescents can include the following:

- Connection between social media cyberbullying and depression
- Poor body image
- Online harassment
- Eating disorders
- Sleep disruption
- Female teens and adolescents identifying as LGBTQ+ are likely to experience harassment and cyberbullying (Annie E Casey Foundation, 2024b)

A recent study found that 82% of adolescent Facebook users had emotional issues in the previous month (National Academies of Sciences, Engineering, and Medicine, 2024). This is in line with the increasing persistence of sadness and hopelessness found in the Youth Risk Behavior Survey (CDC, 2023g). As evidence continues to be gathered, the U.S. Surgeon General has issued a new advisory about the effects of social media use on youth mental health. The warning will indicate that usage of social media can be harmful depending on the amount of time the adolescent spends on the social platform. Adolescence is a time for social relationships, and social media has been linked to adolescents feeling more accepted (58%), supported (68%), and connected (80%) (USDHHS, 2023).

Health Objectives for Adolescents

Healthy People 2030 objectives are focused on improving the health of all Americans. Goals and objectives for adolescent health have been developed (Box 20-7). Because much of the mortality and morbidity in this age group stems from risk-taking behaviors, many objectives address alcohol-related unintentional injuries, violent behaviors, and suicide and mental health issues, as well as more responsible reproductive health.

Emotional Issues and Suicide

The adolescent years are a time of rapid growth and change. Complex developmental changes physically, emotionally, cognitively, and socially may cause a teen to be emotional and unpredictable at times. The influence of peers increases, and peer pressure may influence behavior. Teens test family rules and generally search for their own identity and individuality apart from the family. Most parents/guardians and teens ride out this period with love and understanding and no long-term negative effects. For some children, however, a real or perceived lack of emotional support can lead to temporary or permanent emotional problems. Additionally, increased risk behaviors such as suicide, risky sexual behavior, and mental health disorders are associated with child and adolescent maltreatment. Adolescents may have less contact with the healthcare system than children, and conditions or concerns may go undetected. In recent years, there has been a decrease in risky sexual behaviors, teen births, smoking, use of some substances, and higher academic achievement (Youth.gov, n.d.-a). Currently, youth are experiencing a significant increase in depression, anxiety, and mental issues:

- Depression, anxiety disorders, and eating disorders may first appear during adolescence. It is estimated that one in five adolescents has a mental health disorder that causes some degree of impairment, with 1 in 10 causing significant impairment (ACOG, 2024).
- Prevalence rates of depression vary (Fig. 20-6). About 42% of high school students report feelings of sadness or hopelessness every day for longer than 2 weeks. Of those reporting symptoms, 7% are female and 29% are male (CDC, 2023g).
- Among high school students, 29% reported poor mental health in the past 30 days. Of those reporting, 41% were females and 185 were males (CDC, 2023g).
- Adolescents with mental illness may engage in "acting out" behavior or substance misuse; this may increase their risk for outcomes such as STIs and pregnancy (ACOG, 2024).

Many adolescents are reluctant to seek help for emotional problems or help may not be readily available to them. Most mental health disorders are treatable; however, in 2019, only 16.7% of adolescents received treatment (National Healthcare Quality and Disparities Report, 2022). Barriers to treatment may be social and economic:

- Survey results indicate that the number of children aged 3 to 17 years diagnosed with depression grew 27% between 2016 and 2020 (National Healthcare Quality and Disparities Report, 2022).
- For children, 22% living below the poverty level had a mental or behavioral issue; poverty affected treatment for anxiety and depression. Mental health

BOX 20-7 *HEALTHY PEOPLE 2030*

Objectives to Improve the Health and Well-Being of Adolescents

Core Objectives

AH-01	Increase the proportion of adolescents who had a preventative healthcare visit in the past year
AH-02	Increase the proportion of adolescents who speak privately with a provider at a preventative medical visit
AH-03	Increase the proportion of adolescents who have an adult they can talk to about serious problems
AH-05	Increase the proportion of 4th graders with reading skills at or above the proficient level
AH-06	Increase the proportion of 4th graders with math skills at or above the proficient level
AH-07	Reduce chronic school absence among early adolescents
AH-08	Increase the proportion of high school students who graduate in 4 years

Developmental Objectives

AH-D01	Increase the proportion of trauma-informed early childcare settings and elementary and secondary schools
EMS-D04	Increase the proportion of children and adolescents who get appropriate treatment for anxiety or depression
EMC-D05	Increase the proportion of children and adolescents who get appropriate treatment for behavioral problems

Research Objectives

AH-R02	Increase the proportion of adolescents in foster care who show signs of being ready for adulthood
AH-R04	Increase the proportion of 8th graders with reading skills at or above the proficient level
AH-R05	Increase the proportion of 8th graders with math skills at or above the proficient level
AH-R06	Increase the proportion of youth with special healthcare needs, ages 12—17, who receive services to support their transition to adult healthcare
AH-R07	Increase the proportion of secondary schools with a start time of 8:30 a.m. or later
AH-R08	Increase the proportion of secondary schools with a full-time registered nurse
AH-R09	Increase the proportion of public schools with a counselor, social worker, and psychologist

Reprinted from U.S. Department of Health & Human Services (USDHHS). (2020). *Healthy People 2030: Browse objectives.* https://health.gov/healthypeople/objectives-and-data/browse-objectives

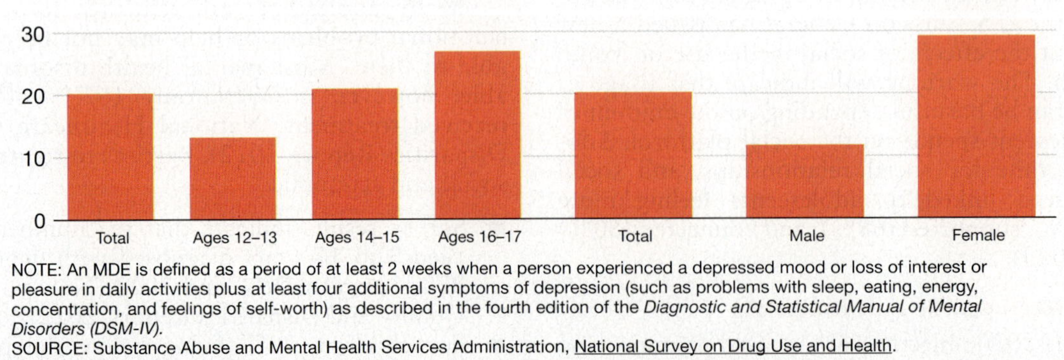

FIGURE 20-6 Percentage of youth ages 12 to 17 who experienced a major depressive episode in the past year by age and gender, 2021. (Reprinted from Child Stats. (2023). *Adolescent Depression.* https://www.childstats.gov/americaschildren/health4.asp)

disorders are a significant economic burden to families; the mean cost of outpatient treatment per episode of a mental health disorder was $2673, with the average number of service encounters at $14.34 (National Healthcare Quality and Disparities Report, 2022). Prices do not include other assessments or services and medications.

- For youth with mental health disorders, 70% to 80% go without care (National Healthcare Quality and Disparities Report, 2022).
- Mental health disorders experienced during adolescence may persist into adulthood, becoming more difficult to treat. It is critical to identify negative adolescent mental health behaviors, provide access to services, and educate teens about healthy physical and mental health skills (Schlack et al., 2021).

Suicide in youth continues to be a serious health concern and is the second leading cause of death in 15- to 24-year-olds (CDC, 2023g). Most adolescents who attempt have depression or mental health concerns. Thoughts of suicide and suicide attempts may be associated with depression but may also be from exposure to violence, aggression, impulsivity, family history of suicide, access to firearms, bullying, feelings of hopelessness, or loss (American Academy of Child & Adolescent Psychiatry, 2024). The Youth Behavior Risk Survey indicates an increase in contemplation of suicide (CDC, 2023g). In 2021:

- Twenty-two percent of high school students seriously considered attempting suicide in the last year. Females (30% from 19% in 2011) were more likely than males (14% from 13% in 2011) to seriously consider suicide. American Indian/Alaska Native (27%) and LGBTQ+ high school students (45%) were more likely than their peers to seriously consider suicide (CDC, 2023g).
- Eighteen percent of high school students in the last year had made a suicide plan (females 24% and males 12%). LGBTQ+ high school students were more likely than their peers to make a plan in the last year (37%) (CDC, 2023g).
- Ten percent of high school students have attempted suicide one or more times in the last year (female 13% and male 7%). American Indian/Alaska Native (16%), Black (14%), and LGBTQ+ high school students (22%) were more likely than their peers to have attempted suicide (CDC, 2023g).

School-based programs to educate adolescents about depression and suicide prevention have been useful. C/PHNs and school nurses often participate in the development or administration of these types of programs.

Suicide prevention programs and direct intervention by counselors or school nurses to determine an adolescent's suicide intentions may be effective school-based interventions. It is important for counselors to identify markers for attempted suicide, such as a precipitating event, intense affective state, suicide ideation or actions, deterioration in social or academic functioning, or increased substance misuse.

Youth suicide has been of great concern over the past several decades. Communities across the nation have been urged to implement effective school-based suicide prevention programs. C/PHNs and community mental health counselors may serve as consultants to schools in developing sound prevention programs.

- The SOS Signs of Suicide program is an evidence-based school-based intervention that educates adolescents about poor mental health, suicide, and coping mechanisms. It has been shown to decrease self-reported suicide attempts.
- Skills training programs that target a broader range of problems (e.g., depression, anxiety, negative self-perceptions) have been effective in teaching adolescents how to monitor feelings, identify triggers, and avoid and reframe negative thoughts. Relaxation skills training, learning how to seek out help from others, and promoting healthier responses to stress have also been successful in impacting internalizing behaviors.
- The Substance Abuse and Mental Health Services Administration (SAMHSA) awards grants in support of youth suicide prevention programs. SAMHSA has also developed a suicide prevention toolkit to help schoos around the nation implement programs (available online at https://store.samhsa.gov/product/preventing-suicide-toolkit-high-schools/sma12-4669#).
- The National Suicide Hotline Designation Act of 2019 designated *988* as the universal number for national suicide prevention and mental health crisis hotline.

A behavior that can sometimes accidentally result in suicide is *self-injury* or *cutting* (Fig. 20-7). Adolescents who overdose, head bang, cut, burn, brand, mark, excessive body pierce, or otherwise dangerously harm themselves are attempting to find relief (desperation, depression,

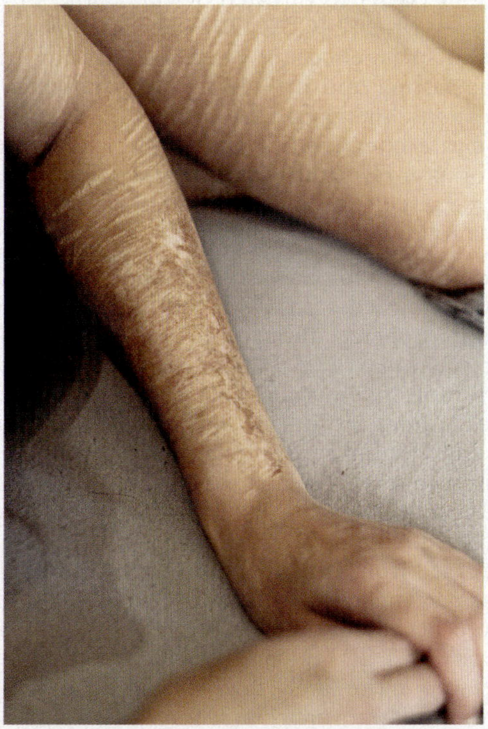

FIGURE 20-7 An adolescent with evidence of "cutting" self-injury.

or anger) from profound psychological pain (depression, psychosis, PTSD, and bipolar disorder). The physical injury distracts them from these painful emotions, often giving them a feeling of control, or providing a means of feeling emotions when they feel emotionally numb (American Academy of Child and Adolescent Psychiatry, 2019).

- Emergency room visits for adolescents with nonfatal injuries have significantly increased in the United States since 2009. Approximately one in 10 youth are seen in an emergency department (ED) for self-inflicted injuries or self-harm with 71% treated for comorbidities (such as self-harm and depression). The majority of those seen in the ED were female adolescents, and 11% had repeated the self-inflicted injury over the past year. Fifty percent of youth were never treated (Peterson et al., 2019).
- For female youth ages 12 to 17, ED visits were 50.6% higher in 2021 as compared to 2019; males had an increase of 3.6% in this same time period (CDC, 2021c). It is more common in those with a family history of suicide or mental illness. Neglect or sexual abuse may predispose an adolescent to this behavior. Depression, anxiety, lack of friendships, and poor family relationships are often associated with self-injury (McEvoy et al., 2023).

C/PHNs and school nurses can educate adolescents and families about this condition and work with schools to promote prevention strategies, such as early detection and referral to mental health providers.

Violence

Youth violence is defined as "the intentional use of physical force or power to threaten or harm others by young people ages 10–24" (CDC, 2024o). The physical, emotional, and social effects of youth violence can be severe and long lasting and include fighting, bullying, threats with weapons, and gang-related violence. Youth violence affects entire communities and is the leading cause of death for non-Hispanic Black youths. The Youth Risk Behavior Surveillance Survey—United States, 2021, indicated the following:

- Seven percent of high school students were threatened or injured with a weapon (gun, knife, club) on school property during the past year. Adolescents who identify as LGBTQ+ or have same-sex partners were more likely than their peers to be threatened. Black, American Indian/Alaska Native, and multiracial high school students were also more likely than their peers to be threatened.
- The percentage of females who were threatened increased from 5% to 6% from 2011 to 2021; males decreased from 10% to 7% in the same time period.
- Nine percent of students in high school did not go to school because of safety concerns. Adolescents who identify as LGBTQ+ and those with same-sex partners were more likely than their peers to feel unsafe on their way to or from school in the last 30 days. Female students were more likely than males to feel unsafe. American Indian/Native Alaskan, Black, and Hispanic high school students were more likely to miss school for safety concerns.
- Sixteen percent of high school students were electronically bullied (texting, Instagram, Facebook, or other social media) in the last year with female students (20%) more likely than males (11%). adolescents who identify as LGBTQ+ (27%) and those have have same-sex partners (37%) were more likely than their peers to be electronically bullied. American Indian/Alaska Native (21%) and White (19%) adolescents were more likely than their peers to be electronically bullied than their peers.
- Fifteen percent of high school students were bullied on high school property in the previous year. Female students (17%) were more likely than male students (13%). Those who identify as LGBTQ+ (23%) and those with same-sex partners (32%) were more likely than their peers to be bullied at school. American Indian/Alaska Native (18%), White (18%), and multiracial (18%) adolescents were more likely to be bullied at school (CDC, 2023g).
- Fifty percent of children sampled have experienced polyvictimization (individuals who have experienced multiple victimizations such as bullying and sexual assault, physical abuse, and intimate partner violence) in the past year, with 66% over their lifetime experiencing two or more types of violence (see ACE information in this chapter and Chapter 4) (U.S. Department of Justice, 2020).
- Homicide is the second leading cause of death for adolescents and youth (aged 15 to 19), with Black youth rates four times higher than White youth rates (Office of Juvenile Justice and Delinquency, n.d.).
- Unfortunately, in the United States, more than 29% of homicide victims are young adults, with 18% having interacted with law enforcement (Office of Juvenile Justice and Delinquency Prevention, n.d.).

Gangs are often associated with teen violence. In the United States, with a rise in gang membership to approximately 30,000 active gangs, gangs are found in all areas of the United States. There is no one risk factor or cause for youth joining a gang, but instead there are an accumulation of factors. However, most youth who join a gang have a history of delinquency; conduct problems can be seen as early as preschool, followed by school failures in elementary and middle school year, and then serious violence and crime (National Gang Center, 2020).

Multiple successful antigang programs have been implemented in communities, including Gang Resistance Education and Training (G.R.E.A.T.). The G.R.E.A.T. program is taught by local law officials to students in middle and high schools. The goal of the program is to teach students how to avoid violence, resist gang pressure, and improve positive attitudes about law enforcement. This promising program has shown promising results as it successfully meets its goals (National Gang Center, 2021).

Although gang members may engage in violence and intimidation, other instances of school violence have captured greater media attention. Incidents of high school shootings are of great concern to parents/guardians, teachers, communities, and the nation. In the last 25 years, there have been 1500 school shootings in the United States. These high-profile events are becoming far too common and bring attention to the need for change (Wisconsin Office of Children's Mental Health, 2024).

- School violence has been linked to bullying and the overall school environment and should be addressed quickly (Sumner et al., 2022). Sumner et al. (2022) found a significant association between those who carried a gun and those who were bullied.
- A meta-analysis of 55 studies determined that the strongest predictor of school violence perpetration was delinquent and antisocial behavior. Other predictors also included ADHD, child maltreatment, peer rejection, moral disengagement, deviant peers, callous unemotional traits, narcissism, exposure to domestic violence, and victimization (Turanovic & Siennick, 2022).
- At least 4.6 million children live in a home where at least one gun is kept loaded and unlocked.
- In 4 out of 5 school shootings, one other person had knowledge of the plans but failed to report.
- Ninety-three percent of school shootings are planned in advance; almost all of the shooters shared threatening or concerning messages (Sandy Hook Promise, n.d.).

Of recent concern is the growing prevalence of school shootings and the effects this can have on students' well-being. Many students and their parents/guardians fear a shooting could occur in their school; gun deaths among U.S. children rose 50% between 2019 and 2021 (Pew Research Center, 2023). School-age children have become involved in the debate surrounding gun violence, where proposals focus on addressing mental illness, assault-style weapon ban, gun regulations, and the use of metal detectors in schools. To address this issue, states and local school districts have implemented a broad range of responses including a school safety and crisis response plan, proactive screening for at-risk students, improving school climate and safety, and addressing bullying and harassment in schools (Sprague & Walker, 2022). Little impact has been seen with harsh disciplinary policies and overreliance on school security as compared to promising approaches from prevention programming (Mayer et al., 2021).

Cultural and environmental influences on youth include the violence to which children and adolescents are exposed. Increased aggressive behavior among children and teens has been attributed to violence in the environment, the home (spousal and child abuse), and the community, and to what children view on screens. The effects of family violence (domestic violence, child maltreatment) can lead to internalizing and externalizing behaviors among youth.

- Personally experiencing or witnessing violence as a child is a risk factor for adolescent behaviors such as school dropout, running away from home, attempting suicide, and delinquency (Brown et al., 2021).
- School climate is important in reducing the levels of violence in this age group, as is adequate parental support. Family cohesion can also be a mediating factor for delinquency due to the childhood effects of violence.
- Promote antibullying in schools through evidence-based programs and training that promote communication, constructive messaging on social media, and advocacy for connectedness and belonging (NASN, 2023).

Substance Use

Substance use is one of the greatest threats to adolescent health (Fig. 20-8).

- In 2021, 16% of high school students said they had used marijuana in the past 30 days; this percentage has decreased since 2011. Use by males in 2021 was 14%, down from 26% in 2011, while use by females was 18% in 2021 down from 20% in 2011 (CDC, 2023g).

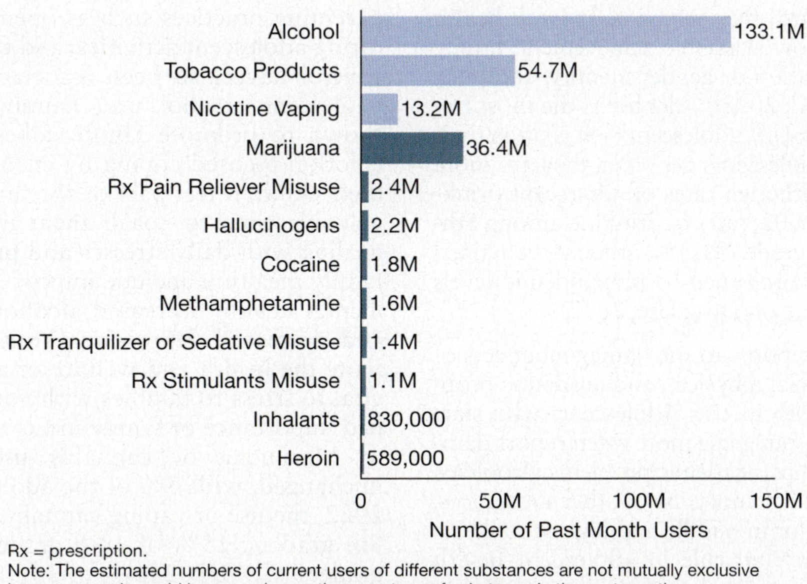

FIGURE 20-8 Past month substance use among people age 12+. (Reprinted from Substance Abuse and Mental Health Services Administration. (2021). *Results from the 2021 National Survey on Drug Use and Health: Graphics from the Key Findings Report.* https://www.samhsa.gov/data/sites/default/files/reports/rpt39443/2021_NNR_figure_slides.pdf)

- In the past 30 days, 23% of high school students reported they drank alcohol (females 27% and males 19%). Alcohol use among American Indian/Alaska Native students was 36% as compared with 26% for White and 13% for Black students (CDC 2023g).
- In the past 30 days, 18% of high school students used electronic vapor products. Female students are more likely than males to use electronic vapor products. Native Hawaiian/Pacific Islander students (25%) were more likely to use electronic vapor products than White (20%) or Black (14%) students. Students who have same-sex partners (44%) were more likely to use electronic vapor products than students who have opposite sex only partners (34%) (CDC, 2023g).
- Among high school students, 13% indicated they had ever used a specific illicit drug (cocaine, inhalants, heroin, methamphetamines, hallucinogenic, or ecstasy). Females (15%) were more likely to use select illicit drugs than males (12%). Asian (7%) and Black (9%) students were less likely to use select illicit drugs than any other race or ethnic group. Students with same-sex partners (39%) were more likely to use select illicit drugs than their peers (CDC, 2023g).
- Among high school students, 12% had ever taken prescription pain medicine (such as codeine, Vicodin, OxyContin, hydrocodone, or Percocet) without a prescription or differently than how they were told to use them. Students who identify as LGBTQ+ (14%) and students with any same-sex partners (34%) were more likely than their peers to use select illicit drugs (CDC, 2023g).
- Youth opioid use is linked to sexual risk behaviors (CDC, 2022i).
- Drug use is associated with sexual risk behavior, experience of violence, mental health issues, and suicide risk (CDC, 2022i).

Risk factors for high-risk substance use in youth include the following: family history of substance use, favorable parental behaviors toward the behavior, mental health issues, childhood abuse, low academic achievement, family rejection of sexual orientation or gender identity, and poor parental monitoring (CDC, 2022i). Alcohol is the most frequently used substance for U.S. adolescents—it is often their first drug of choice. As adolescents get older, they are more likely to drink alcohol. Although rates of adolescent drinking have decreased since 2002, rates of drinking among 8th-grade (15.2%) and 10th-grade (31.3%) students remained stable, but 12th-grade use returned to prepandemic levels (51.9%) (National Institute on Drug Use, 2022).

- The teen brain is susceptible to the damaging effects of alcohol, and many social, physical, and academic problems are associated with its use. Adolescents who start drinking alcohol at a young age more often report damaged family relationships, academic problems, problems with concentration and memory, use of other substances, and delinquent behavior in middle and high school.
- School nurses play a vital role in adolescent health working with students and their families to combat alcohol and drug use (ISM, 2023). It is important to stress education and prevention in late childhood to delay the initiation of alcohol use (Box 20-8).

BOX **20-8** POPULATION FOCUS

Using Evidence-Based Practice to Design Mental Health Concerns and Opioid Overdoses Prevention Strategies

I am a school nurse at a suburban, smaller school district serving over 15,000 students with two high schools, three middle schools, 10 elementary schools, and a continuation high school. Each high school and middle school has a full-time school nurse, and there are five school nurses that share the elementary schools. Each school has one full-time health office specialist. Our focus this year is the mental health issues related to the school closures for 1.5 years due to the pandemic as well as opioid overdoses.

The district school nurses met with our advisory board, parent groups, school administration, and eventually the school board to discuss the problem and address potential interventions. After examining the best research-based methods and partnering with school mental health experts, teachers, and parents, we implemented a Narcan program in our schools. Teachers that were trained received Narcan for their classrooms. In addition, PTSA arranged for their own supply and trained interested parents before giving them two doses of Narcan.

We are seeing an unusual number of students with anxiety and depression since the return to campus. School district mental health officials, school nurses, and administrators meet monthly to develop interventions. Our hope is through these interventions and parent involvement we as a community will help our students get through this time in history.

—*Emma, age 40, School Nurse*

Adolescents who are engaged emotionally and connected to school usually have better outcomes. Positive parenting practices such as open communication, monitoring adolescent activities, and teaching methods of self-control have also been associated with a reduction in adolescent alcohol use. Family mealtimes have been shown to promote family cohesion and problem- and emotion-focused coping by encouraging parents to help their children feel part of the family and allowing them valuable time to coach them in effective methods for dealing with daily stresses and problems. The benefits of family mealtime include improved self-esteem, improved mental health, decreased alcohol and substance misuse, and decreased depression (Youth.Gov, n.d.-b). To promote the health and welfare of adolescent children, it is vital to stress to families with young children the continued importance of family meals throughout adolescence.

Marijuana or cannabis use (Fig. 20-9) remains unchanged, with 6% of the adolescents using it daily. In 2022, the use of vaping cannabis was reported in 6% of 8th graders, 15% of 10th graders, and 20.6% of 12th graders (CDC, 2024p).

- Marijuana use during adolescence has been associated with a much greater likelihood of drug misuse and dependency, poorer mental health, poorer

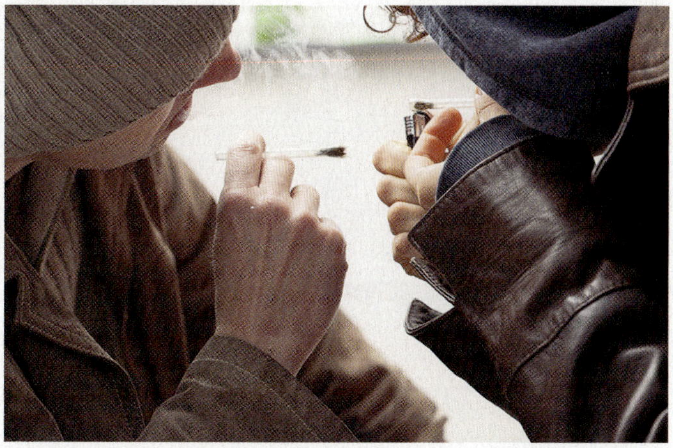

FIGURE 20-9 Marijuana use by adolescents is associated with poorer academic performance.

academic performance, increased delinquency, and neurocognitive deficits (CDC, 2024p).

- Marijuana use has negative health effects, including anxiety, panic attacks, increased heart rate, frequent respiratory infections, impaired memory and learning, and tolerance. Those who regularly smoke marijuana often have respiratory complications similar to those who smoke tobacco—cough, phlegm, respiratory infections, and airway obstruction, and run the risk of cannabis use disorder (CDC, 2024p).

Misuse of inhalants can begin in early adolescence—more 12- and 13-year-olds reported using inhalants than any other illicit drug.

- Inhalants refer to substances that are only taken by inhaling, such as solvents, gases, and nitrites. The most commonly reported inhalants used were shoe polish, glue or toluene, spray paints, and lighter fluid or gasoline.
- Other inhalants commonly used include amyl nitrite "poppers"; locker room deodorizers or "rush"; cleaning fluid, degreasers, or correction fluid; halothane, ether, or other anesthetics; lacquer thinner or other paint solvents; butane or propane gases; nitrous oxide or "whippets"; and other aerosol sprays.
- Inhalant misuse can result in severe nervous system damage or death. Control of legal products, such as spray paint, lighter fluid, household solvents, gasoline, and glue, is difficult, making this problem almost impossible to monitor adequately (National Institute on Drug Abuse, n.d.; U.S. Food and Drug Administration, n.d.).

Another drug used by adolescents is anabolic steroids. The illicit use of anabolic steroids is difficult to monitor; however, 0.7% of high school students reported using steroids (Get Smart About Drugs, 2024). The prevalence of nonprescription steroid use increased between 1999 and 2004 and then decreased from 2005 to 2023 (Statista, 2024).

- Adverse effects of illicit steroid use include irritability, increased risk-taking behavior, extreme mood swings, paranoia, jealousy, and euphoria, as well as psychiatric conditions that may be intensified or induced (Get Smart About Drugs, 2024).
- Because steroids are often readily available through internet pharmacies, policymakers, health educators, and parents must make adolescents aware of the dangers, such as altered serotonin levels and increased aggression.

Adolescents are becoming more involved with prescription drugs, often found in their parents' medicine cabinets, purchased on the internet, or bought from friends at school. Secondary to marijuana and alcohol, they are the most commonly misused substances by teens. Adolescents may mix medications with alcohol, and they may mistakenly believe prescription medications are safer than street drugs when used to produce a high. Prescription drugs are one of the most commonly misused substances by all Americans age 14 years and older (National Institute on Drug Abuse, 2022).

Tobacco products are also easily acquired, often from parents.

- In 2021, approximately 80.2% of high school students and 74.6% of middle school students who used tobacco in the previous 30 days reported using a flavored tobacco product. In 2022, 90.3% of high school students and 87.1% of middle school students who used e-cigarettes in the past 30 days reported using flavored e-cigarettes at that time (CDC, 2023m). Between 1991 and 2023, the overall rates of adolescents currently using cigarettes significantly decreased from 27.5% to 2%.
- In 2023, 1.5% of teens reported using smokeless tobacco such as chewing tobacco, snuff, dip, snus, or dissolvable products, and 1.8% of students reported smoking cigars.
- In 2023, 12.7% of high school students reported using multiple tobacco products (CDC, 2023m).

Social disapproval and heightened perception of health risks are thought to help contribute to the downward trend of smoking and smokeless tobacco use, along with price increases and advertising bans. But tobacco marketing continues to be problematic, as the tobacco industry has joined with convenience stores to more prominently display tobacco products, and even though state and federal taxes comprise about half the cost of a pack of cigarettes, states have not always sufficiently invested these funds in adolescent tobacco prevention (American Lung Association, 2024). Flavored nicotine products are marketed to youth, luring children with such flavors as bubble gum and cotton candy (CDC, 2022j).

Risk factors associated with cigarette smoking include being an older adolescent, male, and White. Other factors include having parents without a college education and adolescents not having college education plans (CDC, 2023m).

C/PHNs and community health nurses can provide information to teens about smoking cessation programs and promote primary prevention by educating children and adolescents to choose not to smoke or engage in other health risk behaviors. They can also encourage physicians and parents to question and monitor adolescents about smoking and the use of tobacco products.

STIs and Pregnancy

Teenage pregnancies, sexually transmitted infections (STIs), and HIV/AIDS are public health concerns associated with the sexual activity of adolescents.

- In the 2021 YRBSS, 30% of high school students reported ever having sexual intercourse, and 52% used a condom during their last sexual intercourse.
- About 6% reported having had sexual intercourse with four or more persons, and 33% used birth control pills to prevent pregnancy (CDC, 2023g).

Adolescent birth rates differ by age, racial and ethnic group, and country region. The downward trend in teen birth rates has continued over the past 25 years; however, the rate in the United States remains higher than many other developed countries.

- In 2020, the teen birth rate (aged 15 to 19) was 15.4% per 1000, down 75% from its peak in 1991 of 61.8%.
- In 2020, American Indian/Alaska Native adolescents had the highest teen birth rates at 27.5 births per 1000 females aged 15 to 19. Black adolescents had a teen birth rate of 24.4, Hispanic adolescents 23.5, and White adolescents 10.4 (Office of Population Affairs, n.d.-b).

Preventive teenage pregnancy factors include being engaged in learning and after-school activities, having a positive attitude toward learning and school, academic excellence, and living in a neighborhood with higher income levels. Teenage pregnancy is associated with increased health risks to both the birthing parent and the child. These risks include increased risk of illness and death, increased risk of birthing parent's death from violence, and increased developmental concerns of the child. In addition, young parents are more likely to live in poverty and to be delayed in their own education. The children of adolescent parents are at risk of several social and health challenges, including lower academic achievement, health problems, incarcerations during adolescence, teenage pregnancy, and young adult unemployment (CDC, 2024r).

As such, it would be appropriate for U.S. society to provide effective sexuality education. There is often debate about the virtues of comprehensive versus abstinence-only educational programs. Despite the controversy about the subject, in 2014, 72% of private and public schools in the United States taught pregnancy prevention as part of required health education. Most adolescents (aged 15 to 19) received education about STIs and abstinence, with 38 states and the District of Columbia mandating sex education and HIV education in school; twenty-one of these states require information on contraception to be provided. Thirty-nine states and the District of Columbia require information on abstinence be provided (Guttmacher Institute, 2023).

Comprehensive sex education has been shown to reduce teen pregnancy with broad-based, abstinence-only programs being ineffective (Mark & Wu, 2022). Besides formal education through schools, adolescents note that peers, the media, and parents are also sources of information on sexual health. Pregnancy prevention programs can be effective in reducing teen pregnancy and birth rates (Fig. 20-10) and in reducing the number of second births to adolescent parents. Research regarding the effectiveness of a multicomponent, community-wide teen pregnancy prevention (TPP) program focusing on 15- to 19-year-old African American and Latino/Hispanic youth found that key elements influenced the success of a community mobilization program. Learnings included the following:

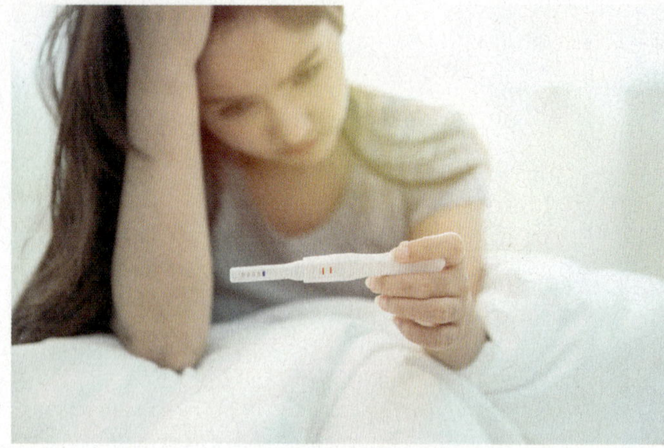

FIGURE 20-10 Pregnancy prevention programs can be helpful in decreasing rates of adolescent pregnancy.

1. Communities are generally willing to "face the issue of adolescent pregnancy."
2. Support of the program by key stakeholders was critical to success.
3. Collaboration of health and human service agencies strengthened the program.
4. Education of and establishing trust within the community was essential.
5. Engagement of youth teams and extensive training for youth leaders was imperative (Youth.gov, n.d.-c).

Primary care providers often miss opportunities to provide counseling on the prevention of pregnancy, HIV, STDs, and other risk factors for unintentional injury. Nurses can provide information and counseling on birth control and emergency contraception to adolescent clients and collaborate with schools to promote effective pregnancy prevention programs. It is important for C/PHNs to provide education and health counseling on these subjects.

Sexually Transmitted Infections

STI and HIV infections are epidemic among adolescents worldwide. An estimated 333 million new cases of curable STIs occur worldwide (WHO, 2024).

- STIs do not always show symptoms and screening is needed for timely diagnosis and treatment. These diseases include syphilis, gonorrhea, chlamydia, HPV, HIV, and herpes simplex virus.
- Almost all sexually active people will get an HPV infection in their lifetime. HPV infections can lead to several types of cancer and other health-related problems (CDC, 2024s).
- Chlamydia, gonorrhea, and syphilis are other STIs found in the adolescent population.

- Of the 20 million new cases of STDs annually, about half were among adolescents (15 to 24 years old) in 2019.
- Only 5% of high school students were tested for STIs (other than HIV) in the previous year. That number has decreased for females since 2019 when 10% were tested as compared to 6% in 2021; males remain unchanged at 5%.

For 2022, chlamydia was the most reportable STI, with 57.7% in the 15 to 24 age range infected (CDC, 2024s). About one in four sexually active adolescent females has an STI. Compared with adults, adolescents (10 to 19 years) and young adults (20 to 24 years) are at increased risk for acquiring STIs. Reasons for this may include a greater likelihood of multiple sex partners, unprotected intercourse, and selection of higher-risk partners. Immature biology makes adolescents more vulnerable to infection and earlier sexual initiation.

- Barriers to prevention and care include social and cultural conditions such as lack of health insurance and transportation, concerns about confidentiality, and lack of quality STD prevention services.
- Adolescent females also have a physiologically amplified susceptibility to chlamydia infection because of increased cervical ectopy.
- Serious complications from STDs include pelvic inflammatory disease, sterility, increased risk of cancers of the reproductive system, and with syphilis, blindness, mental illness, and death. There are also complications for the unborn children of those infected with STDs (CDC, 2024s).

Even though death rates from HIV/AIDS have dramatically fallen, new HIV infections reported annually do not reflect the same steep decline.

- In 2021, 19% of all new HIV diagnoses were in young people 13 to 24 years of age (HIVinfo, n.d.). While adolescent sexual activity has declined since 2011, fewer youth are using condoms, and substance misuse is still prevalent leading to risky sexual activity. Adolescents who identify as LGBTQ+ have disproportionally higher rates of STIs including HIV compared to their heterosexual peers (CDC, 2024g).
- The CDC granted approximately $216 million per year over 5-years to 90 community-based organizations to deliver HIV prevention strategies for those most at risk. The goal of these grants is to identify undiagnosed HIV infections and connect those diagnosed with HIV to appropriate healthcare resources (CDC, 2019).

Poor Nutrition and Eating Disorders

Poor nutrition and obesity are common among adolescents, whose diets often consist of snacks with limited nutritional value interspersed among unhealthful meals. Adolescents' nutritional needs increase as their growth rate and body composition change with puberty. Psychosocial factors, family and peers, the availability of fast food, and mass media marketing influence adolescents' eating behaviors. Adolescents may not be aware of dietary needs, sources of nutrients, and the relationship between diet and disease.

- Females are more likely to struggle with eating disorders than males. Approximately 13% of adolescents will develop an eating disorder by the time they are 20 with the majority being female. Issues with body image and control are at the heart of anorexia nervosa and bulimia nervosa, common problems for youth (Eating Disorder Hope, 2024).
- **Anorexia nervosa** is an eating disorder with an emotional etiology that is characterized by body image disturbance (i.e., young females with this condition perceive themselves as fat, although they may be extremely thin), an intense fear of becoming fat or gaining weight, and refusal to maintain adequate body weight.

Bulimia nervosa is an eating disorder characterized by recurrent episodes of binge eating with repeated compensatory mechanisms to prevent weight gain, such as vomiting (purging type) and fasting or exercise (nonpurging type). **Binge eating**, also a recognized eating disorder, involves recurrent episodes of binge eating without fasting, self-induced vomiting, or other compensatory measures. Self-esteem, depressive symptoms, and emotional eating are very sensitive predictors of binge eating. Low levels of support from peers can also be linked to binge eating, and binge eating is associated with an increased risk of becoming overweight or obese (Substance Abuse and Mental Health Services Administration, 2024). These diseases affect both male and female adolescents. Research indicates that they are caused by multiple factors including genetics, biological, behavioral, psychological, and social elements. Nutrition education, psychological counseling, and cognitive–behavioral techniques that teach clients how to control stimuli, substitute alternative behaviors, and use positive visualization are all part of treatment; the development of a support network is also important. Family and individually based treatments are most often used for severe cases of adolescent eating disorders and have been studied most often. Medications (e.g., antidepressants) have been used to treat some adolescents with eating disorders, when co-occurring illnesses exist (Substance Abuse and Mental Health Services Administration, 2023).

HEALTH SERVICES FOR SCHOOL-AGE CHILDREN AND ADOLESCENTS

Many programs serve the health needs of school-age children and adolescents. Community health nurses play a major and vital role in delivering these services. Such programs fall into three categories that approximate the three practice priorities of community health nursing practice: illness prevention, health protection, and health promotion.

Preventive Health Programs

Among programs to prevent physical illness and other health problems among adolescents are immunizations, tuberculosis (TB) testing, and school- and community-based education, and support programs. Private and public counseling programs and other social services are also geared to promote health and prevent illness.

Immunizations and Tuberculosis Testing

C/PHNs are deeply involved in each preventive activity of immunizations and TB testing. Health departments and schools often work collaboratively to provide immunization services. Compulsory immunization laws are helpful in carrying out these preventive services, but recent survey results reveal that not all adolescents are fully covered.

It is important for adolescents, as well as adults, to get a single dose of Tdap to protect themselves and infants who may be around them from whooping cough. Although pertussis in adolescents or adults often manifests as an upper respiratory infection with a chronic cough, for infants who have not yet been fully immunized, it can lead to serious complications.

In the recent past, adolescents were only given "catch-up" vaccinations (those missed in childhood), except for a tetanus/diphtheria booster. Recommended immunizations now include Tdap, meningococcal vaccine, pneumococcal polysaccharide vaccine, hepatitis A and B vaccine, influenza vaccine, and HPV vaccine for both males and females. Additionally, any missed vaccines such as polio and varicella are recommended.

School-based clinics are a great place to catch adolescents who need updated immunizations. Additionally, vaccinations are becoming more available at retail pharmacies; however, higher levels of medical and health needs are met when children and adolescents have an annual visit with a healthcare provider. Routine visits give the healthcare provider an opportunity to discuss risk behaviors and health concerns with adolescents and to intervene early as problems arise. Annual TB testing is often recommended for children and adolescents from high-risk populations. Targeted TB skin testing identifies adolescents and children at risk for latent TB who could benefit from treatment to prevent the progression of the disease (CDC, 2024t). See Chapter 8 for more on TB skin testing.

Education and Social Services

The health education of school-age children and adolescents includes a wide variety of approaches and can range from the basics of handwashing for elementary school students to health-risk behavior for adolescents. Parental support services are commonly available through many public and private agencies, including churches. These services can have long-range effects on the health of school-age children because emotionally healthy parents and stable families offer a healthy environment and support system for children and can facilitate their progress in school. In most states, C/PHNs provide teaching and counseling services to parents in their homes and in groups. School nurses, school mental health counselors, and school psychologists also organize parent support groups in local schools. This is particularly important during periods of transition (e.g., from elementary to middle school, from middle to high school). Discussing parenting concerns and increasing parents' understanding of typical child growth and development helps to allay fears and prevent problems. Through such efforts, family violence and abuse can be averted. Reduction in rates of divorce and the attendant consequences may also be a benefit of strengthening family resilience.

Family planning programs, often stationed strategically in urban areas, near schools, or in school-based clinics, provide birth control information and counseling to young people.

- In some communities, the school-based clinic dispenses condoms. In many states, adolescents have the right to consent to sexual and reproductive healthcare without parental permission. It is important that healthcare providers be aware of local and regional options for counseling.
- C/PHNs, in collaboration with an interdisciplinary team, are usually the primary care providers in these programs. Their major goals are to prevent teenage pregnancy, educate teens about reproduction and contraception, and encourage responsible sexual behavior.
- Schools can foster evidence-based health education and create healthy, safe, and nurturing school environments, especially when implementing policies and programs regarding reproductive health and health risk behaviors.
- Collaborative efforts by the student, family, school, community, and society are essential to promoting adolescent health. Developing healthy and safe health education environments will influence adolescent health and academic achievement (CDC, 2024r).

Children and adolescents can be influenced by adults smoking in the home. C/PHNs should educate parents about the effects of smoking in the home and its relationship to adolescent smoking. Youth tobacco use is also associated with peer approval, mental health (strongly associated with depression, anxiety, and stress), lower socioeconomic status, lower academic achievement, accessibility, and tobacco advertising.

Multiple programs to reduce and prevent teen smoking have been implemented in recent years. Successful activities include higher tobacco costs, indoor smoking prohibition, raising the minimum age of tobacco sales, social media, and community antitobacco programs (CDC, 2023m).

C/PHNs must work with law enforcement officials, school district administrators, and other community agencies to ensure compliance with local regulations and prevent or delay the use of tobacco products. The CDC and the Foundation for a Smokefree America provide information on smoking cessation and resources to help prevent tobacco use by children and adolescents.

Health Protection Programs

Safety and Injury Prevention

Accident and injury control programs serve a critical role in protecting the lives of school-age children and adolescents. They are cost-effective: seat belt laws, child safety seats, and helmet laws have saved millions of dollars in medical care. Efforts to prevent MVAs, a major cause of adolescent death, include driver education programs, better highway construction, improved motor vehicle design and safety features, and continuing research into what causes various types of crashes.

- Injury prevention and reduction have been addressed through multiple strategies. These include state laws requiring the use of safety restraints; installation of driver and front passenger airbags; substitution of other modes of travel (air, rail, or bus); lower speed limits; stricter enforcement of drunk driving laws; graduated driver's licenses for teenagers; safer automobile design; and helmets for motorcyclists, bicycle riders, and skaters.
- The CDC's "Parents are the Key" campaign focuses on the influence of parents, pediatricians, and communities as safety features for teens (CDC, 2024u).

Safety programs also seek to protect school-age children and adolescents from the hazards of poisonings, ingestion of prescription or over-the-counter drugs, product-related accidents (unsafe toys, bicycles, skateboards, skates, playground equipment, and furniture), and recreational accidents, including drowning, sports-related injuries, and firearms. Safety services assume various forms. Poison control centers in many localities offer information and emergency assistance. Whereas the federal Consumer Product Safety Commission monitors the safety of products, education programs in schools or through local fire or police departments teach school-age children about bicycle and water safety, fire dangers, and hazards related to poisoning. Generally, the C/PHN can educate families to recognize potentially hazardous situations and encourage efforts to eliminate them. Gun safety toolkits provide families with resources to make safe decisions regarding guns in the home. Working with school nurses and school district officials to reduce playground hazards can contribute to the reduction of school-related injuries.

Infectious Disease Prevention

Programs that protect school-age children and adolescents against infectious diseases encompass such efforts as closing swimming pools that have unsafe bacteria counts, conducting immunization campaigns in conjunction with influenza or measles outbreaks, and working with hospital pediatric units to reduce the incidence and threat of iatrogenic disease. Prevention of community-acquired MRSA is a new challenge for public schools, and C/PHNs may work with school nurses or others to provide educational programs covering a variety of infectious diseases. Epidemiologic investigations, especially with school sports teams, may be necessary to determine the cause of outbreaks (WHO, 2022).

Child Protective Services

The Children's Bureau collects and analyzes information on child abuse and neglect, serves as an information clearinghouse, publishes educational materials on the subject, offers technical assistance, and conducts research into the problem (Administration on Children and Families [ACF], 2024).

- In 2022, 4.276 million child maltreatment referrals were made; 74.3% were neglect, 17% were physical abuse, 10.6% were sexual abuse, 6.8% were psychological maltreatment.
- Over 3 million children received prevention and postresponse services.
- The highest rate of abuse is in children less than 1 year old (22.2 per 1000).
- In 2022, 1990 children died from abuse and neglect.
- Child abuse crosses all socioeconomic and education levels, religions, and ethnic and cultural groups.
- Fourteen percent of all men and 36% of all women were abused as children (America, SPCC, 2024).

Consequences for affected children include lower self-esteem, depression, suicide, self-abuse, substance misuse, eating disorders, less empathy for others, antisocial behavior, delinquency, aggression, violence, low academic achievement, and sexual maladjustment. Long-term emotional, social, cognitive, and physical consequences are well documented and often follow children who have been abused into adolescence and adulthood. Posttraumatic stress disorder, poor attachment and problems with trust, difficulties with language development and abstract reasoning, high-risk health behaviors, and abusive or violent behavior may be seen later in life (ACF, 2024). These findings were first noted in a large-scale, landmark research study, the Adverse Childhood Experiences study (Felitti et al., 1998) (see Chapter 4).

In some areas, C/PHNs are working together with social workers, mental health workers, and substance misuse counselors as part of a team that provides services to families. Improved training of mandated reporters, such as teachers and physicians, has led to better reporting of abuse; as professionals and the public become more aware of the problem, an increase in reporting has occurred. Child abuse prevention programs can be found in many public health departments and through some school districts as a primary preventive intervention. Primary prevention of child maltreatment can also occur through home visiting programs utilizing C/PHNs. These visits can also help to connect high-risk families to the community and promote better child outcomes when an appropriate curriculum is followed (Nurse-Family Partnership, 2024). Programs that target at-risk families, especially adolescent birthing parents and young couples prone to partner violence or harsh parenting practices, may help to prevent later child abuse. C/PHNs and school nurses must be vigilant for signs of family stress, harsh parenting practices, family violence, and other risk factors for child abuse and neglect, and must provide resources and respite as needed (for additional information, see Chapters 18 and 19).

Oral Hygiene and Dental Care

Fluoridation of drinking water, school-provided fluoride rinse or gel, and dental sealant programs are cost-effective and can reduce dental caries.

- Fluoride makes teeth less susceptible to decay by increasing the resistance of tooth enamel to the bacterially produced acid in the mouth. School-based programs that provide fluoride rinses and dental sealants and promote tooth brushing and nutrition education for dental health can be found in most areas of the country.

- Fluoridation of community water supplies is considered the most effective, safe, and low-cost means of protecting the dental health of children and adolescents.
- Although most dental care is focused on children, adolescents remain in need of dental health services. In addition to regular dental care, good nutrition, and proper oral hygiene, C/PHNs can promote public water fluoridation as an important program for protecting children's dental health. Nurses can also recommend that parents talk with their primary healthcare provider and dentist about fluoride varnish or supplements (CDC, 2023k).

Health Promotion Programs: Nutrition and Exercise

Nutrition and weight control programs form another important set of health promotion services. Children need to learn sound dietary habits early in life to establish healthy lifelong patterns. Being overweight during childhood or adolescence may persist into adulthood and may increase the risk for some chronic diseases later in life.

- A number of weight control programs for children and adolescents who are overweight are available through schools, health departments, community health centers, health maintenance organizations, and private groups (National Institute of Diabetes and Digestive and Kidney Diseases [NIDDK], 2023).
- Children and adolescents are particularly vulnerable to media and peer pressures with regard to their food choices. Because of increased rates of childhood obesity and a greater awareness of the need for better nutrition in adolescence, district-level policies to increase the availability of healthy foods at public schools are growing (Micha et al., 2018).

The C/PHN plays a significant role in promoting children's health through nutrition education, reinforcement of positive practices, and policy advocacy.

CASE STUDY 10 ESSENTIAL PUBLIC HEALTH SERVICES

How Much Trauma Can a School Population Endure?

Many students in a public combined middle school and high school in a small community on the coast of southern California experienced trauma-related PTSD and anxiety due to two disasters the community experienced in a short period of time: a wildfire and COVID-19.

In 2018, a wildfire ripped through the community, destroying over 400 single-family homes. The community is accustomed to weather-related hardships, such as floods and mudslides closing the only road in and out of the area, and fires are not new either; however, the fire storm in 2018 was one of the worst in California history. Residents had only enough time to collect a few belongings before they had to evacuate. Teachers and staff who lived in the area lost homes and their belongings as well. Phone lines went dead, powerlines went up in flames, and families had limited warning as the blaze drew closer. Residents in the 400 homes that were destroyed had to move out of the area as homes were rebuilt; children went to nearby school districts, or families moved out of state to live with relatives. Then, after many had returned and school had resumed as usual, the COVID-19 pandemic closed the school once again.

The school nurse found that their major role was addressing mental health issues for a variety of concerns and to return students to their classes as soon as possible. Due to anxiety, one sixth grader had an accommodation to sit quietly in the health office during a stressful class. They had lost everything their family knew and loved in the fire, and their grandmother had passed away from COVID-19. Many other students spent time in the health office as well due to stress- and anxiety-related issues.

1. ***Recognize Cues:*** *Which findings require immediate follow-up, are unexpected, or are most concerning?*
2. ***Analyze Cues:*** *What information is noted or needed for interpreting findings?*
3. ***Prioritize Hypotheses:*** *Based on the information that you have, what is happening?*
4. ***Generate Solutions:*** *What intervention(s) will achieve the desired outcome?*
5. ***Take Action:*** *What actions should you take or do first?*
6. ***Evaluate Outcomes:*** *Were outcomes achieved? Why or why not?*
7. *Which Essential Public Health Services influence this situation? (See Box 2-2.)*

SUMMARY

- The physical and emotional health of children and adolescents can affect their academic achievement and society's future. Children and adolescents need the guidance and direction provided by community health nurses.
- Poverty is a significant social determinant of health that has been shown to contribute to many physical, psychological, and behavioral problems in children and adolescents. There is concern that government assistance programs are not meeting the needs of children and adolescents who come from families with a low income.
- Health problems that affect learning and achievement in school-age children include chronic diseases, behavioral and learning problems, disabilities, injuries, communicable diseases, dietary and physical activity concerns, and poor dental health.
- The federally and state-mandated immunization program for school-age children and adolescents is one measure to prevent communicable diseases. Among vaccines given on schedule throughout childhood are those that prevent polio, smallpox, diphtheria, tetanus, typhoid, and many other diseases.

- Mortality rates for children and adolescents have decreased dramatically since the early 1900s, but morbidity rates remain high. Children and adolescents are vulnerable to many illnesses, injuries, and emotional problems, often due to a complex and stressful environment.
- Violence against children and deaths because of homicide occur in the United States at alarming rates. Unintentional injuries, suicide, and homicide are the leading threats to life and health for adolescents.
- Other health problems include alcohol and drug misuse, unplanned pregnancies, STIs and HIV/AIDS, and poor nutrition. All of these problems create major challenges for the C/PHN who seeks to prevent illness and injury among children and adolescents and to promote their health.
- *Healthy People* objectives for children and adolescents provide key goals for the reduction of alcohol-related unintentional injuries; declines in violent behaviors, suicide, and mental health issues; and more responsible reproductive health behaviors. Barriers to achieving these goals vary and include economic inequities; lack of sufficient immunization, educational, and community-supported health programs; and the presence of risk behaviors typical among developing youth.
- C/PHNs play a large role in promoting the health of adolescents, their families, and communities, through education programs and by developing strategies to support healthy growth and development and prevent risky behaviors that lead to injury, teen pregnancy, and sometimes death.
- Health services for children and adolescents span three categories: prevention, health protection, and health promotion. C/PHNs play a vital role in each.
  - Preventive services may include immunization programs, parental support services, family planning programs, services for those with STIs, and alcohol and drug misuse prevention programs.
  - Health protection services often include accident and injury control, programs to reduce environmental hazards and control infectious diseases, and services to protect children and adolescents from child abuse and neglect.
  - Health promotion services may include programs in nutrition and weight control, along with HIV/AIDS prevention and smoking, alcohol, and drug misuse education.
- C/PHNs are integral to the health and well-being of children and adolescents, through their work with families, schools, and other community agencies.

ACTIVE LEARNING EXERCISES

1. Your school district is searching for ways to improve adolescent nutrition and diet. What influencing factors should you consider (e.g., student behaviors, environment/cultural influences, school policies)? What key stakeholders should you include as you research and develop a health improvement plan? Describe an evidence-based program that you could implement to increase physical activity and improve nutrition for school-age children and adolescents; indicate levels of prevention addressed with the program. (Objectives 1 and 6)
2. Apply "Utilize Legal and Regulatory Actions" (1 of the 10 Essential Public Health Services; see Box 2-2), to the following: Your school district allows personal exemptions for vaccination (i.e., parents can refuse to get mandatory vaccinations for their children based on personal, not solely religious, beliefs). The public health department has informed you that there is a measles epidemic in your county. What information do you need to promote a safe and healthy school environment? Outline your concerns and formulate a health intervention for your school; indicate what levels of prevention are used. (Objectives 2 and 6)
3. COVID-19 changed the way schools functioned across the nation. What challenges did students in your local and state experience? Compare your findings to the national statistics. Interview school officials and a student to compare and contrast their opinions on the challenges. (Objective 2)
4. You are a public health nurse leader working in a department of health for a large state. You've been asked by the substance use prevention team to testify at the state capital on the impact of the opioid epidemic on the youth of your state. What data sources might you use to frame the issue? How does substance use impact youth academic achievement in your state? Finally, what would be your top three recommendations for how the state legislature should allocate funds for youth opioid use prevention? (Objectives 2 and 3)
5. You are working in a rural health department and are researching the leading causes of death among children and adolescents. Where can you find national and state data for your search? What evidence-based public health interventions have been successful in preventing childhood deaths? Select one intervention for children or adolescents and describe how you and a group of community health professionals might develop effective preventive measures. (Objective 4)
6. You are a school nurse working in a suburban school district that has four large high schools. There have been two youth suicides in the community in the past 4 months; teachers and parents are very concerned about this "epidemic" and unsure of what to do. A *Healthy People 2030* objective is to reduce suicide attempts by adolescents—MHMD-02. What are some public health partnerships you might engage with to address the issue in your schools? (Objectives 4 and 5)

CHAPTER 21

Adult Health

"Wellness is not a 'medical fix' but a way of living—a lifestyle sensitive and responsive to all the dimensions of body, mind, and spirit, an approach to life we each design to achieve our highest potential for well-being now and forever."

—Greg Anderson

KEY TERMS

Adult
Alcohol use disorder (AUD)
Anorexia nervosa
Binge eating
Bulimia nervosa
Cancer
Cardiovascular disease (CVD)
Chronic lower respiratory disease (CLRD)
Diabetes
Erectile dysfunction (ED)
Gynecologic cancer
Health disparity
Life expectancy
Menopause
Myalgic encephalomyelitis/chronic fatigue syndrome (ME/CFS)
Osteoporosis
Perimenopause/menopausal transition
Prostate
Substance use disorder (SUD)
Transgender
Unintentional injuries

LEARNING OBJECTIVES

Upon mastery of this chapter, you should be able to:

1. Identify major chronic illnesses found in adults throughout the lifespan.
2. Examine the concepts of life expectancy and health disparities, and how they apply to adults living in the United States.
3. Discuss factors affecting the health of adults in the United States.
4. Identify primary, secondary, and tertiary health promotion activities designed to improve the health of adults across the lifespan.
5. Identify the *Healthy People 2030* objectives for adults.
6. Appraise the role of the community health nurse in promoting the health of adults across the lifespan.

INTRODUCTION

Mr. Alvin Mason worked in the fields since age 10 in a rural and racially/ethnically diverse sugarcane farming region in south central Florida. He eventually became a cane cutter and then a truck driver transporting the cane from the field to the factory over 50 times daily. His wife Eula, with 12 years of education compared to Alvin's 8, became a "burner"—someone who manages the controlled burns of the sugarcane fields, depending on the wind direction and weather prediction. Both Alvin and Eula developed asthma at some point in the last 5 years. Alvin was diagnosed several years ago with type 2 diabetes, high BMI, and hypertension during his first visit to a medical provider. Alvin, age 51, had never been screened for cancer, but reported pain, difficulty, and occasional bleeding on urination. His wife noted that he had developed some "memory issues" and was rather unsteady and short of breath occasionally when he walked long distances. They both are life-long members of their local church, which is their only means of socialization, other than visits from their son. They raise chickens and have a vegetable garden, do not drink alcohol, and are eager to learn what they can do to age in place in their 1800 square feet home, gifted to them by the farming industry in the 1950s. What is the C/PHN most concerned about regarding Alvin and Eula's health? How can the Masons best care for themselves as they age?

Mr. Fernandez is a relatively healthy middle-aged individual, with no chronic health conditions. He has a family history of type 2 diabetes, cardiovascular disease, and colon cancer. He tries to adhere to a healthy diet, but a moderately stressful career and busy family make it difficult to find time to eat healthy and exercise. Over the past few years, he has noticed weight gain and is concerned that this, along with his family history, may lead to the development of chronic disease. What are the considerations for Mr. Fernandez based on his age, risk factors, and current health status? What preventative services and screenings might he need?

Community and public health nurses (C/PHNs) are in a key position to educate clients like the Masons and Mr. Fernandez on health promotion and disease prevention and inform them of United States Preventive Services Task Force recommendations (USPSTF, 2023). This teaching impacts community health by improving the health of individuals.

The term **adult** has many different meanings in society. To children, an adult is anyone in authority, including a 14-year-old babysitter. As people age, they tend to redefine the term upward in age. It is not unusual, for example, to hear an older person describe a couple in their mid-30s as "kids." The U.S. criminal justice system distinguishes between adults and juveniles for purposes of delimiting types of crimes and possibilities for punishment, and labor legislation provides different protections for children than for adult workers. Even hospitals and healthcare systems vary somewhat as to the ages at which they distinguish pediatric and older adult clients from middle-aged adults.

How would you characterize an adult? Does your definition rest solely on age, or is it influenced by other factors, such as marital status, employment status, financial independence, amount of responsibility for self and others, and so on?

- For the purposes of this chapter, an adult is defined as anyone 18 years of age or older. Obviously, there are tremendous differences in health profiles and healthcare needs as people age.
- As adults enter their middle years (35 to 65), they experience many normal physiologic changes. However, some changes are the result of disease, environment, or lifestyle and can be modified through behavior change.

Many health promotion and health protection programs are designed specifically for males or for females,* as the examples below illustrate.

- Mammography screening programs and prenatal clinics are designed with female health in mind.
- Teaching about testicular self-examination (TSE) and prostate cancer screening is typically included in health promotion programs for males.
- Programs in many areas, such as cardiac rehabilitation, stress management, and dating violence prevention, may have initially targeted one gender but are now established as programs for all genders.

This chapter examines mortality and morbidity statistics, historical development of research foci, workforce change, the healthcare needs of males and females, as well as the health of adults in general.

*In this chapter, "male" means a person assigned male a birth, and "female" means a person assigned female at birth.

MORTALITY AND MORBIDITY STATISTICS

Examining mortality statistics provides key information to understand changes in the health and well-being of a population. In 2022, a total of 3,273,705 people died in the United States. The age-adjusted death rate decreased by 5.3% from 879.7 in 2021, to 832.8 in 2022, per 100,000 for all ages (Ahmad et al., 2023). This decrease may have been in part due to the slowing of the COVID-19 pandemic related to the first year of global vaccinations (Watson et al., 2022a). Causes of death varied by age, sex assigned at birth, and ethnicity; the 10 leading causes of death for all people in rank order are shown in Table 21-1.

Since the beginning of the 21st century, the major causes of death have remained fairly consistent. This was a major shift from the turn of the 20th century, when communicable diseases, such as tuberculosis and pneumonia, were the leading causes of death. The shift from communicable to chronic illness can be attributed to the significant advances in public health, prevention, technology, pharmacotherapy, and biomedical research (see Chapters 1 and 7). However, with the new threat of novel viruses such as COVID-19 impacting morbidity and mortality on a global scale, a return to public health measures, including vaccination programs, is again playing a vital role in combating communicable diseases. The Centers for Disease Control and Prevention (CDC) recommends the following vaccine schedule for adults: https://www.cdc.gov/vaccines/adults/rec-vac/index.html

Changes in recent leading causes of death include the following:

- In 2021, nine of the top 10 causes of death remained unchanged from 2020. The leading cause in 2021 was heart disease, followed by cancer and COVID-19.

TABLE 21-1 The 10 Leading Causes of Death for All Ages in 2021

Cause of Death (in rank order)	Number of Deaths
1. Diseases of the heart (heart disease)	695,547
2. Malignant neoplasms (cancer)	605,213
3. COVID-19	416,893
4. Unintentional injuries (accidents)	224,935
5. Cerebrovascular diseases (stroke)	162,890
6. Chronic lower respiratory diseases	142,342
7. Alzheimer disease	119,399
8. Diabetes	103,294
9. Chronic liver disease and cirrhosis	56,585
10. Nephritis, nephritic syndrome, and nephrosis (kidney disease)	54,358

Source: National Center for Health Statistics (2023); https://www.cdc.gov/nchs/fastats/leading-causes-of-death.htm

- Influenza and pneumonia dropped from the list of 10 leading causes in 2021, likely due to mask wearing and quarantine practices related to COVID-19 (CDC, 2021a).
- Chronic liver disease and cirrhosis moved up as the 9th leading cause of death in 2021.

The remaining leading causes in 2021 (unintentional injuries, stroke, chronic lower respiratory diseases, Alzheimer disease, diabetes, and kidney disease) remained unchanged from 2020 (Xu et al., 2022). Other statistics of importance to public health nurses include the following:

- Cerebrovascular diseases (stroke) are the third leading cause of death for females (Office of Women's Health, 2023).
- Unintentional injuries (accidents) are the leading cause of death for all adults aged 25 to 44 years and the third leading cause of death for males (CDC, 2022a).
- Cancer is the leading cause of death in adults aged 45 to 65 years (Siegel et al., 2022).

LIFE EXPECTANCY

Life expectancy is the average number of years that a person is projected to live. It is another standard measurement used to compare the health status of various populations and is typically calculated based on age-specific death rates. Health statistics often report life expectancy figures at birth and at 65 years of age (see Table 21-2), and also at 75 years of age.

- The U.S. ranks lowest in life expectancy for both males and females among countries with high GDP per capita (Ho, 2022; see Table 21-3).
- Females have a higher life expectancy than males, but the gap narrowed from 7.0 years in 1990 to 5.0 years in 2018. However, these differences are now doubled for those without a college education, regardless of race or ethnicity (Case & Deaton, 2021).
- Other differences in life expectancy based on race and ethnicity in the United States reflect disproportionate burden of morbidity and mortality. In 2021, people of Hispanic origin had a life expectancy of 77.7 years, whereas the life expectancy for White individuals was 76.4 years and for Black individuals was 70.8 years (Hill et al., 2023).

HEALTH DISPARITIES

The overarching goal of the *Healthy People* initiative is to eliminate health disparities and improve the health of all people living in the United States. A **health disparity** is defined as a difference in health status that occurs by gender, race/ethnicity, education or income, disability, geographic location, or sexual orientation (CDC, 2022b). Health disparities occur when one segment of the population has a higher rate of disease or mortality than another or when survival rates are less for one group when compared with another (National Institutes of Health [NIH], 2019). Often, people with the greatest health burden have the least access to healthcare services, adequate healthcare providers, information, communication technologies, and supporting social services. Interdisciplinary,

TABLE **21-2** Life Expectancy at Birth and 65 Years of Age: United States, Selected Years, 1900–2018

	At Birth (Expected Years Overall)			At 65 Years (Expected Years Remaining)		
Year	**Total**	**Male***	**Female***	**Total**	**Male**	**Female**
1900	47.3	46.3	48.3	—	—	—
1950	68.2	65.6	71.1	13.9	12.8	15.0
1960	69.7	66.6	73.1	14.3	12.8	15.8
1970	70.8	67.1	74.7	15.2	13.1	17.0
1980	73.7	70.0	77.4	16.4	14.1	18.3
1990	75.4	71.8	78.8	17.2	15.1	18.9
2000	76.8	74.1	79.3	17.6	16.0	19.0
2010	78.7	76.2	81.0	19.1	17.7	20.3
2016	78.7	76.2	81.1	19.4	18.0	20.6
2017	78.6	76.1	81.1	19.4	18.0	20.6
2018	78.7	76.2	81.2	19.5	18.1	20.7

*In this table, "male" refers to a person assigned male at birth, and "female" refers to a person assigned female at birth.

—, data not available.

Reprinted from National Center for Health Statistics (NCHS). (2022). *Health, United States 2023.* https://www.cdc.gov/nchs/data/hestat/life-expectancy/life-expectancy-2018.htm

Kochanek, K.D., Anderson, R.N., Arias, E. (2020). *Changes in life expectancy at birth, 2010–2018. NCHS Health E-Stat.*

TABLE 21-3 Life Expectancy at Birth, in Years, of the United States and Comparable Countries, 2022

Country	Male[a]	Female[a]
Australia	81.2	85.3
Austria	78.8	83.5
Belgium	79.6	83.9
Canada	79.1	83.6
France	79.4	85.2
Germany	78.3	83.2
Japan	81.1	87.1
Netherlands	80.3	83.2
Sweden	81.5	84.8
Switzerland	81.6	85.4
United Kingdom	79.0	82.9
United States	**74.8**	**80.2**
Comparable Country Average	**80.8**	**84.4**

[a]In this table, "male" refers to a person assigned male at birth and "female" refers to a person assigned female at birth.
Adapted with permission from Rakshit, S., McGough, M., & Krutika Amin, K. F. F. (2024). *How does U.S. life expectancy compare to other countries?* © 2024 PETERSON-KFF Health System Tracker. All Rights Reserved. Retrieved September 5, 2024, from https://www.healthsystemtracker.org/chart-collection/u-s-life-expectancy-compare-countries/#Life%20expectancy%20at%20birth%20by%20sex,%20in%20years,%202022

collaborative, public, and private approaches as well as public–private partnerships are needed to develop strategies to address the health disparity goal of *Healthy People 2030*. Chapter 23 discusses health disparities in more detail.

MAJOR HEALTH PROBLEMS OF ADULTS

Morbidity and mortality among adults vary substantially by age, sex assigned at birth, and race/ethnicity. Several leading causes of death are presented in this section. Heart disease is the first leading cause of death in adults and is presented along with stroke. Malignant neoplasms, COVID-19, unintentional injuries, chronic lower respiratory diseases (CLRDs), and diabetes are among the top 10 leading causes of death and are discussed separately. Other selected major causes of death are covered in detail in other chapters: suicide (Chapter 25), Alzheimer disease (Chapter 22), and homicide (Chapter 18).

Coronary Heart Disease and Stroke

Cardiovascular disease (CVD) describes a group of heart and blood vessel disorders including hypertension, coronary heart disease (CHD), stroke, arrhythmias, valvular heart disease, peripheral vascular disease, and cardiomyopathies (Tsao et al., 2023). Over the last three decades, cardiovascular mortality in the United States has declined by about 50% (Tsao et al., 2023). These gains are attributed to the increased use of evidence-based medical therapies for secondary prevention and reduction in risk factors associated with lifestyle and environment (see Fig. 21-1). Despite these improvements, approximately one third of all deaths in the United States are still due to CVD. Currently, an estimated 92.1 million adults are living with one or more types of CVD, and over half of these people are 60 years of age or older. It is estimated that every 33 seconds an American will die from CVD (CDC, 2023a).

In the United States, underrepresented racial/ethnic populations continue to encounter more barriers to CVD diagnosis and care, receive lower-quality treatment, and experience worse health outcomes. Such disparities are linked to complex factors such as income and education, genetic and physiologic factors, access to care, and communication barriers. Although it appears as though the disparity gap may be declining, this is in part due to gains made by underrepresented racial/ethnic populations and worsening cardiovascular health in White populations (Javed et al., 2022). Furthermore, evidence is linking climate change to worsening health outcomes in underrepresented racial/ethnic groups (Berberian et al., 2022). To tackle inequalities in CVD morbidity and mortality, actions that focus on the social determinants of health are needed. This includes the development and implementation of health and social policy interventions that improve access to and quality of healthcare services and a reduction in poverty and unemployment (Javed et al., 2022).

Risk factors for CVD can be separated into three categories: major nonmodifiable, modifiable, and contributing (Tsao et al., 2023).

- Major risk factors that cannot be modified or treated include heredity (family history, race), increasing age, and sex assigned at birth.
- Risk factors that can be modified, treated, or controlled include high blood cholesterol, high blood pressure, smoking tobacco, physical inactivity, diabetes, and obesity/overweight.
- Risk factors that are known to contribute to heart disease are stress, alcohol consumption, and diet and nutrition.

Heart Disease

- Heart disease is the number one killer of females, causing the death of 310,661 American females in 2021 (CDC, 2023b). The most common heart problem, CHD, is underdiagnosed, undertreated, and under-researched in females.
- In addition, females have a higher mortality rate after a heart attack and poorer outcomes than males, and this may be related to delayed diagnosis and treatment.
- Risk factors for heart disease in females are age, family history, race/ethnicity, physical inactivity, sleep apnea, obesity, diabetes, high blood pressure,

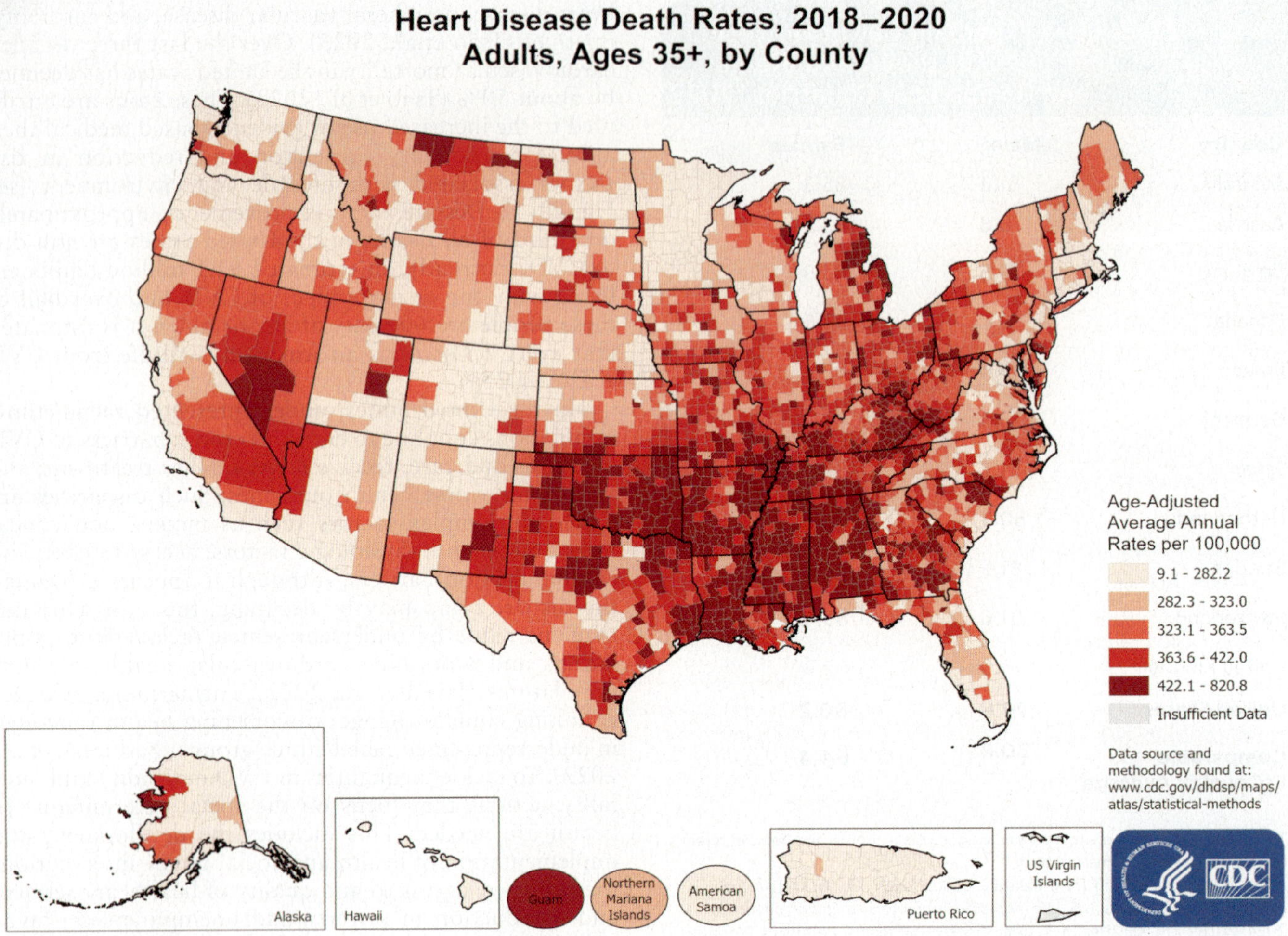

FIGURE 21-1 Heart disease death rates, 2018–2020 adults, ages 35+ by county. (Source: Centers for Disease Control and Prevention, Division for Heart Disease and Stroke Prevention. (2022). *Quick maps of heart disease and stroke*. Retrieved from https://www.cdc.gov/dhdsp/maps/quick-maps/index.htm)

high cholesterol, and cigarette smoking. Nine of 10 females have at least one risk factor for heart disease (Office on Women's Health, 2023).

Family history, race/ethnicity, and advancing age cannot be changed, but females can make lifestyle changes to alter other risk factors. The remaining risk factors are issues that the community health nurse can discuss with female clients in this age group. Community health nurses can help raise awareness regarding heart disease when working with patients at the individual, family, or aggregate levels. Some important facts that can be shared are as follows:

- Heart disease accounts for 1 in 5 female deaths in the United States, yet less than half (44%) of females recognize that heart disease is their number one cause of death (CDC, 2023a).
- Almost two thirds of females who suddenly die from heart disease have had no previous symptoms (CDC, 2023a).
- Hispanic females are more likely to develop heart disease 10 years earlier than non-Hispanic females (AHA, 2023).
- Nearly 60% of non-Hispanic Black females have heart disease (AHA, 2023).
- The average age for the first heart attack in females is 72.0 years (Tsao et al., 2023).
- In all age groups, mortality rate for females following a heart attack is higher than in males (Office on Women's Health, 2023).

An excellent resource is "*Go Red for Women*," a public awareness program of the American Heart Association (AHA) to help improve knowledge (AHA, 2023). Also, *Well-Integrated Screening and Evaluation for Women across the Nation* (WISEWOMAN), a CDC program that helps females with little or no health insurance reduce their risk for heart disease, stroke, and other chronic diseases (located in 21 sites across 19 states), can be helpful. The program assists females ages 40 to 64 in improving their diet, physical activity, and other behaviors (see Fig. 21-2). Locally, this program also often provides cholesterol and other screening tests (AHA, 2023).

Cardiovascular Disease. Heart disease is the leading cause of death in males across most racial/ethnic groups.

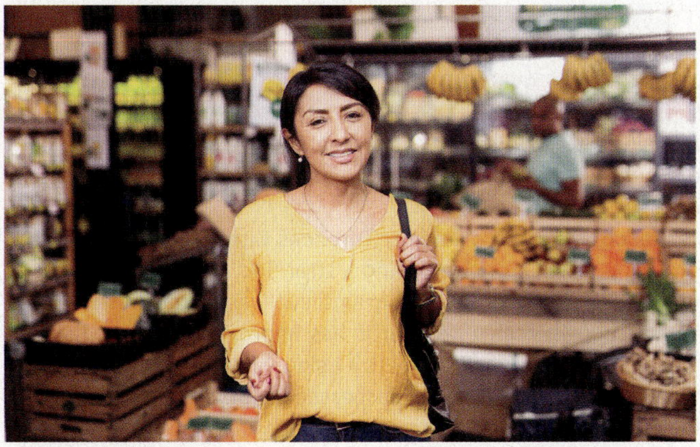

FIGURE 21-2 A healthy diet is an important part of health promotion.

Despite a decline in the overall death rate from CVD, the burden of disease among males remains high.

- In 2021, CVD caused 384,886 deaths in males, or about 1 in 4 male deaths (CDC, 2023b).
- Of those CVD-related fatalities, 50% of these patients have no previous symptoms of the disease.
- The average age for a first heart attack among males is 64.5 years, but one in five heart attacks now occur in men under age 40.
- Age-adjusted heart disease rates per 100,000 for men (CDC, 2022):
  - Non-Hispanic Black: 267.5
  - Non-Hispanic White: 210.7
- It is interesting to note, if all forms of major CVD were eliminated, life expectancy among all people would increase by almost 7 years (Virani et al., 2021).

Major risk factors for heart disease in males include hypertension, hyperlipidemia (high LDL), tobacco use, diabetes, obesity/overweight, lack of physical activity, excessive alcohol consumption, stress, and low daily fruit and vegetable consumption (Boxes 21-1 and 21-2). When working with adult males, the community health nurse should educate them about the importance of modifying factors that increase their risk of developing CVD (CDC, 2020a). C/PHNs should discuss the signs and symptoms of a heart attack and how to access emergency medical treatment with adult males.

About half of all Americans (49%) have at least one of the three key risk factors for heart disease: high blood pressure, high cholesterol, and cigarette smoking. The likelihood of heart disease or stroke multiplies with the increasing number of risk factors present (CDC, 2023b).

Stroke ranks fifth among all causes of death in the United States and is a leading cause of serious, long-term physical and cognitive disability in adults (Box 21-1).

- Approximately 795,000 Americans experience a new or recurrent stroke each year—610,000 of these are first attacks and 185,000 are recurrent attacks. On average, someone in the United States has a stroke every 40 seconds.
- Stroke-related death rates increased from 38.8 per 100,000 in 2020 to 41.1 per 100,000 in 2021 (CDC, 2023c).

BOX 21-1 EVIDENCE-BASED PRACTICE

Landmark Research on Cardiovascular Disease

The hallmark Framingham Heart Study identified major risk characteristics associated with the development of CVD and the effects of related factors such as blood triglycerides, gender, and psychosocial issues. The study began in 1948 under the direction of National Heart Institute, now known as the National Heart, Lung, and Blood Institute (NHLBI). At that time, the death rates from CVD were rising, but little was known about the general causes of heart disease and stroke. The Framingham Heart Study researchers recruited 2336 males and 2873 females between the ages of 30 and 62 in an effort to identify common factors or characteristics that contribute to CVD. All participants lived in the town of Framingham, Massachusetts. Every 2 years, these people were scheduled for an extensive medical history, physical examination, and laboratory tests. In 1971, the study enrolled 5124 of the original participants' adult children and their spouses (offspring cohort) (Framingham Heart Study, 2018).

In an effort to reflect the changing demographics that occurred in the town of Framingham since the original cohort was enrolled, researchers implemented a new study in 1994. This study included people of Black, Hispanic/Latino, Asian, Indian, Pacific Islander, and Native American origin (Omni cohort). In 2002, a third generation (the children of the offspring cohort) was recruited and a second group of Omni participants was enrolled in 2003. Over the last several years, investigators expanded their research into the role of genetics and CVD. The Framingham Heart Study celebrated its 70th anniversary in 2018, with 15,447 participants covering three generations and 3698 peer-reviewed research articles since it began in 1948. Fortunately, findings from the Framingham Heart Study will continue to make important scientific contributions about the causes and treatment of CVD and related health issues (Framingham Heart Study, 2018).

Source: Framingham Heart Study (2018).

- Disparities exist among people who are at risk for having a stroke. For example, females have a higher lifetime risk of having a stroke compared with males, with approximately 55,000 more females than males experiencing a stroke each year.
- The risk of having a first stroke is nearly twice as high for Black people than White people, and Black people are more likely to die following a stroke than are their White counterparts. The risk for stroke among Hispanic/Latino individuals falls between that of White and Black populations, with stroke mortality increasing in this population since 2013.
- In the Southeastern United States (the "Stroke Belt"), stroke death rates are higher than in any other part of the country. Strokes cost the United States $56.8 billion in 1 year alone. This total includes the cost of healthcare services, medications, and missed days of work (Tsao et al., 2023).

BOX 21-2 EVIDENCE-BASED PRACTICE

SDOH in Black Males

Hypertension is a significant disorder among Black males in the United States who develop hypertension-related complications at an earlier age as compared with other racial/ethnic groups. A clinical review (Abrahamowics et al., 2023) looked at the disparities in the epidemiology of hypertension and the impact of social determinants of health (SDOH) on quality care and outcomes. Many SDOH factors impact blood pressure control such as health literacy, socioeconomic status, access to healthcare, health awareness, and dietary habits, which can influence hypertension control. Barriers that impede hypertension control might include inadequate access to healthy food and the presence of food deserts. These dietary patterns are important for hypertension management and are directly related to income, access, and literacy. Additionally, medication and treatment adherence can be difficult due to provider access and understanding of the disease process.

Recognizing the diverse differences within populations and groups is crucial for developing a stratified approach. Community-based management programs such as Cedar-Sinai's L.A. Barbershop is cost-effective; it has improved blood pressure in non-Hispanic Black males by using pharmacists to deliver hypertension care in local barbershops (Bryant et al., 2021). Inclusion of ethnic pharmacologic/nonpharmacologic treatment plans by providers, use of telehealth or mobile monitoring, and community access to healthy foods can address known disparities and the impact of SDOH on health and hypertension in Black males (Abrahamowics et al., 2023).

Cancer

Cancer is a major chronic illness comprising over 200 different diseases and remains the second leading cause of death in the United States after heart disease (Siegel et al., 2022).

- In 2022, there were approximately 18.1 million Americans living with cancer and that number is projected to increase by 24% to 22.5 million by 2032 (National Cancer Institute [NCI], 2023).
- In the next 10 years, the number of people living 5 or more years after a cancer diagnosis is projected to increase approximately 30%, to 16.3 million (American Cancer Society [ACS], 2023a).
- Approximately 87% of all cancers are diagnosed in people 50 years of age and older, and as people age, they are more likely to develop cancer.
- Among ethnic groups, Black people are more likely to develop and die from cancer.
- Over their lifetime, males living in the United States are more likely to develop cancer than females.
- The Agency for Healthcare Research and Quality estimated the total expenditures for cancer in 2020 to be $208.9 billion, an increase of 10%, most likely due to the increase in aging and growth in the United States (National Cancer Institute (NCI), 2022).

Cancer is caused by internal and external factors.

- Internal factors are inherited gene mutations, hormones, immune conditions, and gene mutations that occur from metabolism.
- External factors include tobacco and alcohol use, chemicals, radiation, infectious organisms, and poor lifestyle choices.
- Exposure to agricultural environmental factors such as inhaling polluted air, drinking contaminated water, and working with pesticides also increase cancer morbidity/mortality (Melanda et al., 2022). See Chapter 9 and 27 for more information.
- These factors can occur in isolation or together to initiate illness.
- Screenings can reduce the cancer mortality rate, especially malignancies associated with the breast, colon, rectum, cervix, and lung (ACS, 2023b).

Lung Cancer

While the lung cancer death rate continues to decline, it remains the number one cause of cancer deaths among adults in the United States. In 2023, there will be an estimated 238,340 new lung cancer cases and 127,070 deaths, attributing to 20% of all cancer deaths in the United States. This is a decrease of 5% from 2018 (ACS, 2023a). However, reductions in cancer screening and diagnosis related to the initial COVID-19 quarantine restrictions are associated with lower 2020 cancer incidence rates (NCI, 2023).

Cigarette smoking is the predominant risk factor for lung cancer. The number of cigarettes smoked and the number of years a person smoked both increase a person's risk of developing lung cancer. Other risk factors include occupational or environmental exposure to secondhand smoke, radon, or asbestos; genetic susceptibility (disease at an early age); and a history of tuberculosis. Annual screening for lung cancer using low-dose computed tomography scan is recommended for people 55 to 74 years of age who currently smoke or have smoked in the past 15 years and have at least a 30-pack history. Shared decision making in screening and smoking cessation counseling for current smokers are key factors in the success of screening and prevention (Lopez-Olivio et al., 2021).

Colon and Rectal Cancers

Colon and rectal cancers are the third most common cancers in adults. In 2018, an estimated 97,220 cases of colon and 43,030 cases of rectal cancers were expected to occur, resulting in 50,630 deaths (Siegel et al., 2023).

- The risk of developing colorectal cancer increases with age, and 90% of all cases are diagnosed in people 50 years of age or older.
- There are several modifiable factors associated with the increased risk of colorectal cancer. These factors

include obesity, physical inactivity, a diet high in red or processed meat, alcohol consumption, long-term smoking, and low intake of whole grains, fruits, and vegetables.

- Other risk factors include certain inherited genetic mutations, personal or family history of polyps or colorectal cancer, and personal history of chronic inflammatory bowel disease.
- The U.S. Preventive Services Task Force (USPSTF, 2023) recommends that for people of all genders who are at average risk, screening for colon and rectal cancer should begin at age 45 years and end at age 75.

Chronic Lower Respiratory Diseases

Chronic lower respiratory disease (CLRD), the sixth leading cause of death, refers to conditions characterized by shortness of breath due to airway obstruction, and it is not curable (WHO, 2023). CLRD includes chronic bronchitis, emphysema, asthma, occupational lung diseases, and pulmonary hypertension. Risk factors include exposure to tobacco smoke, including second-hand smoke, air pollution, occupational vapors, dust, and chemical fumes (Syamlal, 2022).

The term chronic obstructive pulmonary disease (COPD) accounts for the most deaths from CLRD, and it includes emphysema and chronic bronchitis. In 2020, COPD was the 6th leading cause of death, affecting older adults in the United States. A staggering $800 billion is the projected cost of caring for people with COPD over the next 20 years (Zafari et al., 2021). An important note is that females are more vulnerable to lung damage from cigarette smoke and other pollutants because their lungs are smaller, and research has found that estrogen plays a role in worsening the disease (American Lung Association [ALA], 2023).

- The exact cause of asthma is unknown, but research indicates that both genetic and environmental factors contribute to its cause. In the United States, nearly 21 million adults suffer from asthma. The prevalence of asthma is higher in females (9.7%) than in males (6.2%) and highest among Black adults (Asthma and Allergy Foundation of America, 2023).

The COPD National Action Plan includes strategies to prevent, diagnose, and treat this disease (National Institute of Health [NIH], 2021), including education, environmental controls, and pulmonary rehabilitation.

COVID-19 (SARS-CoV-2)

A mysterious new virus appeared on the world stage in 2019, and impacted countries on a scale not seen since the 1918 H1N1 Influenza pandemic. The devastation from this disease stemmed largely from its high communicability and illness severity among those with a vulnerable or compromised health status, such as older adults and those with comorbidities. Over 30 million people worldwide were infected, and close to 1 million died in the first 6 months, with 200,000 of those deaths in the United States (Wang et al., 2022). On March 11, 2020, the World Health Organization (WHO) declared COVID-19 a pandemic. Between March 2020 and October 2021, COVID-19 became the third leading overall cause of U.S. deaths (Shiels et al., 2022), with most occurring in the underserved groups of non-Hispanic American Indian/Alaskan Native, non-Hispanic Black or African American people, and lower socioeconomic communities (USDHHS Office of Inspector General [USDHHS OIG, 2022]). However, public health programs to supply masks, vaccinations, and education aided in diminishing this disparity in 2022. In May 2023, the Department of Health and Human Services declared the end of the COVID-19 public health emergency, noting the vital role that public health initiatives played in combating this illness (USDHHS, 2023).

Unintentional Injuries

Unintentional injuries refer to any injury that results from unintended exposure to physical agents, including heat, mechanical energy, chemicals, or electricity. They are the fourth leading cause of death overall and the leading cause of death for people 44 years of age and younger (see Fig. 21-3).

In 2020, deaths from unintentional injuries increased by 11.1% (Ahmad & Anderson, 2021), with deaths per 100,000 population = 67.8, and over 24 million visits to the emergency departments for unintentional injuries (CDC, 2022a).

In 2021, total costs of all preventable injury-related incidents equaled $1255.4 billion. This included fire and vehicle damage, employers' uninsured expenses, medical bills, wage and productivity loss, and administrative expenses (National Safety Council, 2022a).

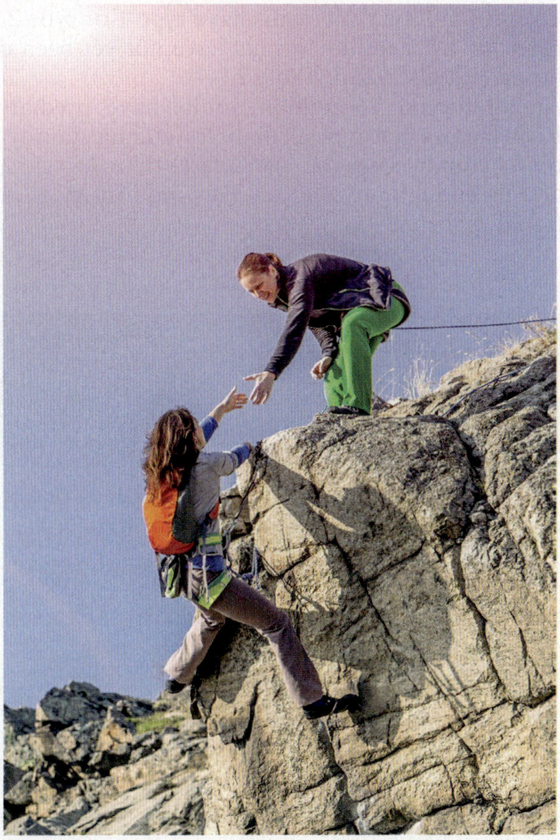

FIGURE 21-3 Unintentional injuries such as falls are the leading cause of death for those aged 44 years and younger.

The top three causes of unintentional injuries include motor vehicle crashes, unintentional drownings, falls, and unintentional poisoning (overdoses) (National Safety Council, 2022a). The CDC advocates for preventing opioid overdose by improving opioid prescribing, reducing exposure to opioids, preventing misuse of opioids, and improving treatment modalities for opioid use disorder (CDC, 2022c). See Chapter 25 for more on substance use.

In the United States, motor vehicle accidents are a leading cause of death. In 2017–2018, an average of 3.4 million people visited an emergency room due to injuries from motor vehicle accidents (Davis & Cairns, 2021).

- The costs of medical care and productivity losses due to motor vehicle accidents in a 1-year period exceeded $75 billion in 2017 (Davis & Cairns, 2021).
- Efforts to decrease motor vehicle injuries are directed toward the prevention of motor vehicle crashes through education and policies related to seat belts, impaired driving, distracted driving, older adult drivers, teen drivers, and motorcycle and bicycle safety.

Diabetes

Diabetes is the eighth leading cause of death in the United States. This chronic health condition puts people at risk for other serious health conditions, including heart disease, stroke, hypertension, blindness, kidney disease, and nervous system disease (i.e., neuropathy, which is a loss of sensation or pain in the feet or hands).

- Over 37 million Americans have type 1 or type 2 diabetes, and 8.5 million adults have not yet been diagnosed (CDC, 2023d; Table 21-4).
- An additional 96 million adults have prediabetes. Risk factors for type 2 diabetes include family history, being overweight, age greater than 45 years, not getting enough physical activity, and history of gestational diabetes.
- People of African American, Hispanic/Latino, non-Hispanic Black, American Indian, Alaska Native, and non-Hispanic Asian race/ethnicity are at greater risk for developing type 2 diabetes than White people (CDC, 2023d).
- Screening for diabetes for all people is recommended beginning at age 45 years and repeated every 3 years if test results are normal and for asymptomatic adults who are overweight and obese. People with more than one risk factor may need to be screened more frequently (CDC, 2023d).

TABLE 21-4 Estimated Diagnosed and Undiagnosed Diabetes Among People Ages 18 Years or Older, United States, 2017–2020

Group*	Number Who Have Diabetes and Rate per 1000
Ages 18–44 years old	4.2%
Ages 45–64 years old	17.5%
Ages 65 years or older	26.8%
Males	14%
Females	12%

*In this table, "male" refers to a person assigned male at birth, and "female" refers to a person assigned female at birth.

Source: National Diabetes Statistics Report. Center for Disease Control https://www.cdc.gov/diabetes/data/statistics-report/diagnosed-undiagnosed-diabetes.html

Confounding Health Concerns

In this next section, several of the most common maladies that contribute to leading causes of death are examined. Others are examined in-depth in other chapters in this text.

Obesity

Obesity is a contributor to or exacerbates many of the leading causes of mortality and morbidity discussed in this chapter. Obesity is defined as having a body mass index (BMI) of 30 or greater and is recognized as a national health threat and a major public health challenge in the United States. This condition is a major risk factor for CVD, along with certain types of cancer, type 2 diabetes, obstructive sleep apnea, and premature death (CDC, 2022d; Watson et al., 2022b).

- The *National Health and Nutrition Examination Survey* highlighted that between 2017 and 2020, the prevalence of obesity among adults was 41.9%. Middle-aged adults (40 to 59 years old) had a higher prevalence of obesity at 44.3% than young adults (20 to 39 years old) at 39.8%. The prevalence of obesity in adults over the age of 60 years was 41.5%.
- People from lower socioeconomic and education levels have a higher prevalence of obesity, as do non-Hispanic Black and Hispanic adults.
- Additionally, certain geographic regions have higher obesity rates than others in the United States. The South (32.4%) and Midwest (32.3%) have the highest prevalence of obesity, and at least 36% of adults in Alabama, Arkansas, Iowa, Louisiana, Mississippi, Oklahoma, and West Virginia have obesity (CDC, 2022e).

Obesity can have serious health consequences; it contributes to the leading cause of death in the United States and worldwide (CDC, 2022d; Watson et al., 2022b), and it is associated with reduced quality of life and poorer mental health outcomes. In addition, those that have obesity are at increased risk for mortality, hypertension, elevated LDL, dyslipidemia, stroke, type 2 diabetes, gallbladder disease, osteoarthritis, CHD, sleep apnea, some cancers, and difficulty with physical functioning (CDC, 2022d; Watson et al.., 2022b). There are also economic and societal consequences from obesity, including medical costs associated with related health issues and productivity concerns related to absenteeism, as well as premature mortality and morbidity (CDC, 2022d). Healthy behaviors that include healthy diet patterns and regular physical exercise should be incorporated into lifestyle habits.

BOX 21-3 HEALTHY PEOPLE 2030

Select Objectives Related to Obesity

OA-01	Increase the proportion of older adults with physical or cognitive health problems who get physical activity
NWS-03	Reduce the proportion of adults with obesity
NWS-05	Increase the proportion of healthcare visits by adults with obesity that include counseling on weight loss, nutrition, or physical activity
PA-02	Increase the proportion of adults who do enough aerobic physical activity for substantial health benefits
PA-04	Increase the proportion of adults who do enough muscle-strengthening activity

Reprinted from Office of Disease Prevention and Health Promotion (ODPHP). (n.d.-a). Obesity. *Healthy People 2030.* U.S. Department of Health and Human Services. https://health.gov/healthypeople/search?query=obesity

Community environments that are safe and offer healthy food and places for physical activity are also necessary (Watson et al., 2022b; Box 21-3). *Healthy People 2030* has several objectives targeting obesity, some of which are shown in Box 21-3.

It is recommended that adults engage in a minimum of 150 minutes (2.5 hours) of moderate intensity or 75 minutes of vigorous aerobic exercise every week, in addition to 2 days of muscle-strengthening exercises (WHO, 2020). However, studies have revealed that even 11 minutes a day of activity can assist with lowering the risk of cardiovascular disease and diabetes (Garcia et al., 2023). Community health nurses play an important role in combating obesity through educating adults on the importance of maintaining a healthy weight, or weight reduction if indicated, through physical activity and proper nutrition.

Substance Use

A **substance use disorder (SUD)** occurs when the recurrent use of alcohol and drugs causes clinically and functionally significant impairment such as health problems, disability, and failure to meet major responsibilities at work, school, or home (National Survey on Drug Use and Health, 2021).

- In 2021, an estimated 35.5 million Americans (61%) aged 26 or older had a SUD related to their use of alcohol or illicit drugs (SAMHSA, 2023).
- Although the prevalence of SUD is higher in males, females are less likely to enter treatment (Fonseca et al., 2021).
- The misuse of opioids, leading to opioid use disorder, has become a national epidemic and public health concern. The number of drug overdose deaths increased by nearly 30% from 2019 to 2020, and most (75%) of those 91,799 drug overdose deaths in 2020 involved an opioid.

Alcohol Use Disorder

The medical diagnosis of **alcohol use disorder (AUD)** refers to a chronic relapsing brain disease characterized by compulsive alcohol use, loss of control over alcohol intake, and a negative emotional state when not using. To be diagnosed with AUD, a person must meet certain criteria as delineated in the Diagnostic and Statistical Manual of Mental Disorders (DSM) (National Institute on Abuse and Alcoholism [NIAAA], 2023). Under the current version of the DSM (DSM-V), anyone meeting 2 of the 11 criteria during the same 12-month period can be diagnosed with AUD. The severity of AUD is outlined as mild, moderate, or severe based on the number of criteria met (NIAAA, 2023).

Tobacco Use

Tobacco use is another major public health problem and the leading cause of preventable diseases and deaths in the United States.

- Despite the evidence that smoking causes cancer, heart disease, stroke, lung diseases, diabetes, and COPD, over 28 million Americans smoked cigarettes in 2021 (CDC, 2023e).
- It is encouraging that cigarette smoking among adults has declined to the lowest recorded prevalence since 1965 (42%) (CDC, 2023f).
- However, e-cigarette use increased from 1920 to 1921 (from 3.7% to 4.5%) mostly among people aged 18 to 24 years (Cornelius et al., 2022).
- Furthermore, troubling disparities in those who still smoke remain, which are those with less education and lower income; American Indians and Alaska Natives; residents of rural areas; the South and Midwest; gay, lesbian, or bisexual adults; and those battling anxiety or depression. Adults enrolled in Medicaid or are uninsured smoke twice as much as those with private health insurance or Medicare (CDC, 2023g).
- Cigarette smoking is responsible for more than 480,000 deaths per year in the United States, including more than 41,000 deaths resulting from secondhand smoke exposure. This is about 1300 deaths every day (CDC, 2023e).
- The cost of cigarette smoking reached a staggering $600 billion in 2018. Over half of that amount came from lost productivity, and $240 billion was a result of healthcare spending (CDC, 2023h).
- When examining cigarette smoking based on sex assigned at birth, males (13.1% of them) are more likely to smoke cigarettes than females (10.1% of them) (CDC, 2023g).
- E-cigarettes (also known as e-cigs, e-hookahs, mods, vape pens, vapes, tank systems, and electronic nicotine delivery systems) are used by 4.5% of adults in the United States (Cornelius et al., 2022).
- E-cigarette use consists of inhaling aerosolized nicotine that is produced after heating. However, the aerosolized product also contains additional potentially harmful substances such as heavy metals and cancer-causing agents. Although adults may use e-cigarettes to reduce craving for regular cigarettes that contain tobacco, the FDA has not approved e-cigarettes as an aid to quit smoking (CDC, 2023i).

Because of the significance of the problem, 24 of the *Healthy People 2030* objectives are related to tobacco use (Office of Disease Prevention and Health Promotion [ODPHP], n.d.-b).

Opioid Use

The illegal use of prescription opioids, synthetic opioids (fentanyl), and heroin is a major public health concern in the United States. A serious national crisis exists due to the misuse of and dependency on. This rise in opioid overdose deaths began with increased prescribing of opioids in the 1990s, the rise in heroin use beginning in 2010, and synthetic opioid (such as fentanyl) abuse stemming from 2013 (CDC, 2022c).

- Every day, at least 136 people die due to opioid overdose in the United States (National Center for Drug Abuse Statistics, 2022).
- In 2021, twice the number of people died from drug overdoses (98,268) as compared to 2017 (47,600) (National Safety Council, 2022b).
- This all-time high is partially related to stress and isolation caused by the COVID-19 quarantine restrictions: Preventable opioid overdose deaths increased by 41% in 2020 and an additional 18% in 2021 (National Safety Council, 2022b).
- Economic costs during the COVID-19 pandemic reached nearly $1.5 trillion (Joint Economic Council [JEC], 2022).
- This economic crisis from prescription opioid misuse in the United States includes costs of healthcare, treatment to overcome dependency, criminal justice management, and lost productivity (Congressional Budget Office [CBO], 2022).

The full extent of the damage of the opioid crisis goes beyond economics, influencing family and community life and placing an extreme strain on community resources, including first responders, emergency rooms, hospitals, and treatment centers.

In 2018, the NIH launched HEAL (Helping to End Addiction Long-term) Initiative, an aggressive, trans-agency effort to increase scientific solutions to positively impact the national opioid public health crisis (NIH, 2023). HEAL is focusing efforts on 1) understanding, managing, and treating pain and 2) improving prevention and treatment for opioid misuse and dependency.

SEXUAL ORIENTATION, GENDER IDENTITY, AND SEXUAL HEALTH

When determining appropriate preventative and healthcare needs, it is important that in addition to recognizing people's biologic characteristics we also take into account the designations with which they identify. Awareness of sexual orientation and gender identity (SO/GI) can assist the C/PHN in caring for all adults while providing necessary healthcare services, which might include appropriate healthcare screenings, assessment and risk for sexually transmitted infections, behavioral health concerns and effective interventions, and parenting discussions (CDC, 2022f; see Fig. 21-4).

People may question their sexuality and gender identification at any time during their life. Sexual orientation and gender identity are not the same; sexual orientation describes a person's pattern of emotional, romantic, and sexual attractions (APA, 2022a; CDC, 2022f), whereas gender identity describes what gender a person identifies as representing their person. **Transgender** is a term for people whose gender identity or expression does not conform with the sex to which they were assigned at birth. People who do not identify as either male or female may identify as gender nonbinary or genderqueer (American Psychological Association [APA], 2022a).

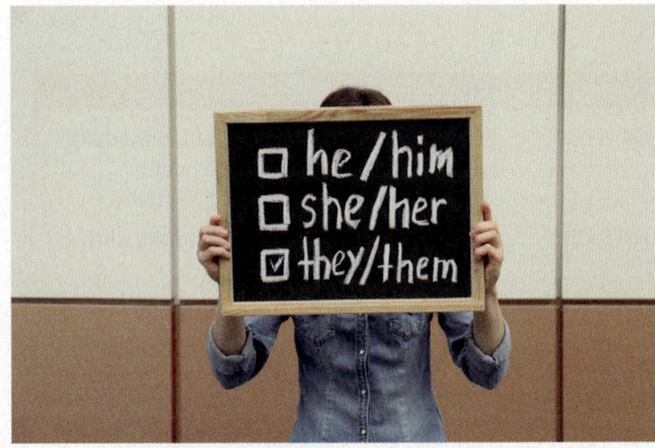

FIGURE 21-4 One example of a person's gender identity and identified pronouns.

Regardless of sexual orientation or gender identification, when taking a sexual and reproductive history, C/PHNs must ask all patients questions regarding risky behaviors, unprotected sex, multiple partners, STIs, family planning, health screenings, and intimate partner violence (CDC, 2022f; Guttmacher Institute, 2020). Discrimination and lack of cultural competence and training for LGBTQ+ populations preclude effective care. Additionally, LGBTQ+ populations are more at risk for violence, harassment, trauma, and targeted injustices (National Sexual Violence Resource Center, 2021).

Sexual Health and STIs

Sexual health and STIs are important health concerns for adults. Sexual activity typically commences in adolescence and continues throughout the lifespan. STIs are epidemic in the United States, with 20 million new cases every year; this number is astounding given that many STIs are treatable (Office of Disease Prevention and Health Promotion [ODPHP], n.d.-c; see Chapter 8).

- Human papillomavirus (HPV) is the most common STI in the United States. Approximately 56 million Americans are infected with HPV, resulting in 13,545 cases of cervical cancer and over 47,000 HPV-associated cancers (26,000 among females and 21,000 among males) (CDC, 2022g). Gardasil 9 is a two or three dose vaccine that can prevent 90% of cervical cancers, as well as anogenital warts, and is approved for all people 9 to 45 years old (CDC, 2020b).
- Chlamydia and gonorrhea are also common STIs; statistics indicate prevalence is underreported and delay in treatment occurs due to limited symptomatology. Rates for both these STIs have increased in adults in

recent years. Chlamydia is the most reported nationally notifiable disease in the United States, with more than 1.6 million cases in 2021 (CDC, 2023j).

- The rate of gonorrhea is lower than chlamydia, but in 2021, there were 710,151 cases reported, making it the second most nationally reported notifiable disease in the United States. Rates of gonorrhea have increased in males and females since 2013. Although gonorrhea is treatable, antibiotic resistance remains an issue (CDC, 2023j). See Chapter 8 for more information on communicable diseases.
- In 2022, more than 38,000 people were diagnosed with human immunodeficiency virus (HIV) in the United States (CDC, 2024). Despite advances in the prevention and treatment of HIV, the disease continues to disproportionately impact males, with 80% of new infections in the United States affecting gay and bisexual men (CDC, 2024). An additional impact of HIV is evident in Black/African American and Hispanic/Latino communities (HIV.gov, 2023). The percentage of people diagnosed with HIV varies by geographic region in the United States. It is therefore important that prevention, testing, and treatment interventions be tailored for each area's distinctive needs (CDC, 2024): https://www.cdc.gov/hiv/statistics/overview/incidence.html
- The CDC (2021b) recommends routine STI screening for all people who are sexually active; visit their website for the most current recommendation)

C/PHNs working with adults should provide factual information to increase the adult's knowledge of STI risk. This information should be a part of frank discussions regarding condom use, gender of sexual partners, type of sexual activity (oral, anal, vaginal), life-threatening consequences of an undiagnosed STI, and undesirable pregnancy outcomes. Outside of abstinence, condom use is the first line of prevention against STIs. See Chapter 8 for more on communicable diseases.

Female Health

Females (see Fig. 21-5) have not been the focus of medical attention throughout history. Exclusion and underrepresentation in studies and treatments have impeded care affecting morbidity and mortality for this group (Office of Women's Health, 2020). Advances in female health are very recent and primarily an advantage for females living in Western countries, where the feminist movement has made major inroads.

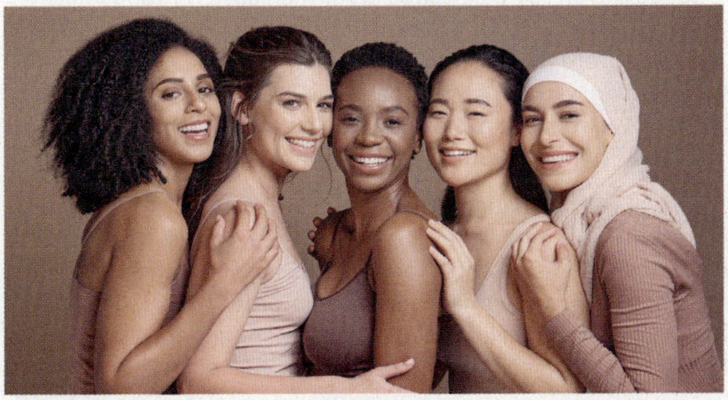

FIGURE 21-5 Female health has not historically been the focus of healthcare research.

Overview of Factors Influencing Female Health

Female rights in the United States started in the second half of the 19th century and over time addressed issues directly or indirectly impacting the health of this population, including voting rights, labor laws, reproductive rights, and intimate partner violence (International Women's Day, n.d.). Female health is still overlooked in much of the world. Only in the past few decades has the health of females been a formidable issue in the United States, coming not so coincidentally with the modern feminist movement that began in the 1960s.

- The landmark 1963 publication *The Feminine Mystique* helped launch the modern feminist movement by critically examining the role of females in American society (Foster, 2015; Friedan, 2013). The Boston Women's Health Book Collective *Our Bodies, Ourselves* (initially released in 1970 with the title *Women and their Bodies*) represented the first book to explore female health issues, exclusively written by and for females. In addition, this publication served as a model for those who wanted to learn about themselves, communicate their findings with doctors, and challenge the medical establishment to change and improve the care that females received (Our Bodies Ourselves, n.d.).
- To further expand the dialogue regarding female health, consumer activists created the National Women's Health Network in 1975, primarily to shape health policy and support consumer health decisions (National Women's Health Network, 2022). These historical occurrences likely contributed to more female researchers and participants in research.
- Feminists paved the way for females to have their voices heard on many health, social, and political issues. Females sought out higher education opportunities in greater numbers and entered workplaces once solely occupied by males, especially during and after World War II.
- These positive changes escalated females toward greater equality, and with equality came the freedom—and pressure—for females to compete with males in their social and work settings. Issues related to female health were discovered as a result of research that now more regularly includes females.
- The importance of female health research was reaffirmed in the NIH's Revitalization Act of 1993, Subtitle B—clinical research equity regarding females and underrepresented groups to "identify projects for research on female health that should be conducted or supported by the national research institutes; identify multidisciplinary research relating to research on females that should be so conducted or supported …" (NIH, 1993, section 486). Yet more work in this area is needed.
- Despite advances in female rights, gender discrimination and bias continue. In many places within the United States, females continue to make 0.78 cents for every $1 dollar earned by a male, while Black females

and Latina females make even less. Equal economic opportunities, educational equity, and gender-based violence are public health concerns (American Civil Liberties Union [ACLU], 2023).

Female Health Research

In response to changing priorities, researchers have designed and implemented major studies that focus exclusively on females. Five significant studies have provided and continue to provide important health information about this population:

- The *Women's Health Initiative* (WHI) was a major research program addressing the most common causes of death, disability, and poor quality of life in postmenopausal females—CVD, cancer, and osteoporosis (WHI, 2023).
- The *Women's Health Study* (WHS) evaluated the effects of vitamin E and low-dose aspirin therapy in primary prevention of CVD and cancer in apparently healthy females (WHS, n.d.).
- The *Nurses' Health Study (NHS) I* involved investigating risk factors for cancer and CVD, and the *NHS II* researched diet and lifestyle risk factors in a population younger than the original NHS cohort (NHS, 2016).
- The *NHS III* is currently investigating female health issues related to lifestyle fertility/pregnancy, environment, and nursing exposures (NHS, 2016; NIH, 2020).
- For a discussion of how research in genomics and pharmacogenomics is being applied to female health, see Box 21-4.

The WHI addressed CVD, cancer, and osteoporosis and was one of the largest prevention studies of its kind in the United States, starting in 1991 and spanning 15 years. This study was sponsored by the NIH and the NHLBI, involved 161,808 females ages 50 to 79 years, and was considered to be one of the most far-reaching clinical trials for female health ever undertaken. To date, more than 616 publications have been associated with findings from this study, which address coronary artery calcium, breast cancer risk, colorectal cancer, venous thrombosis, peripheral arterial disease risk, risk of CHD, dementia and cognitive function, and the effects of estrogen alone in reducing the risk of CHD (WHS, n.d.; National Center for Biotechnology Information, 2023).

The WHS was a randomized, double-blind, placebo-controlled clinical trial sponsored by the NHBLI and the NCI. It was the first large clinical trial to study the use of low-dose aspirin to prevent heart attack and stroke in

BOX 21-4 EVIDENCE-BASED PRACTICE

Genomics and Pharmacogenomics

A person's genome consists of their entire set of DNA, including all genes. Genomics considers how a person's genes interact with each other, the person's environment, and their behaviors, such as diet and exercise, to influence growth, development, and health (CDC, 2023q). This is different from genetics, which considers the function and composition of a single gene. Discoveries made in the field of genomics allow healthcare providers to translate research to clinical practice. For example, genomics has increased understanding of why people with the same disease may not respond similarly or have the same treatment outcomes, guiding individualized treatment. It also assists in the identification of people with increased risk for the development of certain diseases based on gene mutation, gene interaction, and environment, to develop individualized prevention and treatment strategies. These advances in science and technology have allowed healthcare to increase its focus on the delivery of individualized care and prevention, known as precision medicine (CDC, 2023q; NIH, 2022; NIH, NCI, 2021).

Nurses and other healthcare providers use genomics routinely in practice. In the community setting, the nurse may educate females about breast cancer and risk factors, providing information about genetic testing for those with a family history. Healthcare providers partner with patients who have BRCA1 or BRCA2 gene mutations to individualize breast and ovarian cancer prevention and screening. The same is true for those with a strong family history of heart disease. Careful family and personal health histories may guide healthcare providers to recommend testing for familial hypercholesterolemia (FH). People with gene mutations causing FH need targeted treatment to prevent adverse cardiac events (Diboun et al., 2022). Nurses play a key role in patient education to assist the person with FH in reducing or eliminating modifiable risk factors that could also contribute to cardiovascular disease.

Another important aspect of genomics is pharmacogenomics, which considers information about a person's genome to guide decision making in medication and dose selection. The utilization of pharmacogenomics to guide treatment has become routine for some disease states and medications. Examples of utilizing pharmacogenomics to guide treatment include the following:

- Avoiding primaquine and other medications known to cause acute hemolytic anemia in people with G6PD deficiency, caused by an alteration of the G6PD gene
- Choosing an HIV medication other than abacavir for people with an HLA-B*57:01 allele due to increased risk for developing a severe hypersensitivity reaction
- Adjusting warfarin dose in people with CYP2C9 or VKORC1 gene variations to avoid increased bleeding risk (Dean, 2018; FDA, n.d.; NORD, 2023; Zhang et al., 2024)

Individualizing patient care based on genomics and pharmacogenetics will continue to increase as the availability of genomic data expands. It is essential for nurses to have an understanding of genomics and pharmacogenomics in order to answer questions appropriately and provide appropriate and individualized health promotion and disease prevention education.

Source: Centers for Disease Control and Prevention (2023q); Dean (2018); Diboun et al. (2022); Food and Drug Administration (FDA) (n.d.); National Institutes of Health (NIH) (2022); National Institutes of Health, National Cancer Institute (NIH, NCI) (2021); National Organization for Rare Diseases (NORD) (2023).

females 45 years of age and older. This study began in 1991 and continued through March 2009 for additional observation and follow-up of the original 28,345 participants. Findings indicated that low-dose aspirin does not prevent first heart attacks or death from cardiovascular causes in females; however, stroke was found to be 17% lower in the aspirin group. More than 110 professional articles are associated with this investigation. Recent publications address the association of dietary fat intake with the risk of atrial fibrillation in females and the novel protein glycan biomarker and future CVD events (WHS, n.d.).

The NHS (three separate phases) represents the longest-running study related to female health in the world, investigating factors that influence the health of this group.

- The *NHS I*, a prospective study that began in 1976, enrolled registered nurses aged 30 to 55 years. Every 2 years, participants received a follow-up questionnaire with questions about diseases and health-related topics including smoking, hormone use, and menopausal status. Later in the study, questions regarding diet, nutrition, and quality of life were added.
- The *NHS II* represented females who started using oral contraceptives in adolescence, a population with long-term exposure during early reproductive years. Females aged 25 to 42 years were enrolled and followed forward in time. Every 2 years, participants received a follow-up questionnaire and were surveyed about diseases and health-related topics including smoking, hormone use, pregnancy history, and menopausal status.
- The *NHS III* began recruitment in 2010 and will continue until 100,000 nurses (registered and licensed practical, 22 to 45 years of age) are enrolled. Also, nurses from Canada are participants, and the study aims to be more representative of the diverse backgrounds of nurses. These studies are supported by major nursing organizations, with more than 280,000 participants to date (NHS, 2016).

Female Health Promotion Across the Lifespan

What healthcare needs do females have that are different from those of males? Is there a need to look at health promotion throughout the life cycle of adult females? How is the health of an 18-year-old female different from that of a 50-year-old female? Females have different healthcare needs that must be considered, and these concerns vary with age. Knowing what the needs are is essential to knowing how to help females promote their health.

***Healthy People 2030* Goals for Females.** As a nation, we have been focusing on improving the health of all people living in the United States through the *Healthy People* initiatives, commencing with the 1979 Surgeon General's report, *Healthy People: The Surgeon General's Report on Health Promotion and Disease Prevention*, providing measurable population objectives. In the nation's fourth generation of health planning, 35 objectives pertain to the health of females (Box 21-5). As the community health nurse works with people at various stages in the life cycle, the objectives in *Healthy People 2030* can give structure to program planning and services offered to females in the community at the primary, secondary, and tertiary levels of prevention (USDHHS, 2020a).

Young Adult Females (18 to 35 Years). Females in the earlier years of adulthood have different tasks to accomplish and issues to address than females in later adulthood, and the transition from adolescence to adulthood can be stressful. There are major developmental tasks that young females need to accomplish such as forming an identity and the development of intimacy. Behaviors associated with young adulthood may include

BOX 21-5 *HEALTHY PEOPLE 2030*

The Objectives for Females*

Core Objectives—Targets Below Benchmark

MICH-04	Reduce maternal deaths
MICH-05	Reduce severe maternal complications during delivery hospitalizations
MICH-06	Reduce cesarean births among low-risk women with no prior births
MICH-07	Reduce preterm births
MICH-08	Increase the proportion of pregnant women who receive early and adequate prenatal care
MICH-13	Increase the proportion of women who had a healthy weight before pregnancy
FS-03	Reduce infections caused by Listeria
STI-03	Reduce the syphilis rate in females
STI-04	Reduce congenital syphilis
TU-15	Increase successful quit attempts in pregnant women who smoke

*In this box, "females" and "women" refers to people assigned female at birth.

Reprinted from Office of Disease Prevention and Health Promotion (ODPHP). (n.d.-c). Women. Healthy People 2030. U.S. Department of Health and Human Services. https://health.gov/healthypeople/objectives-and-data/browse-objectives/women

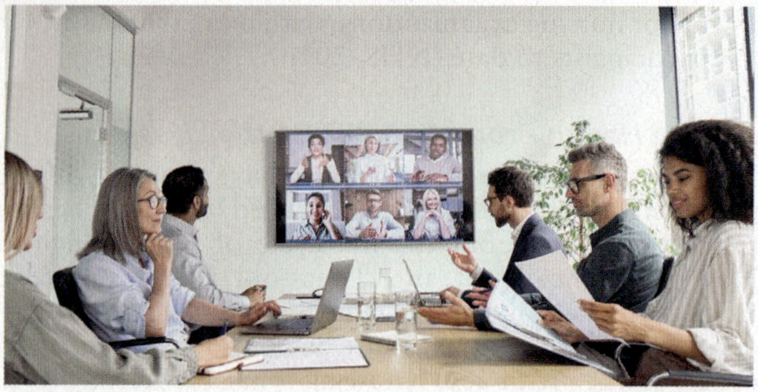

FIGURE 21-6 Choosing a career path is one developmental task for young adults.

postsecondary education, choosing and establishing a career (see Fig. 21-6), military service, choosing a partner, establishing independence, and family planning (decision to have/not have children; timing for having children whether through childbirth, adoption, or foster parenting). During this time, females also develop a personal philosophy that encompasses meaningful and comforting spiritual beliefs that are consistent with day-to-day living (Berk, 2018).

Females in this age group tend to be healthy. Unfortunately, during this period, many females engage in less healthy behaviors such as physical inactivity, poor eating habits, unprotected sex, and smoking (Box 21-6). Some, if not all, of these behaviors may have been established in adolescence and represent modifiable behaviors. If not addressed, poor lifestyle choices can contribute significantly to the leading causes of morbidity and mortality: diseases of the heart and vascular systems, cancers, chronic respiratory diseases, and diabetes (Li et al., 2020). The majority of health concerns for many females in this age group are related to eating disorders, reproductive health and STIs, physical activity, mental health and mood disorders, and substance use.

Reproductive Health

During the reproductive years, it is important for females to be as healthy as possible (see Fig. 21-7; CDC, 2023k). During this time, healthy habits can be initiated, and unhealthy habits resolved to ensure the best health during the years people focus on having children and for the outcome of their babies when pregnant. Preconception health is important for all females of reproductive age, not just for those planning to become pregnant, because it focuses on getting healthy and staying healthy (CDC, 2023l).

BOX 21-6 WHAT DO *YOU* THINK?

Fad Diets

Each year, approximately 45 million Americans begin a diet. Fad diets have been around for centuries and don't seem to be going anywhere. Every year new diets promise results, but do they work and are they safe?

In 2018, the ketogenic diet (keto) made its way back into the mainstream. This is a high-fat, low-carbohydrate diet that eliminates sugar, grains/starches, fruits, beans/legumes and encourages high-fat foods such as eggs, nuts, meats/fish, full-fat dairy and cheeses, and healthy oils. Low-carb vegetables are also encouraged. The goal is to reach ketosis by replacing dietary carbs with fats. Benefits may include weight loss and decreased glucose and insulin levels. There are conflicting studies reporting benefits and risks of the ketogenic diet. While people adhering to this diet lose weight, once carbohydrates are reintroduced, the resulting side effect is often weight gain. Research has shown both increase and decrease in LDL cholesterol, as well as the development of insulin resistance, and nonalcoholic fatty liver disease.

The paleolithic diet is known by a few different names and continues to be a popular option among people trying to lose weight. This is a low-carbohydrate, high-protein diet that encourages high consumption of lean meats and vegetables, moderate consumption of fruits, nuts, and seeds, and abstinence from dairy, legumes, and grains. While it has many of the same attributes of keto, it is higher in protein and lower in fat. Evidence suggests that maintaining a low carbohydrate diet, such as the paleo or ketogenic diet, long term may increase mortality from cardiovascular disease, stroke, and cancer, when compared to higher carbohydrate diets. However, the source of carbohydrate intake, whole-food versus highly processed, must be considered and whole-food sources recommended as an individual's main carbohydrate intake.

The plant-based, or vegan, diet has gained momentum in recent years and eliminates all animal products including meat, eggs, and dairy. It is rich in fruits, vegetables, nuts, seeds, legumes, and plant proteins. While there are variations of veganism, such as whole-food plant-based or raw, there are many vegan "junk foods" or processed vegan replacement foods that can cause more harm than good. Adherence to a plant-based diet that is not heavily based on processed vegan foods may reduce weight and help manage or eliminate chronic disease.

Other recent dieting trends include intermittent fasting, juicing, detoxing, and gluten-free diet. Whether people ask about the health benefits or adverse effects of diets they are following or considering, it's important to encourage them to research potential nutritional deficiencies certain diets may cause. This allows for intentional monitoring for dietary deficiencies and supplementation if needed. For example, people following a ketogenic diet may not be consuming sufficient amounts of fiber or vitamins and minerals found in fruits and vegetables. Vegans may need to supplement or be intentional about consuming vitamins B12 and D3, omega-3 fatty acids, iron, and calcium.

Do you know someone who seems to always be trying the latest diet? Is that person successfully losing weight or in a constant weight loss/weight gain cycle? As a C/PHN, how would you approach this subject?

Source: American College of Cardiology (2023); Healthline (2023); T. Collin Campbell Center for Nutrition Studies (2023).

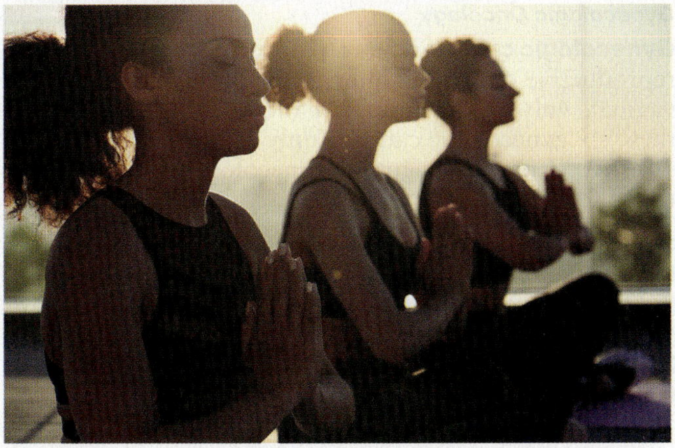

FIGURE 21-7 Good health is important during pregnancy.

Although preconception care is addressed in *Healthy People 2030*, many of the preconception objectives are related to family planning and maternal health. The CDC has developed a checklist for females of reproductive age to commit to healthy preconception activities including the following (CDC, 2023l):

- Make a plan and take action.
- See a healthcare provider.
- Take 400 µg of folic acid every day.
- Stop smoking, using drugs, and drinking excessive amounts of alcohol.
- Avoid toxic substances.
- Avoid environmental contaminants.
- Reach and maintain a healthy weight.
- Seek help if living in a stressful environment or experiencing intimate partner violence.
- Learn family history.
- Get mentally healthy.
- When ready, plan pregnancy.
- Stay current on immunizations.

Community health nurses have been at the forefront of maternal and child healthcare for decades, and they must continue to strive to incorporate components of preconception care into their practices. Nurses must also advocate for clients to influence public policy, which has the potential to improve access to care for many females and improve pregnancy outcomes.

Adult Females (35 to 65 Years). Females in the adult age group of 35 to 65 years have established patterns of living that have served them well or ill (Li et al., 2021). During this period, the results of years of choices may present themselves in the form of chronic illnesses. Nevertheless, many females in this age group have time to change health habits to possibly reverse encroaching chronic illnesses. For other females, lifestyle choices and undetected diseases have shortened their lifespans, and large numbers of females in this age group are dying prematurely.

Adult female demographics are shifting. An increasing number of educated female are having children, and they are having them later in life; they are also spending more time in the workforce before they have children. Births within the United States are decreasing. Additionally, one in four birthing parents is a solo parent, raising children on their own. Stereotypes are shifting as working female face pressure to be more involved as parents, while males are more involved in childcare and housework than in the past (Pew Research Center, 2023). Females between 35 and 65 years of age may face challenges such as follows:

- Caring for aging parents
- Supporting young adult children
- Family–work role conflict
- Financial vulnerabilities
- Shrinking social and healthcare safety net
- Changing mental and physical health
- Gender/racial gap
- Parenting pressures (Infurna et al., 2020)

Menopausal Transition

- **Perimenopause**, or **menopausal transition**, is the period of time leading up to the last menstrual cycle and is characterized by cycle changes and irregularity. Females typically begin to notice symptoms of perimenopause in their 40s. Menstrual flow may be light or heavy, and spotting may occur, depending on varying estrogen and progesterone levels. Females may also have vasomotor symptoms such as hot flashes (flushes) or night sweats, as well as sleep disturbances and vaginal and urinary tract changes (American College of Obstetricians and Gynecologists [ACOG], 2020; Martin & Barbieri, 2023). The average length of perimenopause is 4 years but may last up to 10 years.
- **Menopause** is a time that marks the permanent cessation of menstrual activity (last menstrual period). The average age is 51 years (range = 45 to 58); however, it can occur earlier (Office on Women's Health, 2021). Natural menopause is defined as cessation of menstrual periods for 12 consecutive months, and the person can no longer become pregnant (Office of Women's Health, 2021).
- Menopause symptoms differ among females and may last months to years. They range from hardly noticeable in some individuals to very severe in others. Symptoms include nervousness or anxiety, hot flashes (flushes), chills, excessive sweating (often at night), excitability, fatigue, mood disorders (apathy, mental depression, crying episodes), insomnia, palpitations, vertigo, headache, numbness, tingling, myalgia, urinary disturbances, and vaginal dryness (ACOG, 2020; Office on Women's Health, 2021).
- According to the *Study of Women's Health Across the Nation* (SWAN), hot flashes and some of the other menopausal symptoms last an average of 7.4 years, persisting 4.5 years once menopause is reached. However, these symptomatic menopausal transitions may persist, as noted in a study with Chinese females who had excess weight or obesity (Tang et al., 2022).

Recommendations for females in the menopausal transition include discussions about menopausal symptoms, osteoporosis, cancer screening, and assessment for CVD along with a determination of the need for appropriate menopausal hormone therapy (MHT) (Martin &

Barbieri, 2023; Office of Women's Health, 2021). Additionally, postmenopausal risks associated with osteoporosis should be assessed; ACOG provides recommendations for osteoporosis management (ACOG, 2022).

- Females who choose natural or herbal supplements for symptomatic relief should be counseled on lack of evidence supporting efficacy and long-term safety, as well as potential side effects and drug interactions (Women's Health Concern, 2022).
- Other complementary health approaches females may choose for menopausal symptom relief include hypnotherapy, meditation, yoga, and acupuncture (Johnson et al., 2019).
- Combined estrogen and progestin therapy for primary prevention of chronic conditions in postmenopausal people is not recommended (U.S. Preventative Services Task Force, 2022).
- Estrogen alone for primary prevention of chronic conditions in postmenopausal people who have had a hysterectomy is not recommended (U.S. Preventative Services Task Force, 2022).

Osteoporosis

- A gradual loss in bone density is known as **osteoporosis**. Typically, bone mass stops increasing around age 30 years. As females age, bones may weaken and easily fracture as estrogen levels decrease.
- In the United States, 1 in 4 females over the age of 65 years has osteoporosis (CDC, 2022j). Therefore, it is important for females to build strong bones early. Bone density is influenced by many factors such as heredity, race/ethnicity, physical activity, and nutrition. It is important for females of all ages to maintain a healthy diet that is rich in calcium and vitamin D, engage in physical activity, and avoid smoking (see Fig. 21-8).
- There are several classes of medications that can be used to treat osteoporosis (Endocrine Society, 2022; Office of Women's Health, 2021).
- Screening for osteoporosis in females over the age of 65 years or in postmenopausal women under age 65 years with increased risk for osteoporosis-related fractures is recommended (Bone Health and Osteoporosis Foundation, 2022). See Chapter 22 for more on osteoporosis in older females.

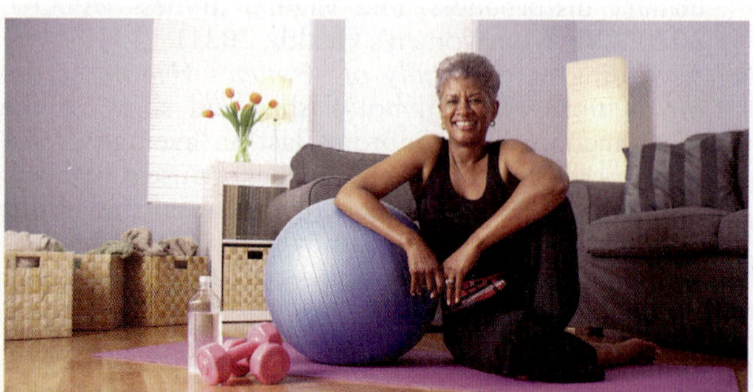

FIGURE 21-8 Menopause is a transitional period in a female's life.

Gynecologic Oncology

Gynecologic cancer refers to cancers that start in female reproductive organs including cervical, ovarian, uterine, vaginal, vulvar, and fallopian tube (CDC, 2023m). Of these six gynecologic cancers, only cervical cancer can be screened. Common signs of gynecologic cancer include the following:

- Abnormal bleeding or discharge (except for vulvar)
- Feeling of fullness or bloating
- Back or abdominal pain
- Dysuria
- Constipation (ovarian and vaginal cancers)
- Skin changes, itching, burning, sores, rash in vulvar region (vulvar cancer) (CDC, 2023m)

Cervical cancer screening has improved early detection and prevention of cervical cancer dramatically. Both the incidence and the death rates for cervical cancer have been stable from 2010 to 2019 because of treatment of preinvasive cervical lesions. The major risk factors for this disease are infection with certain types of HPV, unprotected intercourse at an early age, and multiple sex partners. In 2023, it is estimated that 13,960 new cases of invasive cervical cancer will be diagnosed in the United States, contributing to 4310 deaths among females from this disease. The 5-year survival rate for this cancer, if prompt treatment is initiated, is 67.2% for all stages (SEER, 2023b). The CDC (2023m) published the following cervical cancer screening recommendations:

- Females age 21 to 29 years: cervical cytology; if normal, may wait 3 years.
- Females age 30 to 65 years: every 3 years with cervical cytology alone, or every 5 years with high-risk human papillomavirus testing (hrHPV), or every 5 years with hrHPV and cytology combination.
- Females older than 65 years: recommend against screening with adequate screening previously and not at high risk.

C/PHNs can continue to improve screening and early diagnosis through education and advocating for low-cost screening, which will allow at-risk females with low incomes or rural location access to regular cervical cancer screenings. In addition to screening, educating patients about the HPV vaccine is an important strategy to reduce the incidence of cervical cancer. The Gardasil 9 vaccine protects against 9 HPV virus types that may cause cervical cancer and anogenital warts. It is started as early as age 9 and given as two (age 9 to 13) or three doses (age 14 and older) over 6 months.

Ovarian cancer contributes to more deaths than any other cancer of the female reproductive system and accounts for 2.2% of cancer deaths among females. In 2023, a total of 19,710 cases were anticipated, and 13,270 deaths were expected.

- The primary risk factor for this disease is a strong family history of breast or ovarian cancer. The 5-year survival rate is 50.8% compared to cervical (67.2%) and breast (90.8%) cancers.
- The USPSTF recommends against routine screening for ovarian cancer in people who do not have

symptoms. However, people considered at high risk should receive a pelvic exam, a transvaginal ultrasound, and a blood test for the tumor marker CA 125. Therefore, C/PHNs need to continue to stress the importance of early detection (SEER, 2023c).

Myalgic Encephalomyelitis/Chronic Fatigue Syndrome

- **Myalgic encephalomyelitis/chronic fatigue syndrome (ME/CFS)** is a chronic and debilitating disease characterized by fatigue lasting for 6 or more months, worsening of symptoms after exertion, and unrefreshing sleep. Other symptoms may include cognitive impairment, orthostatic intolerance, frequent sore throat, headache, painful muscles, and joint pain. It is estimated that between 836,000 and 2.5 million people in the United States have ME/CFS, with females affected up to four times more than males.
- Symptoms may last for months or years, waxing and waning, and are difficult to validate objectively, but they are subjectively debilitating. Because the cause is unknown, there is no specific treatment and no prevention suggestions.
- Treatment is focused on supportive care for the associated pain, depression, and insomnia.
- The community health nurse can assess activity level and degree of fatigue, emotional response to the illness, and coping ability. Emotionally supportive family members and healthcare providers are helpful. Referring patients to mental health counseling or a local support group is useful for many patients and within the role of the community health nurse (CDC, 2021c).

Health Issues that Predominantly Affect Females

Eating Disorders

Eating disorders are estimated to affect over 5 million people in the United States (4.4 million females and 1.1 million males) (APA, 2022b). There is a high comorbidity association of eating disorders with mental health disorders affecting all biopsychosocial domains of people's lives, posing medical complications and quality of life issues. The three most common eating disorders are anorexia nervosa, bulimia nervosa, and binge eating (National Institute of Mental Health [NIMH], n.d.).

- **Anorexia nervosa** is characterized by marked weight loss, emaciation, a disturbance in body image, and a fear of weight gain. People affected lose weight either by excessive dieting or by purging themselves of ingested calories. People have a distorted body image; inability to maintain body weight can be life-threatening due to electrolyte disturbances, anemia, and secondary cardiac arrhythmias. Low body weight can impair the person's health impeding insulin production, leading to amenorrhea (absent menstrual periods) and decreased bone density (National Eating Disorders, 2022).
- **Bulimia nervosa** is characterized by recurrent episodes of binge eating, self-induced vomiting and diarrhea, misuse of laxatives or diuretics, excessive exercise, strict dieting or fasting, and an excessive concern about body shape or weight. Bulimic people have a fear of gaining weight and are unhappy with their body image, yet they may fall within normal parameters for their weight (NIMH, n.d.).
- **Binge eating** is the most common eating disorder in the United States, with typical onset in late adolescence and early 20s. It is characterized by repeated episodes of uncontrolled eating including eating large amounts quickly, when not hungry, and until comfortably full. Obesity is common because purging is not a characteristic of this disorder. This disorder results in increased risk for type 2 diabetes, high cholesterol, osteoarthritis, kidney disease or renal failure, heart disease, and hypertension (NIMH, n.d.).

The community health nurse can play a vital role in identifying affected people and refer these people to appropriate healthcare providers, mental health counselors, and self-help groups. Screening tools that may help identify people requiring referral for further assessment are available (NIMH, n.d.).

Breast Cancer

Although breast cancer overwhelmingly affects females, 1 out of every 100 cases is diagnosed in a male CDC, 2022h (CDC, 2022h). Overall, females' death rates from breast cancer have declined since 1990 (Table 21-5); this can be attributed to early detection and improvements in treatment. The sooner breast cancer is discovered, the more successfully it is treated. Obtaining regular clinical breast exams and mammograms, eating a diet low in fat and high in fruits and vegetables, breastfeeding (if possible), and avoiding prolonged use of menopausal hormonal therapy (MHT) all promote breast health. It was estimated in 2023 that there would be 297,790 new cases of breast cancer in females diagnosed in the United States, contributing to 43,170 deaths among females. The 5-year survival rate for this cancer, if prompt treatment is

TABLE 21-5 Breast Cancer Death Rates Among All People Assigned Female at Birth: 2016–2020

	Rate (%)
Age-Adjusted Rates per 100,000	
All races	19.6
Black	27.6
White	19.7
American Indian/Alaska Native	20.5
Hispanic	13.7
Asian/Pacific Islander	11.7

Source: Cancer Statistic Center (2023); Estimated deaths. https://cancerstatisticscenter.cancer.org/#!/cancer-site/Breast

initiated, is 90.8% (SEER, 2023a). Risk factors are similar for males and females:

- Genetic mutations (BRAC1 and BRAC2)
- Getting older
- Radiation therapy
- Hormone therapy
- Reproductive history
- Personal/family history of breast cancer
- Obesity (CDC, 2022h, 2022i)

For females, breast density, exposure to the drug diethylstilbestrol, physical inactivity, and alcohol use are added risk factors. For males, liver disease, Klinefelter syndrome, and conditions that affect the testicles are additional risk factors. For those at risk, genetic testing for BRAC1 and BRAC2 mutations might be recommended (CDC, 2022h, 2022i and National Cancer Institute n.d.). For females, the breast self-examination (BSE) is no longer a routine screening recommendation. However, it is important that all adults are familiar with their breasts. This allows them to recognize any overt changes in their breasts, especially changes related to size, shape, symmetry, nipple discharge, as well as skin changes. The C/PHN has many resources available to provide information and to teach adults breast awareness in their homes, small groups in clinics, or in various other community settings to enhance knowledge of breast health (ACS, 2022).

For females, breast cancer screening is important for early detection when tumors are likely to be smaller and confined to the breast. Early detection is associated with better prognosis for survival. The American Cancer Society (ASC, 2022) published the following breast cancer screening recommendations for females of average risk:

- Females between 40 and 44 years: should be an individual decision, and the patient's context (risk for disease) should be taken into account.
- Females 45 to 54 years: yearly mammogram.
- Females 55 years and older: may choose to have mammograms every other year or may continue yearly based on their risks.
- Screening continues while the female is in good health and expected to live at least 10 more years.
- Clinical breast exams are not recommended for breast cancer screening among average-risk females of any age.

Male Health

Males (see Fig. 21-9) have a higher mortality after 60 years, with health habits formed in their earlier years influencing health outcomes as they age. Males are therefore more likely to die earlier from a chronic illness or risky behaviors than females (Zarulli et al., 2021). This is evidenced by the difference in life expectancy between males and females in the United States; females survive an average of 5 years longer than males. Additionally, males of color are disproportionately affected by life expectancy as compared to their White counterparts (CDC, 2021c; Kaiser Family Foundation, 2023; Zarulli et al., 2021).

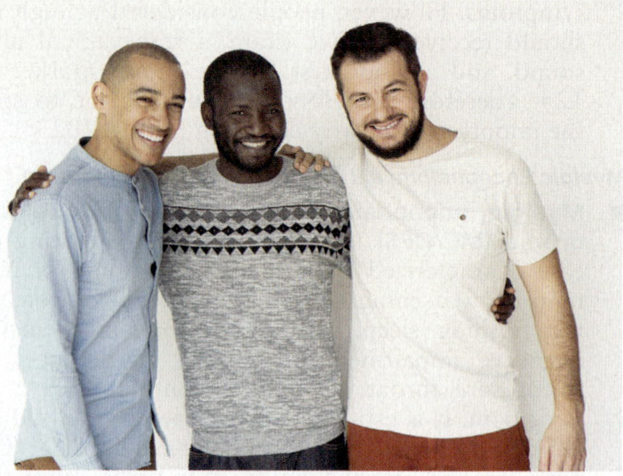

FIGURE 21-9 Males have different healthcare needs at various stages of life.

Overview of Factors Influencing Male Health

Historically, males have been less likely to seek healthcare for physical or mental health concerns. The past decade has expanded males health to include specialty health centers and healthcare specific to such areas as endocrine, reproductive, sexual, physical performance, surgical, and psychological issues (Houman et al., 2020). How the male identity is maintained can include high-risk activities, resulting in a higher death rate. Examples of these activities may include substance use, use of firearms, poor eating habits, inactivity, obesity, excessive alcohol consumption, and smoking (CDC, 2021e; Li et al., 2021).

Male Health Promotion Across the Adult Lifespan

In the early years of young adulthood (between 18 and 35 years), males continue to grow and mature. Adult males aged 35 to 65 years have reached maturity, the peak of their physical and intellectual development, and their greatest earning power. What specific needs do males in these age groups have? Are their needs being met through provided services?

***Healthy People 2030* Goals for Males.** *Healthy People 2030* addresses male health through family planning, STD, LGBTQ+, and adult health issues such as mental health, substance misuse and opioids, tobacco, nutrition, physical activity, chronic diseases, and cancer (Box 21-7).

Young Adult Males (18 to 35 Years). The young adult male has many tasks to accomplish including:

- Acquisition of training/education leading to a personally rewarding career
- Selecting a compatible partner and establishing a life together (see Fig. 21-10)
- Practicing and internalizing a belief and value system that brings comfort and meaning to existence
- Actively planning for having or not having children
- And participating in the betterment of the greater community

Young males may choose work that involves skills or a trade, office work, or a variety of other endeavors,

BOX 21-7 *HEALTHY PEOPLE 2030*

The Objectives for Males*

Core Objectives

C-07	Increase the proportion of adults who get screened for colorectal cancer
C-08	Reduce the prostate cancer death rate
STI-02	Reduce gonorrhea rates in male adolescents and young men
STI-05	Reduce the syphilis rate in men who have sex with men
HIV-03	Reduce the number of new HIV diagnoses
LGBT-01	Increase the number of national surveys that collect data on lesbian, gay, and bisexual populations
LGBT-02	Increase the number of national surveys that collect data on transgender populations
PA-02	Increase the proportion of adults who do enough aerobic physical activity for substantial health benefits
TU-01	Reduce current tobacco use in adults
SU-03	Reduce drug overdose deaths
SU-13	Reduce the proportion of people who had alcohol use disorder in the past year
SU-15	Reduce the proportion of people who had drug use disorder in the past year
NWS-03	Reduce the proportion of adults with obesity
MHMD-08	Increase the proportion of primary care visits where adolescents and adults are screened for depression

*In this box, "males" and "men" refers to people assigned male at birth.
Reprinted from Office of Disease Prevention and Health Promotion (ODPHP). (n.d.-d). Healthy People 2030. U.S. Department of Health and Human Services. https://health.gov/healthypeople/objectives-and-data/browse-objectives

including active duty military. They may also be veterans of military service.

In 2019, the Behavioral Risk Factor Surveillance System reported 53.8% of young males had at least one chronic health condition, with 22.3% reporting more than one chronic condition. The most prevalent conditions are obesity, depression, and high blood pressure with a higher prevalence in young males with a disability or who are unemployed (Watson et al., 2022). There is a concerted effort by C/PHNs nurses to raise awareness so young males ages 18 to 35 can manage and treat these chronic issues. Health prevention activities for this age group include the following:

- Blood pressure screening
- Diabetes screening
- Cholesterol screening
- Dental examination
- Eye examination
- Immunizations (National Library of Medicine, 2023)

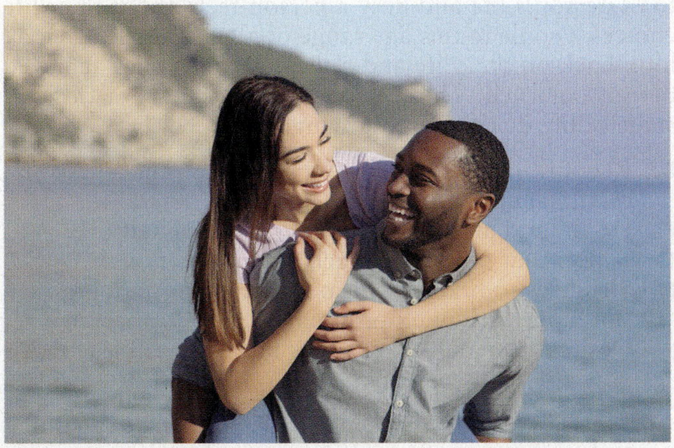

FIGURE 21-10 Choosing a significant other is a developmental task of young adulthood.

Young males may engage in risk-taking behaviors without thinking about the consequences. Depending on their attitudes and practices before entering young adulthood, they may or may not be enticed to experiment or continue with the use of tobacco, alcohol, or illicit drugs. This is an important age group for the C/PHN to reach with health information because decisions made in these formative years may affect how these individuals live the rest of their lives. The nurse can meet with people in this populations in work settings, college campuses, military bases, health clubs and bars, and at single-adult groups sponsored by religious communities and other organizations.

Reproductive Health

Another issue to address is the young male's attitudes and beliefs about sex. Males who are sexually active can reduce the possibility of being infected with an STI by limiting the number of sexual partners and using condoms consistently and correctly. Condoms also serve as a form of birth control. Monogamy (having sex with only one partner) and abstinence can further reduce or eliminate the chance of contracting an STI. Male involvement in reproductive health and contraceptive decision making has been shown to increase effectiveness in prevention of pregnancy and STI (CDC, 2023n). C/PHNs can serve as a resource and can help patients obtain free or low-cost condoms and treatment for STIs.

During the reproductive years, especially when a male has decided that their family is complete (see Fig. 21-11), they may choose a permanent form of birth control through a surgical procedure called *vasectomy*. A vasectomy entails the following:

- Block/cut/removal of all or a segment of the vas deferens
- Sperm cannot be released
- Routinely conducted on an outpatient basis
- Minimally invasive
- Takes about 30 minutes (CDC, 2023o)

Compared to tubal ligation (a surgical form of contraception for females), vasectomy is equally effective in preventing pregnancy, but vasectomy is simpler, faster, safer, and less expensive. A vasectomy does not protect against STIs and may be reversed depending on the procedure (CDC, 2023i). Because these methods, however, are intended to be irreversible, patients of all genders should be counseled about the permanency of these procedures (CDC, 2023o).

The choices a young adult male makes during these years establish healthy eating, work, rest, and exercise habits that will be beneficial for a lifetime. People should follow the dietary food guidelines that are recommended by the U.S. Department of Agriculture (2020–2025). Establishing a pattern of rest that allows the body to recover and refresh from a day full of meaningful activities will help the individual look forward to each day. The person should establish an exercise routine that meets personal needs, fits skills and talents, and includes some physical activities that involve the family (see Fig. 21-12). These choices provide the knowledge that they are doing everything they can to keep themselves healthy and to prevent the two major killers of males—heart disease and cancer (Li et al., 2020). Typically, young adult clients have few interactions with healthcare providers in any given year. It is important for people in this age group to have regular health checkups, be assessed for early signs of disease, and engage in health promotion activities.

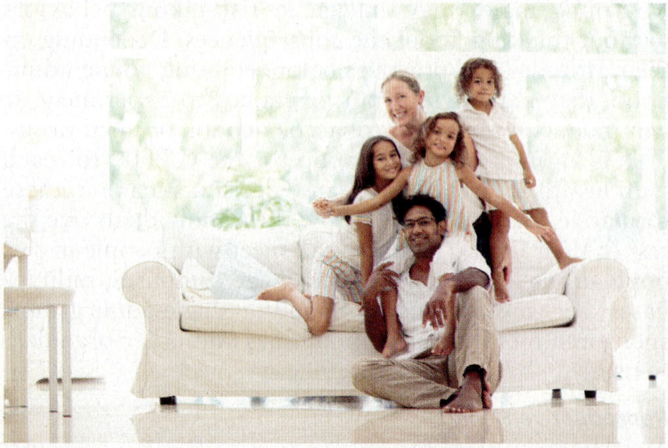

FIGURE 21-11 Reproductive health is an important consideration for males.

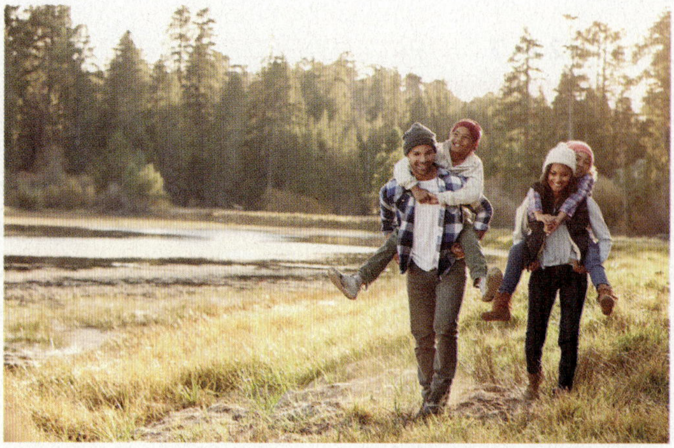

FIGURE 21-12 Adult males are encouraged to maintain good health through eating a healthy diet and getting regular exercise.

Adult Males (35 to 65 Years). Males in the developmental stage between 35 and 65 years of age face many challenges as well as opportunities. Challenges might include the following:

- Caring for their own families and children
- Caring for aging parents and in-laws
- Economic burdens of putting children through college
- Adjusting to the reality that their career path is probably set, and many life choices have been made

The term "midlife" is applied to the age period 40 to 60 years, during which terms such as "midlife crisis" have been used to describe tension or emotions related to a person's life and how a person feels about their life choices. People in this age range of all genders range may look back on their life and reflect on milestones achieved or not achieved. This period of time can be a difficult stage of life due to the following:

- Reappraisal of values, priorities, and personal relationships
- Doubt and anxiety realizing that life is half over
- Beliefs that one has not accomplished enough
- Struggles to find new meaning or purpose in life
- Boredom with one's personal life, job, or partners
- Desires to make life changes in personal life, job, or partners

Males in midlife are at higher risk for suicide than the general population (SAMHSA, 2023). It is important to distinguish a reappraisal of life priorities from depression, which is not a normal part of mid-life behavior (CDC, n.d.; Center for Men's Health, 2022).

Males in this age range may also experience andropause, also known as male menopause or a decrease in testosterone levels. Hormone levels for males may change as they age, and it is important to know symptoms of low testosterone:

- Loss of energy
- Low libido (decreased sex drive)
- Erectile dysfunction
- Hot flushes or sweats
- Weight gain
- Breast discomfort or swelling
- Infertility
- Reduction in bone density (CDC, 2023p; Center for Men's Health, 2022)

As males age, continued good health habits are important such as adequate sleep, healthy foods, and regular exercise. Earlier health behaviors may influence health later in life, leading to chronic conditions such as diabetes, heart disease, high blood pressure, and obesity (Li et al., 2021). Not all treatments are appropriate for low testosterone, and having the correct diagnosis for symptomatology is important. The C/PHN has a role to play in reinforcing good lifestyle choices and stress management for males.

The later years in this stage, ages 50 to 64, involve preparation for retirement. In anticipation of retirement, these years are marked by the following:

- Expanded social relationships
- Pursuit of new hobbies to fill increased leisure time
- Finishing a career and accumulation of the best retirement benefits
- Making life altering decisions
- Potential health problems
- Loss of loved ones, particularly a spouse or long-term companion

Successful navigation of this stage can be fulfilling but may require enhancement self-care skills. This includes having a positive attitude toward aging, one that examines the benefits of maturity, finds a balance between work and home, and maintains a healthy lifestyle by eating balanced meals and obtaining regular exercise. The community health nurse can provide anticipatory guidance to males approaching this stage and provide them with information on ways to manage life more effectively.

Reproductive Health

Erection problems are common among males of all ages but especially as individuals age. **Erectile dysfunction (ED)**, sometimes called impotence, is the repeated inability to get or keep an erection firm enough for sexual intercourse. The word impotence may also be used to describe other problems that interfere with sexual intercourse, such as lack of sexual desire and problems with ejaculation or orgasm. Using the term *erectile dysfunction* makes it clear that these other issues are not involved (National Institute of Diabetes and Digestive and Kidney Diseases [NIDDK], n.d.; Urology Care Foundation, 2023a). The vascular, nervous, and endocrine symptoms can cause or contribute to ED (NIDDK, n.d.). Some causes of ED include the following:

- Over 50
- Diabetes
- High blood pressure
- Cardiovascular disease
- Smoking
- Drug use
- Excessive alcohol
- Obesity
- Lack of exercise (Urology Care Foundation, 2023a)

In addition, there can be physical reasons for ED such as blood flow to penis, nerve signals from brain to spinal cord, cancer treatment, and medications. Emotional causes can include stress or worry (Urology Care foundation, 2023a). Treatments for ED may include lifestyle changes, counseling, changing medications, medications specific for ED, vacuum erection devices, penile implants, and surgery (NIDDK, n.d.; Urology Care Foundation, 2023a). The C/PHN should counsel males with ED symptoms to seek sound medical advice and be cautious of gimmicky products.

Testicular Cancer

- Testicular cancer occurs most often in males older than 65 years of age and rarely occurs in those younger than 40, but the chance of prostate cancer rises significantly after 50 years of age (ACS, 2023c).
- A few risk factors have been identified that increase a young adult's chance of developing testicular cancer including a personal history of an undescended testicle, abnormal testicular development, family history of testicular cancer, race/ethnicity (White), and age, (ACS, 2023c).
- It is a rare form of cancer and is not on the list of objectives for males in *Healthy People 2030*. If detected early, this cancer is highly curable.
- According to the Testicular Cancer Society (2023), it may be beneficial to the overall health of a young adult to know how to perform a testicular self-examination. For more information on TSE, visit the following website of the Testicular Cancer Society: https://testicularcancersociety.org/pages/self-exam-how-to

Prostate Health. Prostate health is another concern that may occur later in this life stage. The **prostate** is a doughnut-shaped gland located at the bottom of the bladder, about halfway between the rectum and the base of the penis. The prostate encircles the urethra. The walnut-sized gland produces most of the fluid in semen. Males can experience infection (prostatitis), prostate enlargement (benign prostatic hyperplasia [BPH]), and prostate cancer (American Cancer Society [ACS], 2023d).

- BPH is very common.
- The primary risk factor for developing BPH is age. Nearly 50% of men over 50 years of age

report symptoms that are related to prostate gland enlargement.

- Symptoms of BPH are caused by an obstruction of the urethra and gradual loss of bladder function, which results in incomplete emptying of the bladder. The most commonly reported symptoms of BPH involve lower urinary tract symptoms (LUTS), such as hesitant, interrupted, or weak urinary stream, urgency or leaking of urine, and more frequent urination, especially at night.
- Patients often report the symptoms of BPH before the primary provider diagnoses it through a digital rectal examination (DRE).
- Treatment for BPH can include medication or surgery to reduce the size of the prostate (Urology Care Foundation, 2023b).

Prostate cancer is the most frequently diagnosed cancer in males and is the second leading cause of cancer deaths.

- According to the ACS (2023b, 2023d), 1 male in 8 will get prostate cancer during their lifetime, and 1 male in 41 will die from the disease.
- However, most prostate cancers grow slowly and do not cause any health problems.
- More than 3.1 million males in the United States who have been diagnosed with prostate cancer at some time in their lives are still alive today.
- Prior to age 40, prostate cancer is very rare, but the chance of having prostate cancer rises rapidly after age 50.
- About 6 cases in 10 are diagnosed in men 65 years of age and older.
- Although age is the strongest risk factor for prostate cancer, family history and ethnicity also need to be considered. Prostate cancer occurs more often in Black males than in those of other races and occurs less often in Asian and Hispanic/Latino males.

The reasons for these racial and ethnic differences are not clear. Starting at age 50, all males should talk to their healthcare provider about the pros and cons of screening for prostate cancer. This discussion should start at age 45 if a man is Black or has a biological father or brother who had prostate cancer before age 65. Having a biological father or brother diagnosed with prostate cancer doubles a patient's risk. ACS (2023b, 2023d) recommends a discussion about screening:

- For males 50 years old at average risk of prostate cancer and are expected to live at least 10 more years
- For males 45 years old at high risk for prostate cancer including Black males and those who have a biological father or son (first-degree relative) diagnosed with prostate cancer at an early age (younger than 65)
- For males 40 years old at higher risk (more than one first-degree relative diagnosed with prostate cancer at an early age)

Following a discussion, those who want to be screened should get a prostate-specific antigen (PSA) test; a digital rectal examination (DRE) may also be done (ACS, 2023e). Screening recommendations can be found at (ACS, 2023e): https://www.cancer.org/cancer/types/prostate-cancer/detection-diagnosis-staging/tests.html

Treatment for prostate cancer ranges from management through monitoring of PSA tests, biopsy, or watching for symptoms, to invasive procedures such as surgery (ACS, 2023f). Options may include the following:

- Treatment options may include surgery to remove all or part of the prostate (prostatectomy), radiation, and hormone therapy.
- Surgery, radiation, and hormone therapy all have the potential to disrupt sexual desire and performance, temporarily or permanently.
- Urinary dysfunction and incontinence are common side effects that occur after surgery or radiation.
- Radiation therapy, including internal and external treatments.
- Other procedures may include cryotherapy, ultrasound, chemotherapy, and immunotherapy (ACS, 2023d; CDC, 2023e).

A C/PHN can reinforce or clarify information shared with the patient by the healthcare provider, discuss treatment options with the patient and their family, and provide the support they may need if prostate cancer is diagnosed.

ROLE OF THE COMMUNITY HEALTH NURSE

The community health nurse works with adults in all age groups using the three levels of prevention—primary, secondary, and tertiary—as a guide. Interventions are conducted at the individual, family, group, and aggregate levels to make progress toward the *Healthy People 2030* objectives (Box 21-8).

Client teaching by the community health nurse is a major factor in preventing and managing chronic diseases. The challenge to the nurse is to be prepared to discuss issues, backed up with knowledge of and access to the appropriate community resources, to meet client needs. What the nurse can accomplish can be quite dramatic in terms of reducing days in the hospital because of chronic disease, improving quality of life for the person with a chronic illness, and preventing a combination of unhealthy habits from becoming causative factors in new cases of chronic disease. A nursing care plan matrix can guide the community health nurse in discussing areas of health promotion and protection with the client. An example of a nursing care plan matrix for young adults can be found in Box 21-9.

Primary Prevention

- Primary prevention activities focus on education to promote a healthy lifestyle. Much of the community health nurse's time is spent in the educator role.
- When working with people, the C/PHN should encourage routine health examinations, healthy eating habits, adequate sleep, moderate drinking, and no smoking. Among aggregates, the community health nurse focuses on community needs for services and

BOX 21-8 LEVELS OF PREVENTION PYRAMID

Breast Cancer

SITUATION: Breast cancer.
GOAL: Using the three levels of prevention, avoid or promptly diagnose and treat negative health conditions and restore the fullest potential.

Tertiary Prevention

Rehabilitation	*Health Promotion and Education*	*Health Protection*
▪ Recovery at home with return to activities of daily living within 2 wk	▪ Maintains periodic follow-up with healthcare provider, follow-up mammogram at 6 and 12 mo, and as recommended by healthcare provider ▪ Education regarding risk for other cancers (cervical, ovarian, uterine, etc.)	▪ Practices breast awareness and receives mammograms as recommended; receives screening for ovarian cancer—transvaginal ultrasonography and blood test for tumor marker CA 125

Secondary Prevention

Early Diagnosis	*Prompt Treatment*
▪ Identification of lump in left breast, appointment made with healthcare provider for evaluation ▪ Receives mammogram and sonogram	▪ Needle aspiration of lump followed by cytologic studies ▪ Lumpectomy with removal of two suspicious lymph nodes ▪ Low-dose radiation

Primary Prevention

Health Promotion and Education	*Health Protection*
▪ Education regarding breast awareness and mammograms, as needed ▪ Education regarding environmental exposure and breast cancer (smoking, alcohol, chemicals) ▪ Education regarding low-fat diet and maintaining a body mass index <29	▪ Avoidance of environmental exposures that may contribute to cancer ▪ Maintains breast awareness and obtains mammogram when appropriate

programs that will keep that population healthy, such as providing flu vaccine clinics, teaching sexual responsibility, and preventing STIs.

The community health nurse may collaborate with community leaders and other stakeholders in designing programs, work with committees to secure funding, or approach the state legislature to lobby for needed changes to state laws and policies governing the health of adults. At other times, the nurse works with small groups of adults who could benefit from making healthy choices in diet, relaxation, and physical activity. Likewise, it is not unusual for the C/PHN to work with an individual to promote healthy living.

Secondary Prevention

- Secondary prevention focuses on screening for early detection and prompt treatment of diseases. Throughout the lifespan, screening tests can help adults identify disease early; currency on immunizations is recommended to protect yourself and loved ones, as well as prevent serious illness.
- A significant amount of the community health nurse's time is spent in assessing the need for planning, implementing, or evaluating programs that focus on the early detection of diseases.
- This is followed by teaching to prevent further damage from the disease in progress or to prevent the spread of the disease if it is communicable. Examples of secondary prevention programs include establishing mammography clinics, teaching breast and TSE, and screenings—blood pressure, blood glucose, BMI, and Cholesterol (see Box 21-10).

Tertiary Prevention

- The tertiary level of prevention focuses on rehabilitation and preventing further damage to an already compromised system. Many adults with whom a

BOX 21-9 Nursing Care Plan Matrix for Health Promotion, Young Adults: 18 to 35 Years

Community health nurses can use this matrix to individualize teaching, services, and care to young adult clients. Use the questions to stimulate the development of an individualized approach that is client focused and client driven with the community health nurse acting as the catalyst. In any or all of these areas, the community health nurse may (1) discuss issues and commend the client for positive attitudes and behaviors (e.g., when the client is making healthful decisions, such as condom use for their health and the health of significant others); (2) discuss the issues and guide the client to resources that will enhance more positive behaviors and decisions (e.g., flu shot clinic or healthy lifestyle program for adults); or (3) discuss the issues and inform the client that immediate changes must be made to protect the health of self or others and inform/utilize the appropriate resources as soon as possible (e.g., follow-up for symptoms related to suspected STI).

1. *Life partner.* Ascertain whether the client is looking for a life partner or is choosing to live a single life. Discuss how the single life is satisfying for the client and ways to make it richer.
   Discuss settings in which client can meet others (male or female, based on sexual preference) with similar interests, philosophy, and outlook, such as work settings, school settings, faith communities, recreational communities, and the like.
   Discuss what the client is looking for in a potential life partner, expectations for the relationship, what the client contributes, how the client compromises and resolves conflict, and other issues. If in a relationship, what is good, what needs improving, and how to initiate change.
2. *Life's work.* How is the client preparing for their life's work (education, formal training, on the job training)? Will the life's work provide resources for client's life plans? Will the work choice provide long-term satisfaction? Is the work choice a "stepping stone" to another work role? How will/do they handle work and rearing children? What needs changing or can be improved in the work/children arrangement?
3. *Planning for children.* What knowledge do they have about family planning? What methods fit best with their philosophy, religious beliefs, and lifestyle? What are the long-term effects of the choices? How many children is the client planning to rear? Have they thought through the ramifications of this number? If choosing not to have (or unable to have) children, how will they deal with this? Do they want alternative suggestions for raising a child (adoption, foster parenting) or information about interacting with children (volunteering)?
4. *Maintaining physical and mental health.* In this area, the community health nurse needs to explore all areas of health promotion and protection. This will include discussions regarding primary and secondary prevention. Primary prevention discussions could include the following:
   - Diet and nutrition
   - Physical and leisure activities
   - Safe sex practices
   - Periodic health examinations
   - Personal safety—seat belts, protective helmets, dating violence, etc.
   - Immunizations
   - Regular use of sunscreen
   - Stress reduction activities

   Secondary prevention discussions could include the following:
   - Screening for sexually transmitted infections
   - Testicular self-examination
   - Smoking cessation
   - Pelvic examinations and Pap smears
   - Counseling and support at times of stress
5. *Developing a life's philosophy.* Discuss client's personal life satisfaction, which may include religiosity and spirituality, living in congruence with cultural/ethnic/family beliefs and expectations, and coming to a comfortable level of satisfaction with life choices, having few regrets.

community health nurse works have chronic diseases, conditions resulting from another disease, or long-standing injuries with resulting disability.

- Ideally, negative health conditions can be prevented. If not, the next best thing is for them to be diagnosed early, without damage to an individual's health. But if negative health conditions have not been treated or brought under control, then the person is at a tertiary level of prevention. At this level of prevention, the nurse focuses on maintaining quality of life.

Caring for people at the tertiary level of prevention can become quite complicated because many body systems may be involved. In addition, all people function within many social systems, which may include family expectations, roles people have within the family, expected behaviors, community system knowledge and involvement, personal expectations, motivation, and support. Working at the tertiary level involves all of the nurse's skills in addition to community resources and a client who can be or wants to be motivated.

BOX 21-10 Secondary Prevention of STIs Among Nonpregnant Adults Experiencing Homelessness

Adults experiencing homelessness are at increased risk of negative health outcomes, including an increased incidence and prevalence of sexually transmitted infections (STIs), compared to the general population (Williams & Bryant, 2018). A 2019 study estimates that the prevalence of sexually transmitted infections (STIs) among adults experiencing homelessness ranges from 2.1% to 52.5%. A nurse-led clinic exclusively serving people experiencing homelessness (PEH) identified that it was likely underscreening for STIs. Ethical and theoretical principles were applied to research, and a protocol was developed to better guide the clinicians at a clinic to screen for STIs in adults experiencing homelessness and who are without symptoms and not pregnant.

The clinic lead identified that when serving PEH, a vulnerable population, it is important to account for how their prior lived experiences affect their health and health beliefs (O. Ridgway, personal communication, September 13, 2022). Therefore, Leininger's (1988) Sunrise Model was adapted to create a protocol that addressed Spiers' (2000) emic and etic principles of vulnerability and address the person as a whole being. Special consideration was taken to use inclusive terminology in relation to gender, religion, social, cultural, political, economic, education, and technologic factors (Leininger, 1988). The protocol was developed using a web-based tool so that it could be easily modified as the state of the science changes. It first approached the emic principles of culturally competent, trauma-informed, and gender-inclusive care and outlined how to take a detailed sexual history to determine risk. Then it addressed the etic principle to provide guidance on how to appropriately screen for STIs. It outlined screening intervals, appropriate screening tests, whether the infection was reportable in the state where the clinic is located, and whether retesting is necessary. This was broken down by patient population (people with a cervix, people with a penis who have intercourse with a person with a cervix (MSW), people with a penis who have intercourse with a person with a penis (MSM), people with a neopenis or neovagina, and people living with HIV) and then by STI (chlamydia, gonorrhea, hepatitis B, hepatitis C, herpes, HIV, human papillomavirus [HPV], syphilis, and trichomoniasis). PEH are vulnerable, underserved, and experience higher rates of STIs compared with the general population. Strategies are needed to address STI risk for this population. This project is a small step in improving the care of PEH at one clinic but may be transferable to other clinics who serve PEH. Future protocols may include partner testing, symptomatic testing, and STI treatment.

Kelsi Keyek, RN

Source: Leininger, M. (1988). Leininger's theory of nursing: Cultural care diversity and universality. *Nursing Science Quarterly, 1*(4), 152–160. https://doi.org/10.1177/089431848800100408

Spiers, J. (2000). New perspectives on vulnerability using emic and etic approaches. *Journal of advanced nursing, 31*(3), 715–721. https://doi.org/10.1046/j.1365-2648.2000.01328.x

Williams, S. P., & Bryant, K.L. (2018). Sexually transmitted infection prevalence among homeless adults in the United States: A systematic literature review. *Sexually Transmitted Diseases, 45*(7), 494–504. https://doi.org/10.1097/OLQ.0000000000000780

CASE STUDY 10 ESSENTIAL PUBLIC HEALTH SERVICES

Tertiary Prevention in the Community

Depending on the client's age, tertiary prevention can be simple or very complex. A 19-year-old person who breaks their leg while skiing needs information about using crutches safely, a reminder to eat protein foods for bone healing, and an appointment to return to their healthcare provider if they experience various symptoms and to get the cast removed. They generally need no additional help from others. Tertiary prevention in this case is uncomplicated. On the other hand, a 62-year-old who has 70 pounds of excess weight and with out-of-control blood glucose levels, symptoms of congestive heart failure, and difficulty walking more than 20 ft has much to accomplish in order to feel healthy.

1. ***Recognize Cues:*** *Which findings require immediate follow-up, are unexpected, or are most concerning?*
2. ***Analyze Cues:*** *What information is noted or needed for interpreting findings?*
3. ***Prioritize Hypotheses:*** *Based on the information that you have, what is happening?*
4. ***Generate Solutions:*** *What intervention(s) will achieve the desired outcome?*
5. ***Take Action:*** *What actions should you take or do first?*
6. ***Evaluate Outcomes:*** *Were outcomes achieved? Why or why not?*
7. *Which Essential Public Health Services influence this situation? (See Box 2-2.)*

SUMMARY

- Despite the shift in the 20th century in the leading cause of death from communicable to noncommunicable, there appeared on the world stage in 2019 a new virus not seen since the 1918 H1N1 Influenza pandemic. On March 11, 2020, the World Health Organization (WHO) declared COVID-19 (SARS-CoV-2) a global pandemic.
- The leading causes of death in adults in 2021 are diseases of the heart, malignant neoplasms, COVID-19, unintentional injuries, cerebrovascular diseases, and CLRDs. Obesity and substance use contribute to or exacerbate many of the leading causes of mortality and morbidity discussed in this chapter.
- Caring for our community requires recognition of people and the designations in which they identify as well as the biologic characteristics of a person for appropriate prevention and healthcare needs. Awareness of sexual orientation or gender identity (SO/GI) can assist in caring for all adults while providing necessary healthcare services.
- The healthcare needs of adults are of great concern. Many needs are the same for males and females, with important differences addressed in this chapter.
- Adults have healthcare needs that change as they age. Diet and exercise, obesity, substance use, safety, and healthy lifestyle choices are issues that adults must consider throughout their lives.
- Genomics refers to how a person's genetic makeup and environment predispose a person to the development of disease. Understanding a person's genetic risk and environmental factors that may further influence and increase risk allows community health nurses to provide targeted education on disease prevention. Heart disease and cancers remain important concerns for people of all genders, and health decisions made as a young adult can have a major impact on people as they age.
- Chronic illness is an issue of increasing concern as life expectancies increase. C/PHNs should use the three levels of prevention to promote health across the lifespan. Primary prevention activities focus on education to promote a healthy lifestyle and vaccination programs. Secondary prevention focuses on screening for early detection, and tertiary prevention focuses on prompt treatment of diseases.
- The C/PHN role at this stage is to assess needs; to plan, implement, or evaluate programs that focus on the early detection of diseases; and to educate clients to prevent further damage from or spread of disease. The tertiary level of prevention focuses on rehabilitation and prevention of further damage to an already compromised system. At this level of prevention, the nurse focuses on maintaining quality of life.

ACTIVE LEARNING EXERCISES

1. Using resources, determine what health issues affect adults in your town, city, or neighborhood. How does this affect the lifespan of adults in the community? Consider the socioeconomic impact that this has on members of your community. Who is most affected? What can you use as the C/PHN to promote the health of your community? Identify ways that the C/PHN can provide primary, secondary, and tertiary health promotion activities specific to these issues. (Objectives 3 and 4)
2. Identify a major chronic illness found in adults. Create a program to address this health issue. What steps would you take to develop a successful program? What would be important to emphasize with this age group? What resources (e.g., smartphone apps, online information) might be useful? (Objective 1)
3. Apply "Assess and Monitor Population Health" (1 of the 10 essential public health services; see Box 2-2) as follows: Using nursing and other healthcare databases, research a chronic disease associated with adults aged 35 to 65. Identify selected concerns and discuss both personal responsibility and societal responsibility (consider health equity and health disparities) regarding the management of this health problem. What are health priorities and why? (Objective 2)
4. Using Healthy People 2030, determine screening recommendations for clients who are 50 to 65 years of age. (Objective 5)
5. Complete a health history on an adult, including medical, family, social history, and environmental history. Based on the information collected, determine the individual's personal risk factors. Which risk factors are modifiable? Which are not modifiable? Which chronic diseases are they at risk for developing? What education would you provide to help the person reduce their risk? (Objective 6)

CHAPTER 22

Older Adults

"A healthy community is one in which [older adults] protect, care for, love, and assist the younger ones to provide continuity and hope."

—Maggie Kuhn, founder of the Gray Panthers

KEY TERMS

- Age dependency ratio
- Ageism
- Aging in place
- Alzheimer disease (AD)
- Arthritis
- Assisted living
- Beta-amyloid
- Case management
- Chronic conditions
- Continuing care retirement communities (CCRCs)
- Custodial care
- Geriatrics
- Gerontologic
- Hospice
- Long-term care
- Nursing home
- Older adult abuse
- Osteoporosis
- Palliative care
- Polypharmacy
- Respite care
- Senility
- Tau proteins
- Universal design

LEARNING OBJECTIVES

Upon mastery of this chapter, you should be able to:

1. Describe the global and national health status of older adults.
2. Identify and refute at least three common misconceptions about older adults.
3. Describe the characteristics of healthy older adults.
4. Describe the most common health issues facing older adults.
5. Provide an example of primary, secondary, and tertiary prevention practices in the older adult population.
6. Describe various types of residential living arrangements for older adults.

INTRODUCTION

What age is *old*? For most of us, we think of retirement age or Medicare eligibility age of 65. For people born after 1960, Medicare eligibility will remain at age 65, while Social Security eligibility will begin at age 67. The aging process among older adults is individual, subtle, gradual, and lifelong. One can see remarkable differences among individuals in the rate of aging. Even in a single individual, various systems of the body age at different rates. Therefore, chronologic age cannot readily be a reliable indicator of health needs. Methods for calculating your "real" or biologic age can give you a better picture of your body's true state of health (see http://www.biological-age.com/about.html for a calculator you can use for yourself and your clients).

Some older people are staying in the workforce longer, reflecting their good physical and mental health. Reflect on the difference in age and health of Mrs. Barbara and Frank Mendez. Chronologic age only tells us part of the story.

Ms. Barbara is still in the apartment she and her husband shared for many years after they retired. At 94, Ms. Barbara takes thyroid and cholesterol medications, and occasional Tylenol for her "old knee." She tends her parakeet, Bert, and visits with her neighbors regularly. Because she does not drive anymore, she orders her groceries online for delivery. Her apartment has a universal design with safety bars and a pull string for quick assistance. She loves games and plays Bridge and Scrabble regularly with others in the retirement community. Her health has had its ups and downs, but with the support of an automated pill box and frequent visits from her daughter, Ms. Barbara is able to remain independent in her apartment.

Frank Mendez, 83, lives in an urban apartment complex that is considered affordable housing. He takes medication for heart failure and chronic obstructive pulmonary disease (COPD). He takes care of his grandson after school 2 days a week and plans carefully to afford healthy after school snacks. Frank's rent has increased by $25 each year for the past 3 years, which makes it challenging to balance the budget. His insurance plan covers many costs but does not include any dental. Frank has two loose teeth, which are painful, but he has postponed his dental visit due to health costs. Frank hopes that the cost-of-living increase from his Social Security will offset the rent increase and the higher price of his groceries this year.

Older adults constitute a large and rapidly growing population group in the United States, one that you will join eventually. Perhaps your parents or grandparents are part of that group now. Improved medical care, advances in public health standards, and a focus on prevention have contributed to dramatic increases in life expectancy in the United States.

- In addition to increases in life expectancy, the growth in the number of older adults began when the Baby Boomers (people born after World War II between the years of 1946 and 1964) reached age 65.
- 631,000 of the population was age 95 and older in 2022; an increase of 50% from 2010 (Caplan, 2023).
- Older adults represent 17% of the U.S. population or about one in every six Americans (Administration for Community Living, 2024a).
- Eleven million older adults are either working or actively seeking employment (Administration for Community Living, 2024a).
- One third of those aged 65 and older have a disability such as difficulty walking or vision or hearing loss (Administration for Community Living, 2024a).

Baby boomers bring much to the conversation about aging in place in their communities, including retirement planning and providing for their healthcare needs.

In addition to financial preparation for retirement and older age, 25% of married couples age 65 and older divorced in 2019, highlighting the possibility more baby boomers will be divorced than widowed (Brown & Lin, 2022). This percentage increased to 33% when divorced, and separated/spouse-absent was combined in a study completed in 2023 (Administration for Community Living, 2024a). This percentage has increased since 1980 when approximately 5% of the older population were divorced or separated/spouse absent. Given that many baby boomers are divorced or have never been married, they often have a different opinion about the definition of marriage and children ember (Vera-Toscano & Meroni, 2021).

It is projected that in the next 8 to 10 years, older adults will outnumber children for the first time in U.S. history (Vesper et al., 2020). Racial and ethnic underrepresented populations are projected to constitute 28% of the older adult population by 2030 (ODPHP, n.d.-a). For a variety of reasons, older adults may experience the effects of health disparities more dramatically than any other population group. As noted in Figure 22-1, the life expectancy of all groups dropped between 2019 and 2021, with a higher impact on underrepresented groups, particularly Hispanic people.

Another factor affecting the health of the current generation of older adults is ever-rising healthcare costs in the United States. While Medicare and Medicaid insurance pays for healthcare for older adults, Americans have higher out-of-pocket costs than in other resource-abundant countries (Commonwealth Fund, 2021). When older adults are living on fixed incomes, the research indicates that they may skip healthcare or not fill a prescription or visit the dentist due to cost (Commonwealth Fund, 2021; see Chapter 6).

The growth of the aging population presents opportunities for C/PHN to work with communities to strengthen and expand programs and services targeted to

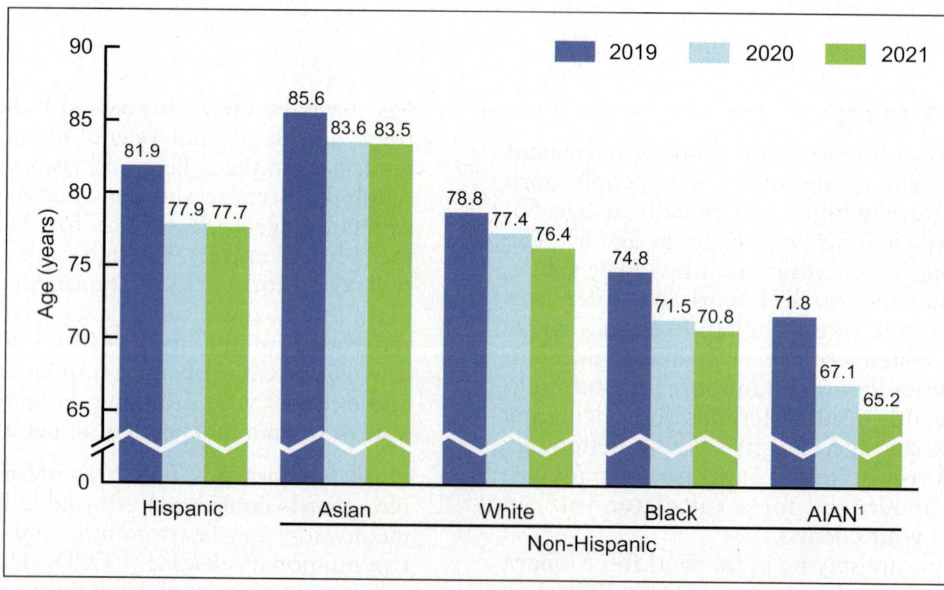

[1]American Indian or Alaska Native.
NOTES: Estimates are based on provisional data for 2021. Provisional data are subject to change as additional data are received. Estimates for 2019 and 2020 are based on final data. Life tables by race and Hispanic origin are based on death rates that have been adjusted for race and Hispanic-origin misclassification on death certificates; see Technical Notes in this report.
SOURCE: National Center for Health Statistics, National Vital Statistics System, Mortality.

FIGURE 22-1 Life expectancy at birth, by Hispanic origin and race: United States, 2019–2021. (Reprinted from National Center for Health Statistics, National Vital Statistics System, Mortality. https://www.cdc.gov/nchs/data/vsrr/vsrr023.pdf)

older adults, to advocate for the needs of the aging population with government agencies and other organizations, and to work toward the Healthy People 2030 goals for older people.

This chapter first examines the characteristics of the aging population in the United States and the global challenge of an aging society.

- Ageism is discussed in the context of misconceptions about older adults.
- The primary, secondary, and tertiary health needs of older adults are explored.
- Diseases common among older adults are reviewed, with a focus on Alzheimer disease (AD) and other dementias.
- Older adult abuse is reviewed with a focus on financial abuse and abuse reporting.
- Population-based health services and nursing interventions applied to the health of the aging population are discussed in light of cost containment and comprehensive care.

GERIATRICS AND GERONTOLOGY

Nurses trained in the specialty of gerontologic nursing are needed to care for our aging population. **Gerontologic** nursing encompasses all aspects of the aging process, including economic, social, clinical, psychological, and spiritual factors. Gerontologic nursing focuses on promoting and improving the health of older adults. This holistic approach includes evaluating the impact of these factors on older adults and society. Health is defined by the person and may include the ability to age in place or sustain maximum functioning.

In contrast, geriatrics is a medical specialty. Like other medical specialties, **geriatrics** focuses on abnormal conditions and the treatment and cure of those conditions. A geriatrician is a medical doctor with specialized training in geriatrics.

A C/PHN works with older adults at the individual, family, and group levels. In one instance, the nurse may work to promote and maintain the health of a vigorous 80-year-old who lives alone in their home. However, a community and public health nursing perspective must also concern itself with the aggregate of older adults.

- There are many groups of older people with whom the nurse may choose to work, such as those who attend a memory daycare center, those who belong to a retirement community, those who live in a nursing home, or members of a caregiver support group.
- Other groups include residents of a 55+ apartment building; those with cognitive, vision, or hearing loss; people experiencing homelessness; and veterans.
- Work with clients can also involve political advocacy.
- The possibilities for C/PHNs to work with older adults are vast and ever expanding.

HEALTH STATUS OF OLDER ADULTS

People are generally living longer as a result of improved healthcare, eradication and control of many communicable diseases, use of antibiotics and other medicines, healthier dietary practices, safer global water supplies, regular exercise, and accessibility to resources. Increased life expectancy reflects, in part, the success of public health interventions. However, C/PH programs must now respond to new challenges, such as the following: the growing burden of chronic illness, physical and cognitive impairments, increasing concerns about future caregiving, coordinating care across providers and settings, and rapidly rising healthcare costs.

Chronic diseases, often referred to as **chronic conditions**, affect older adults at a disproportionately higher rate.

- They contribute to disability, diminish quality of life, and increase healthcare costs.
- Chronic conditions can be addressed in public health work, as many factors that lead to poor health—like obesity, substance use, and sedentary behaviors—are modifiable.

C/PHNs are positioned to address key challenges faced by the older population. They can work to meet the long-term needs of people with cognitive and physical disabilities coordinate care across providers, oversee the adequacy of services, and support family caregivers in the plan of care. In this way, C/PHNs can help older adults live in the communities, a more cost-effective and desirable outcome.

Global Aging and Health

The unprecedented growth in the number of older adults is happening worldwide, due to increasing levels of life expectancy and lower fertility rates. Between 2020 and 2050, the number of older people is expected to double in all areas of the world (United Nations, 2023). In addition to changes in life expectancy and fertility, the following factors affect older populations:

- Changes in family composition—single person living alone versus intergenerational housing
- Cohabitation or divorce and rural-to-urban migration
- Living alone—older women are more likely than older men to live alone, or to live with extended family, which may provide support; research indicates that living arrangements around the world impact the health and mortality of older people (United Nations, 2023).

Worldwide between 2020 and 2021, adults 60 years and older had the highest mortality rate of any age group, at 80%. Among the 154 countries that reported vaccination rates, rates were as high as 76% in resource-abundant countries and as low as 33% in resource-limited countries (Harris, 2023).

National Aging and Health

As a result of demographic transitions, including a decrease in child births, improvements in adult health, and the pandemic, the shape of age distribution is changing. In many states in the United States, the death rate has outpaced the birthrate. Between July 1, 2020 and June 30, 2021, more deaths occurred in the following regions:

- 78% of the Northwest
- 65% in the South
- 33% in the Midwest (Johnson & Sabo, 2022)

Maine, Rhode Island, and West Virginia were the only three states that saw more deaths than births in two consecutive years of 2019 and 2020 (Johnson, 2021).

The Age Dependency Ratio

The **age dependency ratio** consists of three groups: people from 0 to 14 years old, people 15 to 64, and people 65+. These data capture the dependency ratio of younger and older populations compared to the working-age population group. Governments and those between 15 and 64 bear the dependency burden of the other two age groups (Central Intelligence Agency, n.d.).

- For those between age 0 to 14, this means schools and child services.
- For those between 65+, this means healthcare and pensions.

In 2020, about 1 in 6 people were age 65 and over. One hundred years ago, less than 1 in 20 people were 65 and older. From 2010 to 2020, the 65+ population experienced its largest-ever percentage growth from 13% to 16.8% (U.S. Census, 2023).

The growth of the nonworking aging population (13%) is outpacing the growth of working-age people (3.1%) (Rogers & Wilder, 2020). This is often represented by an age dependency ratio.

- By looking at Figure 22-2, you can see an increasing number of younger, working-age adults are needed to provide support for older adults.
- This figure shows the age dependency ratio in 2010 as compared with 2019 (Rogers & Wilder, 2020).
- These data could be interpreted as alarming, but as C/PHNs, you should consider these data from a public health lens.
  - Policies that support health across the lifespan can increase healthy years, including those working years.
  - Not all older adults want complete or even partial retirements.
  - Encouraging employment opportunities for all working age people can help with the age dependency ratio.
- Finally, C/PHNs can educate and advocate for policies that support health, such as decreasing smoking and substance use disorders, and increasing access to and quality of care. By addressing social and economic factors, C/PHNs can help improve life expectancy and reduce the age dependency ratio.

However, more interesting is that the labor force participation rate for the age 75+ population is the only age group that is expected to grow from 8.9% in 2020 to 11.7% in 2030 (Bureau of Labor Statistics, 2021). This may reflect the improved health status of the age group or be necessary due to economic reasons.

Until the COVID-19 pandemic, the national trend was toward longer life expectancy. Between 2019 and 2021, the U.S. life expectancy declined 2.7 years, from 78.8 to 76.1, which represents the largest decline in life expectancy in one hundred years (Hill & Artiga, 2023). Some analysis identifies the COVID-19 pandemic as the primary driver of life expectancy decline, with the pandemic disproportionately affecting people of color as compared with White people (Hill & Artiga, 2023).

Despite the overall trend toward increased life expectancy, disparities exist among various subgroups in the population. Life expectancy is highest for White Americans and lowest for Black Americans, who have the highest death rates of any of the racial and ethnic groups in the United States (Hill & Artiga, 2023).

To help address these health disparities, the Racial and Ethnic Approaches to Community Health (REACH) (CDC, 2023a) (Box 22-1) program supports community-based coalitions in the design, implementation, and evaluation of innovative strategies to reduce or eliminate health disparities among racial and ethnic underrepresented groups. The goal of REACH is to achieve health equity, eliminate disparities, and improve the health of all groups (CDC, 2023a).

Growth in the number of older adults will significantly affect healthcare resources, housing options for older adults, and national longevity statistics. As the number of older people increases, so, too, will their need for assistance with activities of daily living (ADLs) and other services, especially those people with AD and other dementias. Many will serve as caregivers to family members who need assistance in attending to ADLs such as dressing, eating, toileting, and bathing, and researchers are seeking effective methods for providing respite to caregivers and reducing costs. Laws pertaining to healthcare and social services are being passed to better address the needs of older adults, most of whom will remain in the community. The Administration on Community Living, along with the National Family Caregivers Support Project Program, provides grants to states and territories to provide five types of services (Administration for Community Living, 2022):

- Information to caregivers about available services
- Assistance to caregivers in gaining access to the services
- Individual counseling, organization of support groups, and caregiver training
- Respite care
- Supplemental services, on a limited basis

These services are designed to work with other state- and community-based services to provide a coordinated set of supports. Studies have shown that these services can reduce caregiver burnout and stress and keep them healthy, delaying the need for costly assisted living or **nursing home** care (Administration for Community Living, 2022).

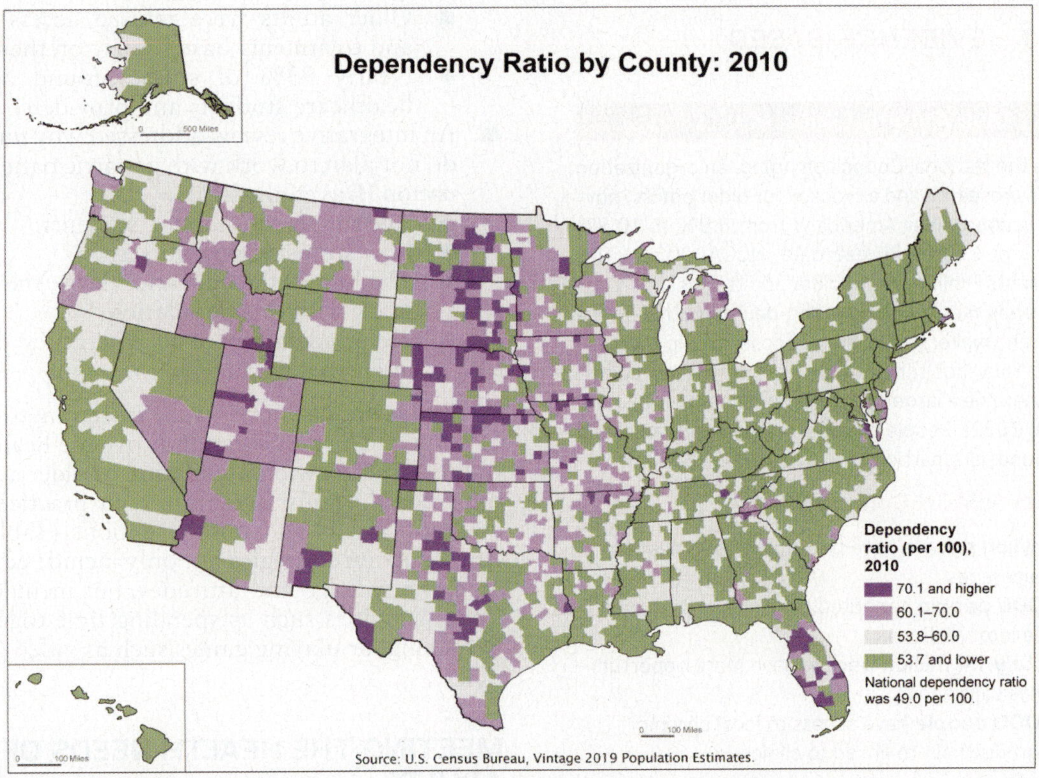

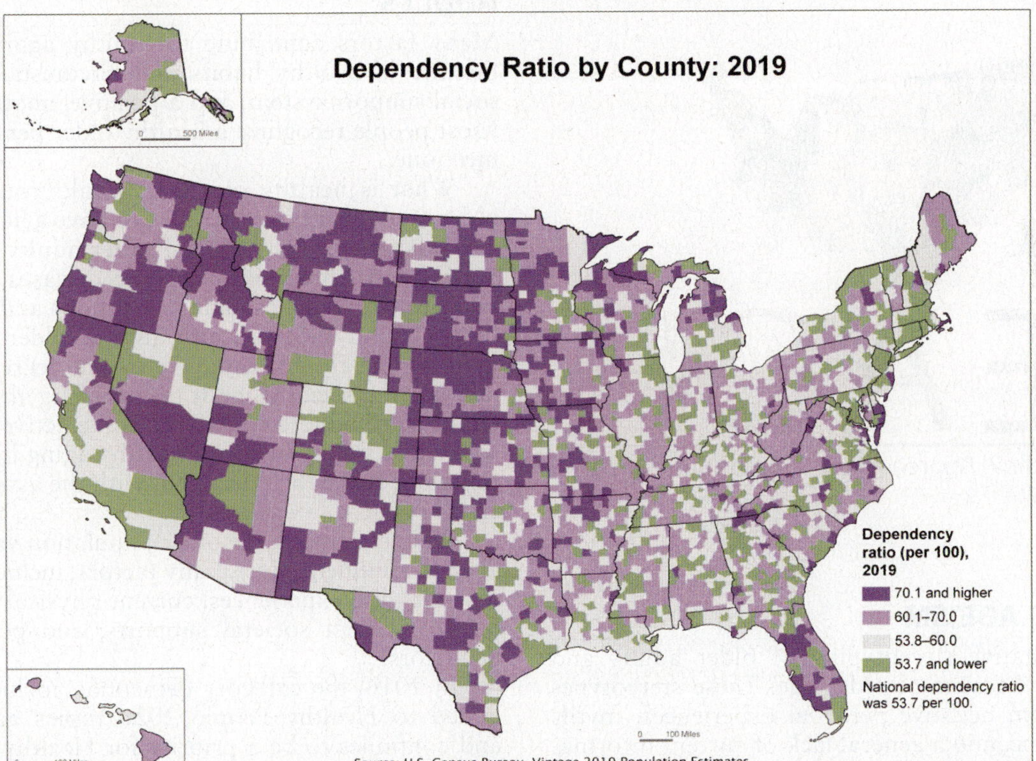

FIGURE 22-2 Age dependency ratio by County in 2010 as compared with 2019. (Reprinted from United States Census Bureau. (2020, June 25). *Shift in working-age populations relative to older and younger Americans.* https://www.census.gov/library/stories/2020/06/working-age-population-not-keeping-pace-with-growth-in-older-americans.html)

BOX 22-1 EVIDENCE-BASED PRACTICE

Poverty Increase Among Older Adults

According to the National Council on Aging, an organization that provides research and advocacy for older adults, poverty increased among older Americans from 8.9% to 10.3% in 2021, looking at Census Bureau data (NCOA, 2022). This increase represents 1 million more older adults who are struggling to make ends meet. Consider the decisions that these older adults might make; would they choose to skip medications, or would they not turn on the heat or the air conditioner? Could there be a large growth in homelessness in older adults? (Bolton, 2022). People of underrepresented racial and ethnic backgrounds are particularly at risk (CDC, 2023a).

Impact Across REACH Communities

- **Over 2.9 million people** have better access to healthy foods and beverages.
- **Over 322,000 people** benefited from smoke-free and tobacco-free interventions.
- **Approximately 1.4 million people** have more opportunities to be physically active.
- **Over 830,000 people** have access to local chronic disease programs that are linked to clinics.

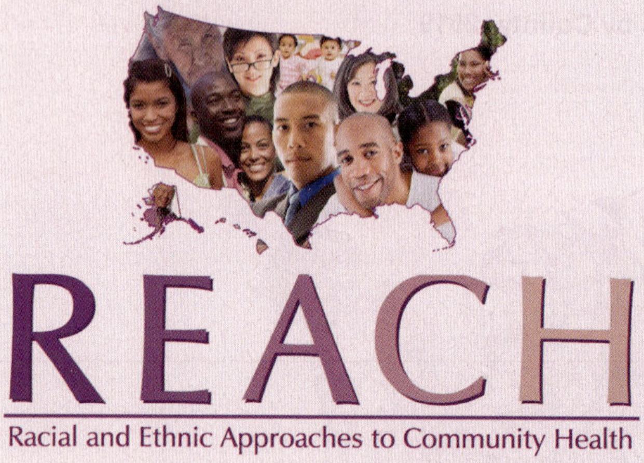

DISPELLING AGEISM

Ageism is negative stereotyping of older adults and discrimination because of older age. These stereotypes often arise from negative personal experiences, myths shared over time, and a general lack of current information.

- Most older adults report having experienced ageism in the form of being patronized, ignored, or treated as if they were incompetent (Martínez-Angulo et al., 2023).
- A systemic review found ageism has a significant effect on health (Chang et al., 2020).
  - Older adults were not included in research studies that would benefit them.
  - Older adults were refused access to healthcare and treatments based solely on their age.
  - Nearly 93% of studies found ageism among healthcare students and providers.
- An integrative review addressed why nursing students do not plan to work with geriatric patients after graduation (Dai et al., 2021).
  - Ageism among nursing students.
  - Low status among nurses.
  - The higher the education level, the least likely to work with this population.
  - Preferred fast pace of emergency department or intensive care unit.

By becoming more aware of the myths and realities of older age, C/PHNs can improve the health and quality of life of the growing population of older adults. C/PHNs must guard against ageism in their practice by dispelling common myths and misconceptions (Table 22-1). Ageism reduction strategies not only include education about aging knowledge and attitudes, but include intergenerational activities such as spending time together cooking, gardening, or playing games such as video games (WHO, 2021).

MEETING THE HEALTH NEEDS OF OLDER ADULTS

Many factors contribute to healthy aging, including a lifetime of healthy habits and circumstances, a strong social support system, and a positive emotional outlook. Most people recognize a healthy older person when they meet one.

What is healthy old age? Would you consider the older adult clients in Box 22-2 to have a healthy old age? The vast majority (94%) of older adults in the United States, even those with chronic diseases or other disabilities, are living outside institutions and are relatively independent. Good health in the older adult means maintaining the maximum possible degree of physical, mental, and social vigor. It means being able to adapt, to continue to handle stress, and to be active and involved in life and living. In short, healthy aging is being able to function, even when disabled, with the assistance of others as needed.

Wellness among the older population varies considerably. It is influenced by many factors, including personality traits, life experiences, current physical and cognitive health, current societal supports, and personal health behaviors.

In 2016, the category dementias, including AD, was added to Healthy People 2020 topics and objectives, and continues to be a priority for Healthy People 2030. Important steps for the care of those with dementia and their caregivers include earlier diagnosis, reduction of severity of both cognitive and behavioral symptoms, and supporting caregivers (ODPHP, n.d.-b).

Other actions that can increase healthy aging include the following:

- Addressing health disparities among older adults
- Encouraging people to plan for end-of-life care and communicate their wishes through advance directives

TABLE **22-1** Myths About Older Adults

Myth	Reality
Senility: *It's normal for older adults to become confused, childlike, and forgetful. They become "senile."*	Certain parts of the brain do shrink, and some blood flow is reduced. Regardless, many older adults continue to think well. **Senility** and dementia are often equated. However, not all older adults develop dementia. Alzheimer dementia is the most common of all dementias (Alzheimer's Association, 2020).
Rocking chair: *As age increases, older adults withdraw, become inactive, and cease being productive.*	People live longer, work later, and live well with chronic conditions. People over 50 are firing up the longevity economy with "encore careers" (Halvorsen et al., 2022)
Homogeneity: *As older adults age, they lose their individual differences and become progressively more alike.*	"Young" and "old" are helpful when one considers living a long or a short period of time. However, despite looking different, older people feel about the same inside as they did when young. The move to slow or stop aging may not be helpful.
The old benefiting at the expense of the young: *Older people are pulling down the economy. We cannot afford longevity.*	The economy profits more from the wisdom of older workers than ever before (Kiger, 2023). Many grandparents care for their children and grandchildren, and Medicare and Medicaid keep older adults independent when younger people raise their families. The federal government established an advisory council to help older adults raise grandchildren in the *Supporting Grandparents Raising Grandchildren Act* (2018). We can provide for healthcare and retirement if we use our resources wisely (Sol Price School of Public Policy, 2023).
Inability: *Older adults are unable to learn new things and are set in their old ways of doing things.*	Learning is a lifetime ability that continues into old age. Although older adults may experience some difficulty with short-term (or working) memory as they get older, their long-term memory generally remains sound. People at any age can learn new information and skills. Studies show learning new things helps memory (National Institute of Aging, 2024).

- Improving oral health
- Increasing physical activity among older adults by promoting environmental changes
- Increasing adult immunization levels
- Preventing falls

Some older adults demonstrate maximum adaptability, resourcefulness, optimism, and activity. Others, often those from whom we tend to draw our stereotypes, present a picture of dependence and resignation. Most older adults are somewhere in between these two extremes.

The goals in community and public health nursing is to maximize the wellness potential of older adult clients and to support their highest level of functional ability. The C/PHN must analyze and build on an older person's strengths rather than focus on the difficulties or deficits.

BOX **22-2** STORIES FROM THE FIELD

Forever on My Heart

When I served as a case manager for the county aging agency, I saw older clients living in their own homes or apartments. While each had their own story, a few are imprinted forever on my memory. One of my clients lived in an old trailer in a mobile home park. She was bitter and still complained about her ex-husband who left her for another woman 50+ years ago. I saw her weekly to provide social support and to manage her health needs. I believe I was the only support she had. She had no family, no children, and no friends in the community. One evening, I went to see her before leaving on a vacation and walked into her small cluttered mobile home, only to find her place smelled like gas. It was discovered she had a gas leak. I shut off the gas and waited for the gas company to make an emergency visit. They were able to fix the gas leak. The client agreed to be evaluated by the local hospital and was released the next day.

Ron was an older adult who began to go blind before I was assigned as his case manager. His story was heart-wrenching. His wife had died while they were sitting on the couch watching TV; his son had died from a heroin overdose. Both these deaths took place in the apartment where I visited him. He lived in Section 8 housing for those with lower income. Previously, he lived in a wealthy area of a metropolitan city where he owned a restaurant. As his eyesight declined and the economy weakened, he was forced to retire and sell the business. In contrast to the previous client, who was bitter with no support, this client had a host of friends. He was giving to the community. He helped others and was generally happy. Once, he told me how beautiful I was, which I responded to laughing saying how could he tell what I looked like since he was blind. We had a good laugh together. Why are people so different? One thing I learned during my employment with the agency is that our clients deserve our care and knowledge. There are clients you will never forget; they leave a permanent mark on our souls that reinforces why we became RNs.

—Charlene, RN, PHN

1. *How would you begin your in-home visit with a client?*
2. *What assessments could be helpful (social, spiritual, mental/cognitive, etc.)?*
3. *What resources and services might be helpful to them?*

LEVELS OF PREVENTION

Older adults, like any age group, have certain basic needs: Physiologic and safety needs, as well as the needs for love and belonging, self-esteem, and self-actualization. Their physical, emotional, and social needs are complex and interrelated. The following sections discuss these needs according to primary, secondary, and tertiary prevention activities. Box 22-3 provides an example of the three levels of prevention.

Primary Prevention

Primary prevention activities involve actions that keep one healthy. Activities such as health education, follow-through of sound personal health practices (e.g., flossing, seat belt use, exercise), and maintenance of an appropriate immunization schedule ensure that older adults are doing all that they can to maintain their health. The following topics are all considered primary prevention strategies.

BOX 22-3 LEVELS OF PREVENTION PYRAMID

SITUATION: Making a healthy transition into a satisfying old age

GOAL: Using the three levels of prevention, prevent or delay chronic diseases, promptly diagnose and treat conditions, and restore to the fullest possible potential.

Transitioning to Older Age

Tertiary Prevention

Rehabilitation

- Adapt to changed roles with spouse and significant others.
- Maintain health while assessing increasing dependency needs, including alternative housing, modifications in transportation, and changing healthcare needs.

Health Promotion and Education

- Periodically review and update will, insurances, and other important documents as needed.
- Keep beneficiaries or executors aware of changes in and location of documents and personal wishes regarding end-of-life care and funeral/burial arrangements.

Health Protection

- Review medications, prescription and over-the-counter, on a regular basis.
- Explore and provide community resources as needs change.

Secondary Prevention

Early Diagnosis

- See Chapter 21 recommendations for screenings for adults.
- Follow the U.S. Task Force Recommendations for regular screening of potential health problems (USPSTF, n.d.-a).
- Focus on results of the Medicare Annual Wellness Visit (Centers for Medicare and Medicaid Services [CMS], 2023) results or screen for cognitive impairment and depression symptoms.
- Assess for social engagement: volunteerism, faith-based activities, family, and support of others.
- Assess for caregiver health and burden levels.

Prompt Treatment

- Provide resources for social engagement: healthy, satisfying, and enriching activities.
- Follow-up on any unexpected findings, keeping any family or caregivers informed.
- Manage vision, hearing problems.
- Provide strategies for behaviors resulting from cognitive problems.
- Provide community resources to prevent caregiver burnout.

Primary Prevention

Health Promotion and Education

- Begin preparations early—emotional, spiritual, and financial.
- Plan ahead for changes in health status and potential need for long-term care.
- Complete documents, such as a will and a living will.

Health Protection

- Regularly assess health status.
- Follow the recommended schedule for immunizations of the Centers for Disease Control and Prevention (2024a; https://www.cdc.gov/vaccines/imz-schedules/adult-easyread.html).
- Medicare Wellness visit.
- Include oral examination in routine medical and nursing visits.
- Implement a health-promoting regimen that includes diet and exercise.
- Assess living environment for comfort and safety hazards.

Nutrition and Oral Health Needs

People who have maintained sound dietary habits throughout their life have little need to change in old age. However, the proportion of adults with obesity is growing as they age, threatening longevity and healthy aging (ODPHP, n.d.-c). Given the linkage of chronic conditions like type 2 diabetes, cardiovascular disease, and some cancers to diet, older adults need to eat a healthy diet. The U.S. Department of Agriculture (USDA, n.d.-a) replaced the food pyramid with MyPlate as a visual to guide the food intake of Americans. Tufts University has modified MyPlate for older adults (see https://hnrca.tufts.edu/myplate). The modifications include an emphasis on drinking plenty of fluids, including water, and consuming a diet high in fiber. Although multivitamins are not meant to replace food as a source of nutrients, taking them as a supplement to food to achieve recommended intakes may be a good idea (Fantacone et al., 2020). USDA (n.d.-b) provides helpful tools and recommendations for older adults on their website at https://www.myplate.gov/life-stages/older-adults.

It is generally believed that older people need to maintain their optimal weight by eating a diet that is low in fats, moderate in carbohydrates, and high in proteins with a daily calorie count of 1200 to 1600 (Fig. 22-3).

Older adults need less vitamin A than younger adults. They need more calcium and vitamin D (for healthy bones), more folic acid, and more vitamins B6 and B12 (for cognitive health).

Many communities offer meals to older people, either at centers for older adults or by way of Meals on Wheels, through grants provided by the Older Adult Nutrition Program (Administration for Community Living, 2024b).

Oral health is integral to general health and well-being throughout one's life. Major advances in the field of oral health—including community water fluoridation, advanced dental technology, better oral hygiene, and more frequent use of dental services—have had a substantial impact on the number of older adults who retain their natural teeth.

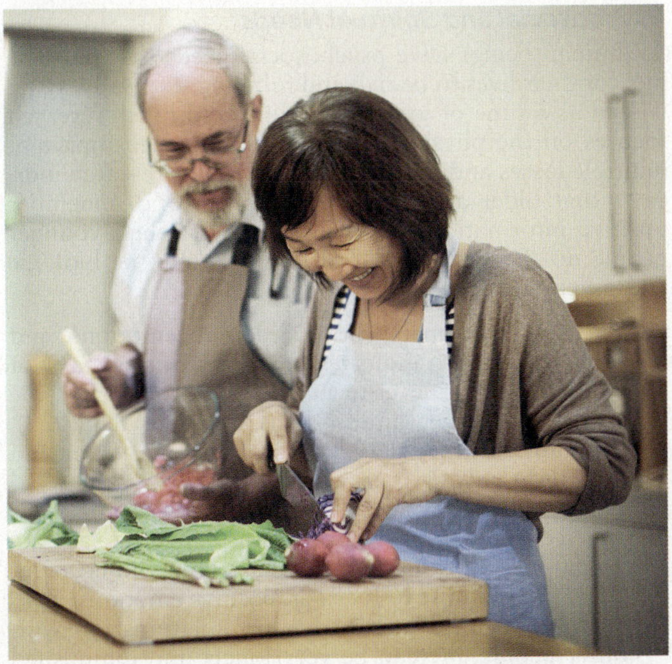

FIGURE 22-3 Preparing and eating meals can be an uncomplicated, natural process that can be shared with others.

- The percentage of adults aged 65 or over with a dental visit in the past year was 65.6% (CDC, 2023b).
- Healthy People 2030 guidelines address oral health and maintenance, with a focus for older adults receiving treatment for root decay (ODPHP, n.d.-d).

Poor oral health has been associated with peripheral vascular disease, diabetes, and risk for death caused by respiratory illness (Kotronia et al., 2021). Even those with dentures must be vigilant in maintaining oral health, as they are still at risk from inflammatory processes leading to diseases such as pneumonia. Many older adults, especially those who have limited incomes, have decreased nutritional and fluid intake, changes in gums, increased periodontal disease, and a higher incidence of dry mouth.

Fluid intake and oral hygiene are appropriate topics for anticipatory guidance from C/PHNs working with older adults. Take the time to assess the older adult's oral cavity, including mucosa, denture fit, and any complaints about chewing or swallowing.

In addition to maintaining a healthy diet, older adults are cautioned to limit their use of alcohol. Researchers noticed that during the COVID-19 pandemic, older people with chronic conditions were drinking at a higher rate. Although this rate has decreased since 2020, screening for unsafe alcohol use would be something a C/PHN could consider (Phillips et al., 2023).

As with all adults, older people should avoid tobacco, drink fluoridated water or use fluoride toothpaste, practice good oral hygiene, and have regular dental checkups. They should also avoid the habitual use of laxatives, instead adding more fluids, fiber, and bulk to their diet with fresh fruits and vegetables. Also, inadequate fluid intake can contribute to bowel and bladder problems. Increased physical activity and exercise help maintain regularity of bowel function in older adults.

Exercise Needs

Older adults need to exercise; in fact, they thrive when exercise is incorporated into their daily routine (National Institute on Aging, 2020). Research demonstrates that exercise and increased physical activity have multiple benefits for older adults, including the following:

- Arthritis relief, restoration of balance and reduction of falls, strengthening of bone, proper weight maintenance, and improvements in glucose control, cognitive and brain function, and overall mortality (Malapaz et al., 2022)
- Healthy cognition, improved sleep, and reduced risk of heart disease (Ghosh et al., 2024; Murray et al., 2023; Song et al., 2024)
- Decreased incidence of osteoporotic fractures due to a reduced risk of falling, with an exercise routine that includes activities to improve strength, flexibility, and coordination, even among the very old

The C/PHN should explore the kinds of activity that appeal to older adults, including walks. A wide variety of activities are appropriate for and benefit older adults:

- A PhD student team designed a walking intervention that tested their theory that older people would be more likely to stick to a 16-week peer-led walking group to promote walking behavior if they walked in small groups. The authors found that motivation, walking self-efficacy, balance, and physical activity improved more in participants who walked in groups than those who walked alone (Kritz et al., 2021).
- Exercise may occur with others in connection with such activities as homemaking chores, gardening, hobbies, or recreation and sports.
- Resistance training (with small dumbbells or resistance bands), along with either Tai Chi or regular walking, has been shown to increase muscle strength, stability, and functional ability among older adults (Healthfinder.gov, 2023).
- Physical disabilities need not be a barrier to exercise, as there are specialized exercise programs (e.g., chair aerobics, wheelchair fitness).

Sleep

Sleep is another area of focus in *Healthy People* and is important to older adults for the following reasons:

- In older adults, adequate sleep is necessary to fight off infection and support the metabolism of sugar to prevent diabetes or to work effectively and safely.
- Sleep timing and duration affect endocrine, metabolic, and neurologic functions critical to individual health maintenance.
- Untreated sleep disorders and chronic short sleep are associated with an increased risk of depression, heart disease, high blood pressure, obesity, diabetes, and all-cause mortality (Koffel et al., 2023).

Some changes in sleep are natural with aging, such as follows:

- Decreased slow-wave or deep sleep due to the body producing lower levels of growth hormone
- Altered circadian rhythms (the internal clock that tells one when to sleep and when to wake up), causing the older adult to want to go to sleep earlier in the evening
- Nighttime wakefulness and interrupted sleep due to pain, the need to void, medications, and snoring, which may worsen with age (Koffel et al., 2023)

The C/PHN can assess and help older adults having sleep challenges:

- Ask them to keep a sleep journal.
- Investigate their nighttime voiding patterns.
- For men, assess for the possibility of an enlarged prostate, which can cause problems with complete bladder emptying and may need treatment.

Objectives for Healthy People 2030 focus on reduction of accidents due to driving while drowsy, providing treatment for those with obstructive sleep apnea, and sufficient sleep (ODPHP, n.d.-e).

Economic Security Needs and Poverty

Economic security is a major need for older adults. Many older adults work beyond retirement age for reasons of enjoyment and purpose, but they may also be concerned about having financial stability through the rest of their lives. Factors affecting economic security in older adults include the following:

- Having to spend retirement resources caring for older parents or grandchildren
- Limited income and reliance on Social Security and Supplemental Security Income, with one fourth of all people on Medicare in 2023 having incomes of <$21,000 (Cottrill et al., 2024).

Fearing the potential cost of major illness and wanting to avoid being a burden on family or friends, many older people conserve their limited finances by practices that may threaten their health:

- Adopting frugal eating patterns
- Skipping or taking only partial doses of medications
- Limiting the use of home heating and cooling
- Spending little on themselves, in general

For older adults today who have lived many years past retirement without sufficient financial security to maintain them throughout these additional years, fears are not unfounded.

Many older adults are not aware that there are important preventive health measures and community-based programs that can maximize function and help older adults maintain health at a higher level (U.S. Preventive Services Task Force [USPSTF], n.d.-b). C/PHNs should be familiar with and share with their clients, local support services that may provide housing, food, and utilities for older people in need, which can do much to help relieve the source of that stress and anxiety.

Psychosocial and Spiritual Needs

All human beings have psychosocial needs that must be met for their lives to be rich and fulfilling. Typically, aging is seen as a time of loss and decline, and much research focuses on the physiologic and psychological impact of multiple losses and decline. However, some research indicates that older adults pay attention to and remember positive information and memories more than younger people do (Barber et al., 2020). There may be biologic and psychological reasons for this:

- The amygdala in the brain reacts to emotions, and biologic research indicates that older adults may not react at a brain level to negative information in the way the younger adults do (Doucet et al., 2023), meaning that they may be more likely to gather and hold onto only their good memories.
- For many, old age may be a time of life reflection, review, and reevaluation of what gives meaning and satisfaction in life. Knowing that they have limited time, older adults may choose to focus on positive emotions.
- However, with a lack of healthy relationships with other people, life can be very lonely and diminished in quality for older people.

Holistic nursing is a hallmark of community and public health nursing. This means a focus on the body, mind, and spirit. The word spirit comes from the Latin meaning "breath" and refers to the core of an individual, the part that gives meaning to life (New World Encyclopedia, n.d.). Although related, religion and spirituality are distinct concepts:

- A spiritual component exists in all people but not everyone is religious.
- Religion is generally recognized to be the practical expression of spirituality or the organization, rituals, and practice of one's beliefs.
- Religion includes specific beliefs and practices, whereas spirituality is far broader.

According to the Pew Forum, belief in God continues to be very important to older adults, including the younger baby boomers, even though religious practices vary (Pew Research Center, 2022). Whereas other sources of well-being decline, religion may become more important over time. People within different cultures have varying philosophies and practices of spirituality but derive similar positive outcomes.

Faith community nursing is one of the community nursing roles that epitomizes this holistic approach of caring for one's clients, many of whom are older adults. More information on this unique role for C/PHNs can be found on the Faith Community Nurses International website https://www.fcninternational.org/Becoming-a-Faith-Community-Nurse. (Roles and settings for C/PHNs can be found in Chapter 2.)

Coping With Multiple Losses and Suicide. Older adults may experience multiple losses, including loss of income and purpose from a career once practiced, loss of the economic stability of employment, and loss of space due to replacement of a larger residence, where the older adult may have raised a family. The loss of a spouse after 50 years of marriage may have a huge impact on the remaining partner. Short- or long-term declines in health may result in pain or limited mobility and may necessitate multiple moves, such as a move to a child's home, a move to an assisted living facility, and a move to a skilled living facility. Repetitive losses occur as significant others, relatives, friends, and acquaintances die. There is no right or wrong way to grieve, but there are healthy and unhealthy ways to cope with the pain. Assisting older adults with handling these losses is an important role of the C/PHN. To do this, C/PHNs need to be aware of some of the facts about grief.

Inadequate coping with compounding losses can make an older person believe that life holds no meaning. Depression may be a difficult problem for older adults. Social and emotional withdrawal can often occur, as can suicide.

- Among the risk factors for suicidal behavior in older adults are the loss of a spouse; having other mental disorders, such as dementia and depression; physical illnesses or decline; and social isolation.
- Although older populations have a much lower rate of suicide attempts than younger age groups do, the rate of completed suicide is high (NCOA, 2022). The rates of suicide may be underreported, given the negative stigma around suicide, especially in older adults.

Community health nurses should be observant of risk factors and be prepared to ask questions, including whether the client is suicidal, as older adults are not likely to talk about the subject. Asking someone whether they are suicidal does not put the idea in the person's head. This is a myth. Most people are grateful that they have been asked. If you think someone is suicidal, do not let them be left alone; seek further services for the older adult. The Brief Geriatric Suicide Ideation Scale is one of several scales for assessing suicide risks (Heisel & Flett, 2022).

Older adults who have maintained good health and developed a supportive system of family and friends have more fulfilling lives (Fig. 22-4). Churches, universities, and older adult service programs often have volunteers who regularly meet with isolated older adults either in their homes or **long-term care** facilities, increasing social support for those who have no family members nearby.

Explore the services for older adults available in your community on the internet. Good examples are the local Area Agency on Aging (AAA), the local health department, community centers for older adults, and the YMCA. Some counties have a resources guide. The Eldercare Locator, available at https://eldercare.acl.gov/Public/Index.aspx, can provide current information on local caregiver services and resources.

Maintaining Independence. The need for autonomy—to be able to assert oneself as a separate individual—is important for all people. Independence helps to meet the need for self-respect and dignity.

- Older adults need to have their ideas and suggestions heard and acted upon, and they ought to be addressed by their preferred names in a respectful tone of voice.
- Respect for older adults is not a strong value in American society, but it is highly valued in Asian, Italian, Hispanic, and Native American cultures.
- Older people represent a rich resource of wisdom, experience, and patience that is often unacknowledged in the United States.

Older adults who are in poverty, underrepresented groups, or veterans and who experience poorer health need support at home to remain independent. Communities work with local, state, and federal agencies to create programs to provide support to older adults who need assistance but want to remain in their home communities.

- A good example of a program supporting older veterans at home is the Veteran in Charge program in Colorado Springs, Colorado.
  - This program allows veterans to receive community-based services to continue living in their homes as long as possible and gives them control of the who, what, when, and how much related to the care (https://www.theindependencecenter.org/veterans/).

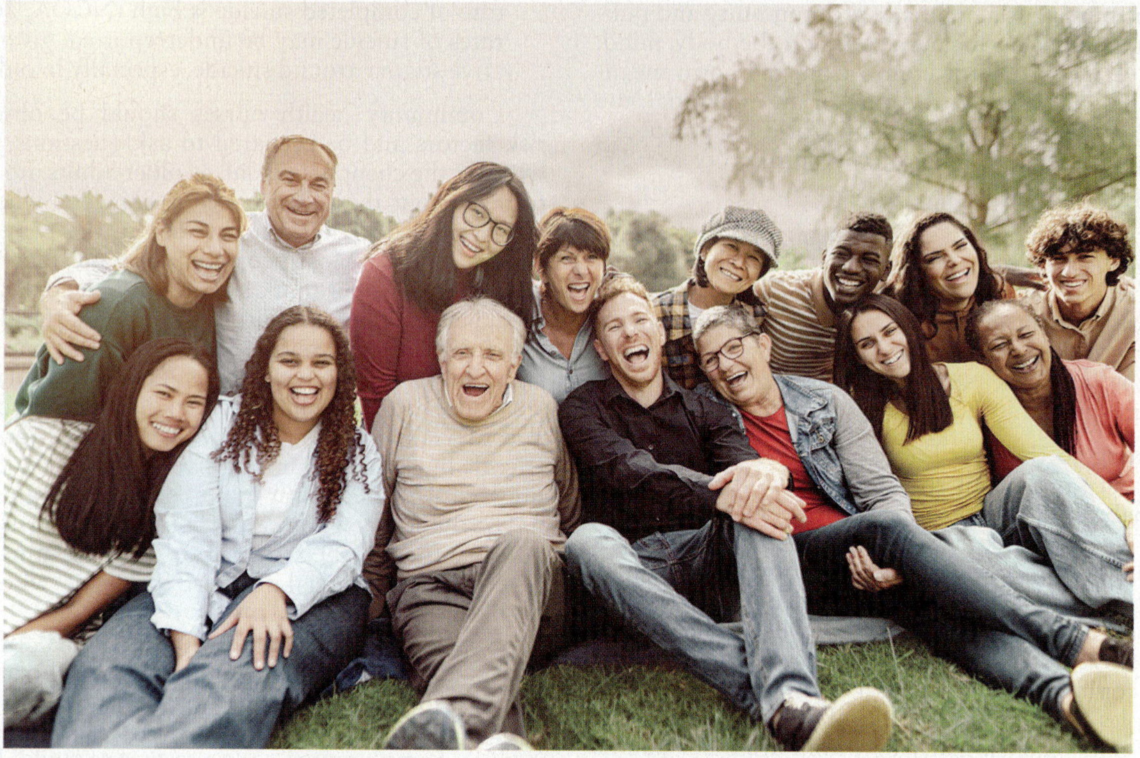

FIGURE 22-4 A supportive system of family and friends helps older adults meet their psychosocial needs.

Interaction, Companionship, and Purpose. Baby boomers turning 65 in 2024 are the largest single group to turn 65 in any given year, and they have changed the face of aging (Kiger, 2023). Many adults at age 65 feel that full-time retirement is not for them. This may be, in part, due to several reasons: job satisfaction or financially unable to retire, or better health than previous generations (Kiger, 2023). As the largest and healthiest aging cohort, they may also be the most engaged. Adults in this generation are known for a strong work ethic, developing relationships, and add value to both the workforce and society in general.

However, not everyone will be employed after the age of 65. Some may be challenged with physical or mental difficulties or caring for spouses or parents. A new phrase in our language is "Grand families." It is possible that grandparents and even great-grandparents may be cutting into their own finances to care for grandchildren whose parents may have been deployed or are struggling with substance misuse.

Programs exist to support older adult caregivers.

- Examples include the federally supported Foster Grandparents and Senior Companions programs, which engage millions of Americans in service (Fig. 22-5).
- These older adults work part-time, offering companionship and guidance to children with disabilities, people with a terminal illness, and other people in need (AmeriCorp, n.d.).
- Depending on each state's Medicaid rules, some family members may be compensated for caregiving, and the need for caregiving support will increase with the growing numbers of older people who will, at some time, need in-home support and services.

In cases where family and social networks have weakened, C/PHNs and others can help to improve their psychosocial health by working at the individual, family, and community levels. The problem is of greatest significance for women, who outnumber men considerably in the later years and who more frequently live alone. Take time to explore activities that older adults can do from home: letter writing, volunteer phone calling, or crafting for others who are ill.

Safety and Health Needs

Safety issues are a major concern for older adults and the C/PHNs who work with them. Several areas of focus are discussed here: personal health and safety, home safety, and community safety.

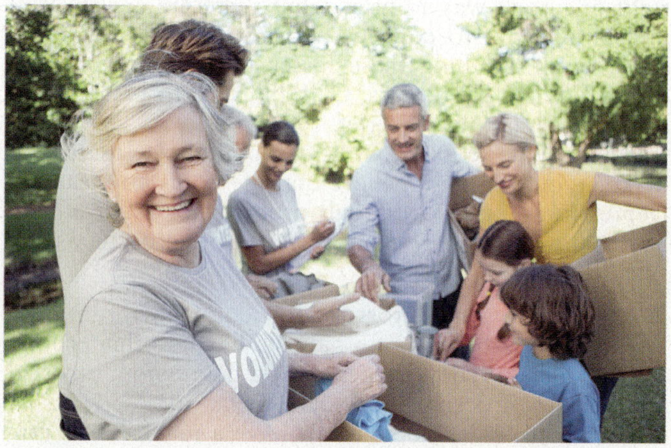

FIGURE 22-5 Volunteering can be a rewarding experience for older adults.

BOX 22-4 C/PHN USE OF THE NURSING PROCESS/CLINICAL JUDGMENT

Falls Among Older Adults in the Community

A C/PHN working part time in an emergency department notices a high incidence of falls among older adults in the community. The nurse discovers that the local center for older adults has expressed a need for an exercise class but does not have the funding to start the class. The average age at the center is 75+, and the participants are mainly women. They have expressed an interest in the exercise class.

Assessment/Recognize Cues

You do the following:

- Meet with older adults at the community center to determine possible risk factors in their living arrangements.
- Meet with older adults to determine their willingness to participate in self-care activities.
- Interview center staff to enlist their feedback on possible risks and solutions.

Diagnosis/Analyze Cues and Prioritize Hypotheses

After completing your assessment, you decide a nursing diagnosis would look at:

- Possible risk for falls related to home environment conditions
- Lack of center financial resources
- Willingness of participants for self-care

Planning and Implementation/Generate Solutions and Take Action

- Contact local nursing programs and public health department to conduct home visits for safety checks.
- Research possible grants to hire instructor at center to conduct class.
- Reach out to community leaders and volunteer groups to update living environments of the older population to ensure safety.
- Implement strategies to prevent falls through dance class, exercise class, stretching class at the center.

Evaluation/Evaluate Outcomes

After 1 month, the emergency department (ED) reported a decrease in visits related to falls in older adults. In addition, C/PHN students at a local university have conducted 25 home visits to conduct safety checks. The center has been raising funds for an exercise bike and has raised over 60% of the needed funds so far. Evaluation of the nursing diagnoses includes the following goals:

- Older adults will have no fall-related injuries.
- Older adults will be free of falls.
- Older adult living conditions will be free from any risk factors that may cause falls.
- Center will offer exercise course for older adults to strengthen gait and mobility.

Personal health and safety include three major areas: immunizations, home safety and prevention of falls, and drug safety (Box 22-4).

Immunizations. Older adults are at increased risk for many vaccine-preventable diseases. Preventable illnesses cause substantial morbidity and mortality in older patients, who tend to have more medical comorbidities and are at higher risk for complications.

- Vaccination rates in the United States do not meet targets for vaccinations that protect against flu and pneumonia, with even greater disparities noted among underrepresented races and ethnicities (Hung et al., 2022).
- Healthy People 2030 objectives target a reduction in hospital admissions due to pneumonia by older adults (ODPHP, n.d.-f)
- Not only do respiratory illnesses contribute to the mortality rates of older adults, but they also exacerbate chronic conditions like congestive heart failure asthma or COPD) (National Foundation for Infectious Diseases, 2023).

In 2022, older people consisted of 16% of the population but comprised 75% of COVID-19 deaths (Harris, 2023). Although vaccinations, boosters, and care helped bring down the death toll during COVID-19, the slow response to COVID-19 booster immunizations led to an increase in the number of COVID-19 deaths the summer and fall of 2022 (Ndugga et al., 2022).

SARS-CoV-2 variants circulating in the population are closely related to the 2023–2024 COVID-19 vaccines. The updated COVID-19 vaccines may be taken with the annual flu vaccine, which improves the likelihood that an older adult will be protected against both respiratory diseases (CDC Newsroom, 2024). Keep in mind that many respiratory illnesses are vaccine preventable. The CDC regularly updates immunization guidelines for older adults (CDC, 2024a). (See Table 22-2 vaccinations available for older adults.)

Racial and ethnic disparities exist among older adults receiving vaccines; therefore, it is important to engage in outreach efforts to these populations, such as culturally targeting communication, reaching out to those providers serving this population, and offering vaccination clinics in underserved sections of the community (Hill et al., 2023). Attempts to improve immunization coverage involve changing provider knowledge, attitudes, and behavior through reminders and standing orders, so that "missed opportunities" when seeing clients are prevented. Additional opportunities for vaccinating people exist beyond the primary care setting, including supermarkets, pharmacies, and planned immunization public health events. Regardless of the site, a method for tracking and communicating vaccinations is needed so that vaccination information may be documented and shared with the client's primary care provider.

- Shingles is caused by the varicella–zoster virus (VZV); this is the same virus that causes chickenpox.
- Anyone who has had chickenpox can develop shingles because VZV remains in the nerve cells of the body after the chickenpox infection clears, and VZV can reappear many years later causing shingles.

TABLE 22-2 Recommended Adult Immunization Schedule

Vaccine	Age >65	Dose/Schedule
COVID-19	Yes	At least one dose of current COVID-19 vaccine
Influenza (inactive or recombinant)	Yes	1 dose annually
Respiratory syncytial virus (RSV)	Maybe >60	Single dose with consultation with the primary provider
Recombinant zoster vaccine (RZV, Shingrix)	Recommended for adults 50 and older	Two doses for immunocompromising conditions
Pneumococcal	Yes	Depends on vaccination history, but at least one dose of PCV 20 at least 5 years after the last dose

Source: Recommended Adult Immunization Schedule (CDC, 2024a). See https://www.cdc.gov/vaccines/imz-schedules/adult-easyread.html for the full table and notes (14 vaccines).

Shingles is a very painful localized skin rash, often with blisters. The disease most commonly occurs in people 50 years or older, people who have medical conditions that keep the immune system from working properly, or people who receive immunosuppressive medications. The current vaccination program for VZV is included in Table 22-2. Shingrix provides strong protection against shingles, and C/PHNs should advise clients to talk with their provider about receiving this vaccine.

Fall Prevention. According to the CDC (2023c) STEADI fact sheet, every 20 minutes an older adult dies from a fall, and one in five falls causes a serious injury, such as head trauma or a fracture. Furthermore, fewer than half of those who fall talk to their primary provider about the fall. Injuries related to falls account for more than 3 million emergency department visits annually, as well as 32,000 deaths yearly. In fact, falls are the leading cause of injury-related deaths for age 65 and above (American Public Health Association [APHA], 2023). The APHA has a policy to address this public health problem which can be found at https://www.apha.org/policies-and-advocacy/public-health-policy-statements/policy-database/2024/01/16/falls-prevention. The policy provides a comprehensive approach to the prevention of falls that addresses multiple risk factors. Technology and wearable monitoring can be used to assist with safety concerns for older adults.

- Smart homes may include environmental, activity, and physiologic sensors, with more affordable systems being developed in a rapidly expanding market (Boxes 22-5 and 22-6). Smart homes are one strategy to safeguard older adult safety through alerts and notification related to falls, first aid, and detection of unattended cooking (Ma et al., 2022).

Risk factors for falls include (CDC, 2023d, para 4) the following:

- Difficulty with walking and balance
- Vitamin D deficiency
- Medications that affect balance such as tranquilizers, sedative, or antidepressants
- Vision problems
- Poor footwear
- Hazards such as throw rugs, clutter, and uneven steps

Medications. Older adults often have multiple chronic diseases for which they take prescription medications. It is not unusual for older people to be taking four to six medications daily. The use of multiple medications, called **polypharmacy**, is defined as using 5 to 10 prescription drugs (Alookaran & O'Sullivan, 2023). For example, an older adult with two chronic diseases, such as heart failure and COPD, is likely to take more than five medications.

A significant safety issue for older adults arises from the combined use of prescription and over-the-counter medications. Problems can arise from a single difficulty or a combination of issues such as follow:

- Number of medications taken daily
- Absorption rate of medications
- Drug interactions
- Side effects

In addition, the more medications taken daily, the higher the rate of nonadherence to the schedule (González-Bueno et al., 2021). This problem is compounded when older adults have visual or cognitive difficulties. That said, a common reason for not taking medications is "forgetting" (Epstein et al., 2022).

Older adults often receive multiple prescriptions from multiple providers and sometimes from multiple pharmacies, including mail-order pharmacies. They are less likely to see the pharmacist in person, and these circumstances put older adults at risk for receiving the same or similar medications in error.

- For example, an older adult living in the community has arthritis and heads to the pharmacy for pain management.
- Many of the pain medications the older adult considers contain acetaminophen (Tylenol).
- However, this older adult is already taking prescribed pain medication that contains acetaminophen and thus is at risk for overdosing.

BOX 22-5 Guidelines for Assessing the Safety of the Environment

Illumination and Color Contrast

- Is the lighting adequate but not glare producing?
- Are the light switches easy to reach and manipulate?
- Can lights be turned on before entering rooms?
- Are night-lights used in appropriate places?
- Are there working flashlights close by (bedroom, kitchen, bath, living room)?
- Is color contrast adequate between objects such as a chair and floor?

Hazards

- Are there throw rugs, highly polished floors, or other hazardous floor coverings?
- If area rugs are used, do they have a nonslip backing and are the edges tacked to the floor?
- Are there cords, clutter, or other obstacles in pathways?
- Is there a pet that is likely to be running underfoot?

Furniture

- Are chairs the right height and depth for the person?
- Do the chairs have armrests?
- Are tables stable and of the appropriate height?
- Is small furniture placed well away from pathways?

Stairways

- Is lighting adequate?
- Are there light switches at the top and bottom of the stairs?
- Are there securely fastened handrails on both sides of the stairway?
- Are all the steps even?
- Are the treads nonskid?
- Should colored tape be used to mark the edges of the steps, particularly the top and bottom steps?

Bathroom

- Are grab bars placed appropriately for the tub and toilet?
- Does the tub have skid-proof strips or a rubber mat in the bottom?
- Has the person considered using a tub seat?
- Is the height of the toilet seat appropriate?
- Has the person considered using an elevated toilet seat?
- Does the color of the toilet seat contrast with surrounding colors?
- Is toilet paper within easy reach?

Temperature

- Is the temperature of the room(s) comfortable?
- Can the person read the markings on the thermostat and adjust it appropriately?
- During cold months, is the room temperature high enough to prevent hypothermia?
- During hot weather, is the room temperature cool enough to prevent hyperthermia?

Overall Safety

- How does the person obtain objects from hard-to-reach places?
- How does the person change overhead light bulbs?
- Are doorways wide enough to accommodate assistive devices?
- Do door thresholds create hazardous conditions?
- Are telephones easily accessible, especially for emergency calls?
- Would it be helpful to use a cordless portable phone or a cellular phone?
- Would it be helpful to have some emergency call system available?
- Does the person wear sturdy shoes with nonskid soles?
- Are smoke alarms present and operational?
- Is there a carbon monoxide detector (if the house has gas appliances)?
- Does the person keep a list of emergency numbers by the phone?
- Does the person have an emergency exit plan in the event of fire?

Bedroom

- Is the height of the bed appropriate?
- Is the mattress firm at the edges to provide enough support for sitting?
- If the bed has wheels, are they locked securely?
- Would side rails be a help or a hazard?
- When side rails are in the down position, are they completely out of the way?
- Is the pathway between the bedroom and bathroom clear of objects and adequately illuminated, particularly at night?
- Would a bedside commode be useful, especially at night?
- Does the person have sufficient physical and cognitive ability to turn on a light before getting out of bed?
- Is furniture positioned to allow safe use of assistive devices for ambulation?
- Is a telephone situated near the bed?

Kitchen

- Are storage areas used to the best advantage (e.g., are objects that are most frequently used in the most accessible places)?
- Are appliance cords kept out of the way?
- Are nonslip mats used in front of the sink?
- Are the markings on stoves and other appliances clearly visible?
- Does the person know how to use the microwave oven and other appliances safely?

Assistive Devices

- What assistive devices are used?
- Is a call light available, and does the person know how to use it?
- Would the person benefit from any assistive devices that are not being used?
- Are assistive devices being used safely and properly, or do they present additional hazards?

Source: Miller (2019).

BOX 22-6 SPOTLIGHT ON ESSENTIAL NURSING COMPETENCIES

Quality and Safety Through Safe and Effective Care

Nurses must deliver safe and effective care. Not only must they be vigilant in the safety of the care they provide, but they are also tasked with proving a safe environment for the patient. In the community setting this can be difficult, because patients and families may need assistance or education regarding home safety. C/PHNs may be able to identify issues or concerns based on home visits and discussions with patients and their families and are positioned to provide support and education.

For example, a C/PHN working in a metropolitan city makes a home visit to Margaret, a 90-year-old living alone, following her hospitalization for a fall. The nurse discovers that despite using a walker, "Maggie" is spry, alert, and attentive. In the 900 square foot home, the nurse notes many small rugs scattered around and furniture cluttered within every room, limiting walking space. Maggie states that she has lived in this house for 70 years and is not moving. The daughter is present for the home visit, and the son lives two blocks away; both check in on their mother daily.

1. *What risks are presented in this situation?*
2. *How would you address safety for the patient and her family?*

Source: Lotas (2021).

Medication side effects or drug interactions can lead to falls and further disability. Older adults need education about the medications they take and their possible interactions and effects. They also need proper supervision of their overall medication intake, including complementary and alternative therapies (e.g., herbal treatments) and over-the-counter medications. It is important for all older adults to keep a list of their current medications and doses and to have this available in the event of an emergency. This is an area in which the C/PHN can intervene effectively (Box 22-7).

Research evidence shows that polypharmacy in older adults is being addressed by appropriate screening tools such as the Beer's criteria and STOPP Screening tool. C/PHNs can help by doing a thorough medication review with older adults (Box 22-7).

Safety in the Community. Safety can involve many things, such as pedestrian and driving issues, crime and fear of crime against older adults, and environmental factors such as sun exposure, pollution, heat, and cold.

Climate Change. Climate change has made exposure a topic of concern for older adults. The increasingly frequent natural disasters worldwide point to high health impacts for older adults who have higher mortality rates from storms, wildfires, heat, and flooding (Carlson et al., 2023). The impact of climate change matters across socio-economic status, where some older people are less adequately sheltered with access to heating, cooling, food, and water in a disaster situation (Carlson et al., 2023). C/PHNs can work with local and state health departments to create and implement action plans for climate crises that affect the health of older people.

Driving Safety. Because of age-related changes in vision, hearing, and mobility and the effects of polypharmacy, older adults are at risk in the community as both pedestrians and drivers. Automobile crashes and pedestrian injuries can be life-threatening events, especially when older people are involved. As pedestrians, older adults must be increasingly vigilant to traffic patterns, sidewalk irregularities, and the possibility of being a victim of street crime.

Often out of necessity and pride, older people may drive longer than their abilities permit. The C/PHN may recommend resources for families who need to talk about driving safety https://www.aarp.org/auto/driver-safety/we-need-to-talk/ (AARP, n.d.-a).

BOX 22-7 Preventing Polypharmacy in Older Adults

Below are some strategies you can use to help patients reduce the risk of polypharmacy.

Recommendations

- Use the correct medication, at the correct dose, and for the shortest duration.
- AMOR
  - **A**ssess medications and review for interaction.
  - **M**inimize nonessential medications.
  - **O**ptimize by noting duplication.
  - **R**eassess patient for function, cognition, clinical status, and medical adherence.
- *Start low and go slow* is recommended for medication prescriptions of older adults.

Nurse's Role

- Implement medication reconciliation.
- Collaborate with healthcare professionals.
- Advocate for healthcare recipients.
- Look for duplications in drugs—same category or drug classification.
- Assess if medication dosages are therapeutic.
- Assess for adverse interactions such as drug–drug, drug–food, or drug–disease.
- Advocate for nondrug therapies if appropriate.
- Conduct a quality improvement to lower rates of polypharmacy.

Source: Cheng et al. (2023); Kim & Parish (2021); Rijal (2022).

BOX 22-8 Simple Steps to Prevent Crime and Identity Theft

- Never open the door automatically; always keep doors and windows locked.
- Use neighborhood watch to keep an eye on your neighborhood.
- Don't leave notes on the door when going out.
- Let someone know when you are away and cancel deliveries.
- Keep the lights on at night and use a timer.
- Keep an inventory of serial numbers and photographs of valuable items; keep copies in a safe place.
- Ask for proper identification of delivery people or strangers. Do not let a stranger in your home.
- Never give out information on the phone letting someone know you are alone.
- Use direct deposit as much as possible, and keep valuables in a safe deposit bank box.
- Be wary of unsolicited offers to fix your home. It could be a scam. If it happens, report it to the police right away.

Crime. Although many older adults are fearful of being victims of crime, rates of nonfatal violent crime and property crime against older adults are lower than in all younger age groups. See Box 22-8 for actions the C/PHN can take to assist older adults with a fear of crime.

Secondary Prevention

Secondary prevention focuses on early detection of disease and prompt intervention (see Chapter 1). Much of the C/PHN's time is spent in educating the community on preventive measures and positive health behaviors. This includes encouraging people to obtain routine screening for diseases such as hypertension, diabetes, or cancer, which, if identified early, can be treated successfully. Many nurses, working in collaboration with community agencies, are in positions to establish screening programs based on the desires and demographics of the community and agency focus, making them accessible to the population being served.

Older adults need to be encouraged to follow the routine health screening schedule prescribed by their clinic or healthcare provider. See Chapter 21 for information on adult screenings and preventative services (see http://www.cdc.gov/vaccines/schedules/hcp/imz/adult.html for a recommended immunization schedule for older adults).

Diseases and Conditions Common in Old Age

Four of five older adults experience at least one chronic condition, and many suffer multiple chronic conditions as they progress into older age. Cardiovascular disease, cancer, diabetes, and obesity are far too common to all adults and are discussed in depth in Chapter 21. The National Center for Health Statistics provides brief data on older adult's health at https://www.cdc.gov/nchs/fastats/older-american-health.htm. Common chronic conditions seen in older adults are as follows:

- Alzheimer disease
- Arthritis
- Cardiovascular disease
- Depression
- Diabetes
- Hearing loss
- Obesity
- Osteoporosis

The prevalence of chronic disease and resulting disability in older adults require health promotion behaviors and guidance.

Alzheimer Disease.

- **Alzheimer disease (AD)** is the most common form of dementia in older adults, first described in 1907 by Dr. Alois Alzheimer, who outlined many of the symptoms that are now known as Alzheimer dementia. AD is the sixth leading cause of death and the only disease among America's top 10 that cannot be prevented or cured.
- Ethnically diverse older adults face a higher risk: African Americans are twice as likely and Hispanics one and one-half times more likely to develop AD than White people (Hale et al., 2020).

Although much is still unknown about this devastating age-related disease, the Alzheimer Association (AA, 2023) annually releases a report of the current scientific findings. To identify AD, a comprehensive examination is needed (see Box 22-9). AD causes more deaths than breast and prostate cancer combined.

Between 2017 and 2025, every state in the United States is expected to see at least a 14% rise in the AD prevalence (AA, 2020b).

- Because of this growth, *Healthy People 2020* designated dementias, including AD, as a focus area.
- *Healthy People 2030* guidelines highlight the need for early identification, reduction in preventable hospitalizations, and communication with a provider regarding care and treatment (ODPHP, n.d.-g).
- The occurrence of AD is not a normal development in the aging process. Damage to the brain from AD can begin 20 years prior to the onset of symptoms.
- One of the major contributors to AD is the slow accumulation of "plaques and tangles" that interfere with brain function. The concentration of **tau proteins** results in tangles and blocks the transport of essential nutrients inside the neurons.
- Plaques result from an excess amount of **beta-amyloid**, which are thought to interrupt neuronal communication at brain synapse.
- The increased presence of tau proteins and beta-amyloid activates the production of microglia, which are charged with clearing these toxins.
- Unfortunately, the microglia are overwhelmed by the amount of proteins and debris left by dying cells, and a harmful chronic inflammatory response ensues. The result is even more cell death and brain atrophy.

Another contributor to decreased brain function is the consequent decreased ability of the brain to metabolize its

BOX 22-9 Annual Cognitive Assessment

Although there is no single test to identify AD (Alzheimer Association [AA], n.d.), annual cognitive assessment is a mandatory component of the Annual Wellness Visit required for all Medicare and Medicaid enrollees (CMS, 2023). The Annual Wellness Visit includes a review of opioid prescriptions, check for cognitive impairment, medical and family history, health risk assessment, and functional ability. Based on results, a prevention plan is developed. A comprehensive assessment is needed because many conditions, including some that are treatable or reversible (e.g., thyroid disease, depression, brain tumors, drug reactions), may cause dementialike symptoms.

C/PHNs are well positioned to initiate a discussion about memory with their clients and family members as the first step of assessment for cognitive decline, followed by a brief 5-minute screening using one of several methods recommended by an AA workgroup (Cordell et al., 2013; Scott & Mayo, 2018), such as Borson's (2013) Mini-Cog, which involves a clock-drawing test and recall of three words. Another tool is the Quick Dementia Rating Scale (Galvin, 2015), which asks family members 10 questions regarding the client's functional ability; the patient's responses give a clear indication of dementia risk. If an AD diagnosis is given, the nurse can provide anticipatory guidance on managing potential behavior changes and help the family to plan for future care needs. Early and accurate diagnosis could save up to 7.9 trillion in care costs by 2050 (AA, n.d.).

—*Dr. Lisa Wiese, Assistant Professor, Florida Atlantic University*

main fuel, glucose. People with diabetes and cardiovascular disease were recently found to have a higher risk for AD and related dementias (ADRD). This led to the additional findings that a combination of a person's health, environmental factors, and lifestyle choices in addition to age-related and genetic factors influence the onset and progression of AD (AA, 2023).

- There is a simple means of describing the difference between the normal forgetfulness of aging and AD. We may forget where we have placed our keys, but upon finding them, we remember why we needed the keys, whereas a person with AD loses immediate recall.
- People in the preclinical Alzheimer stage eventually notice that they are forgetting recent activities or events, or names of familiar things or people (AA, 2023).
- In the mild stage, people may be able to work, drive, and participate in well-known activities but may become lost or forget commonly used words. A typical sign of Alzheimer is the difficulty in creating new memories, as the limbic system where memories are stored is often the area affected first by beta-amyloid plaques and neurofibrillary tangles.
- As the disease advances, the symptoms become serious enough to cause people with AD or their family members to recognize that things are "not right" and that help is needed. The moderate stage is characterized by struggles to complete routine tasks, wandering, and behavior and personality changes. People may become agitated, experience paranoia, and begin to lose the ability to complete ADLs.
- People in the severe stage of Alzheimer dementia become bedbound and cannot communicate in words that can be understood by others (AA, 2023).
- On average, a person with AD lives 4 to 8 years after diagnosis but can live up to 20 years, depending on other factors (AA, 2023). Contrary to the myth, people with AD are still the same person they once were, but their current reality is different.

Several medications have been approved for use with people diagnosed with Alzheimer dementia. Medications called cholinesterase inhibitors are prescribed for mild to moderate AD. Memantine is prescribed for moderate to severe stages, often in combination with donepezil. However, these medications only delay the progression of symptoms for a limited time. At best, available medications "turn back the clock somewhat" with the disease worsening at a slower rate, or the medications control some of the client's behaviors that jeopardize safety, thereby promoting caregiver management.

How does this disease impact the role of the C/PHN? First, the C/PHN can conduct family teaching regarding health behaviors that may reduce the risk of ADRD, such as staying active, exercising, healthy eating habits, adequate sleep, and managing cardiovascular risk factors (diabetes, smoking, obesity, and hypertension; AA, 2023). The C/PHN can stress the importance of completing the Medicare Annual Wellness Visit, including routine cognitive screening to detect early signs and symptoms of mild cognitive impairment, which provides the opportunity to investigate other possible causes of decline. Early detection benefits also include the following:

- Effective management of coexisting conditions
- Appropriate use of available treatment regimens and holistic modalities
- Pursing health-promoting activities; brain games, exercise, improved nutrition, and sleep patterns
- Coordination of care between all members of the healthcare team, including providers and caregivers
- Encouraging the client and family to participate in activities that bring joy/are meaningful
- Accessing support services, day centers, and caregiver support groups

Learning about illness and ADRD management that will decrease care costs is essential, where nearly one in every five Medicare dollars is spent. The average per person Medicare spending for those with ADRD is three times higher than the average per person spending across all other older adults. Medicaid payments are 22 times higher (AA, 2024). In 2023, unpaid caregivers provided an estimated **18 billion** hours of care valued at $346.6 billion (AA, 2024).

- The person with dementia often exhibits depression, agitation, sleeplessness, and anxiety, which disrupt the caregiver's normal routine, greatly adding to caregiver stress. Caregiver burden is multiplied by new or worsening illness, creating a further demand on healthcare resources.
- In many situations, the main caregiver is a spouse who is also older. The C/PHN can make a difference in health outcomes for both the person with ADRD and their caregiver by helping to connect families to community resources (Box 22-10).

Arthritis. **Arthritis** encompasses more than 100 diseases and conditions that affect joints, surrounding tissues, and other connective tissues and is the leading cause of disability for adults in the United States (CDC, 2024b).

Types of arthritis include osteoarthritis (OA), rheumatoid arthritis (RA), gout, and fibromyalgia. With OA, the number of cartilage cells diminishes, cartilage becomes ulcerated and thinned, and subchondral bone is exposed. The bony surfaces rub together resulting in joint destruction with subsequent pain and stiffness (National Institute of Arthritis and Musculoskeletal and Skin Diseases [NIAMS], 2022a).

Gentle exercise is helpful for clients with OA, following treatment for pain. Acetaminophen is the first medication of choice; however, clients often find a combination of medications and daily routines that helps them the most. The nurse can best assist these clients by assessing the safety of a particular regimen and suggesting treatment changes as new research becomes available: new medications, surgical options for joint replacement, and dietary changes, such as vitamins and foods high in essential fatty acids (NIAMS, 2022a).

RA is a progressive chronic condition that begins during young adulthood and becomes disabling as the disease continues, attacking tissues of the joints and causing systemic damage in the later years (NIAMS, 2022b). This form of arthritis is an autoimmune disease that causes inflammation, deformity, and crippling. RA is treated with anti-inflammatory agents, corticosteroids, antimalarial agents, gold salts, and immunosuppressive

BOX 22-10 C/PHN USE OF THE NURSING PROCESS/CLINICAL JUDGMENT

Resources for Managing Alzheimer Disease

Assessment/Recognize Cues

As a home health nurse, you have been asked to assess Mrs. Boxwell regarding her diabetes by Mrs. Boxwell's primary provider. The doctor is concerned because of her high H1C. Mr. and Mrs. Boxwell are in their early 80s and have lived modestly on a fixed income since Mr. Boxwell's retirement. However, their budget has been strained this year because they have had $300 to $400 a month in out-of-pocket expenses for prescription medications. Mrs. Boxwell confessed to you that during some months, they skip medication doses to "make ends meet." Mrs. Boxwell has diabetes, Mr. Boxwell has heart failure, and they both take medications for hypertension. Because of the high cost of the new hypertension medication, Mrs. Boxwell has started giving herself half the insulin dose to save money. They live in a small, older home. Their older model car is seldom driven; they report "the traffic is getting worse" and they have "come close to having a car crash two times." They are receptive to your suggestions and are trying to stay healthy and independent.

Diagnosis/Analyze Cues and Prioritize Hypotheses

- Health status altered as a result of insufficient finances to purchase needed medications for chronic diseases
- Altered safety and diminished driving skills

Planning and Implementation/Generate Solutions and Take Action

- The C/PHN will explore the clients' eligibility for Medicare Part D and Medicaid. It is possible that these clients are eligible yet unaware of these programs. The C/PHN will look at Benefits CheckUp, a service of the National Council of Aging that has information on benefits programs for older adults (benefitscheckup.org).
- The C/PHN will consult with the clients' primary healthcare provider and ask for a change in prescriptions from brand names to generic. Also, ordering some medications in larger doses that come in scored tablets may be less expensive, and the client can safely break the larger pills in half. Mrs. Boxwell will check with her present distributor of supplies for diabetes about getting larger quantities and generic brands of syringes, alcohol pads, etc.
- Mr. Boxwell will look into selling the car and exploring the bus schedule and other shuttle services for older adults that can be used to travel to the doctor and grocery store. Mr. and Mrs. Boxwell's daughter spends a day with them monthly and takes them wherever they want to go, as long as it is "a fun outing," and they will look into coordinating errands with her.

Evaluation/Evaluate Outcomes

- The couple is eligible for Medicare Part D, and this will help defray the out-of-pocket costs for medications. They have reduced medication costs as much as possible and report not missing any prescribed medications. Mrs. Boxwell's H1C is within normal range, and she expresses feeling more in control of her health.
- They sold their car and use bus in good weather and a taxi in the winter or when it is raining (they figure they save $1000 a year [$89 a month] in auto insurance, auto maintenance, and gasoline, whereas the bus and taxi cost them about $22 a month).
- Because the couple is receptive to the help you have provided, you initiate a discussion regarding their long-term plans for housing needs as they get older. They are not opposed to an older adult housing option and have been talking about it with their daughter. They are going to talk with a realtor about selling their house, explore some senior 55+ apartments with their daughter on her monthly visits, and review their budget.

medications. Joint discomfort is often relieved by gentle massage, heat, and range-of-motion exercises.

The C/PHN needs to be aware of the major differences between these two prevalent forms of arthritis. Recommended treatments, including physical therapy, diet, and medication, change as more evidence-based research is conducted on arthritis (NIAMS, 2022a).

Depression. Depression is not a normal part of growing older, yet it is common among older adults (CDC, 2023e). Healthcare providers can miss depression and mistake it for a natural response to grief/loss or illness.

The nurse needs to keep in mind the many potential causes of depression. Medical conditions, such as stroke, cancer, vitamin B_{12} deficiency, diabetes, chronic pain with dependence on prescription painkillers, or insomnia, may lead to depressive symptoms. Many prescription medications can trigger or exacerbate depression. These include blood pressure medications, sleeping pills, calcium channel blockers, ulcers, and pain medications. Screening for depression is within the scope of responsibility of the C/PHN. The Geriatric Depression Scale is available and revised for 2019 (https://consultgeri.org/try-this/general-assessment/issue-4.pdf).

C/PHNs can help older adults prevent the overwhelming signs and symptoms of depression related to losses by working with community groups. Through centers for older adults, adult housing units, daycare centers for older adults, or groups at religious centers, the C/PHN can meet with older adults to offer support, teach strategies to improve the quality and quantity of support systems, invite mental health speakers to discuss the topic of depression prevention, and generally assess the holistic health status of the clients in that setting.

Osteoporosis. **Osteoporosis** is a disease of aging bone in which the amount of bone is decreased, and the strength is reduced. Osteoporosis means "porous bone"; the condition enlarges the holes, and the bones become brittle.

- Of people assigned female at birth in the United States, researchers estimate that one in five has osteoporosis and that half of those over 50 will have a fracture of the hip, wrist, or vertebrae; osteoporosis is considered a major public health threat for approximately 44 million U.S. adults over age 50 (International Osteoporosis Foundation, n.d.).

Proper diet and weight-bearing exercise throughout life are now recognized as the most effective measure to maintain bone health. There is growing evidence that calcium and vitamin D supplementation can help lower rates of fractures and reduce bone loss in older adults. Higher protein intake may also help prevent bone loss (International Osteoporosis Foundation, n.d.). There are many FDA-approved medications to treat osteoporosis that can be prescribed by a primary care provider. Therefore, identification of risk factors and regular screenings is essential to prevent the progression of this debilitating disease (International Osteoporosis Foundation, n.d.).

Sensory Loss. Older adults complain about losing their taste buds and experience deficits in smell. This is why it is not unusual for older adults to over-salt their food or reach for sweet foods they can taste. The prevalence of presbycusis (hearing loss) in those age 75+ is close to 50% (National Institute on Deafness and Other Communications Disorders, 2023), whereas loss of visual perception in those 71+ is close to 30% (Killeen et al., 2023). Most hearing loss happens slowly over time, and the older adult may not recognize their hearing problem. These losses of hearing and vision are correlated with depression, social isolation, physical function, cognitive impairment, and quality of life (Hwang et al., 2022).

There is good news about hearing loss that can help older adults. In August of 2022, the United States Food and Drug Administration (FDA) issued a final rule to improve access to hearing aids over the counter, without examination or prescription (FDA, 2023). This legislation is a significant milestone in making hearing aids more cost effective and accessible to older people.

Dual hearing and vision loss increases the risk of dementia, including AD, threefold (Hwang et al., 2022).

C/PHNs can assess hearing and vision loss using simple tests. For vision, a simple reading of text from a book or newspaper with glasses can suffice. Problems like macular degeneration or glaucoma can cause blindness and need medical care, while presbyopia can be solved with drugstore readers. For hearing, check to see if the older adult uses a well-fitted hearing aid, and that they have a good supply of batteries. A family member may be able to supply information about how well the older adult is hearing, but a referral to a clinic or audiologist may be helpful. Regular eye examinations are essential to diagnose and treat age-related eye and vision changes.

Tertiary Prevention

Tertiary prevention involves follow-up and rehabilitation after a disease or condition has occurred or been diagnosed and initial treatment has begun. Chronic diseases that are common among older adults, such as heart failure, stroke, diabetes, cognitive impairment, or arthritis, cannot always be prevented but can frequently be postponed into the later years of life through a lifetime of positive health behaviors. However, when they occur, the debilitating symptoms and damaging effects can be controlled through healthy choices encouraged by the C/PHN and recommended by the primary care practitioner.

- Although many older adults are considered generally healthy, 95% have at least one chronic condition and 80% have at least two (National Council on Aging [NCOA], 2023).
- A small proportion suffer more disabling forms of disease, such as COPD, cerebral vascular accidents, cancer, or diabetes mellitus, with some requiring extensive care and ongoing medical management.

Heart disease and cancer pose their greatest risks as people age, as do other chronic diseases and conditions, such as stroke, chronic lower respiratory diseases, AD, and diabetes. Influenza and pneumonia also continue to contribute to older adult deaths among older adults, despite the availability of effective vaccines. While the risk for disability from disease clearly increases with advancing age, poor health is not the inevitable outcome of aging. Many older adults manage chronic conditions well throughout the remainder of their lives.

HEALTH COSTS FOR OLDER ADULTS: MEDICARE AND MEDICAID

As the number of older adults grows, so do costs for healthcare (see Chapter 6's discussion of Medicare and Medicaid). Healthcare is a financial burden for 4 in 10 older Americans with 37% unable to pay for needed services. Out-of-pocket expenses increase due to medical needs and inability of Medicare to cover all expenses (Willcoxon, 2022). See Figure 22-6 for total federal outlays for Medicare spending in 2021. With the addition of Social Security, Medicaid, ACA, and CHIP, half of the pie is spent annually (Cubanski & Neuman, 2023).

Medicare or Medicaid does not cover all healthcare costs for older adults. It is predicted that by 2050, the number of older adults, especially those over 85 years of age and those with cognitive impairment, will need support with ADLs. Most care is done by informal unpaid caregivers. This is often done at a heavy physical and financial cost, including lost opportunities for employment, health insurance, and retirement savings. Services for older adults are very expensive.

OLDER ADULT ABUSE

Older adult abuse or mistreatment (i.e., abuse and neglect) is defined as intentional actions that cause harm or create a serious risk of harm to a vulnerable older adult by a caregiver or another person who has a trusting relationship with the older adult.

Signs of older adult abuse may be missed by professionals working with older adults because of lack of training on older adult mistreatment or lack of reporting. In addition, older adults themselves may be unwilling to speak up for fear of retaliation, physical inability to report, cognitive impairment, or they do not want to get the person who is abusing them (90% of whom are a family member) in trouble. See Chapter 18 for comprehensive discussion of all types of older adult abuse and mistreatment. It has been documented that older adult abuse surged during the COVID-19 pandemic (Chang & Levy, 2021). Addressing older adult abuse is a priority for the PHN, who is considered a mandated reporter (NIH, 2023).

It is notable that financial abuse often accompanies one of the other forms of abuse (see Box 22-11). The financial abuse of older adults is a growing problem, often called the "crime of the 21st century."

- An older adult can be financially stable and living independently and may suddenly become destitute and forced out of the home as a result of financial abuse.
- The most common perpetrators of older adult abuse are spouses or partners of older adults, often in a relationship with long-term domestic violence. Family members account for 76% of reported mistreatment.
- The people who abuse older adults, particularly their adult children, are often dependent on the person being abused for financial assistance, housing, or because of personal issues such as mental illness, alcohol use disorder, or substance use disorder (National Library of Medicine, 2023).

In 2021, Medicare Spending Accounted for 10% of the Federal Budget

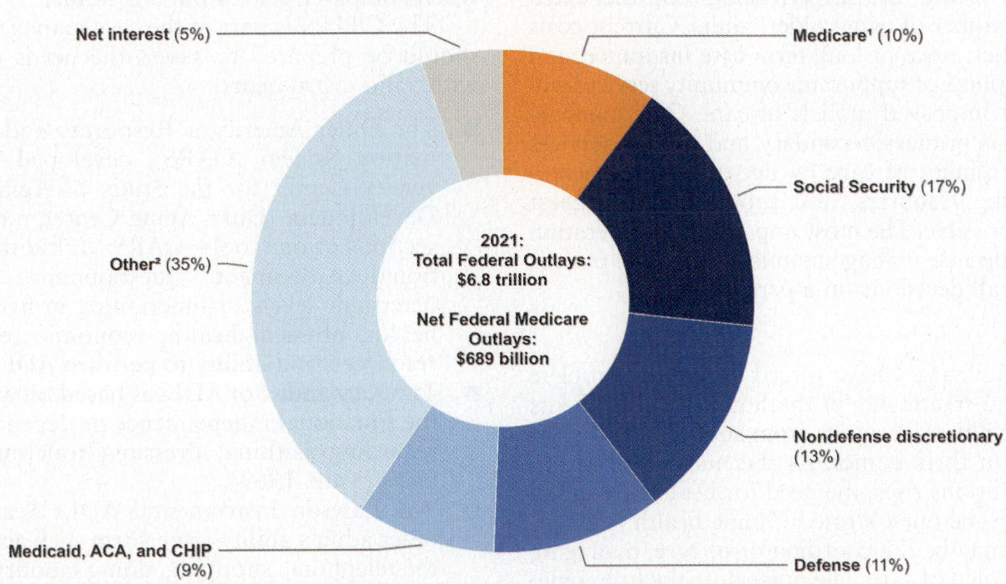

NOTE: All amounts are for federal fiscal year 2021. ¹Consists of mandatory Medicare spending minus income from premiums and other offsetting receipts. ²Includes spending on other mandatory outlays minus income from offsetting receipts. ACA is Affordable Care Act. CHIP is Children's Health Insurance Program.
SOURCE: KFF analysis of federal spending from Congressional Budget Office, The Budget and Economic Outlook, 2022 to 2032 (May 2022).

KFF

FIGURE 22-6 In 2021, Medicare spending accounted for 10% of the federal budget. (Reprinted with permission from KFF, Cubanski, J., & Neuman, T. (2023, January 19). *What to know about Medicare spending.* https://www.kff.org/medicare/issue-brief/what-to-know-about-medicare-spending-and-financing/)

BOX 22-11 WHAT DO *YOU* THINK?

Mrs. Smith's Story

A referral from a home health agency is requesting a home evaluation of an older adult who was recently discharged from the hospital. As the C/PHN for that district, you have been given the referral. The home health nurse was fearful of entering the home because of the adult son's drug use. As you enter the home, you notice Mrs. Smith sitting in the dirty, cluttered living room. She is alert, oriented, and happy to see you. Her dressing change has not been done since her discharge from the hospital 3 days ago. The dressing is dirty with blood stains. She is unkempt, her clothes are dirty, and hair is matted down. The home is an older home in need of repair. There are no screens on the windows and the carpet in the living room is worn with holes. As you enter the kitchen, you notice the adult son standing over the stove cooking his heroin in a spoon as he prepares to inject it. The kitchen is filled with dirty dishes, pots, and bags of stale food on the counter. The son is focused on what he is doing and barely notices you. There is some concern that he is writing checks from his mother's account. What should the C/PHN do? Review the steps for reporting older adult abuse in your state: What is your professional responsibility?

Various state, local, and county agencies investigate and enforce older adult abuse laws. The first agency to respond to a report of older adult abuse in most states is adult protective services (APS).

APPROACHES TO OLDER ADULT CARE

As we noted in the introduction to this chapter, the United States and the world are experiencing unprecedented growth in the number of aging older adults. Current costs of care in facilities, price of long-term care insurance, and the limits on amounts of support in community services will demand new or improved models of care. Case management can focus on primary, secondary, and tertiary services to enhance the quality of care by decreasing fragmentations, maximizing resources, and providing the highest quality of care possible. The most important consideration when considering case management is keeping the patient at the center of all decisions on a person's behalf.

Home Health

Early hospital discharges have forced clients to complete interventions and treatments in the home setting. Clients manage chronic illness, recovery from surgeries, and treat severe illnesses in their homes. As the number of multiple chronic conditions rises, the need for healthcare in the home is critical. The nurse's role in home health is extensive. The nurse may be the coordinator of care, managing and providing a plan of care. The nurse does the following:

- Makes referrals
- Assesses safety of home
- Provides nursing care
- Communicates with family and healthcare team
- Reviews medication regime
- Educate and advocates

Omaha System

The Omaha System is a comprehensive method of utilizing a problem classification scheme with four domains that include environment, psychosocial, psychological, and health-related behavior. Each domain has areas of concern. Next, problems are rated, and interventions are implemented (Omaha System, n.d.). Chapter 12 discusses Omaha System as well.

Case Management and Needs Assessment

Case management involves assessing needs, planning and organizing services, and monitoring responses to care throughout the length of the caregiving process, condition, or illness. Nurses have stepped into the case management role to coordinate and manage patient care across the continuum of health services.

- Following the nursing process, nurses as case managers assure quality outcomes, cost containment, and care coordination.
- They work in an interdisciplinary fashion with members of the healthcare team to ensure coordinated care.

Social workers use case management to address their clients' physical and social needs, including their financial problems. These needs include food, shelter, and access to care. Provisions of the Affordable Care Act support home- and community-based services by providing Medicaid coverage for home services coordinated by a case manager. This funding is available through states that opt in to the ACA Community First Choice (Medicaid.gov, n.d.). When covered by a community program like the First Choice option, case managers and C/PHNs can support the older adult's family members who will be paid for caregiving for their family member, a great cost saving when compared with a nursing home.

The C/PHN is part of the case management team and should be prepared to assess the needs of older adults with valid instruments:

- The Older Americans Resources and Services Information System (OARS), developed by Duke University Center for the Study of Aging and Human Development (Duke Aging Center, n.d.), utilizes two sections of one tool—OARS Multidimensional Functional Assessment Questionnaire (OMFAQ)—to determine levels of functioning in five areas (mental health, physical health, economic resources, social resources, and ability to perform ADLs).
- The Katz Index of ADLs is based on an evaluation of the functional independence or dependence of clients regarding bathing, dressing, toileting, and related tasks (Katz, 1963).
- The Lawton Instrumental ADLs Scale looks at an older adult's ability to perform such activities as using the telephone, shopping, doing laundry, and handling finances (Graf, 2008).
- Timed Up and Go Test (TUG) is a measurement of the time in seconds for a person to rise from sitting from a standard armchair, walk 10 ft, turn, walk back to the chair, and sit down. The person wears regular footwear and walking supports (cane, walker). The test is predictive of falls in older adults (Sears, 2023).

- Cognitive Screens: to screen for the need for further testing, should the client or family be worried. Open this link and try the MiniCog (https://consultgeri.org/try-this/general-assessment/issue-3.1).
- Vision and hearing screens: The test is familiar to older adults. A simple test of reading with corrective lenses if used will suffice to know if the older adult can read directions (i.e., pill bottles). This would not screen for eye problems like macular degeneration. For hearing, the Whisper Test may be used, with hearing aids if the older adult uses them (see https://geriatrics.ucsf.edu/sites/geriatrics.ucsf.edu/files/2018-06/whispertest.pdf)
- Spiritual assessment: Spiritual needs can be assessed using many different instruments or questionnaires. Try FICA (Faith, Importance, Community, Address) for example (Coalition for Compassionate Care, 2023; https://coalitionccc.org/CCCC/CCCC/Resources/FICA-Spiritual-Assessment-Tool.aspx)

HEALTH SERVICES FOR OLDER ADULT POPULATIONS

How well are the needs of older adults being met? To answer this question, other questions must be raised. Do health programs for older adults encompass the full range of needed services? Are programs both physically and financially accessible? Do they encourage clients to function independently? Do they treat older people with respect and preserve their dignity? Do they recognize older adults' needs for companionship, economic security, and social status? If appropriate, do they promote meaningful activities, not just the usual games or activities such as bingo, shuffleboard, and ceramics? Are healthcare services and other social services provided based on evidence and research? Effective services for older adults should be comprehensive, coordinated, and accessible and demonstrate evidence-based quality.

Criteria for Effective Service

Several criteria help to define the characteristics of an effective community health service delivery system. Four deserve attention.

In order to be effective, it should be *comprehensive*. Many communities provide some programs, such as limited health screening or selected activities, but do not offer a full range of services to more adequately meet the needs of their older adults (see Box 22-12). A comprehensive set of services should provide the following:

1. Affordable housing options
2. Adult day and memory care programs
3. Access to high-quality healthcare services (prevention, early diagnosis and treatment, rehabilitation)
4. Health education (including preparation for retirement) and centralized resources for information
5. In-home services that promote aging in place
6. Recreation and activity programs that promote healthy nutrition and socialization
7. Specialized transportation services
8. Safe and outdoor spaces that promote activity and enjoyment

BOX 22-12 WHAT DO *YOU* THINK?

Services in Your Community

Have you wondered if you should intervene if you see an older adult in a situation where they might need help? Or perhaps a neighbor will tell you about someone who might be in trouble. As a nurse, these kinds of situations come to our attention regularly. Silver Key SOS of Colorado Springs, Colorado, offers an SOS (Senior Outreach Service). Anyone can contact Silver Key if there is a concern about an older person who may need help (https://www.silverkey.org/services/senior-assistance/silver-key-sos/). The reporting person need not be identified to the referred older adult. Once notified, a case manager will contact the older person and connect them with appropriate services, if the older adult is willing. Services include counseling for many problems, community resources, and treatment for depression or misuse of drugs or prescriptions. Teach your peers and family to recognize some warning signs: confusion, physical problems, signs of home/person neglect, social isolation, and economic problems.

Look for these kinds of services in your community. Do they exist under city services? Perhaps the County Health Department? How would you go about connecting families or older adults to services?

A second criterion for a community service delivery system is *coordination*. A good example of efforts toward effective and coordinated services is the age-friendly cities and Communities programs (AARP, n.d.-b). Communities that apply for age-friendly demonstrate that the community addresses the points in Box 22-12. By 2024, 12 states and the U.S. Virgin Islands were designated age-friendly (AARP, 2024a). A coordinated information and referral system provides another link. Most communities need this type of information network, which contains a directory of all resources and services for older adults and includes the name and telephone number of a contact person with each listing. An example of this network is 2-1-1 (Help Starts Here). This number connects the caller to services, and many communities have their own (https://www.211.org/).

A third criterion is *accessibility*. Too often, services for older adults are inconveniently located or are prohibitively expensive. Some communities are considering multiservice community centers to bring programs and services for older adults with limited resources closer to home. The Program of All-Inclusive Care of the Elderly (PACE) is one example of this (National PACE Association, 2023). Comprehensive services are offered to people who qualify for nursing home care but could stay in the community with supports, including personal, healthcare, and housing. Other services such as transportation and in-home services (home health aides, homemakers, grocery, and meal delivery) may further solve accessibility problems for many older adults.

Finally, an effective community service system for older people should promote *quality* programs. This means that services should truly address the needs and concerns of a community's older adults and be based on evidence of good outcomes.

- A range of housing types, from retirement communities with all amenities for active and older people to secure and more affordable apartments for independent living, are being built in most communities.
- However, affordable rental apartments and homes for older adults and families with limited resources are in short supply in many communities, putting increasing numbers of older adults in unsheltered situations (Office of the Assistant Secretary for planning and evaluation, 2023).
- Age-friendly communities are focusing on this problem with an array of solutions, including "tiny houses," "granny flats," home shares, and redesigning current homes using **universal design**, that is, usable by anyone of any age, whether they have a disability or not (e.g., wider door frames, fewer steps up).

Services for Older Adults by Level of Care Required

There is increased emphasis on providing needed services for older people at home, the essence of **aging in place**. Today's emphasis on cost control gives added support for providing services at home. Given the increase in longevity, the potential for cost savings appears significant if care for dependent older people can be supported where they live (see Table 22-3).

Maintaining functional independence should be the primary goal of services for the older population. Assessment of needs and ability to function and the use of assessment tools to determine appropriate services are necessary. Outreach programs serve an important function in many communities, as they locate people in need of health or social assistance and refer them to appropriate resources.

- Independent living housing is a general term for any arrangement designed exclusively for older adults. Types of independent living facilities include subsidized housing for older adults, retirement communities, Continuing Care Retirement Communities (CCRCs), and age-restricted apartments (55+). The older adult housing industry is rethinking these older models to come up with intergenerational community models, as some baby boomers tend to be less interested in 55+ communities.
- The concept of **continuing care retirement communities (CCRCs)**, sometimes referred to as total life care centers, allows older people to "age in place," with flexible accommodations designed to meet their health and housing needs (AARP, 2022a). Residents entering CCRCs sign a long-term contract that provides for housing, services, and nursing and dementia care. Many older adults enter into CCRC contracts while they are healthy and active, knowing they will be able to stay in the same community and receive nursing care should this become necessary. Currently, CCRCs are redesigning their homes and apartments to fit the needs of the baby boomers, who want more of a village feel. Dedicated memory care units in long-term and assisted living are part of the redesign. Older adults who invest in a CCRC need to have financial means to support the entrance and monthly fees.
- **Assisted living** communities provide care to residents who need nonmedical support with ADLs (these could include eating, dressing, bathing, mobility, toileting, grooming, and assistance with medications). These communities typically provide cooked meals in a shared dining hall, housekeeping, laundry, and transportation (National Institute on Aging, 2023).
- Memory care units are for people with dementia who require skilled care and supervision. These units or living spaces provide 24/7 supervision by staff who are specifically trained to care for patients with memory loss (AARP, 2024b).
- The growing *Village Concept* is a relatively new, self-supporting cooperative solution for independent living in which older adults live in their own homes, in a neighborhood, or in some cases high-rise city apartment buildings.
- Neighbors share services such as transportation, grocery shopping, or helping with household chores provided by village providers, either professional or volunteer.
- The village encourages socialization with a wide range of activities among the members, and some hold wellness activities. This option requires a membership fee to provide services (Village to Village Network, 2023). Older adults who remain in their homes or apartments may rely on smart home technology to improve their autonomy (Norouzi, 2020). Other older people may live with family members or participate in home sharing (https://homeshareonline.org/). They may attend an adult or memory daycare center during the day. Sometimes being able to stay home or return home includes short-term living arrangements. This could be a rehabilitation hospital for recovery and physical therapy related to a hip fracture or complications of acute care, like a stroke or cardiac event.

Many nurses do not know the difference between a skilled nursing facility (SNF) and a **custodial care** nursing home. They often exist within the same building.

- SNFs are reimbursed for 30 days by Medicare for rehabilitation for conditions such as post stroke, spinal cord injury, IV therapy, and PT, OT, and Speech (CMS, 2023).
- When an older adult has a long-term chronic condition that cannot be managed in the community, a nursing home is an option. There is 24-hour nursing and nursing assistant care in both SNF and nursing homes, but the payment model is quite different (see Table 22-3).

Nursing home reform was legislated in the late 1980s, putting increased demands on facilities to provide competent resident assessment, timely care plans, quality improvement, and protection of resident rights (Omnibus Budget Reconciliation Act, 1987). This increased complexity of services has resulted in increased costs in these facilities. Staffing needs increase as care becomes more complex and the resident population grows.

- The COVID-19 pandemic shined a bright light on staffing needs in long-term care, where deaths from the virus were highest (The White House.gov, 2023).

TABLE **22-3** Residential and Home Healathcare Services for Older Adults

Living facility types (National Institute on Aging, 2023)	**Assisted living** can be a few residents or a large building, great variety in types and services	**Skilled nursing facility (SNF)** Skilled rehabilitation	**Custodial care (nursing home/facility)** There are 15,000 nursing homes in the United States; the majority are for profit. 1.2 million people reside in nursing homes (Office of Inspector General, 2024)	**Home healthcare**
Model	Social housing model	Medical model	Both	Both
Services provided (AARP, 2022b) (National Center for Assisted Living, 2023; Office of the Federal Register Publications, 2024)	• Care and supervision • Room and board • Activities • Assist ADLs • Stores/may provide medication assistance • Dementia care • May have a dementia unit	• 24-hour nursing • Room and board • Assistance with ADLs • Activities • Dispenses/administers medications • Provides rehab care: PT, OT, and speech posthospitalization • No dementia care	• 24-hour nursing • Room and board • Assistance with ADLs • Activities • Dispenses/administers medications • May have a dementia unit	• Homemaker • Home health aide • Nursing services • Provides rehab care: PT, OT, and speech posthospitalization • Limited dementia care
Skilled professionals (National Center for Assisted Living, 2023; Office of the Federal Register Publications, 2024)	Varies by state, with some states. LVNs, RNs may not be required	Nursing staff are required by law RN 24 hours daily within 3 years of new 2024 CMS ruling	RN 24 hours daily within 3 years of new 2024 CMS ruling LVNs 24 hours daily CNAs Dieticians States may have additional requirements	Varies by state: licensure for providers. Can be for profit or nonprofit, or a subdivision of an agency or a hospital
(National Center for Assisted Living, 2023; Office of the Federal Register Publications, 2024)	State-driven: Department of Public Health or Human Services	Federal oversight: U.S. Department of Health and CMS	State Department of Health and Federal CMS	State and federal
Average cost/month (Genworth, 2024; SNF cost is from Goldy-Brown & Clem, 2024; National Center for Assisted Living, 2023)	$5350 for private room	$8029–$10,025	$8669–$9733	$5720 for home health service $6292 for home health aide
Who pays? (National Institute on Aging, 2023)	• Private pay • Long-term insurance • Medicaid in indigent cases is limited by space	• Medicare limited days • Private pay • Medicaid in indigent cases, limited by space	• Medicare limited days • Private pay • Medicaid in indigent cases, limited by space	• Private pay • Long-term insurance • Medicaid in indigent cases

ADLs, activities of daily living; CNA, Certified Nursing Assistant; LVN, licensed vocational nurses; OT, occupational therapy; PT, physical therapy; RN, registered nurses.

- In April of 2023, the Biden administration signed an executive order to increase staffing in nursing homes, including the presence of a registered nurse each 24 hours. This law, which will be managed by the Centers for Medicare and Medicaid (CMS), will go into effect in phases, as the current shortage of long-term care staffing is still acute following the pandemic (The White House.gov, 2023).
- Licensed personnel must be knowledgeable decision makers; managers of unskilled staff, educators, and role models; and efficient and effective administrators in an essentially autonomous practice setting.

END OF LIFE: ADVANCE DIRECTIVES, HOSPICE, AND PALLIATIVE CARE

A final need of older adults is preparing for a dignified death. In her classic work *On Death and Dying*, Elisabeth Kübler-Ross (1969) described death as the final stage of growth and one that deserves the same measure of quality as other stages of life.

- Although death is a natural part of life, many older people fear death as an experience of pain, humiliation, discomfort, or financial concern for loved ones. Sometimes, very aggressive and heroic medical treatments are offered to those near the end of their lives, often at the urging of family members.
- Planning for a dignified death is an important issue for many older people, and C/PHNs can facilitate conversations among family members and provide necessary information and resources. Look up www.theconversationproject.org, which is a very helpful toolkit to help people and families have the conversation about wishes for end of life.

The C/PHN will need to be aware of the laws around physician-assisted suicide and patient self-determination around death. The Death with Dignity website is very helpful: https://www.deathwithdignity.org/learn/access/.

Advance Directives

Living wills and advance healthcare directives, sometimes referred to as *advance directives*, are legal documents that instruct others about end-of-life choices should an person be unable to make decisions independently. The forms for advance directives are available for every state online through AARP (n.d.-c).

An advance healthcare directive only becomes effective under the circumstances specified in the document. This document allows for the appointment of a healthcare agent who will have the legal authority to make healthcare decisions on behalf of the patient and for specific written instructions for future healthcare in the event of any situation in which the patient can no longer speak for himself or herself. Examples include the following:

- The use of dialysis and breathing machines
- Use of resuscitation if breathing or heartbeat stops
- Tube feeding
- Organ or tissue donation

Having such documents prepared and making them known to significant others can ensure that wishes will be honored. These documents can provide clear directions for families and healthcare professionals and are gaining more recognition and importance because of increasing ethical dilemmas and challenges brought on by advances in technology (American Medical Association, n.d.). Advance directives can be revoked or replaced at any time, as long as the person in question is capable of making their own decisions. It is recommended that these documents be reviewed every 2 years or so, or in the event of a change in health status and revised to ensure that they continue to accurately reflect an individual's wishes.

Hospice

Hospice is an option that takes a multidisciplinary approach to end-of-life care and needs. Hospice is more a concept of care than a specific place, although some hospice organizations provide people with a place to die with dignity if they have no home or choose not to die at home. Hospice is an option for people with a "projected" life expectancy of 6 months or less and often involves holistic care as well as pain and symptom relief as opposed to ongoing curative measures. The hospice movement has emphasized four major changes in end-of-life care:

- Care should encompass body, mind, and spirit.
- Death should be discussed and not considered off limits.
- Medical technology should be used only when absolutely necessary.
- Clients should be actively involved in discussions about treatment decisions.

The C/PHN can be a helpful resource in connecting clients with hospice services before the end of life is imminent, and hospice is most beneficial for all.

Palliative Care

Palliative care consists of comfort and symptom management and does not provide a cure. For most chronic ongoing health conditions—such as diabetes, high blood pressure, congestive heart failure, arthritis, and COPD—there are no cures, only symptom relief. Palliative care should not be viewed as synonymous with hospice or end-of-life care. Rather, palliative care should be viewed as any care primarily intended to relieve the burden of physical and emotional suffering that may accompany illness associated with aging.

CARE FOR THE CAREGIVER

The burden of caregiving has received more attention in recent years because it is such a demanding and costly role. More older people are cared for in their homes by a spouse or other family member, often called an informal caregiver, on an unpaid basis.

- Almost 75% of people receiving care at home rely exclusively on informal caregivers, usually women between the ages of 45 and 64 (U.S. Bureau of Statics, 2023).
- Positive aspects of caregiving, such as enriching the relationship between the caregiver and the family member, can give caregivers a sense of accomplishment (Lindeza et al., 2024).

BOX 22-13 Family Caregiving Concerns

Finances

Most caregivers are working women who will not be contributing to their own retirement accounts for possibly long periods of time because of taking time off from work to care for an older adult, which results in loss of income. The Credit for Caring Act 2024 is proposed legislation that would create a tax credit up to $5000 for caregivers who work and care for their parents (Congress.gov, 2024).

Payment for Caregiving

Caregivers are often not paid. Medicaid eligible and veterans may get assistance, which varies by state. Long-term care insurance is often out of the financial reach of many families.

Hospice and End-of-Life Guidance

This concern centers on how to have the conversations with family members.

Caregiver Life Balance

This concern involves the daily work of caregiving, especially when it falls on one family member, can result in depression, anxiety, fatigue, guilt, and anger.

Resources

These include adult day programs, support groups, dementia care, and respite care.

Safety as We Age

These concerns include aging parents' driving as well as home safety (AARP, n.d.-a; AARP, 2023).

- The demands of caregiving exact a toll on the caregiver, who may give up employment income, may miss important screening and healthcare visits for themselves, and risk isolation from others. The AARP provides a host of resources for caregivers at https://www.aarp.org/caregiving/
- Caregivers own decline in health can compromise their ability to be a caregiver unless they get some relief (Box 22-13).

Respite care is a service that is receiving increasing attention. Although there are different approaches to respite care, all have the same basic objective: to provide caregivers with planned temporary, intermittent, substitute care, allowing for relief from the daily responsibilities of caring for the care recipient (AARP, 2024c). Long-term care insurance may cover some costs of respite care. The 2000 Older Americans Act Amendments provided funding for states to work through National Family Caregivers Support Project Program to address respite care specifically on the local level (ACL, 2022). The reality is that finding respite care is costly and out of reach of many people.

CASE STUDY 10 ESSENTIAL PUBLIC HEALTH SERVICES

Beyond the Front Door

A C/PHN received a home visit referral from the VA clinic after the client missed two appointments. The client, Mr. P, was a 77-year-old veteran with a diagnosis of diabetes and right heel ulcer who needed IV antibiotics and wound care twice a day. The C/PHN had the address and circled around the block a couple of times; the house was in a residential neighborhood in the middle of town, a block from an elementary school. The client did not have a phone. The C/PHN parked close to the address and walked; only then did they see the 5-foot weeds in front of the house. The C/PHN knocked on the door and called for Mr. P a couple of times. He finally answered the door. He was an unkempt, unbathed older adult crawling on his knees (due to his inability to put weight on his right foot), with a toothless smile. He let the C/PHN in and sat in an old chair by the door. Introductions were made. The home was very dark and dusty; piles of books, magazines, and newspapers were stacked 3 to 4 ft high in between furniture, leaving a small maze in which to walk through the house. The VA had sent 2 months of supplies, which were in dozens of boxes by the front door. Although the house was dark, the kitchen windows provided some light. The C/PHN noticed that there were no appliances in the kitchen, only piles of books, a Styrofoam ice chest on the floor (inside was warm milk and green lunch meat), and open cans of food in the sink.

Assessment reveals blood glucose of 355, 4-in diameter Stage 3 wound on the right heel, and pain level of 8 out of 10 (Mr. P had not taken prescribed pain medicines). Mr. P is very cooperative and talkative. He has lived alone in the house for over 40 years and never married. Family lives an hour away; he has not seen them in 10 or more years. He has no friends locally because many have passed on. Mr. P has no car; the closest VA clinic is 90 miles away. He purchases food from the corner grocer but says that he has been unable recently to walk to the store.

1. ***Recognize Cues:*** *Which findings require immediate follow-up, are unexpected, or are most concerning?*
2. ***Analyze Cues:*** *What information is noted or needed for interpreting findings?*
3. ***Prioritize Hypotheses:*** *Based on the information that you have, what is happening?*
4. ***Generate Solutions:*** *What intervention(s) will achieve the desired outcome?*
5. ***Take Action:*** *What actions should you take or do first?*
6. ***Evaluate Outcomes:*** *Were outcomes achieved? Why or why not?*
7. *Which Essential Public Health Services influence this situation? (See Box 2-2.)*

SUMMARY

- C/PHNs can make a significant contribution to the health of older adults. The nurse may function as a collaborator, case manager, advocate, and educator to assist older adults and their families to maintain or improve health. Because these nurses are in the community and already have contact with many older adults, they are in a prime position to carry out a comprehensive needs assessment, culminating in a nursing diagnosis and holistic plan for the healthcare needs of this group.
- C/PHNs work with older adults and families in many settings, wherever they find them, and with whatever health needs are present.
- Although the priority of community and public health nursing is health promotion and disease prevention, community nurses work with older adults with chronic health conditions who are aging in place to help them achieve their maximal health potential. C/PHNs need to assess their living situations and find out as much as possible about the community's support systems, available resources, and gaps in services.
- As the number of older adults in America grows, the need for healthcare services and health professionals that serve older people in communities will continue to increase.
- Healthy longevity is the goal for the aging population and is a focus of *Healthy People 2030*. This means being able to function as independently as possible and maintaining as much physical, mental wellness, and social engagement as possible while adapting to chronic conditions and functional impairments.
- The C/PHN can effectively improve the quality of care and the environment for older adults through advocacy, education counseling, case management, and collaboration with clients, families, and health services and providers.
- Older adults generally prefer to age in place and live independently in the community. C/PHNs deliver healthcare services to a large and rapidly growing segment of the population.
- Alzheimer disease is the sixth leading cause of death and the only disease among America's top 10 that cannot be prevented or cured. Between 2017 and 2025, every state is expected to see at least a 14% rise in AD prevalence (AA, 2020b). The C/PHN will support families and caregivers who need support caring for older adults with this devastating disease.
- A variety of living arrangements and care options are available from which to choose and can be tailored to the older person's desires and needs. These include continuing care communities, villages, day and memory care centers, PACE programs, assisted living, skilled and SNF long-term care centers, and hospice.
- The C/PHN perspective includes a case management approach that offers a centralized system for assessing the needs of older people and then matching those needs with the appropriate services. The C/PHN should also serve the entire older population by assessing their needs, examining the available services, and analyzing their effectiveness. The effectiveness of programs can be measured according to four important criteria (targeted to the specific needs of the population): comprehensiveness, effective coordination, accessibility, and quality.

ACTIVE LEARNING EXERCISES

1. Research global, national, and state health statistics of older adults. Compare and contracts findings. Share findings with your peers and notice similarities and differences. Share websites where the data were collected. (Objective 1)
2. Start to take notice of the terms you and others use to describe older adults. Reflect on misconceptions you and your classmates have for this population. The words we use to describe our patients affect how we view them. While this exercise may be difficult, an honest appraisal is the first step to change. Interview an adult age 70 or older and ask what misconceptions related to age have they heard or experienced from others. Is this a population you want to work with? Why or why not? Could your answer be due to any misconception of the population? (Objective 2)
3. Reflect on where you see yourself at age 65, 75, and 85. What healthy characteristics would you want to have? Next interview a person from each of the three age groups. How do they define healthy? Does the definition change based on the age group? (Objective 3)
4. As part of your regular community health nursing workload, you visit a daycare center for older adults one afternoon each week. You take the blood pressure of several people who are taking antihypertensive medications and do some nutrition counseling. The center accommodates 60 clients, and you would like to serve the health needs of the aggregate population. List five potential health needs of this group. Which of the 10 Essential Public Health Services did you address in this assignment? Refer to Box 2-2. (Objective 4)
5. For one of the five potential health needs from #4, develop primary, secondary, and tertiary prevention. Base your decision on the health need to focus on from interviews with the older adults and staff at the center. Implement one of the primary preventions at a center for older adults. With whom did you consult as you planned the intervention? What feedback did you receive? What went well and what would you change? (Objective 5)
6. This chapter discussed several types of residential living arrangements for older adults. Research the costs of each, the type of resident that would qualify for each, the type of nursing care provided, and the socioeconomics of the neighborhoods where these residentials are located. Next, research if any complaints have been made against any living arrangements for older adults that are located in your area. Where did you find that information? (Objective 6)

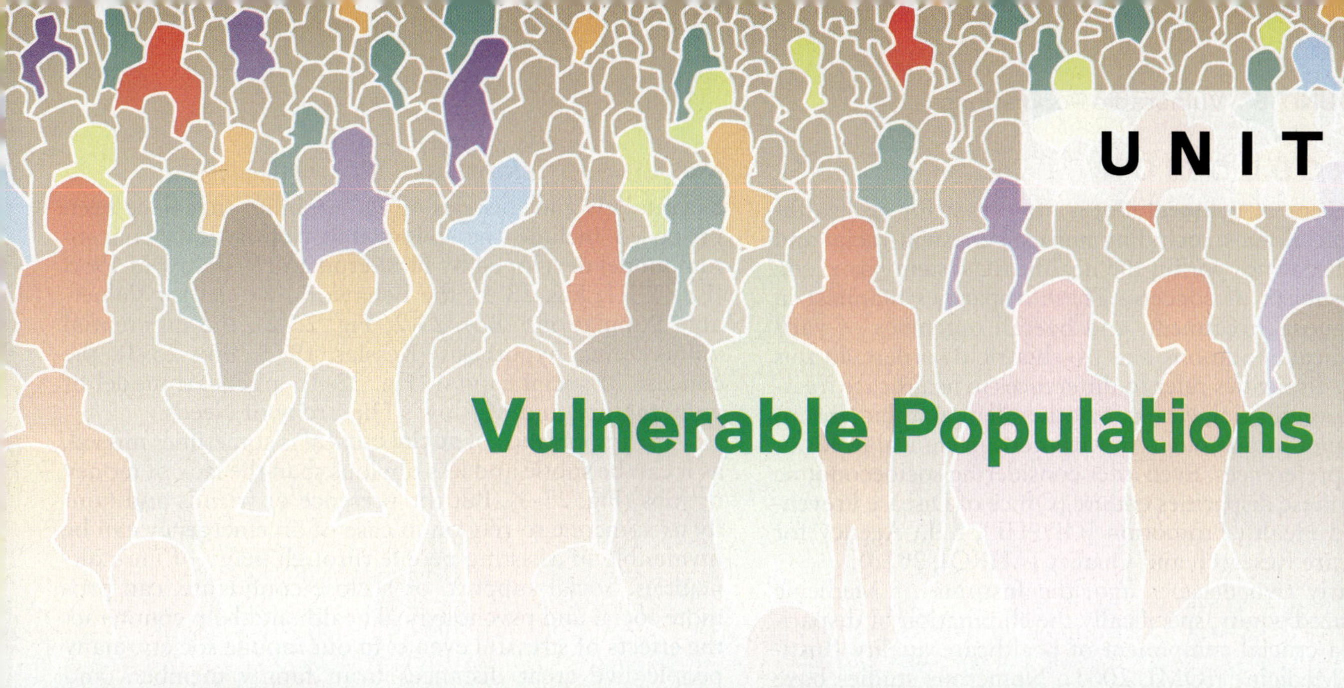

UNIT 6

Vulnerable Populations

CHAPTER 23

Working With Vulnerable People

"How far you go in life depends on your being tender with the young, compassionate with the aged, sympathetic with the striving, and tolerant of the weak and the strong—because someday you will have been all of these."

—George Washington Carver (1860–1943), Botanist and Scientist

KEY TERMS

- Differential vulnerability hypothesis
- Empowerment strategies
- Environmental resources
- Health disparities
- Human capital
- Racial/ethnic disparities
- Racism
- Relative risk
- Social capital
- Social determinants of health
- Socioeconomic gradient
- Socioeconomic resources
- Underrepresented populations
- Vulnerability
- Vulnerable populations

LEARNING OBJECTIVES

Upon mastery of this chapter, you should be able to:

1. Assess the adverse effects of health disparities and the relative risk for various vulnerable populations.
2. Identify interagency groups or committees that address the needs of vulnerable populations in your area.
3. Evaluate evidence-based practices when working with vulnerable groups.
4. Partner with vulnerable populations to evaluate current healthcare programs and services.
5. Describe C/PHN roles or behaviors that help promote client empowerment.
6. Describe the role of the C/PHN in social justice and health equity when working with vulnerable populations to propose policy changes that improve the population's health.

INTRODUCTION

The concept of **vulnerability** is important for all healthcare professionals, including nurses. Persistent racial and ethnic disparities within the healthcare system have long been a subject of concern. These disparities manifest in the diagnosis, treatment, and overall outcomes of various medical conditions and psychiatric disorders. In this context, disparities refer to differences in healthcare treatment among racial, ethnic, or other demographic groups that cannot be attributed to variations in clinical needs or patient preferences. Even after considering socioeconomic factors, these disparities endure (Office of Disease Prevention and Health Promotion [ODPHP], n.d.; Agency for Healthcare Research and Quality [AHRQ], 2023).

Nearly two decades ago, the Institute of Medicine emphasized equity, specifically the elimination of disparities, as a crucial component of healthcare quality (Institute of Medicine [IOM], 2001). Numerous studies have highlighted that people who are economically disadvantaged, lack insurance, or belong to underrepresented groups often receive suboptimal care. Additionally, these populations are more likely to have chronic illnesses such as diabetes and hypertension. In 2009, the AHRQ National Healthcare Disparities Report underscored the persistence of disparities in healthcare quality and access (AHRQ, 2010). The report also revealed variations in the magnitude and patterns of these disparities within different underrepresented subpopulations. Unfortunately, the COVID-19 pandemic and the nationwide racial justice movement of recent years have brought health disparities into sharp focus, shedding light on their deep-seated causes. These issues have led to a heightened emphasis on achieving health equity. It is crucial to recognize that these disparities are not new; they are the result of longstanding structural and systemic inequities deeply rooted in racism and discrimination (Shortreed et al., 2023; Takian et al., 2020; Wiltz et al., 2022).

The origins of healthcare disparities are multifaceted and complex. They encompass challenges such as patients struggling to navigate the healthcare system, difficulties in doctor-patient communication due to language barriers or cultural differences, healthcare providers relying on stereotypes when interacting with patients, patient mistrust of healthcare providers, family structures affecting an person's ability or willingness to seek healthcare services, and varying beliefs about the advantages of alternative or folk medicine across racial and ethnic groups.

In this chapter, we examine popular models and theories of vulnerability, including important concepts and contributing factors. We also briefly discuss health disparities that are more common among vulnerable members of society and the role of C/PHNs working with these groups. This chapter provides an overview of this subject and lays the foundation for other chapters.

THE CONCEPT OF VULNERABLE POPULATIONS

In this section, we consider several key models and theories related to vulnerability, the criteria used to determine who is considered vulnerable, and causative factors linked to vulnerability.

Models and Theories of Vulnerability

Key models and theories of vulnerability that have been proposed include the **vulnerable populations** conceptual model developed by Flaskerud and Winslow in 1998 (Box 23-1; Fig. 23-1), the Behavioral Model for Vulnerable Populations (Box 23-2; Fig. 23-2), the differential vulnerability hypothesis (Kessler, 1979; Box 23-3), the concept of social capital (Fig. 23-3), a general model of vulnerability, and Maslow's Hierarchy of Needs.

The importance of **social capital** is sometimes missed, as it can be subtle and less obvious than the lack of money or jobs (Fig. 23-3). But the presence of friends and family or someone to rely on in case of an emergency can be invaluable in assisting people through many of life's difficulties. Social support, or a close confidante, can promote social and psychological health and help counteract the effects of stressful events. In our mobile society, many people live great distances from family members and have difficulty establishing new friendships. Those who live alone or who are socially isolated are at the greatest risk of vulnerability, increased morbidity and mortality, and decreased overall health (New Jersey Department of Human Services Office of Research & Evaluation, 2023); thus, C/PHNs should be aware of this and strive to provide additional support and resources.

BOX 23-1 Vulnerable Populations Conceptual Model (Flaskerud & Winslow, 1998)

Flaskerud and Winslow (1998) developed a popular conceptual framework of vulnerability (see Fig. 23-1) that contains three related concepts: resource availability, relative risk, and health status. The model provides evidence of the link between poor health status and socioeconomic resource availability through the loss of income, jobs, and health insurance. The following concepts are supported by this model:

- Lack of resources (e.g., socioeconomic and environmental) increases a population's exposure to risk factors and reduces people' ability to avoid illness.
- **Socioeconomic resources** include **human capital** (e.g., jobs, income, housing, education), social connectedness or integration (e.g., social networks or ties; social support or the lack of it, characterized by marginalization), and social status (e.g., position, power, role).
- **Environmental resources** deal mostly with access to healthcare and the quality of that care.
- Limited access or lack of access to care can arise from many sources, including crime-ridden neighborhoods, insufficient transportation systems, lack of adequate numbers and types of providers, limited choices of healthcare plans, or no health insurance.
- **Relative risk** refers to exposure to risk factors identified by a substantial body of research as lifestyle, behaviors and choices (e.g., diet, exercise, use of tobacco, alcohol and other drugs, sexual behaviors), use of health screening services (e.g., mammogram, colonoscopy), and stressful events (e.g., crime, violence, abuse, firearm use).

Source: Flaskerud and Winslow (1998).

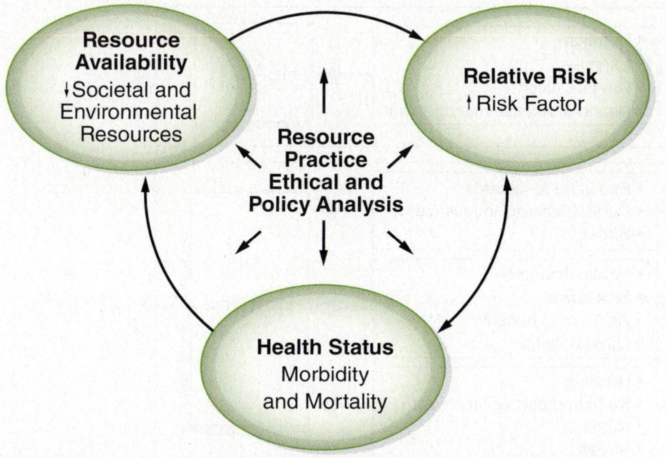

FIGURE 23-1 Vulnerable populations conceptual model. (Adapted from Flaskerud, J. H., & Winslow, B. J. (1998). Conceptualizing vulnerable populations health-related research. *Nursing Research, 47*(2), 69–78.)

A general model of vulnerability helps to explain individual and community risk factors that lead to vulnerability, as well as problems with the access to care and the quality of care received that impact health outcomes on both an individual and community level, as described in a seminal article by Shi et al. (2008). According to this model, vulnerable populations often experience clusters of risk factors, and these are viewed as cumulative. The specific combinations of risks (e.g., low income, low education) are more detrimental to health outcomes, as is the greater number of risk factors that accumulate over time.

Most nursing students are familiar with Maslow's Hierarchy of Needs (Maslow, 1987), with physiologic needs (e.g., water, food, air) as the base of a pyramid, and the needs for safety, belonging, esteem, and self-actualization building from the basic needs. Chronic poverty, environments of crime and violence, or disenfranchisement, racism, and discrimination (vulnerability) can keep people from meeting their higher needs (Bates, 2023). **Racism** is largely defined as believing that race is the primary factor of our capacities and traits as humans and that any racial differences result in feelings of superiority or inferiority.

Who Is Considered Vulnerable?

In her classic book, Aday (2001) included the following factors and populations in the description of who is considered vulnerable:

- Income and education
- Age and gender
- Race and ethnicity
- Chronic illness and disability
- HIV/AIDS
- Mental illness and disability
- Alcohol and substance misuse
- Familial abuse
- Homelessness
- Suicide and homicide risk
- High-risk birthing parents and infants
- Immigrants and refugees
- Military personnel

Other authors considered the uninsured and underinsured as vulnerable populations because of their difficulties with healthcare access and the potential for poor health outcomes, as well as people who had experienced bullying or crimes, children in foster care, those in the LGBTQ+ community, veterans and returning military personnel, and those who had experienced torture and terrorism (Collins, et al., 2022; Hutchison & Cox, 2020; Tolbert et al., 2022). Although many segments of the population may be considered vulnerable at some point in their lives, some population segments are more often identified as vulnerable because of their long-term situations

BOX 23-2 The Behavioral Model for Vulnerable Populations (Gelberg et al., 2000)

Gelberg et al. (2000) advanced another classic model, the Behavioral Model for Vulnerable Populations; this model looks at population characteristics (predisposing and enabling factors and needs) as an explanation for health behaviors and eventual health outcomes (Burg & Oyama, 2016). The following concepts are supported by this model:

- Predisposing factors included demographic variables (e.g., gender, age, marital status), social variables (e.g., education, employment, ethnicity, social networks), and health beliefs (e.g., values and attitudes toward health and healthcare services, knowledge of disease).
- Social structures (e.g., acculturation and immigration), sexual orientation, and childhood characteristics (e.g., mobility, living conditions, history of substance misuse, criminal behavior, victimization, or mental illness) were also considered predisposing factors.
- Enabling factors included personal and family resources, as well as community resources (e.g., income, insurance, social support, region, health services resources, public benefits, transportation, telephone, crime rates, social services resources).
- Perceived health needs and population health conditions also were considered, as were health behaviors including diet, exercise, tobacco use, self-care, and adherence to care.
- The use of health services (e.g., ambulatory and inpatient care, long-term care, alternative healthcare) and personal health practices (e.g., hygiene, unsafe sexual behaviors, food sources) combined with the other factors to produce outcomes such as perceived and evaluated health and general satisfaction with healthcare services.

See Figure 23-2, interrelated pathways linking education to health.

Source: Burg and Oyama (2016); Gelberg et al. (2000).

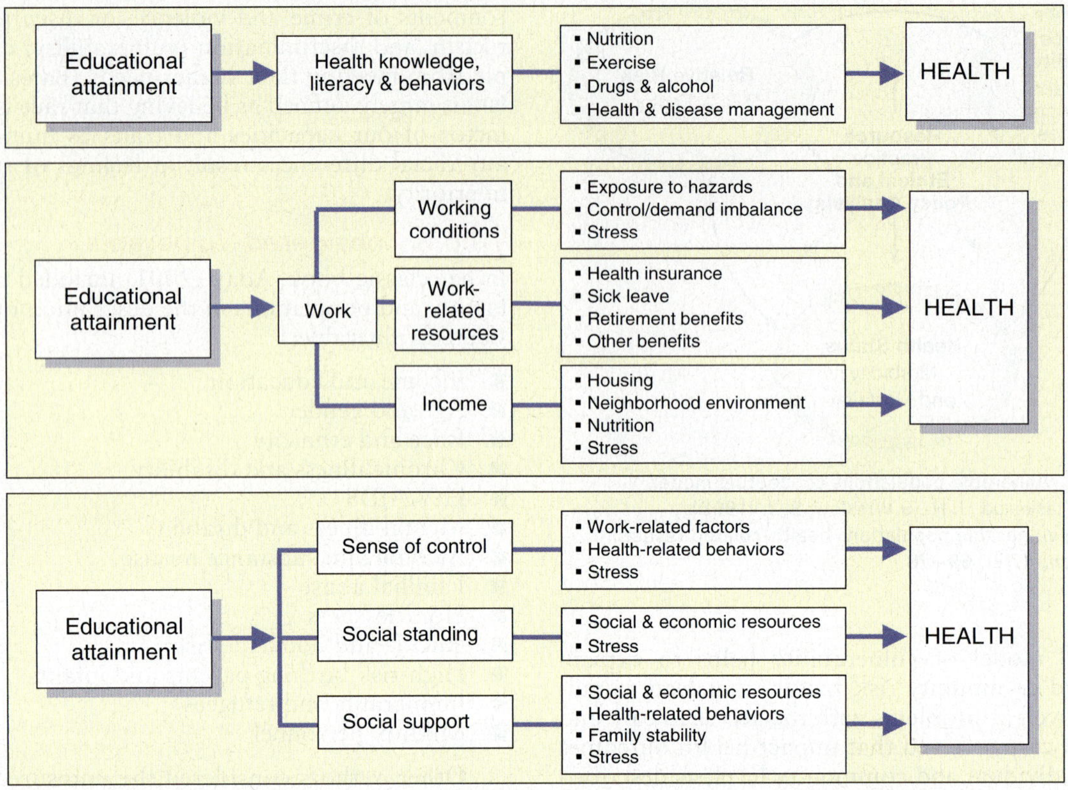

FIGURE 23-2 Interrelated pathways linking education to health. (From Braveman, P., Ergerter, S., & Williams, D. R. (2011). The social determinants of health: Coming of age. *Annual Review of Public Health, 32,* 381–398, used with permission.)

(Hutchison & Cox, 2020). The very young and the very old have particular risk factors that increase their chances of poor health, as well as unique issues with access to healthcare.

- An extensive body of research substantiates the reality of higher morbidity and mortality rates for racial and ethnic populations other than for the White population, thus demonstrating **racial/ethnic disparities** in health (Hutchison & Cox, 2020; Tolbert et al., 2022).

BOX 23-3 The Differential Vulnerability Hypothesis (Kessler, 1979)

Kessler's (1979) **differential vulnerability hypothesis** states that there is a relationship between social status and psychological distress; a person's psychological distress is determined by the impact of the stressor event as influenced by social status (this includes class, sex, marital status, and rural vs. urban). The formula $P_i = V_i\ (S)_i + a_i$ is defined as (Kessler, 1979, p. 101): "(P) Psychological distress is the result of varying exposure to environmental stress events or situations (S) acting on individuals who possess varying vulnerabilities to stress (V); (a) represents the residual influence of constitutional makeup of the mental health of person (i) independent of any environmental stresses he/she might experience" (Kessler, 1979, p. 101).

Kessler (1979).

Prevalence of Vulnerable Populations and Causative Factors

Root causes of vulnerability, such as low socioeconomic status (SES), lack of insurance coverage, racism, and discrimination, have been widely researched. Which cause or causes are considered most important? The exact weight of the interaction of these causes has been difficult to ascertain. The current approach to understanding the complex interrelationships among the causes and factors related to vulnerability is to examine multiple determinants of health (Iorhen, 2021), including the social determinants of health (SDOH) (Box 23-4).

Poverty

If only one indicator is measured—poverty—it is evident that vulnerability touches a large segment of the global population and the population in the United States:

- According to the latest figures from the World Bank (2020), an estimated 719 million people are living in extreme poverty (living on $1.90 or less a day), and 2.1 billion are living in moderate poverty (living on between $1.90 and $3.10 a day).
- The official poverty rate in the United States is 11.6%, which represents an estimated 37.9 million people (Center for Poverty Research, University of California Davis [UCD], 2021).
- Poverty thresholds in the United States are $15,060 for a single person under age 65, $20,440 for a household of two people with a householder 65 years or older with no children, and $27,700 for a family

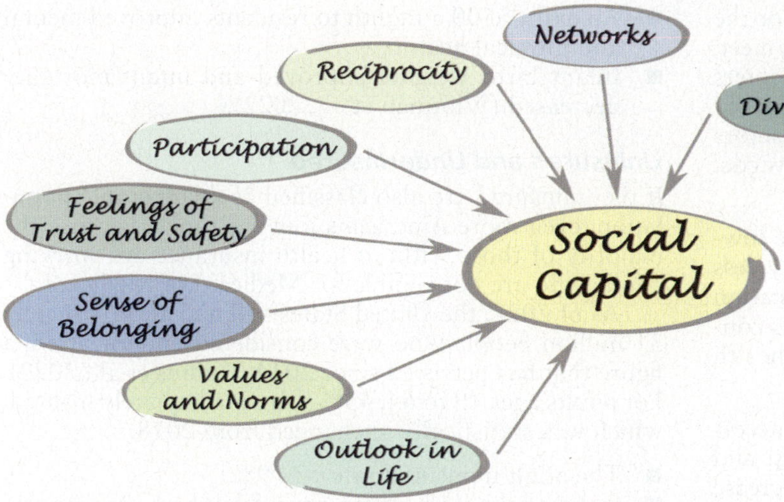

FIGURE 23-3 Social capital is a network of relationships where one lives and works.

of four with two children under age 18 (Healthcare.gov, 2024).

- According to Annie E. Casey Foundation (2023), 31% of the children in poverty are Black or African American, 28% are American Indian or Alaskan Native, 23% are Hispanic or Latino, 11% are Asian or Pacific Islander, 11% are non-Hispanic White, and 19% are two or more races.

How does poverty make one vulnerable to poor health outcomes? The answer to this question is complex:

- One supposition is that having less money means being less able to afford most aspects associated with quality of life, including adequate housing in a safe neighborhood. This living situation may lead to fewer opportunities for exercise, especially if walking outside puts one at risk for experiencing violence.
- Fewer community resources are usually available, such as grocery stores, quality schools, recreation facilities, and healthcare providers. Lower income level is associated with lower levels of education and often results in a person having to work at jobs where

BOX **23-4** POPULATION FOCUS

Teen Pregnancy

Medical complications associated with adolescent pregnancy include poor maternal weight gain, anemia, and pregnancy-induced hypertension. Poverty, lower educational level, and inadequate family support can contribute to a lack of adequate prenatal care, which can lead to higher rates of anemia, preeclampsia, poor nutrition, preterm birth, and low birth weight. Adolescent parents who lack social support and who are at a lower socioeconomic status are less likely to breastfeed. Adolescent partners who maintain active participation in the prenatal, neonatal, and immediate postpartum process have a greater likelihood of ongoing involvement with their children. Birthing parents with higher parenting stress and parent–child dysfunction, have higher rates of depression. The prevalence of intimate partner violence among teen birthing parents is 7%; formal screening for intimate partner violence of adolescent parents during pregnancy and in the postpartum period is important. Additional education should be focused on prevention of child abuse because risk factors for abuse include adolescent pregnancy and low socioeconomic status. Within the first year of a child's life, 63% of teens who gave birth will receive public assistance benefits, and 52% of birthing parents who receive welfare will have had their first child in their teen years (Powers & Takagishi, 2021).

Community-based programs, including school-based and home visitation programs have shown to decrease subsequent pregnancies, use of government assistance, child abuse and neglect, and criminal behavior. The Nurse–Family Partnership is an evidence-based program that pairs young first time birthing parents with trained nurses beginning in early pregnancy and continuing through the child's second birthday. Programs such as Head Start and Early Head Start are designed to address the needs of both parents and children with limited resources. A parent-centered approach utilizing Teen-tot clinics, where the teenage parent or parents and their children are seen by the same provider at the same appointment have shown successful outcomes. Parenting and life skills interventions coupled with medical appointments improved maternal self-esteem and decreased repeat pregnancy (Powers & Takagishi, 2021).

Nurse–Family Partnership is an evidence-based, community health program with 45 years of research showing significant improvements in the health and lives of first-time moms and their children affected by social and economic inequality. Nurse–Family Partnership succeeds by having specially educated nurses regularly visit first-time moms from early pregnancy through the child's second birthday. Moms benefit by getting specialized care and support during pregnancy, and their nurse becomes a trusted source on everything from child safety to taking steps to provide a stable, secure future for their family. Research consistently proves that the mom/nurse partnership is a winning combination that makes a measurable, long-term difference for the whole family.

Source: Powers and Takagishi (2021).

they are exposed to higher risks (e.g., mining), or the need to work at more than one job to make ends meet, and often without health insurance coverage (Centers for Disease Control & Prevention [CDC], 2023a). For further information on the role socioeconomic factors have on health outcomes, refer to https://www.cdc.gov/dhdsp/health_equity/socioeconomic.htm.

Research has shown that those groups with the lowest income and least education were consistently less healthy than those with the most income and education (World Health Organization [WHO], 2020a). SES is considered a consistent and robust variable related to health and death:

- Resource-limited neighborhoods with poor access and poor walkability to fresh fruits, vegetables, and lean proteins are associated with a significant increase in cardiovascular disease mortality and type 2 diabetes (U.S. Department of Agriculture [USDA], 2023). Many of these neighborhoods are termed food deserts due to the lack of available supermarkets (Fig. 23-4).
- Research has shown that fast food restaurants are more prevalent in low-income neighborhoods, and this prevalence has been shown to have a positive correlation with obesity and type 2 diabetes (Institute for Functional Medicine, 2023). Another risk factor for vulnerability that is associated with poverty is exposure to pollution and smoking.
- One finding indicates that the highest amount of pollution is most often found in neighborhoods where there is more poverty, lower education levels, and higher rates of unemployment (American Lung Association, 2023).
- Other researchers note an association between SES and obesity, hypertension, kidney disease, certain cancers, and coronary heart disease (Australian Institute of Health and Welfare, 2022).

At the population level, increases in total income and reductions in poverty levels are known to improve the overall health of a community.

- Health improvements improved with cash incentives.
- Families and people with disabilities received cash payments.

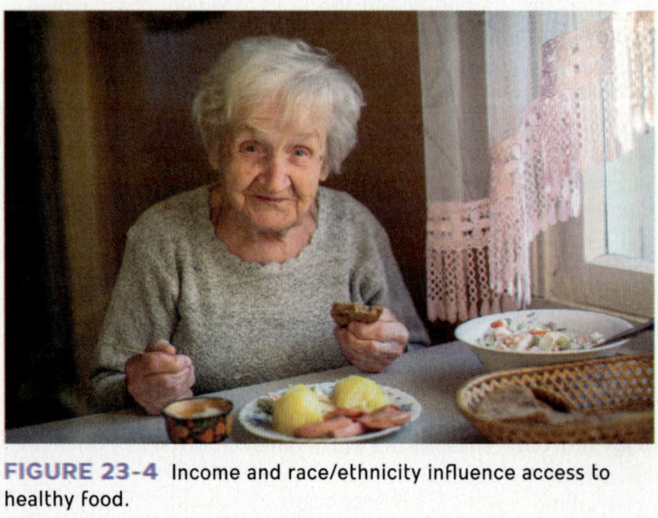

FIGURE 23-4 Income and race/ethnicity influence access to healthy food.

- An extra $500 a month to residents improved mental and physical health.
- Infant birth weights improved and infant mortality decreased (Whitman et al., 2022).

Uninsured and Underinsured

If the uninsured are also classified as a vulnerable population, even more Americans join the ranks, because the majority of those without health insurance are working adults who are not eligible for Medicaid or Medicare.

As of 2022, the United States still had approximately 31 million people who were considered underinsured, a figure that has persisted since 2014 (Collins et al., 2022). For adults ages 19 to 64, 43% were inadequately insured, which was statistically unchanged from 2018.

- The adult uninsured rate was 9%.
- Some adults, 11%, were insured but had a gap in coverage in the past year, and 23% were underinsured.

Despite efforts to address healthcare disparities, many healthcare experts continue to express concerns that disparities in quality, access, and outcomes will persist, particularly for people classified as more vulnerable (National Conference of State Legislators, 2021). Also, most healthcare experts feel that there will still be disparities in quality, access, and outcomes for those who are more vulnerable (Wasserman et al., 2019).

How does having inadequate or no health insurance lead to poor health outcomes? As explained in Chapter 6, those with few or no resources in this area do not use early screenings and preventive measures, and they delay getting treatment in an effort to save money. Those without health insurance receive care only for the problem at hand and not always for underlying causes. They do not get regular physical examinations and may be inadequately immunized against common diseases. Thus, they are at risk for poorer general health. Also, when examination and subsequent treatment are delayed, diseases, such as cancer or cardiovascular illness, may result in earlier death (American Cancer Society, 2022).

Race and Ethnicity

- The United States is a multiracial, multiethnic country. About one-third of the population belongs to an underrepresented racial or ethnic group. The U.S. Census takes place every 10 years with the last one in 2020.
  - White 58.9%
  - Hispanic–Latinx 19.1%
  - Black or African American 13.6%
  - Asian 6.3%
  - Two or more races 3%
  - Pacific Islanders 0.3% (U.S. Census, 2023)
- The U.S. Hispanic population reached 62.1 million in 2020, constituting 19% of the total U.S. population. This demographic group is the second largest racial or ethnic group, following White Americans and surpassing Black Americans, as reported by the U.S. Census Bureau. Moreover, it is one of the most rapidly expanding population segments in the United States, with a 23% growth rate between 2010 and 2020, compared to 50.5 million in 2010. Since 1970, when Hispanics comprised 5% of the U.S. population

at 9.6 million, the Hispanic population has expanded more than sixfold (Nadeem, 2023).

- Data collected from 1999 to 2018 was used to determine the prevalence of hypertension among different races. Sells et al. (2023) found that non-Hispanic Black participants had the highest prevalence of hypertension (48.8%), as compared with 37.6% for non-Hispanic White participants and 27.9% for Hispanic participants. While 7.5% of non-Hispanic White participants lived in poverty, 26% of the Hispanic participants lived in poverty.
- In 2021, Black birthing parents experienced a preterm birth rate of 14.8%, which was approximately 50% higher than the preterm birth rate observed among White or Hispanic birthing parents, which were; 9.5% and 10.2%, respectively (CDC, 2022a).
- Immigrants experience differences when compared with U.S.-born persons.
  - Higher levels of Hepatitis B and TB
  - Less enrollment for health insurance
  - Underserved in healthcare
  - Earn 200% of poverty level
  - Fewer high school graduates
  - Higher prevalence of mental health concerns when the home country experiences war and violence
  - Age faster (Bustamante et al., 2021)

Why does simply being a member of an underrepresented racial or ethnic group make someone vulnerable? The reasons are complex and just beginning to be understood but some key considerations include the following:

- Institutional racism in policies and procedures within social institutions including healthcare (Needham et al., 2023).
- Examples of institutional racism are numerous both toward healthcare providers and patients.
  - Healthcare staff encounter overt and covert racism.
  - Patients experience racism by healthcare staff: inadequate healthcare, scolding by healthcare providers, avoidance of being touched, and lack of respect (Hamed et al., 2022).
- Cultural racism affects economic status and health by creating a policy environment adverse to equal policies.
- Experiences of racial discrimination are a type of psychosocial stressor that can increase health risks.

VULNERABILITY AND INEQUALITY IN HEALTHCARE

Various social factors, known as the **social determinants of health**, including SES, affect a person's vulnerability to poor health. Specific areas in which inequities in health outcomes result from these social factors are known as **health disparities**.

Social Determinants of Health

The WHO has defined the social determinants of health as "…factors such as where we live, the state of our environment, genetics, our income and education level, and our relationships with friends and family all have considerable impacts on health…," including the available health system (WHO, 2020b, para 1). Commonly acknowledged factors, such as social norms or attitudes (e.g., discrimination, racism); exposure to crime, violence, and social disorder; and concentrated poverty, are associated with health outcomes and are recognized as social determinants of health (CDC, 2022b; USDHHS, n.d.).

The unequal distribution of these factors among certain groups is thought to contribute to health disparities that are persistent and pervasive. The IOM report *For the Public's Health: The Role of Measurement in Action and Accountability* called for addressing the underlying factors, not only the data, related to morbidity and mortality (2012). When we address health disparities, we must consider these social determinants and work on all levels—person, aggregate, community, and population—to reduce them.

Social determinants of health are related to both morbidity and mortality. Quantified deaths that could be attributed to social factors in the United States were reported:

- In California, life expectancy declined during the COVID-19 pandemic from 81.4 years in 2019 to 78.37 years in 2021. Life expectancy differences between the highest and lowest income earners increased from 11.52 years in 2019 to 15.51 years in 2021 (Schwandt et al., 2022).
- Publicly funded healthcare and programs to reduce SDOH increased life expectancy by 5 to 10 years (Galvani-Townsend et al., 2022).
- The community's neighborhood conditions and resources available for children at time of birth are associated with life expectancy in adults (Shanahan et al., 2022).
- Hong Kong has a higher life expectancy by 8.3 years when compared to the United States. When compared with similar populous countries, the United States ranked 46th in life expectancy (Woolf, 2023).
- Healthy People 2030 addresses the context in which people's lives influence their health (see the social determinants of health in Box 23-5).

Socioeconomic Gradient of Health

In a series of large-scale, longitudinal studies in England, the now classic Whitehall studies, British civil servants were divided into socioeconomic groups based on their occupational status, from executives to unskilled workers.

BOX 23-5 *HEALTHY PEOPLE 2030*

Social Determinants of Public Health

- Economic stability
- Education access and quality
- Healthcare access and quality
- Neighborhood and built environment
- Social and community context

Reprinted from USDHHS. (2020). *Social determinants of health.* Retrieved from https://health.gov/healthypeople/objectives-and-data/social-determinants-health

What the investigators discovered was an improvement in mortality and morbidity rates as the level of one's occupation and pay increased. Those at the lowest levels had the poorest health, but as they moved up the salary scale and occupational level, their health improved. What makes this so interesting is that all of the workers had basic health insurance coverage and free medical care—no real problems with access to healthcare existed. Although less pronounced, even when the researchers adjusted for diet, exercise, and smoking, the gradient persisted (Marmot et al., 1997).

This direct relationship between social class or income and health has been termed the **socioeconomic gradient** (Hajizadeh et al., 2016). It has been found in populations around the world, although not always unfailingly, and has been related to

- Poor health outcomes regarding cardiovascular disease in South America (Mullachery et al., 2022). In one U.S. study that spanned from 1999 to 2016 researchers discovered that people with higher income had lower prevalence of cardiovascular disease (Abdalla et al., 2020).
- Higher mortality rates in childhood cancers in resource-limited European countries (WHO, 2022).
- Outcomes of adult and child asthma (WHO, 2023) behaviors, such as smoking, are highest among those who have lower income and general educational levels (CDC, 2023b).
- The lower the income or access to resources, the lower the ability of a person to self-manage health concerns in China (Hu et al., 2021).

Health Disparities

Health disparities are differences in the quantity of disease, burden of disease, and other adverse health conditions present in different groups (CDC, 2020).

- Health disparities may be unavoidable, such as health-damaging behaviors that are chosen by a person despite health education and counseling efforts, but most are thought to be due to inequities that can be corrected (Ndugga & Artiga, 2023).
- A long-held belief about health inequities, adopted by the WHO (2017), is that they are unnecessary and avoidable as well as unjust and unfair, so the resulting health inequalities also lead to inequity in health.
- Health disparities can be objectively viewed as a disproportionate burden of morbidity, disability, and mortality found in a specific portion of the population in contrast to another.
- The topic of social determinants of health was added to *Healthy People 2020* (Office of Disease Prevention and Health Promotion [ODPHP], 2020).
- Promoting healthy choices does not eliminate health disparities; action must be taken to improve the conditions within people's environments. That is why Healthy People 2030 has increased its focus on SDOH (USDHHS, n.d.). In fact, one of Healthy People's 2030 goals focuses on SDOH: "Create social, physical, and economic environments that promote attaining the full potential for health and well-being for all" (USDHHS, n.d., para 4).
- Lack of empathy in patient care produces poorer health outcomes. Teaching empathy in a variety of clinical scenarios throughout a nursing program, especially with the vulnerable populations, improves patient outcomes (Zeller et al., 2024).
- Transgender and gender-diverse older adults face verbal harassment by healthcare professionals, have been refused care, and are concerned they will not receive good healthcare in long-term agencies (Velasco et al., 2023).
- Health disparities include lower birth rates of infants among non-Hispanic Black birthing parents (Clay, 2021); lower rates of breast cancer screenings were seen in different races and ethnicity (Ponce-Chazarri et al., 2023); and parts of the country with a high African American population have a higher rate of COVID-19 mortality rate than other parts of the country (Kodsup & Godebo, 2023).

Poor access to quality care and overt discrimination are examples of disparities. Discrimination can occur during service delivery if healthcare providers are biased against a specific group or hold stereotypical beliefs about that group. Providers may also not be confident about providing care for a racial or ethnic group with whom they are unfamiliar. Language may be a problem, as are cultural values and norms that are unfamiliar to providers. The healthcare system must improve on building trust with the population that may be leery of the healthcare system (Griffith et al., 2021).

Access to Care

The landmark IOM (2003) report *Unequal Treatment: Confronting Racial and Ethnic Disparities in Health Care* noted a large body of research highlighting the higher morbidity and mortality rates among all underrepresented racial and ethnic groups when compared with White populations. This report drew attention to an issue that continues today and remains relevant. Differences in healthcare access were also explained, whether due to inadequate or no health insurance, problems getting healthcare, poorer quality of care, fewer choices in where to go for care, or the lack of a regular healthcare provider. For instance, because there are fewer numbers of healthcare providers in neighborhoods with underrepresented populations, finding a primary care provider is more difficult for those living in these areas. Providing low-cost or free clinics within low-income neighborhoods has been shown to improve the management of chronic conditions and decrease rates of hospitalization (Health Resources & Service Administration [HRSA], 2023).

Progress in this area has remained slow. The Institutes of Medicine's Progress Report highlights the following mechanisms to address 21st-century healthcare needs: better coordination of care, nurses to practice to the full extent of their license, increased educational levels of nurses (including more doctorate and bachelor's prepared nurses), increased workforce diversity, and nurse engagement in leadership roles (National Academy of Sciences, 2019).

Healthcare access is also problematic for other vulnerable groups. For example, services and resources for people with mental illness or substance use disorders are often fragmented and inadequate, as are those for families experiencing abuse and people who are unsheltered. Refugees and immigrants may have difficulty finding affordable and easily accessible healthcare, largely because of their lack of health insurance and the need to find care at free clinics or emergency rooms (Kaiser Family Foundation [KFF], 2023). When people from vulnerable populations cannot get appropriate healthcare or treatment for illness or disease, for whatever reason, they are more likely to have health deficits.

Quality of Care

Quality of care is another area in which health disparities persist. One aspect of quality care is the comfort level patients have with their providers. Research indicates that clients from underrepresented racial and ethnic groups may feel more comfortable and satisfied with care from a healthcare provider who comes from the same racial and ethnic group (Fig. 23-5). For example, Spanish-speaking patients had higher levels of patient satisfaction, higher levels of care, and were able to share sensitive medical information when the provider was Spanish speaking (Lopez Vera et al., 2023).

However, a shortage of ethnically diverse healthcare providers exists. Despite underrepresented racial and ethnic groups constituting 37% of the U.S. population, only 19.4% of registered nurses are from underrepresented racial and ethnic groups (American Association of Colleges of Nursing [AACN], 2023). Also, research needs to be more inclusive of underrepresented groups. For example, there is limited acute care stroke research that includes participants with limited English proficiency, even though this population is growing (Zeidan et al., 2023).

Communication can also be a factor in poor quality of care. **Underrepresented populations**, such as people with substance use disorders, at-risk birthing parents and infants, families experiencing abuse, people at risk of suicide or harming others, and people with mental illness or disability, may feel they are treated as "second-class citizens," and cultural barriers and misunderstandings can lead to a discontinuation of recommended regimens.

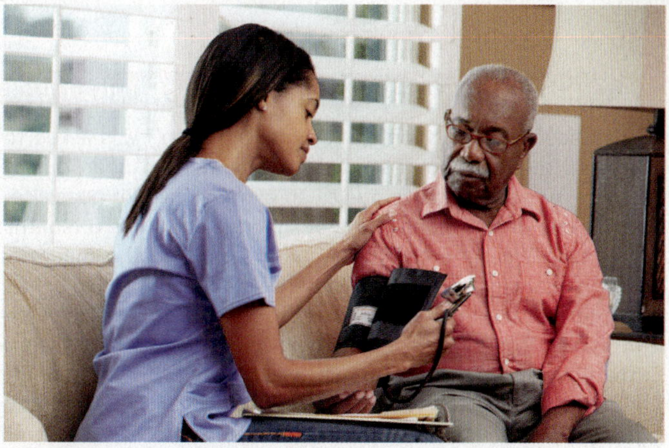

FIGURE 23-5 Clients from underrepresented racial and ethnic groups often prefer healthcare providers from the same racial and ethnic background.

WORKING WITH VULNERABLE POPULATIONS

Through the day-to-day provision of care and participation in larger efforts in the community, the nurse can help improve health outcomes for vulnerable populations (see Box 23-6).

BOX 23-6 Community/Public Health Nurse Actions to Promote Client Empowerment

Which community/public health nursing activities/actions are most effective in promoting empowerment among nurses' vulnerable clients? In Falk-Rafael's (2001) well-known qualitative study of public health nurses (C/PHNs) and their clients, several themes were noted as components of the C/PHN role:

- *Empowerment* is "an active, internal process of growth" that is reached by actualizing the full potential inherent within each client, and this occurs "within the context of a nurturing nurse—client relationship" (p. 4). C/PHNs describe the process of empowerment as a two-way street with clients not only gaining knowledge and skills and "acting on informed choices" but also further empowering the nurse to continue the work of the empowerment (p. 6).
- *Having a client-centered approach*, denoted by flexibility in dealing with clients, for example, "meeting them where they are," "communicating at their level," and "backing off and following client's agenda" (p. 6).
- *Developing a trusting relationship* based on mutual respect and dignity, for example, clients as active partners with the C/PHN assuming more or less responsibility as needed; being empathetic, nonjudgmental, and "creating a safe environment" (p. 7).
- *Employing advocacy*, both at an individual level as well as political advocacy, for example, using their role and power as a professional to cut through bureaucratic red tape, connecting clients with available community resources, supporting clients in reaching their health goals, making their expertise available, and being a client resource as someone who is open and "available" (p. 8).
- *Being a teacher and role model*, using a variety of strategies and providing opportunities for clients to safely practice new skills. For example, using strategies such as teaching classes, providing individual coaching, providing positive reinforcement and support, demonstrating skills such as assertiveness, and encouraging community action/participation are helpful.
- *Capacity building* through encouraging and supporting of clients' work toward attaining health goals, for example, "reflective listening and an empathetic approach" focusing on strengths, not limitations; facilitating client "self-exploration" and providing encouragement for them to "act on their choices" while being "realistic about barriers to success"; or having expectations for client accountability regarding their decisions and actions (p. 9).

Source: Falk-Rafael (2001).

BOX **23-7** PERSPECTIVES

A C/PHN's Viewpoint on Community/Public Health Nursing

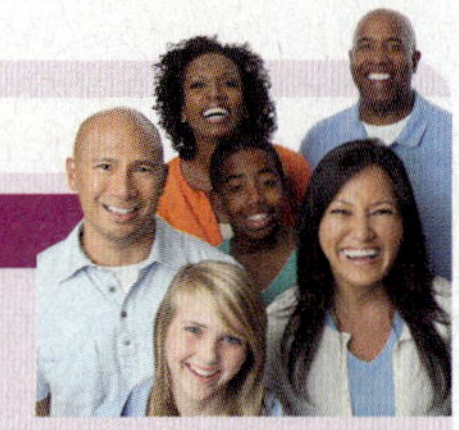

I had been a PHN for only a few months when I was asked to assess the home of a second grader who had been out of school for several weeks due to an extreme case of head lice. It was one of the hottest days of the year and I was 8 months pregnant. When I entered the apartment, I found a family of five in a studio apartment, instead of a kitchen the family had a hot plate that they heated food on. It was always my practice to ask if I could use the bathroom to check for warm water, towels, and soap. The bathroom was extremely dirty. The family earned money by recycling trash, and the small studio had plastic bottles in piles. The father was sleeping on the one mattress on the floor without bed linen. The windows were open but had no screens; flies were everywhere. The mother was more concerned for me and my pregnancy. She offered me a glass of cold water, which I politely accepted. When I returned to the office, I discovered this family was well known by the other PHNs. They had been evicted from several apartments because of unsafe and unsanitary conditions. Unfortunately, this is what happened after this visit. I asked the environmental health officer to assess the safety of the apartment, and it was determined to be uninhabitable. I lost contact with the family, but I think of them often and what we could have done to be more helpful.

Malia, PHN, RN

The Role of Public Health Nurses

C/PHNs can work to improve the health of vulnerable populations by empowerment, facilitating external support from patients' family and friends and engaging in evidence-based practice.

Empowerment

Because vulnerability often equates with feelings of powerlessness, the actions of C/PHNs can either promote engagement or destroy chances for rapport. C/PHNs can use **empowerment strategies** in their work with clients once trust and rapport have been established (Box 23-7). The personal values, experiences, characteristics, and actions of both nurses and clients influence the speed at which this process takes place and the eventual level of connection. Helping clients identify their fears and clearly defining the C/PHN role with the client and family are also important.

Building and preserving relationships with clients is a central focus of C/PHN home visits. It requires building trust and rapport and helping them to feel accepted, engaged, and ready. The building phase involves working with individual clients to improve their social connections, build their strengths, and work toward their goals. Building self-efficacy, motivation, and health literacy are essential in this stage, as are helping them with coping skills and giving encouragement as they build resilience.

While empowering clients, nurses should also remember to empower themselves through collaboration with others (see Box 23-8) and self-care. Working with vulnerable populations can be challenging and exhausting. Often, novice community health nurses feel overwhelmed and suffer "compassion fatigue" when confronted with the crushing realities that their clients

BOX **23-8** SPOTLIGHT ON ESSENTIAL NURSING COMPETENCIES

Interprofessional Partnerships When Working With Vulnerable Populations

C/PHNs work with many vulnerable groups, including individuals and families that are unsheltered. Vulnerable groups within the community may be underrepresented and lack access to quality healthcare services. To provide services, C/PHNs must partner with a variety of agencies, interested parties, and clients. To build rapport and trust, nurses must provide respectful understanding and care while focusing on the needs of the client. How do essential nursing competencies assist C/PHNs in demonstrating interprofessional partnerships when meeting the needs of single parents with young children that reside in a shelter?

Students in a community health clinic spent time working with single parents with young children residing in a shelter. Some students had limited previous exposure to diverse populations and were aware only of stereotypes and misconceptions regarding this population. Single parent heads-of-household and their children made up 60% of the population using this facility. Students were unaware of the variance of demographics and backgrounds regarding this vulnerable group. However, as the students began to learn about the families, they realized that partnerships with the community and other professionals were needed.

In conjunction with the shelter, students identified clients' needs and provided an educational health fair. Partnering with local health clinics, Medicaid providers, advocates for people who have experienced abuse, and local school nurses, the students focused their teaching on the health needs of the adults and the children. Local agencies supplied free needed items; education stations were then created to support health issues surrounding the donated items (e.g., an oral health education station provided free travel-size toothbrushes).

BOX **23-8** SPOTLIGHT ON ESSENTIAL NURSING COMPETENCIES (*Continued*)

While offering health education, students engaged with clients, their families, and other community members, which gave them the opportunity to learn that nothing can be accomplished alone. As they learned the role of C/PHN, they gained insight into the importance of working with interprofessional partnerships. One student had a conversation with a parent about how they came to live in the shelter. The parent shared that after their partner died, there were no family or support systems to help, and the child had severe asthma. The family lost their home and insurance, which caused medical bills to pile up.

1. *Reflect on the role of the C/PHN. What other interprofessional partnerships would be beneficial?*
2. *Why is it important to maintain a collaborative relationship with interprofessional, intraprofessional, and paraprofessional partners?*

face on a daily basis. Feelings of guilt sometimes surface when nurses contrast their own life experiences with those of their clients. To be effective in working with vulnerable populations, it is often more helpful to donate money and items on a group level rather than an individual level and to work for substantial changes in community attitudes and policies. Also, it is vital to remain grounded to continue to have the necessary energy and compassion (Box 23-9).

Patient empowerment implies a shared decision making with the provider. In one literature review, clients who were empowered made positive changes in their health behavior (Cardoso Barbosa et al., 2021). They were better able to seek information and services. Clients' focus became more proactive than reactive, and they felt that they could communicate more effectively to define boundaries or express feelings. Consequently, clients were also better able to collaborate with their healthcare providers, becoming more trusting partners in care by demonstrating ownership for their actions and their health. A large part of C/PHN practice is to encourage their clients to become more self-reliant and responsible for their health in spite of systemic barriers.

BOX **23-9** EVIDENCE-BASED PRACTICE

Caring and Compassion

Campbell et al. (2020) conducted a 5-year longitudinal study from 2013 to 2018, identifying factors that contributed to recruitment, retention, and turnover in C/PHN nurses working in Nurse Family Partnership programs in rural British Columbia. Initially, the C/PHNs were motivated to be part of an evidence-based program for young birthing parents who were economically disadvantaged. While C/PHNs expressed motivation to work for an institution that supported nurse's personal and professional philosophies in providing care to vulnerable populations, as well as autonomy in working to the full extent of their practice, modifiable factors such as organization and geographic factors may influence job satisfaction, making this a "hard job to love." In this qualitative study, C/PHNs expressed the need for support through a culture of connectivity. Team connections and viewing client successes may support job satisfaction and retention in an already fatiguing healthcare role.

Source: Campbell et al. (2020).

Facilitating External Support

The degree of external support clients have, along with their temperament and other individual factors, affects their ability to cope with stress and adverse situations. The support can be from family members, neighbors, friends, teachers, or others. C/PHNs can help clients establish external support at both the individual and population levels (Boxes 23-10 and 23-11). (For an interactive map that provides information on the degree to which specific U.S. communities are affected by external stressors on human health, see the CDC's Social Vulnerability Index (https://svi.cdc.gov/).

Using Evidence to Reduce Vulnerability

Community health nurses can help vulnerable populations, communities, people, and families reduce their vulnerability by using evidence from research, expert opinion, and best practices (see Chapter 4 on evidence-based practice). Often, evidence is embedded in policies, procedures, and clinical guidelines. Thus, the first place to locate evidence for practice is in the specific agency documentation for nursing practice. Sometimes, a community need is discovered that requires creative thinking and evidence-based interventions (Box 23-12).

Many areas for improvement of the lives of vulnerable populations lie in areas related to prevention and health promotion, as described above. Primary prevention is readily available in the form of immunizations for children, adolescents, and adults. Nursing activities to promote increasing immunization levels among these populations will result in greater economic and social returns for the whole community. Similar is the involvement of nurses in smoking prevention and smoking cessation activities. Also, some vulnerable subpopulations require additional insight and experience, such as people who are incarcerated (see the case study at the end of this chapter), American Indian/Indigenous American and Alaska Native Populations (Box 23-13), and people who have experienced human trafficking (Box 23-14).

Improving Health Literacy

Healthy People 2030 has incorporated goals related to personal and organizational health literacy. People who do not understand health information are less likely to get preventative healthcare and more likely to experience health problems. Nurses are in a position to improve out-

BOX 23-10 STORIES FROM THE FIELD

A View of Disasters

When disaster strikes the communities of those who are struggling to survive, the effects are devastating, and the recovery is long and challenging. Communities with poorly built homes, without strong foundations or storm windows, are less safe during tornadoes and hurricanes. Floods impact low-lying, low-income neighborhoods the hardest (Lowrey, 2019). The high cost of living in California has encouraged people with limited resources to migrate to less expensive and remote fire-prone areas (Lowrey, 2019).

In 2018, the most destructive fire in California history incinerated the town of Paradise within a matter of hours. People living below the poverty level were the hardest hit, and 2 months after the disaster, because of inadequate housing for people with limited resources, there were still hundreds living in shelters. Many of those impacted were older and disabled, living in trailer homes. Local hospitals and other healthcare facilities were also incinerated, impacting access to healthcare. A nurse who was interviewed after the disaster, referring to the struggling people with limited resources who were impacted by the devastating fire, likened the incident to a house of cards; when removing a card, the whole house collapses (Lowrey, 2019).

In 2017, Hurricane Harvey caused catastrophic flooding and many deaths in Houston, Texas. The New York Times interviewed a survivor of this disaster 1 year later. She spoke about the experience of losing her home and living in a trailer. The survivor had no savings to use for recovery, and the support she received from the government, nonprofit groups, and volunteers was not enough for her and her family to return to a sense of normalcy. The survivor and her family were left feeling sad, broken, and confused (Fernandez, 2018).

In 2005, Hurricane Katrina broke through the levee system in New Orleans, Louisiana, causing massive flooding. Many of the residents with limited resources could not flee because they did not have a car, and they didn't have money to pay for a hotel and other necessities. Health issues related to the aftermath of the hurricane included concerns about contamination of local waters with solid waste, pesticide use for vector control from an abundance of mosquitoes, and reduction in air quality from mold and dust. People with limited resources bore the brunt of the disaster, and the few facilities that existed to quickly help people experiencing the disaster became miserable and dangerous places (Schake et al., 2019). Moving from large shelters to trailer homes negatively affected the mental health of some survivors and caused a great strain on family relationships. A Hurricane Katrina survivor who was born and raised in a housing project in New Orleans was relocated, as many were, to Houston, where she had no family, social support, nor means of transportation (Voice of a Witness, 2019).

Source: Fernandez (2018); Lowrey (2019); Schake et al. (2019); Voice of a Witness (2019).

comes for people who are underserved and can work to address the structural and institutional factors that produce health disparities in the first place. Nurses can use their unique expertise and perspective to help develop and advocate for policies and programs that promote health equity. Having a broader engagement as every nurse's core activity helps advance health equity nationwide. This focus requires the following (Committee on the Future of Nursing, 2021):

- Support for and the willingness of the nursing workforce to take on new roles in new settings in the community.
- Consistency in nurses' preparation for engaging in downstream, midstream, and upstream strategies aimed at improving health equity by addressing issues that compromise health, such as geographic disparities, poverty, racism, homelessness, trauma, drug misuse, and behavioral health conditions.
- More experiential learning and opportunities to work in community settings throughout nursing education to ensure that nurses have skills and competencies to address people's complex needs and promote efforts to improve the well-being of communities.
- Nursing education that goes beyond teaching the principles of diversity, equity, and inclusion to provide sustained student engagement in hands-on community and clinical experiences with these issues.
- Funding to support new models of care and functions that address health equity, social determinants of health, and population health.
- Evaluation of models to build the evidence needed to scale programs and the policies and resources necessary to sustain them.

BOX 23-11 Foundational Public Health Services (FPHS) Model

The FPHS model is a conceptual framework describing the capacities and programs that state and local health departments should be able to provide to all communities and for which costs can be estimated.

Foundational Public Health Service

Foundational Areas

- Environmental Health
- Chronic Disease and Injury Prevention
- Maternal, Child, and Family Health
- Access Linkage
- Communicable Disease

Foundational Capabilities

- Communications
- Policy Development
- Assessment and Surveillance
- Community Partnership
- Organizational Competencies
- Equity
- Accountability
- Emergency Preparedness

Public Health Accreditation Board (2022).

BOX **23-12** POPULATION FOCUS

Caring for LGBTQ+ People According to *Healthy People 2030*

- Lesbian, gay, bisexual, transgender, and queer (LGBTQ+) youth are more likely to experience homelessness and are two to three times more likely to attempt suicide (Abramovich et al., 2023).
- Lesbians are less likely to get preventive screening services for cervical cancer (Diamant et al., 2020).
- Gay and bisexual men are at higher risk for sexually transmitted infections, especially in communities of color (HIV.org, n.d.).
- Lesbians and bisexual people assigned female at birth are more likely to have excess weight or obesity (Stevens, 2023).
- Transgender people are at increased risk for experiencing violence and have a high prevalence of sexually transmitted infections, mental health issues, and suicide; they are also less likely to have health insurance than heterosexual or lesbian, gay, or bisexual people (AMA, 2019).

Intersectionality, when referring to identities, describes how different facets of identity, including race, gender expression and identity, sexual orientation, socioeconomic class, and other characteristics, are inseparable and affect each other. In healthcare settings, nurses and other healthcare professionals can apply this theory to respond to each patient as a person, not a manifestation of a stereotype, especially not one based on only one aspect of their identity.

Education on communication basics is a crucial aspect of providing compassionate care to LGBTQ+ patients. Nursing professionals should consider the following tips:

- Avoid assuming a patient's sex, gender, gender identity, or sexual orientation. Assumptions based solely on a patient's outward expression may be incorrect and result in malpractice and unintentional disrespect toward the patient's identity.
- If the patient's charted information does not match what they have reported on their forms, never ask for their "real" or given name. Instead, consider asking for the name listed on their insurance and then continue to refer to them by the name they provided.

Lesbian, gay, bisexual, transgender, and queer (LGBTQ+) people are more likely to experience certain health-related challenges and disparities. For example, LGBTQ+ adolescents are especially at risk for being bullied, which can contribute to thoughts of suicide or using illegal drugs (CDC, 2024). Up to 40% of youth who experience homelessness identify as LGBTQ+ (National Coalition for the Homeless, n.d.), and LGBTQ+ youth have a 12% higher risk of experiencing sexual violence (CDC, 2024). *Healthy People 2030* supports improving the health of LGBTQ+ populations through health behavior objectives, objectives that focus on systemic problems, and objectives that increase data collection on both the health and well-being of the LGBTQ+ community.

Research consistently elucidates mental health disparities among LGBTQ+ people when compared to their heterosexual, cisgender counterparts. These disparities are related to social inequalities that affect LGBTQ+ people. Salerno et al. (2020) note the following:

- A greater proportion of LGBTQ+ people lack access to health insurance and face poverty when compared to their non-LGBTQ+ counterparts.
- Poverty figures extend to same-sex parents and single LGBTQ+ parents and their families, who are at least twice as likely to be living near the poverty line when compared to their non-LGBTQ+ counterparts.
- LGBTQ+ people of color face a greater risk of social inequality.
- During the COVID-19 pandemic, the mental health burden to LGBTQ+ people was exacerbated by the psychological impact of concerns with job loss (40% of LGBTQ+ people work in the service industry, and the service industry was impacted greatly during the COVID-19 pandemic) and loss of health insurance.
- LGBTQ+ older adults are twice as likely to be single and living alone, four times less likely to have children, and more likely to be estranged from their biologic families compared with their heterosexual, cisgender counterparts.

Furthermore, older LGBTQ+ people face additional barriers to healthcare because of isolation and a lack of social services and culturally competent providers, and LGBTQ+ people have the highest rates of tobacco, alcohol, and drug use (Velasco et al., 2023).

BOX **23-13** POPULATION FOCUS

American Indian/Indigenous American and Alaska Native Populations

The American Indian and Alaskan Native populations experience more severe health risks and disparities as compared with other racial and ethnic groups in the United States. Members of the 574 federally recognized American Indian and Alaska Native Tribes and their descendants are eligible for services provided by Indian Health Services (IHS). The American Indian and Alaska Native people have long experienced lower life expectancy and a higher disease burden. A lack of education, disproportionate poverty, discrimination in the delivery of health services, and cultural differences are thought to be contributing factors. Cardiovascular disease, malignant neoplasm, unintentional injuries, and diabetes are the leading causes of American Indian and Alaska Native deaths. American Indians and Alaska Natives born today have a life expectancy that is 5.5 years less than the U.S. all-races population. American Indians and Alaska Natives continue to die at higher rates when compared to other U.S. residents in many categories, including chronic liver disease and cirrhosis, diabetes, unintentional injuries, assault, homicide, intentional self-harm/suicide, and chronic lower respiratory diseases (American Indian Services, 2019; Small-Rodriguez & Akee, 2021).

(*Continued*)

BOX **23-13** POPULATION FOCUS (*Continued*)

More than one-quarter of the American Indian and Alaska Native population are living in poverty, a rate that is more than double that of the general population. American Indian and Alaskan natives are likely to experience a range of violent and traumatic events involving serious injury or threat of injury to self or to witness such threat or injury to others. American Indians and Alaskan Natives are 1.3 times more likely to die by suicide using firearms (an increase of 55% between 2019 and 2021), and 3.5 times more likely to commit homicide by firearms (an increase of 24% between 2019 and 2021), than their White counterparts (Davis et al, 2023; Petrosky et al., 2021). Curtin et al. (2024) indicate that accidents are the leading cause of death for people ages 1 to 44, except that for people assigned female at birth ages 10 to 14, suicides are the leading cause of death. American Indian and Alaskan Native children are also exposed to repeated loss related to the high rate of early unexpected and traumatic deaths from injuries, accidents, suicide, homicide, and firearms—all of which exceed the U.S. all-races rate by two times—and due to alcohol use disorder, which exceeds the all-races rate by seven times. The age-related death rate for adults far exceeds that of the general population, with deaths due to diabetes, chronic liver disease and cirrhosis, and accidents occurring at least three times that of the national rate, and deaths due to tuberculosis, pneumonia and influenza, suicide, homicide, and heart disease also exceeding those of the general population (American Indian Services, 2019; Small-Rodriguez & Akee, 2021).

The Indian Health Service (IHS) Innovation Projects initiative supports Tribal and Urban Indian sites by addressing social factors that affect overall health. IHS sites are given federal funds to develop advanced quality improvement projects addressing social determinants. The goal of the Innovation Projects is to improve the link between the clinic and the community and to explore how quality improvement models can address these social factors affecting community health. Nurses have been playing an integral part in initiating these innovation projects and improving healthcare access and outcomes (Indian Health Services, n. d.).

- What prevention services would you prioritize for an American Indian patient?

BOX **23-14** Human Trafficking

Trafficking in persons, "human trafficking," and "modern slavery" are umbrella terms—often used interchangeably, used to refer to a crime whereby traffickers exploit and profit at the expense of adults or children by compelling them to perform labor or engage in commercial sex. When a person younger than 18 is used to perform a commercial sex act, it is a crime regardless of whether there is any force, fraud, or coercion. Globally, an estimated 25 million people are subjected to human trafficking and forced labor, which is responsible for an estimated $150 billion annually in illicit profits. Human trafficking disproportionately impacts some of the most vulnerable and underserved of our society (The White House, 2021).

Some young people are more vulnerable to being trafficked than others. Particularly vulnerable groups tend to share histories of poverty, family instability, physical and sexual abuse, and trauma. The relationship between race and the risk of being trafficked is significant. In some areas, African-American, American Indian, Alaskan Native, Native Hawaiian, and Pacific Islander young people assigned female at birth are also much more likely to be sexually exploited than their nonnative peers. Hispanic youth too are disproportionately affected by human trafficking, especially labor trafficking (National Center for Safe and Supportive Learning Environments, 2023).

Young people who run away from home are often fleeing abusive or neglectful situations. Youth who are homeless can be desperate to address their needs for food, clothing, and shelter. Youth who are homeless are vulnerable to labor traffickers because they need to support themselves. A large study of runaway and youth who are homeless found that 14% of youth receiving services from youth shelters had been trafficked for sex and 8% had been trafficked for labor. Some regional studies have found that up to 40% of youth who are homeless report trafficking experiences. Among youth who are unsheltered, 24% of these identifying as LGBTQ+ reported having been sold for sex or exchanged sex for food (National Center for Safe and Supportive Learning Environments, 2023).

Human trafficking is a public health crisis. Perpetrators of human trafficking gross billions of dollars annually from the sale of human cargo. Due to its pervasive and hidden nature, these crimes are happening at exponential rates but go undetected. Lack of identification of the people experiencing these crimes is seen across numerous disciplines such as law enforcement, social services, education, judicial services, and healthcare. Nurses working in urgent care, emergency departments, and public health or the community are more likely to encounter people held in captivity.

If you suspect that someone is experiencing human trafficking and are unsure how to proceed, call the National Human Trafficking Resource Center hotline: 1-888-373-7888.

- What types of behaviors might lead you to suspect a patient is experiencing human trafficking?

Improving Access to Nursing Services

The benefits of home health are well-known (Olds et al., 1997). Home visiting can be provided from almost any setting that provides services to communities. The usual settings are local health departments, home healthcare agencies, community-based hospice agencies, and visiting nurse associations. In addition, school nurses, ambulatory nurses, parish or faith-based nurses, and other nurses have recently provided limited home visiting services to clients or families seen in a variety of settings, including outpatient clinics, Head Start programs, places of worship, and health centers. Expanding home visiting to all vulnerable groups holds promise for improving the health of many people and communities (Fig. 23-6).

- Prenatal home visits by a C/PHN to expectant birthing parents with limited resources improved birth weight (Shin & Choi, 2023).
- Home visits by nurses and social workers reduce mortality rates among preterm infants (Lewis et al., 2023).

School-based health centers (SBHCs) are considered one of the most effective strategies for delivering preventive care, especially for difficult-to-reach populations such as adolescents. Numerous evaluations have shown that SBHCs achieve marked improvements in adolescent healthcare access when compared with that in other settings (Kjolhede & Lee, 2021). These clinics are included in healthcare reform funding, largely because of their proven record for accessibility and quality.

Nurse-led clinics (NLCs) have also increased access to care for communities and provided care that is more affordable, convenient, and with reduced patient waiting times. The nursing role in such clinics involves patient assessment, admission, health-related education, treatment and monitoring, discharge, and referral to other healthcare professionals. Findings indicate that NLCs enhanced client satisfaction and improved patient outcomes (Connolly & Cotter, 2023).

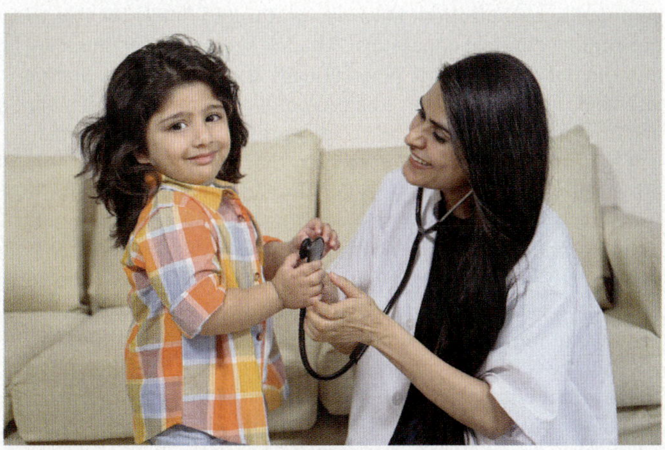

FIGURE 23-6 Home visiting has been shown to have positive outcomes for a variety of vulnerable populations. Results from over three decades of research have demonstrated that home visiting by registered nurses is effective in improving outcomes for birthing parents and children with limited resources.

Improving Health and Public Policy

Policies to reduce vulnerability for people, families, and communities have been shown to be effective at all levels: local, state, and national. Policy based on evidence is an important component of reducing vulnerability for communities and people. This section addresses health and public policy, including policy in schools, cities, counties, and healthcare settings. Policy includes social, economic, environmental, and health aspects. See Chapter 13 for an expansive discussion of policy.

Small changes in policy can make a big difference in outcomes for vulnerable communities. For example, policies to provide healthy foods in school vending machines provide healthier choices for all students, not just those considered vulnerable. Schools provide mental health services at the time when behavioral health concerns are a high priority with school-age children. Mandatory physical activity time for school children contributes to preventing obesity and enhancing learning in all children, and it is essential that future research and policymakers continue to recognize the school environment as a way to improve health for all (CDC, 2021).

SOCIAL JUSTICE AND PUBLIC HEALTH NURSING

Social justice occurs when a society provides for the overall health and well-being of all people by treating people fairly. It involves an equal societal bearing of burdens and reaping of benefits, and it is a widely held view that social justice is the foundation of public health nursing (Matwick & Woodgate, 2017) (see Box 23-15).

- Community health nurses who practice social justice have broad and holistic views of health; they have strong convictions that healthcare is a basic human right and that improving the health of communities is an example of social justice.
- Social justice ensures the distribution of resources that benefit underrepresented populations and holds in check the self-interest of more privileged populations. Impartiality is the goal.
- For instance, C/PHNs concerned with social justice include socially underrepresented and vulnerable populations (e.g., people involved in the criminal justice system, people who are undocumented) in their influenza pandemic planning processes. Not to do so would constitute discrimination and would be morally indefensible.

BOX **23-15** POPULATION FOCUS

Challenges for Community/Public Health Nursing Related to Documented and Undocumented Immigrants

I had always hoped that this land might become a safe and agreeable asylum to the virtuous and persecuted part of mankind, to whatever nation they might belong.

President George Washington

According to the U.S. Census Bureau, there are about 44.8 million immigrants in the United States; this is 13.7% of the U.S. population and 14.6% of these immigrants are living in poverty, while 19.6% do not have healthcare insurance (The White House, 2021). An estimated 10.5 to 12 million of these immigrants are undocumented (3.2% to 3.6% of the U.S. Population) (Kamarck & Stenglein, 2019).

Immigrants may find themselves in vulnerable situations as a result of the conditions that strongly influenced them to leave their country of origin, the circumstances in which they travel or the conditions that they face on arrival, or because of personal characteristics such as their age, gender identity, race, disability, or health status (United Nations Human Rights, 2023).

Immigrant youth coming to the United States may be forced by the journey itself into labor trafficking in order to pay off the debt they or their family members incurred to get to the United States. Children involved in seasonal work crews can be exploited because they travel from place to place and work in relative isolation and some crew leaders may ignore child labor and education laws.

Some immigrant children were born to migrant parents in transit and do not possess documents or have remained in their country of origin while one or both parents have migrated. Women can be especially vulnerable and at risk for workplace violence, harassment, sexual- and gender-based violence, and they are often reluctant to report crimes and transgressions due to a precarious immigration status.

Nurses as Advocates for Immigrants

Individual advocacy is demonstrated when nurses know and implement the highest quality of care possible to immigrant patients. For example, one essential practice is the use of a professional medical interpreter who fluently speaks the immigrant's primary language. Providers should not rely on family members or untrained or informal interpreters. The use of a qualified medical interpreter has a profound effect on positive clinical outcomes and patient satisfaction. In addition to using interpreters, nurses need to self-evaluate their understanding of racial and cultural biases. While cultural competency has been the dominant framework for reducing healthcare disparities, there is neither consistency nor evidence that this is sufficient or results in improved patient outcomes. Instead, Commodore-Mensah et al. (2021) supported a cultural humility where we are "acknowledging the power imbalances in our institutions and implicit bias" (p. e42). Cultural humility implies a willingness to learn and reflect on biases or misconceptions, work in partnership with clients and their families, listen to client's stories, and create an environment for equitable care.

Nurses should engage in critical self-reflection of personal biases and develop an understanding of their own cultural perspectives and the basis for structural health inequalities. Nurses learn skills to ask the right questions and understand the needs of individual patients. This can be as simple as asking patients about their cultural and personal beliefs, their identity, and understanding of their own health. Another way to advocate for immigrants may be uncomfortable for many and involves speaking up when witnessing prejudiced or racist actions or language (Commodore-Mensah et al., 2021).

The Story of Mira

"Mira" is an undocumented immigrant who has lived in the United States for the past 26 years. She had worked steadily in retail and food service jobs for over two decades, despite holding a master's degree in business from her native Bangladesh.

Mira had gone years without seeing a doctor for medical help, even after several injuries on the job. She described an instance in which she slipped from her ladder when stocking a shelf and several heavy goods fell on her:

"I hurt my shoulder very badly from the fall. I couldn't go to the hospital and just took Tylenol for several weeks. My employer wanted me to go to the ER, but I refused since I did not know how I could afford it and if I needed to be a citizen to get help. This was 7 years ago, and I still have trouble carrying groceries and can't do heavy lifting at all."

When she heard about the NYC Care program from a local community organization, Mira was grateful to finally be able to get regular medical check-ups. "I hadn't seen a doctor since my visa ran out 19 years ago. When I finally was able to see a doctor last year, I found out that I had hypothyroidism, hypertension, and recently developed type 2 diabetes." Mira's hypothyroidism had gone untreated for so long that she needed immediate surgery to remove one of her thyroid glands. Mira said, "It takes me anywhere from 3 to 6 months to get an appointment. This is especially difficult when something is causing pain, or if I need an adjustment to my medication. Sometimes, I have to wait in the waiting room for more than 3 hours to be seen for my appointment with no communication from the front desk."

Still, the NYC Care program has made a world of a difference to her. Mira was able to see a primary provider and specialists regularly as well as have her thyroid surgery at Elmhurst Hospital in Queens, which is part of NYC Health + Hospitals.

1. *What do you see as the consequences to the health of undocumented immigrants and access to healthcare?*

Source: Rahman, N. (2021). U.S. *Healthcare Undocumented Immigrants Shut-Out.* CUNY Academic Commons. https://newlaborforum.cuny.edu/2021/04/30/undocumented-immigrants-shut-out/

CASE STUDY **10 ESSENTIAL PUBLIC HEALTH SERVICES**

Correctional Nursing

Correctional nurses provide care to incarcerated populations in various settings that align with community standards. Patients in a correctional setting have unique medical needs with high burdens of chronic conditions, infectious diseases, substance use disorders, and mental health disorders. Patients are afforded timely access to care via ambulatory care services, and patients can also request medical attention for emergent healthcare needs.

Emergency response in correctional settings requires that nursing staff be trained and prepared to respond to emergencies, provide excellent care, and obtain the best clinical outcomes for patients with early interventions. To strengthen the response, there is standardized emergency response equipment, which includes an emergency bag and AED and an emergency comprehensive training curriculum that includes hands-on training, competencies, and drills. Upon notification of an emergency, the nursing healthcare first responders must arrive at the scene of the emergency within 8 minutes. Because of the environment, violence in correctional settings is commonplace, and traumatic injuries account for a large percentage of cases. At one correctional facility housing men, during a 1-month period between December 1st and 31st 2023, a total of 15 out of 62 patients were treated for traumatic injuries.

This case study refers to a patient who presents with blunt trauma status postaltercation. Upon initial survey at the scene, with the use of the **D**anger **R**esponse **C**irculation **A**irway **B**reathing acronym, the severity of the injuries was quickly assessed by the nursing staff. Multiple injuries were noted: approximately 0.2 cm laceration to the right upper eyelid, 0.1 cm laceration to the left lower chin, left earlobe swelling, multiple hematomas to the head, and superficial abrasions to the right deltoid; bleeding of all sites was controlled with direct pressure and dressings placed. A hard cervical collar was placed to protect the cervical spine.

The patient's vital signs were BP: 154/96, HR: 120, RR: 20, T: 36.7, O2: 96% on RA, pain: 2/10, BG: 138 mg/dL, and GCS: 15.

The nurses departed the scene and transported the patient via a gurney to the treatment and triage area for further assessment and treatment. A secondary survey, which includes a complete head-to-toe assessment, was performed to reduce the risk of undiscovered injuries. Multiple injuries were noted: superficial abrasions to the right buttock.

The second set of vital signs obtained was BP: 164/111, HR: 74, RR: 18, T: 36.7, O2: 99% on RA, pain: 10/10, and GCS: 15.

After treatment and stabilization of the patient, the physician on call (POC) was informed of the assessment findings, treatments, and interventions. The nurse received a verbal order to monitor the patient for elevated BP. The POC was called a second time for epistaxis and left facial swelling. The RN staff received an order to transfer the patient to a higher level of care for CT of the head. Supervising nursing and custodial staff were notified, and the patient was transported via ambulance to a local hospital for further trauma evaluation and management. A telephone nursing hand-off report was provided to the receiving hospital ED nurse.

Aimee Young R.N.

1. ***Recognize Cues:*** *Which findings require immediate follow-up, are unexpected, or are most concerning?*
2. ***Analyze Cues:*** *What information is noted or needed for interpreting findings?*
3. ***Prioritize Hypotheses:*** *Based on the information that you have, what is happening?*
4. ***Generate Solutions:*** *What intervention(s) will achieve the desired outcome?*
5. ***Take Action:*** *What actions should you take or do first?*
6. ***Evaluate Outcomes:*** *Were outcomes achieved? Why or why not?*
7. *Which Essential Public Health Services influence this situation? (See Box 2-2.)*

SUMMARY

- Vulnerable populations are at risk for poor health outcomes, including increased risk for morbidity and mortality.
- Various models or theoretical frameworks examine personal and environmental resources and risks relative to vulnerability.
- Leading factors that make aggregates vulnerable are poverty, age, gender, race, or ethnicity, being uninsured or underinsured, being a single parent, and having little or no education.
- Social determinants of health are factors strongly associated with health outcomes and include social norms or attitudes, such as discrimination and racism; exposure to crime, violence, and social disorder; and concentrated poverty.
- The socioeconomic gradient, a direct relationship between social class/income and health, has been repeatedly demonstrated in research conducted around the world.
- Health disparities are defined as differences in access to quality healthcare and in health outcomes, particularly along income/class and racial/ethnic lines, and are usually characterized as avoidable and unfair.
- To be effective, C/PHNs must establish a sense of trust and rapport with their clients by finding common ground.
- Empowerment strategies with individual clients can help them meet their full potential while also providing empowerment to the nurses working with them.
- Community health nurses can provide person support as well as support and leadership for vulnerable communities.
- Nurses can use evidence-based practice when addressing health disparities among vulnerable populations.

- C/PHNs should be concerned with improving health literacy, access to healthcare, and health outcomes through political action.
- C/PHNs must be aware of the value of cultural, racial, and socioeconomic differences and that these differences are often turned into discrimination in healthcare services and policies. With a focus on social justice, they must be determined to ensure equitable access to care for all.

ACTIVE LEARNING EXERCISES

1. Assess four vulnerable groups within your local community. Using one of the models of vulnerability depicted in this chapter, determine the health status for each of these groups. Describe the relative risk for each group. (Objective 1)
2. Check with the health department about any interagency groups or committees that may be addressing the needs of vulnerable populations in your community. What issues are most important to this group? Who are the members? Note the agencies represented. Are there any community members present? If possible, attend a meeting or access minutes of a recent meeting and determine the types of issues being discussed. Is there a sense of community involvement and participation? (Objective 2)
3. Search for a current evidence-based article on vulnerable populations based on ideas from this chapter. Discuss the main points of each article and how they may relate to vulnerable populations (e.g., health disparities, socioeconomic gradient), as well as individual clients you may be seeing in your clinical rotations (e.g., empowerment, health literacy). Based on the research findings, what interventions might be most helpful? Are they feasible in your area? With your specific populations? (Objective 3)
4. Using one of the 10 Essential Public Health Services (Box 2-2), find available community resources for each of the groups you identified in exercise 1. Where are the resources located? How easily accessible are they? What outreach services do they provide for the vulnerable population they serve? Describe some socioeconomic resources. What areas are most deficient? (Objective 4)
5. Talk to two expert C/PHNs and discuss the concept of empowerment with them. What strategies have they used with clients? Ask them to share examples of when they felt that they made a real difference in the lives of their clients. Note any similarities between these nurses' responses and the roles and behaviors of C/PHNs and client empowerment strategies described in this chapter. (Objective 5)
6. Reflect on the terms "social justice" and "health equity." Do the local agencies take these concepts and put them into practice? Evaluate policies in your area that relate to your four vulnerable populations. What policies need to be reevaluated or developed? What are some advocacy strategies you can do to improve the population's health through policy? (Objective 6)

CHAPTER 24

Clients With Disabilities

"I'm officially disabled, but I'm truly enabled because of my lack of limbs. My unique challenges have opened up unique opportunities to reach so many in need."

—Nick Vujicic

KEY TERMS

Activity limitations
American Sign Language
Americans with Disabilities Act (ADA)
Assistive devices and technologies
Disability
Environmental factors
Family and Medical Leave Act
Impairments
Individuals With Disabilities Education Act (IDEA)
International Classification of Functioning, Disability, and Health (ICF)
Medical home
National Council on Disability
Participation restrictions
Respite care
Secondary conditions
Social Security's Supplemental Security Income (SSI)
Temporary Assistance for Needy Families (TANF)
Universal design

LEARNING OBJECTIVES

Upon mastery of this chapter, you should be able to:

1. Identify various disabilities and impairments, noting functional patterns and health concerns, for different age groups.
2. Compare and contrast the local, national, and global implications of disabilities to recognize health, social, and economic patterns.
3. Recognize the social determinants of health and how these factors impact the healthcare outcomes and the well-being of people with disabilities and their families.
4. Explain the role of the C/PHN when working with clients with disabilities.
5. Describe the laws and policies that protect people with disabilities and their families.
6. Identify resources for persons with disabilities during manmade and natural disasters.

INTRODUCTION

Currently, an estimated 61.4 million (25.7%; Fig. 24-1) of noninstitutionalized American adults live with disabilities, consisting of vision, hearing, mobility, self-care, cognitive, and independent living deficits (Centers for Disease Control and Prevention [CDC], 2023a). Globally, that number jumps to 1.3 billion (World Health Organization [WHO], 2023). **Disability** is an overarching term to describe limitations in activities, **impairments**, and restrictions in one's ability to participate. "Disability refers to the negative aspects of the interaction between people with a health condition (such as cerebral palsy and depression) and personal and **environmental factors** (such as negative attitudes, inaccessible transportation and public buildings, and limited social supports)" (WHO, 2011, p. 7). Conditions such as an aging population and a higher risk for disabilities in older people, as well as a global increase in chronic health conditions, have led to a greater prevalence of disabilities.

Across the world, people with disabilities have fewer educational opportunities and higher unemployment. These factors alone increase the risk of poverty, thus exacerbating health concerns and gaps in services (WHO, 2023). Stigma and discrimination may cause a reluctance for the population to seek healthcare services. Moreover, healthcare providers may have implicit biases toward the population (WHO, 2023). These difficulties are exacerbated in less advantaged communities.

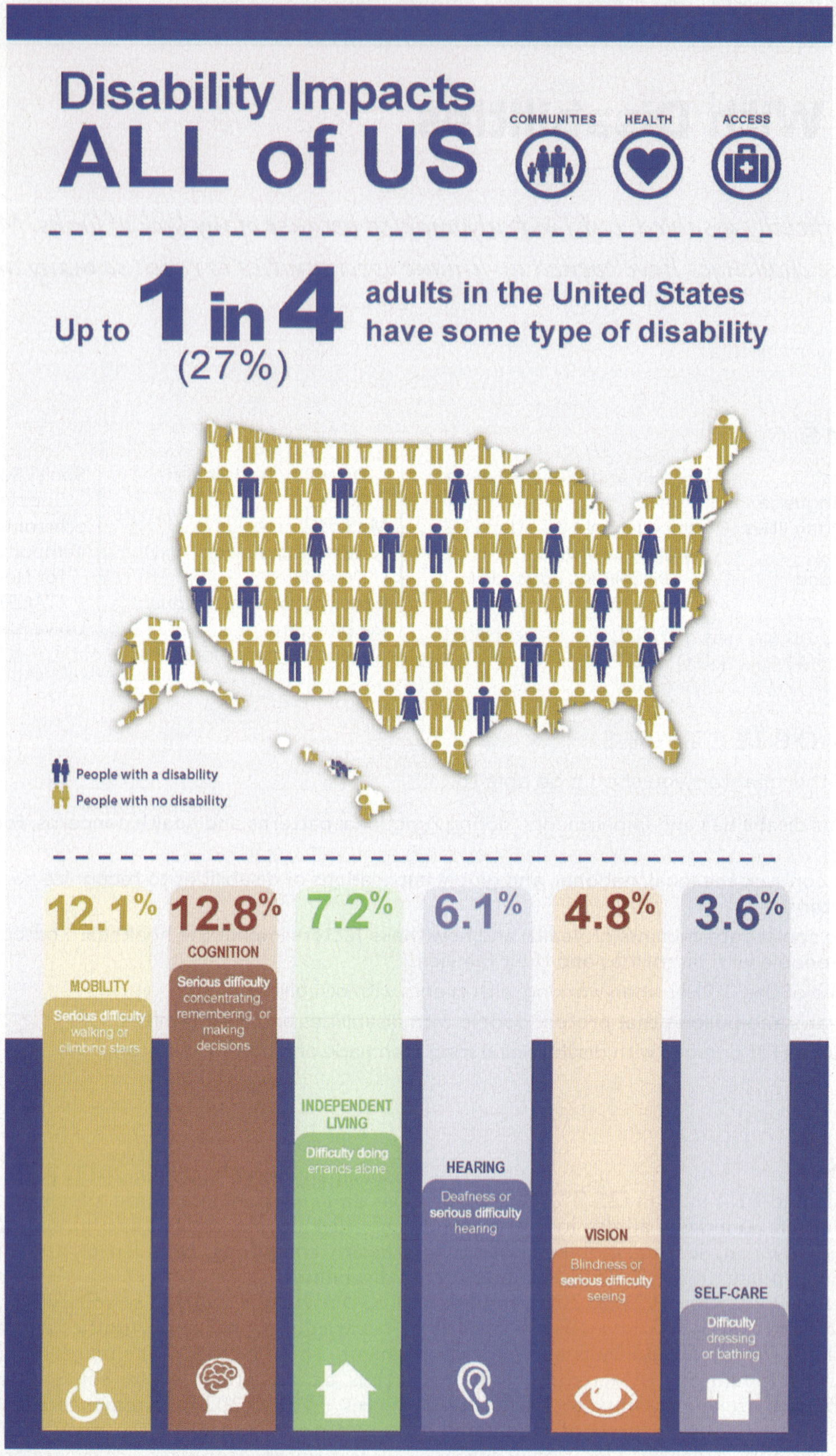

FIGURE 24-1 Disability impacts ALL of US. (Reprinted from Centers for Disease Control and Prevention. (n.d.). *Disability impacts all of US.* https://www.cdc.gov/ncbddd/disabilityandhealth/infographic-disability-impacts-all.html)

According to the Census Bureau, disability status is determined by difficulties in any one or more of these six areas:

- Hearing
- Vision
- Cognitive
- Ambulatory
- Self-care
- Independent living

In the United States, arthritis is the main cause of disability in adults, whereas asthma is the leading cause of disability in children (CDC, 2020a). When comparing urban and rural sections of the United States, rural parts of the country have only 20% of the population, yet they have a higher rate of the population with disabilities (U.S. Census Bureau, 2023). Moreover, southern states have a high rate of disabilities, followed by the mid-west, the mid-east, and finally the western portion of the United States. The southern states' disability rates are due to several risk factors, with the most prevailing attributed to the areas' high percentage of strokes, thereby coining the term "Stroke Belt," and the subsequent disabilities associated post stoke (U.S. Census Bureau, 2023).

Globally, 16% of the world's population has a disability (WHO, 2022). Worldwide, behavioral and mental health issues are the single largest reason for disabilities (Chen, 2022; PAHO, 2019):

- Depression
- Anxiety
- Dementia
- Substance use disorder
- Alcohol use disorder

In addition to the human burden of disability, the related financial costs of direct medical care and associated indirect costs have a significant impact on public and private payers of health and behavioral health insurance.

- Those living with disabilities are at a greater risk of poverty due to the high cost of medical care directly related to the disability, as well as the costs associated with secondary conditions, lower educational attainment, and a higher rate of unemployment or low-paying employment (American Psychological Association, 2019).
- Children living in poverty are at risk for development delays and chronic illness, while older adults are at an increased risk of disability (ODPHP, n.d.).
- Costs related to disabilities vary depending on the severity of the disability, the person's age, the comorbidities, and the need for caregiver services and household composition (Morris et al., 2022).
- Employment status varies depending on the type of disability.

People with hearing disabilities have the highest percentage of employment, and those with self-care disabilities have the lowest rate of employment (Erickson et al., 2024).

In 2022, 21.3% of those with disabilities were employed compared with 65.4% of persons without disabilities (Bureau of Labor Statistics, 2023). This chapter begins with an overview of disabilities, followed by a discussion of current national and global trends in addressing these issues. The various organizations that focus on improving the well-being of those affected by disabling conditions, the impact of these disabilities on families, and the role of the community/public health nurse (C/PHN) in addressing the related needs of people, families, and aggregates are also reviewed in this chapter. The benefits of universal design and issues of easy access for all ages and abilities are introduced.

PERSPECTIVES ON DISABILITY AND HEALTH

Health outcomes differ between those without and those with disabilities. According to the WHO (2022), there are three key indicators:

- Mortality: People with intellectual disabilities die at a younger age
- Functioning: People with disabilities have higher rates of functional limitations
- Morbidity: People have a higher rate of chronic diseases.

People with disabilities face negative societal views and stereotypes of disability. Many people, however—along with their families, allies, and advocates—have challenged these views. New and more positive approaches continue to emerge that view people and their needs from a more person-centered, holistic standpoint. October is National Disability Employment Awareness Month (NDEAM). During the month of October, contributions of American workers with disabilities, past and present, are recognized and policies and practices that are inclusive are highlighted (U.S. Department of Labor, 2023). The diverse personal narratives of people living with disabilities emphasize the individual circumstances. The CDC offers stories of victory and hope in *Disability and Health Stories from People Living with a Disability* (2020b). Unfortunately, not everyone is so fortunate. The Civil Rights Division of the U.S. Department of Labor presents 114 civil rights cases regarding disability violations.

People living with a disability must be included in population health strategies and policies to improve and maintain their health and wellness.

- Several studies have highlighted the importance of outdoor space and parks with facilities for older adults. Parks provide social interaction and physical activities, which are important in maintaining physical, psychology, and social well-being (Perry et al., 2021; Veitch et al., 2022).
- The landmark U.S. Surgeon General's *Call to Action to Improve the Health and Wellness of Persons with Disabilities* placed the health of persons living with disabilities equal in importance to the health of the nation as reflected in the *Healthy People 2030* goal: Improve health and well-being in people with disabilities.

BOX 24-1 *HEALTHY PEOPLE 2030*

Disability and Health—Objectives

Core Objectives

DH-01	Reduce the proportion of adults with disabilities who delay preventive care because of cost
MICH-18	Increase the proportion of children with autism spectrum disorder who receive special services by age 4 years
A-01	Reduce the proportion of adults with arthritis who have moderate to severe joint pain
DH-04	Increase the proportion of homes that have an entrance without steps
DH-05	Increase the proportion of students with disabilities who are usually in regular education programs
V-09	Increase the use of assistive and adaptive devices by people with vision loss

Research Objectives

DH-R02	Increase the proportion of state and DC health departments with programs aimed at improving health in people with disabilities

Reprinted from Office of Disease Prevention and Health Promotion (ODPHP). (n.d.). *Healthy people 2030: People with disabilities*. https://health.gov/healthypeople/objectives-and-data/browse-objectives/people-disabilities

- Box 24-1 offers a partial list of HP2030 objectives related to improving the health of those with disabilities (ODPHP, n.d.).

One area in which further development is needed to better meet the needs of people with disabilities is that of health and wellness apps, such as medical text messaging or mHealth. C/PHNs can assist their clients by providing them with helpful app resources. Internet searches on health and wellness apps yield a multitude of links. The following are some resources that may be helpful:

- 25 Life-Changing Apps for People with Disabilities offers a variety of helpful apps (Ishbia, 2024).
- Top 10 Apps for Visually Impaired People offers helpful information on apps (Keck Medicine of USC, 2023).
- Partnering with people with intellectual and developmental disabilities, the University of Rhode Island produced an R3 app that helps people recognize, respond, and report abuse they may experience (2023).
- Digital technology (DT) advances were exploding prior to the COVID-19 pandemic.
  - The importance of DT in education, health, and social inclusion took on new urgency during the pandemic. This was especially true for persons with disabilities.
  - Technology provided the ability to work from home, created new employment opportunities, made provisions for educational advances, provided essential services, and promoted social inclusion (United Nations [UN], 2021).
- While these advances had a positive effect, there are negative ramifications as well.
  - There is a gap between people who are nondisabled and those who are disabled.
  - People with disabilities own fewer desktop or laptop computers, cell phones, and tablet computers (Perrin & Atske, 2021).
  - Accessing digital technology takes certain skills that people may lack due to certain disabilities or the platform is not inclusive. Parts of the county may not have Wi-Fi connections or the connection is unstable.
  - Affordability is a huge concern given the already high cost of assistive devices and for those who are unemployed or underemployed (UN, 2021).

Healthy People 2030

The evolving United States perspectives on disability and chronic illness have been reflected in the changing focus of the Healthy People series. A comparison among Healthy People plans since its inception underscores the emergence of new approaches to both identifying priority areas and planning to improve the health of people with disabilities and chronic illness. In *Healthy People 2030*, the section "Disability and Health" further strengthens *Healthy People*'s approach to disability to emphasize the principles of health promotion and disease prevention for those currently experiencing disabilities and chronic illnesses.

- Rather than narrowly defining people with disabilities or chronic illnesses through their limiting conditions, *Healthy People 2030* developers understand that people with disabilities or chronic illnesses have the potential to meet and exceed health promotion and disease prevention goals set for the nation's population as a whole.
- This approach is consistent with the multifaceted national goal of improving parity across all groups and among all people. For example, the goal of "Disability and Health" in *Healthy People 2030* is to engage those with disabilities of all ages to maintain the optimal state of health and prevent chronic conditions so that the highest quality of life can be maintained (ODPHP, n.d.).

Healthy People 2030 indicates a growing realization that healthy life years for people with disabilities equate to decreased health costs at local, state, and national levels, just as they do for persons without disabilities (ODPHP, n.d.; Box 24-2). The goal of HP2030 is to improve the health and well-being of people with disabilities through the following:

- Provide support and services for the school, work, home, and healthcare services.

BOX 24-2 PERSPECTIVES

Focus on Persons With Disabilities

Recent events from the COVID-19 pandemic and rolling electrical outages in California to prevent wildfires highlight the isolating effect events can have on the health and well-being of those with a disability, specifically those with limited mobility. Living independently can be difficult for those using wheelchairs and walkers and for those relying on care providers. The recent pandemic provided other aspects of care to consider such as good hygiene, cleaning and disinfecting, and preventing the spread of infection, as well as having plans for if the direct support provider gets sick, ways to ensure enough prescription medication is on hand, and how to obtain assistance with purchasing household items and groceries. Electrical outages required patients in the community to have backup medical equipment, generators, batteries, nonperishable food, and flashlights or lanterns. It is imperative that clients with mobility limitations have a plan in place to support their care and well-being during these isolating events. A C/PHN's disaster preparedness plans must address such crises and provide resources for clients and their families so they are not forgotten.

Mark, a C/PHN case manager in the field

- Make healthcare more affordable.
- Improve access at home, work, school, healthcare services, and environment.

There are 34 objectives related to disability and health under several headings in HP2030.

- 12 objectives at baseline.
- 7 objectives have little or no detectable change.
- 4 objectives are improving.
- 5 objectives are getting worse.
- 3 objectives are met or exceeding.
- The remaining objectives address research or developmental interests.

More can be found under People with Disabilities in Healthy People 2030. https://health.gov/healthypeople/objectives-and-data/browse-objectives/people-disabilities

International Classification of Functioning, Disability, and Health

The **International Classification of Functioning, Disability, and Health (ICF)** supports the more positive, emerging approaches to understanding disabling conditions (WHO, 2019). The ICF (WHO, 2019) is a universal classification system using standardized language that views the domains of health from a holistic viewpoint. It takes into account body functions and structures, activities and participation, environmental factors, and personal factors. This multidimensional approach supports a complex evaluation of a person's circumstances in terms of functioning, disability, and health. By combining the "medical model" with the "social model," the ICF provides a biopsychosocial approach for assessing people with disabilities. Its approach emphasizes that no two people with the same disease or disability have the same level of functioning. The aims of the ICF are to provide a scientific basis for understanding and research, improve communication among providers and those with disabilities, allow for data comparisons, and provide a coding system for health information systems (WHO, 2019).

The following concepts and related definitions further clarify the ICF view of health:

- Body functions: physiologic functions of the body
- Body structure: anatomic parts of the body
- Impairments: problems in body function or structure
- Activity: task or action
- Participation: to be involved in a life situation
- **Activity limitations**: difficulty a person may have with an activity
- **Participation restrictions**: limitations in involvement
- Environmental factors: the physical and social environments where people live and conduct their lives (WHO, 2019)

For public health nursing practice, the application of the ICF reinforces that disability and disease are additional factors to be considered in planning and implementing a care plan for individual clients and for population groups in the community.

For individual clients, the ICF guides and facilitates assessment across a wide range of variables.

- Although two people may have the same apparent disability, such as a below-the-knee amputation, their health status and personal well-being can be quite different.
- One may have a more positive outlook, more social supports, or fewer additional health issues that complicate rehabilitation than another.

The C/PHN must always consider the totality of the situation, including the biologic, psychological, sociocultural, and environmental realms of the whole person.

The World Health Report

The landmark World Report on Disability (WHO, 2011) addressed the barriers for people with disabilities and the role of the environment in facilitating or restricting participation for those with disabilities.

- The barriers include inadequate policies and standards, negative attitudes, lack of provision of services, problems with service delivery, inadequate funding, lack of accessibility, lack of consultation and involvement, and lack of data and evidence (WHO, 2011, pp. 9–10).

- According to the report, when those with disabilities encounter barriers, results may include poorer health outcomes, lower educational achievements, less economic participation, higher rates of poverty, and increased dependency and restricted participation.
- The WHO challenged the global community to address barriers and inequalities for those with disabilities in regard to health, rehabilitation, support and assistance, environments, education, and employment (WHO, 2011).

In addressing the barriers to healthcare, the following provided for a more patient-centered care approach for people who are disabled:

- Use of equipment with universal design, communication of information in appropriate formats, and using alternative models of service delivery providers.
- Health service providers must have education and training to know how to provide care to those with disabilities.
- Services for care should focus on efficiency and effectiveness; increasing access to assistive technology increases independence and participation and may reduce costs.

Those who are disabled must be empowered to manage their health and advocate on their own behalf. Additionally, policy responses must emphasize early intervention, benefits of rehabilitation, and provision of services close to where people live (WHO, 2011).

The United Nations Convention on the Rights of Persons With Disabilities (CRPD)

An estimated 1.3 billion people across the globe live with disabilities, with 240 million of these children (WHO, 2022). Factoring in the over 2.6 billion family members affected by disability, the WHO stressed that almost one third of the world population is directly impacted by disabilities. The sheer magnitude of this issue and the recognition that people with disabilities are significantly overlooked across the world led to the 2006 United Nations (UN) Convention on the Rights of Persons with Disabilities (CRPD). The Conference of States Parties to the Convention on the Rights of Persons with Disabilities (COSP) meets yearly in New York to discuss the implementing the CRPD.

The June 2022 COSP round table meeting discussed the following (UN, 15th Session, 2022):

- Innovation and technology advancing disability rights
  - Increase remote learning platforms
  - Decrease cost of technologic devices
- Economic empowerment and entrepreneurship of people with disabilities
  - Corporations are obligated to prompt social engagement within the work environment.
  - Provide mentorship for entrepreneurs.
- Participation of people with disabilities in climate action, disaster risk reduction, and resilience against natural disasters
  - Importance of disaster management and universal design.
  - Include people with disabilities in policymaking.

(Conference of States Parties to the Convention on the Rights of Persons with Disabilities, 15th session 2022)

This document remains the standard for considering the rights of those with disabilities, regardless of age, race, gender, or other demographic considerations. Some of the key principles include respect for dignity and autonomy, nondiscrimination, inclusion into society, and acceptance. To learn more information, refer to the United Nation's Department of Economic and Social Affairs site on disability: https://social.desa.un.org/issues/disability.

The World Report on Disability

In 2011, the WHO and the World Bank reassessed global progress on disability since the 2006 CRPD (UN, 2016). The *Convention* provided guidance to governments globally and communicated that it was their responsibility to improve the lives of people and families living with disability. Citizens of every country must and need to participate in their country's development. People living with disabilities must advocate for the removal of barriers that prevent their full participation in their communities, including access to health, education, employment, transportation, and information services. To ensure full participation of people with disabilities in their communities, stakeholders in each country—and globally—must establish an inclusive world characterized by enabling environments, rehabilitation and support services, adequate social protection, and relevant policies, programs, standards, and legislation (WHO, 2023).

Specific recommendations follow:

- Address unmet healthcare needs.
- Assess health risks for those with disabilities (such as comorbidities or engagement in health-risk behaviors).
- Advocate for those who have barriers to care (WHO, 2023).

CIVIL RIGHTS LEGISLATION

Legislation is vital to ensure that every person's rights are protected and that there is legal recourse to secure needs that have been denied. As is often true for other issues of equality, legislation is only one of many steps that must be taken. The movement to achieve civil rights for persons with disabilities in this country has gained momentum and continues to seek the influence and public attention that will improve the health and lives of those with disabilities.

- The **Americans with Disabilities Act (ADA)** was signed into law in 1990 and continues to be updated.
- In 2017, movie theaters were required to provide captioning and audio descriptions for movies that are produced with those features (United States Department of Justice [USDOJ] Civil Rights Division, n.d.-a).
- Section 504 of the Rehabilitation Act of 1973.
- People with Disabilities Education Act in 1990.

People with disabilities and their advocates made their voices heard by an unwavering demand for an end to inferior treatment and lack of equal protection under the law. The ADA has set the standard for a number of subsequent laws that, together with pre-ADA legislation, have

TABLE **24-1** Disability Rights Laws

Law	Summary	Contact
Americans with Disabilities Act (ADA) (1990)	Prohibits discrimination in employment 1. State and local government 2. Public accommodations, commercial facilities, transportation, and telecommunications	▪ U.S. Equal Opportunity Commission ▪ Civil Rights Division ▪ U.S. Department of Justice (USDOJ) ▪ Office of Civil Rights, Federal Transit Administration
Telecommunications Act of 1996	Telecommunication equipment and services are accessible	Federal Communications Commission
Fair Housing Act (amended 1988)	Prohibits housing discrimination	U.S. Department of Housing and Urban Development
Civil Rights of Institutionalized Persons Act (CRIPA) 1997	Right to receive care in the least restrictive setting	USDOJ
Individuals with Disabilities Education Act (1990)	Make available free public education in the least restrictive environment for all children with disabilities	U.S. Department of Education, Office of Special Education Programs
Accessible Design (2010 Standards)	Standards required for new construction and alterations under Title II and Title III	U.S. Architectural and Transportation Barriers Compliance Board
Revision of the ADA Title II and Title III regulations to implement the requirements of the ADA Amendments Act of 2008 (2016)	To clarify the meaning and interpretation of the ADA definition of "disability"	Civil Rights Division, U.S. Department of Justice (USDOJ)
Provide appropriate auxiliary aids and services for people with disabilities (2017)	Movie theaters provide closed captioning and audio description when showing a digital movie	Civil Rights Division, U.S. Department of Justice (USDOJ)

Source: U.S. Department of Justice Civil Rights Division, Disability Rights Section (2020b).

become a broad spectrum of protections for people with disabilities (USDOJ Civil Rights Division, 2020). Some of these laws are listed in Table 24-1 and cover a variety of issues, including telecommunications, architectural barriers, and voter registration. To learn more regarding these laws and others in more detail, go to Guide to Disability Rights Laws at https://www.ada.gov/resources/disability-rights-guide/. Examples of violations of these laws are found under press releases of the Disability Rights Section News at https://www.justice.gov/crt/disability-rights-section (USDOJ Civil Rights Division, n.d.b)

The ADA protects those with a disability, which is defined as "…a person who has a physical or mental impairment that substantially limits one or more major life activities, a person who has a history or record of such an impairment, or a person who is perceived by others as having such an impairment. The ADA does not specifically name all of the impairments that are covered" (U.S. Department of Justice Civil Rights Division, 2020, paragraph 2).

- The ADA does not list specific diagnoses but focuses on the impact the disability has on daily living, such as on the ability to care for self, perform manual tasks, see, hear, eat, sleep, walk, stand, lift, bend, speak, breathe, learn, read, concentrate, think, communicate, and work.
- In addition to the uncertainty about who is actually protected by the ADA, there can also be confusion about who is required to comply with the provisions of the Act and what specific remedial actions are necessary.

People who believe that their legal rights under the ADA have been violated may seek remedy by filing a lawsuit or submitting a complaint to one of four federal offices, depending on the specific type of alleged violation: (1) the USDOJ, Civil Rights Division; (2) Equal Employment Opportunity Commission; (3) Department of Transportation; or (4) Department of Housing and Urban Development (USDOJ, Civil Rights Division, n.d.c). The process for filing a complaint is not a simple task, and many people seek the assistance of attorneys, legal aid societies, or various private organizations, some of which are discussed later in this chapter (Box 24-3).

The USDOJ published *A Guide to Disability Rights Laws* (2020). The guide provides information on federal civil rights laws for those with disabilities and is available in large print, CD, and Braille. The laws included are as follows:

- Americans with Disabilities Act (ADA)
- Telecommunications Act
- Fair Housing Act

BOX 24-3 Office of Civil Rights: Compliance With the Americans With Disabilities Act

The responsibility of the U.S. Department of Justice, Office of Civil Rights (OCR), is to investigate complaints of alleged violations of the Americans with Disabilities Act (ADA). An example of one of those complaints involved a 22-year-old Connecticut woman with cerebral palsy. She had been placed in a nursing home because of changes in her living situation and healthcare status but wanted to move back into the community. The OCR intervened to ensure that the woman secured appropriate housing and that counseling and intensive case management services were in place when she moved back into the community. Another example involved a man with traumatic brain injury who was told he must remain in a hospital when he requested home healthcare services. OCR intervened and secured physical, occupational, and speech therapy for the client, as well as physical modifications needed for his home. A 32-year-old man with quadriplegia had lived independently in his own apartment with a health aide's assistance, but suddenly lost his apartment and was transferred against his will to a facility. He was able to get a wheelchair-accessible apartment but could not get health aide services. OCR intervened on his behalf and secured a personal care assistant so that he could live in his new apartment. Without the protection afforded under the ADA, the outcome could have been much different.

Source: USDHHS, Office for Civil Rights (September, 2006).

- Air Carrier Access Act
- Voting Accessibility for the Elderly and Handicapped Act
- National Voter Registration Act
- Civil Rights of Institutional Persons Act
- **Individuals with Disabilities Education Act (IDEA)**
- Rehabilitation Act
- Architectural Barriers Act

The most common and challenging barriers to providing services for persons with disabilities are stereotyping, stigma, and prejudices. These attitudes contribute to other barriers such as communication, transportation, social, and policies that people with disabilities face (CDC, 2020c). The perspective of one community member offers one such example (Box 24-4).

The **National Council on Disability (NCD)** (n.d.) is an independent federal agency charged with advising the President, Congress, and other federal agencies regarding policies, programs, practices, and procedures that affect people with disabilities. Its policy areas include civil rights, cultural diversity, education, emergency management, employment, financial assistance and incentives, healthcare, housing, international issues, long-term services and support, technology, transportation, and youth issues. NCD's website has publications dating back to 1986 on civil rights. Information can be found at https://www.ncd.gov/policy-areas/civil-rights/index.html

BOX 24-4 PERSPECTIVES

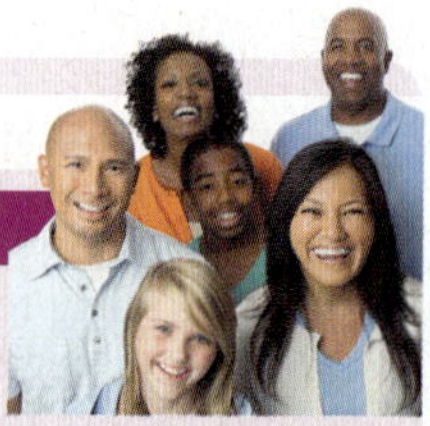

A Community Member Viewpoint on Hearing Loss

I lost my hearing as a young adult. By the time I was 28 years old, I had no natural hearing left. I received a cochlear implant when I was 32. Around the time I decided to have the implant, I was struggling so much to survive in the hearing world (phone usage, conversations with hearing people, etc.). The decision to receive a cochlear implant changed my life. I could now communicate with the hearing world again. While the cochlear implant has some amazing benefits, there are some negatives still. For one, I still do not have perfect hearing. I have enough hearing, though, for people to not realize I am deaf. This "hidden disability" can be problematic. Many people assume I am just stupid. It happens all the time. What they don't know is that I am actually well-educated and very intelligent. Often, I hear my friends, family, and fellow students talk about how smart I am, but when I don't hear something I sound stupid. I might mishear the beginning of a conversation and respond with something totally off topic. This particular trait should be a red flag that the person may have a hearing loss. It is very demoralizing for people to treat you like you are stupid, when the reality is you just can't hear well. Another very difficult thing about having a cochlear implant is that when you can't wear it for some reason (dead battery, loss, medical procedure, etc.), you feel absolutely powerless, and often fearful, in the hearing world. I've most often experienced this in the healthcare environment. When I had to have surgical procedures that required removing my implant, I could not hear the instructions provided to me in preop. I could not hear the words that were intended to calm or comfort me. Instead, I was in a constant state of panic wondering if I was missing important information related to my health and safety. Hearing people should also realize that deaf people are extremely attuned to the visual world. We see your frustrated eye rolls, side glances, and facial expressions very acutely. It is very hurtful and frustrating to see this and not be able to do anything about it. Like many "hidden disabilities," imagining yourself in someone else's shoes would probably facilitate a more beneficial and pleasant interaction.

Veronica Russell, Nursing Student

HEALTH PROMOTION AND PREVENTION NEEDS OF PERSONS WITH DISABILITIES

Two ways that C/PHNs and other healthcare providers can better address the healthcare needs of people with disabilities are to take advantage of every opportunity to promote their quality of life and to work to eliminate disparities between their level of healthcare access and quality and that of people without disabilities.

Missed Opportunities by Healthcare Providers to Affect Quality of Life

All of us, whether with or without disabilities, require basic elements to maintain health, including clean air and water, a safe place to live, sunshine, exercise, nutritious food, socialization, and the opportunity to be successful in life's pursuits. As self-evident as these health-promoting elements may seem, for the millions of persons who deal with disability, such basic needs too often take second place to other issues. It is equally problematic that health promotion and disease prevention measures, most notably at the primary and secondary levels, are often nonexistent or lacking (Fig. 24-2).

- People with disabilities are more likely to experience difficulties accessing healthcare, dental services, mammograms, Pap tests, and fitness activities and are more likely to use tobacco, have excess weight or obesity, have hypertension, and have lower employment rates (ODPHP, n.d.).
- Key to addressing these barriers is for people with disabilities to have an opportunity to participate in public health activities, receive appropriately timed health interventions, engage with the environment without restrictions, and be able to participate in life without limitations (Fig. 24-3; ODPHP, n.d.).

The CDC is making an effort to reduce health disparities among persons with disabilities. Surveillance, or use of surveys, helps to determine the needs and problems that people with disabilities experience, and research programs help to prevent the development of **secondary conditions**. The CDC provides *Disability & Health U.S. State Profile Data* that provides disability healthcare costs, the percentage of adults with functional disability types, and a comparison of certain comorbidities. To learn more about your state go to https://www.cdc.gov/ncbddd/disabilityandhealth/impacts/index.html

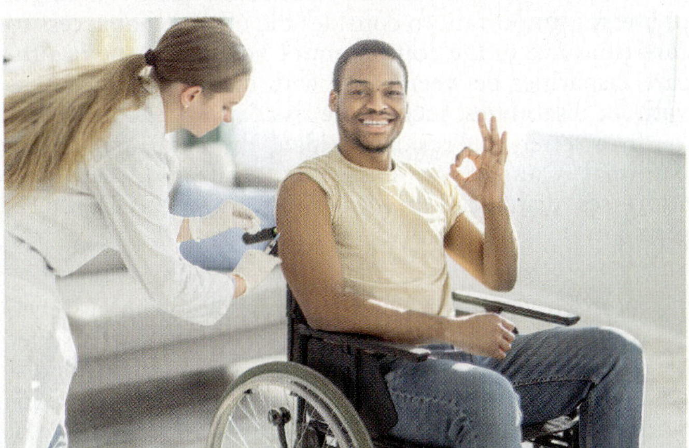

FIGURE 24-2 Preventive services, such as immunizations, are sometimes forgotten in the care of people with disabilities.

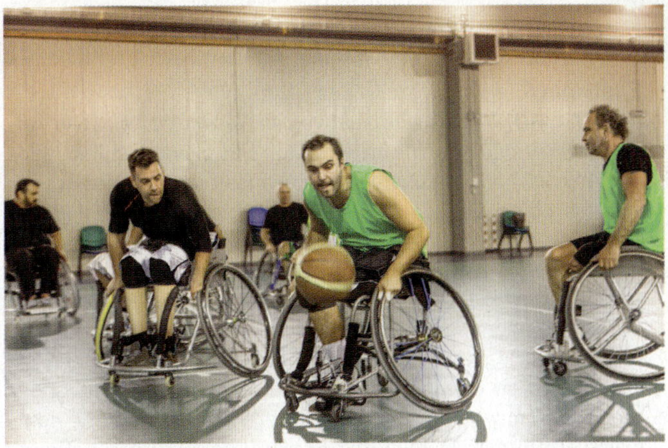

FIGURE 24-3 People who use wheelchairs playing basketball.

The focus of the healthcare delivery system is increasingly skewed toward secondary and tertiary prevention efforts, and limited emphasis is placed on the primary prevention needs of this population. Healthcare providers often fail to address many issues related to health promotion and prevention with people with disabilities, unlike those without disabilities, which is a grave concern (CDC, 2020d).

- For example, issues such as sexuality are often not explored with people with disabilities.
    - Coulter et al. (2023) discovered that young adults with developmental disabilities had the same needs of intimacy and sexual relationships as other young adults.
    - Societal attitudes need to change.
    - Sex education for these young adults needs to be individualized and taught by experienced health educators.
    - For this population, expressing sexuality was difficult.

Disability often serves as the presenting reason for a person's encounter with the healthcare community, including the C/PHN. As a result, the disability often drives the selection of prevention efforts, to the possible exclusion of other, equally important health issues. Box 24-5 offers several examples of missed opportunities in the areas of primary and secondary prevention. It is of particular concern to the practice of C/PHN that the broad range of health promotion and prevention needs of all clients be addressed.

A study published in 2022 documented the lack of knowledge U.S. primary providers have regarding the laws around disabilities.

- The majority of primary providers felt they were at risk for lawsuits regarding ADA violations.
- Roughly 36% had insufficient knowledge regarding their legal responsibilities of ADA.

BOX 24-5 Missed Opportunities

Example 1

HP2030 A-01 and A-02 objectives address joint pain and limited activity due to arthritis. Although this client is still an adolescent, A-01 and A-02 are used because there are no juvenile arthritis objectives. Sally is a 16-year-old high school junior who was diagnosed with polyarticular juvenile idiopathic arthritis rheumatoid factor negative in elementary school. The high school is built on a hill that has many outdoor steps to get to classrooms, administration (including health office), and food services. During a typical day, students move often between the different levels of campus. Due to Sally's academic load, she is required to move between levels several times a day. She complains of hip pain from sitting in class too long; has difficulty walking up the numerous stairs on campus; requires daily eye drops but does not have a safe place to self-administrate; and misses school days because of joint pain in the morning. The school nurse has met with the student and parents throughout the academic year. Special seating has been provided to ease Sally's hip pain from sitting too long in class. Based on the missed opportunity, what other needs and services do you think she may experience in the community, at home, at school, and in the healthcare environment? What resources could be used to help Sally move around campus?

Example 2

HP2030 V-09 Increase the use of assistive and adaptive devices by people with vision loss. Joseph, a 20-year-old with a distance vision of 20/200 and learning disabilities, is employed at a local factory part-time. He receives a regularly scheduled physical examination but does not have vision insurance at work. The employer is happy with the job Joseph is doing and is interested in offering Joseph full-time work. The company provides full-time employees medical, dental, and vision care at a small cost. However, because of his learning disability and poor vision, Joseph is unable to complete the forms for insurance or read the policy on vision care. Apparently, he didn't complete the forms correctly, and he was afraid to ask for help from his employer. As the occupational health nurse for the company, what assistance could you provide to assist Joseph and other employees with these forms? What resources are available in the community to help pay for glasses or other assistive devices?

Example 3

HP2030 NWS-04 Reduce the proportion of children and adolescents with obesity. Sam, age 12, is fearful to participate in physical education because he would have to change into gym clothes in a common area. He gets very little exercise at school or home because he tires easily and dislikes changing clothes. The pediatrician has advised parents to prepare healthy foods and take family walks together. Although the family and Sam have tried their best, there has been little weight change. Recently, it has been discovered Sam is hiding in the school bathroom during recess and lunch because of teasing by peers. He is going all day without eating and spends a great deal of time in the library. He no longer wants to see his pediatrician because he feels like he is being lectured to and told he is not doing enough. There is no encouragement for the work Sam and his family are doing. Furthermore, weights are done in the office hallway, and there is no privacy. Sam has noticed the medical assistant roll her eyes when Sam gets on the scale. This situation could have been handled in a compassionate manner, recognizing the painful experience that weighing is for many people and suggesting alternatives, one of which could have been simply to bypass the scales until after the interview and examination. What changes could you make in the doctor's office to help Sam be more comfortable? What interventions/policies could the school implement to help with Sam's embarrassment and bullying taking place on campus?

- A barrier to caring for the population focused on the lack of knowledge and training in medical schools (Iezzoni et al., 2022).
- People with physical disabilities were less likely to receive a cervical cancer screening than their counterparts who are not disabled (Baruch et al., 2022).

As of 2024, the U.S. Department of Health and Human Services (USDHHS) took a stronger stand against the discrimination of people with disabilities. Titled *Discrimination on the Basis of Disability in Health and Human Service Programs or Activities*, the rule was approved in May 2024 and took effect July 8, 2024. This rule updates and strengthens Section 504 of the Rehabilitation Act of 1973 and the Americans with Disabilities Act (USDHHS, 2024). See https://www.hhs.gov/about/news/2024/05/01/hhs-finalizes-rule-strengthening-protections-against-disability-discrimination.html for more information.

Healthcare Disparities

People living with disabilities, along with their families and advocates, have embraced concerns about the type and quality of the health-related services to which they have access and the referral process they face. They also have concerns about the care they receive being appropriate to their individual circumstances. Lack of access to individualized, quality healthcare can result in increased illness and disability, as well as potentially decreased quality or length of life. It is important to consider the impact that access to care can have in the continuum of health and the healthcare disparities between those with disabilities and those without disabilities, such as the risk for unmet care needs.

In a letter to President Biden, the chairman of the National Council on Disability, Andrés J. Gallegos, addresses disparities in dental coverage (NCD, 2022, para 1):

> Dear Mr. President, People with Intellectual and Developmental Disabilities (I/DD) in the United States suffer significant health disparities compared to their nondisabled counterparts and report unmet medical, prescription and dental needs. With respect to dental needs, Medicaid does not uniformly provide adults with I/DD dental coverage and in 12 states no basic Medicaid dental benefits are provided for adults with I/DD, aside from

limited waiver programs available in seven of those states. As a result, people with I/DD in those jurisdictions often forego preventative and routine dental care and seek emergency dental care in hospital emergency rooms at significantly greater costs.

Those with disabilities should be afforded with a continued and coordinated care approach that addresses the special health needs and disabilities of the client. For children, care coordination through a medical home can provide families with a comprehensive and coordinated approach for their child's health and disability concerns. According to the American Academy of Pediatrics (2024), a **medical home** should have the following features:

- Care is easy to obtain.
- Family-centered.
- Continuous.
- In partnership with family and provider.
- Concern is for a child's well-being.
- Culturally based care.
- Provide all levels of care.

A medical home can improve healthcare outcomes, enhance access and continuity, provide consistency in health management and coordination, reduce health disparities between those with and without disabilities, and provide an opportunity for maximal health of those with disabilities and the general U.S. population.

Primary, secondary, and tertiary prevention activities are essential aspects of quality care for all persons. According to a recent study, researchers found that people with disabilities face obstacles in accessing healthcare:

- Lack of physical accommodations at the provider's office
- Lack of communication accommodations for those with vision and hearing loss
- Lack of knowledge, experience, and skill of the provider regarding disabilities
- Lack of ADA knowledge of the provider
- Structural barriers such as not enough time to provide care within the 15-minute structure
- Negative attitudes on the part of the provider (Lagu et al., 2022)

C/PHNs are in a prime position to advocate for needed changes for those with disabilities. Such changes include increased attention to health promotion and disease prevention needs, accessible and appropriate delivery of those services, and specialized treatment plans that incorporate the latest knowledge of a specific illness or disability (Box 24-6).

BOX **24-6** PERSPECTIVES

Living Our Best Lives Together

I am a mother of a 27-year-old daughter with Down syndrome. She was my firstborn. I remember her weak cry and her soft nursing. When we were about to be discharged, a nurse present at my delivery came to my room and said, while watching my daughter sleeping, "Whenever you have any concerns, please come and ask for help." I had no idea what she meant at that time. But one month later, when we received the diagnosis of Down syndrome, the nurse's gentle eyes and her words came back to my mind. The memory of her kindness comforted me countless times over the last 27 years, and still today it gives me strength.

My daughter has been healthy, without any serious conditions. However, she seems to have passed the peak of her cognition and physical strength. We have begun worrying about aging-related issues such as cataracts or Alzheimer disease. In addition, I have an even greater concern, which is how healthcare providers treat my daughter. When my daughter was receiving pediatric care, healthcare providers were all kind and patient with her. However, after she transitioned to adult care, the way they interacted with her became more "rough."

Recently, my daughter had an ophthalmologist appointment. Her pupils were dilated, and a primary provider examined her with a bright light. This examination would be difficult for anyone. My daughter had difficulty following the primary provider's instructions and he became impatient, loud, and abrupt, demanding, "Left! Look left! Don't move! Keep your eyes open! Left! Top left!!!" His behavior increased the fear of my daughter who was already frightened. This made it even more difficult for her to cooperate. He diagnosed her with a retinal tear and said she would need immediate laser treatment that day. However, we did not feel comfortable and could not trust this doctor. We went to another clinic for a second opinion.

In the second office, the primary provider was very gentle and patient. He explained each process to my daughter. He also asked how she was doing and if she needed a break at every step. The examination went very smoothly because of his clear explanation and kind attitude. The diagnosis was the same. However, the doctor gave a detailed description of the different types of tears. He said her type of tear does not require immediate treatment and suggested close regular monitoring. We had the same examination with two doctors, with two different experiences, and two treatment plans. It was a simple matter to choose the second clinic for my daughter's care.

I hope that primary providers consider their patients' mental age, which may greatly differ from their chronologic age. I hope they meet their patients "where they are" and adjust accordingly. A little extra effort affords both the primary provider and patient a more pleasant experience as well as better quality care. Unfortunately, the frequency of seeing a doctor will increase as my daughter ages. My mission is to find primary providers, nurses, and staff who understand my daughter's needs.

As my daughter ages, I too am getting older. We have lived our lives together as well as we could. We do not know how much time we have left together. No matter how much, we will continue living our best lives together—the life my daughter thinks, "I am happy to be born," and I think, "I am happy that she was born my daughter."

Miwa Hasegawa, Mother. Translated from Japanese

DISABILITIES AND DISASTERS

The recent human-caused and natural disasters have brought to the forefront the need to improve disaster response for all people. According to the National Centers for Environmental Information (NCEI), from January 2024 to April 2024, there were seven natural disasters in the United States that caused 70 deaths and cost an estimated 13 billion dollars. In 2023, there were a total of 28 natural disasters that caused 492 deaths and cost over 90 billion dollars (NCEI, 2024).

- Between 21% and 31% of people who had vision loss or a physical disability had to leave their homes during disaster versus only 1% for people who were not disabled.
- Furthermore, people who were disabled were more likely to live in unsafe and unsanitary conditions 1 month after the disaster (Sisson, 2023).

In 2006, Federal Emergency Management Agency (FEMA) was required to appoint a disability coordinator. This was based on the death of the 91-year-old Ethel Freeman, who relied on a wheelchair and who died outside the New Orleans Convention Center because of a lack of accessible buses during Hurricane Katrina. Currently, agencies and advocacy groups are working together on ways to improve disaster relief for the population with disabilities. Issues addressed include improving communication, involving people with disabilities in emergency planning, ensuring shelters are accessible to all, and improving FEMA resources.

Resources

FEMA (2023) offers several valuable tips for people with disabilities. These tips are provided in 11 languages. They include the following:

- Get informed.
- Make a plan.
- Get your benefits electronically.
- Build a disaster supply kit.
  - Tips for medications.
  - Tips for people who are deaf and hard of hearing.
  - Tips for people who are blind or have low vision.
  - Tips for people with speech disability.
  - Tips for people with Alzheimer and related dementia.
  - People with intellectual or developmental disabilities.
- People at risk for experiencing extreme heat/heat exposure.
- Details can be found at: https://www.ready.gov/disability.

FEMA provides videos with open captions and American Sign Language (ASL) for wheelchair users and those that are hard of hearing or blind. For older adults, FEMA provides a wealth of information on how to prepare for disasters. Take Control in 1, 2, 3-Disaster Preparedness guide for older adults can be found at https://www.ready.gov/older-adults

When working in the community, it is imperative that the C/PHN understand the risk factors of prior natural and human-caused disasters that affected the community. Understanding the community's strengths and vulnerabilities provides a starting point for community partnerships. FEMA offers numerous online courses for disaster management. FEMA's course *IS-368: Including people with disabilities and others with access and functional needs in disaster operations* is a helpful course for C/PHNs. Learn more at https://training.fema.gov/is/courseoverview.aspx?code=IS-368&lang=en

Other resources include the following:

- Substance misuse and mental health service administration provides a Disaster Behavioral Health Information Series Resources Center. Resources cover disaster planning for persons with disabilities and information for those responsible for disaster management. For information, see https://www.samhsa.gov/resource-search/dbhis?rc%5B0%5D=populations%3A20181
- The CDC provides resources from State Disability and Health Programs, as well as federal resources.
- The American Red Cross has disaster planning recommendations planning for people with disabilities (https://www.redcross.org/content/dam/redcross/atg/PDF_s/Preparedness___Disaster_Recovery/General_Preparedness___Recovery/Home/A4497.pdf).
- The American Red Cross and the CDC offer resources for first responders and those responsible for disaster management.

VIOLENCE

Violent crimes committed against persons with disabilities are four times greater than persons without a disability (Harrell, 2021). Furthermore, they are less likely to report a violent crime including rape, robbery, and simple assault. Whereas people with a cognitive disability experienced violent crime at a higher rate than any other disability type, people with hearing loss had the lowest rate (Harrell, 2021).

Violence and abuse on children with disabilities include physical violence, emotional violence, sexual abuse, and neglect, with emotional violence being the most reported form of abuse (Fang et al., 2022). Children with complex needs can drain a family's finances and cause caregiver burdens on parents. A meta-analysis found 33% of children with disabilities have experienced violence (Fang et al., 2022). Children with mental and behavioral health disabilities had the highest prevalence of child maltreatment. While 40% of children with disabilities were bullied by their peers, children with sensory impairment had the highest rate of being bullied (Fang et al., 2022).

Although violence against children and older adults is well documented, there needs to be more evidence-based prevention and intervention for these families. School prevention programs to address peer bullying are imperative. A thorough review of current policies for both populations cannot be delayed. Discovering where policies fall short is the first step for improvement. Caregivers of both populations need to be followed by in-home C/PHN case managers to assess strengths and risk factors (Fang et al., 2022).

In response to the college shootings, universities provide training to staff, faculty, and students on actions to take if there is an active shooter on campus. This training is meant to assist the population on what to do should an event occur. However, the training may have unexpected outcomes for people with disabilities (Box 24-7).

BOX 24-7 PERSPECTIVES

A Community Member Viewpoint on Active Shooter Response by Persons With Disabilities

With the recent news reports of gun violence, the safety of those with disabilities must be included in the planning. The following discusses an exercise the writer and I were mandated to attend due to threats at our campus.

—Dr. Charlene Niemi

I went to the "Active Shooter Response" workshop at work to stir things up. As a wheelchair user, I knew the currently popular "Run. Hide. Fight." model didn't take people like me into consideration. I was prepared to draw attention to every point that didn't apply to people with various disabilities and put the facilitator on the spot for alternative solutions. I wanted to make people think, but I quickly realized I had a lot of thinking to do myself.

The facilitator shared some interesting tactics that seemed useful, like creating obstacles between yourself and the shooter, finding a hiding place, and the difference between cover and concealment. Then it was time to test our new skills. I felt surprisingly good about adapting what I'd learned.

The first drill began with a police officer rushing in, screaming for everyone to "get down." I stood out like a spire when everyone else collapsed to the ground. My glaring vulnerability felt like a gut punch. I could drop out of my chair, but then I'd be stranded. My only hope to save myself is to stay in my chair, but where does that leave me with the officer? I'm at the mercy of his training and ability to quickly evaluate the situation.

We reset and drilled again. The "shooter" stormed in, and my colleagues ran from the room slinging furniture behind them, slowing down the faux assailant...and me! Their impromptu barricades effectively trapped me with an armed aggressor.

In that moment, my cautious optimism melted into terror. The well-intentioned light I meant to shed on the need for inclusive emergency preparedness seemed so petty when people were running for their lives. The ADA, accessibility, inclusion, even the kindness of strangers, all the social strategies I had come to rely on for helping me navigate life were suddenly off the table, and I can't even be upset.

My friends and neighbors have families they desperately want to go home to and lives they want to go on living just like I do. You can't really know how a person will react in a crisis, and I have no right to expect anyone to put themselves in danger for me. I don't even want that. In a world where active shooter drills have become necessary, and weather events are becoming more and more extreme, have I finally met my match?

My fellow disabled citizens and I will continue to keep an eye out for ways to disappear in a wheelchair and fight off attackers with crutches and canes, but we all must learn how to be aware of the people around us and create protocols that give everyone at least a chance to survive.

Amanda Timpson, who was diagnosed with bilateral spastic diplegia cerebral palsy as a toddler and who has used a wheelchair since the age of 22 due to a car accident

FAMILIES OF PERSONS WITH DISABILITIES

Families that include a member with a disability face many challenges. Below we consider factors affecting families' ability to cope with the disability and the impact of caregiving on families.

Factors Affecting the Family's Ability to Cope

Families may also have little understanding of what services they are entitled to because of language barriers, difficult agency policies, or disjointed service delivery. These challenges may be magnified when a family member is newly diagnosed with a disability.

- The C/PHN is usually not the first healthcare professional that the family encounters. They may already have been through a lengthy struggle to receive assistance. In these circumstances, the nurse may be confronted with a frustrated family, reluctant to trust yet another healthcare provider.
- Nurses must earn the trust and confidence of the family by practicing consistency, following through with promised actions, and always being truthful.
- Families may also have little understanding of what services they are entitled to because of language barriers, difficult agency policies, or disjointed service delivery. These challenges may be magnified when a family member is newly diagnosed with a disability.
- Not all problems that the family faces can be remedied, and even for problems that do have solutions, time and effort may be needed to obtain the desired result.

Nageswaran and Golden (2018) uncovered four themes in the relationship between the caregivers (parents) and the home health nurse:

- The relationship developed over time.
- Trust and communication were crucial.
- Boundaries were difficult to maintain.
- A good working relationship between the nurse and the caregiver decreased caregiver stress, lowered stress for the healthcare provider, and improved care of the child.

Additionally, when working with an older child and the family, the C/PHN needs to remain respectful to both parties.

The Impact of Caregiving on Families

Parents face financial difficulty when caring for a child with disabilities. The age of the child and the severity of disability places a larger financial strain on the family. Often, mothers of children with disabilities work fewer hours, are unemployed, or make less money than mothers with children who are not disabled (Wondemu et al., 2022). Although, the fathers did not experience fewer work hours, many times they are paid less (Wondemu et al., 2022).

- Caring for a family member who is disabled, whether a child or an adult, is stressful. High levels of stress are often reported in families (Bedewy, 2021). Physical strain occurs due to lack of sleep, round-the-clock care or the need to be available 24/7, and traveling to appointments.
- Emotional strain is due to perceived guilt, blaming self, worry about the loved one's future, and thoughts of not doing enough or handling the situation well.
- Socioeconomic strain is due to feeling alone, lack of social and friend group, lack of childcare, and constant worry about finances (Bedewy, 2021).

Policy changes are needed to ensure case managers are well-versed in the caregivers' overall stress levels and assess strains placed on families (Bedewy, 2021). Parents' education and resources ensure a buffer to difficulties that may be in their future. C/PHNs should provide an up-to-date list of support groups to increase social involvement of caregivers and decrease family isolation.

Nurses need to be aware of the caregiver's mental and physical well-being during office or home visits. Some helpful suggestions for the families include the following:

- Self-care habits such as a healthy diet, regular sleep patterns, an exercise routine, and seek medical care if ill.
- Delegate duties and care where and when possible, ask for help, and reach out.
- Realize that striving toward perfect caregiving can cause stress. Do your best, and set realistic expectations.
- Spend time with significant loved ones including other children. Have routine date nights (CDC, 2020e).

Parents of children with disabilities have a higher prevalence of behavioral health issues when compared with parents of children without disabilities. Some reasons include the increase in financial expenses and the lack of social time with family and friends. Another reason is the lack of intimacy between parents when caring for a young child with disabilities that requires more care, leaving less time for intimacy among couples (Chen et al., 2023).

Although the incidence of Alzheimer disease and other dementias have begun to decline due to better control of known risk factors and education, it is estimated that 6.7 million people in the United States have the disease (Alzheimer's Association, 2023). What's more, there are over 11 million unpaid caregivers providing care to people with these disabilities (Alzheimer's Association, 2023).

- The majority of people (80%) with Alzheimer disease and other dementias are cared for in the home.
- Two thirds of caregivers are women.
- Thirty-four percent of caregivers are over 65 years old.
- Twenty-five percent are the "sandwich" generation, caring for older parents and younger children.
- Close to 60% have provided care for 4 years or more.
- Over 60% expect to provide care for the next 5 years (CDC, 2023b).

Many caregivers experience emotional, psychological, and physical strain. Moreover, they are subject to anxiety, depression, and a low quality of life (Alzheimer's Association, 2023).

C/PHNs working with this population should provide caregivers with community resource referrals such as respite care, support services, and local classes for training. For more information on Alzheimer and other dementias, go to *2023 Alzheimer's disease facts and figures* at https://www.alz.org/media/documents/alzheimers-facts-and-figures.pdf. The Centers for Medicare & Medicaid Services (CMS) provides resources for healthcare agencies to improve access to healthcare for people with disabilities as well as an educational guide for people on accessing care (CMS.gov, 2023):

- Modernizing Healthcare to Improve Physical Accessibility
  - Explains method on how to improve accessibility, needed resources to be in compliance with ADA, and a training video
- Modernizing Healthcare to Improve Communication Accessibility
  - Explores how to provide effective communication to those with sensory disabilities
- Navigating Healthcare with a Disability—Our Stories: Video Vignettes
  - Provides testimonial videos on personal experiences of the healthcare system
- Data Highlights
  - Discusses how disabilities affect Medicare and Medicaid eligibility
- Issue Briefs
  - Examines how to improve healthcare and physical accessibility to healthcare facilities

More detailed information can be found at https://www.cms.gov/priorities/health-equity/minority-health/resource-center/health-care-professionals-researchers/improving-access-care-people-disabilities

For people with disabilities, CMS developed a guide with tools and resources to assist people in receiving the care they are entitled to. The guide is available in eight languages as well as Braille (CMS, 2023). The guide "Getting the care you need" is found at https://www.cms.gov/files/document/getting-care-you-need-guide-people-disabilities.pdf

Although *Healthy People 2030* directly addresses delays in receiving primary and preventative care, the obstacles to obtaining **assistive devices and technologies** may improve due to the 2024 rule *Discrimination on the Basis of Disability in Health and Human Service Programs or Activities* previously discussed. **Temporary Assistance for Needy Families (TANF)**, **Social Security's Supplemental Security Income (SSI)**, and Medicaid are three government assistance programs nurses should familiarize themselves with.

- TANF is a time-limited federal program that provides assistance to families that cannot meet basic needs. Each state determines how to use the funds (USDHHS, n.d.).

- SSI is a federal program that provides income to persons with disabilities who have little or no income to meet their basic needs (Social Security Administration, n.d.).
- Medicaid provides affordable coverage as well as services not normally covered by provider insurance (Medicaid.gov, n.d.).

Those with disabilities and their families often are unaware of eligible programs and confused about the rules and regulations of each program. CHNs working with this population need to educate themselves on government resources and nonprofit agencies that assist the family in attaining equipment and supplies. Advocating for clients and providing case management provide a welcome relief to families.

Respite care is another resource of great importance for families. Due to the constant demands of providing care 24 hours per day, 7 days per week and the stress associated with numerous demands, respite care provides relief to caregivers of adults or children with disabilities. When focus is placed on the needs of one family member, other children may feel that their own needs are not as important, which can lead to behavioral and health-related problems (Box 24-8).

BOX 24-8 C/PHN USE OF THE NURSING PROCESS/CLINICAL JUDGMENT

Supporting a Family With a Child With Autism

Assessment/Recognize Cues

The local public health department received a referral from the school nurse requesting a home visit with the Adams family. The youngest of the three children was diagnosed with level 3 autism spectrum disorder (ASD) when he was 3 years of age. The child has limited vocabulary; aggressive, restricted social skills; runs away from class; and has a difficult time dealing with changes in his routine. The school nurse expressed concern because the child's behavior has become more aggressive toward staff and other children since his father is away on a business trip. Furthermore, he runs out of class and bangs his head against the wall. The other two children are late to school every morning; they arrive to school hungry and are not up-to-date on homework.

The C/PHN arrives at the home unannounced in order to assess the home life. During the interview, the C/PHN realizes the father is out of the country on a business trip and the mother is overwhelmed caring for the children on her own. Because of the youngest child's problems at school, the mother has been called into school frequently and is at risk of losing her job. The older children, ages 15 and 13 years, are playing video games as the mother attempts to prepare dinner for the family. The youngest is in the corner screaming and hitting his head on the floor. The three-bedroom home is clean, and family photos and children's drawings adorn the walls and refrigerator. The mother, Joanne, expresses being overwhelmed and depressed since her husband is on a business trip overseas. Because the job is new and requires him to be away on numerous business trips, he is not able to help as much as he wishes. Finances are tight, but they are able to pay the bills.

The two older children are sick with colds and have productive coughs. They have missed 4 days of school and are falling behind in their studies. The mother expresses her concern for the children but is uncertain where to seek medical care since the family health insurance has not taken effect yet. While speaking with the C/PHN, the mother starts to cry, and the two older children come to comfort her. The oldest child tells the nurse they feel sad when they see their mother cry, but they do not know how to help. It is apparent to the nurse the family members care deeply for each other.

Diagnosis/Analyze Cues and Prioritize Hypotheses

- Family unit is overwhelmed while one parent is on business trip.
- Youngest child, with ASD, has increased difficulty at school and home. Misses father but does not have verbal skills to express feelings.
- Although the older children want to help, they feel helpless and are unsure how to help.

Planning and Implementation/Generate Solutions and Take Action

- Respite and emotional support for mother arranged through an autism support group.
- Older children receive weekly free counseling through the school services.
- School arranged for daily morning video calls with father and youngest child and when behavior escalates.
- Family hold evening meetings to provide emotional support and express love to each other.
- Older children given chores to help mother and feel a part of the solution.

Evaluation/Evaluate Outcomes

The C/PHN conducted follow-up visits every 2 weeks to check on family progress. The children have video calls with father nightly when he is on business trips. To help the youngest child with the father's absence, the father has video calls nightly at the same time no matter the time zone to allow the youngest to keep to a routine. Although the child is nonverbal, it is clear by his excitement he is very happy to be on a video call with his father. The school nurse arranges for the child to speak to his father during the day as well. The child's behavior has greatly improved at school, and he has stopped hitting his head on the floor.

The two older children and the parents have gone to the park twice using a free respite service provided through a local church. The children are attending school and are doing well. The parents have joined a support group for parents with children with disabilities and have made friends with group members. The mother is observed playing with the children.

The C/PHN informs the parents the family is doing well and that the C/PHN will decrease their visits to monthly. The nurse encourages the parents to contact them if they have any questions or concerns.

- Unfortunately, 85% of families do not use formal respite services due to costs of services, waitlists, or lack of knowledge of respite services (Utz, 2022).
- The benefits of respite care became clear during the COVID-19 pandemic when formal and informal respite services ceased. Families and caregivers felt overwhelmed, anxious, and dealt with social isolation (Utz, 2022).

Respite care is vital to the family's health and should be considered a priority in the overall treatment plan. ARCH National Respite Network and Resource Center provides a list of respite services nationwide.

The issue of employment is generally of great significance to families, as employment options may be quite limited when a family member has functional needs.

- The family may have to remain in a particular location to access needed health and social services, reducing the possibility of increased earning potential at a different location or in another field of employment.
- Although some legal protections are provided under the **Family and Medical Leave Act** of 1993, it does not apply in all situations. For instance, it is only available in companies with more than 50 employees and is most often used for the birth and care of a newborn or newly adopted child or for temporary care of a family member with a serious health problem (spouse, parent, or child). More importantly, it allows only for time off; it does not mandate that employers continue a salary during those periods (U.S. Department of Labor [USDOL], n.d.).
- Family members may have to choose between taking unpaid time off and continuing to work while dealing with the needs of the family member as best they can.

At a time when many families need two wage earners to help meet financial commitments, families engaged in caregiving may have to rely on only one income. Limitations in income are particularly challenging considering the myriad needs of those who have disabilities, needs that may not be covered by any insurance.

Families may experience financial difficulties, poor physical or mental health, and a variety of other challenges. For instance, during the COVID-19 pandemic, over 50% of persons with disabilities had difficulty paying household expenses, whereas only one in four who were nondisabled had difficulty (Friedman, 2022). One in three people earned less than $25,000 yearly, whereas 88% of those who were not disabled earned more than $25,000. When considering the cost of living, people with disabilities must consider direct and indirect costs. Indirect costs include healthcare costs and personal assistance needs such as follows:

- Car modifications so that person can drive
- Increased cost of homes that have universal design
- Living in neighborhoods with universal design
- Dictation devices, hearing devices, speech assistance
- Ramps, wider hallways/door
- Adaptive equipment: assistive technology and durable medical equipment

These costs, plus other expenses, increase expenses by 30% or $18,000 more a year (Goodman et al., 2020).

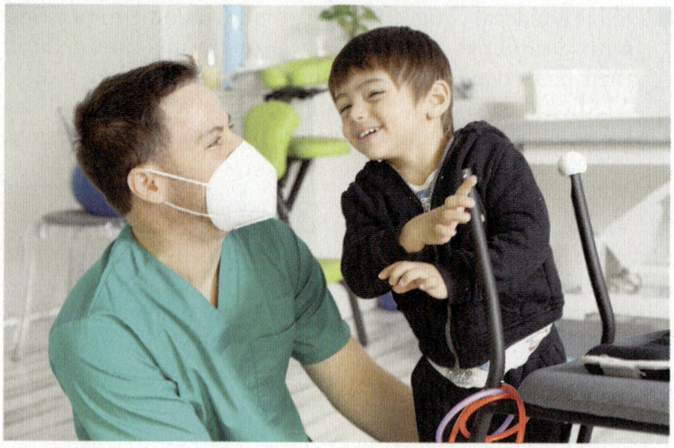

FIGURE 24-4 Child with cerebral palsy with community health nurse.

Furthermore, as children grow or older people decline, these direct and indirect costs continue to increase.

Families are often ill prepared to deal with the complicated systems that must be accessed to obtain needed care. The C/PHN is in an optimal position to interpret those systems to the families and to advocate for the needed care, services, and equipment (Fig. 24-4). The nurse must view the family holistically, recognizing additional needs that may develop as a result of the situation currently faced, and include an assessment of caregiver and family work patterns when caring for families with a family member who is disabled.

Organizations Serving the Needs of People With Disabilities and Their Families

Many governmental and privately funded organizations are dedicated to serving people with disabilities and their families as well as educating the public on disabilities.

- These organizations provide nurses with a starting point for exploring specific topics pertinent to practice.
- As clients and families may also be accessing online content through personal or public internet access, it is important for nurses to prescreen and make recommendations to clients and families about reliable and accurate sites.

Numerous organizations provide websites to assist people with disabilities and their families. Disabled World, updated in 2023, listed in Table 24-2, provides a thorough list of services for people with disability within the United States.

The C/PHN student is encouraged to explore these resources and to learn more about specific disabilities that can impact clients and their families. For example, 40 million adults age 18 years and older have hearing loss. Hearing loss is only expected to grow as the population ages.

- This disability increases the risk of dementia and, if left untreated, affects employment opportunities and pay (Everett, 2023).

TABLE **24-2** Websites to Assist People With Disabilities and Their Families

Organization	Description	Website
Disabled World	Provides a thorough list of disabled services within the United States	https://www.disabled-world.com/disability/foundations/us-organizations.php
Special Olympics	Uses sports and activities to inspire and reach those with disabilities	https://www.specialolympics.org/
Special Needs Alliance	National organization of attorneys who specialize in public benefits law and assist those with disabilities	https://www.specialneedsalliance.org/
National Center on Disability and Journalism	Provides links to many resources and services	https://ncdj.org/resources/organizations/#neurological-disorders-and-injury

- While exact numbers of children are unclear, it is estimated 16% of children between 6 and 19 years have some hearing loss or deficit (CDC, 2023c).
- Nursing students are encouraged to reach out to their local school districts and inquire if the schools conduct hearing and vison screenings.
- When hearing concerns are discovered early, interventions are implemented to lessen consequences to educational goals.

Fortunately, there are screening tools, treatments, and interventions for those that are deaf or hard of hearing. In addition to technology such as hearing aids and cochlear implants, many people learn alternate ways to communicate such as sign language. Box 24-9 offers a brief summary of the purpose and use of **American Sign Language** and other signed languages, and Box 24-10 discusses Braille.

UNIVERSAL DESIGN

For those living with a disability or chronic disease and their family members, the issue of access is of utmost importance. **Universal design** is the concept of purposely creating environments in a way that they are accessible to all without the need for modifications. The term universal design has been attributed to Ron Mace, founder of the Center for Universal Design, based out of North Carolina State University. Mace, who had polio as a child, died suddenly in 1998, leaving behind a long legacy of advocacy on behalf of accessibility in design (Center for Universal Design, 2016). While universal design is at the core of the ADA, it is important to note the relationship between inclusiveness and reduction of barriers to access (Office of Disability Employment Policy, n.d.). Universal design is for everyone, not solely for those with disabilities.

The issue of accessibility is not new. The ADA, as discussed earlier, addresses issues of access in employment, governmental building, and public accommodations. The Fair Housing Accessibility Guidelines, effective beginning in 1991, provide for design and construction of multifamily dwellings (four or more units) in accordance with accessibility requirements (United States Department of Housing and Urban Development [USDHUD], n.d.).

Provisions mandate that doorways be wide enough to accommodate wheelchairs, dwellings be readily accessible to and usable by people with functional disabilities, and accessible routes be throughout buildings (Fair Housing Accessibility First, n.d.; see Figs. 24-5, 24-6, and 24-7). Answers to multiple questions on accessibility guidelines may be found at https://www.hud.gov/program_offices/fair_housing_equal_opp/faq_accessibility_first

BOX **24-9** Sign Language in Brief

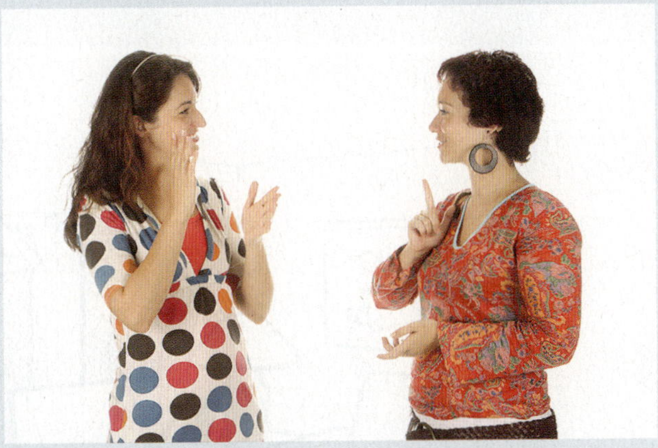

- Sign language is the use of "handshapes" and gestures to communicate ideas or concepts.
- American Sign Language is a unique language with its own rules of grammar and syntax.
- American Sign Language is primarily used in America and Canada and is the natural language of the deaf community; in Britain, British Sign Language is used.
- Sign languages are not universal.
- International Sign Language (Gestuno) is composed of vocabulary signs from various sign languages for use at international events or meetings to aid communication.
- Systems of Manually Coded English (i.e., Signed English, Signing Exact English) are not natural languages but systems designed to represent the translation of spoken language word for word.

Source: ASL University (n.d.); National Institute on Deafness and Other Communication Disorders (2021).

BOX 24-10 What Is Braille?

Braille takes its name from Louis Braille, an 18-year-old blind Frenchman who created a system of raised dots on paper for reading and writing by modifying a system used on board sailing ships for night reading. The six raised dots of each Braille "cell" vary to form palpable letters and punctuation. Persons experienced in Braille can read at speeds of 200 to 400 words per minute, comparable to print readers. Braille text can be written (1) by hand with a slate and stylus; (2) with a Braille writing machine; or (3) with specialized computer software and a Braille-embossing device attached to the printer.

Source: National Federation of the Blind (n.d.)
Note: More information about Braille is available at: https://www.afb.org/blindness-and-low-vision/braille/what-braille

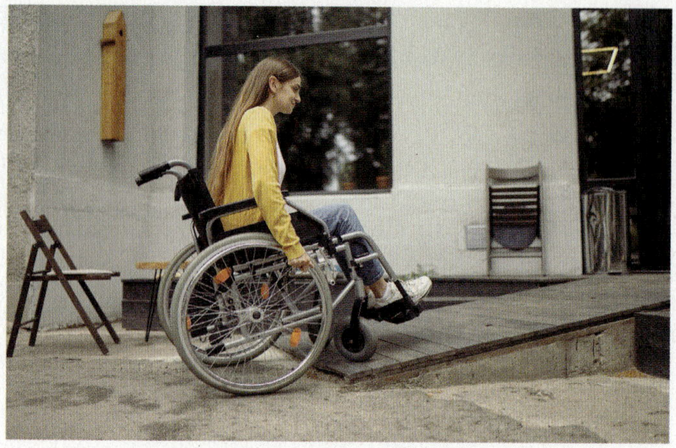

FIGURE 24-5 Person with a spinal cord injury using a wheelchair ramp.

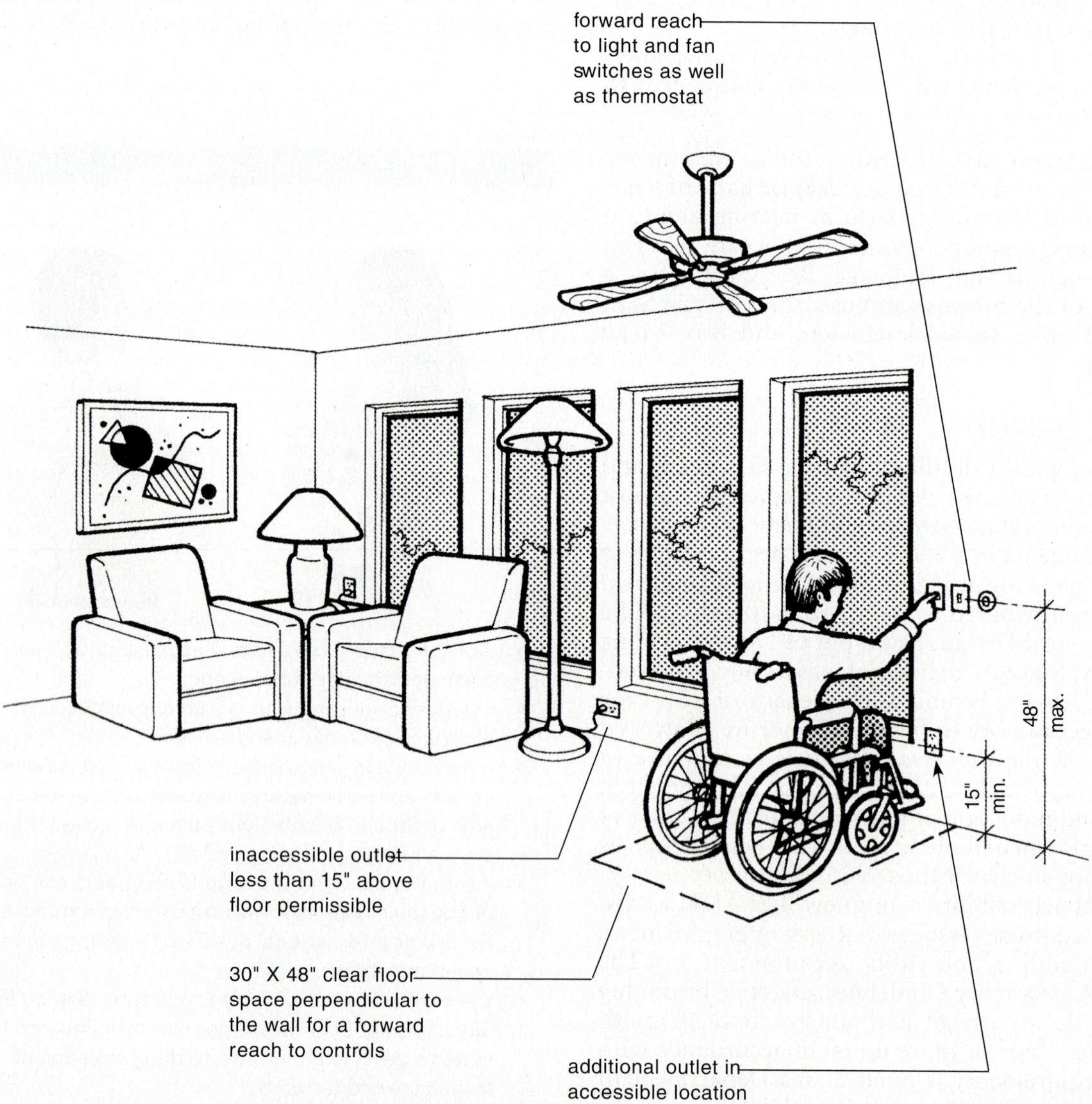

FIGURE 24-6 Recommended height of electrical outlet for ease of access for a person using a wheelchair. (Reprinted from Office of Policy Development and Research. (2008). Fair housing use design manual (p. 5.2). https://www.huduser.gov/portal/publications/destech/fairhousing.html)

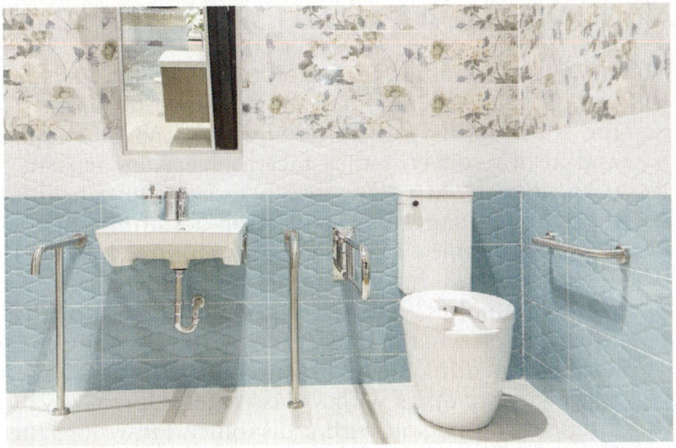

FIGURE 24-7 Toilet for older adults and people with functional disabilities, with bars on both sides to support the body and provide slip protection.

For those with existing disabilities and as the population ages, ensuring easy accessibility for all in businesses, housing, and places of recreation is of paramount importance. Having the opportunities for healthy participation in physical activity may forestall or prevent the development of illness. For the community, having an environment that promotes rather than restricts a healthy lifestyle can be economically advantageous (Fig. 24-8). A healthier population may be achieved with attention to the environmental barriers that impede healthy lifestyles for all persons, including those with disabling conditions.

THE ROLE OF THE COMMUNITY/PUBLIC HEALTH NURSE

This section considers the various roles of the C/PHN working with this population. It is important to review these roles in the context of multilevel practice: the person, the family, and the community. Chapter 2 first examined the broad spectrum of roles that the C/PHN assumes within the community (i.e., clinician, educator, advocate, manager, collaborator, leader, researcher), as well as the 10 Essential Services of Public Health. Consider an example of the variety of roles with respect to a 55-year-old client who uses a wheelchair. The client has difficulty obtaining a gynecologic examination because of the lack of accessible examination tables at the local clinic; as a result, she has not had an examination for more than 20 years. Recognizing the need for a complete examination, the C/PHN arranges with the clinic to find appropriate alternatives that will aid the client in receiving the needed examination, possibly by ensuring that additional personnel are provided. The C/PHN is an advocate at the individual level, providing the essential services of monitoring health. Because this solution is temporary and less than optimal, the nurse contacts a number of clinics in neighboring communities and finds one that has appropriate equipment for people who have difficulty transferring to a standard examination table. Unfortunately, this clinic is an hour away. The nurse then contacts a number of other C/PHNs and discovers that they also have a significant number of clients with this problem who have not received a gynecologic examination in many years. The C/PHN discovers a need at the community level through research. Essential services provided include monitoring health and diagnosis and investigation at the community level.

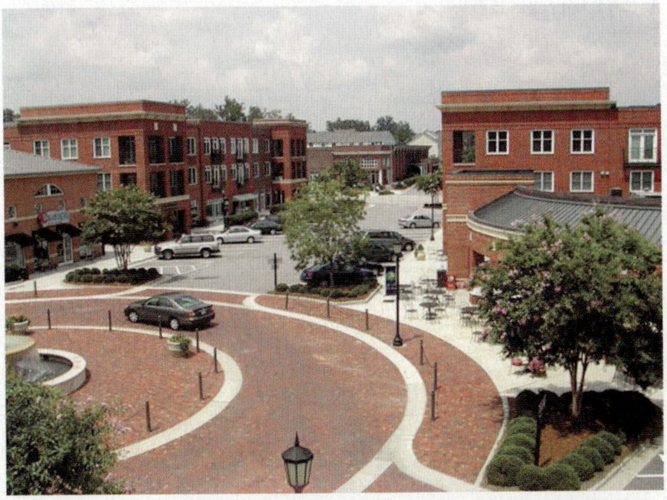

FIGURE 24-8 Planned, mixed-use development with curb cuts, well-marked crossings, sidewalks, and accessible commercial and public spaces. (Source: Center for Universal Design. *CDC Image Library*. https://phil.cdc.gov/Details.aspx?pid=9104)

Through a coordinated effort, the nurse is able to develop partnerships with a local transportation company and the clinic to arrange a twice-yearly gynecologic screening program for people in the community who require special accommodations. Acting as an advocate and coordinator at the community level, the C/PHN mobilizes community partnerships, develops policy, and links the population to needed services. Information sheets that discuss the need for annual gynecologic examinations and advertise the program are distributed to area C/PHNs, employers, and health clinics. Functioning in the educator role at the community level, the C/PHN is providing the essential services of informing, educating, and empowering others. Data collection on examinations provided over the next few years shows a 65% increase in the number of people with functional needs who have received a gynecologic examination within the past year. Continuing in the role of researcher at the community level, the C/PHN practices the Essential Services of evaluating the services and reaching new solutions.

This is not an uncommon scenario in the practice of community/public health nursing. Often, the needs of a person may open the door to areas of concern for many in a community and provide a basis for intervention that can benefit a larger population. The complexity of issues surrounding these conditions requires creativity, tenacity, honesty, and, most of all, knowledge. C/PHNs who are informed about the issues that affect people with disabilities at local, state, and national levels are prepared to offer assistance to their clients and to their communities.

Although successes at the individual level are laudable, the extent to which the health and well-being of those affected are improved must be the ultimate goal. Forming partnerships within the community places the C/PHN in a prime position to initiate and support efforts to improve the health status of those populations.

- It is important for C/PHNs to consider population health among those with disabilities. Our U.S. population is living longer, and the older population is set to outgrow the younger population by 2035 (Cacchione, 2020).
- Nursing and interprofessional interventions are needed to meet the requirements of this aging population.
- Models of care highlighted by Cacchione (2020) describe the development and role of nurses and advanced practice nurses in the prevention of secondary disabilities, the improvement of health behaviors, and in addressing health concerns (Cacchione, 2020).

SUMMARY

- The issues of disability are of growing importance in public health and to community/public health nursing, both nationally and internationally.
- Through the efforts of the WHO, the international community has been challenged to provide increased attention to health promotion and disease prevention.
- The aging of the U.S. population and the rise in lifestyle-related illnesses such as diabetes and obesity are often linked with increasing rates of disability. Health disparities and differing access to services are a focus of *Healthy People 2030*.
- *Healthy People 2030* has placed increasing focus on people's well-being, helping those with disabilities to get support and services within the healthcare system, at work, home, and school. To improve quality of life, accessibility in our homes, schools, and workplaces is essential.
- Legislation is but one step toward equality for those affected by disabilities and chronic illnesses. The IDEA and ADA secured many improvements in accessibility and specific legal protections for people with disabilities, but it is only the beginning.
- C/PHNs are in a prime position to advocate for the health needs of people who are disabled or chronically ill. With a long history of serving those who are most vulnerable, C/PHNs can help make needed changes at the individual, family, and community levels.

ACTIVE LEARNING EXERCISES

1. Using the six areas of disabilities as defined by the U.S. Census Bureau, interview a person from one of the six disability areas; inquire into the functional and health concerns they face in everyday activities (Objective 1). https://www.census.gov/topics/health/disability/guidance/data-collection-acs.html
2. Develop a table listing the socio-cultural, political, economic, and health factors influencing persons with disabilities locally, nationally, and globally. After completing the table, did you discover any similarities and differences? Research why that might be. Share your findings with a classmate. (Objective 2)
3. Interview an person with a disability. How does the Social determinants of health (SDOH) impact healthcare outcomes and well-being specific to economic stability, education access and quality, healthcare access and quality, neighborhood and built environment, and social and community context. How do these determinates impact their health outcomes and well-being? (Objective 3)
4. Conduct a family assessment (Chapter 14) that consists of a family caregiver and a child or an older adult who is disabled. What action plan would you implement? What resources would you recommend? Follow-up with the family during the course and evaluate if your interventions are successful. Describe which of the 10 Essential Public Health Services (Box 2-2) you utilized. (Objective 4)
5. Educate a group of concerned community members on the various laws and policies that protect people with disabilities. (Objective 5)
6. Research a recent natural or human-caused disaster in your area. Based on the current disaster plan in your area, was it sufficient for people with a mobility disability? Address how people were notified, evacuation plans, shelters in the area that are equipped for people with disabilities, and accommodations that were needed during the disasters. Explore possible changes that should be implemented services. (Objective 6)

CHAPTER 25

Behavioral Health in the Community

"We must stop criminalizing mental illness."

—Elyn Saks

KEY TERMS

- Behavioral health
- Gambling disorder
- Harm reduction
- Integrated behavioral health
- Mental disorders
- Mental health
- Substance use disorders
- Toxic brain injury

LEARNING OBJECTIVES

Upon mastery of this chapter, you should be able to:

1. Identify key behavioral health disorders and describe their effect on people and the community.
2. Assess commonly used substances and their effect on health.
3. Follow the steps of the nursing process in detection of behavioral health concerns and management of that risk.
4. Use incidence and prevalence data to inform the development of individual- and community-level interventions that address substance use disorders.
5. Implement universal prevention activities to promote the behavioral health of the community.

INTRODUCTION

The United States faces pronounced behavioral health issues within our communities and populations. High levels of anxiety and depression in youth, jails serving as mental health facilities, the rise in suicide rates, and an increasing death toll from drug overdoses add to our already overburdened mental health system (Insel, 2023). Discussion around mental health has included simplistic pundits as a guide for complex behavioral health issues. Our stance on mental health has negatively impacted the seriousness of this crisis. Health strategies must move past criminalization of mental health and prioritize mental health as part of our population's overall health and wellness. This chapter gives an overview of behavioral health, a term referring to mental health and substance use. A comprehensive approach to behavioral health recognizes a continuum of care, from promotion to prevention, treatment, and recovery. Community/public health nursing practice is discussed, with a focus on individual-, community-, and policy-level interventions. The community/public health nurse (C/PHN) has a key role in working with people, families, and communities to promote optimal behavioral health and thereby decrease the prevalence and incidence of mental and substance-related disorders (Box 25-1).

CONTEMPORARY ISSUES

From concerns over the mental health of the population due to the COVID-19 pandemic, the opioid crisis, and alcohol use and controversies over supervised injection sites and the legalization of marijuana to the integration of behavioral health services and the emergence of anti-stigma strategies, behavioral health issues have undeniably preoccupied the United States in recent years.

Opioid Crisis

While to the numbers remain provisional, more than 107,000 people died in the United States from a drug overdose with 70% of these deaths due to fentanyl-type drugs in 2023 (Centers for Disease Control and Prevention [CDC], 2024a). In 2022, the Drug Enforcement Administration issued a Public Safety Alert regarding fentanyl mixed with xylazine, a powerful sedative. C/PHNs have crucial roles to play in addressing this

BOX 25-1 Behavioral Health Terminology

- **Behavioral health:** This term, which is used to refer to both mental health and substance use, looks at a comprehensive approach, recognizing a continuum of care, from promotion to prevention, treatment, and recovery.
- **Integrated behavioral health:** Integrated care blends medical and behavioral health factors in one setting. The advantage of an integrated system is coordination of care and team communication of all healthcare providers as they work toward person-centered health goals (Agency for Healthcare Research and Quality, n.d.).
- **Mental health:** *Healthy People 2030* addresses increased treatment for those with mental health disorders. In addition, screening and early identification is essential for all including youth and people who are homeless (ODPHP, n.d.-a).
- **Mental disorders:** "any condition characterized by cognitive and emotional disturbances, abnormal behaviors, impaired functioning, or any combination of these. Such disorders cannot be accounted for solely by environmental circumstances and may involve physiological, genetic, chemical, social, and other factors." (American Psychiatric Association, 2018).
- **Substance-related and addictive disorders:** This category consists of **substance use disorders** (SUD) and **gambling disorder**. SUD are classified as mild, moderate, and severe each with certain criteria that must be met. Gambling was added because of the similarity in clinical presentation, origin in the brain, comorbidity, physiology, and treatment (American Psychiatric Association, 2013).

Source: Agency for Healthcare Research and Quality (n.d.); American Psychiatric Association (2013); ODPHP (n.d.-a).

public health problem, including identifying persons at risk because of opioid use and providing education, support, and resources for this population (Fig. 25-1).

Supervised Injection Sites

Supervised injection sites, also known as safe consumption sites, have been found to mitigate overdose-related harms and unsafe drug use as well as facilitate the acceptance of treatment and other health services (Levengood et al., 2021). These services are available in Europe, Australia, and Canada and are beginning to emerge in the United States. The first supervised injection sites in North America were established in Vancouver, Canada, and the experience gained from them has informed

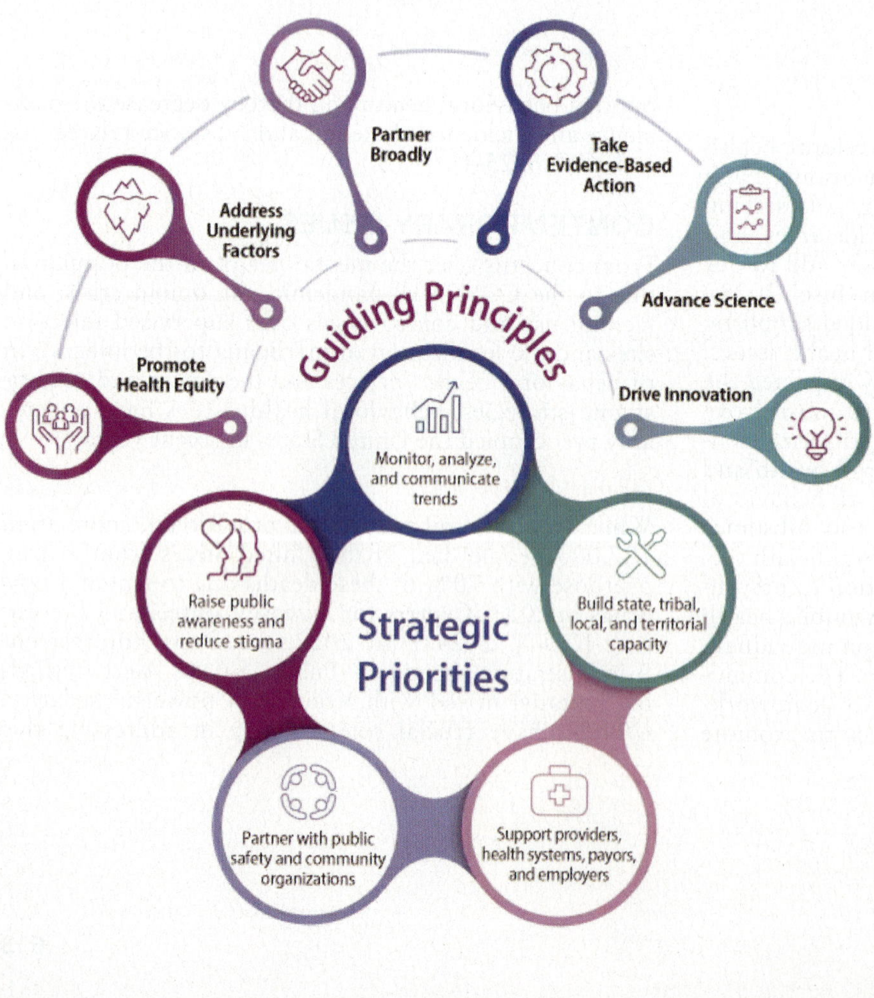

Partner Broadly
Take Evidence-Based Action
Address Underlying Factors
Advance Science
Guiding Principles
Promote Health Equity
Drive Innovation
Monitor, analyze, and communicate trends
Raise public awareness and reduce stigma
Build state, tribal, local, and territorial capacity
Strategic Priorities
Partner with public safety and community organizations
Support providers, health systems, payors, and employers

FIGURE 25-1 The CDC's work is guided by six principles and five strategic priorities to address the overdose crisis. (Reprinted from Centers for Disease Control and Prevention. (2024). https://www.cdc.gov/overdose-prevention/media/images/Guiding-Principles-Infographic.png)

the expansion of this harm reduction approach elsewhere. **Harm reduction** reduces the negative consequences of drug use (SAMHSA, 2023a). Proponents of these services view them as beneficial to public health and the community. Opponents believe that these sites do nothing to deter drug use or help people stop opioid use. Contentious legislative battles are ensuing as federal law prohibits these services, and if such sites are opened, they will face action by the U.S. Department of Justice to close them. Box 25-2 identifies some of the tensions between harm reduction and public safety. Informed by the evidence related to health outcomes for persons who use these services and areas in which they are situated, C/PHNs will be able to advocate for best practices to promote the health of this population and society.

Legalization of Marijuana/Cannabis

Paralleling the opioid epidemic, there has been a rapid expansion of the legalization of cannabis in the United States, for both medical and recreational use. Since November of 2023, 24 states, 3 territories, and the District of Columbia have legalized recreational cannabis use by adults. Although marijuana remains illegal at the federal level, there is a move toward legalizing it at the federal level as well (Fig. 25-2). Although recreational use is permitted in many states, the product is costly. Licensed dispensaries pay a sale tax, plus an excess tax that can range between 15% and 37% (Hansen et al., 2023). These taxes are passed on to the consumer, which can make the price of marijuana expensive. During the pandemic, sales of marijuana increased as cannabis stores remained open and people were homebound (Schauer et al., 2021).

Marijuana helplines have been established to assist people seeking information and help in several of these

BOX 25-2 Safe Consumption Sites: Tensions Between Harm Reduction and Public Safety

Harm Reduction

- Do safe consumption sites reduce drug overdose deaths?
- Do safe consumption sites encourage people who use opioids to seek help/treatment?

Safety Concerns

- Do safe consumption sites create social problems in neighborhoods?
- Do safe consumption sites encourage more people to use drugs?

Source: European Monitoring Centre for Drugs and Drug Addiction (EMCDDA). (2024).

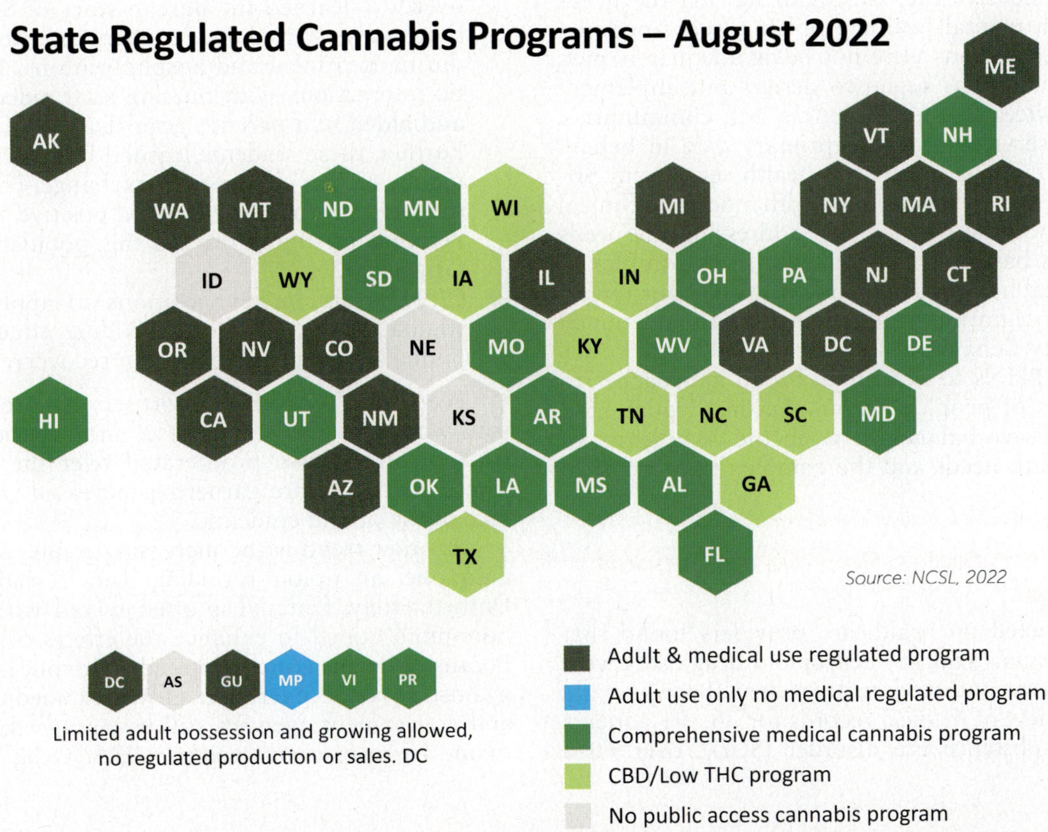

FIGURE 25-2 State Regulated Cannabis Programs—August 2022. (Reprinted with permission from National Conference of State Legislatures. (2022). *State medical marijuana laws.* https://documents.ncsl.org/wwwncsl/Health/NCSL-PH-and-Cannabis-Policy.pdf)

states. In their assessment of such helplines in four states, Carlini and Garrett (2018) reported that helpline staff had no knowledge about the effects and interactions of marijuana's two main components (tetrahydrocannabinol and cannabidiol), nor could they explain the differences in risk between smoking, eating, and vaporizing marijuana. It is essential for C/PHNs to have basic knowledge about marijuana components and methods of use. Educating individuals or the public with this information does not imply endorsement of marijuana use, but rather is an essential role that C/PHNs should assume.

Alcohol Use

The emphasis on the opioid crisis has in some ways overshadowed concerns over alcohol use, which, according to the World Health Organization (WHO), contributes to 3 million deaths annually (WHO, 2023). C/PHNs can provide evidence-based strategies to address this significant problem and help achieve the WHO goal of 10% reduction in the harmful use of alcohol globally by 2025 (WHO, 2023) and the alcohol-related Healthy People goal of reducing alcohol use in the United States (Fig. 25-3).

Integration of Behavioral Health Services

For decades, primary care, mental health, and substance use services have been separated, requiring patients to seek services among multiple sites and providers to obtain comprehensive care. Recognizing that the needs of people with mental health problems, substance use, and physical conditions were not being adequately met, provider organizations began to design and implement integrated services in their practices and communities. These model services provided primary care in behavioral health clinics or behavioral health services in primary care. Integrated behavioral health models of clinical integration guide the providers in addressing the needs of populations based on the behavioral risk/complexity and the physical health risk/complexity. The Four Quadrant Clinical Integration Model by the National Council for Community Behavioral Healthcare (2009) serves as a guide for C/PHNs to determine broad approaches to meet the needs of people and populations. Figure 25-4 depicts the relative balance between the complexity of behavioral health needs and the complexity of physical health needs.

Anti-Stigma Strategies, Peer-Based Support, and Naloxone

A study conducted on healthcare providers found that those with a stigma against illicit opioid drug users were less likely to treat and refer to treatment (Brown et al., 2023). In a review of medical records for 30,391 patients admitted for substance use disorder (SUD), over 60% were found to have stigmatizing language (SL) in the records (Weiner et al., 2023). The patients with the highest amount of SL in the records included people assigned male at birth and older adults. The majority of offenders were primary provider assistants; nurses displayed the least amount of SL (Weiner et al., 2023). Stigma is a key barrier to those who seek treatment for behavioral health conditions (Brown et al., 2023); while some research has been done in this area, more is needed. Corrigan and Nieweglowski (2018) proposed anti-stigma strategies that could be incorporated into public health programs targeting opioid stigma. Such strategies may be relevant for C/PHNs to help resolve the stigma that has persisted for decades. Stereotypes, prejudice, and discrimination underlie stigma, factors that, in part, can be confronted through education that dispels myths with facts.

- A study by Siddiqui and Rutherford (2023) reported that the biologic explanation (i.e., genetic) of SUD has done nothing to decrease the high level of stigma toward people with SUD. Society and social norms have "dehumanized" those with SUD. This "us" versus "them" mentality hampers proper treatment (Siddiqui & Rutherford, 2023). Interventions suggested to rehumanize this population include challenging the stereotypes surrounding people who have SUD, highlighting similarities between those with SUD and those without, and engaging in interpersonal contact (Siddiqui & Rutherford, 2023).
- Students who heard the lived experience of someone in recovery and a parent who lost a child to a drug overdose learned the human story of SUD. The presenters also shared their encounters with nursing staff during treatment and hospitalizations. The therapeutic interactions with nursing staff aided in recovery and aided in a parent's grief (Dion & Griggs, 2020). Further, these students learned harm reduction techniques such as clean needle exchange. The attitudes of the nursing students exhibited positive changes and a decrease in stigma toward this population (Dion & Griggs, 2020).
- C/PHNs are in key positions to apply these anti-stigma strategies when providing education to the public and engaging people in recovery.

Peer-based recovery support services provided by persons who have lived experiences and experiential knowledge of SUDs have proliferated over the past decade. These peer roles are garnering increased support in the face of the opioid epidemic.

Another trend is the increasing public availability of naloxone, an opioid-reversing drug (USDHHS, 2018). Unfortunately, fentanyl is often mixed with xylazine, a nonopioid added to enhance the effects of the fentanyl. Because xylazine is not an opioid, naloxone is not effective against xylazine overdose. However, medical providers and government agencies still encourage the use of naloxone to reverse an overdose (U.S. Drug Enforcement

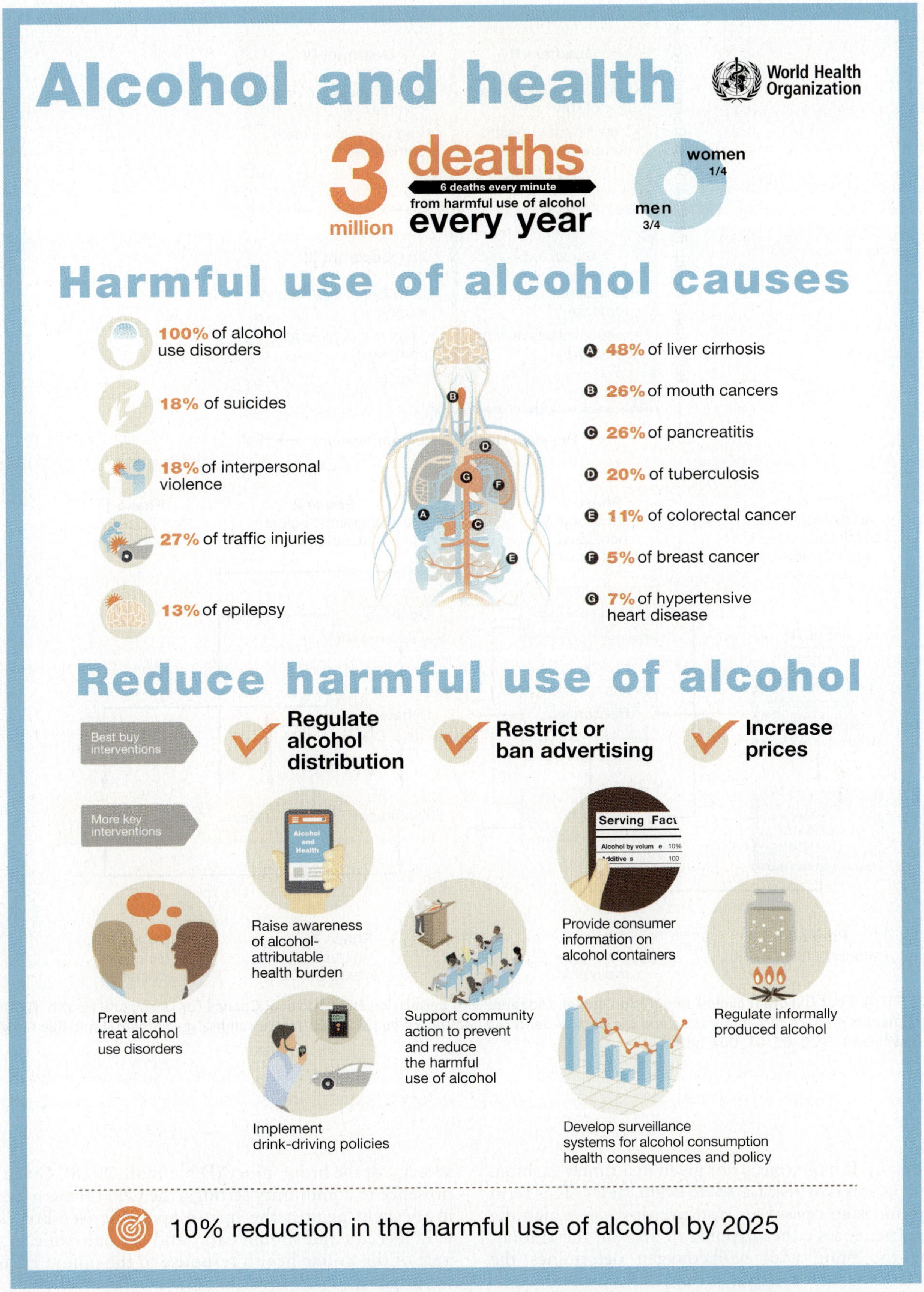

FIGURE 25-3 Alcohol and health. (Reprinted with permission from World Health Organization. (2018). *Global status report on alcohol and health*. https://www.who.int/images/default-source/departments/substances-abuse/alcohol/infographics/alcohol-3-million-death-every-year.png?sfvrsn=8062967_2)

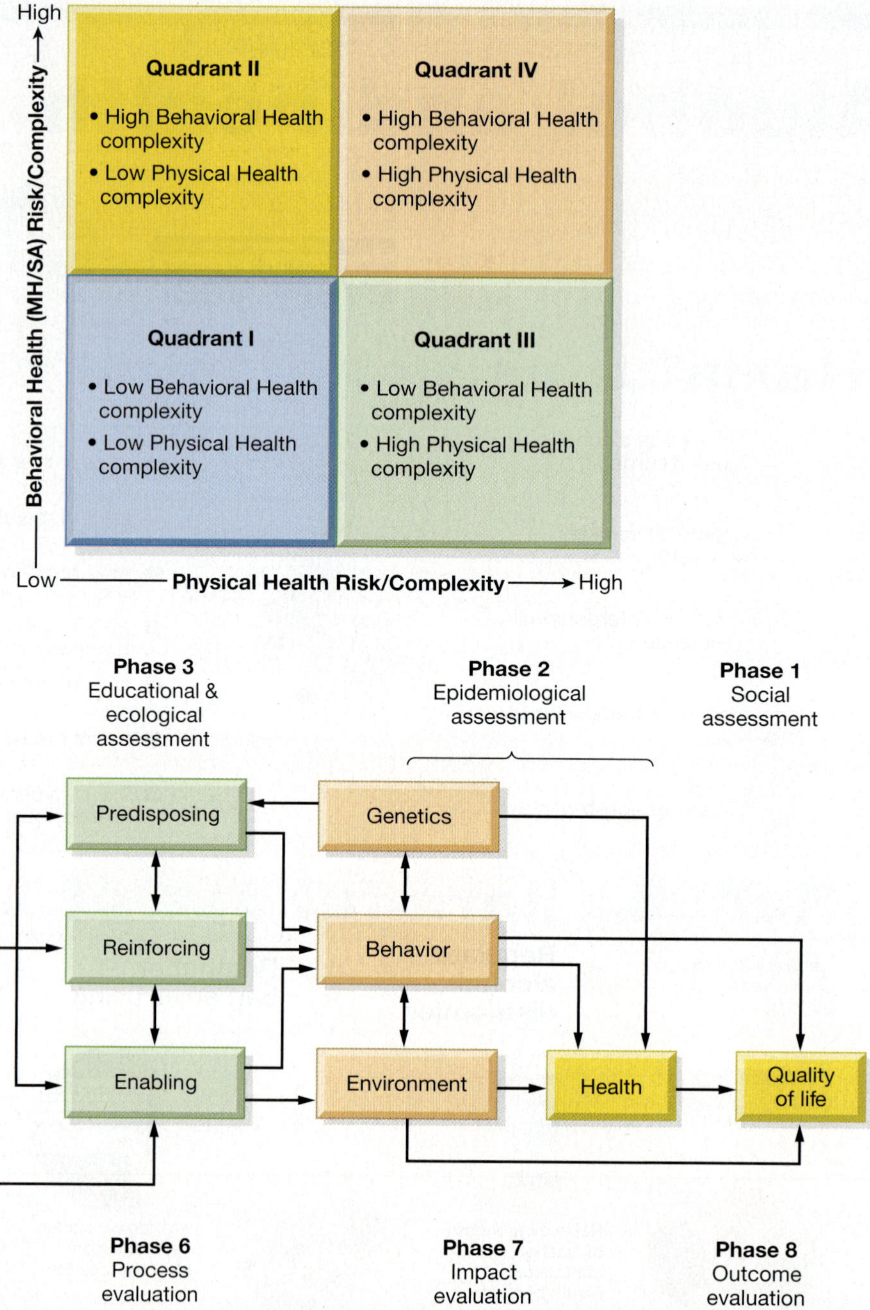

FIGURE 25-4 Four Quadrant clinical integration model. (Adapted with permission from National Council for Behavioral Health. (2009). *Behavioral health/primary care integration and the person-centered healthcare home.* https://store.samhsa.gov/sites/default/files/SAMHSA_Digital_Download/PEP20-02-01_004.pdf)

Agency, n.d.). If naloxone is not given in a timely fashion, then the person is at risk for **toxic brain injury**. This term came about from opioid use and overdoses in which the person experiences either hypoxia or anoxia; the amount of time the brain goes with oxygen determines the severity of the brain injury (Dane et al., 2018). Given their presence in community settings, the C/PHN has a key role in the fight against the opioid epidemic (see Box 25-3). C/PHNs can and should carry and use naloxone as a key part of the public health response to the opioid crisis.

BOX 25-3 The C/PHN's Role in the Fight Against the Opioid Epidemic

The Department of Health and Human Services declared a public health emergency and proposed strategies to combat this opioid epidemic. The accompanying community burdens associated with the loss of life, productivity, and healthcare treatment dollars as well as increased demands on criminal justice systems were deemed unsustainable. In response, the American Nurses Association (ANA) emphasized the nurse's role in the assessment and formulation of plans to decrease the impact of this epidemic while still advocating for appropriate treatment for painful conditions (ANA, 2018).

As frontline caregivers to the opioid-using population, Cleveland Clinic nurses have taken lead roles in the opioid task force established in early 2017. The task force has multiple focus areas designed to change harmful behaviors (Consult QD, 2017).

First, nurses are studying the clinical settings and describing patterns of those with opioid use disorder. Integral to the improvement of clinical care is incorporating alternative treatments to chronic pain as well as the provision of rescue medications in cases of overdose (Consult QD, 2017).

Next, health policy and laws that impact the availability of naloxone to first responders and pharmacists are addressed. In addition, policy is needed to facilitate treatment of pregnant people with SUD and address associated child custody matters (Consult QD, 2017).

Finally, nurses provide prevention education in the community with nurse-led information sessions within public gathering facilities. In addition, nurses develop curricula and educate peers on how to avoid "compassion fatigue," which frequently develops when providing care for those with SUD (Consult QD, 2017).

Source: American Nurses Association (ANA) (2018); Consult QD (October 16, 2017).

PREVENTION OF SUBSTANCE USE AND MENTAL DISORDERS

Relevant to behavioral health, the Healthy People 2030 leading health indicators focus on mental health and mental disorders, substance misuse, and tobacco (ODPHP, n.d.-a). The overarching goals follow:

- Improve mental health through prevention and by ensuring access to appropriate quality mental health services.
- Reduce substance misuse to protect the health, safety, and quality of life for all, especially children.
- Reduce illness, disability, and death related to tobacco use and secondhand smoke exposure.

Across these three major priority areas, C/PHNs can use evidence-based interventions to address the targeted outcomes. Interventions can be categorized according to the three levels of preventive behaviors, as shown in Box 25-4.

A comprehensive approach to behavioral health means seeing prevention as part of an overall continuum of care. The Behavioral Health Continuum of Care Model (Strategic Prevention Technical Assistance Center, n.d.) recognizes multiple opportunities for addressing behavioral health problems and disorders. The components of the model include promotion, prevention, treatment, and recovery. More information can be found at https://www.samhsa.gov/sites/default/files/resourcefiles/sptac-continuum-of-care.pdf

- Promotion strategies reinforce the entire continuum of behavioral health services. These strategies are designed to create the environments and conditions that support behavioral health and help people overcome challenges.
- Prevention strategies, as characterized by Gordon (1983) in a classic article on prevention, may be grouped into three different categories, according to the level of risk that each addresses: universal, selective, and indicated.
  - *Universal prevention* includes those strategies delivered to broad populations wherein the benefits outweigh the costs and risks for everyone. Examples of this include public health campaigns related to suicide prevention, legislation related to impaired driving, and a minimum age for the purchase of alcohol.
  - *Selective strategies* are indicated when a person's risk of becoming ill is elevated. Through detection of risk, vulnerable subgroups of people can be identified. As a result, programs and practices can be provided to reduce the risk.
  - *Indicated strategies* address specific risk conditions, focusing efforts on individual risk factors or behaviors that put people at high risk for developing a behavioral disorder.
- Treatment begins with case identification, which entails the ability to correctly identify those people who have a behavioral disorder with minimal false positives. Once identified, people who are at risk need to be referred for evidence-based treatments.
- Recovery focuses on promoting a high-quality and satisfying life in the community for all people. By engaging with people in recovery, C/PHNs can provide support and help them achieve their recovery goals, monitor progress toward and recognize when they are moving away from goals, and support their transitions throughout the recovery process. C/PHNs can foster activities that contribute to wellness and a meaningful life, enhancing ways that people in recovery can connect with others in their communities.

BOX 25-4 LEVELS OF PREVENTION PYRAMID

The C/PHN Works With High-Risk Populations for Mental Disorders and Substance Misuse

SITUATION: Community and public health nurses play a key role in affecting the social determinants of health in vulnerable populations. The main goal of the C/PHN is to improve the population's health through highlighting prevention and addressing the determinants of health within that population.

GOAL: To provide examples of the three levels of prevention when working with high-risk populations for mental disorders and substance use. These examples are meant to provide a starting point for the C/PHN's practice and will vary based on the population served. The first step in working with any aggregate is the development of trust.

Tertiary Prevention

- Provide classes on mental health and mental disorders to people and families.
- Provide resources and referrals to communities affected by substance use.
- Develop community partnerships to address these issues.
- Focus on the strengths of the community when developing interventions.

Secondary Prevention

Early Diagnosis

- Provide screening programs for the early detection of mental health concerns such as depression, suicidal thoughts, and substance use.
- Ensure that all adolescents receive screenings in schools.
- Increase referrals to inpatient and outpatient treatment programs.
- Provide harm reduction by needle exchange programs.

Prompt Treatment

- Provide referrals and treatment that are culturally sensitive and in native language of the client.
- Provide anticipatory guidance and ensure referrals are operational.
- Provide educational material that is culturally sensitive and literacy appropriate.
- Offer clinic hours that meet the needs of the community such as after-work hours or weekends.

Primary Prevention

Health Promotion and Education

- Ensure that educational material and health promotion take into account the health literacy level of the population and the person.
- Provide education and health promotion activities in partnership with the community members. Education topics should be relevant to the intended age group and community needs. Topics may include coping skills, nutrition, exercise, wellness tips, mental health, and stress reduction.

Health Protection

- Assess the community's social determinants of health and how they affect mental health.
- Hold town meetings to gain insight into the needs of the community.
- Meet with community partners to decrease number of liquor stores in lower-income neighborhoods.
- Assist the population in navigating sign-ups for a medical home.
- Achieving higher education has been shown to improve health and decrease poverty. Provide mentoring to middle school and high school students.
- Nurse-run clinics in areas with low percentage of healthcare providers.

MENTAL HEALTH

Improving mental health is a key goal of *Healthy People 2030* (Box 25-5). Mental health is essential to personal well-being, family and interpersonal relationships, and the ability to contribute to community or society (ODPHP, n.d.-b). C/PHNs should understand the risk factors that challenge and undermine the health of people across the lifespan, such as adverse childhood experiences (Swedo et al., 2023) and social determinants of health (Jeste & Pender, 2022). Early and regular mental health screenings are important for detecting emerging mental health problems. C/PHNs can engage the community in health-promoting activities and help establish community conditions to support health behaviors. These strategies are important for the prevention of mental disorders, which are associated with significant distress or disability in social, occupational, or other activities (American Psychiatric Association [APA], 2022).

Suicide

Two Healthy People 2030 objectives related to mental health improvement are to (1) reduce the suicide rate and (2) reduce suicide attempts by adolescents (U.S. Department of Health and Human Services, 2020). Suicide is one of the leading causes of death in the United States. According to the CDC (2024b), suicide was the 11th leading

BOX 25-5 *HEALTHY PEOPLE 2030*

Selected Mental Health and Mental Disorders Objectives

Core Objectives

MHMD-01	Reduce the suicide rate.
MHMD-03	Increase the proportion of children with mental health problems who get treatment.
MHMD-04	Increase the proportion of adults with serious illness who get treatment.
MHMD-05	Increase the proportion of adults with depression who get treatment.
MHMD-06	Increase the proportion of adolescents with depression who get treatment.
MHMD-07	Increase the proportion of people with substance use and mental health disorders who get treatment for both.

Research Objectives

MHMD-R01	Increase the proportion of adults who are homeless with mental health problems who get mental health services.

Reprinted from Office of Disease Prevention and Health Promotion (ODPHP). (n.d.-b). *Healthy people 2023: Browse objectives.* https://health.gov/healthypeople/objectives-and-data/browse-objectives

cause of death overall during a 2-month period in 2024. The majority of which were people assigned male at birth. Figure 25-5 displays the Suicidal Thoughts and Behaviors among Adults in 2022.

Firearms

The National Violent Death Reporting System collects data regarding violent deaths, including those resulting from suicide. Recognizing at-risk groups is an important first step in reducing suicide rates. C/PHNs can use report summaries to develop, implement, and evaluate programs and policies to prevent suicides and other violent deaths.

The method of suicide and location of the injury can also be important data for C/PHNs developing prevention strategies. For adults, firearms have been reported to be used in nearly half of suicides, followed by hanging/strangulation/suffocation, and poisoning (CDC, 2024c). For children between the ages of 5 and 14 years, hanging and suffocation in the child's bedroom was the leading method of suicide; with death by firearms second (Ruch et al., 2021).

- Firearms are the leading means of suicide among people with dementia. It is believed that 60% of those with dementia live in a home with firearms. However, conversations with caregivers regarding the risk of firearms rarely take place. Healthcare providers need to provide education regarding this risk (Pallin & Barnhorst, 2021).
- Other populations that have a high risk of firearm suicide are veterans, people with serious untreated mental illness, those in chronic pain, and heavily intoxicated people who have had suicide ideation in the past (Pallin & Barnhorst, 2021).
- Often the act of suicide is an impulsive action (Pallin & Barnhorst, 2021). If firearms are in the home, interventions may include changing the lock code, removing the firing pin, or dismantling the gun.
- Conversation regarding guns in the home should not include politics or the C/PHN's opinion. If a C/PHN suspects a person may be suicidal and there are firearms in the home, contact your local police department. C/PHNs have a role to play in firearm safety through education, safe storage, research agendas, and evidence-based advocacy through policy change (Dowdell, 2023).

Youth Suicide

Results from the 2021 Youth Risk Behavior Surveillance System highlight the need for reducing suicide attempts by adolescents. Gaylor et al. (2023) reported that of U.S. high school students assigned female at birth who were surveyed, 30% had seriously considered attempting suicide in the previous 12 months, 13.3% had attempted suicide, and 23.6% had made a plan about how they would attempt suicide. Although this student population saw an increase in suicidal attempts and ideation since the 2019 data, the rates for U.S. high school students assigned male at birth remained unchanged. The CDC has developed a technical package that provides evidence-based strategies for preventing suicide (CDC, 2022). C/PHNs can lead programs to provide children, youth, and adults with skills to resolve problems and negative influences that are associated with suicide

Major Depressive Episode

In the United States, 22.5 million adults (those aged 18 years or older) reported experiencing at least one major depressive episode (MDE). Young adults aged 18 to 25 years have the highest percentage of MDE followed by 26- to 49-year-olds, and 50 years and older with the least percentage (SAMHSA, 2023b). The number of adults with MDE is higher than the populations of 47 states within the United States.

Among adolescents, in 2022, 4.8 million, close to 20%, of the U.S. population aged 12 to 17 years reported at least one MDE. 24.7 million reported SUD or MDE (SAMHSA, 2023b).

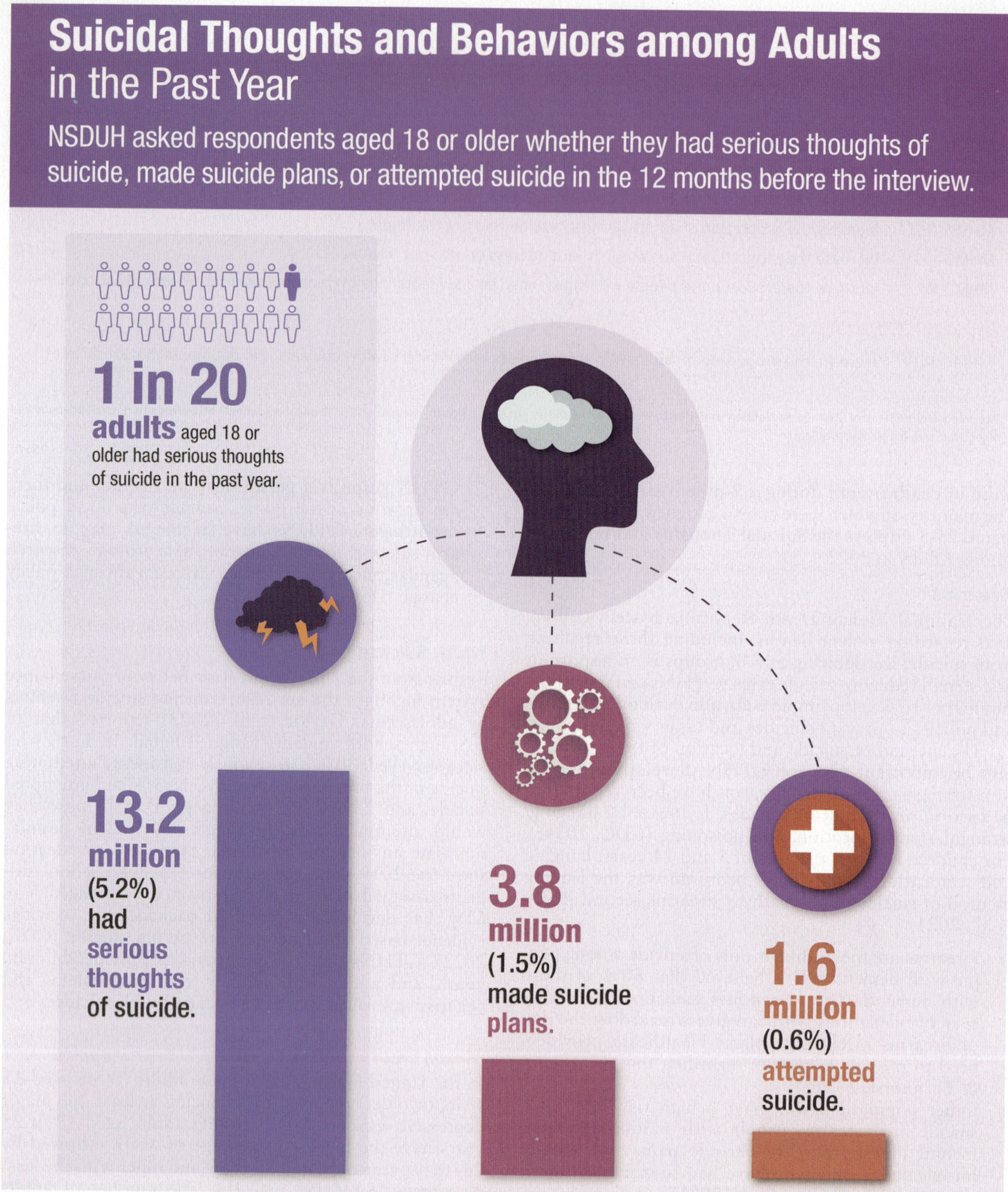

FIGURE 25-5 Suicidal thoughts and behaviors among adults in the past year. (Reprinted from Substance Abuse and Mental Health Services Administration. (2023). *Results from the 2022 National Survey on Drug Use and Health: A companion infographic* (SAMHSA Publication No. PEP23-07-01-007). Center for Behavioral Health Statistics and Quality, and Substance Abuse and Mental Health Services Administration. https://www.samhsa.gov/data/sites/default/files/reports/rpt42730/2022-nsduh-infographic-report.pdf)

What can C/PHNs do to help reduce the proportion of people who experience MDEs and increase the proportion who receive treatment?

- A systematic review and meta-analysis by Chan et al. (2022) reported that a range of eHealth cognitive–behavioral programs (CBP) have positive effects on symptoms reduction for depression and anxiety. However, eHealth CBP did not improve the overall quality of life for people (Chan et al., 2022). The authors suggest that eHealth has potential to be an adjunct of other treatments.
- A Cochrane Review by Thabrew et al. (2018) reported that a range of eHealth CBP were not effective in decreasing depression or anxiety in adolescents and children, especially those under 10 years (Thabrew et al., 2018).
- Technology-supported interventions for depression, such as Step-by-Step, developed by the WHO, are feasible to deliver to communities, adaptable, evidence-based, and scalable in multiple settings (WHO, 2022b). This online psychological intervention is directed toward people with depression, includes informational and interactive exercises, and is designed to be a minimally guided self-help intervention.
- C/PHNs can assist clients with barriers to use or navigation of eHealth technology (Fuller-Tyszkiewicz et al., 2018; see Chapter 10)..

National Depression Screening Day is held annually during Mental Illness Awareness Week in October (http://screening.mhanational.org/screening-tools). C/PHNs can be actively involved by hosting an event in the community, conducting screenings, and providing information to help youth and adults identify the signs and symptoms of depression in themselves, their family members, and their peers. The Patient Health Questionnaire-9 (PHQ-9) is one of the most commonly used and comprehensive tools used to screen for depression (APA, 2020). The PHQ-9 comes in English as well as 30 other languages; containing only nine questions, it provides healthcare providers with quick information on the client's emotional state. Immediate referrals ensure a better prognosis (Elansary et al., 2023). C/PHNs should document a list of resources in the community where adults and adolescents can be evaluated and treated for major depression.

SUBSTANCE USE

The *Diagnostic and Statistical Manual of Mental Disorders*, 5th Edition (APA, 2013) provides diagnostic criteria for substance-related disorders encompassing 10 classes of drugs: alcohol; caffeine; cannabis; hallucinogens; inhalants; opioids; sedatives, hypnotics, and anxiolytics; stimulants; tobacco; and other or unknown substances. *Healthy People 2030*, as shown in Box 25-6, focuses on substance use. C/PHNs should know how to detect the level of risk associated with alcohol and other drug use and the skills to intervene accordingly. The sections below address the scope of the problem associated with each substance, how to screen for risk, and how to intervene accordingly.

BOX 25-6 *HEALTHY PEOPLE 2030*

Selected Substance Use Objectives

Core Objectives

SU-01	Increase the proportion of people with a substance use disorder who got treatment in the past year.
SU-03	Reduce drug overdose deaths.
SU-05	Reduce the proportion of adolescents who used drugs in the past month.
SU-07	Reduce the proportion of adults who used drugs in the past month.
SU-09	Reduce the proportion of people under 21 years who engaged in binge drinking in the past month.
SU-10	Reduce the proportion of people aged 21 years and over who engaged in binge drinking in the past month.
SU-11	Reduce the proportion of motor vehicle crash deaths that involve a drunk driver.
SU-12	Reduce the proportion of people who misused prescription drugs in the past year.
SU-13	Reduce the proportion of people who had alcohol use disorder in the past year.
SU-15	Reduce the proportion of people who had drug use disorder in the past year.

Developmental Objectives

SU-D01	Increase the number of admission to substance use treatment for injection drug use.

Research Objectives

SU-R01	Increase the proportion of adolescents who think substance abuse is risky.

Office of Disease Prevention and Health Promotion (ODPHP). (n.d.-b). *Healthy people 2030: Browse objectives*. https://health.gov/healthypeople/objectives-and-data/browse-objectives

Alcohol Use

Although the opioid crisis continues to loom and rightfully command attention, alcohol contributes to the death of more than 3 million people each year (WHO, 2022b). The most recent published data show 137.4 million people aged 12 years and older reported drinking alcohol in the past month. While the data reflect a wide age range, 15% of these people are between the ages of 12 and 20 years (SAMHSA, 2023b). The 2022 National Survey on Drug Use and Health (NSDUH) collected information from people in the United States aged 12 years or older on past month alcohol use, binge alcohol use, and heavy alcohol use (SAMHSA, 2023b). Figure 25-6 displays the prevalence for each category and its definition.

The percent of alcohol varies by beverage. In screening for alcohol use, it is important to explain the definition of a standard drink. An infographic available from the National Institute on Alcohol Abuse and Alcoholism (n.d.-a) is useful for providing this information (Fig. 25-7).

The National Institute on Alcohol Abuse and Alcoholism (NIAAA) has established low-risk alcohol consumption limits as 2 drinks or less in a day for healthy adults assigned male at birth and 1 drink or less in a day for healthy adults assigned female at birth (United States Department of Agriculture, 2020). There are no safe limits for youth, and various health conditions and activities may warrant lower limits or no alcohol consumption at all. For example, alcohol consumption is contraindicated at any time during pregnancy (CDC, 2024d).

- Binge drinking is defined as follows:
  - For people assigned male at birth: 5 or more alcoholic drinks at the same occasion in 1 day within a 30-day period
  - For people assigned female at birth: 4 or more alcoholic drinks at the same occasion in 1 day within a 30-day period
- Heavy drinking is defined as binge drinking for 5 days within a 30-day period (SAMHSA, 2023b).

Grounded in an understanding of the nursing process, the definition of a standard drink, and recognition of the alcohol consumption limits for healthy adults, C/PHNs can promote the reduction of alcohol use by delivering evidence-based interventions. The NIAAA publications, *Planning Alcohol Interventions Using NIAAA's College AIM* and *Alcohol Screening and Brief Intervention for Youth: A Practitioner's Guide*, provide step-by-step guidance and tools for the delivery of this set of clinical strategies. To learn more about NIAAA's strategic plan for 2024 through 2028 NIAAA (n.d.-b), go to https://www.niaaa.nih.gov/about-niaaa/strategic-plan-fiscal-years-2024-2028/introduction-strategic-plan.

At the community level, C/PHNs can organize and actively engage in the National Alcohol Screening Day. This annual event, an initiative of the National Institutes of Health, is conducted to provide information about alcohol and health, as well as free anonymous screening. C/PHNs can help identify and address gaps in the treatment system by observing the types of specialty treatment that are provided in the community and assessing the time to access treatment as well as other factors affecting one's ability to receive timely and affordable treatment.

Drug Use

The annual NSDUH for persons in the United States aged 12 years or older obtains information on drugs including marijuana, cocaine, heroin, hallucinogens, inhalants, and methamphetamine (SAMHSA, 2023b). C/PHNs should remain up-to-date on the prevalence of drug use in the community.

Screening, Brief Interventions, and Referral to Treatment (SBIRT) provides help in the early stages of substance misuse:

- Screens for the risk of serious substance misuse
- Brief interventions offer insight and self-awareness into substance use
- Referral for treatment support if a client needs extra support and more intense treatment or counseling (SAMHSA, 2023c)

Marijuana

The drug that survey respondents most reported as having used in the past month is marijuana, used by 42.3 million people aged 12 years or older (SAMHSA, 2023b). Seventy-eight million Americans report that they have tried marijuana at least once in their lifetime (National Center of Drug Abuse Statistics [NCDAS], 2023).

Among high school students, 40% report having tried marijuana (NCDAS, 2023; SAMHSA, 2023b). With the emerging context of legalization of marijuana, it will be important for C/PHNs to continue to monitor the prevalence of marijuana use in their communities. Given the adverse health effects and harms associated with marijuana use, C/PHNs need to educate the public on its impact on health (SAMHSA, 2023d; see Boxes 25-7 and 25-8). Visit https://www.samhsa.gov/marijuana to review SAMHSA (2023d) "Learn about Marijuana Risks."

Cocaine and Crack

In 2022, 5.3 million people aged 12 years and older reported current use of cocaine in the past year. Young adults—people aged 18 to 25 years—had the highest amount of use at 1.3 million. The same year, 918,000 people aged 12 years and older used crack for the first time (SAMHSA, 2023b). According to the United Nations Office of Drugs and Crime (2023), over 2000 tons of cocaine was produced in 2020. One ton is worth $30 million wholesale. Two thousand tons is a figure difficult to imagine. This profitable drug for manufacturers has caused a world health problem.

Heroin

Heroin use has increased in recent years. Roughly 1.1 million people aged 12 years or older reported heroin use in 2022, with one million people aged 26 years and older as the majority of users (SAMHSA, 2023b). Until 2002, methadone was the primary medication used to treat people with heroin use disorder and was dispensed through licensed treatment facilities. The introduction

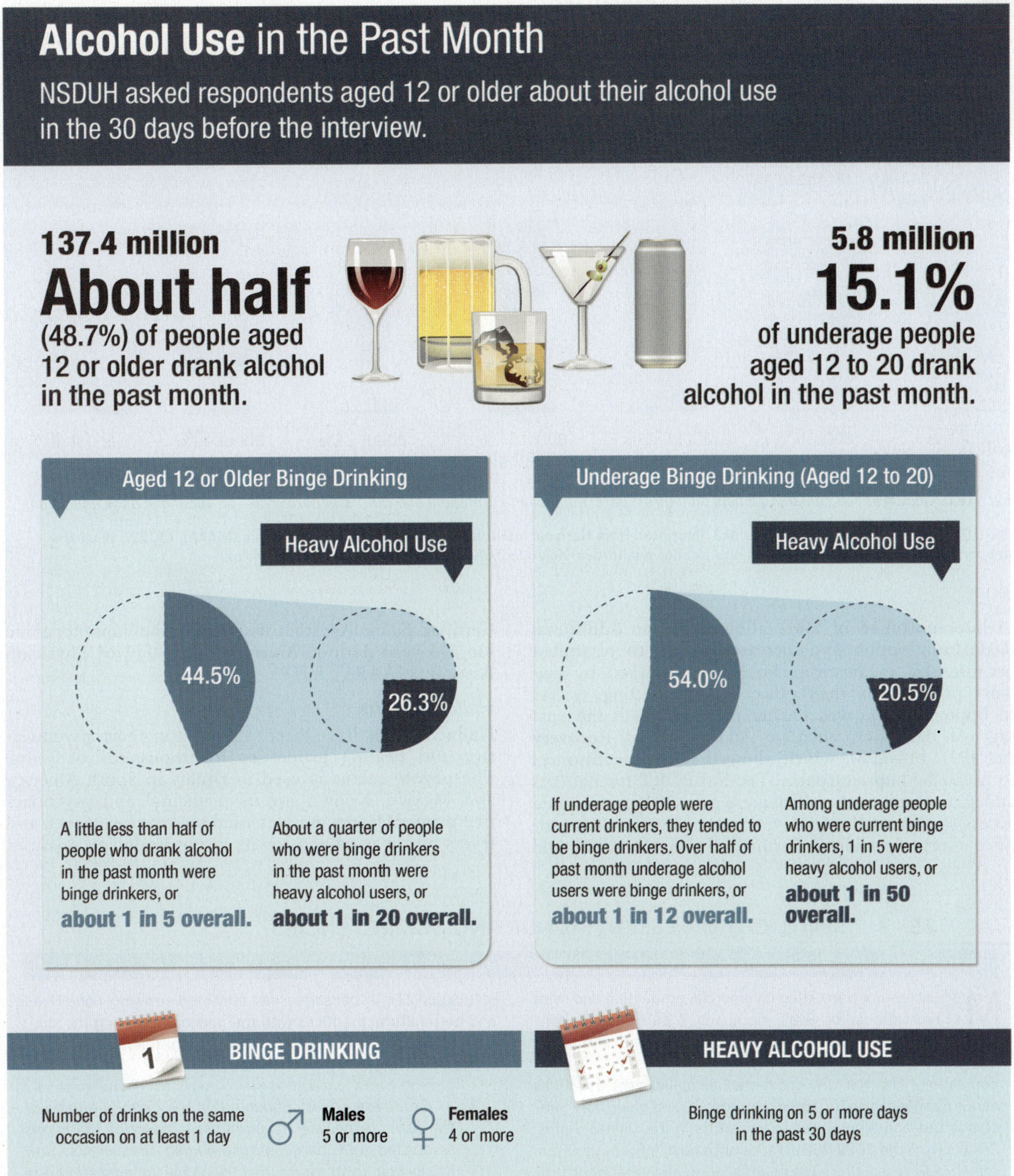

FIGURE 25-6 Alcohol use in the past month: NSDUH asked respondents aged 12 years or older about their alcohol use in the 30 days before the interview. (Reprinted from Substance Abuse and Mental Health Services Administration. (2023). *Results from the 2022 National Survey on Drug Use and Health: A companion infographic* (SAMHSA Publication No. PEP23-07-01-007). Center for Behavioral Health Statistics and Quality, and Substance Abuse and Mental Health Services Administration. https://www.samhsa.gov/data/report/2022-nsduh-infographic)

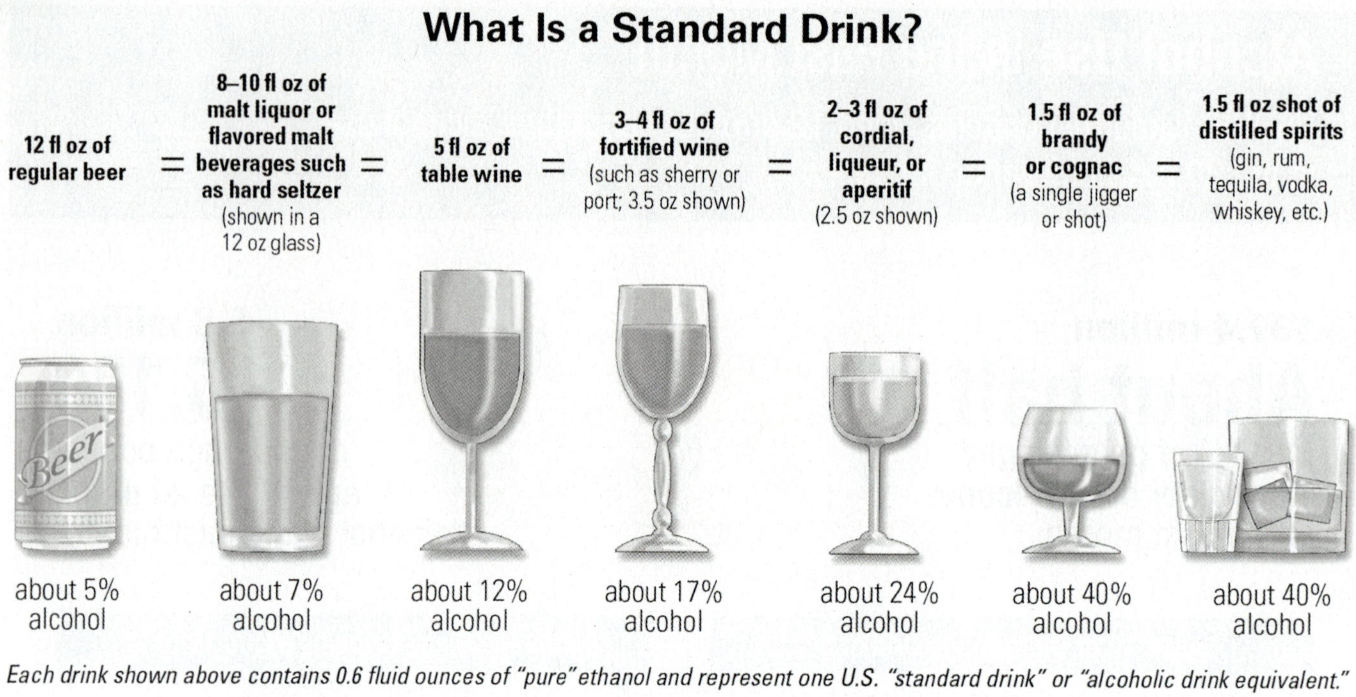

FIGURE 25-7 What is a standard drink? (Reprinted from National Institute on Alcohol Abuse & Alcoholism (NIAAA). (2022). *What is a standard drink?* https://www.niaaa.nih.gov/alcohol-health/overview-alcohol-consumption/what-standard-drink)

of buprenorphine in 2002 allowed for an additional medication option and increased access to treatment because this medication could be prescribed by primary providers in their office or clinic setting. Access to buprenorphine was further increased with the passage of the Comprehensive Addiction and Recovery Act (P.L. 114-198), which allowed nurse practitioners to prescribe buprenorphine. The SUPPORT for Patients and Communities Act (Congress.gov, 2018) expanded access to this medication even further by allowing Certified Nurse Specialists, Certified Nurse Midwives, and Certified Nurse Anesthetists to prescribe buprenorphine for a 5-year period (American Academy of Physician Assistants [AAPA], 2018).

Hallucinogens

Hallucinogens have been valued for their psychoactive and healing properties for thousands of years. The peyote cactus is used in rituals in South America and Mexico. Known for its medicinal and psychoactive properties, peyote was used to treat headaches and fevers and was valued for its vison-producing qualities

BOX 25-7 SPOTLIGHT ON ESSENTIAL NURSING COMPETENCIES

Using Evidence to Guide Education and Health

More states are permitting commercial production and sales of recreational, or retail, marijuana. A public health concern is a potential increase in adolescents' access to and use of marijuana, given the evidence of negative health effects on this population. The NSDUH, conducted annually, asks questions about marijuana use for Americans ages 12 and older (Key Substance Use and Mental Health Indicators in the United States: Results from the 2022 NSDUH at samhsa.gov). Information from the NSDUH is used to support prevention and treatment programs, monitor substance use trends, estimate the need for treatment, and inform public health policy. In Colorado, the commercialization of medical marijuana allowed the proliferation of consumable marijuana products including candies, lozenges, baked goods, and beverages, with little attention paid to standardized dosing levels, guidance for novice users, food safety, and contamination issues. The legalization of marijuana cultivation for dispensaries has impacted growing conditions and horticultural practices with the goal of increasing the supply and the potency of the psychoactive ingredient tetrahydrocannabinol (THC).

1. *As more research is conducted on the harmful effects of marijuana, especially in young users, describe the harms associated with marijuana use among adolescents. How would you incorporate that evidence in educating the public?*
2. *What areas of the healthcare system should be under surveillance to monitor the impact of increased access to marijuana? How would data collected from those systems be used to inform public awareness campaigns or support policies and regulations to protect children, youth, and the community at large?*

BOX 25-8 Marijuana Use in the United States

It is estimated that 52.5 million Americans between the ages of 12 and older used marijuana in 2021 (SAMHSA, 2023b). *Delta-9-tetrahydrocannabinol* (THC) is the main psychoactive chemical found in the *Cannabis sativa* plant. Although usually smoked, it can be brewed in tea or mixed in foods called *edibles*. The THC content has steadily increased since 1976 when the THC content averaged 1% to 3%. In 1995, marijuana had an average THC content of 3.96, and in 2021, the average THC content increased to 15.34% (NIDA, 2022).

Over the past 47 years, the THC content has steadily risen, escalating health problems for long-term and chronic users (Freeman et al., 2021).

Marijuana use disorders (MUD) account for about 30% of all users. Frequent users prior to age 18 and adults who use marijuana frequently are at a greater risk of developing MUD (CDC, 2020). Roughly 16.3 million people in the United States have MUD (NIDA, 2023). Cannabis use in adolescents and children affects the prefrontal cortex, which regulates executive functioning and decision making (Backman, 2023). Students will find it difficult to concentrate, have short-term memory loss, and have learning difficulties (CDC, 2023).

Researchers found an increase in cardiac arrest and tachycardia among frequent users. Furthermore, they discovered the number of emergency room visits was related to the number of dispensaries in the area (Backman, 2023).

Frequent use and long-term use are associated with mental health problems including depression, increased anxiety, and psychosis (Backman, 2023).

Infants born to people who frequently used cannabis while pregnant were at risk for impaired cognitive functioning, stillbirth, or premature birth (SAMHSA, 2023d).

In 2022, the Medical Marijuana and Cannabidiol Research Expansion Act was signed into law, enabling scientists to conduct research on the effects of THC. New research will discover the short- and long-term effects of THC and how it affects the hippocampus and the orbitofrontal cortex.

Teens and young adults' perception of the risks of the drug have decreased partially due to the legalization of the drug for medical and recreational use in some states and advertisers targeting younger users through crafty advertising (Backman, 2023). Research continues to shed light on the benefits and dangers of marijuana use. C/PHNs need to stay up-to-date on the community trends and research in order to serve their communities.

—*Charlene Niemi, PhD, RN, PHN*

Source: National Institute on Drug Abuse (NIDA) (2022); Substance Abuse and Mental Health Services Administration (SAMHSA) (2023d); Freeman et al., (2021); CDC (2023); Backman, (2023).

(U.S. Forest Service, n.d.). Ololiuqui, a member of the morning glory family, is found in Cuba, Central America, and the North American Gulf. Valued for its medicinal and psychoactive properties, ololiuqui was used by shamans for visions. In the 1960s, researchers discovered the active alkaloids in ololiuqui were similar to LSD (U.S. Forest Service, n.d.).

Approximately 3% of those aged 12 years or older reported the use of hallucinogens. Furthermore, in 2021, hallucinogen use increased by 7.7%, the largest increase seen among inhalant and methamphetamine use (SAMHSA, 2023b).

Inhalants

Some examples of inhalants include paint thinner and remover, gasoline, glues, and spray paint. Users may soak a sock in the substance, place the sock in a plastic bag, and place their mouth on the bag and inhale. Others may spray the substance directly into their mouth. Respondents of the NSDUH survey are asked to report the use of inhalants to get high but not to include accidental inhalation of a substance. In 2022, approximately 2.3 million people aged 12 years or older reported use of inhalants. Use was more common among adolescents aged 12 to 17 years than among people in other age groups (SAMHSA, 2023b).

Methamphetamine

Most of the methamphetamine in the United States is produced and distributed illicitly, creating a serious public health and safety problem in the United States. The drug is one of the most addictive substances and can cause permanent damage to the brain. Long-term methamphetamine users develop brain atrophy, an accelerated aging of the brain, and white matter lesions (Petzold et al., 2024). Although only 1% of the population people aged 12 years or older reported current use of methamphetamine, 2.7 million people used the substance over the past year, with those aged 26 years and older having the highest percentage of use (SAMHSA, 2023b).

Prescription Drugs

In the NSDUH, respondents report on any use of a stimulant, sedative, or tranquilizer prescription drug that is not used as directed, including use without a prescription of one's own. This type of prescription drug use was reported by 14.2 million of the population aged 12 years or older. In 2022, the following was reported among different prescription drug categories:

- Prescription tranquilizers and sedatives: 4.8 million people aged 12 years or older reported having used them in the past year.
- Prescription stimulants: 4.3 million people aged 12 years or older reported having used them in the past year.
- Prescription benzodiazepines: 3.7 million people aged 12 years or older reported having used them in the past year.

Pain relievers were the most commonly reported, with 8.5 million people aged 12 years or older reporting having used them in the past year. Hydrocodone was the most misused pain reliever with almost half of the 8.5 million people aged 12 years or older reporting having used hydrocodone in the past year (SAMHSA, 2023b). Of greatest concern are synthetic opioids, namely fentanyl, which contributed to 70% of the 106,000 drug overdose deaths in 2022 (NIDA, 2024). C/PHNs can assume important roles in providing education to the public on the crisis and ways to mitigate it.

Box 25-9 illustrates the application of the nursing process to care for a patient with a SUD involving fentanyl, including the standard steps of screening, brief intervention, and referral to treatment (SBIRT). This example illustrates how SBIRT can be used in public health nursing to help meet the Healthy People 2030 goal of reducing substance use.

TOBACCO USE

Although tobacco use has declined in recent years, 50.9 million Americans still use tobacco products (SAMHSA, 2023b). Across the United States, tobacco consumption was the leading risk factor in terms of disability-adjusted life years (Institute of Health Metrics and Evaluation, 2023). The 2023 Annual National Youth Tobacco Survey found that 10% of high school and middle school students use some of tobacco products with e-cigarettes the most commonly used (FDA, 2023; Fig. 25-8).

Electronic Cigarettes

The use of electronic cigarettes is rapidly emerging among adolescents, along with concerns about its impact on the health of both the individual and the public. The U.S. Surgeon General (2023) reports e-cigarettes

BOX 25-9 C/PHN USE OF THE NURSING PROCESS/CLINICAL JUDGMENT

Detection and Management of At-Risk Opioid Misuse

As the local public health nurse, you notice a high number of opioid deaths in your community. You are concerned because two students at the local high school have overdosed on fentanyl within the past month.

Assessment/Recognize Cues

You do the following:

- Contact local stakeholders in the community consisting of church leaders, school officials, after-school programs, concerned parents, and law enforcement to determine youth who are at risk.
- Speak with student leaders regarding their thoughts on the main issues.
- With parents' permission, screen high school students on their use of opioids.
- Evaluate substance use education in school settings.

Diagnosis/Analyze Cues and Prioritize Hypotheses

After speaking with local community stakeholders and student leaders, and after completing a focused assessment, you decide a nursing diagnosis would look at:

- Thirty percent of the high school students have tried opioids in the past 30 days.
- Emergency departments report an increase in near-deaths.
- Students receive little to no health education regarding use of substances.
- The community offers no after-school activities.

Planning and Implementation/Generate Solutions and Take Action

In the past 30 days, a total of 250 high school students have used opioids. Two local emergency departments have seen a 20% increase in fentanyl overdoses. School personnel have given five students naloxone over the past week. Parents are concerned about the lack of resources in the community.

You plan to work with parents and school officials to decrease opioid use in the adolescent population. A meeting is scheduled to provide possible interventions and to hear feedback from community stakeholders. You discuss some possible interventions the schools and community leaders can put into place:

- Provide after-school activities such as sports and help with homework.
- Meet with teachers and administrators to plan education on opioid misuse and risk factors.
- Apply for local grants to purchase naloxone.
- Train students, parents, church leaders, and school officials in the use of naloxone.
- Organize support groups for students with opioid use to help with recovery.
- Offer counseling referrals for students and families so individuals can discuss feelings in a safe environment.

Evaluation/Evaluate Outcomes

After 6 months, the emergency department (ED) reported a decrease in visits related to opioids. The schools have developed an education plan and will present it to the school board for approval at the next meeting. Funding was reallocated for after-school activities, and church leaders have started a mentoring program with adults and students. Evaluation of the first two nursing diagnoses includes the following goals:

- The community will see a decrease in risk of opioid misuse.
- Parents, students, and stakeholders will be trained in the proper use of naloxone.
- ED visits related to opioid use will continue to decline.
- After-school programs will provide alternative resources to students and families.
- Stakeholders will continue to meet regularly to evaluate outcomes.

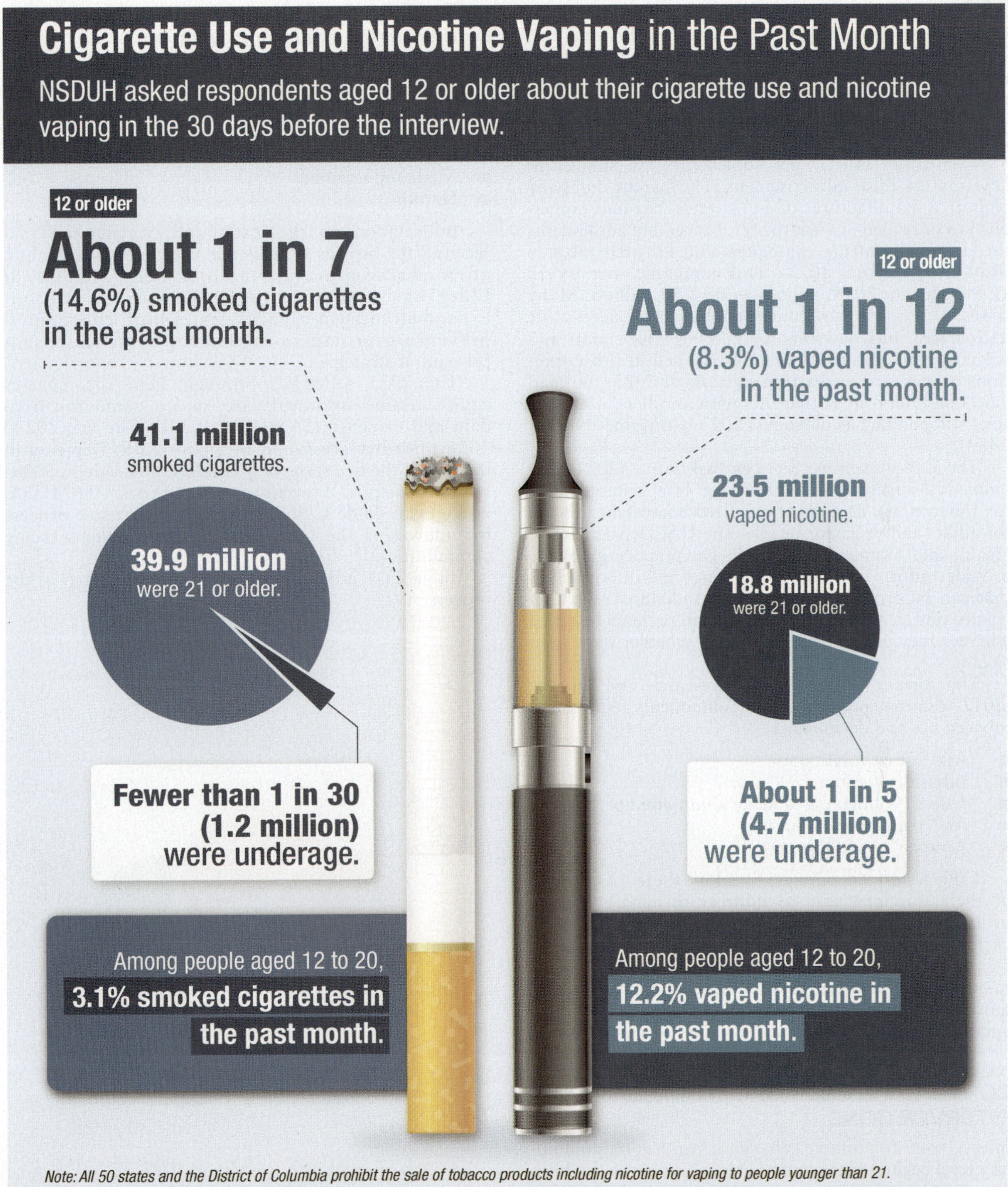

FIGURE 25-8 Cigarette use and nicotine vaping in the past month: NSDUH asked respondents aged 12 years or older about their cigarette use and nicotine vaping in the 30 days before the interview. (Substance Abuse and Mental Health Services Administration. (2023). *Results from the 2022 National Survey on Drug Use and Health: A companion infographic* (SAMHSA Publication No. PEP23-07-01-007). Center for Behavioral Health Statistics and Quality, Substance Abuse and Mental Health Services Administration. https://www.samhsa.gov/data/report/2022-nsduh-infographic)

contain high doses of nicotine, ultrafine particles, flavorants that cause lung cancer, heavy metals, and volatile compounds. Other studies found high levels of environmental toxins and formaldehyde that exceed federal safety levels; carcinogens in the vapor; and diacetyl, an additive for certain flavors that causes lung damage (Ebersole et al., 2020).

Companies that target adolescents are subject to lawsuits for false advertisement. The parent company of Juul, a manufacturer of e-cigarettes, has had numerous lawsuits filed against them for targeting adolescents through social media campaigns and flavored tobacco (Rajesh & Pierson, 2023). This company, once worth 12.8 billion in 2018, is now worth 250 million. Many states, U.S. territories, and school districts across the nation have filed lawsuits for making false claims and targeting minors; people who developed health conditions have joined case action suits. As of 2023, Juul had paid one billion in settlements with another 5400 lawsuits still pending as of August 2023 (Consumer Notice, 2023).

The U.S. Preventive Services Task Force (2021) recommends screening and providing brief interventions for tobacco use as part of standard routine healthcare for adults and pregnant people. The U.S. Department of Health and Human Services clinical practice guideline provides information about screening and interventions that can be provided based on the individual's willingness to quit. It is recommended that all patients be asked whether they use tobacco and, if so, whether they want to quit.

The Agency for Healthcare Research and Quality (2012) recommends five major components for treating tobacco use and dependence:

- "Ask" about tobacco use
- "Advise" to quit
- "Assess" willingness to make a quit attempt
- "Aid" the person in quitting
- "Arrange" for follow-up

C/PHNs are encouraged to adopt these 5As as part of their standard care to address this major health problem in the United States and globally. Strategies for various populations are provided on the smokefree.gov website, including strategies for those who are willing to quit, those unwilling to quit, those who have recently quit, and specific populations (e.g., veterans, women, and those age 50 or older).

COMMUNITY- AND POPULATION-BASED INTERVENTIONS

Interventions to promote behavioral health at the community level begin with a community assessment to establish a community diagnosis, followed by interventions that can address the specific public health issue identified in the diagnosis. The Healthy People 2030 objectives serve as a starting point in developing an intervention. Community interventions move beyond single interventions and outcomes at individual levels of health behavior change. The 2023 Strategic Prevention Framework-Partnerships for Success granted 42.6 million in awards to states and communities for the prevention of substance use.

- Underage drinking
- Cannabis
- Tobacco
- E-cigarettes
- Opioids
- Methamphetamine
- Heroin

Information on the states and communities that received the awards is available at https://www.samhsa.gov/newsroom/press-announcements/20230928/biden-harris-administration-awards-42-million-expand-strengthen-capacity-states-local-community-prevention-providers-implement-evidence-based-prevention-strategies.

The 2023 SAMHSA Strategic Plan encompasses equity, trauma-informed care, and a commitment to data and evidence (SAMHSA, 2023e). The five 2023–2026 priorities are found in Figure 25-9. Depicted in the figure, the five steps of SAMHSA's A Guide to SAMHSA's Strategic Prevention Framework (SAMHSA, 2023e) can guide C/PHNs in a comprehensive process for addressing the behavioral health problems facing communities.

Table 25-1 provides descriptions of each step of the process.

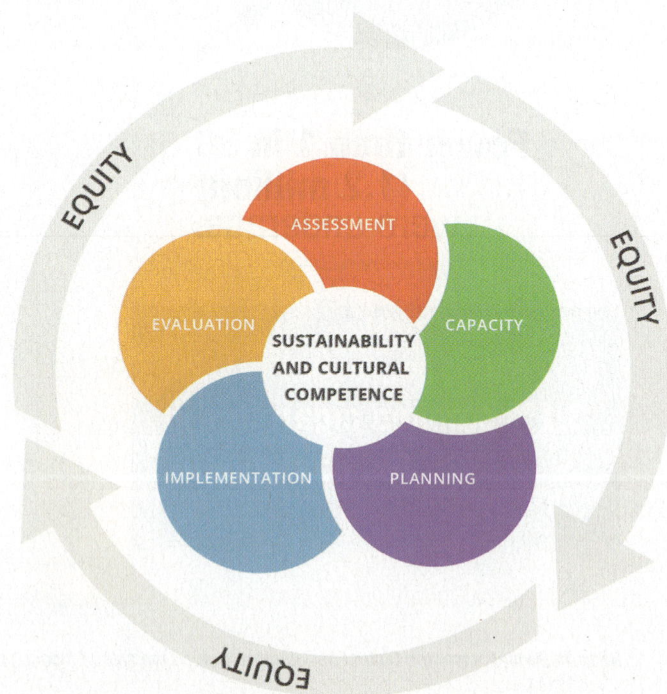

FIGURE 25-9 Steps and guiding principles. (Reprinted from Substance Abuse and Mental Health Services Administration. (2023). *Strategic prevention framework*. https://www.samhsa.gov/sptac/strategic-prevention-framework#:~:text=The%20SPF%20includes%20these%20five,the%20communication%20of%20prevention%20science%3F)

TABLE **25-1** Strategic Prevention Framework: Step-by-Step Guidance for the C/PHN

Step	Description	Questions to Address	Information That Can Help Address the Questions
1. Assess	Assess the problem and related behaviors including risk and protective factors.	What substance misuse problems occur in the community? How often, where, and to which populations is this occurring?	State and local data collected within the community Identified risk and protective factors within the community Identify gaps given current community resources and their capacity
2. Capacity	Build local capacity to address prevention.	Who are your stakeholders, and what information do they need? How can they be motivated to be involved? Who should be part of the prevention team? Can partnerships be created?	Identify all possible stakeholders within the community to raise awareness and support
3. Plan	Formulate a plan and prioritize risk and protective factors.	How are risks and protective factors prioritized? Does the community have the resources to address the problem?	Create a plan that aligns to your logic model
4. Implement	Delivery of evidence-based interventions and programs.	Can the community provide evidence-based solutions for required levels and needs within the community? What support is necessary for implementation?	Create evidence-based program and treatments that meet the needs of your community
5. Evaluate	Conduct a process evaluation, looking at both process and outcomes.	How successful were the programs and practices? What was the effect of the program? Did changes occur, and if so, what were those changes? Were stakeholders included in the evaluation process with respect for all groups?	Create report based on process and outcomes of programs Evaluation designs, instruments, and methods of evaluation used

Source: Substance Abuse and Mental Health Services Administration (SAMHSA) (2023e).

SUMMARY

- Contemporary issues identify the surge of behavioral health concerns in the United States (opioid crisis, injection sites, legalization of cannabis, alcohol use) affecting communities and populations.
- Firearms are reported in half of all suicides; youth suicide remains a public health crisis.
- Stigma toward those with mental health remains a barrier for those most needing treatment.
- Substance use disorders are linked to health problems. *Healthy People 2030* focuses on strategies to prevent substance misuse and provide access to treatment to mitigate health problems and deaths.
- At the individual level, C/PHNs can detect the person's level of risk via screening instruments, assess the person, and intervene accordingly.
- The Strategic Prevention Framework serves to guide C/PHNs in community-level interventions to address behavioral health problems.

ACTIVE LEARNING EXERCISES

1. What are the suicides rates in your community and state? Compare the data with national and global statistics. What effect does suicide have on a family and the community? Which of the 10 Essential Public Health Services (Box 2-2) might you use to educate your community on your findings? (Objective 1).
2. Research the effects of marijuana. Interview siblings and friends regarding their knowledge of these effects. Is their understanding based on evidence or social media? Develop an infographic on the harmful effects of marijuana with classmates and share in class. (Objective 2)
3. Complete a focused community assessment on substance use in college students. Speak with college partners to determine the use of substances on campus. How did you gather your information? What is the college's policy on students who are caught using illegal substances? If a student seeks help, what kind of support and counseling does the college provide? (Objective 3)
4. Gather information on fentanyl overdose deaths within your local community and state. Who are the stakeholders in your community to address this problem? Work with these partners to develop policies and strategies to implement education and distribution of naloxone to community members. Did you encounter any opposition and, if so, how was it handled? (Objective 4)
5. National Depression Screening Day is held the 1st week of October. To highlight the importance of this day, work in small groups with classmates and create a 5-minute skit that implements universal prevention activities. Post to your class learning management system or share in class. What did you learn from researching activities? Reflect on how this video would help you, your loved ones, and your community in screening for depression. (Objective 5)

CHAPTER 26

Unsheltered Populations

"A castaway in the sea was going down for the third time when he caught sight of a passing ship. Gathering his last strength, he waved frantically and called for help. Someone on board peered at him scornfully and shouted back, 'Get a boat!'"

—Daniel Quinn, 1999, *Beyond Civilization: Humanity's Next Great Adventure*

KEY TERMS

Chronically unsheltered
Continuum of care
Deinstitutionalization
Doubling up
Homelessness
Housing first
Literally homeless
Point-in-time counts
Period prevalence counts
Single-room occupancy (SRO) housing
Survival sex
Trauma-informed care (TIC)
Unaccompanied youth
Unsheltered (hidden) homelessness

LEARNING OBJECTIVES

Upon mastery of this chapter, you should be able to:

1. Discuss factors predisposing people to homelessness.
2. Examine the effects of homelessness on health.
3. Provide empathy and compassionate care based on knowledge
4. Compare and contrast the unique challenges confronting subpopulations of homelessness, including demographic characteristics of each subpopulation.
5. In collaboration with stakeholders, propose community-based nursing interventions to facilitate primary, secondary, and tertiary preventions in addressing the problem of homelessness. Advocate for these preventions.

INTRODUCTION

What was once considered unthinkable in a prosperous nation is now an expected occurrence in towns and cities across the United States. Drive through an inner city or suburban community on any given day, and you will see people on street corners holding signs that say, "Hungry and homeless." Where is the public outcry in response to this scene? Has the American conscience been anesthetized to this form of human suffering? Or is the need simply too overwhelming and the problems too far reaching to mount an effective campaign to prevent such a tragedy?

The purpose of this chapter is to define the concept of homelessness, examine the factors contributing to homelessness, analyze the major issues confronting people experiencing homelessness, and examine the role of the public health nurse in addressing the needs of populations experiencing homelessness.

The McKinney-Vento Homeless Assistance Act (Title 42 of the United States [U.S.] Code) defines as homeless a person who lacks a fixed, regular, adequate nightly residence including supervised public or private shelters that provide temporary accommodations (Fig. 26-1). People experiencing homelessness may also reside in institutional settings providing temporary shelter or in public or private places that are not designed for or used as a regular sleeping accommodations for human beings (e.g., cars, parks, campgrounds). Such people are often called **literally homeless**. People who are incarcerated are not considered homeless under this definition (McKinney-Vento Homeless Assistance Act, 1987).

The education subtitle of the McKinney-Vento Homeless Assistance Act expands on the definition of **homelessness** when addressing children and youth experiencing homelessness. The Act includes as homeless

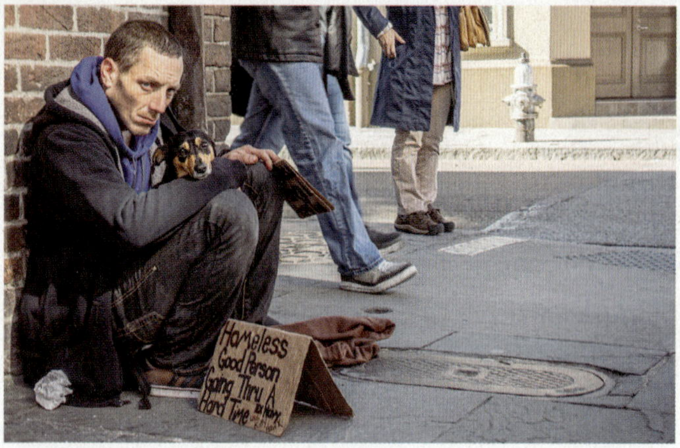

FIGURE 26-1 A person experiencing homelessness in New Orleans.

those children who share housing with others because of economic hardship or loss of housing, are abandoned in hospitals, are awaiting placement in foster care, or are living in motels, trailer parks, or camping grounds. Children awaiting foster care placement were removed from the definition of homeless in 2016 (National Center for Homeless Education [NCHE], n.d.). Box 26-1 outlines selected *Healthy People 2030* goals that relate to populations experiencing homelessness.

SCOPE OF THE PROBLEM

It is difficult to estimate the number of people who are unsheltered, because homelessness is a temporary condition. Rather than trying to count the number of people experiencing homelessness on a given night, or **point-in-time counts**, it may be more prudent to gauge the number of people who have been homeless over a longer time frame such as over the course of a year, or **period prevalence counts** (National Institute of Mental Health [NIMH], n.d.; United States Department of Housing and Urban Development [USDHUD], 2022a).

It is also difficult to locate and account for populations experiencing homelessness. Most estimates of homelessness are based on the number of people served in shelters or soup kitchens or the number of people who can easily be located on the streets. People who spend time at places that are difficult to reach (e.g., cars, campgrounds, caves, boxcars, wooded areas) are experiencing **unsheltered** or **hidden homelessness**. Many people are unable to access shelters because of overcrowding and limited capacity (Box 26-2). In rural areas, there are fewer housing options and resources for people experiencing homelessness. As a result, people may be forced to live temporarily with friends or family (a practice known as "**doubling up**"). While still experiencing homelessness, these people are not always counted in homeless statistics or considered eligible for homeless services (National Healthcare for the Homeless Council [NHCHC], 2022).

The United States Department of Housing and Urban Development (USDHUD), in its Annual Homeless Assessment Report to Congress, publishes the latest counts of homelessness nationwide. In 2021, on a single night in January, there were an estimated 582,500 sheltered and unsheltered people experiencing homelessness across the nation (Fig. 26-2). Approximately 40% of people experiencing homelessness were unsheltered. Sixty percent of unsheltered people were living in urban areas. The number of people experiencing homelessness increased by less than 1% between 2020 and 2022 with the number of people in unsheltered locations increasing by 3% and the number of people in sheltered locations declining by 2%.

BOX 26-1 *HEALTHY PEOPLE 2030*

Objectives Related to Homelessness

Mental Health	
MHMD-R01	Increase the proportion of homeless adults with mental health problems who get mental health services
MHMD-07	Increase the proportion of people with substance use and mental health disorders who get treatment for both
Social Determinants of Health	
SDOH-01	Reduce the proportion of people living in poverty
SDOH-04	Reduce the proportion of families that spend more than 30% of income on housing
Healthcare Access and Quality	
AHS-02	Increase the proportion of people with dental insurance
AHS-04	Reduce the proportion of people who can't get medical care when they need it
AHS-05	Reduce the proportion of people who can't get the dental care they need when they need it
AHS-06	Reduce the proportion of people who can't get prescription medicines when they need them
AHS-07	Increase the proportion of people with a usual primary care provider
AHS-08	Increase the proportion of adults who receive appropriate evidence-based clinical preventive services

Reprinted from Office of Disease Prevention and Health Promotion (n.d.).

BOX 26-2 PERSPECTIVES

A Population Health Perspective on Caring for People Experiencing Homelessness

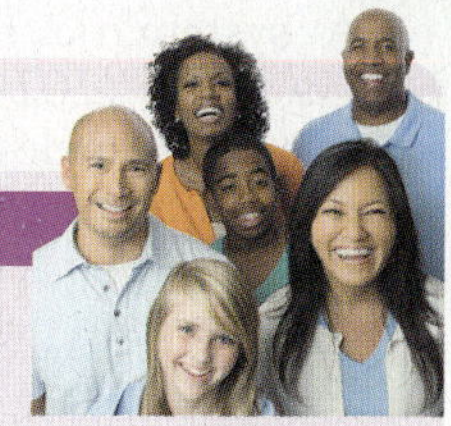

I can't believe I am sitting at this table. What am I doing here? How did I end up on the Board of Directors of an organization that houses one of the largest residential substance use disorder recovery programs for men experiencing homelessness in the country? I have been a public health nurse for years. I know how to take care of patients struggling with homelessness. But this is a whole different ball game. I'm looking at budgets and learning about capital campaigns. I even testified before a gubernatorial commission to advocate for funding for homeless services. And now I am chairing a board-level committee that is analyzing census tract data to determine the impact of its wellness center on public health. We are looking at emergency department utilization rates and rates of hospitalization for substance-related illnesses to see if our Wellness Center has an impact on our clients and the surrounding community. If we can demonstrate that our programs reduce hospitalizations and emergency room visits, we may be eligible to apply for population health funding and to partner with local hospitals in much bigger ways to make a positive impact in our community. This is exciting stuff!

Anika James PHN

Between 2021 and 2022, the number of people in sheltered homelessness increased by 7%, which may be due to eased restrictions in sheltered housing following the COVID-19 pandemic and the increase in COVID-19–related funding for noncongregate shelter-based housing. Housing during the pandemic was also affected by the increase in rental costs, which drove homelessness higher and the investment of federal dollars in housing assistance through the American Rescue Plan, which drove homelessness downward (USDHUD, 2022a).

Approximately 72% of people experiencing homelessness are adults in households with no children. The remaining 28% are part of families with children (USDHUD, 2022a). Because of the transient nature of homelessness and the difficulty involved in locating and counting people experiencing homelessness, it is unlikely that researchers will ever be able to estimate the exact magnitude of homelessness in the United States.

There is a direct relationship between poverty and homelessness. In general, homelessness is not significantly increasing due, in part, to the strides made over recent years to increase federal funding for homeless prevention and assistance programs. Still, only 36 affordable homes exist for every 100 renter households with extremely low incomes (households with incomes at or below the federal poverty guideline or 30% of area median income) (National Low Income Housing Coalition [NLIHC], 2022a). Housing programs for people experiencing homelessness have moved many people off the streets, but the lack of affordable housing continues to present formidable challenges to eliminating homelessness (NLIHC, 2022b).

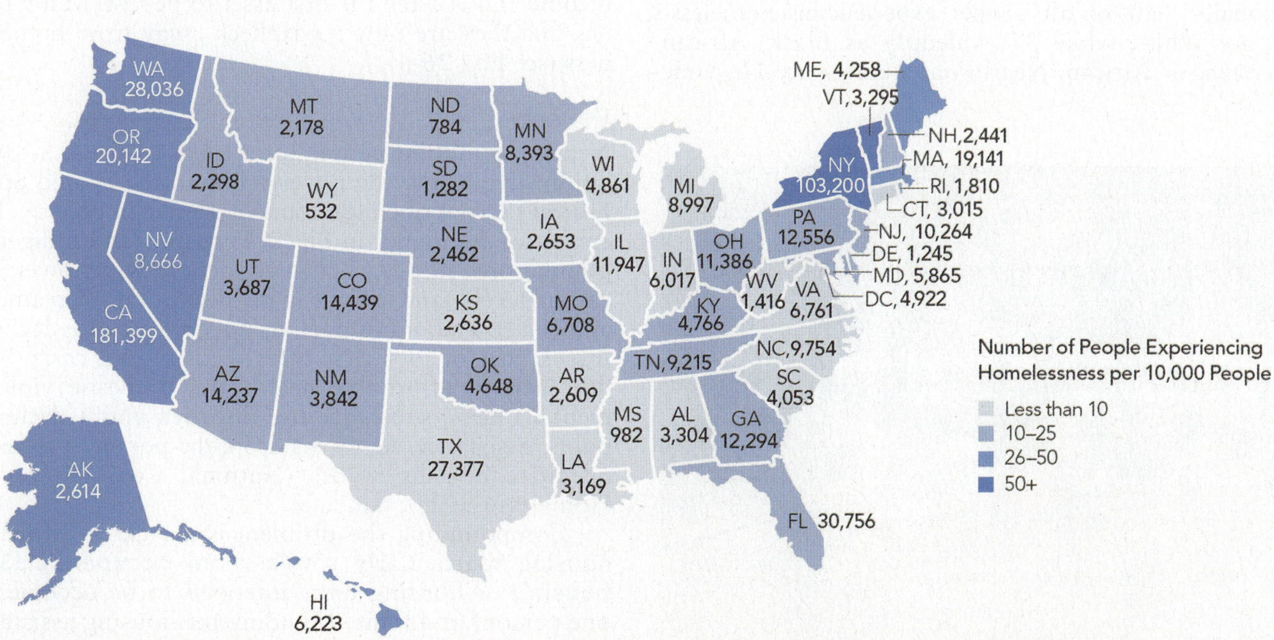

FIGURE 26-2 Estimates of People Experiencing Homelessness by State, 2023. (Reprinted from U.S. Department of Housing and Urban Development (USDHUD). (2023). *The 2023 Annual Homelessness Assessment Report (AHAR) to Congress.* https://www.huduser.gov/portal/sites/default/files/pdf/2023-ahar-part-1.Pdf)

A systematic review and meta-analysis conducted by Liu et al. (2021) found nearly 90% of adults who experience homelessness had at least one adverse childhood experience (ACE). Furthermore, over 50% of this population experienced four or more ACEs in their lifetime. These data need to be in the forefront of prevention planning.

Demographics

Poverty is directly linked to homelessness (Fig. 26-3). Demographic groups more likely to be poor are also at greater risk of becoming homeless.

Age

In 2021, 92% of people experiencing homelessness were adults over 24. Approximately 7% were between 18 and 24, and less than 1% were under 18 years of age. Among the unsheltered population experiencing homelessness, 94% are over 24 and less than 1% are under 18 years of age (USDHUD, 2022a).

Gender

Approximately 61% of people experiencing homelessness are men, and 30% are women (USDHUD, 2022a). Between 2020 and 2022, homelessness increased by 6% among women and 1% among men. Slightly over 1% of people experiencing homelessness identify as transgender, questioning, or a gender that is not singularly male or female. Of these, 63% are living in unsheltered situations. Between 2020 and 2022, the number of people experiencing sheltered homelessness who identified as transgender, not singularly male or female, or questioning increased by 93% (USDHUD, 2022a).

Ethnicity

The racial and ethnic makeup of populations experiencing homelessness varies based upon geographic location. Nationally, half of all people experiencing homelessness are White, while 37% identify as Black, African American, or African. Nearly one quarter are Hispanic or Latinx. When compared to the U.S. population, people who identify as Black, African American, or Indigenous (Native American, Pacific Islanders) are overrepresented in populations experiencing homelessness (USDHUD, 2022a).

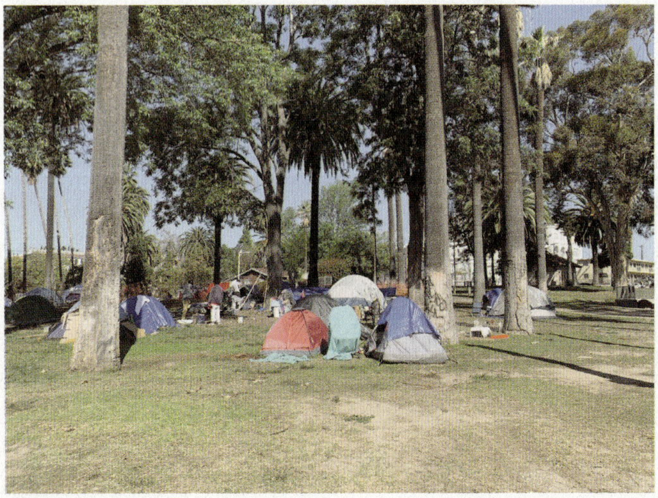

FIGURE 26-3 An encampment of people without housing in downtown Los Angeles, California.

Families

Families with children represented 28% of the population experiencing homelessness in the United States in 2021. Over 20% of people experiencing homelessness are children. Approximately 59% of people who are homeless in families are children under 18 years of age. More than 90% of children under 18 who are homeless in families reside in shelters compared to 57% of children who are homeless as people. Family homelessness declined by 6% between 2020 and 2022 (USDHUD, 2022a).

Only 10% of sheltered families experiencing homelessness are headed by men (USDHUD, 2022b). During recessions and periods of economic decline, more two-parent families and families headed by single partners of the birthing parent are likely to become homeless. Since organizations serving families experiencing homelessness are generally geared to serving single women with children, it may be difficult for intact families and families headed by men to access shelter. Moreover, little research has been done on single men with children and homelessness (Andrade et al., 2020).

Contributing Factors

People are predisposed to homelessness because of a complex array of factors that result in people having to choose between the necessities of daily living (Box 26-3). Scarce resources limit choices. What would you do if you had to choose between eating and buying your child's medication? Housing consumes a huge portion of one's income and is often the first asset to be lost. Many families find they are only a paycheck away from homelessness (see Box 26-4).

Poverty

Nearly 38 million people (or 11.6% of the U.S. population) live below the poverty line in the United States. Fifteen percent of children under 18 live in poverty. Poverty rates are higher in Black, Hispanic, and Indigenous populations, non-U.S. citizens, people with lower education levels, and people with disabilities (Creamer et al., 2022). Factors impacting poverty include declining wages, loss of jobs that offer security and carry benefits, lack of affordable healthcare, domestic violence, mental illness, substance use disorder, and a decline in public assistance. As wages drop, the potential to secure adequate housing wanes (National Coalition for the Homeless [NCH], n.d.).

Compounding the problem is a lack of affordable housing (particularly **single-room occupancy (SRO) housing** or housing units intended to be occupied by one person) and limited funding for housing assistance. A household seeking to afford a modest two-bedroom rental home in the United States must earn at least $25.82 per hour, over 3.5 times the federal minimum

BOX **26-3** PERSPECTIVES

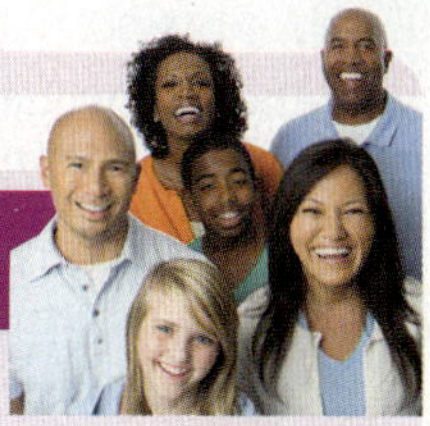

Voices From the Community: A Couple Experiencing Homelessness Who Calls Their Car "Home"

My husband and I have been homeless for 6 months... maybe longer. I lose track of time since we've been on the streets. We became homeless when my husband showed up to work wasted on alcohol. It was his second time so they fired him that day and he hasn't been able to find work since. We haven't had a good shower in several weeks and our clothes smell. After a month of looking, one has no hope of finding work. I receive some disability money for my low back pain but it's not enough. Lately, I'm finding it hard to get out of the car, and it's more difficult to walk. With no work, eventually, we were unable to pay our rent and were evicted from our apartment. We park in the local SuperMart lot at night. This place is great. It is located in a safe area of town, and it is open 24 hours a day, so we always have access to restroom facilities. We stayed in a county shelter for a while. The social worker there tried to help us find housing, but we were afraid to go into the parts of town where the subsidized housing was located. Plus, it was a 2-year waitlist. She said that it was common to wait that long because the need is so great. To be honest with you, I don't think I'll be able to live on the streets that long. Is there nothing that can be done? When we tried to apply for food stamps, we were told we needed to produce our rent and gas and electric bills, or we would be ineligible to receive this benefit. I kept telling them that we live in our car. We don't pay rent! We don't have a gas and electric bill! Many times, we were turned down from housing and other benefits, because we did not meet the eligibility criteria. We were not single parents. We had no children. Neither of us suffer from a severe mental health or substance use disorder. We were not veterans. It is so frustrating. There are resources, but there are so many barriers to accessing them. I feel like an outcast. If this goes on much longer, I'm not sure what will happen to us.

wage of $7.25. Although many states have minimum wages that exceed the federal minimum, an average minimum wage worker would need to work 96 hours a week to be able to afford a two-bedroom rental home (NLIHC, 2022b). The Raise the Wage Act of 2021, legislation introduced in Congress, proposes to increase the federal minimum wage to $15 an hour through a schedule of annual increases over time (United States 117th Congress, 2021–2022).

When rental costs increase and the number of available low-rent units decline, the housing gap widens. Moreover, federal support for housing assistance is unable to keep pace with the high demand for housing (National Alliance to End Homelessness [NAEH], 2023a). As a result, many people must pay high rents to obtain shelter. This situation leads to overcrowding and substandard housing. Since the demand for housing assistance exceeds federal housing assistance resources, there are often long waiting lists. Waitlists may close when demand for housing exceeds the supply of subsidized units available for occupancy (USDHUD, n.d.).

BOX **26-4** WHAT DO *YOU* THINK?

Personal Values

Many of us ask why there are so many people experiencing homelessness who choose not to use shelters. Becca Savransky (2021) gives these reasons: (1) strict hours that make it difficult to hold down a job and return to the shelter in time to secure a bed; (2) rules that prohibit family members or pets from staying together; (3) concerns regarding safety including fears of assault and theft; (4) restrictions on securing belongings; (5) transportation obstacles to and from the shelter; (6) concerns regarding exposure to contagious illnesses and bedbugs, (7) the inability to adhere to sobriety requirements for people with an active substance use disorder; and (8) medical, mental health, or trauma issues that make it difficult to sleep in shared spaces with strangers.

1. *What do you think might be other reasons a person would choose to sleep outside rather than in a homeless shelter?*
2. *How could some of these issues be effectively addressed?*
3. *How does your city address these issues and the overall problem of homelessness?*

Savransky (2021).

Lack of Affordable Healthcare

In the absence of affordable healthcare coverage, a serious illness or disability can lead to job loss, savings depletion, and even eviction. In 2021, 27.5 million Americans who are not eligible for Medicaid (10.2% of the population) were without healthcare coverage. The Affordable Care Act has expanded Medicaid coverage to millions of previously uninsured people, reducing the number of uninsured Americans from 44 million in 2013 to 27.5 million in 2021 (Tolbert et al., 2022).

The uninsured are less likely to receive preventive care or care for chronic health conditions. They are more at risk for preventable hospitalizations and missed diagnoses (Tolbert et al., 2022). Those who qualify for medical assistance may be reluctant to seek employment, fearing termination of benefits. Many others have limited coverage that requires higher co-pays or deductibles and does not cover major catastrophic illnesses. A catastrophic adverse health event can plunge one into a homeless condition.

Employment

Low-income wage earners may hold jobs with nonstandard work arrangements. Temporary employees, day laborers, independent contractors, and part-time employees are examples of work arrangements that tend to pay lower wages, offer little or no benefits, and have less job security. For people with little or no job skills, it is virtually impossible to compete for jobs that offer a living wage. Barriers to employment among people experiencing homelessness may include lack of education and job skills; lack of transportation, childcare, or other supportive services; lack of access to technology; history of incarceration; and chronic physical and mental health and substance misuse issues that make it difficult to pursue or retain employment. To overcome homelessness and maintain employment, one must not only obtain a job that pays a living wage but must also have access to supportive services such as child care and transportation (Lassiter, 2021).

Intimate Partner Violence

Intimate partner violence is a leading cause of homelessness among women (Yakubovich et al., 2022; Zhao, 2022). Of the 7 million people experiencing intimate partner violence in the United States, approximately 500,000 identify the need for housing due to a history of violence (USDHUD, 2022b). For people experiencing domestic violence, the choice is often between living in an abusive situation or leaving and facing life on the streets. Such individuals are often isolated from social support networks and financial resources, rendering these people especially vulnerable. They may lack a steady income or a stable employment record and often suffer from anxiety, depression, or substance use disorders. A major challenge facing service providers of people experiencing domestic violence who are homeless is the need to ensure a safe and secure environment and to protect client confidentiality (NAEH, 2022a; Yakubovich et al., 2022).

Mental Illness

Untreated mental illness may precipitate homelessness, and homelessness is a significant risk factor for poor mental health (Padgett, 2020). Approximately 123,000 people experiencing homelessness across the United States were reported to suffer from a severe mental illness in 2022 (USDHUD, 2022c). **Deinstitutionalization** (being released from institutions into the community) has contributed to the number of people with severe mental illness represented in populations experiencing homelessness (Padgett, 2020).

Some people with a mental illness self-medicate to alleviate their symptoms using street drugs, placing them at increased risk of substance use disorder and diseases transmitted through injection drug use. Mental illness and substance misuse are often comorbid conditions which, coupled with poor physical health, make it especially difficult to secure employment and safe, affordable housing (NIMH, 2021).

Substance Use Disorders

Rates of alcohol and drug misuse are disproportionately high among people experiencing homelessness. In 2022, nearly 123,000 people experiencing homelessness had a serious mental illness, and approximately 95,000 suffered from a chronic substance use disorder (USDHUD, 2022c). For a person already at risk for homelessness, the behaviors associated with a substance use disorder can create instability and jeopardize family and employment support nets. Once homeless, people may resort to drugs or alcohol to dull the pain of being homeless and ease the feelings of hopelessness that accompany such a desperate state. They may also turn to chemical substances to self-medicate to alleviate symptoms of an untreated mental illness. Fragmentation of services, limited access to care, lack of health insurance, difficulty engaging providers, and complex treatment needs make it difficult to receive the services needed to achieve a successful recovery (NAEH, 2022b).

Many shelters require sobriety to access services. Low levels of health literacy and extended wait times create additional barriers to accessing treatment. There may be long waiting lists for treatment for substance use disorder, and people experiencing homelessness who do not have a phone and are difficult to locate may be dropped from the waiting list. Lack of transportation and lack of documentation needed to access programs (i.e., birth certificate, Social Security card) further exacerbate the problem. The possible denial of Supplemental Security Income or Social Security Disability Insurance to people residing in public institutions such as shelters, correctional faculties, or substance misuse treatment centers creates a huge barrier to achieving recovery support, proper medical care, and housing and income assistance (Social Security Administration, 2024). Moreover, the federal programs targeting homelessness, mental health, and substance use disorders lack the extent of funding necessary to exert an impact that would effectively address this problem on a national level (Rizzo et al., 2022).

Additional Variables

Additional variables impacting homelessness include personal or financial crisis, natural disasters, immigration and refugee crises, or personal choice. For example, natural disasters or immigration crises may displace previously independent and self-sufficient people and families, rendering many homeless and in need of emergency shelter. See more on disasters and their aftermath in Chapter 17.

Subpopulations Experiencing Homelessness

Although many of the struggles facing unsheltered people are universal, there are subpopulations within this community that are uniquely vulnerable (Box 26-5). Often, these groups face additional burdens because of their special needs and challenges.

Men Experiencing Homelessness

Approximately 61% of people experiencing homelessness are men (USDHUD, 2022a). The majority of men experiencing homelessness are single adults. Some men find themselves in a cycle of intermittent homelessness as they move back and forth between prisons, treatment centers, shelters, temporary housing, and the streets. Other men are at risk for becoming **chronically unsheltered**.

One third of people experiencing homelessness demonstrate chronic patterns of homelessness. A person with

BOX 26-5 POPULATION FOCUS

Tent Cities and Solutions for People Experiencing Homelessness

After the Great Recession of 2007 to 2008, tent cities began springing up across many larger cities in the United States, some of them with mutually determined codes of conduct and social structures. These temporary communities were a similar phenomenon to the shantytowns of the Great Depression, and many cities have responded to these temporary encampments by criminalizing them, citing concerns for public health and safety (Herring, 2015; National Law Center on Homelessness & Poverty [NLCHP], 2017).

Imagine a world where it is illegal to sit down. Could you survive if there were no place you were allowed to fall asleep, store your belongings, or to stand still? People experiencing homelessness, like all people, must engage in activities such as sleeping or sitting down to survive. Yet in communities across the nation, these harmless, unavoidable behaviors are treated as criminal activity under laws that criminalize homelessness (NLCHP, 2017).

The USDHUD, in a study of homeless encampments in four major cities across the United States, found that the total cost of the encampments in fiscal year 2019 ranged from $3.3 million to nearly $8.6 million. Encampments cost the cities studied between $1600 and $6200 for each unsheltered person per year (USDHUD, 2020). Encampments have been reported in every state across the nation and in the District of Columbia. Most of these temporary communities are illegal and under constant threat of eviction. The dramatic increase in encampments is a reflection of the growth in homelessness and the lack of accessible shelter.

Why do people live in tent cities? Most cities in the United States do not have sufficient shelter beds to accommodate the number of people experiencing homelessness in need of shelter. Many shelters limit admission based on gender. Others do not allow children. Some shelters do not allow personal belongings or have no provision for their safe storage. Other shelters are unable to accommodate people with disabilities. Many shelters have strict curfews that may make it difficult to hold down a job. Very few shelters allow pets (NLCHP, 2017).

Some states have adopted more tent city–friendly policies. Innovations in addressing the tent city crisis include hosting permanent encampments with colocated service centers, engaging religious organizations to temporarily host tent cities on their properties, and providing permits for temporary encampments on city property (NLCHP, 2017).

Herring, C. (2015)

1. *Have you seen tent cities in your community? How do you feel when you see them?*
2. *What do you think could be done to address some of the issues raised by the proliferation of tent cities? Debate the issue with classmates.*
3. *How could PHNs be involved in helping to design feasible population-focused interventions?*

Source: National Law Center on Homelessness and Poverty (2017); United States Department of Housing and Urban Development (2020).

a chronic pattern of homelessness is someone with a disability who has been continuously homeless for at least a year or has experienced repeated episodes of homelessness in the last 3 years totaling at least 12 months of homelessness (USDHUD, 2022b). In 2021, the Annual Homeless Assessment Report to Congress recorded nearly 128,000 people who are chronically homeless in its point-in-time count. Two thirds of these people were unsheltered (i.e., living on the street or in places not fit for human habitation) (USDHUD, 2022a).

Men experiencing homelessness are vulnerable to public disdain and maltreatment. Some people perceive them as largely to blame for their plight, believing they are able bodied and should be able to work. Moreover, men experiencing homelessness may not suffer from disabilities severe enough to warrant eligibility for health and social services. Often health and social programs give priority to women and children (Myrick, 2016).

Women Experiencing Homelessness

Women as single parents lead most families experiencing homelessness in the United States (Fig. 26-4). Ninety percent of sheltered families experiencing homelessness are led by women (USDHUD, 2022b). Domestic violence is a major cause of homelessness among women (Zhao, 2022). Lack of affordable housing forces many women to choose between living in an abusive home or facing life on the streets. Landlords have a duty to provide a safe environment for their tenants. But does that include changing the locks even if the person committing the abuse resides in the home? In some states the answer is yes. For instance, a California civil code requires landlords to change the lock

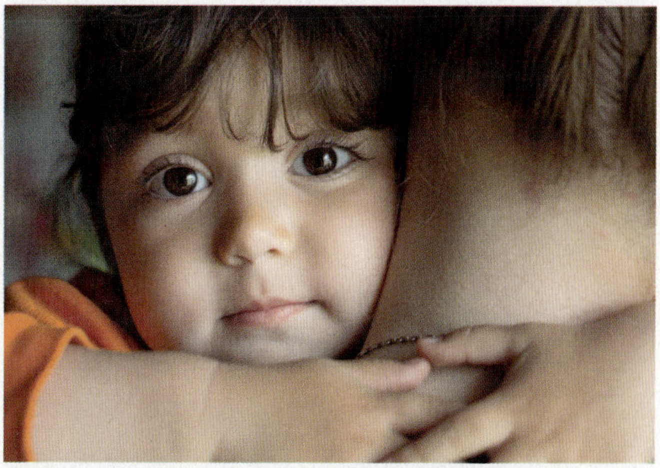

FIGURE 26-4 A child hugging their parent while in a shelter for families with small children. Most families who are unsheltered are headed by single women.

within 24 hours upon request of the person experiencing intimate partner violence as long as that person provides a restraining order or a police report. If the landlord does not comply within 24 hours, the person can legally change the lock themselves (National Housing Law Project, n.d.). If violence is discovered in the home and the person committing the abuse is on the rental agreement, landlords may face legal challenges for changing the lock to deny that individual entry (Kesselman, 2021). A Uniform Lock Change Law would protect the person experiencing intimate partner violence from the person committing the abuse as well as the landlord from litigation (Kesselman, 2021). People experiencing intimate partner violence often have poor credit and employment records due to the disruption caused by family violence. Once on the street, a woman faces the risk of greater abuse. Moreover, the potential for exposure to violence and sexual assault on the streets increases the risk of sexually transmitted infections and traumatic injuries.

Children Experiencing Homelessness

In 2022, children under 18 represented 59% of people in families with children experiencing homelessness in the United States (USDHUD, 2022a). On a single night in 2022, slightly over 30,000 unaccompanied youth were reported to experience homelessness in the United States. Of these, 9% were under 18 years of age (USDHUD, 2022a). In 2021, 15.3% of U.S. children under 18 were living in poverty (Creamer et al., 2022; Fig. 26-5).

Most families experiencing homelessness are headed by single women (USDHUD, 2022b). Poverty, lack of affordable housing, domestic violence, economic recession impacts, racial disparities, and the challenge of single parenting contribute to the growing trend in family homelessness (NAEH, 2023).

Most children and youth experiencing homelessness live in shelters, share housing with friends or relatives, or live in motels or campgrounds. When compared to their housed counterparts, these children are more likely to become ill, to go hungry, and to suffer from emotional and behavioral disorders. Children in families experiencing homelessness are more likely to experience parental separation, either by being placed in foster care or by being placed in the care of friends or relatives. To hear in the words of a child what homelessness is like go to Parents and Kids Talk About Homelessness at https://www.youtube.com/watch?v=CX4TzWdDAFY (NAEH, 2023; Soucy et al., 2024).

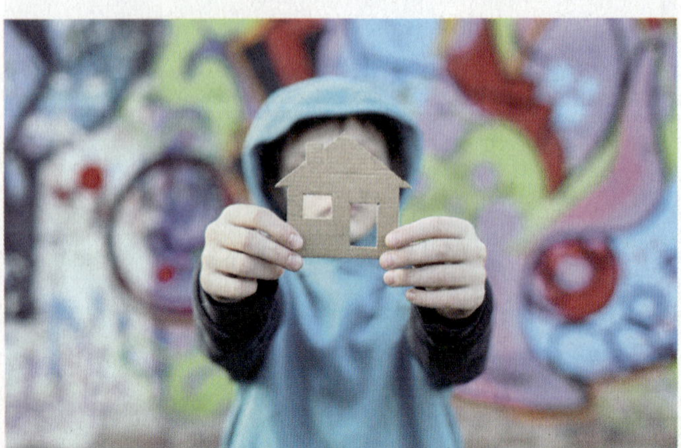

FIGURE 26-5 A child experiencing homeless who is holding a cardboard house.

Education is compromised when one is homeless. Children experiencing homelessness are more likely to repeat grades in school and to drop out or be suspended or expelled (NAEH, 2023). Barriers to education include transportation to and from the shelter, lack of academic and medical records required for registration, unstable living arrangements necessitating multiple moves, and urgent needs for food and shelter that take priority over education (Murran & Brady, 2022).

Children experiencing homelessness are more likely to get sick than other children. While acute and chronic health problems are more severe in these children, they are less able to access medical and dental care. Asthma, mental health, and behavioral problems are more prevalent in children experiencing homelessness than in the general population (Gultekin et al., 2020).

Youth Experiencing Homelessness

On a single night in January 2022, over 30,000 unaccompanied youth were experiencing homelessness in the United States (USDHUD, 2022a). **Unaccompanied youth** are defined as people under 25 years of age who are not accompanied by either a parent or guardian and are not themselves a parent (USDHUD, 2022a). These youth may have run away from home or been evicted by their parents. There may be conflicts in the home that make it dangerous for them to return home. Many have experienced abuse and have spent time in foster care. They may be overlooked during homeless counts as they are often difficult to locate (National Conference of State Legislators [NCSL], 2023).

Children who are part of the foster system are reviewed at age 17, 19, and 21 to determine how they transition from the system. These data are used to determine the needs of this population (Children's Bureau, 2023). According to the survey done by the Children's Bureau (2023), 68% had experienced at least one episode of homelessness; 60% had been incarcerated; and 46% had received a referral and or counseling for substance use by the age of 21. Moreover, some youth who are discharged from residential or foster care with inadequate housing or income support may find themselves homeless (Orsi-Hunt et al., 2024).

Adolescents experiencing homelessness may have difficulty accessing emergency shelter because of shelter policies that prohibit older youth from the facility or because of a lack of bed space. Due to lack of education or job training skills, many resort to prostitution or **survival sex** (exchanging sex for food, shelter, or other basic necessities) (Youth.gov, n.d.). As a result, youth experiencing homelessness are at higher risk for sexually transmitted infections. They also suffer disproportionately from mental health disorders (Youth.gov, n.d.; see Box 26-6).

It is not uncommon for youths experiencing homelessness to be arrested for running away, breaking curfews, or being without supervision. As young people age

BOX **26-6** PERSPECTIVES

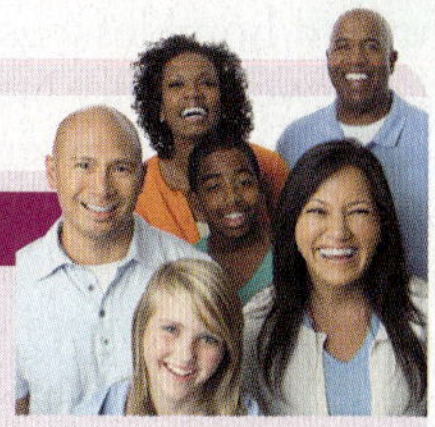

Prostitution as a Survival Tool

If you were to ask me 10 years ago what my hopes and dreams were, I would have told you I wanted to be a forest ranger or an actor. But not this. I can't recall how many men I had sex with just to get enough money for my heroin habit or how many drug dealers I manipulated for free drugs. All I know is it was not part of the plan. Growing up, I had everything I needed. We lived in a nice home. At 16, I had my own car. I attended nice schools. But I grew up in a family where my parents fought all the time. While they never hurt us, we had many holes in walls. I was always ashamed to go outside after one of these fights as their voices carried. I started using drugs at a young age, which progressed to heroin when I was in the 9th grade. How I graduated high school I have no idea. I lived in hotel rooms, my car, on couches, or in abandoned buildings. One day, I saw and felt the sorrow in my mother's eyes, and my life changed.

Things are getting better. My family and lifelong friends are returning. I'm going to a community college and working full-time. While my story includes difficult times, I realized several years ago that my past does not define me. Ask me what my hopes and dreams are today!

Anonymous client of a C/PHN

1. *How could trauma-informed care help this person?*
2. *What resources are available for this population? How long is the waitlist to access these resources?*
3. *Are there barriers to accessing these resources for certain groups that are experiencing homelessness?*
4. *To provide client-centered care, C/PHNs must be aware of any implicit biases they may have regarding the population they work with. Self-reflect on any biases you may have. Research the truth about the population. This is the first step toward freedom from biases.*
5. *What would you want to include in your assessment to identify risks and to implement treatment planning for clients living on the streets with substance use disorder?*

out of the foster care system, they find themselves on the street with inadequate support systems and little opportunity for housing or employment (Orsi-Hunt et al., 2024; Youth.gov, n.d.).

Families Experiencing Homelessness

Poverty and the lack of affordable housing place families at risk for becoming homeless. Risk factors for families with children include if the parent had a history of foster care, moved frequently as a child, experienced sexual or physical abuse as a child or as an adult, and multiple stays at short-term shelters. The majority of these families are young women of underrepresented groups with small children (Farrell et al., 2023). Declining wages, changes in government assistance programs, unstable employment, domestic violence, and a struggling economy all contribute to the problem of family homelessness.

While homelessness often breaks up the family unit, many families attempt to stay together. Whether living in shelters or on the street, children are negatively affected. Children experience social, behavioral, and academic issues (Murran & Brady, 2023). Social networks and friends are lost, shame and stigma due to housing situations, increased school absenteeism and drop-out rates, poor nutrition, and behavior health issues are difficulties these children face. Furthermore, because of stress associated with homelessness, the parent–child relationship is strained (Murran & Brady, 2023).

Children experiencing homelessness are at a high risk of being placed in foster care, and a personal history of foster care predicts family homelessness during adulthood (Orsi-Hunt et al., 2024). To assist families experiencing homelessness, attention must be focused on promoting affordable housing; supporting education, job training, and childcare for parents; promoting access to school; expanding violence prevention and treatment services; and preventing unnecessary separation of families (U.S. Department of Health and Human Services, 2024).

Veterans Experiencing Homelessness

According to the 2022 Annual Assessment Report to Congress, 7% of adults experiencing homelessness are veterans (USDHUD, 2022a). Women represent approximately 10% of the veteran homeless population (USDHUD, 2022a). Homelessness among veterans declined 55% between 2009 and 2022 (USDHUD, 2022a). The U.S. Department of Veteran Affairs (VA) administers programs that provide residential and medical care, shelter, housing, employment assistance, and other supportive services to help end homelessness for all veterans and their families (United States Department of Veteran Affairs, n.d.). Unfortunately, these programs often lack the capacity to keep pace with existing needs (Green Doors, n.d.). See Chapter 28 for more information on veterans.

People Experiencing Homelessness in Rural Areas

On a single night in 2022, 18% of people experiencing homelessness were classified in largely rural continuum of care (CoC) categories. Homelessness in largely rural areas increased by 6% from 2020 to 2022 (USDHUD, 2022a). Because there are fewer shelters in rural areas, people experiencing homelessness living in rural areas are less likely to live in shelters or on the streets and more likely to live in cars, substandard housing, or "doubled up" with friends and family. As a result, they may not be considered "homeless" for reporting purposes. Moreover, the communities in which they live may not be able to access as much federal funding, because the statistics do not adequately reflect the magnitude of the problem. Like urban homelessness, rural homelessness is largely a result of poverty and lack of affordable housing. While housing costs are lower in rural areas, incomes are also lower (Davis et al., 2023; Housing Assistance Council [HAC], 2022).

Homelessness in rural areas may be precipitated by structural or physical housing problems that force families to relocate to safer but more expensive housing. In addition, the lack of job opportunities, the distance between low-income housing and job sites, the lack of transportation, rising rents, geographic isolation, and lack of resources compound the problem. To address the needs of people experiencing homelessness in rural areas, the definition of homelessness needs to be expanded to include people living in temporary or substandard housing (Davis et al., 2023; HAC, 2022).

Older Adults Experiencing Homelessness

Eighteen percent of sheltered people experiencing homelessness were 55 or over in 2020, an increase of 1% from the prior year. Four percent of sheltered people experiencing homelessness were 65 and over (USDHUD, 2022b). Some researchers define the "older homeless" as unsheltered people 50 and older because of the declining physical health that accompanies street living (NAEH, 2022c).

Many older people live on a fixed income. At the same time, housing has become increasingly unaffordable. Moreover, the cost of healthcare continues to rise, leaving older adults at higher risk of poverty. Their restricted income renders them more vulnerable to unexpected financial crisis and even homelessness. Isolation also contributes to homelessness. Many older people live alone and lack a support network. Adults ages 50 to 62 who are experiencing homelessness have health issues like housed adults who are 10 to 20 years older. Older adults experiencing homelessness, when compared to the general population, are also more likely to have difficulty with instrumental activities of daily living at a younger age (Henderson et al., 2023). Many homeless and housing resources are not equipped to meet the needs of older adults (NAEH, 2022c). Shelter conditions, such as the use of bunk beds and shared bathing facilities, may increase the risk of falls and injury. The Social Security benefits to which many are entitled may be inadequate to cover housing costs. Moreover, the waiting list for affordable housing for older adults is often years (3 to 5 years if not longer) due to the demand and limited housing available (Henderson et al., 2023).

Lesbian, Gay, Bisexual, Transgender, Questioning People Experiencing Homelessness

Over 60% of all people experiencing homelessness who identify as transgender, not singularly male or female, or questioning are in unsheltered locations. Four percent of unaccompanied youth experiencing homelessness identify as transgender, not singularly male or female, or questioning (USDHUD, 2022a). Lesbian, gay, bisexual, transgender, and questioning (LGBTQ+) people often have difficulty finding shelters that accept them. Transgender people may be turned away from shelters or subjected to physical, sexual, or verbal abuse. These individuals are more likely to experience violence, abuse, and exploitation than their heterosexual/cisgender peers. The factor that is most frequently cited as contributing to homelessness among the LGBTQ+ population is family rejection based on sexual orientation and gender identity (NCH, 2022a).

HEALTHCARE FOR PEOPLE EXPERIENCING HOMELESSNESS

Acute and chronic health problems are prevalent among populations experiencing homelessness. Conditions such as HIV/AIDS, diabetes, and heart disease are three to six times more prevalent in populations experiencing homelessness than among the general population (NAEH, 2022b). Chronic health conditions require ongoing monitoring and are often difficult to treat in a population that is transient and lacks stable housing (NCH, 2022b). Other barriers to healthcare include lack of medical insurance, lack of transportation, clinician bias, and poor quality of healthcare (Saldua, 2023; Thorndike et al., 2022).

People experiencing homelessness or housing instability have higher rates of HIV and mental illness than people living in stable housing conditions. They are also more likely to engage in activities that lead to a higher risk of HIV transmission (CDC, 2022). Healthcare costs associated with treating HIV can exact an enormous financial burden on a resource-limited family. Insufficient funds to adequately house people living in poverty with HIV/AIDS may also contribute to homelessness among HIV-infected people. Substance misuse and sexual exploitation among people experiencing homelessness increase the risk of HIV infection. Moreover, it is difficult to adhere to complex HIV/AIDS medication regimens without access to good food, bathrooms, refrigeration, and clean water (Mermin, 2023).

Poverty, substance misuse, poor nutrition, smoking, and coexisting medical and psychiatric illnesses also predispose people experiencing homelessness to severe oral health problems. Oral health may take a back seat to other priorities such as safety and food. Additional barriers to maintaining optimal oral hygiene include lack of access to dental care, dental hygiene supplies, and nutritious food and clean water (Yusuf et al., 2023).

It is difficult for people experiencing homelessness to adhere to complex treatment regimens. For example, where does a person with no place to call home find a refrigerator to store insulin? Where would someone keep supplies for dressings? How could someone with no access to transportation keep regular appointments with healthcare providers? How does a person experiencing homelessness keep track of multiple appointment dates? How is a shelter resident who receives the typical shelter diet high in carbohydrates, fats, and sodium to adhere to a low salt or diabetic diet?

"Healthcare for the Homeless" was a model for healthcare developed through a 19-city demonstration project funded by the Robert Wood Johnson Foundation and the Pew Memorial Trust. In 1987, federal legislation (the McKinney-Vento Homeless Assistance Act) was passed that authorized federal funding for these programs. Grants are awarded to community-based organizations that deliver high-quality healthcare to populations

BOX **26-7** EVIDENCE-BASED PRACTICE

Smartphone Application Plus Brief Motivational Intervention Reduces Substance Use and Sexual Risk Behaviors Among Young Adults Experiencing Homelessness

Thompson et al. (2020) examined the feasibility and effectiveness of a smartphone application to self-monitor substance use and sexual risk behaviors and a brief motivational intervention in reducing substance use and sexual risk behaviors among young adults experiencing homelessness. Participants were randomized into treatment and control groups and were evaluated at baseline and at 2-, 4-, and 6-week intervals to assess for changes in substance use and sexual risk behaviors. Brief motivational sessions were conducted at baseline and at 2- and 4-week intervals to encourage the use of the smartphone application, encourage risk reduction, and provide personalized feedback on the self-monitoring data. Results revealed that people in the treatment group were significantly less likely to drink, use marijuana, or engage in unprotected sex than the control group. The researchers concluded that the smartphone application coupled with the brief motivational intervention was an effective strategy for reducing substance use and sexual risk behaviors in this population.

1. *What new technologies might be used to assist people experiencing homelessness to self-monitor and potentially modify their risk behaviors?*
2. *What ethical considerations need to be addressed when using self-monitoring technology in a highly vulnerable population?*
3. *How might the C/PHN use research evidence to make a case for funding technologies that enhance treatment outcomes in populations experiencing homelessness?*

Source: Thompson et al. (2020).

experiencing homelessness. Healthcare for the Homeless projects exist across the nation to provide comprehensive primary care and supportive services, including substance misuse treatment, to medically underserved populations (NHCHC, 2022; see Box 26-7).

RESOURCES TO COMBAT HOMELESSNESS

Both public and private sectors have promoted various initiatives to address homelessness. These initiatives are intended to impact homelessness on the local, state, and national level and to ensure a coordinated, comprehensive, and systematic approach to addressing the problem of homelessness.

Public Sector

The McKinney-Vento Homeless Assistance Act (PL100-77) was the first and only major piece of federal legislation intended to address the problem of homelessness on a national level. This landmark legislation, passed by Congress in 1987, originally consisted of 15 programs to address the major, pressing needs of people experiencing homelessness. These needs included emergency shelter, transitional and permanent housing, job training, primary healthcare, and education (GovInfo.gov, n.d.).

The current Act has been amended over the years to expand its scope and strengthen its impact. In particular, the amendments made to the Act in 1990 represented significant milestones in advocating for the needs of people experiencing homelessness.

- These amendments included the creation of the Shelter Care Plus program, which provided for housing assistance for people with disabilities, mental illness, AIDS, and alcohol use disorder and substance use disorder.
- Another amendment created a demonstration program within the Healthcare for the Homeless program to provide primary care and outreach to children who are at risk and homeless. In addition, the Community Mental Health Services Program was amended and re-titled: Projects for Assistance in Transition from Homelessness.
- Finally, the amendments made in 1990 strengthened access to public education for children and youth experiencing homelessness.

The McKinney-Vento Act authorized the U.S. Department of Education to administer the Education for Homeless Children and Youth program, which provides grants to schools to assist in identifying children who are homeless and to provide services to help them succeed in school. States are required to provide grant funding to local educational institutions to ensure access to a free, appropriate education for children and youth experiencing homelessness. The child is eligible for free transportation to and from school, the right to attend the same school prior to homelessness, immediate enrollment even if the family is unable to produce proof of residence, and immunizations, and school staff should be trained on the child's rights (Institute for Children, Poverty, & Homelessness, 2024; United States Department of Education, 2018).

The U.S. Department of Housing and Urban Development (USDHUD) provides funding to state and local governments and to nonprofits to assist populations experiencing homelessness (USDHUD, 2022c). This federal agency oversees a number of programs that provide rental, homeownership, and supportive housing for older people with low income and disability. The Department also manages grants through the Community Development Block Grant Program for community development initiatives that help to strengthen the housing market (USDHUD, 2024). In many communities, housing is based on a **Continuum of Care** model where programs are developed to assist people to transition from emergency to transitional to permanent housing. Emergency shelters provide temporary overnight shelter while transitional housing provides up to 24 months of housing and supportive services. Rapid rehousing programs provide short-term rental assistance and supportive services, while permanent housing provides long-term housing and supportive services (NAEH, 2022d).

In recent years, a **Housing First** philosophy has guided many of the publicly funded housing initiatives. In a Housing First approach, housing is viewed as an immediate priority. The goal of Housing First is to end homelessness by providing stable, permanent housing as soon as possible and to provide supportive services to enable people to maintain their housing. Housing or supportive services are not contingent upon adherence to rigid rules or policies or to the maintenance of sobriety (NAEH, 2022d). See the previous feature on tent cities and successful approaches to Housing First.

The Homeless Emergency Assistance and Rapid Transition to Housing Act of 2009 expanded the availability of permanent housing, authorized funding for rapid rehousing, established coordinated entry systems for housing and homeless services, and established system-wide performance measures for homeless assistance programs. This legislation was instrumental in providing federal support for Housing First initiatives (Leopold, 2019).

On March 23, 2010, President Barack Obama signed into law the Affordable Care Act, federal legislation that extended health insurance coverage and gave states the option to expand Medicaid coverage to people with limited resources regardless of disability or family status. This landmark legislation enabled people experiencing homelessness in many states to secure healthcare coverage (NAEH, 2022e; USDHHS, n.d.; see Chapter 6).

In 2010, the U.S. Interagency Council on Homelessness published the nation's first comprehensive federal strategic plan to prevent and end homelessness. The document, entitled "Opening Doors," outlined a comprehensive and ambitious plan aimed at eliminating homelessness on a national level. The goals of the plan included ending chronic homelessness in 10 years, preventing and ending homelessness for families, youth, and children in 10 years, preventing and ending homelessness among veterans in 5 years, and establishing a path to end all types of homelessness (United States Interagency Council on Homelessness [USICH], 2015).

- This plan has been updated and amended over the years. "All In," the most recent federal strategic plan to prevent and end homelessness, established an ambitious goal to reduce homelessness by 25% by January 2025.
- The plan calls for promoting equity, addressing racial disparities, using data and evidence to inform policy making, promoting collaborative leadership and information sharing, increasing the supply of safe, affordable housing, improving effectiveness of homelessness response systems, and reducing the risk of housing instability for households at risk for homelessness (USICH, 2022).

The American Rescue Plan of 2021 provided relief legislation to address the needs of communities across the nation arising from the COVID-19 pandemic (USICH, 2021). Included in the legislation was over $21 billion in emergency rental assistance for families struggling to afford rent and utilities. "House America," a federal initiative spearheaded by the USDHUD, was launched in 2021 to address the nation's homelessness crisis (Box 26-8).

- As part of this initiative, the USDHUD and the USICH collaborated to address the crisis of homelessness through a Housing First approach.

BOX 26-8 PERSPECTIVES

Homelessness and the COVID-19 Pandemic

Mosites et al. (2022) outlines important lessons learned on the national level to address the threat of COVID-19 among populations experiencing homelessness. During the COVID-19 pandemic, multiagency partnerships were found to be critical to strengthening the public health infrastructure. Federal and state agencies worked together with community partners to better understand the reality of the situation from "boots on the ground" and to provide guidance, education, and technical assistance to community organizations serving people experiencing homelessness. It became clear that tailored and nuanced approaches were needed to reduce the spread of the virus. For example, prevention guidance differed in shelters and encampments based on demographic characteristics and facility types. In some communities, noncongregate shelter was provided in hotels that partnered with local jurisdictions to enable compliance with isolation protocols. Vaccination programs were adapted to ensure multiple access points for vaccination and to avoid registration systems that required internet access and home addresses. Due to the difficulties in conducting person contact tracing, the CDC recommended location-based contact tracing, with the understanding that, if someone tested positive in a homeless shelter, it was likely that many people would be exposed. Public health authorities worked to ensure that public health recommendations did not limit access to homeless services (i.e., requiring negative COVID-19 tests or proof of vaccination to access care). Structural barriers to prevention included lack of access to sinks for handwashing, lack of racial and ethnic equity to vaccine access, and medical mistrust among underrepresented populations.

1. *What ethical considerations need to be addressed when considering vaccine hesitancy and supply shortages among underrepresented populations?*
2. *What is the C/PHN role in balancing divergent public health and homeless service goals in the context of a global health crisis?*

Mosites et al. (2022).

- These government agencies sought to partner with state, local, and tribal leaders to rehouse 100,000 households by the end of 2022.
- Investments provided through the American Rescue Plan were used to rehouse people experiencing homelessness and to promote affordable housing throughout the nation (USDHUD, 2022d).

Table 26-1 summarizes the nine titles of the McKinney-Vento Act.

Table 26-2 presents selected federally sponsored programs for addressing the needs of populations experiencing homelessness.

Private Sector

The private sector has made a concerted effort to organize communities in the battle against homelessness by forming coalitions, alliances, and memberships that champion the causes of people experiencing homelessness. These organized efforts are carried out at the national, state, and local level to positively impact the problem of homelessness in communities across the nation. Table 26-3 presents a list and description of selected resources in the private sector to combat homelessness.

ROLE OF THE COMMUNITY HEALTH NURSE

Community health nurses maintain a long tradition of providing care to vulnerable populations and play a vital role in addressing the health needs of people experiencing homelessness. Settings for care include shelters, clinics, soup kitchens, churches, community centers, social service agencies, and even the streets.

Trust is an essential ingredient in the development of a therapeutic relationship with populations experiencing homelessness. However, it is sometimes difficult to establish trust with clients who have experienced negative encounters with the healthcare system. Often these negative perceptions are intensified by limited resources, inadequate access to care, or prejudicial views. As with other vulnerable populations, the people experiencing homelessness struggle with feelings of powerlessness, loss of control, and low self-esteem.

Behaviors that would ordinarily be considered lawful in the privacy of one's home become criminal activity when they are exhibited in public. For example, people experiencing homelessness can be arrested for loitering, sleeping, urinating, or drinking alcohol in public. These behaviors can trigger a criminal record and jeopardize future employment or housing opportunities. Moreover, parents can be incarcerated for failing to pay child support (NCSL, 2022). Consider a person who is laid off from a low-wage job. Because they are unable to pay child support, they are arrested. This violation generates a criminal record and compromises this individual's ability to secure employment in the future. They become trapped in a cycle of poverty and homelessness that is difficult to escape.

To effectively address the multifaceted problems associated with homelessness, a comprehensive and holistic approach is needed. As such, the C/PHN is responsible for

TABLE 26-1 McKinney-Vento Homeless Assistance Act Titles I to IX

Title I	Statement of findings by Congress and definition of homelessness
Title II	Establishes the Interagency Council on Homelessness, a Council comprised of 15 heads of federal agencies to address the needs of homeless populations
Title III	Authorizes the Emergency Food and Shelter Program, administered by the Federal Emergency Management Agency
Title IV	Authorizes the emergency shelter and transitional housing programs administered by the Department of Housing and Urban Development (HUD) including the Emergency Shelter Grant Program, the Supportive Housing Demonstration Program, Supplemental Assistance for Facilities to Assist the Homeless, and Section 8 Single Room Occupancy Moderate Rehabilitation
Title V	Requires federal agencies to make available federal land and buildings to states and local governments to assist people experiencing homelessness
Title VI	Authorizes programs to provide healthcare services to people experiencing homelessness, including the Healthcare for the Homeless program, Community Mental Health Services Block Grant Program, and two demonstration programs providing substance misuse and mental health treatment services to populations experiencing homelessness
Title VII	Authorizes the Adult Education for the Homeless Program, the Education of Homeless Children and Youth Program (administered by the Department of Education), the Job Training for the Homeless Demonstration Program (administered by the Department of Labor), and the Emergency Community Services Homeless Grant Program (administered by the Department of Health and Human Services)
Title VIII	Amends the Food Stamp Program to facilitate access by people experiencing homelessness and expands the Temporary Emergency Food Assistance Program (administered by the Department of Agriculture)
Title IX	Extends the Veterans Job Training Act

Source: GovInfo.gov (n.d.).

TABLE 26-2 Federally Sponsored Programs for People Experiencing Homelessness

The U.S. Interagency Council on Homelessness	The United States Interagency Council on Homelessness coordinates the federal response to homelessness and creates a national partnership with public and private sectors to reduce and end homelessness in the United States. The Council is responsible for reviewing the effectiveness of federal initiatives and programs to assist people experiencing homelessness, promoting better coordination of services between programs, and informing state and local governments and private sector organizations about sources of federal homeless assistance (www.usich.gov).
Substance Abuse and Mental Health Services Administration Center for Mental Health Services	The Center for Mental Health Services, a Center of the federal Substance Abuse and Mental Health Services Administration (SAMHSA), supports states in facilitating access to mental health services and supports outreach and case management for people experiencing homelessness and mental illness (SAMHSA, 2022b). SAMHSA also operates the Homeless and Housing Resource Center, which provides training on evidence-based housing and treatment models for addressing the problem of homelessness (SAMHSA, 2022c).
Projects for Assistance in Transition from Homelessness (PATH)	PATH is a SAMHSA grant program created under the McKinney-Vento Act to provide treatment and supportive services to people with severe mental illnesses, including those who are homeless or at risk for becoming homeless. The grants support outreach, mental health and substance misuse treatment, and rehabilitation for those with severe mental illness (SAMHSA, 2022d).
Healthcare for the Homeless (HCH)	The HCH program (a provision of the McKinney-Vento Act) awards grants to community-based organizations that seek to provide quality, accessible healthcare to people experiencing homelessness. The HCH program is administered by the United States Department of Health and Human Services Health Resource and Service Administration. HCH projects provide comprehensive primary care and supportive services to low-income populations in medically underserved communities (NCH, 2022b).
The U.S. Department of Housing and Urban Development (HUD)	HUD provides funding for supportive housing for low-income people and families, including low-income older adults and people with disabilities. Funds can be used for housing development or rental assistance. Grants are also provided to public housing agencies to renovate or replace dilapidated public housing. (www.hud.gov)

TABLE 26-3 Private Sector Initiatives to Combat Homelessness

National Coalition for the Homeless (NCH) National Center on Family Homelessness	The National Coalition for the Homeless is the nation's oldest advocacy and direct service organization for people experiencing homelessness. The mission of the Coalition is to prevent and end homelessness while ensuring that the immediate needs of people experiencing homelessness are met and their civil rights protected. (https:// nationalhomeless.org) The National Center on Family Homelessness partners with the homeless service system to provide research, programs, training, and technical assistance in addressing issues surrounding homelessness and its impact on children, youth, and families. See https://www.air.org/centers/national-center-family-homelessness
National Coalition for Homeless Veterans	The National Coalition for Homeless Veterans is a 501(c)(3) nonprofit organization that provides resource and technical assistance to service providers and local, state, and federal agencies that assist veterans experiencing homelessness. The Coalition advocates for the needs of these veterans and for increased funding for federal homeless veteran assistance programs. See https://nchv.org/
National Alliance to End Homelessness (NAEH)	The National Alliance to End Homelessness seeks to end homelessness by advocating for policies that promote solutions to homelessness, providing technical assistance to local communities, and advancing data and research on best practices and solutions for combating homelessness. See https://endhomelessness.org.
Commission on Homelessness and Poverty, American Bar Association	This Commission is committed to educating the public and the legal community about the issue of poverty and homelessness and trains members of the legal community on how best to advocate for those in need. The Commission also advocates for public policies that protect and provide for the needs of people suffering from poverty and homelessness. See https://www.americanbar.org/groups/public_interest/homelessness_poverty/about_us/
National Low-Income Housing Coalition	The National Low-Income Housing Coalition is dedicated to establishing housing stability and expanding the supply of low-income housing in the United States. A major priority of the coalition is to promote public policy that provides funding for housing for people with extremely low incomes. See https://nlihc.org.

BOX 26-9 C/PHN USE OF THE NURSING PROCESS/CLINICAL JUDGMENT

Addressing Women and Children Experiencing Homelessness

Sheila Hendricks, a public health nurse for the Manchester City Health Department, and her colleagues were brainstorming ideas for how to reach the growing population of women and children experiencing homelessness in their jurisdiction. They arranged a meeting with the director of a local rescue mission in the area. The mission provided emergency shelter to 100 women and children each night. The community health nurses negotiated with the rescue mission to establish an on-site nursing clinic twice a week that would provide health education, screenings, and referrals on a drop-in basis.

Assessment/Recognize and Analyze Cues

After the clinic was in operation for 2 weeks, Sheila identified poor nutrition, lack of primary care services, depression, high rates of sexually transmitted infections, and substance use disorders as priority health issues in the population.

Diagnosis/Analyze Cues and Prioritize Hypotheses

- Unable to access health and social services offered in the community
- Education needed on the prevention of STIs
- High priority for mental health and SUD treatment

Planning and Implementation/Generate Solutions and Take Action

- Primary care services provided by nurse practitioner at the shelter.
- Healthcare for the Homeless Clinic referrals made for more extensive follow-up.
- Social worker engaged to assist clients in applying for housing and public assistance.
- Referrals to local community mental health center for counseling.
- Nurse-led health education and counseling sessions, and on-site screenings with referrals to health department clinic as needed.

Evaluation/Evaluate Outcomes

Outcomes after 3 months of the clinic being in operation were a success. Evaluation of nursing diagnoses includes the following goals:

- Clients in the clinic will receive health promotion teaching and a resource packet for further reference.
- Clients that require referrals to outside agencies will be successful in accessing care.
- Clients will be followed by the nurse practitioner for acute or chronic health conditions.
- Clients will apply for social service benefits.

implementing primary, secondary, and tertiary preventive measures to prevent homelessness or to assist those who are homeless to obtain needed services (see Box 26-9).

Primary Prevention

Primary prevention includes advocating for affordable housing, employment opportunities, and better access to healthcare to prevent the downward spiral into homelessness. Strategies for preventing homelessness may include financial counseling to assist clients to better manage their money, assistance in locating sources of legal or financial aid to prevent eviction (i.e., loans or grants for emergency funds to help pay for rent, utilities, etc.), or assistance in accessing social services, temporary housing, or healthcare to avoid a housing, health, or family crisis (Kushel et al., 2023; Box 26-10).

Health education that addresses primary prevention may focus on positive parenting skills, child development, violence prevention, anger management, coping skills, healthy eating, or principles of basic hygiene. Immunization programs will help to prevent communicable disease in this high-risk population. Counseling people who have experienced intimate partner violence and helping them to locate safe shelter can also aid in the prevention of homelessness (Kushel et al., 2023). Treatment for substance use disorder is also important to prevent the consequences if it is left untreated, which can include death, incarceration, admission to a mental health facility, or homelessness.

Secondary Prevention

The focus of secondary prevention measures is on the early detection and treatment of adverse health conditions. This requires a thorough assessment of client needs including the need for housing, healthcare, education, social services, and employment (Box 26-11). Clients will also benefit from secondary prevention measures such as screening for communicable and chronic diseases (i.e., hepatitis, TB, STI, HIV, hypertension, diabetes, cancer). Of importance is screening for ACE since 90% of this population has had at least one ACE in their lifetime (Liu et al., 2021).

Barriers to accessing services and the extent of community resources available to people experiencing homelessness also need to be assessed (Kushel et al., 2023). Resources such as shelters, soup kitchens, medical clinics, social service agencies, and supportive housing should be readily accessible to people experiencing homelessness. Providers servicing populations experiencing homelessness should be educated in **trauma-informed care (TIC)**, a service delivery model that recognizes the widespread impact of trauma, understands the paths for recovery, recognizes the signs and symptoms of trauma, and responds by integrating knowledge about trauma into policies, procedures, and practices. Developed in 2014 and widely used still today, the key principles of a trauma-informed approach to care are safety, trust and transparency, peer support, collaboration, empowerment, and attention to cultural, historical, and gender issues (SAMHSA, 2014).

BOX 26-10 WHAT DO *YOU* THINK?

Sleeping on the Streets

Every nurse encounters new situations with prior assumptions, biases, and preunderstandings. When considering working with populations experiencing homelessness, it is important to clarify one's own beliefs and values about poverty, homelessness, substance use disorders, and mental health disorders.

1. *What has been your experience with people experiencing homelessness?*
2. *Have you ever observed a person asking for money or holding up signs at a busy intersection?*
3. *What thoughts and feelings do encounters such as these provoke?*

It may be helpful to interview people who work with populations experiencing homelessness or to visit clinics, shelters, or other settings where people experiencing homelessness congregate or access services.

1. *How are these people treated?*
2. *What is a typical day like for someone who is experiencing homelessness?*
3. *How often do people hear their names?*
4. *How often are they touched in a way that is therapeutic, respectful, and affirming?*

By reflecting on your personal values and by allowing yourself to get closer to the people and places that are a part of the experience of homelessness, you will gain a deeper understanding of the homeless condition and be better equipped to serve those suffering from homelessness.

BOX 26-11 PERSPECTIVES

A Nurse's Viewpoint on Working With Persons Experiencing Homelessness

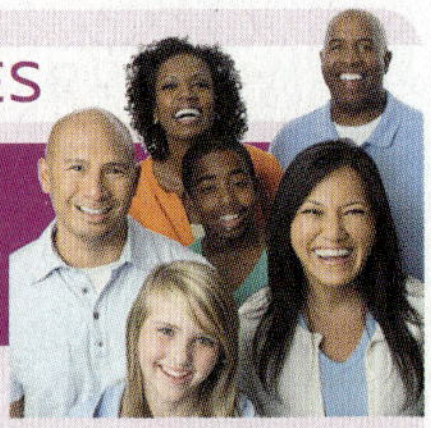

When I first decided to visit the overnight shelter for men experiencing homelessness, I was scared to death. Here I was, a new PHN just out of nursing school wanting to change the world. But what I learned was so much more... I changed.

The shelter offers a medical clinic in the local park, so I went to volunteer. I didn't know the area, and the clinic took place at night. The healthcare providers were volunteers from a local medical center; the support staff were college students from a variety of academic programs at a large university.

No child has the dream of growing up to be homeless; no parent wishes it for their child. Yet, here they are. The simple act of asking someone their name shows you care and respect them. When I use a person's name, they are no longer "homeless"; rather they become a person.

A hot meal and a sack lunch for the following day were provided to each person. The meals build trust and camaraderie with the clinic. Building trust is the first step with this population, and food was a way to gain that trust.

While the stories differ, there are many similarities such as estrangement from family and friends, shunned by others, aching feet, and weather-worn skin. I felt helpless at times, the needs so great. We did what we could and hope they return next week. One man shared he felt human and respected by the volunteers, something he had not felt for years. I challenge the reader to spend time with those that are unsheltered or homeless. Give your time and talents, you will not leave disappointed.

Anne PHN

Lack of transportation can be a major barrier to accessing care. Some programs have responded to this need by adopting mobile health vans that provide care for medically underserved populations on street corners and in neighborhoods (Gupta et al., 2022). Clinics have also been established in shelters to facilitate client access (Ramirez et al., 2022; Winiarski et al., 2020). Nurse-managed clinics that engage students in providing care to medically underserved clients represent another best practice for addressing access to healthcare for vulnerable populations (Saude et al., 2020). Finally, shelter-based telehealth services are an effective alternative for promoting healthcare access, particularly in the wake of the COVID-19 pandemic (Bekasi et al., 2022).

The community health nurse should also consider the role of faith-based communities in providing physical and spiritual support to people experiencing homelessness. Many places of worship have responded to the crisis of homelessness by offering food, shelter, counseling, medical care, and social services within the context of the faith community. Clinics have been built within faith communities to promote access to care (see Box 26-12).

Advocacy

Advocacy is a vital dimension of the community health nurse's role in working with populations experiencing homelessness. The community health nurse acts as an advocate at each level of prevention to effect positive change (Boxes 26-13 and 26-14). For example, the nurse may advocate (1) for mental health and substance misuse services to promote mental health and prevent homelessness (primary prevention) (2) for healthcare institutions and providers to screen clients for SUD and ACE (secondary prevention); and (3) for legislation to fund supportive housing, healthcare, or social services to benefit the person who has a chronic mental illness and is experiencing chronic patterns of homelessness (tertiary prevention). The C/PHN can also assume an advocacy role by becoming involved in local, state, or national coalitions or organizations devoted to protecting the rights of people experiencing homelessness or by speaking out on legislation that impacts this vulnerable population.

BOX 26-12 STORIES FROM THE FIELD

Faith-Based Outreach

As a faith community nurse working in a large church congregation, you are invited to develop an outreach program to minister to the needs of an inner-city mission that is receiving financial support from the church. Approximately 500 men experiencing homelessness who are in recovery from chemical substance use disorders frequent the mission daily. Staff and residents have expressed concerns regarding a recent outbreak of boils among residents.

Assessment data reveal the following issues:

- Approximately 80% of clients have a history of injection drug use.
- Clients sleep in dormitory-style accommodations and share bathroom facilities.
- An on-site barbershop operated by the residents provides haircuts for a nominal fee.
- Clients have access to a small recreational area with donated exercise equipment.
- Laundry is typically washed in cold water and, at times, the laundry runs out of detergent.

Questions

1. *What additional data would you wish to gather to address the outbreak of boils at the shelter? How would you collect these data?*
2. *What host, agent, and environmental factors may have contributed to the outbreak of boils?*
3. *Discuss appropriate nursing interventions to address the outbreak. Consider the following levels of prevention: primary, secondary, and tertiary.*
4. *What advocacy role might the C/PHN play in addressing this issue?*

BOX 26-13 LEVELS OF PREVENTION PYRAMID

Preventing Illness Among Men Who Are Homeless and Have a Substance Use Disorder

SITUATION: Promoting health and preventing illness among men experiencing homelessness and substance use disorder
GOAL: To apply the three levels of prevention to avoid adverse health conditions, promptly diagnose and treat disorders, and assist this vulnerable population to maintain or regain optimal health

Tertiary Prevention

- Provide case management of chronic health conditions.
- Advocate for expansion of counseling, rehabilitative services, and substance use disorder treatment programs for people experiencing homelessness.
- Advocate for supportive and transitional housing to enable people experiencing homelessness and substance use disorders to successfully transition back into the community.

Secondary Prevention

Early Diagnosis and Treatment

- Conduct mass screenings for diseases commonly found in populations of men experiencing homelessness (TB, HIV, hepatitis, prostate cancer, colorectal cancer).
- Develop programs for health screening and early diagnosis and treatment in the community that are culturally sensitive and accessible to people experiencing homelessness (i.e., mobile vans, faith community, or shelter-based clinics).

Primary Prevention

Health Promotion and Education

- Support employment and job training opportunities that assist clients to obtain jobs with livable wages and benefits.
- Advocate through housing coalitions and legislative efforts to promote affordable housing, employment opportunities, and better access to healthcare.
- Develop culturally sensitive health education programs that promote healthy coping, positive parenting, communication and relationship building, mental health, and injury and illness prevention.
- Promote programs that offer counseling and support to prevent continued high-risk behaviors as a result of untreated substance use disorder.

Health Protection

- Advocate for legislation to protect citizens from environmental toxins and industrial wastes common to low-income areas.
- Provide immunization services to prevent communicable disease transmission.
- Counsel clients on proper nutrition, exercise, and basic hygiene to promote healthy lifestyles and prevent disease transmission.
- Advocate for funding for nutrition programs for people experiencing homelessness and for homeless shelters that would allow for the purchase of nutritious foods.

BOX 26-14 SPOTLIGHT ON ESSENTIAL NURSING COMPETENCIES

Quality Improvement through Faith-Based Programs

Every day you are in a patient care environment, you probably evaluate the quality of the care given to your patients. Biomarkers such as improvements in blood pressure and hemoglobin A1C levels, reduction in pain, or changes in function such as improvement in activities of daily living may serve as indicators of success when measuring the effectiveness of one's nursing interventions. But how is success measured when one is caring for large and diverse population groups?

To measure change in this context, one must first define what is meant by "success." For example, what are the markers for success when working with a population of teen parents experiencing homelessness? What about a population of adults experiencing homelessness with decades-long histories of active substance use disorder? Literature reviews, surveys, or focus groups may help point to measures of success. Interviews with key stakeholders also provide insight as to the most important measures for evaluating program effectiveness in a population. Success could also be measured on the population level by considering the social or financial impact of a program or service on the surrounding community or region.

Lashley (2020) examined the economic impact of a faith-based residential substance use disorder recovery program on men experiencing homelessness and chemical substance use disorders. To compare costs and savings at different program intervals, program data were examined for over 5000 men experiencing homelessness before, during, and following completion of a 1-year residential, faith-based substance use disorder recovery program. The study found that each person who participated in the program for 1 year saved state and local governments over $14,000, and each person who completed the program saved state and county governments more than $5000 per year postgraduation. Each individual who worked for 1 year following graduation and reallocated spending from illicit drugs to goods and services in the economy was estimated to support 1.5 jobs and generate over $240,000 in additional revenue and economic output. The findings from this study affirmed the value of a faith-based residential substance use disorder recovery program in promoting economic productivity in the surrounding community and region.

1. *What outcomes do you believe are most important to track when caring for populations experiencing homelessness?*
2. *How might you engage a target population to actively participate in the evaluation process?*

Source: Lashley (2020).

SUMMARY

- Poverty, lack of housing, domestic violence, mental illness, substance use disorders, personal crisis, and natural disasters are factors that may predispose people to homelessness.
- Acute and chronic health problems plague people experiencing homelessness and are difficult to treat because of the challenges associated with being homeless.
- Both the public and private sectors have launched concerted efforts to combat the problem of homelessness through the passage of federal legislation and through the formation of national, state, and local coalitions and alliances to champion this important cause.
- The community health nurse delivers primary, secondary, and tertiary preventive measures to prevent homelessness or to assist those who are homeless to obtain needed services.
- The community health nurse serves as a case manager to coordinate care and to assist clients to negotiate the bureaucracy of multiple agencies and services.
- The C/PHN acts as an advocate to promote the rights of people experiencing homelessness and to speak out on legislation impacting homelessness.

ACTIVE LEARNING EXERCISES

1. Interview a family, a single man, or a LGBTQ+ young adult experiencing homelessness. What factors in their lives led to homelessness? How does this person's experience compare to national statistics? (Objective 1)
2. Interview healthcare providers working with people who are homeless. What are the health issues most encountered? Where is their practice located? Is the health clinic in a shelter, on the street, or in a park, or in a mobile van? Ask the providers their most rewarding experience working with this population. Are they able to provide all services needed and, if not, what road blocks do they encounter? Are health concerns reflective of what is seen on the state and national levels? (Objective 2)
3. Volunteer to work at a soup kitchen or shelter for people experiencing homelessness. Observe the faces, sounds, attitudes, and activities. What is it like there? What would it be like to receive rather than give service? Listen to some of the life stories of people who are now in this situation. Interview a parent of young children and an older person. Reflect on the experience; were their stories what you expected? Did the stories fit into your worldview? Did your

view change? How will your patient care change when working with those who are unsheltered since this experience? (Objective 3)

4. Analyze online census data to determine the rates of homelessness in your county, state, or region. How many people are experiencing homelessness? What is the age and gender distribution? What subpopulations exist within your county, state, or region? How do these compare with other counties or states? (Objective 4)
5. Perform a windshield survey in an area with a high density of people who are homeless or unsheltered. What resources are lacking? Where is the nearest bank, school, foodbank, grocery store, or health clinic? What are the conditions of the roads, homes, and other buildings? Interview key stakeholders regarding what needs to be done and what they are doing to help. What are some primary, secondary, and tertiary preventions you would consider in addressing the unsheltered population? List your stakeholders. Describe how collaborating with stakeholders broadens the opportunities for preventions. What did you learn from working with others? Which 10 Essential Public Health Services did you utilize in this activity (Box 2-2)? (Objective 5)

CHAPTER 27

Rural, Migrant, and Urban Communities*

"I grew up with my family in Bellas Gate, in a big old ramshackle house. Deep rural. Mountainous. Mist-covered after the rain. Beautiful. Isolated. No radios. No telephones. Life was sweet. Life was harsh."

— Trevor Rhone, *Bellas Gate Boy*

"Give me your tired, your poor, your huddled masses yearning to breathe free. The wretched refuse of your teeming shore. Send these, the homeless, tempest-tost to me. I lift my lamp beside the golden door!"

— Emma Lazarus, "The New Colossus"

KEY TERMS

Built environment
Critical access hospitals (CAHs)
Federally qualified health centers
Frontier area
Health professional shortage areas (HPSAs)
Medically underserved areas
Medically underserved population
Migrant farmworkers
Migrant streams
Nomadic migrant workers
Pesticide drift
Population density
Rural
Rural health clinics
Seasonal farmworkers
Sustainable communities
Urban
Urban health
Urbanized area
Urban planning
Urban sprawl

LEARNING OBJECTIVES

Upon mastery of this chapter, you should be able to:

1. Compare and contrast the health problems of adults residing in rural, migrant, and urban communities.
2. Develop a plan of action to address the health problems of adults residing in rural, migrant, or urban areas.
3. Describe environmental toxins in the rural, migrant, and urban communities and their effect on children.
4. Advocate for children affected by toxins in rural communities through social awareness and policy change.
5. Demonstrate respect for the communities of the rural, migrant, and urban populations.

INTRODUCTION

Rural and urban life can be vastly different. About half of the population lives in the suburbs, but the rest live in one of two diametrically opposed areas: in a very densely populated, bustling urban area (Fig. 27-1) or in a sparsely populated, somewhat isolated rural area. Public health nursing in urban and rural areas requires not only general public health nursing knowledge and skills but also a unique understanding of how these distinctive environments affect the health of the populations living there. Where you live can and does markedly affect your health outcomes, with rural and urban areas having distinctive problems and issues.

*In this chapter, "male" refers to a person assigned male at birth, and "female" refers to a person assigned female at birth.

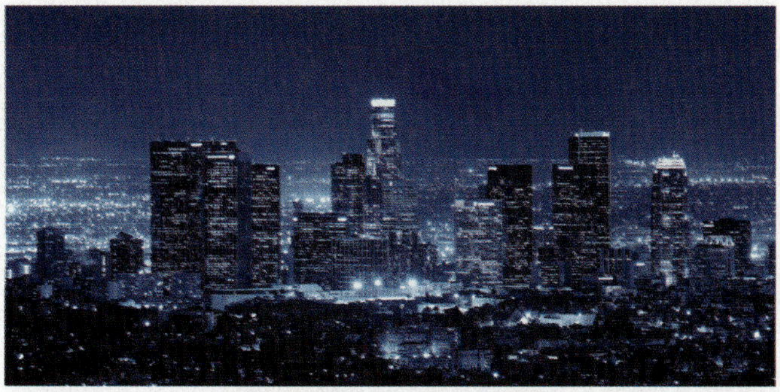

FIGURE 27-1 Los Angeles is a bustling urban area.

Rural nursing practice offers many opportunities. C/PHNs may live and work in rural parts of the United States. The pace in rural America may be slower and everyone, typically, knows one another. Nurses are respected members of the rural community—their judgment and opinions count. As key members of the healthcare team, rural C/PHNs often struggle to help clients gain access to quality healthcare and deal with the inherent transportation problems found in rural and isolated areas.

Urban C/PHNs often specialize in particular areas of interest. They deal with different types of problems, such as homelessness, overcrowding, bioterrorism threats, and violent crime. They are often called upon to advocate for their most vulnerable clients, and they develop collaborative relationships with other professionals. While there are unique challenges in rural and urban healthcare, both are filled with rewards.

In these community settings, migrant workers are an aggregate population most at risk for higher frequency of illness, greater complications, and more long-term debilitating effects as this population works many of the dangerous and laborious jobs within a community. Exacerbated by a magnitude of environmental and work stressors, the health of migrant families is also compromised by limited access to healthcare, mobility, language and cultural barriers, low educational levels, and few economic and political resources. Because migrant health needs are largely manageable within community settings, C/PHNs are ideal health providers. C/PHNs must advocate for the health of migrant workers, who have very little economic or political power, and also guide them through the complexities of a changing healthcare system.

This chapter addresses the special health needs and concerns of rural, migrant, and urban clients and the ways in which a C/PHN can address those needs. After reading the chapter, you may come to appreciate the many advantages that rural nurses enjoy and consider rural nursing as a practice choice, or you may find that being a C/PHN in an urban area offers you more opportunities for specialization and networking. Either way, your contributions can improve the health of populations living at both extremes.

DEFINITIONS AND DEMOGRAPHICS

Definitions

The U.S. government provides several definitions of *rural*. It is important to understand the terms and how they are used in federal programs and grant funding. The National Center for Health Statistics (NCHS) (n.d.) examines metropolitan and nonmetropolitan areas based on counties and provides data apart from census reports. The updated NCHS Urban-Rural Classification Scheme for Counties will be published in 2024. Nonmetropolitan areas have some combination that includes "open countryside," rural towns (less than 2500 people), urban clusters (greater than 2500 to less than 50,000 people), and urban areas (2500 to 49,999 people; Fig. 27-2; Rural Health Information Hub [RHIH], 2022a).

The U.S. Census Bureau determines the classification of rural in an official capacity and defines it as "all territory, population, and housing units located outside urban areas" (RHIH, 2022a). State and federal agencies recognize county-level jurisdictions and governments and depend on employment, income, and population data available annually. Many states have offices of rural health or other agencies dealing with issues specific to rural populations.

- For the purposes of this chapter, rural areas are defined as *communities with fewer than 10,000 residents and a county* **population density** *of less than 1000 persons per square mile*. This definition of rural is arbitrary because rural clients do not merely consider population density or community size when defining their *ruralness*. Those in rural communities may consider other attributes for being rural such as distance from a large city, major occupations in the area (e.g., agriculture), or number of students in the local schools (USDA, n.d.-a).
- The term **frontier area** is used to designate sparsely populated rural places that are isolated from population centers and services, but specific definitions vary (RHIH, 2023a). A common definition of a "frontier and remote area" (FAR) is one with six or fewer persons per square mile, but other definitions include not only population density but also distance and travel time to market service areas. For instance, 60 miles or 60 minutes of driving on paved roads to the nearest 75-bed (or greater) hospitals could constitute a frontier area. The USDA (2024a) has developed FAR codes based upon urban–rural census data and delineated by Zone Improvement Plan (ZIP) codes. There are four levels of FAR codes:
  - Level 1 includes a good number of people living far from city areas where higher-level goods are available (e.g., regional airport hubs, stores with major household appliances, advanced medical care).
  - Level 4 includes fewer people with a more significant level of remoteness (e.g., decreased access to stores selling gas or groceries; access to basic medical care).
  - The other two levels may also have access to movie theaters, car dealerships, and clothing stores.
  - The use of levels is helpful to researchers and public health agencies in determining rural–urban status and designing programs to meet specific needs.

It is estimated that 3 million people (4% of the population) live in frontier areas that comprise 56% of the U.S. land areas. States with more than 30% of their

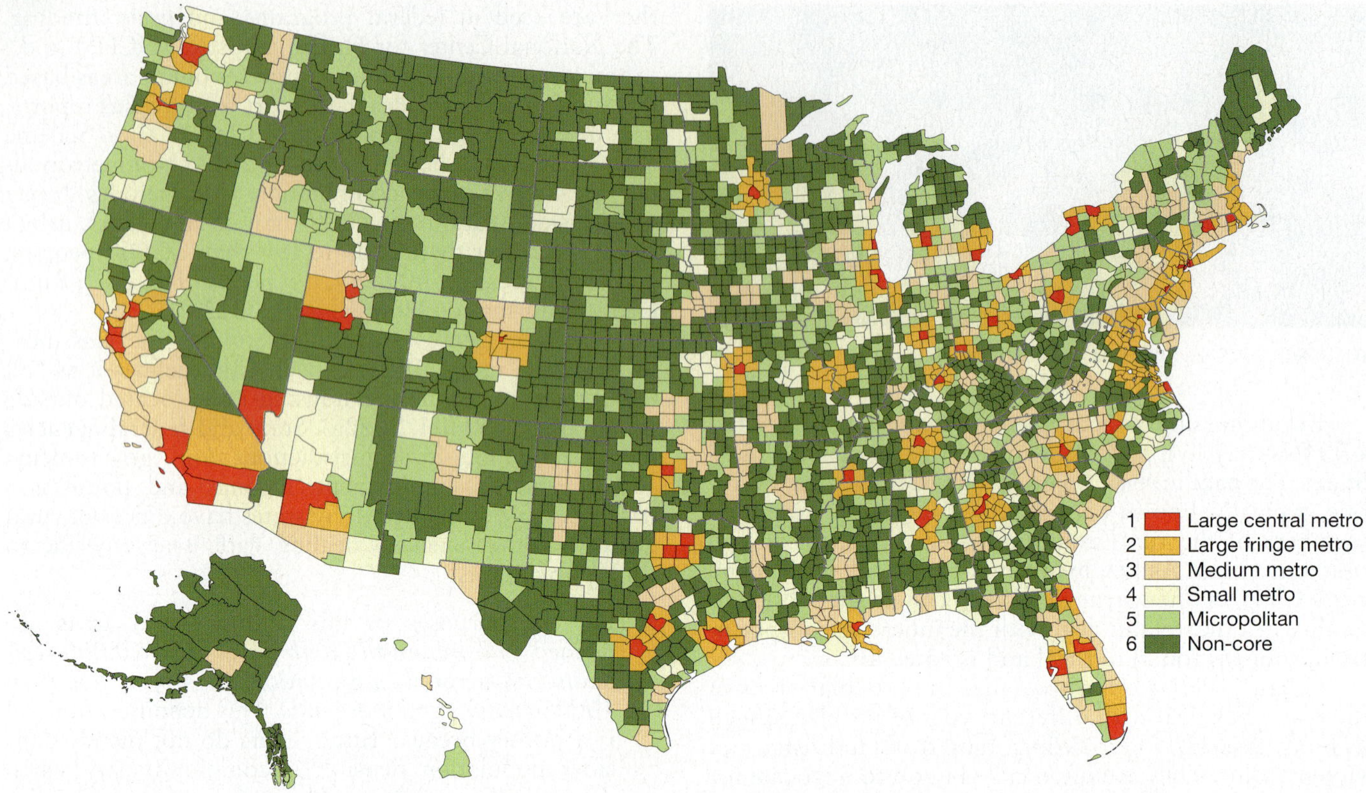

FIGURE 27-2 2013 urban–rural classification schemes for counties, 2017. (Reprinted from Centers for Disease Control and Prevention, National Center for Health Statistics. (2020). https://www.cdc.gov/nchs/images/popbridge/URv3.png)

population in a frontier area include Alaska, Arizona, Montana, New Mexico, North Dakota, and South Dakota. Wyoming leads the list with nearly 74% of its population in a frontier area (National Center for Frontier Communities, 2020).

Health issues of concern in rural areas may be of even greater concern for frontier areas. Sparsely populated areas may be less able to attract healthcare professionals.

- The term **health professional shortage areas (HPSAs)** is used to identify urban or rural geographic areas, population groups, or facilities with chronic shortages of medical, dental, or mental health professionals. The federal government determines which areas are HPSAs, based upon a scoring system including the following: population/provider ratio, percent of the population below 100% federal poverty level, and travel time to the nearest healthcare source outside an HPSA (HRSA, 2023).
- In **medically underserved areas**, residents experience a shortage of health services; these areas are determined by the federal government using a score based on the shortage of primary care providers, high infant mortality rates, high percentage of the population living below the poverty level, and a high proportion of residents over age 65.

Population Statistics

The number of people living in urban areas of the United States has tripled since the mid-1800s, to almost 60 million in 2000, and grew 10.8% from 2000 to 2010 (Table 27-1). About 80% of the total population can be found in urban areas (U.S. Census, 2022). The total U.S. population today is 331,449,281, a 7.4% increase since the 2010 U.S. Census (Dobis et al., 2021). In the United States, 12.3% of those living in urban areas are at the poverty level, while 15.4% of those living in rural areas are at the poverty level (RHIH, 2023b).

An all-time high of 51% of the population live in the suburbs.

- Less than 20% of the U.S. population is characterized as rural.
- Rural areas are caught in a vicious cycle of people moving away to find jobs and businesses reluctant to relocate to rural areas because of a smaller pool of potential workers. Vermont has the highest percentage of its population residing in rural areas. States with the largest percentage of rural population are Texas, North Carolina, Pennsylvania, and Ohio (U.S. Census Bureau, 2022).
- Rural areas in the United States have higher rates of poverty (USDA, 2023a).
- People in rural areas were less likely to have a bachelor's degree, but the number of people in rural areas without a high school degree or equivalent decreased from 2000 to 2018 (USDA, 2021).
- Many Americans living in rural communities continue to face barriers that prevent them from attaining the quality of life they deserve. Access to adequate transportation is difficult for many rural Americans.

TABLE **27-1** A National Rural Health Snapshot: Rural Versus Urban

National Rural Health Snapshot	Rural	Urban
Percentage of population	19.3%	80.7%
Number of primary providers per 10,000 people	13.1	31.2
Number of specialists per 100,000 people	30	263
Population aged 65 years and older	18%	12%
Average per capita income	$45,482	$53,657
Non-Hispanic White population	69%–82%	45%
Adults who describe health status as fair/poor	19.5%	15.6%
Adolescents who smoke	11%	5%
Male life expectancy in years	76.2	74.1
Female life expectancy	81.3	79.7
Percentage of dual-eligible Medicare beneficiaries	30%	70%
Medicare beneficiaries without drug coverage	43%	27%
Percentage covered by Medicaid	16%	13%

All information in this table is from the Health Resources and Services Administration and Rural Health Information Hub.
National Rural Health Association. (n.d.). *About rural health care.* https://www.ruralhealthweb.org/about-nrha/about-rural-health-care

Insufficient access to medical care can lead to health problems; this can be exceptionally hard to overcome for Americans living in rural areas. In addition, too many rural Americans do not have the necessary broadband access needed to engage in the modern economy (USDA, n.d.-b).

- A rural e-connectivity program provides loans and grants to facilitate broadband internet services in rural areas to support long-term economic development and opportunities in rural United States (Federal Register, 2023). A large majority of people in the United States have the moderate-speed or high-speed broadband internet service needed for high-quality video calls available in their census blocks. However, only 72% of rural residents and only 63% of rural residents in persistent poverty counties had moderate- or high-speed broadband available in their census blocks (Dobis et al., 2021).
- Rural residents are less likely to receive recommended preventive services, and they make fewer visits to healthcare providers. They also have fewer primary providers (10% of total), and there is continuous concern about the recruitment of healthcare professionals in rural areas of the United States and other countries beyond what incentives (e.g., scholarships, forgivable loans) can offer. As of September 2022, 65.6% of Primary Care HPSAs were in rural areas (RHIH, 2024a).
- Specialized medical care is rarely found in rural areas. Of the 2000 rural hospitals, 75% have 50 or fewer beds; most are designated **critical access hospitals (CAHs)** as they have 25 or fewer beds (RHIH, 2024b).

Recent solutions have been formulated to address these issues:

- The National Health Service Corp Program addresses long-standing shortages of primary care health professionals by providing primary providers, advanced practice registered nurse (APRN), and other health professionals with scholarships and repayments of student loans in return for at least 2 years of service in communities facing shortages.
- Area Health Education Centers were developed by Congress in 1971 to recruit, train, and retain healthcare professionals committed to underserved populations, which include rural areas. Many work collaboratively with medical schools, nursing programs, and allied health schools to improve health for underserved and underrepresented populations.
- Increased broadband internet access to better support telehealth services in rural areas.
- **Federally qualified health centers** make up one of the largest healthcare systems for rural America and are frequently the only source of primary and preventive services in their communities. Fifty-three percent of these community health centers are in rural and frontier areas. Nurses play a central role in all three of these initiatives, providing both direct primary and preventive care (RHIH, 2024c).

CHANGING PATTERNS OF MIGRATION

Rural counties have seen an increase in population due to COVID-19 concerns and the increase in remote work. Persistently resource-limited rural counties have only seen a slight population decline (Davis et al., 2023). Employment in the rural counties has returned to 99% of prepandemic levels. In fact, more people moved into rural areas than people who moved into urban areas (Davis et al., 2023). Housing insecurity remains a problem in rural areas (Davis et al., 2023). Residents who live in smaller and more isolated rural settings often face greater difficulties accessing goods and services or commuting to work, among other challenges. Population trends have many implications for the health services needed by rural people. The patterns of rural migration have been changing since the pandemic, adding to the challenge of planning resources for rural communities.

- Today, rural areas are more economically diverse than in the past, reflecting the national trend of a greater reliance on clean-energy jobs. Other employment opportunities involve coal, petroleum, and natural gas (Davis et al., 2023). While traditional rural occupations, such as agriculture, employ less of the rural population than before, they continue to play a major source of economics in many communities. Rural employment opportunities are growing in manufacturing plants, clean air employment, and recreational activities (Carnevale et al., 2024).
- Figure 27-3 shows the Percentage of People in Poverty in the United States and Puerto Rico (U.S. Census Bureau, 2023).

Demographics

Migrant farmworkers constitute a mobile population with a shifting composition, and it is difficult to determine their number or origins precisely. These estimates also vary because of the influx of undocumented workers. In addition to male workers, who make up the majority, you may also see female workers bring infants (strapped to their backs) and young children to work with them, and the children spend their days playing among the pesticide-laden fields.

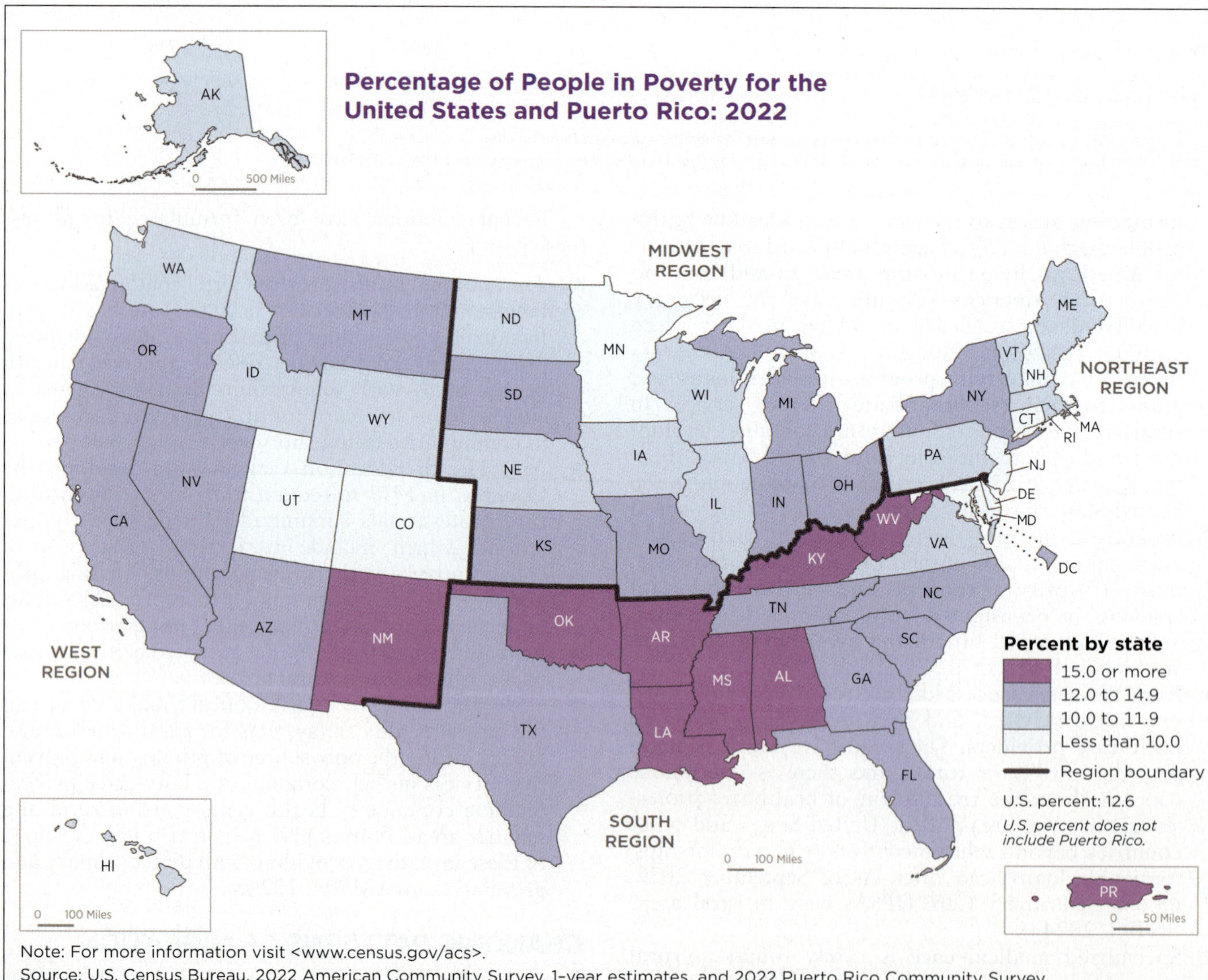

FIGURE 27-3 Percentage of people in poverty for the United States and Puerto Rico: 2022. (Reprinted from U.S. Census Bureau. (2023). *Poverty in states and metropolitan areas: 2022.* https://www.census.gov/content/dam/Census/library/publications/2023/acs/acsbr-016.pdf)

- **Seasonal farmworkers** generally live in one geographic location or housing and are temporarily employed in agriculture, whereas migrant farmworkers meet that classification while moving to find agricultural work throughout the year, usually from state to state, and establishing temporary residences (JBS International, 2022).
- Some live apart from their families, forming groups of single males; others travel with their entire families. The average migrant farmworker spends from June to September doing seasonal harvesting, with about 8 weeks on the road traveling from farm to farm for work, and is then unemployed unless other work, such as hauling or canning, is found.
- Workdays on the farm (Fig. 27-2) begin before dawn and often last 12 hours or longer. Farmworkers cannot be paid for overtime, as federal laws exclude this category of work. Seventeen states do not require workers' compensation insurance for agricultural workers, 14 states require workers' compensation for all agricultural workers, and the remainder require it but provide exceptions for small employers (National Center for Farmworkers Health [NCFH], 2023a).

Migrant farmworkers represent some of the most economically disadvantaged people in the United States. According to the 2019 to 2020 National Agricultural Workers Survey results, 43% of migrant worker families had total family income levels below the national poverty guidelines. Seventy-eight percent of the workers identified themselves as of Hispanic ethnicity, 60% as Mexican, 10% as Mexican American, and 8% as Chicano, Puerto Rican, or other Hispanic.

Eighty-five percent of foreign-born farmworkers have been in the United States for at least 10 years. Over half the farmworkers have work authorization (56%), and 36% of those are American citizens, with the remainder lawful permanent citizens. Sixty-five percent of the farmworkers were born in Mexico, 30% were born in the United States or Puerto Rico, and 5% in Central America. Fifty-seven percent were married, and 50% had children, although 69% were unaccompanied (living apart from the nuclear family). The average level of formal education was 9th grade, and 62% reported Spanish as their primary language. The majority of farmworkers reported compensation as an hourly wage at an average of $13.59 per hour at their current farm job. Thirty-eight percent stated that they worked in fruit and nut crops, 20% in vegetable crops, and 24% in horticulture (JBS International, 2022).

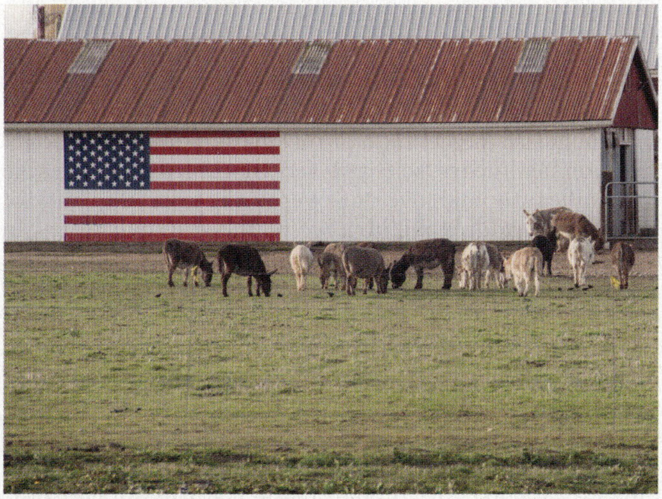

FIGURE 27-4 An American farm.

Migrant Streams and Patterns

From their home base, migrant farmworkers move to locations where new crops are ready for harvest, following the harvest seasons as they move from place to place along predetermined routes called **migrant streams** (Fig. 27-5). Some migrant farmworkers are multigenerational; their families have been farmworkers for several generations, traveling the same streams for many years. Globally, an estimated $647 billion was sent by migrants to people in their home countries in 2022 (Fried, 2024). More specifically, more than 63 billion dollars was sent from the United States to Mexico by migrant workers (Rivera, 2024).

Three principal streams formulate the agricultural routes that migrant laborers follow.

- The *eastern stream* originates in Florida, where most of their time is spent, and extends up the East Coast through North Carolina, Tennessee, Kentucky, Virginia, and other states east of the Mississippi, as far as north as Ohio, New Jersey, New York, Connecticut, Massachusetts, New Hampshire, Vermont, and Maine.
- The *midwestern stream* begins in southern Texas or northern Mexico and fans out across the United States, ending in the Northwestern and Midwestern states bordering Canada, both east and west of the Mississippi.
- The *western stream* originates in California and moves up the West Coast to all Western states and from central California into Oregon and Washington (JBS International, 2022).
- California, Florida, and Texas are regarded as *sending states*, as they are often home states with long growing seasons where migrant streams begin and end. Workers move from areas with cotton, tree fruits and nuts, and vegetable crops to other areas where they harvest strawberries, cherries, watermelons, cantaloupes, or potatoes (Fig. 27-6).

Nomadic migrant workers travel away from home for several years, working from farm to farm and crop to crop and relying on word of mouth about job opportunities. Some of these workers eventually settle in the areas to which they have migrated, whereas others return to their home base. A given ethnic group usually follows its own particular stream and pattern of migration. New growth states, like Utah, Minnesota, Wisconsin, Nebraska, Kansas, Tennessee, and Arkansas, have seen immigrant populations increase. Some migrant workers find work in service sector jobs, and others labor in construction or landscaping, thus ending their need to move constantly with the crops. Married males who do not live

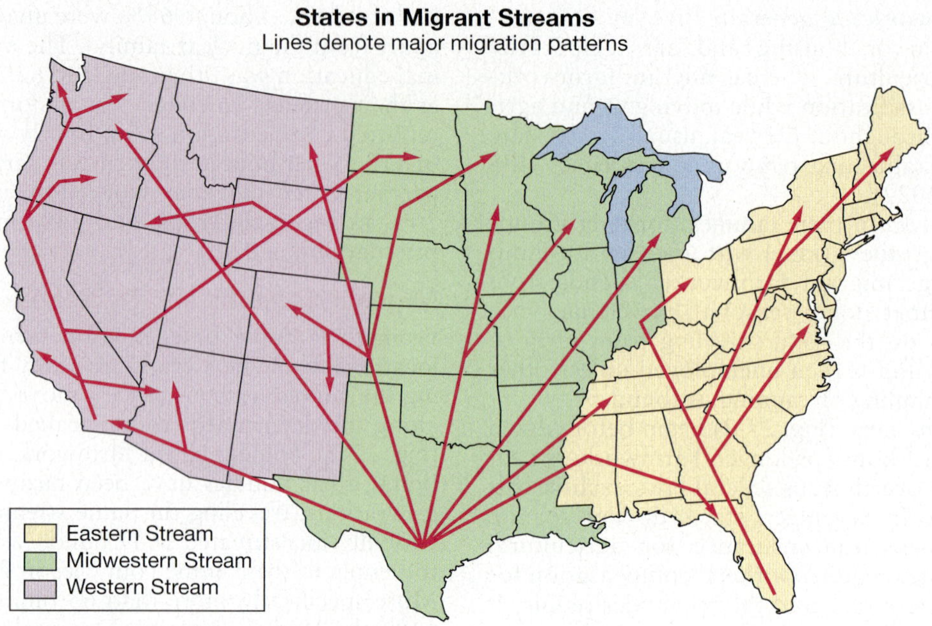

FIGURE 27-5 Migrant streams. (Source: Migrant Head Start Program, USHDHUD.)

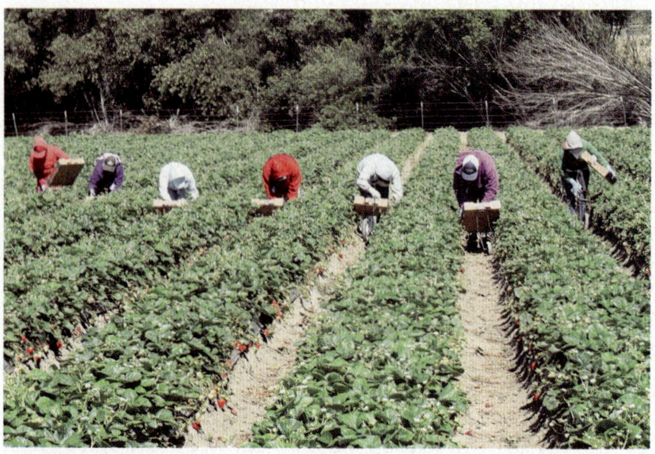

FIGURE 27-6 Migrant farmworkers pick and package strawberries directly into boxes in the Salinas Valley of central California.

with their families are more likely to migrate than those living with their families, often because of the need to send money back home.

RURAL HEALTH

Rural areas have 15% of the U.S. population (CDC, 2024a). Rural areas have historically had less racial diversity than urban areas. However, that is rapidly changing. More recently, rapid Hispanic growth areas are found in the South and Metropolitan areas (Fig. 27-7; JBS International, 2022). In rural counties, the White population has decreased, and other ethnic groups have increased in size, but still, only 11% of rural counties are majority non-White (Johnson & Lichter, 2022).

Urban and rural disparities have changed over time. The CDC (2024a) identifies rural communities as having a higher mortality rate than their urban counterparts from cancers, strokes, cardiovascular disease (CVD), unintentional injuries, and chronic respiratory diseases. Yet life expectancy has shifted, with those in rural areas living slightly longer than those in urban areas (Table 27-1). Health concerns of populations in rural areas, when compared to urban areas, are related to an older population, higher tobacco use, obesity, poverty, less seat belt use, injuries, and distance from healthcare providers (CDC, 2024a). Population trends directly relate to the kinds of health services needed in rural communities. Growing families with young children need maternity, pediatric, family health medical services, dental care, and mental health services. They also can benefit from health promotion and disease prevention activities. The older population, on the other hand, needs healthcare to manage an increased number of chronic health conditions. Rural communities need to provide access to nursing homes, home health, and rehabilitative services, as well as to hospitals, clinics, and health promotion programs that serve older adults and the entire community.

The Built Environment in Rural Areas: Relationship to Health

Even with the advances in medicine and genomics and the staggering percentage of our gross domestic product spent on healthcare, scientists feel that we will not be able to significantly improve our overall health and quality of life without addressing how we plan our living spaces. In a study conducted by Nguyen et al. (2019), areas characterized by street view images as "rural" (having limited infrastructure) had higher obesity, diabetes, fair/poor self-rated health, premature mortality, physical distress, physical inactivity, and teen birth rates but lower rates of excessive alcohol use. This is also further impacted by less access to quality healthcare. The **built environment** consists of the development of housing, highways, shopping areas, and other human-made features added to the natural environment.

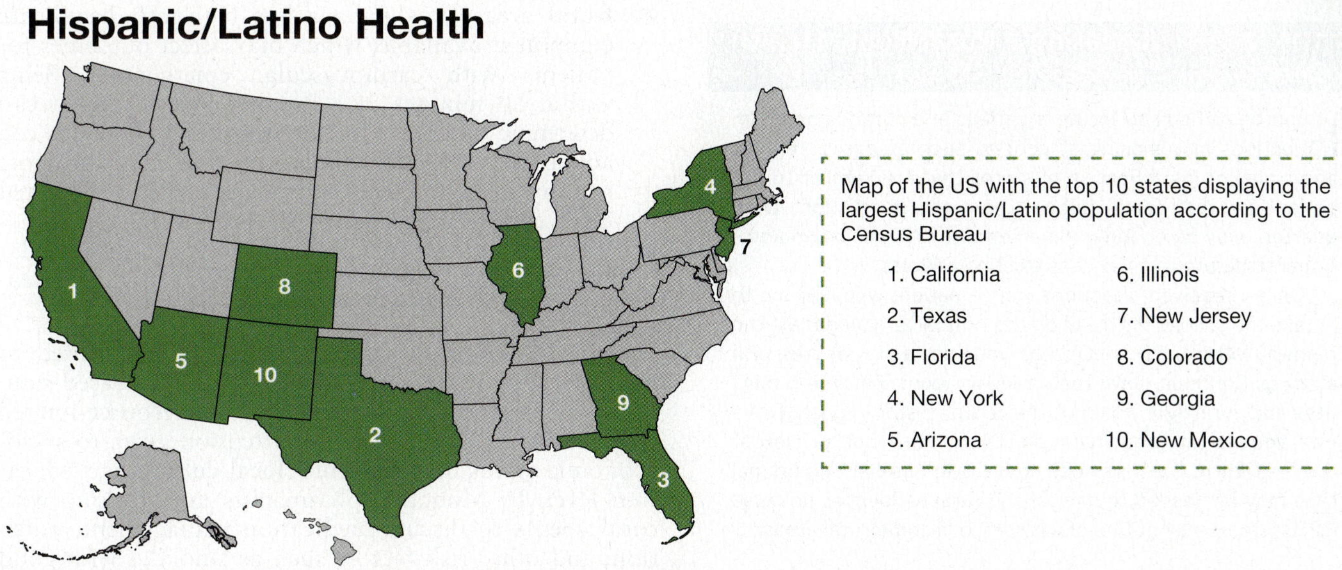

FIGURE 27-7 States with the largest Hispanic/Latinx populations. (Reprinted from U.S. Department of Health and Human Services Office of Minority Health. (n.d.). *Hispanic/Latino health*. https://minorityhealth.hhs.gov/hispaniclatino-health)

Encroachment of housing areas into natural habitats or farmlands can lead to wider human exposure to pesticides, herbicides, and other hazards such as mosquito-borne illnesses. Mass transit is not often available in suburban areas and is almost never found in rural areas. Opportunities for health-promoting behaviors are often more limited in rural areas. Deteriorating (or no) sidewalks can be a barrier to walking in rural areas. Exercise or fitness facilities, bike paths, jogging trails, and other incentives for physical activity are also often lacking in rural communities. Rural roads are another concern because they are often narrow, without streetlights, and poorly maintained. Slow-moving farm equipment traveling on rural roads, along with speeding and failure to use safety restraints, are often fatal conditions for drivers in rural areas.

Self, Home, and Community Care in Rural Areas

Historically, self-management of healthcare problems has been the most common way for rural people to cope with illness (Fig. 27-8). This can be viewed as a type of strength or as a limitation.

- Rural residents are often viewed as hardworking, traditional, hardy, self-reliant, and resistant to accepting help or services from outside agencies regarded by them as welfare-type programs.
- Rural clients often take care of illnesses or injuries on their own or have a supportive network to help them get their health needs met.
- Small communities commonly have strong social networks, but this type of familiarity may lead to problems with privacy and confidentiality, as well as stigma regarding mental health or substance misuse treatment.
- Because cost, travel, weather, and distance are barriers to obtaining health services from formal healthcare providers, rural clients may employ a variety of folk treatments and home remedies before consulting a nurse or a primary provider; such clients tend to visit providers at a much later stage than do people in urban areas.
- Rural residents may utilize primary providers who are more likely to provide care that is outside their specialty areas.
- Compared with hospitals that are less rural, CAHs have significantly higher patient mortality rates.
- Patients living in rural areas are known to have a higher risk for poor health outcomes, are more likely to smoke, and consume less healthy diets. These factors may contribute to higher mortality rates.
- The low population density in rural areas makes service delivery more difficult, especially for those with special health needs. The greater treatment barriers when living in an isolated area are geography and lack of adequate transportation.
- Home healthcare (HHC) is particularly difficult for both patients and nurses in sparsely populated areas. Locating addresses in very rural areas often takes

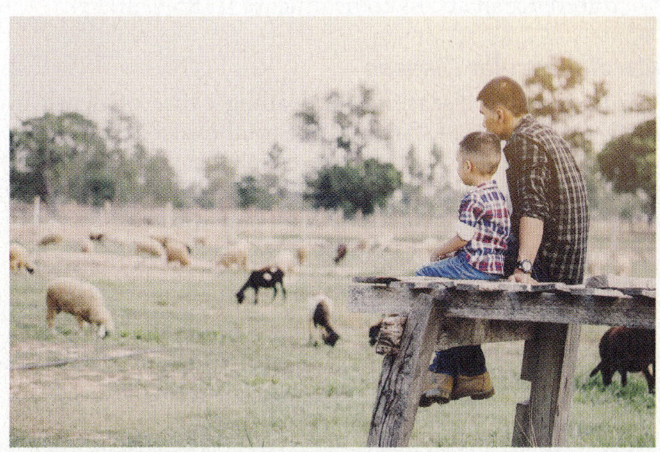

FIGURE 27-8 Life in a rural area may seem idyllic, but there are some significant risks associated with a rural lifestyle.

BOX 27-1 Locating a Rural Home Health Client

It can be difficult to locate a patient in a rural community. Directions may include structures such as barns, fences, and trees, or identification of stores that are familiar to the patient and their family but not the nurse. In addition, living quarters may be on long unmarked dirt roads or be an additional structure to an already existing address.

Once I received directions from a patient who told me to "...take the second dirt road on the right after you get off the highway (after the Dairy Queen), you'll see a big oak tree with a swing. Continue down that road for about 5 maybe 6 minutes and turn right again at the red one-story house. Drive until you see the green barn, don't turn there, but turn left at the next barn. You'll see our house over the hill." Additional time may be needed to navigate to rural residences because GPS systems may not be of assistance in some rural areas.

additional skills. (See Box 27-1 for the story of a home health nurse trying to locate a client's home.) HHC allows people to stay at home, supports their hardiness, and compensates for the long distance between home and formal healthcare.

Major Health Problems in Rural Communities

- Among major health problems affecting people in rural areas are cardiovascular disease, diabetes, and COPD. Geography, economics, and rural lifestyle factors may account for the higher rate of these major health problems. Rural populations also face greater barriers to diagnosis, treatment, and follow-up care. Some compliance issues with prescribed medication regimens may relate to the lack of health insurance and low-income levels in rural areas but could also be due to lower health literacy and education levels.
- Other problems with accessing care may involve transportation and weather. A lack of access to quality healthcare services has been a long-standing problem for rural Americans because of the significant difference in access to healthcare (HRSA, 2023).

Cardiovascular Disease

Cardiovascular disease is the leading cause of death in the United States (42%), and the total direct and indirect costs of CVD and stroke were estimated at over $239.9 billion between 2018 and 2019 (CDC, 2024b). Research demonstrates that geography may play a role.

- Mortality due to heart disease is highest in the southern United States, especially Alabama, Mississippi, Louisiana, Arkansas, and Oklahoma (CDC/NCHS, 2022). Regional variations have been noted in the prevalence of CVD and stroke. Studies have found increased stroke mortality in the South (stroke belt), and many researchers are focusing on the possible underlying risk factors related to geographical variations.
- Rural areas usually have less high-tech healthcare equipment available, which may affect outcomes for patients with cardiovascular emergencies. Being within 60 minutes of a Primary Stroke Center can determine outcomes for many patients. C/PHNs can advocate for better access to care and promote healthy lifestyle choices as well as population-targeted interventions to reduce stroke and CVD.
- Rural residents may ignore early cardiovascular symptoms and give little heed to preventive interventions such as exercise and low-fat diets.

Several models of care are being implemented to address rural CVD. In Maine, community-based education is targeting the specific needs of resource-limited residents who have CVD, with attention given to socioeconomic status and residents' local culture and education level. In Montana, pharmacists are working with rural clients to discuss medication management, nutrition, and other risk factors such as smoking with good success. In rural East Colorado, community health workers meet clients in local community facilities such as libraries and schools to provide screenings, referrals, services, and education (RHIH, 2022b).

Diabetes

Compared with urban populations, rural populations demonstrate a 16% higher prevalence of type 2 diabetes. In addition, there was a higher obesity prevalence in rural areas than in urban areas (Li & Whitacre, 2022).

Obesity

Although it is estimated that approximately 15% of the U.S. population resides in a rural area, the prevalence of obesity is 6.2 times greater than urban areas.

- Obesity prevalence was significantly higher among adults living in rural counties than among those living in metropolitan counties.
- Obesity is a leading cause of mortality in the United States and significantly impacts quality of life, vulnerability to CVD and stroke, renal failure, and blindness.
- West Virginia accounts for the highest national prevalence of obesity due to an aging population, physical inactivity, geography, lack of access to healthcare, and cultural mistrust of the healthcare system (Okobi et al., 2021).

C/PHNs, especially in rural and frontier areas, often provide follow-up for clients with diabetes who may be unable to regularly access their healthcare providers because of problems with distance or transportation. Home visits to check on their diet/exercise, blood glucose monitoring, and foot care are important safeguards for this population. Also, interventions targeted to behavior change can be helpful.

Chronic Obstructive Pulmonary Disease

Prevalence of COPD in rural counties was almost twice that of urban areas with high concentrations occurring in the Appalachia and the southern geographic regions (RHIH, n.d.-a).

- Cigarette smoking has a greater prevalence among rural adults than those adults residing in large and small urban areas.
- Decreased access to care, limited transportation, decreased specialty services, and fewer treatment options increase the disparity of COPD in rural versus urban areas.
- In addition, occupational exposures account for approximately 15% of COPD cases. Typical rural occupations expose people to very dusty or dirty air, chemicals, environmental pollutants, and occupational activities such as farming and coal mining.
- Even nonagricultural rural workers are much more likely to be exposed on the job to high levels of mold, nitrogen dioxide, and toxic dust (RHIH, 2023c).
- Rural people may have to travel longer distances to receive care and treatment, and rural areas may not have the healthcare infrastructure or workforce to provide pulmonary rehabilitation, oxygen therapy, or other specialized services and equipment.

Agriculture and Health

Although farming is not characteristic of all rural areas where agricultural production occurs, both direct and indirect effects on health can exist (Box 27-2). According to the Rural Health Information Hub (2023c), the following can affect the health of rural populations:

- Exposure to farm chemicals such as pesticides, fertilizers, and toxic gases, which can also affect surrounding water, air, and soil.
- Exposure to high dust levels, which contain mold, bacteria, and animal feces.
- Falls from farm equipment and ladders.
- Exposure to ultraviolet rays from the sun, resulting in skin cancer.
- Exposure to loud noise from machinery resulting in hearing loss.
- Stress from environmental factors (droughts, floods, fire), working long hours, and financial concerns.
- Risk of extreme weather conditions affecting health such as heatstroke, frostbite, or hypothermia.

BOX 27-2 Agricultural Accidents

Farm Tractor Accidents

Prior to the invention of mechanical farming equipment, a farmer might be injured by one of their horses or mules, or accidentally stabbed with a pitchfork. Today, tractors are involved in the majority of injuries and deaths. A rollover protective structure (ROPS), which is a roll cage over the tractor seat, can save lives; these structures were standard on every tractor manufactured in the country since 1985 (1959 in Sweden). If a farmer uses the seat belt and the tractor equipped with ROPS turns over, there is a good chance that they will survive the accident. Unfortunately, many farmers don't use seat belts, and many use older tractors without ROPS protection. There are many potential hazards on farms (e.g., falling bales of hay, heat stroke, dangerous equipment like hay balers, choppers, combines), but tractor rollovers and children falling from tractors are much too common and can often be prevented.

1. As the C/PHN in a farming community, you notice a high incidence of children severely injured from falls off tractors. Describe primary prevention techniques you could take.
2. You realize that you need to enlist the help of community members in order to make lasting changes. What community members and stakeholders could you develop partnerships with?

Death on the Farm

Agricultural deaths are not uncommon. Older males, youths, and hired hands are the most affected. Tractor rollovers are preventable; ROPS along with seatbelt use can eliminate these injuries. Engineering controls along with policies, practices, and protective equipment can control agricultural workplace accidents. There are 4.8 million tractors in use today, with only 50% equipped with ROPS. Injuries and fatalities have devastating effects: 1 in 7 farmers are permanently disabled, and 70% of

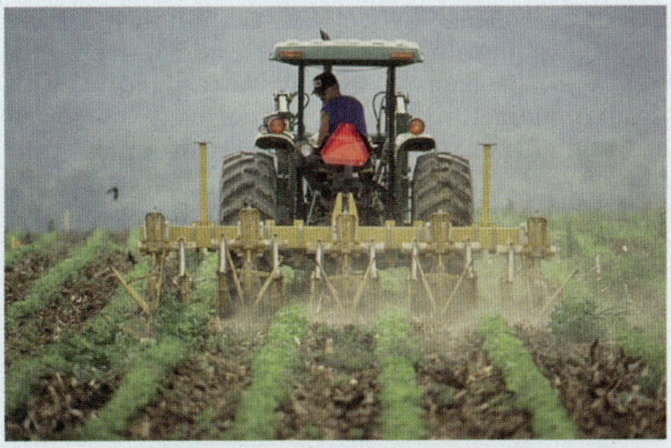

fatalities result in the farm closing within 5 years (Murphy, 2022). Retrofitting of equipment is an option, but cost, special clearance, tractor housing, and personal preferences are barriers for many farmers. Between 2012 and 2021, the highest percentage of agricultural worker fatalities occurred in 2019. Although the fatalities overall have declined, the populations most at risk are males age 55 and older. In 2021, 25 of the 133 fatal injuries that occurred in agricultural regions took place on nonpublic roadways (U.S. Bureau of Labor Statistics, 2023). Fatal injuries to agricultural workers in 2021 were the second lowest in a decade (https://www.bls.gov/opub/ted/2023/fatal-injuries-to-agricultural-workers-in-2021-were-the-second-lowest-in-a-decade.htm).

Telling the Story Project provides first-hand accounts of farm-related injuries and deaths told by farmers, agriculture workers, and family members. The website also includes vignettes, discussion guides, and resources. Go to https://tellingthestoryproject.org to learn more about the Telling the Story Project injury prevention program.

Photo by Keith Weller, USDA Agricultural ResearchService. https://www.ars.usda.gov/oc/images/photos/k5197-3

- Risk of injury related to operating farm machinery or working with livestock.
- Behavioral and mental health issues, including anxiety, depression, substance misuse, and suicide due to environmental, financial, and social factors.
- Child hazards from animals, farm equipment, vehicles (including all-terrain vehicles (ATVs)), grain bins, ponds, and chemicals/gases.
- Toxicity can develop due to pesticides and air pollutants. Other environmental hazards include the following: physical factors from machine-related injuries; biologic factors related to exposure to viruses, bacteria, parasites, and fungi; and social factors related to inadequate access to services, housing and food insecurity, and lack of social and workplace protections (Castillo et al., 2021). Exposure to synthetic pesticides may be associated with adverse health outcomes, including certain cancers, DNA damage, oxidative stress, neurologic disorders, respiratory diseases, metabolic disorders, and thyroid effects (Curl et al., 2020).

Pesticides are linked to disease and environmental risks through various routes (e.g., residues in food and drinking water). More on pesticides is discussed under migrant health. Many rural residents depend on their own well water for drinking, and water quality is monitored only sporadically by well owners and then usually only for heavy metals, contaminants, and microorganisms (Leys, 2023). Runoffs from chemicals and byproducts from manufacturing plants and farms get into well water. Another hazard is the placement of septic tanks in proximity to well water. About 24 million rural residents obtain drinking water from very small water systems without the monitoring and regulations associated with large urban water suppliers (Leys, 2023). Testing of small water systems should be done regularly to get a true picture of water quality.

Access to Healthcare in Rural Areas

Insurance, Managed Care, and Healthcare Services

Health insurance in today's market is costly, especially for individual purchasers. Some people, therefore, forego health insurance for themselves and their families. Depending on their income, people may or may not be eligible for Medicaid or State Children's Health Insurance Programs (S-CHIPs).

Historically, a traditional fee-for-service model delivered healthcare in rural and urban communities. However, that is changing, and it is challenging for rural providers to deliver the cost-effective, complex healthcare that people who live in rural areas need in small practices.

- Patients who live in rural areas often utilize family practice clinics.
- The managed care model, which attempts to control costs and improve healthcare delivery, has slowly diffused into rural communities. In addition, rural practitioners are reluctant to become part of organizations that negotiate to reduce their payments, as many of them already see a disproportionate number of Medicaid and uninsured patients that impact their bottom line.
- Low population density makes this type of healthcare insurance less profitable.
- More states are moving to Medicaid-managed care models, and Medicare offers this option to beneficiaries. This puts rural residents at a disadvantage, as they may have poor access to services because of distance and travel time (see Box 27-3).

BOX **27-3** PERSPECTIVES

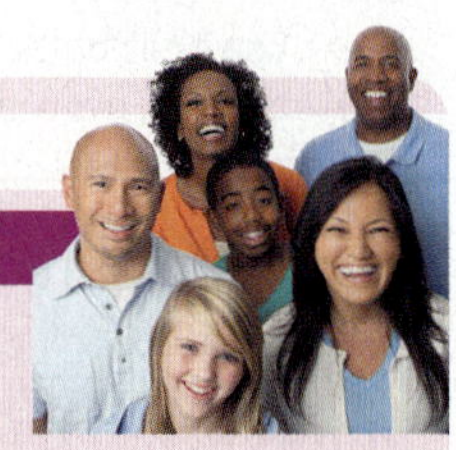

A Nursing Student Viewpoint on Rural Transportation

I live in a relatively large city of 450,000 people. When I started my community health nursing rotation, I was assigned to a rural county public health department in an adjoining county over 50 miles from my house. When I arrived for my first clinical day, my professor told me that I was assigned to see clients in an isolated community another hour away from the health department! There was nothing but farmland between the county seat and this small town.

After I got over my frustration about traveling such long distances, I began to visit some of my families and started to enjoy my time with them. They were so appreciative and open to my suggested interventions. I really seemed to be making a difference. One older gentleman, Armando, who had diabetes spoke very little English. He lived with his wife of 50 years, who spoke almost no English. Their children had moved away in order to go to school and get better jobs. His diabetes was not well controlled, and the rural health clinic (RHC) FNP suggested that he see a specialist (actually an internist) in the largest city in the county. I helped him arrange for an early afternoon visit with the doctor and made sure he could catch the county bus between the smaller communities and the county seat.

When I came back for a follow-up visit the next week, I was shocked to learn that Armando's appointment had been pushed back to 4:30 p.m. because of the doctor's involvement in hospital emergencies, and by the time Armando was finished with his appointment, the county bus service had ended. Armando, with no money and no one to call for a ride, began walking back to his home—over 52 miles away! About halfway home, a farm truck driver gave him a lift to the large cotton farm a few miles from his home. I never realized how difficult it was for rural people to get to their medical appointments. I thought that the bus would not be a problem, but I learned my lesson. Now, I make sure that the primary provider's office understands the patient's circumstances and the importance of getting them back to the bus stop in time to make the last bus.

—*Andrea, senior nursing student*

Building provider networks in rural communities is both time- and effort-intensive because rural providers are often inexperienced with managed care organizations. The federal government provides support for **rural health clinics** in areas designated as underserved and nonurban; differences in effectiveness and efficiency have been noted in larger clinics versus smaller clinics (RHIH, 2023d). These clinics have served rural clients for more than 30 years, and they are an important source of healthcare.

- **Rural** areas are characterized by a lack of core healthcare services (e.g., primary care, hospital care, emergency medical services, long-term care, mental health and substance misuse counseling services, dental care, and public health services).
- Shortages were noted for primary providers and dentists. Ninety percent of rural counties are designated as HPSAs with a limited number of or no providers, and 83% of areas lack dentists. Unfortunately, the number of providers entering rural health is declining, whereas the number is increasing in urban areas. Rural areas with a higher population and a hospital had a higher percentage of providers than areas with fewer people and no hospital (Patterson et al., 2024; Pender et al., 2023).
- Family nurse practitioners and primary provider assistants are providers who can care for rural populations.

Several factors have a role in the recruitment and job satisfaction of family primary providers in rural health: increase of medical schools that offer residencies in rural health, growing up or vacationing in a rural area, broad scope of practice and autonomy, and the natural environment (Patterson et al., 2024; Pender et al. 2023). Unpredictable weather adds to potential barriers for rural clients. Snow, ice, wind, flash floods, and rain can make travel dangerous, even over short distances.

- Parents may decide not to risk driving on poorly maintained roads to get their children immunized or to have their own hypertension evaluated (Fig. 27-9).
- Older people may choose to delay healthcare when long travel times, especially in isolated rural areas, are involved.
- Rural populations have disproportionately high injury mortality rates from motor vehicle accidents (Governors Highway Safety Association, 2022).
- The high mortality rates from motor vehicle accidents are due to driving under the influence, speeding, not wearing seat belts limited number of emergency medical services, and lack of nearby hospitals with emergency departments (Governors Highway Safety Association, 2022).

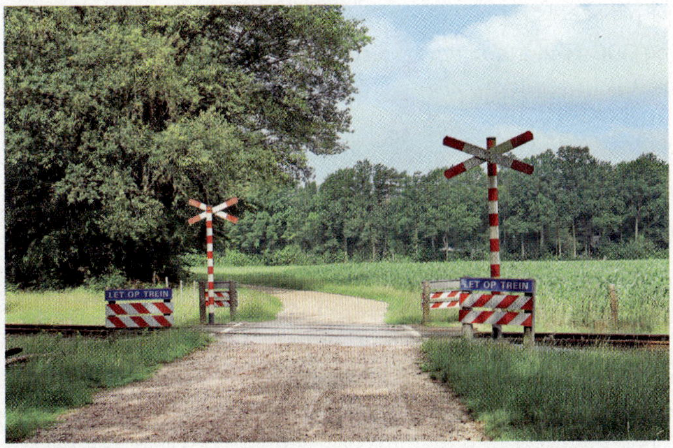

FIGURE 27-9 A railroad crossing along a dirt road across farmland.

New Approaches to Improve Access

The *Healthy People 2030* document mandates improvements in access, health education, health screening, immunizations, environmental health, and disease morbidity for the United States. Creative ways of delivering these and other services to rural clients need to be explored. Access to care is a social justice issue; clients who live in rural areas should receive quality healthcare, regardless of where they choose to live. The *Healthy People 2030* plan of action includes investment in health and well-being for all people. The first three overarching goals of *Healthy People 2030* focus on the elimination of health disparities, improving health access, and creating healthy environments.

Faith community nursing has been a staple in rural areas, as well as in some urban communities, but is gaining momentum as more formal interventions are developed. These nurses' partner with religious leaders and community members to improve the health of parishioners. The setting is a trusted environment, which fosters spiritual care. Nurses conduct screenings and education on chronic diseases, nutrition, and coping strategies. Faith community nurses are instrumental in integrating one's religious beliefs with medical interventions (Kruse-Diehr et al., 2021).

Another approach that has been successful in numerous rural areas is the use of *mobile clinics*. These clinics bring healthcare providers to remote places for health screenings, immunizations, dental care, mental health visits, and other services.

- Mobile health clinics are frequently staffed by NPs and can improve access to healthcare for resource-limited residents.
- They are often available to residents on evenings and weekends, offer culturally sensitive and bilingual outreach, and care for uninsured clients.
- Although the aim of the Affordable Care Act (ACA) includes increasing the number of insured people in the United States and overcoming health disparities, it has no provisions for mobile medical clinics, which appear to serve as an important component of healthcare delivery, especially to vulnerable populations.
- In addition, mobile dental clinics are an innovative solution to providing care and improving physical access to dental care for the **medically underserved population** in resource-limited urban and remote rural communities.
- Many mobile clinics provide existing dental services at lower or no cost to the user.

School-based clinics can improve access for schoolchildren (and sometimes their families) but may be less prominent in rural areas. These clinics provide available, community-based, affordable, and culturally acceptable care to well and sick children. Often, grant-supported, school-based clinics facilitate the receipt of health education and primary care by children who are otherwise without easy access to health services. In addition, school-based health centers are associated with improved educational status, including higher grade point averages and higher rates of high school completion (U.S. Department of Health and Human Services National Advisory Council on Migrant Health [NACMH], 2023).

Telehealth, another approach to increasing access to care, provides electronically transmitted clinician consultation between the client and the healthcare provider. It is also useful for patient and professional health education, public health applications, and health administration. Specialty healthcare also may be accessed, with patients and providers connected via two-way audiovisual transmission over telephone lines or the internet, thus obviating the need for patients to leave their residences. Online counseling and remote counseling link rural clients with urban behavioral health services. Counseling services can also be provided online in Spanish.

Telehealth is especially critical in rural and other remote areas that lack sufficient healthcare services, including specialty care. The range and use of telehealth services have expanded over the past decades, along with the role of technology in improving and coordinating care. Grants and other funding are available to promote the use of this technology (RHIH, 2024d). Go to the Rural Health Information Hub at https://www.ruralhealthinfo.org/topics/telehealth-health-it# to learn more about the benefits of telehealth in rural communities.

Healthy People 2030 Goals

Because of the unique health issues facing rural America, *Healthy People 2030* identifies broad areas of concern such as access to health services, environmental health, and health communication/information technology (Box 27-4). There are data to substantiate continued problems with access to healthcare and insurance, as well as emergency services, in rural areas. As discussed previously, there is a higher rate of CVD and diabetes, along with obesity and tobacco use among rural populations.

- Primary care providers, dentists, and specialty providers are lacking in rural America.
- Teens living in rural areas have a higher rate of tobacco and alcohol use than their urban counterparts (Egan et al., 2024).

BOX 27-4 *HEALTHY PEOPLE 2030*

Health Issues in Rural America

Access to Health Services

AHS-01	Increase the proportion of people with health insurance
AHS-02	Increase the proportion of people with dental insurance
AHS-05	Reduce the proportion of people who can't get the dental care they need when they need it
AHS-08	Increase the proportion of adults who get recommended evidence-based preventative health care
AHS-R02	Increase the use of telehealth to improve access to health services
ECBP-D06	Increase the number of community-based organizations providing population-based primary prevention services

Diabetes

D-09	Reduce the rate of death from any cause in adults with diabetes
D-D01	Increase the proportion of eligible people completing CDC-recognized type 2 diabetes preventative programs

Environmental Health

EH-06	Reduce the amount of toxic pollutants released into the environment

Health Communication and Health Information Technology

HC/HIT-06	Increase the proportion of adults offered online access to their medical record

Heart Disease and Stroke

HDS-01	Improve cardiovascular health in adults

Reprinted from Office of Disease Prevention and Health Promotion (ODPHP). (n.d.-c). *Healthy People 2030 browse objectives.* https://health.gov/healthypeople/objectives-and-data/browse-objectives

- Unintentional overdose deaths due to nonopioid use disproportionately impact rural over urban settings in the United States. When comparing causes of death due to substances, methamphetamine was the only substance that killed more people in rural areas than in urban communities (Indiana Department of Health, 2024). Unknown to people who use this substance, methamphetamine may be mixed with fentanyl to enhance the effect, thus increasing the risk of drug overdose and death.

Opioid-related mortality rates have reached epidemic levels in rural and urban communities, killing more people than any other substance (Indiana Department of Health, 2024). Rural areas lack many of the treatment services urban areas may have. Drug treatment programs within rural areas come with challenges. Rural areas are often small, close-knit communities, which raise concerns about privacy. The limited number of treatment facilities may require long commutes and waitlists; local care providers may not be aware of current treatment options outside their area (Stopka et al., 2024).

Cancer disparities are found in rural populations. Recent research has shown a lower incidence rate of cancers in rural areas when compared with urban communities. However, the mortality rate in rural communities is higher than the mortality rates of urban and nonurban areas combined. Death from lung and colorectal cancers is higher than in urban areas (National Cancer Institute [NCI], n.d.). This may be due to fewer cancer screenings than in urban areas, inadequate cancer care, and a higher prevalence of obesity and tobacco use. Rural areas have fewer primary care providers and even fewer specialty providers. In fact, only 3% of oncologists practice in rural areas, and 70% of rural communities do not have an oncologist (NCI, n.d.). Fortunately, some urban teaching hospitals are partnering with rural clinics to provide services in communities (Association for American Medical Colleges [AAMC], 2023). Additionally, the USDHHS (2023) provided $11 million to expand residence programs in rural areas.

Mental and behavioral health is another concern in rural settings as 20% of rural residents aged 18 years and older have a mental health issue and the incidence of anxiety and suicidal thoughts has increased since the pandemic (RHIH, 2024e). The prevalence of mental health issues is similar between rural and urban; yet, there are limited services available to address these issues in rural communities. Accessibility of services, availability of services, and acceptability are all barriers for those residing in rural areas (RHIH, 2024f).

Rural C/PHNs need to consider the *Healthy People 2030* objectives' priority areas as guides for improving the health status of clients in rural communities.

Community/Public Health Nursing in Rural Settings

Rural areas promote a broad scope of C/PHN practice, as these nurses deal with a wide variety of issues—immunizations, home health, school nursing, maternal–child health, emergency preparedness, as well as communicable disease/epidemiology. Rural health departments are often lacking in technological and communication systems, but there is an even greater need for reliable communication capability and training opportunities for rural C/PHNs who provide the majority of care in rural and frontier communities (Knudsen & Meit, n.d.).

Rural C/PHNs most often grew up in rural areas or lived for a time in small communities. They frequently have extended family, are active members of their community, and are highly respected professionals.

The rural community health nurse plays many roles:

1. *Advocate*: Assists rural clients, families, and populations in obtaining the best possible care
2. *Coordinator/case manager*: Connects rural clients with needed health and social services, often assisting with information on transportation
3. *Health teacher*: Provides education to people, families, or groups on health promotion and prevention or other health-related topics
4. *Referral agent*: Makes appropriate connections between rural clients and urban service providers
5. *Mentor*: Guides new community health nurses, nursing students, and other nurses new to the rural community
6. *Change agent/researcher*: Suggests new approaches to solving patient care or community health problems based on research, professional literature, and community assessment
7. *Collaborator*: Seeks ways to work with other health and social service professionals to maximize outcomes for individual clients and the community at large
8. *Activist*: With a deep understanding of the community and its population, takes appropriate risks to improve the community's health

Rural C/PHNs can use autonomy in daily practice. Nurses must rapidly assume independent and interdependent decision-making roles because of the small workforce and large workload. Rural C/PHNs may experience the challenge of physical isolation from personal and professional opportunities associated with urban areas. Rural nurses may also feel isolated in their clinical practices because of the scarcity of professional colleagues (Box 27-5).

There are benefits to rural nursing when one considers lower housing costs, less traffic to contend with, slower pace of life, and open spaces. From a professional standpoint, C/PHNs who practice in rural communities have a broader scope of practice, higher level of independence, and need the skills to make do with less resources.

MIGRANT HEALTH

Have you ever thought about the people who harvest the fruits and vegetables that you eat? Have you ever thought about who they are, where they come from, where they live, or what their health is like? Whatever your political, social, or ethical views on this subject, migrant workers and their families often cross paths with C/PHNs, and we need to understand them in order to effectively provide care (Box 27-6).

BOX 27-5 STORIES FROM THE FIELD

Frontier Nursing: Then and Now

As described in Chapter 2, Mary Breckinridge founded the Frontier Nursing Service in 1925, with nurse-midwives providing care to clients in their own homes. Nurses traveled by horseback and on foot into the sparsely populated hollows of Kentucky (American Association for the History of Nursing, 2018). Today, NPs working in nurse-managed clinics in rural Appalachian communities in Virginia were interviewed about their practices, in a classic study by Caldwell (2007), and spoke about their connections to the people and communities they serve. One said, "Here you get to know the whole family and that is rewarding...you know what is important to them...what their worries and concerns are....so you probably get closer to your patient in this area than you might outside here. It becomes an extended family, which is very rewarding" (p. 76).

Another NP described a man with severe COPD who visited her clinic. He was also a patient of another area provider, but when the NP examined the man, she noticed the gauze 4 × 4 he had on the back of his neck and enquired about it. The man said he "cut himself shaving." The NP pressed the man to see the wound and found that he had "cancer with the bone exposed," describing it as "the most awful thing that I had ever seen in my life. I could put my fist in there. And you could see his carotids pulsating." She told the patient how serious this was and arranged for a plastic surgeon to see him right away. He had a total neck resection and recovered completely. She reflected, "What if I had accepted his story about the sore and it being all right? It was not what he was coming to see me for...I look at more than just the chief complaint" (p. 77).

1. *What factors are important to consider when caring for clients in a rural setting?*
2. *What situations have you seen in rural settings?*
3. *Knowing more about rural health, would you do anything differently in this scenario?*

Migrant farmworkers are an integral part of the farming community in the United States and across the world. The agricultural industry relies heavily on migrant workers to harvest the almost endless array of fresh produce that appears year-round in supermarkets across the United States as fresh, frozen, and canned fruits and vegetables.

- Opponents of immigration restrictions predict that imposing them would jeopardize the supply of labor available to farmers during critical plant and harvest seasons (USDA, 2023b).
- Nearly 3 million seasonal and migrant farmworkers (NCFH, 2022a) provide labor for the $28 billion vegetable and fruit crops of the United States (USDA, 2024b).
    - Sixty-three percent were born in Mexico (NCFH, 2022a).
    - Fifteen percent of agricultural workers are migrant farmworkers (NCFH, 2022a).
    - It is estimated that 41% of farmworkers are undocumented (USDA, 2023b).

BOX 27-6 WHAT DO *YOU* THINK?

Undocumented Migrant Workers

There are many critics of undocumented migrant workers. Some feel that their willingness to work for low wages keeps overall wages lower for everyone working in agriculture, while others feel that migrant workers are taking jobs away from Americans. The United Farmworkers, an agricultural worker union, introduced the *Take Our Jobs* program in 2010 to address these issues. Unemployed Americans were invited to work in the fields along with migrant farmworkers, but very few accepted this invitation; those that did attempt it had a difficult time keeping up with the grueling pace of work. Stephen Colbert, a television show host and comedian, picked beans and packed corn as part of the challenge, and filmed some of his workday experiences for his late-night show. He also gave testimony to Congress on the need for better wages, living conditions, and visa programs for these workers.

What do you think about the issue? You can view this testimony first-hand in the following video (https://www.youtube.com/watch?v=0TYyeNU8Wvc). You can also view Charlie LeDuff taking this migrant challenge in the San Joaquin, California, fields (https://www.youtube.com/watch?v=J7TGWaHaUeU).

In addition, a government project was trialed in 1965, when the Bracero Agreement between the United States and Mexico, providing Mexican agricultural workers in the U.S. fields, expired. Farmers complained, stating that crops would rot in their fields. Therefore, project A-TEAM was created—Athletes in Temporary Employment as Agricultural Manpower. A nationwide call was placed to recruit high school males, providing field labor as their summer job. Although initially 18,000 were registered, only 3300 actually worked in the fields. Ironically, even though the initial intent was to recruit "jocks," many of the recruits were not athletes but just young males looking for summer jobs. For filling crates with fruits or vegetables, they were paid minimum wage—$1.40 per hour at that time—plus a small stipend (i.e., 5 cents for every crate filled with 30 to 36 cantaloupe). Work was hard, the days were long, temperatures were hot, and the workers were not allowed to return home until summer's end. Many of them did not last the entire stint. A university history professor, Lori Flores, was quoted as saying, "The A-TEAM reveals a very important reality: It's not about work ethic for undocumented workers. It's about the fact that this labor is not meant to be done under such bad conditions and bad wages" (Arellano, 2018. p. 7). The A-TEAM was considered a giant failure and was never tried again!

AGRICULTURAL LABOR AND IMMIGRATION POLICIES CHANGING

Despite their importance to American agriculture, migrant workers often go unnoticed beyond the fringes of the camps and farms to which they travel in order to pursue their livelihood. The number of migrant agricultural workers in a particular region, state, or even in the nation is difficult to estimate due to high mobility, language and cultural differences, and varying levels of citizenship status (RHIH, 2024f). California (49%), Washington (9%), Florida (7%), and Texas (5%) currently have the highest number of migrant farmworkers (Center for Migration Studies [CMS], 2022). All endure backbreaking, menial labor for low wages and are often deprived of basic rights to safe working conditions, adequate sanitation/housing, healthcare, and quality education for their children (see Boxes 27-7 and 27-8).

The United States has passed legislation affecting agricultural workers. States across the nation have implemented strict policies and laws to address growing numbers of unauthorized workers, whether they work on farms or elsewhere. One such law went into effect in Florida, which makes it a felony to transport undocumented workers into the state, employers of 25 people or more must verify legal residency, and hospitals that accept Medicaid must report the cost of care of patients that are undocumented (Daly, 2023). Farmers and ranchers who hire more than 25 people are concerned about the new law and its effect on business; some have hired lawyers to help with documentation paperwork. The C/PHN must be aware of and understand the stress and fear undocumented workers experience in order to provide the care needed.

The H-2A Temporary Agricultural Program provides a legal means to bring foreign-born workers to the United States to perform seasonal farm labor on a temporary basis; these consist of crop farmers and producers of livestock. Employers must demonstrate, and the U.S. Department of Labor must certify, that efforts to recruit U.S. workers were unsuccessful. Employers must also pay a state-specific minimum wage, provide housing, and pay for transportation. In April 2024, the "Improving Protections for Workers in Temporary Agricultural Employment in the United States," also called "The Worker Protection Rule" went into effect. This rule further protects the agricultural workers' rights and offers protection against retaliation for whistleblowing—i.e., advocating for themselves and others. To learn more about "The Worker Protection Rule" go to https://www.dol.gov/agencies/eta/foreign-labor/programs/h-2a (U.S. Department of Labor [DOL], 2024).

Migrant Farmworkers: Profile of a Nomadic Population

Maintaining a low public profile, migrant workers are often underrepresented in mainstream society. Common ailments include infectious diseases (e.g., TB, parasites), gastrointestinal disorders, dermatitis, pesticide exposure, emotional distress and depression, vision and eye

BOX 27-7 U.S. Migrant Worker Demographics

Origin and Nationality
- Most are foreign-born (73%), with about 61% from Mexico.
- Seventy-one percent have been in the United States 15 or more years, while 5% for 1 year.
- Fifty-eight percent of the crop workers are authorized, 38% are citizens, and 20% have work visas or green cards.

Age
- The age of agricultural workers in the United States has been increasing since 2000.
- Seventy-one percent are between the ages of 14 and 19.
- Eleven percent are between 20 and 24 years.
- Twenty-five percent are between 25 and 34 years.
- Twenty-two percent are between 35 and 44 years.
- Eighteen percent are between 45 and 54 years.
- Thirteen percent are between 55 and 64 years.
- Five percent are 65 years or more.

Sex/Marital Status/Offspring
- Sixty-eight percent of agricultural workers are male, and 32% are female.
- Sixty percent are married.
- Forty-nine percent are parents, of those 69% have one to two children, and 19% have three children, and 12% had four or more children in the household.

Education
- Four percent have no formal education.
- Thirty percent have completed grades 1 to 6.
- Twenty-three percent have completed grades 7 to 9.
- Twenty-seven percent have completed grades 10 to 12.
- Sixteen percent have completed education beyond grade 12.

English Language
- Ninety-eight percent speak Spanish well.
- Twenty-seven percent cannot speak English "at all."
- Thirty-six percent speak English "a little" or "somewhat."
- Thirty-seven percent speak English "well."

Migrant Status and Seasonality
- Approximately 15% of farmworkers are considered migrant (traveling 75 miles to obtain farm jobs).
- Many travel to multiple farm sites within a year.
- About 85% are considered seasonal agricultural workers.
  - Most (38%) work in fruit and nut crops.
  - Others (24%) work in horticulture (23%) and vegetables (20%) (JBS International, 2022).

Compensation
- Mean and median personal income is $20,000 to $24,999. Mean and median family income is $30,000 to $34,999.
- Wages increase with years at the same farm: Starting at $13.73 and increasing to $15.56.
- Forty-one percent of migrant workers have a family income below the poverty level.
- Twenty-eight percent of employers offer health benefits, 45% are covered under unemployment insurance, and 72% have workers' compensation.
- The majority are paid low hourly wages (85%).

Source: JBS International (2022).

BOX 27-8 STORIES FROM THE FIELD

A Case of Active Tuberculosis in a Rural Community

As the C/PHN in a rural community, I received many types of referrals for families including maternal, child, older adults, child abuse, or communicable disease cases. The small public health district office was located in a small agricultural town of approximately 20,000 people, with a large Spanish-speaking population. One day, I responded to a new, active tuberculosis (TB) case. A 20-year-old Hispanic male had been in the county hospital and was in respiratory isolation. I would need to examine his living conditions and his contacts.

Gregorio explained that he and his brothers had traveled from his home country of Chiapas, Mexico, to the United States. There were 20 names in total that were close contacts and needed follow-up. They lived in a two-bedroom home, without furniture, and each man took a spot on the floor to sleep at night. One by one, each was interviewed for TB risk assessment and a TB skin test was placed. On my return to the home 2 days later, skin tests were read, and those who had positive tests were referred to the community health center for chest x-rays.

Gregorio was hospitalized until he was no longer communicable. The county health department instituted daily directly observed therapy and assisted with transportation to medical appointments.

1. *What do you see as the role of the community health nurse in this situation?*
2. *Discuss how communicable disease control and surveillance looks different in a rural setting.*

—Judy H. Pedro, MSN, RN, APHN-BC

problems, cancer, and chronic illnesses, such as asthma, bronchitis, diabetes, and hypertension.

- They are often affected by poverty, poor nutrition, substandard housing conditions, extended working hours, and grueling, often unsafe, working conditions.
- Although migrant families are in dire need of health resources, various economic, cultural, and language barriers prevent this aggregate from accessing available health services.
  - Poverty, frequent mobility, low literacy, and language and cultural barriers impede farmworkers' access to cost-effective healthcare and social services.
- Fifty-one percent of agricultural workers reported being covered by workers' compensation insurance (NCFH, 2022a).

Migrant workers often live and work in areas where healthcare practitioners are in short supply. Among Latino/Latinx immigrants, common barriers to utilizing the healthcare system include access to insurance, limitations in the type of healthcare utilized, discrimination in healthcare services, immigration fears, stigmas, lack of social and financial capital, communication problems, and long waiting periods for access to healthcare (Migrant Clinicians Network, n.d.). Additional barriers include limited transportation, prejudice because of immigrant status, mistreatment because they are "undocumented," lack of time-efficient healthcare delivery methods, increasing cost of healthcare, and needing services not being offered (NCFH, 2023a).

Historical Background

Both historically and internationally, farmers have rarely been able to permanently employ the large workforce needed to harvest their crops.

- During the 1920s, over half a million Mexicans migrated to the United States, many drawn to work in seasonal agriculture. With the great depression, many of the small, independently run farms went bankrupt, and citizens were concerned about limited employment opportunities.
- The United States has experienced farm labor shortages for the past century, becoming more severe during World War II (WWII). To meet the demand for farm laborers, the Bracero Program was created in 1942, which allowed over 4 million guest workers to come in from rural, poor areas in Mexico due to agricultural worker shortages in the United States.
- In 1964, the program was replaced by the H2 Temporary Guest Worker program, with H-2A being agricultural workers and H-2B being guest workers who perform nonagricultural work.
- Some studies have noted an increase in the agricultural worker population over the last decade, and the presence of agricultural workers has been shown to increase the overall economic output of the regions in which they work. In fact, research conducted about the agricultural economy of Michigan found that agricultural workers contributed over $23.3 million to the state's economy annually by enabling farmers to produce higher-value crops after wages and housing were deducted. Stringent immigration laws passed in Arizona and Georgia demonstrated the devastating impact of farm labor shortages (NCFH, 2022a).

Living apart from society, the plight of migrant farmworkers was largely ignored until exposure in a 1960 television documentary—Edward R. Murrow's *Harvest of Shame*—created a national outcry. This led to the passage of the Migrant Health Act of 1962, which addressed the specific health needs of migrant workers for the first time in U.S. history. This act authorized the delivery of primary and supplementary health services to migrant farmworkers (NCFH, 2022a).

Primary and preventive healthcare services are provided to migrant workers and their families throughout more than 500 clinic sites. However, funding is often inadequate, and many clinics are not sufficiently staffed or operated to meet the health needs of this aggregate and their dependents. Additionally, although these clinics exist throughout the United States, large geographic regions are not served well or at all. Other services, such as *promotora programs*, employ members of the aggregate and act as the bridge between the community and the healthcare system. Promotoras are trusted and share the same culture as the aggregate. One role they serve is providing health education regarding the health risks surrounding farmwork (RHIH, n.d.-b).

Migrant Lifestyle

To understand the health needs of migrant farmworkers and their families, it is important to realize their lifestyle. Migrant workers and their families endure a transient and uncertain life, with long hours, stressful working conditions, low wages, and poor healthcare. Substandard housing, unsafe working conditions, and language barriers make life even more difficult (USDHUD, n.d.). Over 70% have not graduated from high school, and 42% do not speak English. While 71% have been in the United States for a decade or more, many have only been in the United States for under a year (CMS, 2022). Migrant workers are exposed to environmental hazards such as pesticides, extreme temperatures, and chemicals.

- Up to 20,000 pesticide injuries are reported yearly by the 2 million agricultural workers in the United States (Stoklosa et al., 2020).
- Those in agriculture and farming are at risk for musculoskeletal injury. In addition, limited or no PPE may be provided (Stoklosa et al., 2020).
- Workplace demands such as pressure to work without breaks and jobs that are physically demanding coupled with fear of job insecurity and deportation affect workplace stress (Porru & Baldo, 2022).

Depending on the economy and the crop, a migrant farmworker's income varies widely. Federal poverty guidelines for people are $13,590 and $27,750 for a family of four. Ninety-three percent of migrant workers fall below the federal poverty level (NCFH, 2022b). Even so, despite their poverty, most farmworkers are not eligible for social services. Less than 1% of all farmworkers use general assistance welfare, 2% use social security, and fewer than 15% are Medicaid recipients (NCFH, 2022b).

Migrant Hero

César Chavez founded the National Farm Workers Association (later changed to United Farm Workers), the first union in agricultural labor history to successfully organize migrant farmworkers.

- As a child, he traveled with his family to harvest crops, but they rarely had enough food to eat and often lived in shacks.
- Work was frequently scarce, and wages were low.
- Chavez attended as many as 65 different schools and dropped out of school upon completing eighth grade to help support his family by working full time in the fields (Biography, 2019).
- Chavez organized many successful strikes and boycotts, the most famous being the boycott of California grapes against the indiscriminate use of spraying by growers in 1968.
- His legacy is an example of how people can unite to build power together.
- Throughout his life, he ignored personal hardships to continue the struggle with union victories and losses. Chavez and his union won several victories for migrant farmworkers when many growers signed contracts with the union.
- As a labor leader, Chavez employed nonviolent means to bring attention to the plight of farmworkers. He led marches, organized boycotts, and went on several hunger strikes (Biography, 2019).

Health Risks of Migrant Workers and Their Families

Poverty, transient lifestyle, low literacy, language barriers, and cultural barriers impede migrant workers' access to social services and cost-effective healthcare (RHIH, 2024f). In addition, migrant workers who use health services must overcome other issues: limited means of transportation, lack of time-efficient healthcare delivery methods, and the medical referral system. According to National Center for Farmworker Health (NCFH) (2022b) data, the most common diagnoses reported by these Health Centers for migrant workers included the following:

- Overweight/obesity
- Diabetes
- Hypertension
- Anxiety
- Substance misuse disorders

Migrant workers who are lawfully in the United States (including H-2A workers) may receive coverage under the ACA. Legal farmworkers whose income is below 138% of the federal poverty line may receive healthcare through Medicaid. Unauthorized workers cannot receive health insurance (RHIH, 2024f).

Notably, compared to their documented working peers, undocumented migrant farmworkers are less likely to utilize private health clinics and are even less likely to rely on migrant health centers, even when these providers are their most viable sources of health services (Ornelas et al., 2020). National statistics on migrant seasonal workers are sparse, with much of the data regional and only sporadically collected. Some of the statistics include the following:

- Migrant workers are a vulnerable and underserved population, with an average life expectancy of 49 years, compared to 77.2 years for most Americans. They have a greater disease burden than other populations and work in occupations with high hazard levels.
- TB rates remain high for migrant workers who are at increased risk for contracting viral, fungal, bacterial, and parasitic infections (MCN, 2024a).
- Migrant children may be delayed in immunizations due to the constant moving or overimmunized due to no lack of records and may lack consistent education due to migration. Health concerns are commonly related to food insecurity and overcrowded housing (MCN, 2024b).
- Migrant children of farmworkers experience the same environmental health-related problems as their parents. One extra burden of these children is the fear of deportation of an undocumented parent (MCN, 2024b).
- The data indicate that HIV/AIDS is escalating among migrant farmworkers, and in some areas, it is 10 times higher than the national average. Recommendations

are provided for improving health outcomes among migrant workers, preventing HIV transmission, and providing continuous comprehensive care and support for HIV-infected migrant farmworkers (Rojas et al., 2020).

- Poverty, migration patterns, lack of knowledge regarding HIV, lower educational level, and language barriers may make it harder for some Hispanic/Latinx individuals to get HIV testing and care. Hispanic/Latinx individuals who are undocumented may be less likely to use HIV prevention services, get an HIV test, or get treatment for HIV because of concerns about being arrested and deported (Rojas et al., 2020).
- Migrants disproportionately suffer from the effects of COVID-19 due to economic hardships brought on by shutdowns and social distancing; contagion risk due to overcrowding, predisposed health issues, lack of access to healthcare, and uninsured status; and as targets for hate and discrimination (Migrant Policy Institute, 2020).

Occupational Hazard

The hazards of agricultural employment, coupled with limited legal protection, jeopardize the migrant farmworker's health.

- Migrant workers have higher rates of adverse job-related exposures and working conditions, which lead to poor health outcomes, musculoskeletal injuries, lacerations, falls, exposure to pesticides, and weather extremes.
- Migrant and seasonal farmwork typically requires stooping, long hours working in wet clothes, working with sometimes contaminated soil and water, climbing, carrying heavy loads, and exposure to the sun and the elements. Failure to perform these activities on a rigid timetable dictated by seasons and weather can result in crop loss. As this population ages, the physical demands of work increase the risk of injuries and long-term musculoskeletal problems.
- According to the U.S. Department of Labor (n.d.-a), motor vehicle accidents are the number one cause of injuries and fatalities in agricultural workers. In 2020, there were 589 fatal injuries, of which 271 were related to transportation.

Pesticide Exposure

Migrant farmworkers may be at higher risk for exposure to cancer-causing chemicals than the general population (Fig. 27-10). They are exposed to pesticides used routinely in the fields: picking produce that has been sprayed; walking behind farm equipment that is mobilizing dirt that has been treated; contact with pesticide spray from a neighboring field; bringing home pesticide residue on their clothes and shoes; or exposure to chemical residues in the soil, air, food, and well water (de-Assis et al., 2021).

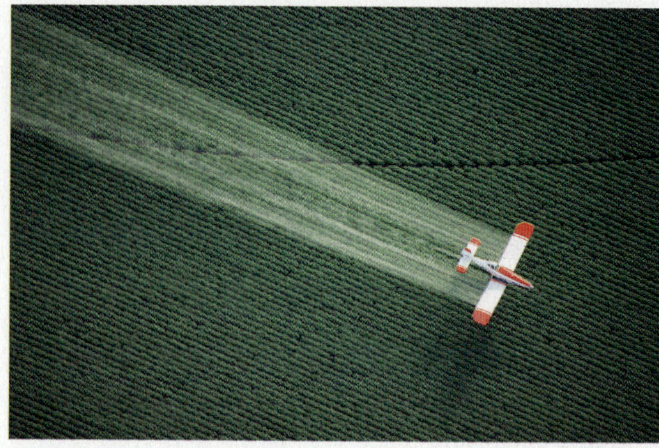

FIGURE 27-10 A crop duster applies chemicals to a field of vegetation.

- A large body of evidence exists on the role of pesticide exposures in the increased incidence of human diseases such as cancers, Alzheimer disease, Parkinson disease, amyotrophic lateral sclerosis, asthma, sleep apnea, bronchitis, infertility, birth defects, ADHD, autism, diabetes, and obesity (Ahmad et al., 2024; de-Assis et al., 2021).
- While research shows that pesticide-associated cancers are higher in farmworkers, data strongly suggest that cancer is even higher in farmworkers' children. This is due to several factors, including the developing organs (Novoselov, 2022), living next to the fields that have been sprayed, and exposure to dust and chemicals on parents' clothing (Cheney et al., 2022).

Pesticide exposure levels in reproductive-age farmworkers consistently exceed levels in the general population. It is estimated that thousands of farmworkers suffer pesticide poisoning each year, but exact counts are not possible because of inadequate surveillance systems and the reluctance of farmworkers to report injuries (Cheney et al., 2022). Surveillance systems are only in place in 13 states. The Sentinel Event Notification System or Occupational Risk is a means of reporting pesticide-related injuries as well as other occupational illnesses and injuries (CDC/National Institute for Occupational Safety & Health, 2024). Some farmworkers, primarily those without H-2A visas, were less likely to be provided pesticide safety equipment and often were not notified when pesticides were applied. Reporting of pesticide-induced morbidity and mortality is not required in every state. California has the oldest and most thorough pesticide surveillance system in the United States, which began in 1971; the system requires healthcare providers to contact their local health department (LHD) whenever they suspect an illness or injury is related to pesticide exposure. The health department then alerts the county agricultural commissioner and also completes a Pesticide Illness Report (California Department of Pesticide Regulation, n.d.).

But, even with reporting laws, many cases are never recognized because workers do not seek medical care. Pesticide burns and rashes often go untreated because of a lack of education about the dangers of pesticides and a lack of available services. Migrant workers are often unaware of the hazards of pesticides.

- **Pesticide drift** can impose health risks when sprays and dust are carried by wind and then deposited in other areas such as homes, schools, playgrounds, adjacent fields, plants, and bodies of water (U.S. Environmental Protection Agency [EPA], 2023a).

- Even though it may be required of healthcare providers to report pesticide poisoning, it is often misdiagnosed because the symptoms can mimic those of viral infections or heat-related illnesses.
- Symptoms of pesticide exposure include sore throat, runny nose, headache, fatigue, red/swollen/watery eyes, drowsiness, itchy skin, abdominal pain, and nausea or vomiting.
- More severe symptoms may include sweating, salivation, blurred vision or pinpoint pupils, fever, severe thirst, muscle twitching or weakness, and incontinence (especially with organophosphate or carbamate exposures).
- Finally, with the most severe exposures, seizures, respiratory depression, and unconsciousness or coma can occur. There are over 19,000 pesticide products registered with the EPA and more than one thousand active ingredients (U.S. Environmental Protection Agency [EPA], 2024).
- Only a few categories of pesticides account for more than half of the cases of acute illness; these include inorganic compounds, carbamates, pyrethroids, and organophosphates. Although the impact of acute pesticide poisoning is widely recognized, little is understood about the long-term effects of the repeated low-level exposures to which migrant farmworkers are constantly subjected.
- Today, it is more common for farmworkers to be exposed to "nonpersistent" pesticides that are metabolized in the body within days. High levels of nonpersistent pesticides were found in male adolescents' urine. High levels can cause behavioral and social behavioral health issues (Rodríguez-Carrillo et al., 2022).

The Environmental Exposure History, I PREPARE is a helpful assessment tool for community health nurses working with migrant and seasonal workers to use to determine pesticide exposure. When a client presents with symptoms that may be suggestive of pesticide exposure, mnemonic prompts may help to clarify common symptoms (Box 27-9).

Pesticide exposure can be a single event, may occur multiple times, or can even be continuous. Health effects are thought to be a function of the frequency of exposure and the dose.

U.S. Laws Enacted to Protect the Migrant Farmworker

Below are some laws enacted to protect migrant farmworkers and their families. Even so, despite difficult working conditions, farmworkers in the United States are excluded from many federal-level labor protections.

- The Migrant and Seasonal Agricultural Worker Protection Act (1992/revised in 2015) protects migrant and seasonal agricultural workers through the establishment of standards relating to wages, housing, transportation, disclosures, and record-keeping. This act also mandates that farm labor contractors register with the U.S. Department of Labor (n.d.-b).
- Occupational Safety and Health Standards for Agriculture specifies that agricultural employers with 11 or more employees who conduct hand labor operations in a field must provide drinking water at a suitable drinking temperature, toilet and handwashing facilities within a reasonable, accessible distance, and the employee must be notified by the employer of the location of such facilities (Occupational Safety and Health Administration [OSHA], n.d.).
- Agricultural Worker Protection Standard: Enforced by the U.S. EPA, this standard is primarily focused on the safe handling of pesticides. It now prohibits children under the age of 18 from handling pesticides, requires that workers do not enter areas recently sprayed with pesticides, and improves protection for workers from retaliation if they make complaints about standard violations (EPA, n.d.).
- Immigration and Nationality Act: The H-2A portion of this act offers protections for H-2A workers concerning the following: pay rate; written notification of a work contract with beginning and end dates; the three-fourths guarantee (employee must guarantee employment for at least 75% of the contract period); housing will be provided at no cost to the employee; and the employer will be responsible for transportation to and from work as well as to and from their country of origin (U.S. Citizenship and Immigration Services, n.d.).
- Title VII of the Civil Rights Act of 1964: This act initially involved the prohibition of employment discrimination based on race, sex, color, national origin, and religion. Multiple amendments to this act are especially significant for female migrant farmworkers. Title VII protects employees against sexual harassment such as quid pro quo, hostile environments, and retaliation (U.S. Equal Employment Opportunity Commission, n.d.).

BOX 27-9 Mnemonic Prompts to Determine Cholinergic Symptoms of Organophosphate Exposure

Sludge

Salivation
Lacrimation
Urination
Defecation
Gastric secretions
Emesis

Dumbbels

Defecation
Urination
Miosis
Bronchorrhea
Bradycardia
Emesis
Lacrimation
Salivation/seizures/sweating (the four most acute symptoms: bradyarrhythmias, bronchospasm, muscle weakness, and bronchorrhea).

Source: Open Anesthesia (2020); Katz (2023).

Substandard Housing and Poor Sanitation

Quality of housing affects farmworker health and safety. Formal demographic data on farmworker housing are often lacking. Migrant worker housing is often substandard or nonexistent. Even though the federal government requires H-2A migrant housing to be inspected, the oversight can be minimal. This may lead to poor living conditions such as little or no hot water, rodent and insect infestations, or nonworking smoke detectors (Chadde & Hettinger, 2022).

Over the last decade, governmental agencies and nonprofit groups have become more interested in the improvement of agricultural worker housing conditions. Information on the improvement of housing conditions can be found on the U.S. Department of Agriculture's Rural Housing Service, the U.S. Department of Labor, and the U.S. Department of Housing and Urban Developments websites.

Migrant farmworkers move frequently and often have great difficulty securing adequate housing. Farmers who hire workers on H-2A visas are required to provide free housing, but this accounts for only 2% to 5% of the workers. Some states, though, have adopted statutes and administrative codes governing the rules, providing minimum sanitation and health standards related to the construction, operation, and maintenance of migrant labor camps and residential housing for migrants (Florida Department of Health, 2023). Although data on migrant housing are scant, surveys have uncovered the following:

- Over 30% of all housing units were overcrowded (JBS International, 2022).
- Some workers and their families live in substandard living conditions. They may lack access to clean running water, inadequate plumbing, mold, and rodent and pest infestations (Castillo et al., 2021).
- Agricultural workers mainly reside in single-family homes (56%), mobile homes (21%), apartments (20%), and 3% live in dormitories, barracks, cars, tents, garages, or other types not meant as living quarters (JBS International, 2022).
- Housing may lack electricity, placing residents at risk of food borne illness due to unsafe food storage.
- Overcrowding limits access to bathroom use which affects personal hygiene.
- Poor sanitation increases the risk of pest and rodent infestation.
- Unsafe or lack of water limits drinking water and hygiene (National Center for Farmworkers Health, n.d.).

Substandard housing is not the only concern. Crowding is also a problem, as many farmworkers, unable to find sufficient numbers of rental units, share housing—sometimes paying per person costs. When housing cannot be found, workers and families may have to resort to paying rent to live in garages, barns, sheds, chicken coops, or they may be forced to stay in their cars. A Guide for Safe and Adequate Housing for Agricultural Workers National Center for Farmworkers Health's (n.d.) provides valuable resources, recommendations, and housing safety and hygiene assessments at https://www.ncfh.org/uploads/3/8/6/8/38685499/a_guide_for_safe_and_adequate_housing_for_ag_workers-final.pdf

Poor Nutrition, Overweight, and Obesity

Migrant and seasonal farmworkers and their families have higher rates of obesity and are more likely to be overweight or have obesity (Lopez-Cavellos et al., 2019). Despite often working among fruit and vegetable crops, migrant families often have difficulty procuring food and maintaining a sufficient supply. Farmworkers constitute a vulnerable population with several characteristics that put them at risk for poor dietary quality: low income, food insecurity, rural isolation, poor housing, and lack of access to food subsidy programs. Food-related practices of migrant farmworkers require change to improve the inclusion of fresh produce and other nutrient-dense foods. Common health problems of migrant children are similar to those of their parents and include general poor nutrition, anemia, and vitamin A deficiency.

Risks to Social, Emotional, and Behavioral Health

- Migrant children are often called upon by their families to stay home from school to care for younger children, attend to other household chores, or even work alongside their parents in the fields. Many children of farmworkers report beginning as early as age 10 (MCN, 2024b).
- They may feel socially estranged, be constantly moving, have difficulty finding health-promoting recreational activities, and have difficulty assimilating (MCN, 2024b). This causes stressors related to immigration status.

Migratory patterns for farmworker's children make it difficult to complete credits and stay in school. The transient nature of farm working means children may leave the school year early or receive partial instruction for an academic year. Organizations like Head Start Migrant and Seasonal Head Start (2022) programs provide alternative programs to help. School districts offer services as well. Migrant children are less likely to graduate from high school because of educational interruption and difficulty "catching up." An average child of migrant farmworkers attends three schools in 1 year. While most students plan to graduate from high school, very few do (Los Angeles Unified School District, n.d.).

Intimate Partner Violence

Intimate partner violence is a serious public health problem with substantial consequences for female physical, sexual, and mental health. Migrant farm-working females are particularly at risk in intimate relationships because of cultural beliefs and environmental factors, which include challenges with the migratory lifestyle, limited finances, as well as poor working and living conditions. In addition, female migrant workers are often less aware of resources to advocate for themselves within the healthcare system, making interventions difficult (Pacific Northwest Agricultural Safety and Health Center, n.d.; MCN, 2024c). What makes farmworker domestic violence so significant is the fact that female farmworkers often experience language barriers, lack adequate access to healthcare, live isolated lives with little social support, and have economic constraints, cultural issues, and fear of deportation if they report the abuse—all factors that lead them to endure their violent situation in silence (Pacific Northwest Agricultural Safety and Health Center, n.d.; MCN, 2024c). The Violence Against Women Act affords protection for people who are undocumented and experiencing domestic violence by allowing them to seek legal immigration

BOX 27-10 LEVELS OF PREVENTION PYRAMID

Domestic Violence in the Migrant Population

SITUATION: Although the migrant lifestyle can be difficult for the entire family, when there is family violence, females and children suffer most. Research is scant; however, informal discussions occur among individuals and healthcare providers. Outreach workers sometimes possess lists of people who are abusive and the people they abuse. Isolation and subjugation to a patriarchal system usually prohibit female migrant workers from seeking help if they are abused. Fear of consequences and difficulty expressing negative views about their husbands prevent such individuals from speaking out (MCN, 2024c).

GOAL: Prevent intimate partner violence.

Tertiary Prevention

Rehabilitation	*Health Promotion and Education*	*Health Protection*
▪ Promote family rehabilitation, with or without person conducting the abuse in the home. ▪ Encourage ways to eliminate or reduce social and geographic isolation among vulnerable females.	▪ Alleviate stressors of the migrant lifestyle, such as overcrowding and substandard living conditions. ▪ Provide emotional support and educate on what constitutes abuse. ▪ Promote self-esteem and encourage females to take control of their situation.	▪ Encourage people experiencing intimate partner violence to contact healthcare providers as they migrate. ▪ Encourage people experiencing intimate partner violence to find appropriate lay community outreach workers for support. ▪ Encourage people experiencing intimate partner violence to unite and create an environment that allows them to speak out while supporting one another against abuse.

Secondary Prevention

Early Diagnosis	*Prompt Treatment*
▪ Promptly identify people experiencing intimate partner violence—through self-identification or by other family members or professionals—remove from the dangerous situation.* ▪ Keep communication lines open, be culturally sensitive, and examine for injuries.	▪ Secure people experiencing intimate partner violence in a safe shelter. ▪ Assist people experiencing intimate partner violence to regain self-esteem.

*Secondary prevention is difficult because of limited financial resources, lack of transportation, no nearby friends or relatives for support, language barriers (e.g., non–English speaking), and limited safe shelters for people experiencing intimate partner violence in rural areas.

Primary Prevention

Health Promotion and Education	*Health Protection*
▪ Create awareness of the harsh living conditions that migrant families endure. ▪ Advocate for improved and safe living conditions on state and national levels.	▪ Train bilingual and bicultural people in the community on the issues of spousal abuse and help them form support groups. ▪ Provide opportunities for people in the community to improve self-esteem that will change attitudes toward each other.

status without the help of the person who is abusing them (American Immigration Council, n.d.; MCN, 2023). C/PHNs must be aware of these issues and what resources are available in the community (Box 27-10).

Infectious Diseases

- TB is a common infectious disease among farmworkers.
- Seventy-one percent of TB cases in the United States are non–U.S.-born people (MCN, 2024a).
- Migrant farmworkers are at risk for TB due to poor ventilation in housing, strict work schedules, and cultural and language barriers (MCN 2024a).
- Research conducted with migratory workers near the U.S.–Mexico border found that 55% of the 109 workers tested positive for a latent TB infection (NCFH, 2023b). Because of their migrant patterns, it is difficult to be accurately diagnosed and to complete treatment regimens; they endure poor access to healthcare and social isolation.
- Many factors may prevent them from successfully completing a treatment regimen, and language barriers, along with cultural differences, may preclude them from fully understanding the impact of their disease on themselves and others. Not completing

the treatment regimen places a person at risk for multidrug-resistant TB.

- Migrant workers are at greater risk for HIV infection due to inconsistent condom use; heterosexual contact with an infected male; use of commercial sex workers due to the shortage of potential partners in rural communities; and use of lay injections, where untrained peers will inject a migrant with vitamins and antibiotics and reuse needles (NCFH, 2023c; Rojas et al., 2020).
- HIV-positive status may be misunderstood and, because of stigmatization and fears of deportation, may be purposely hidden from health officials. Other infectious diseases (e.g., hepatitis, enteric diseases, and parasites) may commonly afflict migrant workers, often because of inadequate sanitation and hygiene facilities.

Whatever your viewpoint on this issue, it is important to the public's health that basic healthcare services be available to vulnerable populations. Continued efforts must be made to conduct research assessing risks and hazards, especially those of pesticide exposure. Migrant workers are a mobile population and difficult to study; they represent an important, integral part of our economy; infectious disease among this population increases health risks for all (NCFH, 2023c).

Unique Methods of Healthcare Delivery and Primary Prevention

Because migrant health centers do not adequately meet the health needs of the entire migrant community, several innovative methods of healthcare delivery have been developed and implemented by community health nurses.

- Several programs are using promising models to intervene to address some of the social determinants of child health by utilizing existing programs and also linking community partners to better serve the community.
- Mobile health vans staffed with bilingual medical providers, community health nurses, and promotoras can travel to migrant camps; this provides an effective strategy for outreach health screening and education. By going to migrant camps and delivering care during nonwork hours such as evenings and weekends, the team increases health access and overcomes barriers. A viable alternative to traditional medical clinics, the mobile clinic provides primary care to an underserved population through health promotion, disease prevention, and early treatment (Tulimiero et al., 2021).
- Mobile dental vans can provide services to migrant workers' children, often with arrangements made through school nurses and dental care provided by dental schools or through partnerships. Barriers to good oral health include lack of insurance, high cost of services, language, immigration status, socioeconomic status, and fear/trust (Adekug & Ibeh, 2024).
- Mobility impedes continuity of care, and the inadequate system of medical record-keeping for the migrant population is frustrating and challenging. Data information systems are vital components for monitoring the health status of individual farmworkers as they migrate, as well as essential for generating research and follow-up care for long-range health planning. Data also helps justify the appropriation of monies to migrant health agencies.

The medical histories of migrant children are often unknown to current providers. The U.S. Department of Education (n.d.) now offers the Migrant Student Information Exchange (MSIX) that permits states to transfer health and educational information on migrant students. The MSIX system was a part of the amended No Child Left Behind Act that was enacted by Congress to assist states in developing an effective method of tracking educational and health information as well as the number of migratory children in each state. However, the ability to track these children in the migratory lifestyle from one work location to another is often inconsistent. Early intervention for migrating children is not always feasible, but it can greatly improve outcomes.

Community Health Nursing in Migrant Settings

Beyond barriers to healthcare, the migrant lifestyle is troubled with challenges. Because of the insecurity and instability inherent in a mobile lifestyle, long-term health goals are difficult to establish, and long-term follow-up of any chronic illness is problematic. Nonetheless, C/PHNs provide much-needed services using community resources, innovative thinking, tenacity, and sensitivity.

Strategies for improving the health status and resource use of migrant workers and their families include the following:

- Improving existing services
- Advocating and networking
- Practicing cultural sensitivity
- Using lay personnel for community outreach
- Utilizing unique methods of healthcare delivery
- Employing information tracking systems

Community health nurses are the major providers of migrant health services and have a crucial role in the development and management of interventions. In response to the growing need for available, accessible, and affordable healthcare for migrant farmworker families, C/PHNs are called on not only to understand the migrant lifestyle but also to help migrant families overcome the barriers to healthcare (Box 27-11).

Added attention must be given to family members exposed to the hazards of the migrant lifestyle. Even as many migrant workers settle into communities, the cycle of poverty continues as other workers arrive from impoverished countries. With a paucity of health resources, the C/PHN is sometimes the only health provider who provides care for this population.

BOX **27-11** PERSPECTIVES

Nurse and Nursing Instructor Viewpoints on Migrant Health

"I spoke with one of my students after clinical last week, and she told me about her work this semester with a 35-year-old single mother of two who had been discharged from the hospital following a lupus flare-up. The student felt her client was a devoted mother, but she let her 8- and 12-year-old children stay home from school to help with family farm tasks to make ends meet. After weekly visits with her client for almost 2 months, she told me—I was finally able to get her to trust me enough to help her trust others. She has reached out to her neighbors and asked for help and they are more than willing to lend a hand. Now, her children can return to school and go back to being children instead of day laborers! I told her that sometimes, it takes a strong person to reach out for help and that she is a strong woman!"

—Kevin, nursing faculty member, faith-based college, western Massachusetts

"I was having a conversation with students about how to 'break the ice' when making home visits to families who have never had home health services. One student mentioned that at the beginning of the semester, she was afraid that her shyness would be her downfall. But in the week that followed, it occurred to her that the best way to establish trust with anyone is to express an interest in answering questions they have before you pose your own. The student now makes it a habit to ask every patient the three things they would like her to know about them that will help her to personalize their care. During week 8 of the clinical semester, the student stated—This was a real 'icebreaker' and my patients have been much more open to listening and learning from me once I listen and learn about them!"

—Betsy, community health nursing instructor in a northern California school of nursing

"First of all, a nurse should expect the unexpected. Because of the migratory way of life...clients do not always know where they will be next week or next month. Therefore, we must understand that they do not always have their medical records, immunization records, or income records. Hours are very irregular, depending on what time the workers get in from the fields and what time the shifts are. Because of the distances we travel, we work anywhere from 8 to 12 hours a day. The most rewarding part of the job is bringing health services to the underserved and uninsured. The people are so gracious and appreciative of whatever services we provide."

—J. S., RN, Michigan

"Since farmworkers come to our area for only 4 months of the year, it is rare that I care for a migrant woman through her entire pregnancy. I may diagnose her pregnancy, I may see her for three or four prenatal visits, or I may meet her only once before she goes into labor and delivers her baby. I struggle with the desire to make a difference in a short period of time and with the disappointment of not being able to follow through."

—C. K., CNM, RN, Pennsylvania

"I worked as a Head Start nurse for many years in an agricultural area of California. One of my assignments was a state/county migrant farm labor housing project. I was asked to make a home visit to check on a 4-year-old who hadn't come to preschool in a few days. When I arrived at the family's duplex, I found the sixth grader there, caring for all five of her younger siblings, including the 4-year-old and an 8-month-old baby. When I asked why she was home with all of the children, she guardedly informed me (after some coaxing) that her parents had been picked up in an immigration raid at the tree farm where they worked and had been taken back to Mexico. The children were now alone, with no family nearby. I worked with a nun at Catholic Social Services to provide care for the children until the parents returned to the United States so that the children, who were all U.S. citizens, would not be placed in foster care. The parents had not been allowed to contact their children before being placed on the bus to Mexico, but other workers, who were not undocumented, had seen them go and told the children about their plight. It was heartbreaking to see the fear in their eyes. I quickly went to work looking for resources for them."

—Holly, Head Start nurse, California

Providing care for migrant workers presents a challenge, requiring nurses to be innovative and to go beyond the boundaries of traditional health services (Box 27-12). Although many resources and programs exist to help migrant families, the needs are still overwhelming. By aligning with the goals of Healthy People 2030 to improve the health of one of the most underserved populations, the community health nurse will also improve the health of the nation.

BOX **27-12** C/PHN USE OF THE NURSING PROCESS/CLINICAL JUDGMENT

Working With Migrant Families

Analysis/Recognize Cues

Tom Reynolds is a community health nurse in central Montana. He has three migrant camps in his service area that are homes for primarily Mexican residents. The males in the community primarily work in strenuous construction jobs—masonry, landscaping, and agriculture (cherry orchards, dairy farms, and ranches). The females in the community work as housekeeping staff in private homes, motels, and hotels in the area.

Tom did the following: the evenings, he would stop by the camps to catch up with residents and assess any current health concerns. At the end of a 3-week period, Tom had met with the residents in each of the three camps.

Diagnosis/Analyze Cues and Prioritize Hypotheses

The feedback from these informal conversations assisted Tom in the formulation and implementation of a nursing plan of care

(Continued)

BOX 27-12 C/PHN USE OF THE NURSING PROCESS/CLINICAL JUDGMENT (*Continued*)

Working With Migrant Families

targeting the health promotion needs of this unique population of residents.

- Changes in the family health status secondary to language, transportation barriers, and health literacy barriers
- Fear as it relates to deportation and separation from family members
- Occupational and situational injury, illness, and stress because of extended work hours and poverty-level living conditions

Planning and Implementation/Generate Solutions and Take Action

Tom and the community developed possible interventions. Tom researched funding options for a project that was sponsored by the local health department. The director of the health department agreed to support the project for 6 months if Tom could find matching funds for the project from a local foundation, recruit the needed personnel, and the results were positive.

Tom recruited three other community health nurses, one of whom was bilingual and familiar with the migrant workers' cultural values and practices. In addition, Tom reached out to the university's undergraduate nursing program, and the community health instructor agreed to utilize the three camps as clinical sites for the upcoming semester.

The nurses, students, and staff social workers from the health department coordinated weekly evening and weekend visits to each of the three camps. The teams completed a family assessment for each family, established health records, completed a community-based assessment for each of the three camps, administered immunizations, assisted with arranging transportation to and from medical appointments, and enrolled families in the Women, Infants, and Children Supplemental Food Program. In addition, the teams completed short teaching sessions on topics such as oral care, hand hygiene, family planning, and infant safety.

The local farmworkers heard about all the activities at the camps and began to organize food and clothing drives to help the residents meet the challenges of the warm Montana summers and snowy winters.

Evaluation/Evaluate Outcomes

The evaluation of the interventions was so positive that the program became a permanent health department service. In the months that followed, a nurse practitioner and volunteer dentist were added to the team to provide on-site care and evaluations. With optimal health and a decrease in issues related to health disparities, several families were able to leave the camps and establish permanent homes in the local community.

Evaluation of the three nursing diagnoses includes the following goals:

- Family health status will improve.
- Family members will not experience fear of deportation and separation from family members.
- Workers will not experience injury, illness, and stress.

URBAN HEALTH

Urban health is influenced by the interactions of citizens in three areas:

- Where they reside
- Where they work
- Where they gather for daily life events

According to the World Health Organization's (WHO) (2024) *Operational Framework for Monitoring Social Determinants of Health Equity*, the social determinants of health (SDOH) and their subdomains with the focus on **urbanized area** settings are as follows:

- Economic security and equality include the subdomains of employment, food insecurity, and poverty. Often, urban households experiencing poverty may be hidden in urban areas of higher wealth. Many people are also likely to be pushed into poverty due to higher prices of essential commodities in urban areas.
- Physical environment includes climate, air quality, disasters, housing, drinking water and sanitation, and urbanization. Eighty-eight percent of the urban population is exposed to particulate matter levels in the air that exceed WHO Air Quality Guideline values.
- Education subdomains contain access to education, the quality of that education, and the educational outcomes.
- Social and community context encompasses crime and violence, incarceration, discrimination, gender equality, and healthy aging.
- Health behavior addresses substance use and misuse, nutrition, and physical activity.
- Healthcare incorporates healthcare access and the healthcare system. A range of acute and chronic health concerns and risk factors has emerged in urban settings, and these realities offset earlier gains. Noncommunicable diseases are pervasive in urban living.

The urbanization component under the physical environment of the SDOH focuses on safe and affordable housing; a public transportation system that meets the needs of the community; adequate solid waste management that ensures environmental safety; the establishment of green and public spaces that encourage exercise and recreation; and the development of partners between urban and rural communities for economics, social, and environmental betterment (UN, n.d.).

There is a direct relationship between the health of urban residents and the physical environment, the social influences within the environment, and access to services that support physical health and social well-being. Urban health considers those characteristics of the environment as they relate to the health of the population living within large cities. Characteristics that define **urban** areas, such as size, density, and complexity, come with advantages and disadvantages; large size in cities may mean that the public health system can efficiently reach large numbers of people for interventions but may also lead to incomplete coverage for services due to larger populations.

According to the UN (n.d.), over 55% of the world's population resides in urban areas. Summer heat that breaks temperature records can place vulnerable populations and those living in urban areas at greater risk for heat-related illness and deaths (CDC, 2024c). Federal Emergency Management Agency (FEMA) conducts a national risk index for the effects of disasters on U.S. counties, taking into account expected annual loss, social vulnerability, and community resilience (FEMA. n.d.). The city and county of Los Angeles, California, received the highest rating of any other area in the United States at 100. Other urban areas at risk include Houston, Texas (99.97); Miami, Florida (99.81); and Seattle, Washington (99.65) (FEMA, n.d.). While disasters have negative effects on any area, urban areas experience some of the most devastating effects of disasters based on population density, vulnerability, and lack of resources. To discover the National Risk Index in your area, go to https://hazards.fema.gov/nri/. U.S. urban areas account for 80% of the population and have grown denser (U.S. Census Bureau, 2024). Three cities in California have the most densely populated urban areas in the United States, followed by the New York area (U.S. Census Bureau, 2024).

In 2000, the Johns Hopkins University founded the Urban Health Institute as a means to bolster support among an urban population. The mission of the Institute includes the following:

- *Facilitate collaborations* between communities, universities, and healthcare delivery systems to build collective capacity for achieving health equity in Baltimore
- *Mobilizing resources* in support of promising strategies to achieve substantial gains in health and well-being in Baltimore residents
- *Advancing understanding* and dialogue by including community voices to build trust and enhance pathways to health, well-being, and social justice in Baltimore (Johns Hopkins Urban Health Institute, n.d.)

The New York Academy of Medicine (2020) has organized the Institute of Urban Health and sponsors the *Journal of Urban Health*, a publication that focuses on population-based research with resource-limited and at-risk populations living in urban areas.

History of Urban Healthcare Issues

An examination of urban healthcare issues requires an in-depth analysis of the vulnerabilities of urban dwellers that have existed for centuries. The following list provides a historical summary of these unique issues:

- Housing: During the mid-1800s and early 1900s, the U.S. population increased dramatically due to the influx of millions of immigrants from large European and Eastern European countries. Groups of people and families began to congregate in urban tenements and ghetto housing buildings.
- Poverty: Today, Haitian and Middle Eastern families inhabit some of the same neighborhoods that were inhabited by Eastern European immigrants during the early 1900s. However, many of the same buildings continue to provide less than optimal shelter for this new group of immigrants.
- Access to healthcare remains inequitable due to cultural, economic, and health literacy barriers that were not adequately addressed by many healthcare organizations.

Two connected disciplines, urban planning and public health, have addressed housing and healthcare issues from the 19th century to the present. **Urban planning** has improved the welfare of people and communities by supporting the growth of healthy, effective, appealing, and accessible places.

- *The American Public Health Association* (APHA, n.d.) describes the mission of public health to "promote and protect the health of people and the communities where they live, learn, work, and play."
- Together, these disciplines addressed the needs of the identified vulnerable populations. Initially, these two systems were linked in promoting health by facilitating physical activity through the creation of green space.

The objectives of specialists in urban planning and public health are to support sustainable urban development in resource-abundant nations to mitigate climate change, minimize energy consumption, reduce pollution, protect natural areas, and provide a safe and healthy environment for the citizens, particularly those who comprise the most vulnerable populations. Leaders at the CDC are concerned with factors that affect people and their environments and support efforts that address the improvement of both physical and social environments as related to places to live, work, and play. The CDC's *Built Environment* describes the components involved: interaction between environment and health, poorly planned growth leading to sprawl, increased use of vehicles, and healthy community design that promotes health and well-being (CDC, 2022).

- WHO provides education and information regarding strategies that will optimize the health of cities and their citizens (WHO, n.d.-a).
- WHO recognizes the opportunities that exist for urban residents regarding health, education, and safety while acknowledging the unique risks that face urban residents (WHO, n.d.-b).
- Issues of overcrowding and lack of available sanitation facilities and clean water increase the risks of communicable diseases for urban residents who reside in urban ghettos and tenement housing projects.

The *Healthy People 2030* document addresses societal determinants of health and the environments in which we live, work, and play. Notwithstanding the complexity of urban areas, particularly in large metropolitan cities, health promotion efforts and a focus on healthier environments are key components of this national health effort.

Emerging Issues in Access to Health Services

Access to healthcare in the United States is regarded as "unreliable" because many people do not receive the appropriate and timely care they need. The U.S. healthcare system, which was already overwhelmed, has faced an even greater influx of patients because healthcare reform was fully implemented in 2014. While 92% of Americans have gained health insurance coverage in 2022 (Keisler-Starkey et al., 2023), millions still lack coverage. Healthcare issues that should be monitored over the next decade include the following:

- Increasing and measuring insurance coverage and access to the entire care continuum (from clinical

preventive services to oral healthcare to long-term and palliative care)
- Addressing disparities that affect access to healthcare (e.g., race, ethnicity, socioeconomic status, age, sex, disability status, sexual orientation, gender identity, and residential location)
- Assessing the capacity of the healthcare system to provide services for newly insured people
- Determining changes in healthcare workforce needs as new models for the delivery of primary care become more prevalent, such as the patient-centered medical home and team-based care
- Monitoring the increasing use of telehealth as an emerging method of delivering healthcare (ODPHP, n.d.-a).

Urban Populations and Health Disparities

The majority of the world's populace now lives in cities (Fig. 27-11). An analysis of the mortality rate differences between high-poverty urban and high-poverty rural areas suggests that place characteristics influence health and health outcomes above and beyond the impact of the social determinants of health for those populations. However, it is important to note that these populations are not static in their residence, and the dynamic nature of urban living directly influences the health of populations over time.

In the United States, in 2023, 83% of the population was urban (over 286,900,000 people), which is expected to increase to 89% by 2050 (Center for Sustainable Systems, 2023). In 2020, 19% of the population lived in rural areas, 12% were urban residents, and 69% lived in the suburbs (Anderson, 2020). Rural county populations have lagged in recent years, with one half having fewer residents now than in 2000 due to young adults finding employment in urban areas and the aging of baby boomers.

One example of how changes in population can adversely affect large cities can be found in Detroit, Michigan. At one time, the city was the wealthiest in the country with the fourth largest population. Prosperity was due to the city's manufactory plants, including the American-produced automobiles General Motors and Ford. Riots during the 1980s occurred throughout the city due to a long history of inequality and racism. In 2009, General Motors filed for bankruptcy, and the city followed suit. Workers lost their pensions, and in 2013, the city had the highest unemployment rate of all the cities in the country. The recent revitalization of the city means that large companies are investing and setting up headquarters in Detroit. An automobile plant that sat vacant for 56 years is in the final stage of demolition; 24,000 abandoned homes have been demolished (Briscoe, 2024; Rahal, 2024). If Detroit is to become a story of success, the past mistakes must be addressed. Population loss leads to a smaller tax base and a greater proportion of residents who live in poverty, yet the city had the same maintenance expenses for sewers, water lines, and streets.

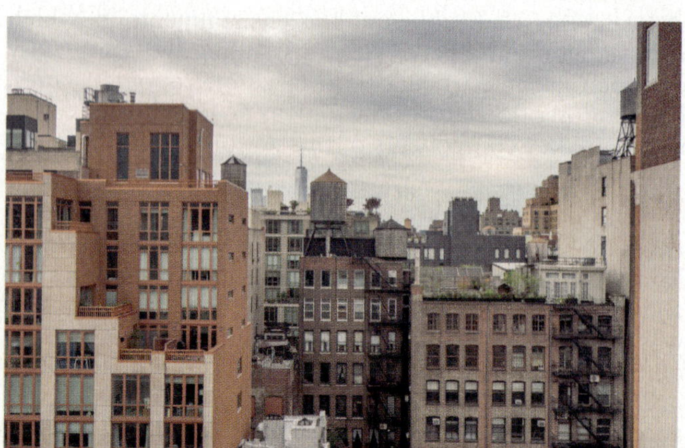

FIGURE 27-11 An example of urban housing: buildings, water tanks, and other structures in the Chelsea neighborhood of New York.

- Historically, movement to the suburbs began with the housing boom and highway expansion occurring after WWII.
- People moved from large cities to more suburban areas, and shopping malls and schools followed.
- Cars became even more essential because public transportation did not always extend into suburban areas, thereby leading to long commute times and traffic congestion.

Although not all suburban areas have remained attractive and vital, an income gap persists between city and suburban residents.

Today, the declining urban situation is not confined to a few large cities. To achieve the vision of creating "social, physical, and economic environments that promote full potential for health and well-being for all" as an overarching goal of *Healthy People 2030*, more must be done to promote health and prevent disease in urban areas (ODPHP, n.d.-b). The primary reason for health disparities is the disproportionate burden of certain health and social problems among different populations—in this instance, urban areas. Environmental exposure to air pollution contributes to illness and mortality, including heart disease, cancer, and respiratory diseases. Some researchers consider urban areas to be food deserts due to the high volume of fast-food restaurants and liquor stores. In a study conducted by Taylor et al. (2024) on the "food desert" of Flint, Michigan, they found alternatives through healthy food options at ethnic food stores, community gardens, food banks, and mobile food vans. Consumer products—such as fast food, alcohol, and tobacco—are more readily available in urban and low-income areas, yet many communities find alternative means to healthy foods (Taylor et al., 2024).

Other environmental issues, such as extreme heat events where temperatures rise and lead to climate-related deaths, may amplify public health stressors and profoundly affect vulnerable populations. When examining urban form and its relationship to this weather phenomenon, exposure to dangerously high temperatures is a public health threat expected to increase with global climate change (CDC, 2024c).

- Heat waves can exacerbate the risks associated with heat exposure, and urban residents are more vulnerable to these threats due to the urban heat island effect. Extreme heat events not only lead to increased ED visits for heat-related illnesses, but they can also lead to increased hospitalizations for those with asthma and other chronic conditions, as well as death for older and other vulnerable populations (CDC, 2024c).

- Cities provide interventions such as extreme heat warnings and cooling centers but not all residents use these services.

Urban health equity depends on the political empowerment of the people to strongly represent their interests and needs to challenge unfair resource distribution. Further, with most of the world living within the built environment, this poses a major opportunity to improve urban health and equity (APHA, 2020). Poor social conditions and health inequalities have been recognized in urban areas around the world. Urban areas in low- and some middle-income countries provide social exclusion for many living in poverty and threaten development. For example:

- The Zika virus was, and continues to be, a disease that mainly impacts resource-limited areas. Characteristics such as poor water and sanitation, crowding, and poor structural quality of housing offer ample opportunities for mosquitoes to breed and spread the Zika virus (Touchton & Wampler, 2023).
- People in cities are also at risk for infectious disease outbreaks (e.g., COVID-19 infections) based on risk factors such as household overcrowding, race, ethnicity, low income, and underlying health conditions such as diabetes and obesity (Zhang & Li, 2024).
- Noise and light from urban environments had a negative effect on children's night-time sleep (Yeo et al., 2023).
- Indoor air pollutants have been associated with long-term health issues in children (e.g., asthma and allergies), and reducing indoor allergens and pollutants have shown improvements in asthma symptoms (Nardocci et al., 2023).
- Urban indoor environments in multifamily housing units pose challenges as pollutants may be seen in many of the units and residents have limited ability to make changes (EPA, 2023b).
- There is a significant correlation between urban environment and mental health. Adults living in urban environments are at risk for apathy, fatigue, loneliness, depressed mood, irritability, stress, and anxiety (Xu et al., 2023). According to the WHO, about 4.2 million deaths per year occur due to exposure to outdoor air pollution (WHO, 2022). Denser populations, such as urban areas, experience more air pollution. While global data have often suggested that urban residents have better health on average than their rural counterparts, this benefit may only be greater for those at the high end of the income scale.

In 2021, crime rates were higher in urban areas; 24.5 out of 1000 people aged 12 years and older in urban areas reported being victims of violent crimes and 157.6 victims of property crimes, while crime rates in rural settings were 11.1 and 57.7, respectively (USAFacts, 2023). Urban areas are often thought to be places with resource-limited residents living in large, poorly maintained government housing projects. Dilapidated housing in central cities exposes residents to cracks in walls and ceilings, peeling paint, broken windows, leaking pipes, and pests such as cockroaches and rats. There is often limited access to adequate rental properties, and rent is often higher in large cities, making it difficult for resource-limited residents to find adequate housing.

Nationwide, about one third of households live in rentals, but 43% of rental properties are in central cities. In order to rent a two-bedroom apartment in California, the most expensive state for renters, a person needs to earn $7098 a month or $87,800 a year. Conversely, in Arkansas, the least expensive state, for a two-bedroom rental, the renter must earn $2730 a month or $33,800 yearly (Chapman, 2023). The standard percentage of salary required to pay for housing remains at 30%; however, if one lives in New York City, it may cost 68% of one's monthly income, and in Miami, it will cost 42% of a person's monthly income (Scott, 2023). The median cost for other expenses after housing costs is $310 a month for those in the lowest income brackets (Joint Center for Housing Studies of Harvard University, 2024). This leaves limited monthly income for food, transportation, or other expenses.

Sociologists Wilson and Kelling first proposed the *broken window theory* in 1982, noting that if a broken window goes unrepaired, soon more windows are broken, and this sends a powerful message to residents that no one cares. A classic research study by Keizer et al. (2008) tested this theory in six-field experiments where neighborhoods—characterized by broken windows, litter, unreturned shopping carts, and graffiti—were studied. They found that when residents see others violating social norms or rules (e.g., disorderly or petty criminal behavior), they are then more likely to also violate norms and rules and that this is a cause for the spread of disorder.

Urban areas are associated with population density, complexity, and racial/ethnic diversity. In the 21st century, America has evolved into a metropolitan nation, with more than 8 out of 10 Americans living in metropolitan areas of varying sizes. In 2023, the fastest-growing U.S. states/areas were South Carolina, Idaho, Maryland, and seven cities in Florida (realestate.usnews.com, 2023). Conversely, the states with the greatest rates of decline were Mississippi, Missouri, Utah, Louisiana, and California (Businessinsider.com, 2023).

Working-class urban residents can no longer find industrial jobs, and a concerted effort to improve conditions in urban America is needed in the form of urban policy development. Over the past 25 years, cities and their suburbs have become more alike, and the demographic and health profiles that were previously uniquely urban are now shared by "edge cities" and suburbs populated by resource-limited and underrepresented families. Political power has shifted to more affluent suburban areas, where the tax base and spending practices are greater, at the expense of these cities.

Urban health disparities present a challenge that can be addressed only by the joint effort of public health and urban planning bodies. Coalitions of public health professionals, planners, builders, and architects, along with transportation engineers and government officials, are needed to promote healthy, sustainable communities (Fig. 27-12).

There is a move to make cities and their suburbs **sustainable communities**. These are seen as healthy places where both natural and historic resources are protected, employment is available, **urban sprawl** is contained, neighborhoods are safe, air pollution is minimized, lifelong learning is promoted, healthcare and transportation are easily accessible, and all citizens have the opportunity to improve their quality of life.

As with all good plans, the sustainable plan requires that the recipient of the planning be involved. Democratizing the practice of urban planning is vital to its success. Communities that have been victimized through ineffective planning must be included in the decision-making process. This process will require the inclusion of the practical experience that residents bring to the table, alongside expert input. A framework to ensure such justice requires that all people and communities have the right to work, play, and live in environments that are safe and healthy. It also requires that polluters be punished and required to provide compensation for damages and renovation.

Community Health Nursing in Urban Settings

Urban C/PHN can be very rewarding, and many nurses are drawn to urban areas where salaries are higher and there are greater opportunities for advancement or additional education. In urban areas, there are a larger number of nurses, more schools of nursing, and more intensive recruitment efforts than in rural areas, although urban areas, much like rural settings, can have problems filling C/PHN vacancies.

- RN workforce studies reveal a higher rate of nurses and a greater proportion of nurses with a bachelor's in science degree (BSN) in urban areas than in rural areas (Odahowski et al., 2021).
- The current healthcare education system tends to be urban-centric, with the exception of online education programs. These online programs provide an opportunity for rural nurses with an associate degree (ADN) education to achieve a BSN. Thus, closing the gap between ADN and BSN nurses in rural areas.
- Earnings in hospitals and outpatient clinics are significantly higher in urban areas when compared to earnings in rural areas (Odahowski et al., 2021).

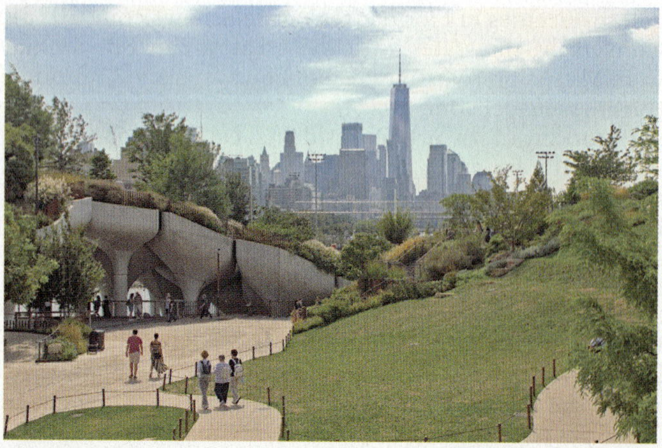

FIGURE 27-12 Central Park, a green area interspersed among densely populated areas, is an example of good urban planning.

C/PHN practice is population-focused care that requires unique knowledge, competencies, and skills. Primary prevention (health promotion) is a major focus. C/PHNs have a key role in working with populations to improve the health and social conditions of vulnerable populations. These nurses practice in diverse settings such as community nursing centers, home health agencies, housing developments, local and state health departments, neighborhood centers, churches, street outreach programs, schools, and worksites. C/PHNs can develop sustainable programs and build community capacity for health promotion in collaboration with community members. By utilizing a community-based participatory research model (National Institute on Minority Health and Health Disparities [NIMHHD] 2024), C/PHNs can partner with community members, leaders, and stakeholders to identify resources and solutions to problems. Specific public health roles include advocate, collaborator, educator, partner, policymaker, and researcher. Community health nurses collaborate with their clients to develop their facility for long-term health promotion and improvement of their quality of life. Their ultimate goal is to empower clients to be self-sufficient. C/PHNs must remember to listen to the community and have cultural humility.

Nurses provide services in deteriorating urban areas, with those living in poverty in all settings and among all vulnerable populations. Nurses first need to assess themselves for their attitudes and preconceptions. Although access to care can be improved for many people with low income in urban areas, many clients simply need an advocate. Our ability to envision solutions and join with clients helps us create a healthier environment for all. Urban communities—and the people with low incomes or vulnerable people living in them—need strengthening and interventions that can be initiated by C/PHNs using the nursing process as a guide.

Self-Assessment

Confronting poverty and caring for vulnerable people from diverse backgrounds, whether in rural or urban areas, necessitates a reflective assessment of one's own assumptions and beliefs. Because poverty may be prevalent over a lifetime, nursing students may have personal or family experiences of living in poverty. However, because the stigma is so great and fault-finding so pervasive in American society, acknowledging and reflecting on this experience may be painful. In contrast, because poverty is so hidden and frequently denied, some nursing students have lived apart from any knowledge of the human experience of poverty. They may have come to believe many of the negative stereotypes about people who live at or below the poverty level. Nursing students and practicing nurses need to ask such questions as

BOX 27-13 PERSPECTIVES

C/PHN Instructors' Viewpoints on Urban Health Nursing

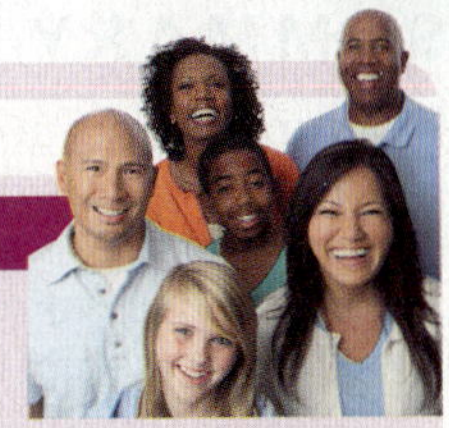

- Ann, a nursing faculty member at a small Roman Catholic college, had a one-to-one postclinical conference with a student and relays this conversation. The student had made many visits to an African American teen mother of two thriving children. The young mother lived in a dangerous housing project, and, although she locked her abusive ex-boyfriend out of her second-floor apartment, had been known to climb up the drainage pipe and over the porch roof to gain entry. Sometimes, he forced open a window and beat her. The mother worked every day at a fast-food establishment; her grandmother took care of the children. After a couple of months of weekly visits, the student exclaimed, "When I read her chart, I saw her as an immoral girl—a slut—and I expected her to be a loser. Now, I can't believe what I've learned about how strong she is. She just keeps fighting for herself and for her kids to survive! She's a great mom, and I told her so!"
- Another faculty member, Sharon, who taught community health nursing in a Midwestern school of nursing, was having an informal discussion with a student who related her experience of trying to get comfortable making home visits to a pregnant patient who was about her age and lived in the deteriorating outskirts of a major city. She thought she had established a rapport and was making headway in developing trust with the client. One day, the client asked the student, with concern in her voice, if she had "broken off her engagement." The flustered student then had difficulty explaining the absence of her engagement ring, which she had never mentioned, but the client had obviously noticed. During the previous week, she had suddenly realized she was wearing this special ring in neighborhoods with a high crime rate and thought it best to leave it at home. Of course, she thought that she had to fabricate another reason to tell the client but felt bad for being so judgmental when the client was identifying with the student and believed they had something in common.
- Lynn, a new public health nursing faculty member from a large state university in the West, was shocked and repulsed by the comment of one of her students during a lecture one day. When discussing vulnerable populations in urban centers and rural areas, the point was made that poverty can be a generational phenomenon and that many clients may find it difficult to dig out of this circumstance. Social justice was discussed, along with the need for C/PHNs to become social activists to change political and socioeconomic factors that keep the status quo. A Hispanic female stduent stated, "They should all get jobs at McDonald's." This comment spurred further discussion about population-focused versus individual-focused interventions and approaches, and the need for all of us to be aware of our prejudices and stereotypical viewpoints.

"How have my judgments been shaped? How can I open myself to caring for those from whom most of society turns away?"

We learn from one another's stories (Box 27-13). First, learn from your classmates, friends, and neighbors who are courageous enough to tell you their own experiences of living in poverty. Ask them and listen intently. Then, let your clients teach you. One honor that nurses have is the opportunity to work with people from all walks of life.

Improving Access

- Even with ACA and government-sponsored health insurance and services, extensive barriers prevent many people from accessing services. The community health nurse serves as an advocate and bridge for families who need to gain access.
- Barriers to access associated with the clients themselves include reluctance to seek coverage because of feelings of powerlessness, ignorance that such services exist or are worthwhile, lack of resources such as a telephone or transportation, illiteracy, and preoccupation with meeting survival needs and competing life priorities instead of health needs.
- Barriers associated with applying for health insurance include a system that is unfriendly and complicated. The process may require a car, a phone, and appointments at inconvenient times. Also, service interruptions are not uncommon, as wages vary over time. The nurse can intervene as a coach and guide, interpreting the system to the client and the client to the system. Likewise, nurses can serve as change agents to improve the system whenever possible.

Strengthening Communities

We are all connected. Society is impacted when adults are incapable of providing nurturing environments for their children. In addition, the alienation of many groups in society erodes our sense of community as a nation. Community health planning should seriously consider an organizing process that builds community and that focuses on developing neighborhood competence to solve problems and create solutions for itself.

SUMMARY

- Rural clients are a unique aggregate, and community health nurses are key to ensuring the delivery of appropriate health services to this population. There are numerous definitions of the term *rural*. In this chapter, some characteristics of rural communities include the following:
  - Communities with fewer than 10,000 residents.
  - A county population density of fewer than 1000 people per square mile.
  - Rural areas often have less diversity than urban cities but that is changing in many areas.
  - Rural clients generally have lower educational levels than urban clients, due in part to less access to higher education and lower-paying jobs.
  - Income levels and housing costs are frequently lower in rural areas than in larger cities.
  - Many at-risk populations live in these communities, where there are often fewer employment opportunities, a lack of adequate housing, and limited access to health and social services.
  - Older adults living in rural areas may have more limited alternatives for housing if they can no longer live alone.
  - Mental health services are inadequate, even though the need may be great. Numerous risks are associated with agriculture.
- Many disenfranchised and underrepresented groups call cities home. Air pollution, poverty, discrimination, substandard housing, crime, substance use disorder, and social inequities often characterize life in urban settings.
- The built environment is an important consideration in urban as well as rural settings and can contribute to greater health risks. Some large cities have had marked decreases in population and significant problems with unemployment, although more people around the world live in urban areas now than in rural areas.
- Migrant farmworkers are an integral part of the agricultural community in the United States and the world but are often barely visible in society. As members of the community with varied and significant health needs, these are complicated by social isolation, occupational hazards such as pesticide exposure, poor working conditions, and working with dangerous farm equipment.
- Migrant workers and their families often endure substandard housing and poor sanitation, while living in high-risk environments. Migrant children are often educationally, socially, and physically disadvantaged. Migrant healthcare centers often do not adequately meet the health needs of the migrant community; therefore, innovative methods of healthcare delivery have been developed and implemented by community health nurses, including mobile health vans and information tracking systems.

ACTIVE LEARNING EXERCISES

1. Identify a health problem for each of the populations discussed in this chapter. Through the lens of social determinants of health, compare and contrast these health problems. Share your findings with classmates. Reflect on the results. Were they similar or different? Why do you think this is? (Objective 1)
2. Based on your findings in the first exercise, develop a plan of care to address the problem within the community. Focus on primary prevention. Review the roles of C/PHN listed in the rural section of the chapter for ideas on interventions. Develop an infographic on the intervention. (Objective 2)
3. Pesticides used in agricultural products have an adverse effect on children. Contact a school nurse or a pediatric nurse (or PNP) who works in children's health. Have they worked with children affected by toxins? What adverse effects did the child experience? What environmental toxins are in your community? What are short-term and long-term adverse reactions in children? (Objective 3)
4. As C/PHNs, we advocate for our patients and communities. Children have no voice in the toxins used within their communities. Research policies that address toxins. What did you learn? Do the policies accomplish what they set out to do? Are updates needed? Which of the 10 Essential Public Health Services (Box 2-2) might you use to advocate for children? (Objective 4)
5. Describe in your own words the definition of respect. Do you have the respect of your peers? How do you show respect to others? As you read this chapter, reflect on the importance of respect we have for our clients. How do you demonstrate respect to the rural, migrant, and urban populations? Why is this important in the care we provide to our communities? (Objective 5)

CHAPTER 28

Veterans Health

"But I fear they do not know us. I fear they do not comprehend the full weight of the burden we carry or the price we pay when we return from battle. This is important because a people uninformed about what they are asking the military to endure is a people inevitably unable to fully grasp the scope of the responsibilities our Constitution levies upon them... We must help them understand, our fellow citizens who so desperately want to help us."

—Admiral Michael Mullen, U.S. Navy, Chairman, Joint Chiefs of Staff

KEY TERMS

Active duty
Disability
Homelessness
Mental health
Post-traumatic stress disorder (PTSD)
Substance use disorders
Suicide
U.S. Armed Forces
U.S. Uniformed Services
Veteran
Veteran benefits
Veterans Administration
Veterans Health Administration

LEARNING OBJECTIVES

Upon mastery of this chapter, you should be able to:

1. Differentiate the term veteran with key cultural characteristics of the population.
2. Assess the unique physical health priorities and challenges faced by veterans.
3. Assess the unique mental health priorities and challenges faced by veterans.
4. Describe the difficulties veterans have in accessing services.
5. Compare and contrast health disparities among the veteran and the civilian communities.

INTRODUCTION

As we look at the veteran community, it is important to understand that the United States has been engaged in armed conflict for decades, and our veteran community bears the scars of those wars. As of 2022, according to demographic reports, there were 16,200,322 veterans in the United States (USAFacts, 2023). This number has been on a steady decline as we see the aging population of many of our World War II (WWII), Korean War, and Vietnam War era veterans, with 1,594,413 still living (U.S. Department of Veterans Affairs [VA], 2023a). The peak of the military population was in 1968 at 3.5 million, which was attributed to the draft-era military. Today, we see an all-voluntary military force composed of just 1% of the adult population in the United States, which is another reason for the decline in the veteran population today (Schaeffer, 2023). The Veterans History Project Collection on the Library of Congress website, which can be found at https://www.loc.gov/collections/veterans-history-project-collection/about-this-collection/, provides information on veterans.

With the decrease in service members and veterans in the United States, the nation is also experiencing a divide between the military/veteran community and the civilian population, mainly due to the fact 67% of adults under the age of 30 are not likely to know a family member who has served in the military (Cleveland-Stout, 2021). With this growing divide, it has become even more critical that those community and healthcare providers who serve our military, veterans, and their families have an even greater understanding of their physical, psychological, and overall well-being.

This chapter introduces the military and veteran community and the important role C/PHNs play in improving and sustaining optimal health for this population. Further engagement with military and veteran communities and education is highly recommended.

DEFINING THE MILITARY AND VETERAN COMMUNITY

As a C/PHN, when dealing with the military/veteran community, it is important to clarify specific terminology, have a general understanding of the military/veteran community, and eliminate some misconceptions or preconceived biases some may have of the military/veteran community. This can be achieved first by defining the term veteran as it is a more complex term than one may expect.

Definition of Veterans

In the civilian community, it is presumed that if a person has served in the military, then they receive **veteran benefits** such as healthcare through the Department of Veterans Affairs. Unfortunately, this is not always the case.

The term **veteran** has various definitions based on the organization/institution and personal experience of the veterans themselves. A veteran is someone who has actively served in the armed services and has received an honorable discharge (VA, 2019). This may not encompass all veterans a C/PHN will interact with, as there are national guard, reserve personnel, and those who were dishonorably discharged who can be considered veterans as well. States, counties, and cities will have their own definition of a veteran for local benefits.

The term **active duty** means the following:

- Full-time duty in the Armed Forces
- Full-time duty as a commissioned officer of the Regular or Reserve Corps of the Public Health Service
- Full-time duty as a commissioned officer of the National Oceanic and Atmospheric Administration or its predecessor organization the Coast and Geodetic
- Service as a cadet at the U.S. Military, Air Force, or Coast Guard Academy, or as a midshipman at the U.S. Naval Academy
- Authorized travel to or from such duty or service (Thomas, 2023)

The term **U.S. Armed Forces** means the U.S. Army, Navy, Marine Corps, Air Force, Space Force, and Coast Guard, including the reserve components thereof.

Historical Context and the Evolution of Veterans: Healthcare Services

Before the federal government became responsible for caring for veterans, the community took responsibility for caring for its soldiers. According to the Department of Veterans Affairs (VA, 2024a), the origins of caring for soldiers who were disabled date back to 1636. At that time, the Pilgrims of Plymouth Colony passed a law stating that the colony would care for soldiers who were wounded and disabled fighting the Pequot Indians. That practice continued, and the responsibility became that of the state and the communities the service members came from.

Today's Veteran Health Administration (VHA) began in the late 1800s, with the establishment of the Soldiers and Sailors Asylum, later renamed the National Home for Disabled Volunteer Soldiers. This asylum was established to care for honorably discharged soldiers who fought for the Union Army. These "military homes" eventually became the blueprint for today's veteran hospitals (Encyclopedia.com, n.d.).

The Veteran's Administration (VA) has the largest healthcare system in the United States and serves nearly half of the veteran population in varying capacities, including but not limited to benefits such as **disability**, direct health services, educational benefits commonly referred to as the GI Bill, job training, home loan guarantees, and burial to name a few (https://benefits.va.gov/benefits/). These earned benefits, distributed by the various administrations within the Department of Veterans Affairs (Fig. 28-1), ease veterans' transition into the civilian community and provide the necessary assistance after military service. However, as in any large federal entity, the system has its own barriers and challenges.

What has become increasingly unclear over the last century, with the increased presence of the federal government in providing care and benefits, and given the military/civilian divide, is the role of the community in ensuring veterans and their families return to communities where they can reintegrate into the civilian world and access appropriate federal, state, and local resources. One way the VA has opened the door for this is through the Community Care program, which allows veterans to receive care and services within the civilian community when not offered at a VA hospital or clinic nearby (VA, 2024b).

THE MILITARY AND VETERANS

Civilians may not be aware of the challenges associated with separation from military service and reintegration into civilian life. Veterans have experience from their military career that may or may not transfer to specific jobs within the community. Family roles may need to be reestablished, as well as reestablishing services, healthcare, housing, and career. Coming from an institution where many necessities are provided and having to reenter civilian life and community can be difficult for veterans. Additionally, veterans may return to their families following difficult combat, affecting both their physical and mental health. C/PHNs can assist veterans with these transitions, acknowledging their service sacrifices while supporting their comprehensive health needs.

Demographics and Characteristics of the U.S. Military

There are six branches of the **U.S. Uniformed Services**. The U.S. Army, Navy, and Marine Corps were established in 1775; the Coast Guard was established in 1790; the Air Force was established in 1947; and the Space Force was established in 2019.

Although not part of the U.S. Armed Forces, due to the nature of overlap and collaborations among the services, some exposures discussed later in this chapter may pertain to the members of the National Oceanic and Atmospheric Administration and the U.S. Public Health Services.

The majority of the U.S. military are White and are men, with the number of service members who are women and who are from underrepresented groups on the rise. Most of the service members are enlisted, and approximately half of active-duty service members are married and a third have children (Figs. 28-2 and 28-3; U.S. Department of Defense [DOD], 2022).

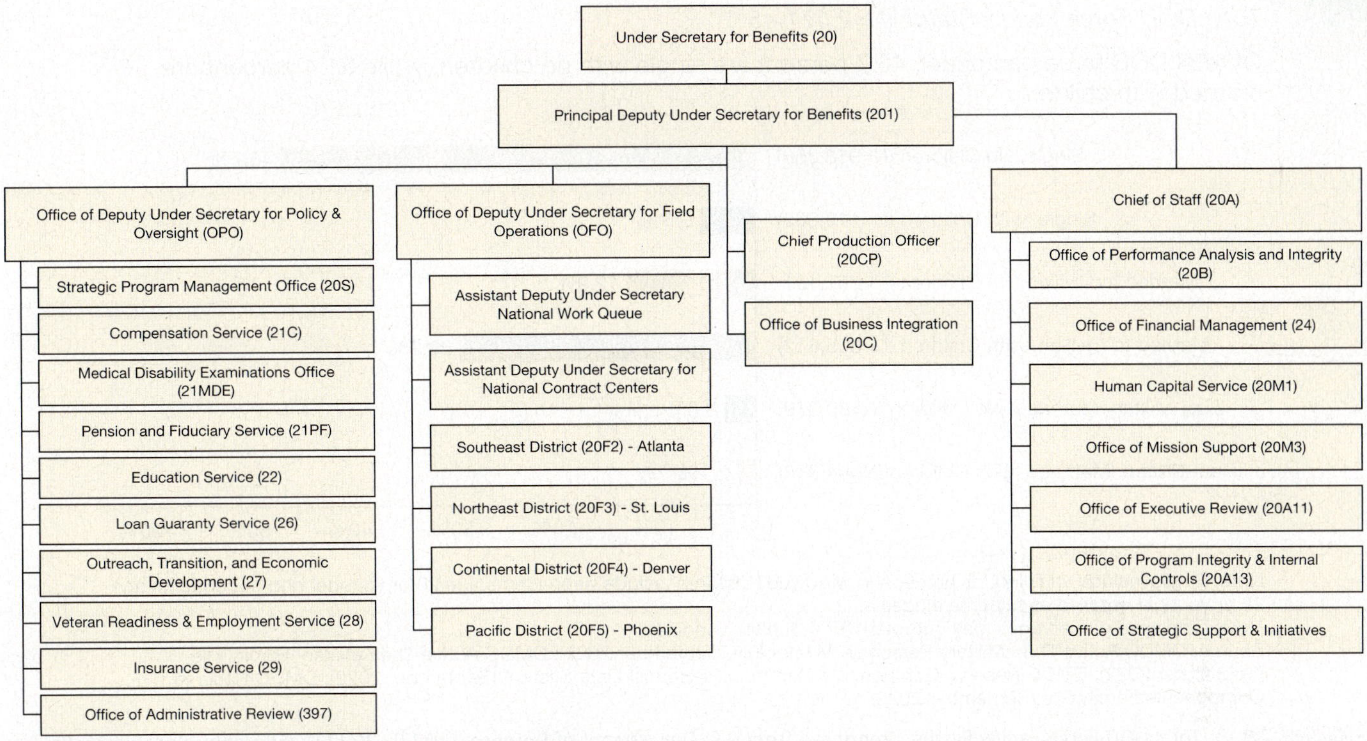

FIGURE 28-1 Veterans Benefits Administration organizational chart. (Reprinted from Department of Veterans Affairs Functional Organization Manual Version 7. (2021). https://www.pathfinder.va.gov/assets/resources/about-va/2021-va-functional-organization-manual-volume-one-administrations.pdf)

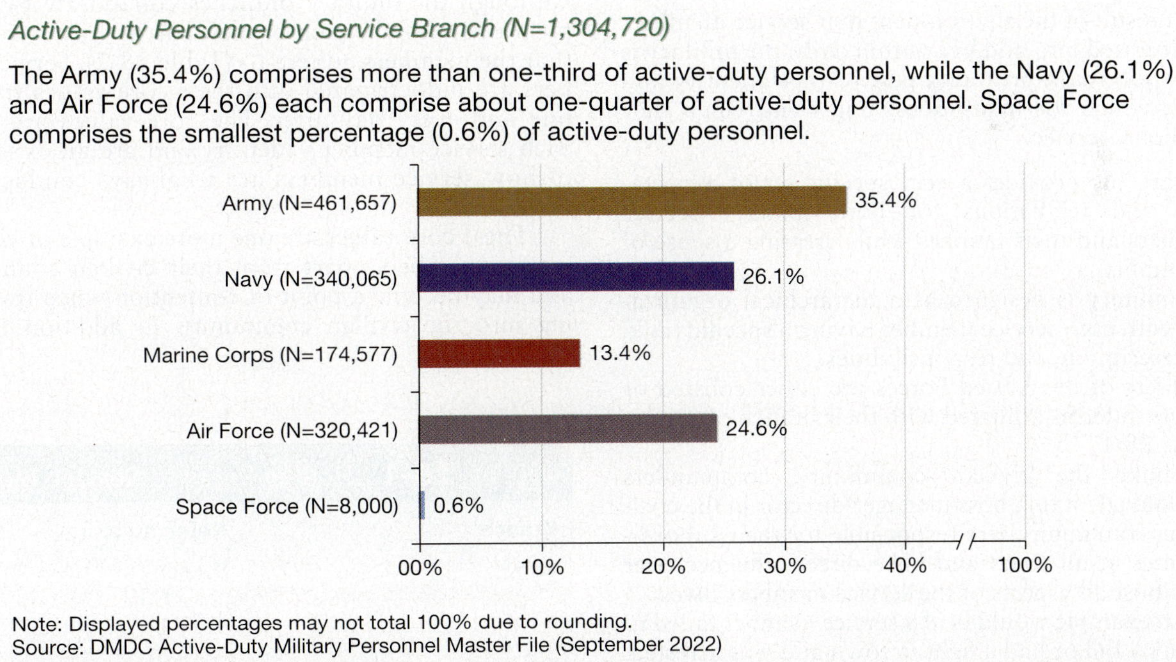

FIGURE 28-2 Active-duty members of the Armed Forces. (Reprinted from U.S. Department of Defense. (2022). *2022 Demographics profile of the military community*. https://demographics.militaryonesource.mil/)

Military Culture

The military is a tight-knit, cohesive community with its own knowledge, stories, language, traditions, and values. The American Psychology Association (APA) described military culture as an iceberg; everything seen above the surface is what the civilian world can see as well, and what is below the surface is the core that makes up a member's link to their military service (n.d.). It is the oaths they take, the creeds they live by, the teamwork and discipline that drive their daily life, their self-sacrifice that sometimes tears them apart from others, and their fighting spirit that keeps them alive. Service

Total DOD Force Family Status (N=2,071,451)

Of total DOD force personnel, 46.7 percent are single with no children, while 31.4 percent are married with children.

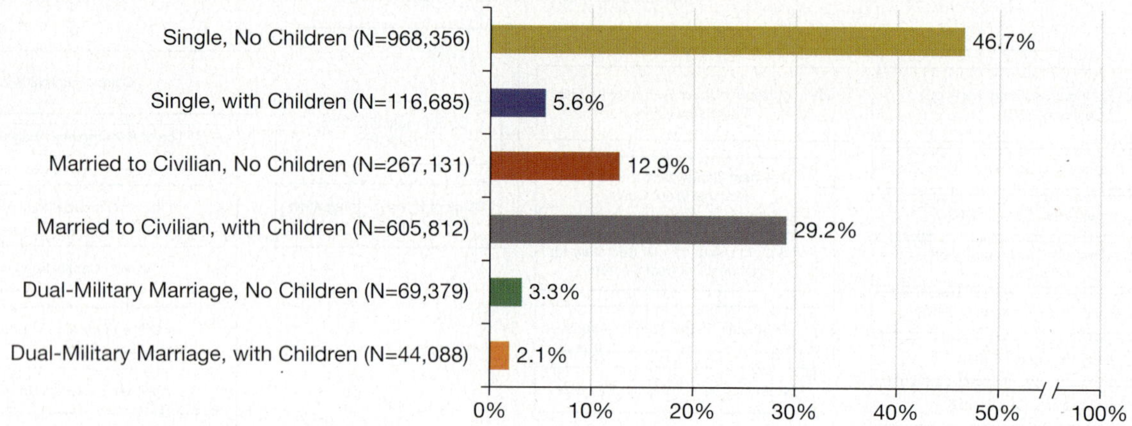

Note: Single include annulled, divorced, and widowed. Children include dependents age 20 or younger and dependents age 22 or younger enrolled as full-time students.
Note: Displayed percentages may not total 100% due to rounding.
Source: DMDC Active-Duty Military Personnel Master File (September 2022); DMDC Active-Duty Military Family File (September 2022); DMDC Reserve Components Common Personnel Data System (September 2022); DMDC Reserve Components Family File (September 2022)

FIGURE 28-3 Total DOD Force Family Status. (Reprinted from U.S. Department of Defense. (2022). *2022 Demographics profile of the military community.* https://demographics.militaryonesource.mil/)

members are goal-oriented, driven, and function in team environments with close ties to their fellow service members. As a result of the environment that service members are enculturated into and live within daily, the military is not just a job but a profound part of their identity and character, which for many doesn't just end when they leave military service.

- Military life provides a very specific set of expectations and regulations for both military service members and their families while creating a sense of community.
- The military is designed as a hierarchical organization, with each service member having a specific rank, job description, and responsibilities.
- Members of the Armed Forces are either enlisted or officers in terms affiliated with their branch of service (Table 28-1).
  - Unlike the civilian community, commanders (equivalent to a boss/manager/director in the civilian community) are responsible for their subordinates at all times and have direct influence over almost all aspects of the service members' lives.
  - An example would be if a service member failed to pay a bill or had a fight in town and was arrested.
- With such oversight and control over the general military population, veterans often face challenges when transitioning to the civilian community.
- The culture change that occurs when veterans transition often leads to isolation as veterans feel comfortable in this isolation and may think the civilian community does not understand their perspectives and questions and may seek out other veterans. So, understanding the military and veteran community is key to engaging with them.

Military Values

Although the military branches collaborate to accomplish the mission, each branch has its own core values that the members adhere to (Table 28-2). Service members are indoctrinated into their core values from day one and every day after. The core values are part of each service member's identity and are an expectation of how service members are to always conduct themselves.

These core values are one more example of what sets service members apart from their civilian counterparts and may become a point of contention when transitioning into the civilian community. In addition to these

TABLE 28-1 How to Refer to Service Members

Branch	Referred to as
Army	Soldier
Navy	Sailor
Marine Corps	Marine
Air Force	Airman
Coast Guard	Coast Guardsman
Space Force	Guardian
Reserve	Reservist

Source: Veterans Employment Toolkit. https://www.va.gov/vetsinworkplace/docs/em_termslingo.asp

TABLE 28-2 U.S. Armed Forces Branch Values

Branch	Values
Army	Loyalty, Duty, Respect, Selfless Service, Honor, Integrity, and Personal Courage (LDRSHIP)
Navy and Marine Corps	Honor, Courage, and Commitment
Air Force	Integrity First, Service Before Self, and Excellence in All We Do
Coast Guard	Honor, Respect, and Devotion to Duty
Space Force	Character, Connection, Commitment, and Courage

Source: Military Leadership Diversity Commission. (n.d.). Department of Defense Core Values. https://diversity.defense.gov/Portals/51/Documents/Resources/Commission/docs/Issue%20Papers/Paper%2006%20-%20DOD%20Core%20Values.pdf

values, specific principles guide the lives of service members, including but not limited to the following:

- Unit cohesion—the camaraderie that exists within a unit and among service members
- Leave no one behind—when in battle or at home
- Stoicism—controlling emotions in the face of stress, danger, and adversity

These values and principles are rewarded and create bonds within the military that may not be understood in the civilian community.

Understanding the Components of Active Duty, the National Guard, and the Reserves

Active duty service members are full-time and stationed worldwide. They are moved based on the military's needs. Based on location, families of service members often can move with the service member and live on or near a military base.

The National Guard is a federally funded entity but is organized and controlled by the state. It contains part-time members who can be deployed across the globe. The National Guard response is often seen during natural disasters and during the height of conflicts, often deployed to war areas. The National Guard is composed of the Army National Guard and the Air National Guard.

Often called the weekend warriors, reserve service members serve one weekend a month and two weeks a year. Reserve units are composed of trained service members who can and are often called to active duty to supplement and fill the gaps. Reserve units are often activated to fill the roles when active-duty service members become deployed overseas. However, after September 11, 2001, many reserve units were also regularly activated and deployed overseas.

The Uniform Code of Military Justice

The military is governed under its own laws known as the "Uniform Code of Military Justice" (UCMJ). The Manual for Courts-Martial United States: 2024 edition's purpose is to promote justice, maintain discipline, and ensure efficiency and effectiveness within the armed services to uphold national security (Joint Service Committee on Military Justice, 2024).

- The UCMJ, a federal law enacted by Congress, applies to all active-duty personnel, including all National Guard and reserve components when activated.
- The system allows commanders within military units to apply administrative punishments for what may be considered lesser offenses.
- The punishments may be a reduction in rank, forfeiture of pay, confinement to quarters, and additional labor.
- Administrative punishments may also include separation from service with a less-than-honorable discharge.
- Less-than-honorable discharges will be further discussed in this chapter as the consequences for veterans after being discharged from the military can be a significant barrier to transition into the civilian community.
- It should also be noted that if service members violate civilian laws while on active duty, the military may also bring additional or equivalent charges within its own justice system.
- The rules of double jeopardy do not necessarily apply in the military.

The second system the military uses for more serious violations of the UCMJ is the use of courts-martial.

- These are the military court systems presided over by military judges, lawyers, and jury pools.
- More severe violations of the UCMJ can result in the service member receiving prison time in the military system and can lead to a lesser discharge.

Military Characterization of Discharge

The military has five levels of discharge. A civilian community/public health system needs to be aware of these discharges because the type of discharge impacts the level of services available to the veteran upon discharge from the military. Administrative discharge levels are Honorable, General, and Other than Honorable. Punitive discharges are Bad Conduct (special and general) and Dishonorable, which are determined through court martial. The characterization of discharge may impact earned benefits (VA, 2024c) and resources available.

Veterans' Return to Civilian Life

As this chapter further explores the veteran community, it is important for the C/PHN to understand that veterans' return to civilian communities and their transition into those communities may be a lifelong endeavor.

- Less than half of veterans access federal **Veterans Administration** (VA) services for healthcare and other benefits (Giefer & Loveless, 2021).
- There are complexities to attaining VA benefits, and not all veterans are eligible for benefits, as previously discussed in this chapter.
- Civilian communities must strive for cultural humility to understand the veteran community and seek to provide appropriate care and services.

The demographics of U.S. veterans are evolving and decreasing due to the continued downsizing of the military; the aging population of our World War II, Korean, and Vietnam era veterans; and other reasons, such as service-related exposures, illness, and suicide. There were 19.5 million living veterans in 2020, with an estimated drop to approximately 13.6 million veterans by 2048 (VA, 2020). However, despite the decreasing numbers (Fig. 28-4), veterans are a significant community within the U.S. population, and their experiences and service are exponentially increased due to the multigenerational impact their service may have.

The U.S. Census Bureau provided the following statistics on veterans in 2021:

- 73.0% non-Hispanic White
- 8.2% Hispanic or Latinx (of any race)
- 12.3% African American
- 1.9% Asian American
- 0.7% American Indian or Alaska Native
- 0.2% Native Hawaiian or Other Pacific Islander
- 2.7% other races
- 24% aged 75 years and older
- 8.2% younger than age 35
- Over a million veterans who are women

Prevalence of Physical and Mental Health Conditions

Physical and mental health conditions are common issues among service members. Due to the nature of the service members' work, the physical demands on their bodies, and exposures to dangerous situations, service members often suffer from physical and mental health issues. Although this chapter will not cover all veteran-related health concerns, some of the most common and concerning issues will be addressed.

- Not all veterans are alike. The various services all have their own subculture within the Armed Forces. Even within each branch of the service, due to various military job assignments, there are different customs, traditions, language, and experiences.
- The experiences of an enlisted service member will differ from those of an officer; a hospital-based medic will have a different experience than a Navy Corpsman stationed with front-line Marines.
- Because of this variation, it is important to truly understand what the veteran does and their exposures because of their service and experience while active duty.

Identifying Health Disparities in Veteran Populations

Identifying and eliminating health disparities for the veteran community should be a priority for C/PHNs. The civilian community often assumes that all veterans are cared for within the VA health system. Unfortunately, that is not true; veterans often go unnoticed in the civilian health systems because those systems do not ask the appropriate questions to identify veterans and veteran-connected families. This leaves many veteran community members underassessed and inappropriately screened for their service-connected disabilities, illnesses, and any needed preventable measures.

For example, diabetes is more prevalent among veterans than in the general population, with 20.5% of veterans diagnosed with diabetes and 3.4% undiagnosed with diabetes. The percentage of veterans with diagnosed diabetes was highest among Black individuals (25.6%), Native Hawaiian and Pacific Islanders (25.3%), American Indians/Alaskan Natives (24.4%), and Hispanics individuals (23 %). Veterans living in rural areas have a higher rate of diabetes (24.3%) when compared to veterans living in urban areas (21.4%). Of note, veterans with 100% service-connected disabilities had a diabetes prevalence of 30.3% when compared to 21.6% for veterans with no service-related conditions (VA, 2022a).

- When obtaining a health history from a veteran, what questions do you believe would be the most important to ask?
- You are coordinating care for a veteran—what services might you suggest or offer?

Veterans in Rural America

There are 4.4 million veterans living in rural areas. When compared with veterans in urban areas, as well as nonveterans in rural areas, these veterans have less formal education, a higher poverty rate, higher unemployment, and are older adults (Patzel et al., 2023). There exist

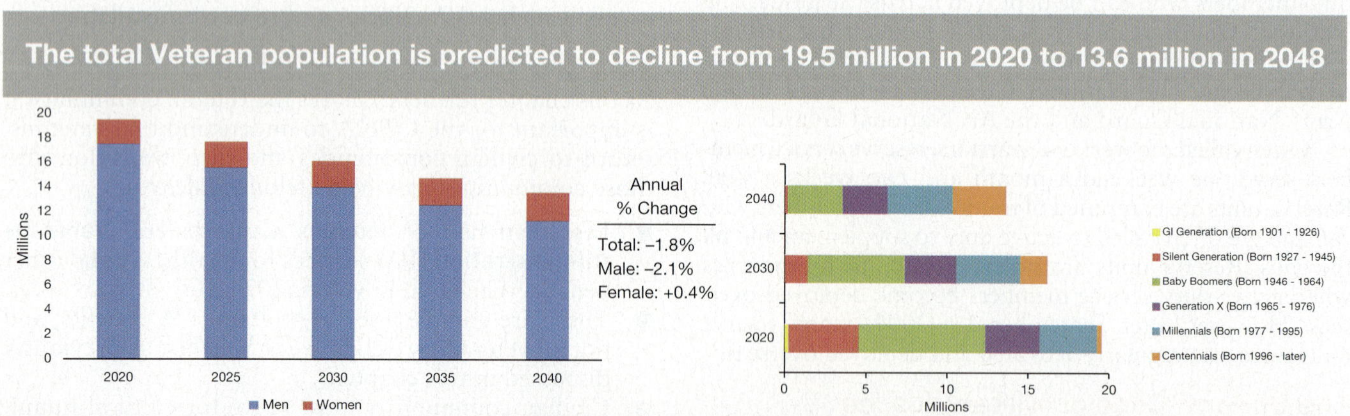

FIGURE 28-4 Veteran population will see a decline from 2020 to 2048. (Reprinted from U.S. Department of Veterans Affairs. (2020). https://www.va.gov/vetdata/docs/Demographics/New_Vetpop_Model/Vetpop_Infographic2020.pdf)

several disparities between urban and rural healthcare for veterans. Rural areas may lack or have inadequate broadband, have fewer VA healthcare providers, civilian providers may not be familiar with veteran needs, and long distances between rural communities and the urban VA medical care facilities (Patzel et al., 2023). The number one concern for rural veterans is the lack of transportation to urban-located VA medical centers and providers. To assist rural veterans, three U.S. Senators proposed a bipartisan bill to increase the funding for transportation to urban VA medical centers and providers (U.S. Senate, 2024). Additionally, the VA has implemented interventions to help this community:

- Education of rural clergy to the signs and symptoms of posttraumatic stress disorder (PTSD) and resources
- Education of rural healthcare providers to the needs of the veterans who are older adults
- Outreach to the community regarding prosthetic care
- Increase home healthcare (Office of Rural Health, n.d.)

To learn more about rural health, refer to Chapter 27, and to learn more about older adults, refer to Chapter 22.

Physical Health Challenges

With improved technology and engineering, more service members survive the brutalities of war. Over the past several decades of conflict and war, veterans have sustained lifelong disabilities related to combat.

- Today, veterans often face polytrauma, in which a person experiences more than one major injury that is either life threatening or can cause impairments or disabilities (VA, 2023b).
- Injuries related to combat could include but are not limited to chronic pain and musculoskeletal (MSK) issues, blast injuries, penetrating injuries, soft tissue and internal trauma, loss or severe injury of a limb, burns, visual and auditory deficits, traumatic brain injuries (TBIs), spinal cord injury, respiratory illness, neurologic deficits, and toxic exposures.

Traumatic Brain Injury

Estimates of TBIs during the conflict in Afghanistan range from 9% to 28% (Reger et al., 2022). Since September 11, 2001, the VA has screened soldiers discharged for TBI. The VA reviews all electronic medical records of soldiers that transitioned to Veterans Affairs for any experiences that placed a solider at risk for TBIs such as a motor vehicle accident, falls, or close proximity bomb blast. If found, the person is referred for further evaluation with a specialist for diagnosis and to be referred for treatment (VA, n.d.-a). TBI leads to serious medical conditions. Symptoms related to TBI include tinnitus, cognitive changes, photophobia, hyperacusis, depression, PTSD, unsteadiness, headaches, alcohol use disorder, and suicidality (Reger et al., 2022; VA, n.d.-b). Treatment options through the VA are the use of medications to help with behavioral health changes, learning better coping strategies, and attending speech therapy, physical therapy, and occupational therapy (VA, n.d.-c).

Exposure to Environmental Hazards

The history of exposure to environmental hazards and toxic exposure for service members goes back over a century (e.g., Agent Orange, burn pits). Today, veterans have various exposures based on the era of their service. Most veterans (7.8 million) served during the Gulf War, which comes with combat exposure and has been linked to a variety of health conditions, including PTSD, arthritis, pain, headaches, TBI, asthma, lung disease, diabetes, heart disease, and stroke. Roughly three quarters (78%) of veterans in 2021 served during wartime, and 22% served during peacetime. Veterans are a vulnerable population because they have higher risks for mental health disorders, substance use disorder, and PTSD and have a higher risk for suicide because of these chronic conditions (Office of Health Equity, 2023).

In 2022, the United States passed a new law known as the PACT Act, the largest expansion of the VA health services, expanding VA healthcare benefits for veterans exposed to burn pits, Agent Orange, and other toxic substances (Congress, 2022). Although this expansion of VA services and benefits is geared toward veterans in the VA health system, more than half of all veterans receive care outside of the VA system. It is crucial for civilian health systems to be aware of the various exposures and appropriately guide veterans to benefits, assessments, diagnostics, and treatments. The VA has comprehensive Level I and Level II military environmental exposure certifications available for civilian healthcare providers in the civilian communities (American College of Preventive Medicine, 2023).

Exposures can include—but are not limited to—burn pits, depleted uranium, toxic embedded fragments, sand and dust particles, Chemical Agent Resistant Coating, Mefloquine-Larium, contaminated water supply, and nuclear/biologic/chemical testing (Fig. 28-5). Additional detailed information and an exposure map (Fig. 28-6) can be found on the VA website for veterans' health issues related to service history. More information can also be found on the Environmental Health Registry site for veterans: https://www.publichealth.va.gov/exposures/benefits/registry-evaluation.asp.

Mental Health Challenges

Veterans' **mental health** remains the top priority for the nation and the VA. This is one area in which the VA is more available to veterans, even if they are not enrolled in the VA healthcare system. Mental health issues such as suicidal ideation, PTSD, psychological effects of military sexual trauma (MST), and substance use disorder (SUD) are areas that the VA and military are trying to address. According to a 2022 study by the Substance Abuse and Mental Health Services Administration (SAMHSA, 2024), over 49% of veterans aged 18 to 25 years had SUD or a form of mental illness.

When looking at the mental health of veterans, gender plays a large role in screening for mental health issues. Compared with veterans who are men, veterans who are women have higher rates of depression, anxiety, and PTSD (Wounded Warrior Project, 2023).

Period of Military Service	Agent Orange	Airborne Hazards and Open Burn Pit	Depleted Uranium Follow-up	Gulf War	Ionizing Radiation	Toxic Embedded Fragments
1940s–1950s					●	
1960s	●				●	
1970s	●					
1990s		●	●	●		
2000s–Present		●	●	●		●

FIGURE 28-5 Environmental health registry evaluation for veterans. (Reprinted from U.S. Department of Veterans Affairs. (n.d.). *Environmental health registry evaluation for veterans.* https://www.publichealth.va.gov/exposures/benefits/registry-evaluation.asp)

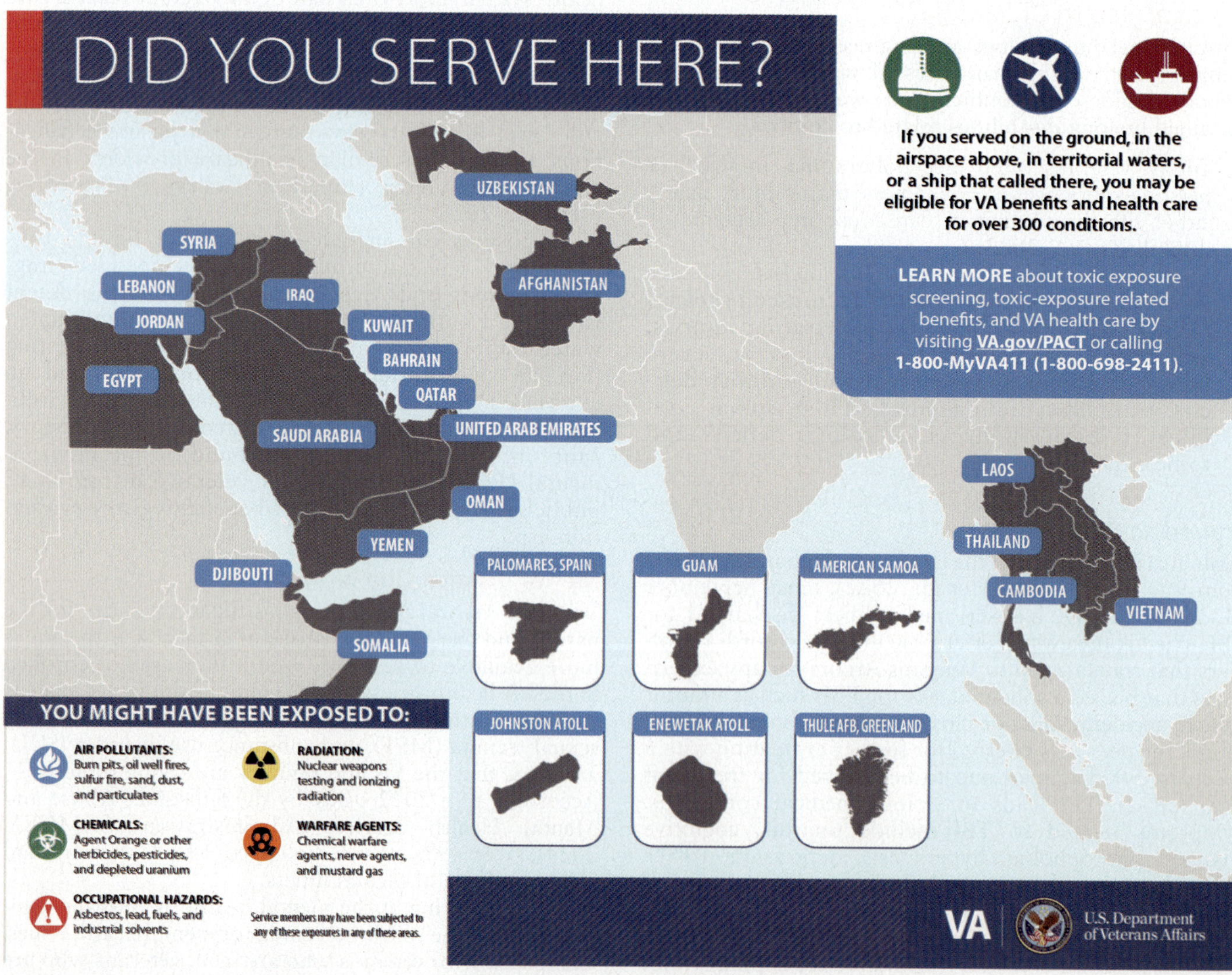
DID YOU SERVE HERE?
If you served on the ground, in the airspace above, in territorial waters, or a ship that called there, you may be eligible for VA benefits and health care for over 300 conditions.
LEARN MORE about toxic exposure screening, toxic-exposure related benefits, and VA health care by visiting VA.gov/PACT or calling 1-800-MyVA411 (1-800-698-2411).
UZBEKISTAN
SYRIA
LEBANON
JORDAN
IRAQ
AFGHANISTAN
KUWAIT
BAHRAIN
EGYPT
QATAR
UNITED ARAB EMIRATES
SAUDI ARABIA
OMAN
YEMEN
DJIBOUTI
SOMALIA
LAOS
THAILAND
CAMBODIA
VIETNAM
PALOMARES, SPAIN
GUAM
AMERICAN SAMOA
JOHNSTON ATOLL
ENEWETAK ATOLL
THULE AFB, GREENLAND
YOU MIGHT HAVE BEEN EXPOSED TO:
AIR POLLUTANTS: Burn pits, oil well fires, sulfur fire, sand, dust, and particulates
RADIATION: Nuclear weapons testing and ionizing radiation
CHEMICALS: Agent Orange or other herbicides, pesticides, and depleted uranium
WARFARE AGENTS: Chemical warfare agents, nerve agents, and mustard gas
OCCUPATIONAL HAZARDS: Asbestos, lead, fuels, and industrial solvents
Service members may have been subjected to any of these exposures in any of these areas.
VA
U.S. Department of Veterans Affairs

FIGURE 28-6 Military toxic exposures map. (Reprinted from U.S. Department of Veterans Affairs. (n.d.). *Did you serve here?* https://www.va.gov/files/2023-06/PACT%20Act%20Exposure%20Map%20V6.21.2023%201030hrs.pdf)

Resource tools for veterans, specifically for mental health, are available at:

- https://www.va.gov/WHOLEHEALTH/veteran-resources/MobileApps-OnlineTools.asp
- https://www.militaryonesource.mil/resources/mobile-apps/

Suicide Among Veterans

Preventing **suicide** among veterans remains the number one health issue in the veteran and veteran health community. More than 46,000 U.S. adults committed suicide in 2023; nearly 6400 were veterans, averaging approximately 17 to 18 suicides per day (VA, 2024d). This figure has been disputed as being significantly low by many in the veteran community due to inconsistencies in reporting among various cities, counties, and states.

Despite the decreasing number of overall veterans over the past two decades, the number of suicides has remained consistent. Between 2020 and 2021, the majority of age groups saw an increase in suicides, except for those aged 75 years and older:

- 18 to 34 years saw an increase of 7.1%.
- 35 to 54 years saw the largest increase of 10.7%.
- 55 to 74 years saw an increase of 7.4%.
- 75 years and older saw a decrease of 8% (VA, 2023c).
- In 2021, the age-adjusted suicide rate among veterans who are women was 166.1% higher than among nonveteran counterparts (VA, 2024d).
- Veteran suicide is a public health issue that must be addressed not only by the federal government but also by the communities veterans return to. Several factors can help reduce veterans' suicide: referrals to the Veterans National Crisis Line (988, then press 1) and programs that are inclusive of the veteran community; proactive outreach; and early identification of veterans at risk, especially during the first year of transition out of military service.

Posttraumatic Stress Disorder

The VA National Center for PTSD is one of the leading research education centers across the globe, with effective treatments being provided throughout VA facilities nationally. **Posttraumatic stress disorder** is a mental health problem that results from the exposure or experience of a traumatic effect (VA, n.d.-d). PTSD has varying levels, and for some people, it can be disabling.

As one can presume, some experiences or events witnessed by service members can have lifelong effects. It also needs to be noted that veteran women experience PTSD at higher rates than do veteran men. In an analysis of a nationally representative sample of U.S. adults, the past-year prevalence of PTSD was nearly 12% for veteran women compared with 6.7% for veteran men. The Veterans Healthcare Administration also screens all veterans who seek care for a history of MST, because 1 in 3 women and 1 in 50 men report having experienced MST in these screenings (VA, 2023d).

Screening for PTSD is important because it has been noted those with PTSD have a higher risk for other health conditions. For example, veterans diagnosed with PTSD have a nearly 50% greater risk for heart failure than those without PTSD. PTSD more than doubles a person's risk for ischemic heart disease. Studies show veterans are more likely than the general population to smoke, and smoking is another risk factor for heart conditions (Hinojosa, 2019).

The VA National Center for PTSD provides resources such as tools for assessment, trauma/PTSD and treatment information, consultation programs, technology integration for mobile mental health applications that can be found at https://www.ptsd.va.gov/appvid/mobile/index.asp, and patient education information (Fig. 28-7). To learn more about PTSD and other behavioral health issues refer to Chapter 25.

Military Sexual Trauma

MST is an unfortunate reality of today's military. MST is any sexual assault that takes during military service (VA, 2023d). Examples include the following:

- Being pressured into sexual activities
- Nonconsensual sexual contact or activities
- Rape
- Being touched or grabbed in a sexual way that made a person uncomfortable, including during hazing experiences
- Comments about a person's body or sexual activities that a person could find threatening
- Threatening unwanted sexual advances (VA, 2023d)

According to VA National data, 1 in 3 women and 1 in 50 men reported they had experienced MST during their military service. MST can have lifelong effects and needs proper care and treatment. However, due to the stigma and self-blame, many victims do not report or seek treatment (Box 28-1; Thelan, 2022). VA centers across the nation have MST services to address both the physical and mental health needs of veterans. To learn more about sexual abuse and violence, refer to Chapter 18.

Substance Use Disorder

Substance use disorders (SUDs) are a major concern both within the Armed Forces and among the veteran community. The cause of substance use varies, from an accepted culture of drinking alcoholic beverages in the military to self-medication for physical or psychological issues. The Armed Forces have strict policies and regulations in place for personnel still engaged with the Armed Forces; however, despite campaigns informing the veteran community of the dangers of SUDs, the numbers of veterans with SUD continue to rise (VA, 2023e); 3.6 million veterans have an SUD, and 1.4 million veterans have both an SUD and a mental health illness (SAMHSA, 2024; Fig. 28-8).

Opioid misuse must also be a consideration when discussing SUDs in the veteran community. Many veterans suffer from MSK issues related to their service and rely on opioids for pain management.

The VA has identified MSK issues as the number one reason that veterans seek treatment and the number one cause of pain in both the active duty and veteran community (VA, n.d.-e). The use of opioids in the treatment of chronic pain related to MSK issues has led to unintended consequences, with SAMHSA (2024) reporting nearly half a million U.S. veterans who misuse prescription pain relievers (Fig. 28-9).

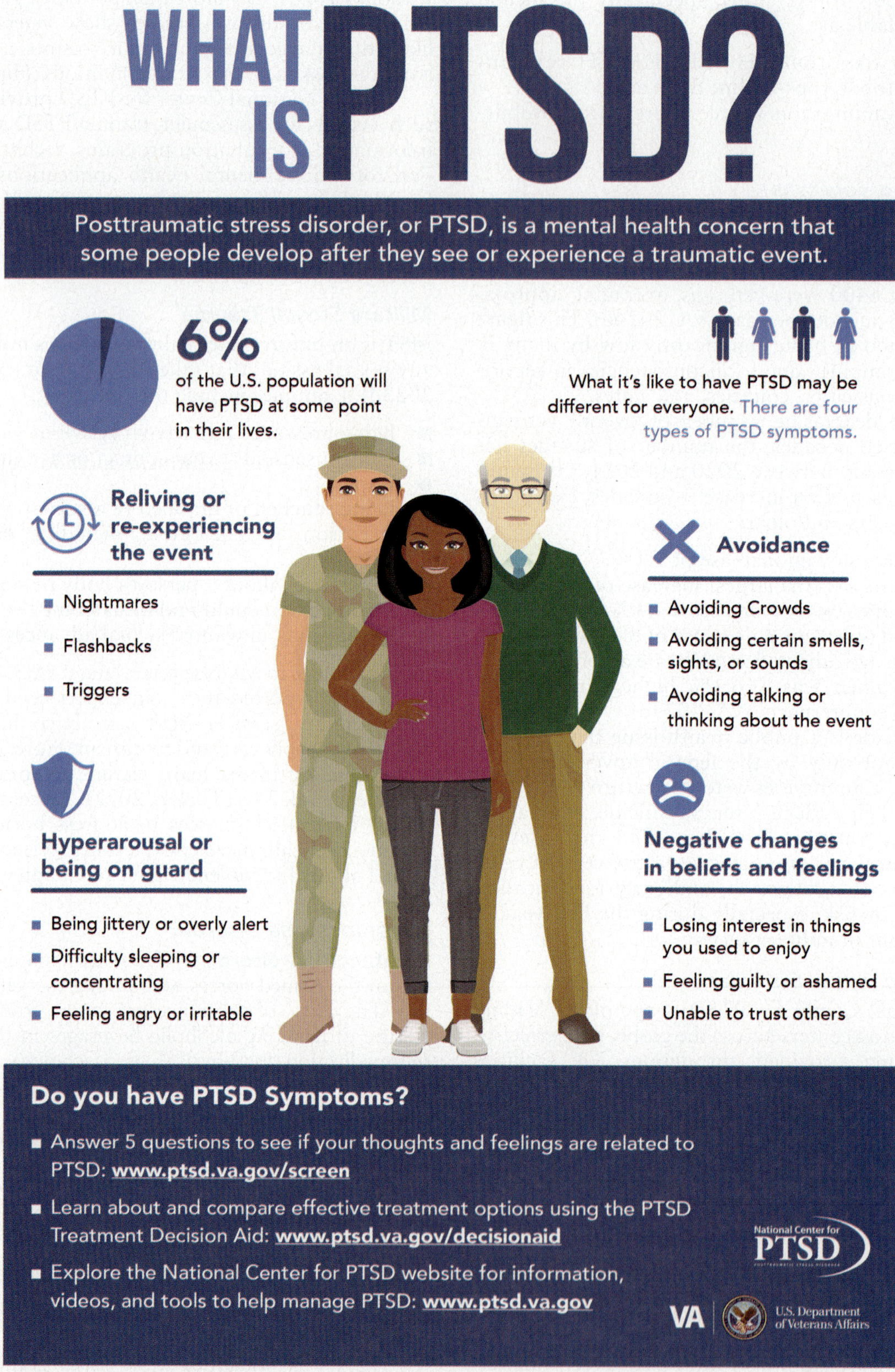

FIGURE 28-7 Patient education flyer about PTSD. (Reprinted from U.S. Department of Veterans Affairs. (n.d.). *What is PTSD?* https://www.ptsd.va.gov/publications/print/NCPTSD-Symptoms-of-PTSD-Infographic.pdf)

BOX 28-1 VA Military Sexual Trauma Fact Sheet (2021)

Difficulties faced due to MST may include:

- **Strong emotions:** feeling depressed; having intense, sudden emotional reactions to things; feeling angry or irritable all the time
- **Feelings of numbness:** feeling emotionally "flat"; difficulty experiencing emotions like love or happiness
- **Trouble sleeping:** trouble falling or staying asleep; disturbing nightmares
- **Difficulties with attention, concentration, and memory:** trouble staying focused; frequently finding their mind wandering; having a hard time remembering things
- **Problems with alcohol or other drugs:** drinking to excess or using drugs daily; getting intoxicated or "high" to cope with memories or emotional reactions; drinking to fall asleep
- **Difficulty with things that remind them of their experiences of sexual trauma:** feeling on edge or "jumpy" all the time; difficulty feeling safe; going out of their way to avoid reminders of their experiences
- **Difficulties in relationships:** feeling isolated or disconnected from others; abusive relationships; trouble with employers or authority figures; difficulty trusting others
- **Physical health problems**: sexual difficulties; chronic pain; weight or eating problems; gastrointestinal problems

Reprinted from VA Military Sexual Trauma Fact Sheet. (2021). https://www.mentalhealth.va.gov/docs/mst_general_factsheet.pdf

Signs and symptoms of SUD include:

- Strong urge to use substances
- Unable to stop use
- Drinking alcohol or using drugs in dangerous situations
- Loss of relationships
- Depressed or anxious about substance use
- Experiencing withdrawal symptoms when stopping use
- Need to use a greater amount for a desired effect (VA, n.d.-f)

To learn more about substance use, refer to Chapter 25.

SUD Treatment

The VA uses evidence-based practices with supported research to provide clinical assistance for veterans seeking assistance for SUD. Using a combination of behavioral therapies and medication, the VA provides comprehensive care for opioid disorder treatment. Veterans not in the VA health system should be provided resources for care with the VA, when eligible, and be provided resources in the community as VA resources may take some time to access. Veterans not eligible for care in the VA health system will need the appropriate level of care in the civilian community.

The VA utilizes the following evidence-based therapies as an effective treatment method for the veteran community:

- **Cognitive–behavioral therapy** uses relaxation techniques, exercises, or socialization to help veterans understand how their behaviors, emotions, and thoughts affect their behavior.
- **Motivational enhancement therapy** helps veterans to strengthen their commitment to recovery through talk therapy (VA, 2022b).

SUD requires medical detoxification and counseling treatments. Detoxification from chronic alcohol use needs medical oversight. To learn more about medical treatment for substances, refer to Chapter 25.

Homelessness and Housing Support

The issue of **homelessness** among U.S. veterans is not just a public health issue but a national one. It is a complex social, economic, and healthcare challenge. It is also a moral imperative to know how this nation provides for those who have served their country (Box 28-2). According to the

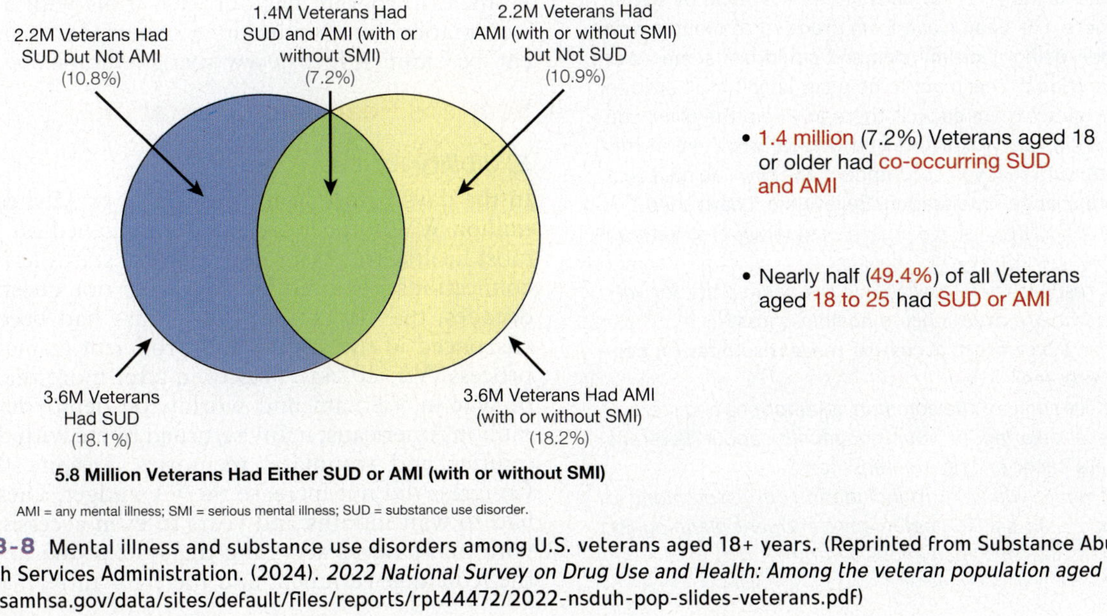

FIGURE 28-8 Mental illness and substance use disorders among U.S. veterans aged 18+ years. (Reprinted from Substance Abuse and Mental Health Services Administration. (2024). *2022 National Survey on Drug Use and Health: Among the veteran population aged 18 or older.* https://www.samhsa.gov/data/sites/default/files/reports/rpt44472/2022-nsduh-pop-slides-veterans.pdf)

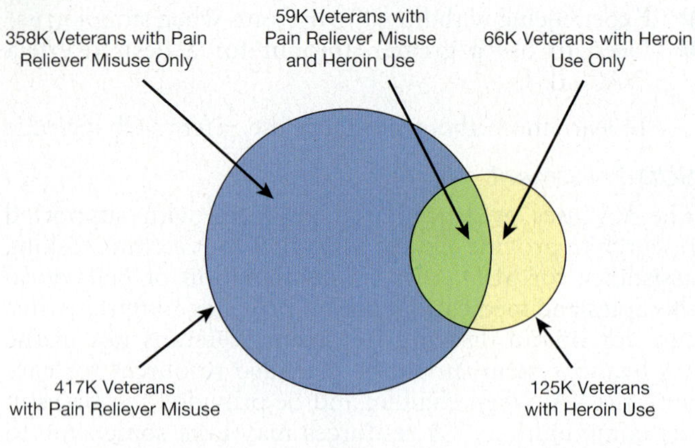

FIGURE 28-9 Opioid misuse and heroin use among U.S. veterans aged 18+ years. (Reprinted from Substance Abuse and Mental Health Services Administration. (2024). *2022 National Survey on Drug Use and Health: Among the veteran population aged 18 or older.* Retrieved from https://www.samhsa.gov/data/sites/default/files/reports/rpt44472/2022-nsduh-pop-slides-veterans.pdf)

BOX 28-2 Dental Care Needs for One Army Veteran

This Army veteran saved his money to travel over 60 miles to have his teeth repaired at a veteran's clinic that provided free medical, vision, and dental care. He barely spoke to anyone, and the Director of Patient Education was asked to see him after the dentist was finished. After 7 hours of dental work, he shared his story with the Director.

"I am an Army veteran and served two deployments in Afghanistan. I joined the military in hopes it would provide me with structure and a place to belong. But after seeing so many of my friends die in battle, I turned to drugs so I could sleep at night. Seven years ago, my Army friend committed suicide; to be honest, I have thought of it as well. I've lived on the street since his death. Sleeping inside a room gave me nightmares of gunshots and screams. Sometimes I think life would be better if I wasn't here. I've been clean from drugs for 6 months now but I've been doing it on my own and could use some help. People have tried to reach out to help but I don't trust anyone and never contact them back. Is there any help the clinic can provide? I know you look at me and wonder why I am in this position. I am sure that you don't understand why I do not seem to be able to change my situation. Believe me, I have tried."

—*Anonymous, Veteran*

1. *What resources are available in the community for veterans who are experiencing homelessness?*
2. *Are there barriers to accessing these resources for certain veterans?*
3. *What are some of the common assumptions and stereotypes circulating in your community about veterans who are experiencing homelessness?*
4. *What would you want to include in your assessment to identify risks and to implement treatment planning for veterans like this anonymous veteran?*

Point-in-Time (PIT) count reported by the VA in January 2023, there were approximately 35,574 veterans experiencing homelessness in the United States, with 20,067 sheltered and 15,507 unsheltered (VA, 2024e). However, this number is often disputed, and critics of the PIT count claim these numbers grossly underreport the actual numbers of veterans who are experiencing homelessness. To learn more about unsheltered populations, refer to Chapter 26.

Overall, there has been a steady decline since 2010 in the number of veterans who are experiencing homelessness; however, between 2022 and 2023, there was a 7% increase (VA, 2023f; Fig. 28-10). In 2023, 35,574 veterans were experiencing homelessness, with the majority being White men followed by Black men (Fig. 28-11).

Housing instability can impact a veteran at many points in their lives. With the many negative consequences for veterans, it can impact finances, physical and mental health, and employment, and can create an increased need for supportive services on local, state, and federal levels. It is also important to recognize that once a veteran becomes homeless, they may further become at risk due to societal criminalization of the unsheltered community, SUD, lost social support, and financial hardships. Never assume a veteran is housed or sheltered because they are receiving VA benefits.

Housing Assistance and Supportive Services

The VA provides street or community-based outreach services directly on the streets, in encampments, in congregate meal sites, and with Community Resource and Referral Centers or with the help of community partnerships. However, housing the veteran community remains a challenge as many VA housing areas are far from services. It has become exceedingly clear the community must step up and fill the gaps in housing and services.

The VA Homeless Program

The National Call Center for Homeless Veterans has staff to assist veterans who are experiencing homelessness or at risk for homelessness (VA, 2023f). Anyone who works or cares for the veterans can call. In addition, the VA Homeless Program has outreach tools with a variety of information for community partners. More information can be found at https://www.va.gov/homeless/.

Veterans Health Administration

Eligibility for Care

In the days before health insurance or Medicare, the 20 million WWII and Korean veterans relied on the VA for most healthcare. As a rule, economic status or line of duty connections, required by law, were not questioned. For decades, the veterans of those wars had become firmly ensconced in the system and proficient at managing the process (VA, 2024a). However, after more than 10 years of war in Vietnam and worldwide deployments of 8.7 million Americans, many returned home with devastating injuries and traumatic memories. Despite this influx, Congress did not increase the VA budget. These veterans had to wait months and years to even access the system, with many never accessing the system due to distrust of the federal government and the era's antiwar movement.

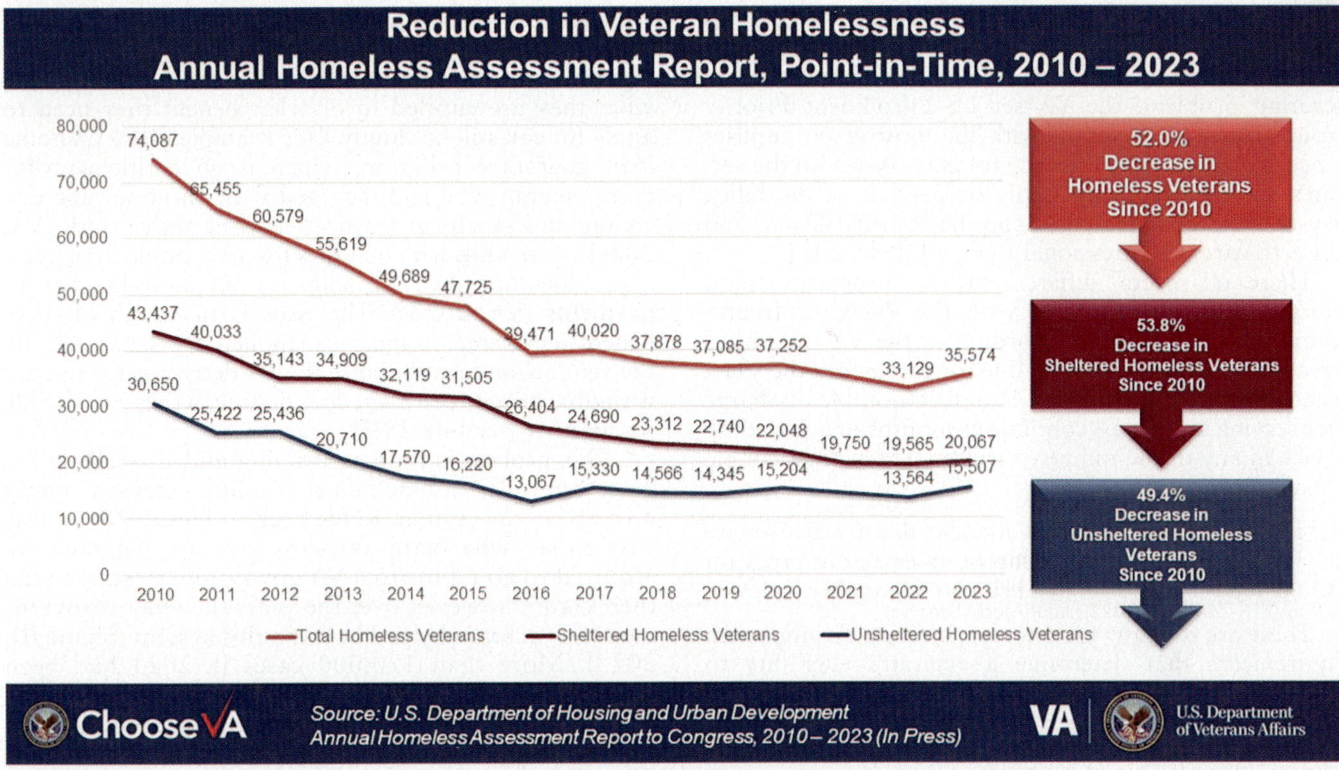

FIGURE 28-10 Between 2022 and 2023, veterans who experienced homelessness increased by 7.4%. (Reprinted from U.S. Department of Veterans Affairs. (2023). *2023 Veteran PIT count results.* https://news.va.gov/126913/veteran-homelessness-increased-by-7-4-in-2023/#)

	All Veterans		Sheltered Veterans		Unsheltered Veterans	
All Veterans	35,574	100%	20,067	100%	15,507	100%
Gender						
Female	3,980	11.2%	1,815	9.0%	2,165	14.0%
Male	31,231	87.8%	18,148	90.4%	13,083	84.4%
Transgender	173	0.5%	74	0.4%	99	0.6%
A Gender that is not Singularly 'Female' or 'Male'	161	0.5%	21	0.1%	140	0.9%
Questioning	29	0.1%	9	0.0%	20	0.1%
Ethnicity						
Non-Hispanic/Latin(a)(o)(x)	30,885	86.8%	18,235	90.9%	12,650	81.6%
Hispanic/Latin(a)(o)(x)	4,689	13.2%	1,832	9.1%	2,857	18.4%
Race						
American Indian, Alaska Native, or Indigenous	1,269	3.6%	461	2.3%	808	5.2%
Asian or Asian American	608	1.7%	183	0.9%	425	2.7%
Black, African American, or African	11,136	31.3%	7,203	35.9%	3,933	25.4%
Native Hawaiian or Pacific Islander	427	1.2%	169	0.8%	258	1.7%
White	20,287	57.0%	11,343	56.5%	8,944	57.7%
Multiple Races	1,847	5.2%	708	3.5%	1,139	7.3%

FIGURE 28-11 Demographic characteristics of veterans experiencing homelessness. (Reprinted from U.S. Department of Housing and Urban Development. (2023). *The 2023 Annual Homelessness Assessment Report (AHAR) to Congress.* Retrieved from https://www.huduser.gov/portal/sites/default/files/pdf/2023-ahar-part-1.Pdf)

It was not until 1986 that Congress enacted legislation that required a "means test" for veterans who did not have "service-connected disabilities." To address this proliferating problem, the VA set up Enrollment Priority Groups to ensure veterans with the most severe injuries or needs were given preference for care. Based on the veteran's specific eligibility status or percent of disability, they become qualified for a specific Priority Group and access to care (Congressional Budget Office, 2021).

There are several different factors in determining a veteran's eligibility for care with the **Veterans Health Administration** (VHA). According to the VA (2024f), a person can be considered eligible for care under the VHA system if they have not received a dishonorable discharge after serving at least 24 continuous months of active-duty service in any of the military services. There are a couple of exceptions to the rules:

1. Discharged under medical disability due to active service
2. Discharged under hardship or an early-out program
3. Served on active service prior to September 7, 1980

There are so many factors after meeting the minimum requirements that determine a veteran's eligibility to receive healthcare from the VHA that the VA recommends that a veteran seek help in applying from their state's Veterans agency (VA, 2024f). Some categories of veterans could qualify for enhanced eligibility status with the VHA and be placed in a higher priority group.

Enrollment priority groups are determined by several factors, with veterans with service-connected disabilities placed in the highest priority group and veterans earning a high income with no service-connected disability in the lowest priority group (VA, 2024g).

Veteran Benefits Versus Entitlements

A veteran can either receive veteran benefits or entitlements from the VA. It can be confusing to know which is which for the veteran. Any service member separating or retiring from the military is required to attend a transition assistance program class (VA, 2024h) prior to leaving their respective services; however, their knowledge of what they are entitled to or what benefit they need to apply for can still be cloudy. One example is the VA home loan guarantee program, which is an entitlement for every veteran who is discharged with an honorable discharge and served at least 90 days of active duty (VA, 2024i). A veteran who qualifies for a VA home loan guarantee does not always qualify for VA disability benefit payments (VA, 2022c). The issue is that each of these benefits/entitlements must be applied for separately by the veteran, and just because the VA determines a veteran is eligible for one program does not mean they are eligible for another (see Box 28-3).

This process is time consuming and frustrating for most veterans, so much so that many veterans simply give up on the system. Refer back to Figure 28-1—it is easy to see why many veterans give up. Veterans are required to go online to a VA.gov system to start to file their claim; however, over the years the federal government has acknowledged holes in this system (Shane III, 2023). More than 120,000 cases in 2023 had been noted to be lost in the system, meaning the veteran filed their claim but it was never processed, and no benefits were ever established. The importance of filing these claims is important for the benefit of medical coverage or supplemental payments. Data from a 2019 to 2021 National Health Interview Survey estimated that 12.8% of veterans aged 25 to 64 years had difficulties paying their medical bills; 38.4% were worried if they got sick or injured, they would have issues paying for the medical bills; and 8.4% just went without medical care due to lack of ability to pay (Cohen & Boersma, 2023).

The VA has made strides to correct the system. However, as of June 2024, there are 962,416 pending claims in their system, 268,390 on the backlog list, and the current average day to claim completion is 154.8 days (VA, 2024j).

BOX 28-3 Benefits/Entitlements Must Be Applied for Separately

Let's look at an example of how a veteran can receive benefits/entitlements:

Jason is an Army veteran who served 36 months and deployed in Operation Enduring Freedom twice. Jason was honorably discharged after the completion of his contract.

Jason wants to buy a house. He must let his lender know he wants to use his VA home loan benefit and qualifies. The lender will then check with the VA to verify that he qualifies. He is approved and can purchase his home.

Jason decides he wants to go back to school. He is already in the VA system from when he applied for his VA home loan; however, it is not automatic that he gets VA education benefits. He needs to speak with the VA representative at his school to apply for benefits. He served after September 11, 2001, and therefore qualifies for education benefits.

Jason has been paying out of pocket at urgent care every time he gets sick, and it is starting to add up. He decides to see if he qualifies for VA healthcare. To qualify, he must start the process online with VA registration. Since he had an honorable discharge and served at least 24 months, he is approved but at a low priority as he is not in a service-connected disability priority category yet.

Jason has recurring nightmares and is easily angered. He suspects he may have PTSD from his combat experiences and decides he may qualify for VA disability. Again, he must go into the VA.gov system and file a claim to see if he qualifies. He files his applications but cannot proceed as he is required to supply evidence that he truly has PTSD caused by active-duty service.

1. *How can the C/PHN assist veterans with benefits and entitlements?*
2. *What resources exist in your community for assisting veterans?*
3. *Does your community offer support to link veterans to benefits and entitlement?*

Military Health History

Pocket Card For Health Professions Trainees and Clinicians

A Veteran's perspective:

"Help me understand my medical condition."

"I had some unique experiences while serving our country, many that civilians would never have. Some of them may be affecting my health, and that is why I am here at VA."

"Please be patient with me. Some of my memories are difficult to discuss."

Asking the questions on this card will clarify a Veterans' medical concerns.

- Ask these questions in a safe and private place.
- Engage with good eye contact.
- Use a supportive tone of voice.
- Thank Veterans if they disclose stressful or traumatic experiences.
- If you suspect someone is actively at risk for suicide, do not leave them alone.

Suicide Prevention Questions

- Would it be okay if I asked you about suicide?
  (self-directed violence includes suicidal thoughts, self-harm, attempts of suicide, etc.)
- Are you having thoughts of suicide? Have you ever exhibited self-destructive behavior, such as drug abuse, risky use of weapons, etc.?

Veterans Crisis Line
Dial 988, then Press 1

OAA Office of Academic Affiliations
Passion to learn. Power to heal.

VA U.S. Department of Veterans Affairs

FIGURE 28-12 Healthcare professional pocket card. (Reprinted from U.S. Department of Veterans Affairs. (n.d.). *Military health history pocket card for health professions trainees and clinicians*. https://www.va.gov/oaa/docs/mhpcmobile.pdf)

C/PHN RESOURCES

Although nursing resources remain scarce in the civilian community, there is a growing movement to better prepare our workforce to care for veterans and their families. Some basic resources available now are the *Military Health History Pocket Card for Health Professions Trainees and Clinicians* (VA Office of Academic Affiliation, n.d.) and *Have You Ever Served in the Military?* (American Academy of Nursing, n.d.; Fig. 28-12).

Nursing organizations are leading efforts to bring veterans' care to the forefront through campaigns and collective work. Exemplars include the American Nurses Association/California Veterans Health campaign and the work of the American Academy of Nursing Veterans Health Expert Panel in pursuing a specialty nursing organization, competencies, and certification in veterans care. These exemplars open opportunities for all nurses to better understand the community of veterans we serve.

SUMMARY

- It is crucial to recognize the veteran community as a population with its own culture, language, and needs.
- Veterans' health, benefits, resources, and reintegration into the civilian community remain complex issues.
- Veterans' mental health, housing, and SUD remain top national priorities.
- The C/PHN specialty must act as knowledgeable partners with the federal, state, and county entities that serve our veteran community.
- It is important to recognize that not all veterans utilize or are aware of the available resources, and some do not qualify for VA resources and benefits.
- The C/PHN is responsible for ensuring the knowledge and information regarding veterans is up to date, accurate, and culturally appropriate when engaging the veteran community.

LEARNING ACTIVITIES

1. The Library of Congress (LOC) Veterans History Project Collection has recorded personal stories of veterans across several eras (World War I, World War II, the Korean War, the Cold War, the Persian Gulf War, and the War in Iraq and Afghanistan). Using the provided link, https://www.loc.gov/collections/veterans-history-project-collection/serving-our-voices/, select at least two veterans from two different eras to listen to. Reflect on any preconceived notions, biases, or stereotypes you might have had about veterans before engaging in this assignment. Discuss how these perceptions have evolved or been challenged based on the reading and any insights gained from the LOC veteran interviews. (Objective 1)
2. Decide on a physical health problem discussed in the chapter. How does it affect the person? How prevalent is the health issue within the veteran community? What challenges does the problem cause within the environment? Identify resources in your community that support the unique healthcare need. Do these resources/support services exist in your area or does the veteran need to travel outside the area? (Objective 2)
3. Decide on a mental health problem within the veteran population discussed in the chapter. Why is it a public health problem? Interview a healthcare provider or C/PHN who works with veterans to discuss the best approach when working with this population and the problem of finding resources. (Objective 3)
4. Assess the community in which you live through the eyes of a veteran. Are you in a rural area or do you live in a city? Based on your assessment, describe the difficulties veterans have accessing care. If possible, speak with a veteran and ask what the difficulties are. Do they access VA-provided services? If not, why not? Share your findings with classmates to gain a broader view of these difficulties. Which of the 10 Essential Public Health Services (Box 2-2) did you employ? (Objective 4)
5. Scenario: You have been invited to be one of the presenters at the local community center regarding health disparities between the veteran and civilian communities. The community has a high veteran population and their families. You are given the option to present on any health disparity discussed in the chapter. Once you decide on the topic, create a poster with the information needed. What information will you include on the poster? What do you hope the community will learn? (Objective 5)

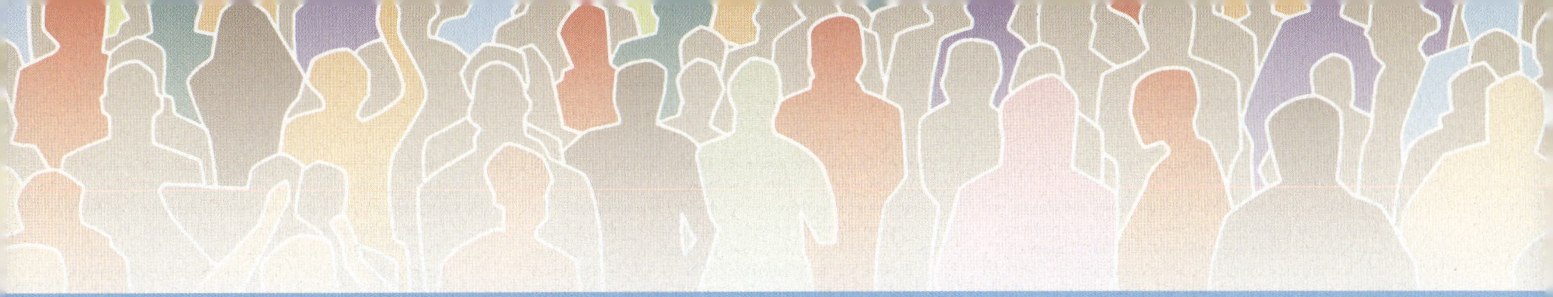

REFERENCES

CHAPTER 1

AbdulRaheem, Y. (2023). Unveiling the significance and challenges of integrating prevention levels in healthcare practice. *Journal of Primary Care & Community Health*, *14*, 21501319231186500. https://doi.org/10.1177/21501319231186500

Alfonseca, K. (2023, August 29). Maui wildfire victims search on land ends, moves to the ocean. *ABC News*. https://abcnews.go.com/US/maui-officials-search-wildfire-victims-ocean-land-search/story?id=102648231

Ali, A., & Katz, D. L. (2018). Disease prevention and health promotion: How integrative medicine fits. *American Journal of Preventive Medicine*, *49*(5 Suppl 3), S230–S240.

American Hospital Association, Center for Health Innovation. (2023). *Community health & well-being. What is community health?* https://www.aha.org/center/community-health-well-being#:~:text=Community%20health%20refers%20to%20non,in%20a%20geographically%20defined%20population

American Nurses Association (ANA). (2022). *Public health nursing: Scope and standards of practice* (3rd ed.).

American Public Health Association (APHA). (2023). *What is public health?* https://www.apha.org/what-is-public-health

American Public Health Association (APHA). (2024). *About APHA*. https://www.apha.org/About-APHA

American Public Health Association (APHA) Public Health Nursing Section. (2024). *About public health nursing*. https://www.apha.org/apha-communities/member-sections/public-health-nursing/who-we-are#:~:text=Public%20health%20nursing%20is%20the,assessment%2C%20assurance%20and%20policy%20development

Anderson, E. T., & McFarlane, J. (2019). *Community as partner: Theory and practice in nursing* (8th ed.). Lippincott Williams & Wilkins.

Bhukhan, A., Dunn, C., & Nathoo, R. (2023). Case report of leprosy in central Florida, USA 2022. *Emerging Infectious Diseases*, *29*(8), 1698–1700. https://doi.org/10.3201/eid2908.220367

Blacksin, A. A. (2022). Case report: Vaccine Brigade Chicago, Illinois: from founding February to July 2021. *Public Health Nursing*, *39*(5), 1034–1040. https://doi.org/10.1111/phn.13072

Butterfield, P. G. (1990). Thinking upstream: Nurturing a conceptual understanding of the societal context of health behavior. *Advances in Nursing Science*, *12*(2), 1–8.

Butterfield, P. G. (2002). Upstream reflections on environmental health: An abbreviated history and framework for action. *Advances in Nursing Science*, *25*(1), 32–49.

Butterfield, P. G. (2017). Thinking upstream: A 25-year retrospective and conceptual model aimed at reducing health inequities. *Advances in Nursing Science*, *40*(1), 2–11.

Campbell, L., Harmon, M., Joyce, B., & Little, S. (2020). Quad Council Coalition community/public health nursing competencies: Building consensus through collaboration. *Public Health Nursing*, *37*(1), 96–112.

Castner, J., Amiri, A., Rodriguez, J., Huntington-Moskos, L., Thompson, L. M., Zhao, S., & Polivka, B. (2019). Advancing the symptom science model with environmental health. *Public Health Nursing*, *36*(5), 716–725. https://doi.org/10.1111/phn.12641

CDC Foundation. (2023). *What is public health?* https://www.cdcfoundation.org/what-public-health#:~:text=Overall%2C%20public%20health%20is%20concerned,or%20region%20of%20the%20world

Centers for Disease Control (CDC). (2011). Ten great public health achievements—United States, 2001—2010. *Morbidity and Mortality Weekly*, *60*(19), 619–623. https://www.cdc.gov/mmwr/preview/mmwrhtml/mm6019a5.htm

Centers for Disease Control (CDC). (2021a). *Division of Scientific Education and Professional Development. Introduction to public health. Winslow's definition of public health.* https://www.cdc.gov/training/publichealth101/public-health.html#:~:text=Public%20health%20is%20"the%20science,and%20individuals."%20—%20CEA%20Winslow

Centers for Disease Control (CDC). (2021b). *Division of Scientific Education and Professional Development. Introduction to public health: Public Health 101 Series. Knowledge check*. https://www.cdc.gov/training/publichealth101/documents/introduction-to-public-health.pdf

Centers for Disease Control and Prevention (CDC). (2023). *What is health literacy?* https://www.cdc.gov/healthliteracy/learn/index.html#:~:text=Personal%20health%20literacy%20is%20the,actions%20for%20themselves%20and%20others

Centers for Disease Control and Prevention (CDC) & National Center for Chronic Disease Prevention & Health Promotion (NCCDPHP). (2022). *Built environment: NCCDPHP's program successes*. https://www.cdc.gov/chronicdisease/healthequity/sdoh-and-chronic-disease/nccdphp-and-social-determinants-of-health/built-environment.htm#:~:text=For%20example%2C%20communities%20with%20parks,determinants%20of%20health%20(SDOH)

Centers for Disease Control and Prevention (CDC) National Center for Health Statistics. (2022). *Life expectancy in the U.S. dropped for the second year in a row in 2021*. https://www.cdc.gov/nchs/pressroom/nchs_press_releases/2022/20220831.htm#print

Chan, M., Shamasunder, B., & Johnson, J. (2023). Social and environmental stressors of urban oil and gas facilities in Loss Angeles County, California, 2020. *American Journal of Public Health*, *113*(11), 1182–1190. https://doi.org/10.2105/AJPH.2023.307360

Corley, J., Okely, J., Taylor, A., Page, D., Welstead, M., Skarabela, B., Redmond, P., Cox, S., & Russ, T. (2021). Home garden use during COVID-19: Associations with physical and mental wellbeing in older adults. *Journal of Environmental Psychology*, *73*, 101545. https://doi.org/10.1016/j.jenvp.2020.101545

County Health Rankings. (2023). *County health rankings and roadmaps: About us*. https://www.countyhealthrankings.org/about-us

Czachor, E. M. (2023a, July 19). Canadian wildfire maps show where fires continue to burn across Quebec, Ontario, and other provinces. *CBS News*. https://www.cbsnews.com/amp/news/map-canadian-wildfires-2023-where-are-the-fires-ontario-quebec/

Czachor, E. M. (2023b, July 27). How did the Maui fire start? What we know about the cause of the Lahaina blaze. *CBS News*. https://www.cbsnews/how-did-Maui-fire-start-cause-Lahaina-Hawaii-wildfire/

Dintica, C. S., Bahorik, A., Xia, F., Kind, A., & Yaffe, K. (2023, July 19). Dementia risk and disadvantaged neighborhoods. *JAMA Neurology*, *80*(9), 903–909. https://doi.org/10.1001/jamaneurol.2023.2120

Dos Santos, O. P., Melly, P., Joost, S., & Verloo, H. (2023). Climate change, environmental health, and challenges for nursing discipline. *International Journal of Environmental Research and Public Health*, *20*(9), 5682. https://doi.org/10.3390/ijerph20095682

Edmonds, J., Kneipp, S., & Campbell, L. (2020). A call to action for public health nursing during the COVID-19 pandemic. *Public Health Nursing*, *37*, 323–324. https://doi.org/10.1111/phn.12733

Environmental Protection Agency (EPA). (2023). *Learn about environmental justice*. https://www.epa.gov/environmentaljustice/learn-about-environmental-justice

Everytown for Gun Safety. (2023). *We have a plan to end gun violence*. https://www.everytown.org/?_gl=1%2Akmuzfs%2A_ga%2AMTAwODI1ODkxMC4xNjkxNjA3NDU4%2A_ga_LT0FWV3EK3%2AMTY5MTcwNDgxNS4zLjEuMTY5MTcwNDkyMS4wLjAuMA

Federal, Provincial, and Territorial Advisory Committee on Population Health. (1999). *Toward a healthy future: Second report on the health of Canadians*. Minister of Public Works and Government Services Canada.

FEMA. (2024a). *Biden-Harris administration leaders to join Hawaii officials and survivors one year following the devastating wildfires on Maui*. https://www.fema.gov/press-release/20240806/biden-harris-administration-leaders-join-hawaii-officials-and-survivors-one

FEMA. (2024b). *One year later, Maui wildfire recovery continues with nearly $3 billion in deferral support*. https://www.fema.gov/fact-sheet/one-year-later-maui-wildfire-recovery-continues-nearly-3-billion-federal-support

Fleszar, L., Bryant, A., Johnson, C., Blacker, B., Aravkin, A., Baumann, M., Dwyer-Lindgren, L., Kelly, Y., Maass, K., Zheng, P., & Roth, G. (2023). Trends in state-level maternal mortality by racial and ethnic group in the United States. *JAMA*, *330*(1), 52–61. https://doi.org/a10.1001/jama.2023.9043

Gaffney, A., Himmelstein, D., & Woolhandler, S. (2020). COVID-19 and US health financing: Perils and possibilities. *International Journal of Health Services*, *50*(4), 396–407. https://doi.org/10.1177/0020731420931431

Galea, M., & van Schalkwyk, M. C. I. (2023). Understanding the US health care industry as a commercial determinant of health. *JAMA Health Forum*, *4*(7), e232795. https://jamanetwork.com/journals/jama-health-forum/fullarticle/2807445

Get Healthy San Mateo County. (n.d.). *Strategies for building healthy, equitable communities*. Retrieved August 7, 2023, from https://www.gethealthysmc.org/sites/main/files/file-attachments/get_healthy_smc_strategic_plan_2015-2020_final.pdf?1485905434

Gramlich, J. (2023, April 26). *What the data says about gun deaths in the U.S. Pew Research Center*. https://www.pewresearch.org/short-reads/2023/04/26/what-the-data-says-about-gun-deaths-in-the-u-s/#:~:text=How%20many%20people%20die%20from,U.S.%2C%20according%20to%20the%20CDC

Granrud, M. D., Anderzen-Carlsson, A., Bisholt, B., & Steffenak, A. K. M. (2019). Public health nurses' perceptions of interprofessional collaboration related to adolescents' mental health problems in secondary schools: A phenomenographic study. *Journal of Clinical Nursing*, *28*(15–16), 2899–2910. https://doi.org/10.1111/jocn.14881

Gwon, S. H., Cho, C. I., Paek, S., & Ke, W. (2020). Public health nurses' workforce factors and population health outcomes in the United States. *Public Health Nursing*, *37*(6), 829–836. https://doi.org/10.1111/phn.12793

Gwon, S. H., Thongpriwan, V., & Kett, P. (2023). Public health nurses' perceptions and experiences of emergency preparedness, responsiveness, and burnout during the COVID-19 pandemic. *Public Health Nursing*, *40*(1), 124–134. https://doi.org/10.1111/phn.13141

Harris, O., Bialous, S., Meunch, U., Chapman, S., & Dawson-Rose, C. (2022). Climate change, public health, health policy, and nurses training. *American Journal of Public Health*, *112*(S3), S321–S327.

Hinton, E. (2023). *A look at recent Medicaid guidance to address social determinants of health and health-related social needs*. Kaiser Family Foundation. https://www.kff.org/policy-watch/a-look-at-recent-medicaid-guidance-to-address-social-determinants-of-health-and-health-related-social-needs/

Horntvedt, J. (2023). *Five ways to think about community*. University of Minnesota Extension. https://extension.umn.edu/community-news-and-insights/five-ways-think-about-community

Institute for Healthcare Improvement. (2023). *Population health*. https://www.ihi.org/Topics/PopulationHealth/Pages/default.aspx#:~:text=Population%20health%20is%20defined%20as,such%20outcomes%20within%20the%20group

Institute of Medicine (IOM). Committee on Assuring the Health of the Public in the 21st Century (2003). *The future of the public's health in the 21st century. Preface*. National Academies Press. https://www.ncbi.nlm.nih.gov/books/NBK221223/

Iriarte-Roteta, A., Lopez-Discastillo, O., Mujika, A., Ruiz-Zaldibar, C., Hernantes, N., Bermejo-Martins, E., & Pumar-Mendez, M. J. (2020). Nurses' role in health promotion and prevention: A critical interpretive synthesis. *Journal of Clinical Nursing*, *29*(21–22), 3937–3949.

Jarvie, J. (2023, August 31). The hunt for bones and closure in Maui's burn fields *The Los Angeles Times*. https://www.latimes.com/world-nation/story/2023-08-31/maui-fire-missing-forenic-experts-dead-identify-closure

Kindig, D., & Stoddart, G. (2003). What is population health? *American Journal of Public Health*, *93*(3), 380–383. https://doi.org/10.2105/ajph.93.3.380

Krishna, P. (2022). Assuring a continuum of care for heart failure patients through post-acute care collaboration: An integrative review. *Case Management Monthly*, *28*(1), 3–10. https://doi.org/10.1097/NCM.0000000000000600

Kuo, C., & Kawachi, I. (2023). County-level income inequality, social mobility, and deaths of despair in the US, 2000–2019. *JAMA Network Open*, *6*(7), e2323030. https://jamanetwork.com/journals/jamanetworkopen/fullarticle/2807161

Lantz, P. M. (2020). "Super-utilizer" interventions: What they reveal about evaluation research, wishful thinking, and health equity. *The Millbank Quarterly*, *98*(1), 31–34.

Leavell, H., & Clark, E. (1953). *Textbook of preventive medicine*. McGraw-Hill.

Lenartowicz, M. (2023). *Prevention of disease in the elderly (levels of prevention)*. Merck Manual: Professional Version. https://www.merckmanuals.com/professional/geriatrics/prevention-of-disease-and-disability-in-the-elderly/prevention-of-disease-in-the-elderly

McDermott, J., & Kelleher, J. S. (2023, August 28). *Hawaii power utility takes responsibility for first fire on Maui, but faults county firefighters*. Associated Press. https://apnews.com/article/hawaii-wildfires-maui-electricity-power-utilities-1741e22bbf955b62103db6b60f5c4853

McKillop, M., & Lieberman, D. A. (2022). *The impact of chronic underfunding in America's public health system: Trends, risks, & recommendations*. Trust for America's Health. https://www.tfah.org/wp-content/uploads/2021/05/2021_PHFunding_Fnl.pdf

McKinley, J. (1979, June). *A case for focusing upstream: The political economy of illness* Proceedings of the American Heart Association Conference: Applying Behavioral Science to Cardiovascular Risk, Seattle, WA.

McMahon, N. E. (2021). Framing action to reduce health inequalities: What is argued for through use of the 'upstream-downstream' metaphor? *Journal of Public Health*, *44*(3), 671–678.

Melariri, H., Osoba, T., Williams, M., & Melariri, P. (2022). An assessment of nurses' participation in health promotion: A knowledge, perception, and practice perspective. *Journal of Preventive Medicine & Hygiene*, *63*(1), e27–e34. https://www.ncbi.nlm.nih.gov/pmc/articles/PMC9121667/

Merriam-Webster. (2023). *Definition of wellness*. https://www.merriam-webster.com/dictionary/wellness

Moen, O. L., & Jacobsen, I. C. (2022). School nurses' experiences in dealing with adolescents having mental health problems. *SAGE Open Nursing*, *6*(8), 223779608221124411. https://doi.org/10.1177/23779608221124411

Moms Demand Action. (2023). *About our story*. https://momsdemandaction.org/about/

Munoz, E., Scott, S. B., Corley, R., Wadsworth, S. J., Sliwinski, M. J., & Reynolds, C. A. (2020). The role of neighborhood stressors on cognitive function: A coordinated analysis. *Health and Place*, *66* art. 102442. https://doi.org/10.16/jhealthplace.2020.102442

Murdaugh, C., Parsons, M. A., & Pender, N. (2019). *Health promotion in nursing practice* (8th ed.). Pearson. ISBN-13 9780134754086.

National Academy of Sciences, Engineering, and Medicine (NASEM). (2021). *The future of nursing 2020–2030: Charting a path to achieve health equity*. National Academies Press. https://doi.org/10.17226/25982

National Council of State Boards of Nursing (NCSBN). (2023). *Next Generation NCLEX: NCLEX Test Plan*. https://www.ncsbn.org/public-files/2023_RN_Test%20Plan_English_FINAL.pdf

National Institute of Environmental Health Sciences (NIEHS). (2023a). *Environmental health disparities and environmental justice*. https://www.niehs.nih.gov/research/supported/translational/justice/index.cfm

National Institute of Environmental Health Sciences (NIEHS). (2023b). *Gene and environment interaction*. https://www.niehs.nih.gov/health/topics/science/gene-env/index.cfm

Nightingale, F. (1859/1992). *Notes on nursing: What it is, and what it is not* [Commemorative edition]. Lippincott Williams & Wilkins.

Office of Disease Prevention & Health Promotion. (2023). *Healthy people 2030 objectives & measures*. https://health.gov/healthypeople/objectives-and-data/about-objectives/healthy-people-2030-objectives-and-measures

Pope, D., Tisdall, R., Middleton, J., Verma, A., van Ameijden, E., Birt, C., & Macherianakis, N. G. (2018). Quality of and access to green space in relation to psychological distress: Results from a population-based cross-sectional study as part of the EURO-URHIS 2 project. *European Journal of Public Health*, *28*(1), 35–38.

Quad Council (now Council of Public Health Nursing Organizations [CPHNO]). (1997). *Tenets of public health nursing*. https://www.cphno.org/wp-content/uploads/2020/08/QCC-tenets.pdf

Quad Council Coalition Competency Review Task Force (now Council of Public Health Nursing Organizations). (2018). *Community/public health nursing competencies*. https://www.cphno.org/wp-content/uploads/2020/08/QCC-C-PHN-COMPETENCIES-Approved_2018.05.04_Final-002.pdf

Ray, R., Lantz, P., & Williams, D. (2023). Upstream policy changes to improve population health and health equity: A priority agenda. *The Millbank Quarterly*, *101*(S1), 20–35. https://onlinelibrary.wiley.com/doi/10.1111/1468-0009.12640

Robert Wood Johnson Foundation. (n.d.). *About the Robert Wood Johnson Foundation*. Retrieved August 7, 2023.

Robertson, D. (2020, December 23). Flint has clean water now. Why won't people drink it? *Politico Magazine*. https://www.politico.com/news/magazine/2020/12/23/flint-water-crisis-2020-post-coronavirus-america-445459

Romero-Collado, A., Baltasar-Bague, A., Puigvert-Viu, N., Rascon-Hernan, C., & Homs-Romero, E. (2020). Using simulation and electronic health records to train nursing students in prevention and health promotion interventions. *Nurse Educator Today*, *89*, 104384. https://doi.org/10.1016//j.nedt.2020.104384

Rudner, N. (2021). Nursing is a health equity and social justice movement. *Public Health Nursing*, *38*(4), 687–691.

Rural Health Information Hub. (2023). *The Hunger Coalition's Bloom Truck and Bloom Markets* (online). https://www.ruralhealthinfo.org/project-examples/1116

Savulescu, J., Persson, I., & Wilkinson, D. (2020). Utilitarianism and the pandemic. *Bioethics*, *34*(6), 620–632. https://doi.org/10.1111/bioe.12771

Scott, S. B., Munoz, E., Mogle, J. A., Gamaldo, A. A., Smyth, J. M., Almeida, D. M., & Sliwinski, M. J. (2018). Perceived neighborhood characteristics predict severity and emotional response to daily stressors. *Social Science & Medicine*, *200*, 262–279.

Seabert, D. M., McKenzie, J. F., & Pinger, R. R. (2022). *An introduction to community and public health* (10th ed.). Jones & Bartlett Learning.

Servadio, J., Lawal, A., Davis, T., Bates, J., Russell, A., Ramaswami, A., Convertino, M., & Botchwey, N. (2019). Demographic inequities in health outcomes and air pollution exposure in the Atlanta area and its relationship to urban infrastructure. *Journal of Urban Health*, *96*(2), 219–234. https://www.ncbi.nlm.nih.gov/pmc/articles/PMC6458195/

Sharifian, N., Spivey, B. N., Zaheed, A. B., & Zahodne, L. B. (2020). Psychological distress links perceived neighborhood characteristics to longitudinal trajectories of cognitive health in older adulthood. *Social Science & Medicine*, *258* art. 113125.

Shen, A., Browne, S., Srivastava, T., Kornides, M., & Tan, A. (2023). Trusted messengers and trusted messages: The role for community-based organizations in promoting COVID-19 and routine immunizations. *Vaccine*, *41*(12), 1994–2002. https://doi.org/10.1016/j.vaccine.2023.02.045

Stout, S., Howard, P., Lewis, N., McPherson, M., & Schall, M. (2017). *Foundations of a community of solutions. SCALE 1.0 synthesis reports*. Institute for Healthcare Improvement. https://www.100mlives.org/wp-content/uploads/2017/07/Foundations-of-Community-of-Solutions-Approach-7.10.17.pdf

Students Demand Action. (2023). *We're young activists committed to ending gun violence in our communities*. https://studentsdemandaction.org

Subu, M. A., Holmes, S., Arumugam, A., Al-Yateem, N., Dias, J. M., Rahman, S. A., Waluyo, I., Ahmad, F. R., & Abraham, M. S. (2022). Traditional, religious, and cultural perspectives on mental illness: A qualitative study on causal beliefs and treatment use. *International Journal of Qualitative Studies on Health and Well-Being*, *17*(1), 2123090.

Sylvers, D., Hicken, M., Esposito, M., Manly, J., Judd, S., & Clarke, P. (2022). Walkable neighborhoods and cognition: Implications for the design of health promoting communities. *Journal of Aging & Health*, *34*(6–8), 893–904. https://doi.org/10.1177/08982643221075509

U.S. Department of Health and Human Services (USDHHS), Office of Disease Prevention and Health Promotion (ODPHP). (2023a). *Healthy People 2030 framework*. https://health.gov/healthypeople/about/healthy-people-2030-framework

U.S. Department of Health and Human Services (USDHHS), Office of Disease Prevention and Health Promotion (ODPHP). (2023c). *Healthy People 2030 overview*. https://health.gov/our-work/national-health-initiatives/healthy-people/healthy-people-2030.

U.S. Fire Administration. (2024a). *Lahaina Hawaii fire timeline report*. https://www.usfa.fema.gov/blog/lahaina-hawaii-fire-timeline-report/

U.S. Fire Administration. (2024b). *Preliminary after-action report: 2023 Maui wildfire*. https://www.usfa.fema.gov/blog/preliminary-after-action-report-2023-maui-wildfire/

van Daalen, K., Romanello, M., Rocklov, J., Semenza, J., Tonne, C., Markandya, A., Dasandi, N., Jankin, S., Achebak, H., Ballester, J., Bechara, H., Callaghan, M. W., Chambers, J., Dasgupta, S., Drummond, P., Farooq, Z., Gasparyan, O., Gonzalez-Reviriego, N., Hamilton, I., ... Lowe, R. (2022). The 2022 Europe report of the Lancet Countdown on health and climate change: Towards a climate resilient future. *Lancet Public Health*, *7*, e942–e965.

Ware, D., Landy, D., Rabil, A., Hennekens, C., & Hecht, E. (2022). Interrelationships between self-reported physical health and health behaviors among healthy US adults: from the NHANES 2009-2016. *Public Health in Practice*, *4*, 100277. https://doi.org/10.1016/j.puhip.2022.100277

Wei, M., Woo, J., & Cui, J. (2023). Factors influencing foot care behavior among patients with diabetes: An integrative literature review. *Nursing Open*, *10*(7), 4216–4243. https://doi.org/10.1002/nop2.1710

Weiss, A., & Jiang, J. (2021, December). *Most frequent reasons for emergency department visits, 2018*. Statistical Brief #286. Healthcare Cost & Utilization Project. Agency for Healthcare Research & *Quality*. https://hcup-us.ahrq.gov/reports/statbriefs/sb286-ED-Frequent-Conditions-2018.pdf

Whitman, A., De Lew, N., Chappel, A., Aysola, V., Zuckerman, R., & Sommers, B. D. (2022, April 1). *Addressing social determinants of health: Examples of successful evidence-based strategies and current federal efforts*. https://aspe.hhs.gov/sites/default/files/documents/e2b650cd64cf84aae8ff0fae7474af82/SDOH-Evidence-Review.pdf

Woolf, S. H. (2023). Falling behind: The growing gap in life expectancy between the United States and other countries, 1933-2021. *American Journal of Public Health*, *113*(9), 970–980. https://doi.org/10,2105/AJPH.2023.307310

World Health Organization (WHO). (2023a). *Constitution of WHO: Principles*. https://www.who.int/about/governance/constitution#:~:text=Health%20is%20a%20state%20of,belief%2C%20economic%20or%20social%20condition

World Health Organization (WHO). (2023b). *Globalization and health* (Meeting 24 October 2008). https://www.who.int/director-general/speeches/detail/globalization-and-health

World Health Organization (WHO). (2023e). *Social determinants of health: WHO called to return to the Declaration of Alma Ata*. https://www.who.int/teams/social-determinants-of-health/declaration-of-alma-ata

World Health Organization (WHO). Regional Office for the Eastern Mediterranean. (2023). *Health promotion and disease prevention through population-based interventions, including action to address social determinants and health inequality*. https://www.emro.who.int/about-who/public-health-functions/health-promotion-disease-prevention.html

Youde, J. (2019). *Globalization and health*. Rowman & Littlefield Publishers. ISBN-13: 978-1538121818.

Zierold, K., Sears, C., Hagemeyer, A., Brock, G., Polivka, B., Zhang, C., & Sears, L. (2020). Protocol for measuring indoor exposure to coal fly ash and heavy metals, and neurobehavioral symptoms in children aged 6 to 14 years old. *British Medical Journal Open*, *10*(11), e038960. https://doi.10.1136/bmjopen-2020-038960

Zota, A. R., & Shamasunder, B. (2021). Environmental health equity: Moving toward a solution-oriented research agenda. *Journal of Exposure Science & Environmental Epidemiology*, *31*, 399–400. https://doi.org/10.1038/s41370-021-00333-5

CHAPTER 2

American Association of Colleges of Nursing (AACN). (2021). *The essentials: Core competencies for professional nursing education.*

American Nurses Association (ANA). (2010). *Nursing's social policy statement: The essence of the profession.* Nursesbooks.org

American Nurses Association (ANA). (2015). *Code of ethics for nurses with interpretive statements.* Nursesbooks.org

American Nurses Association (ANA). (2017). *School nursing: Scope and standards of practice* (3rd ed.). Nursesbooks.org

American Nurses Association (ANA). (2021). *Nursing: Scope and standards of practice* (4th ed.). Nursesbooks.org

American Nurses Association (ANA). (2022). *Public health nursing: Scope and standards of practice* (3rd ed.). Nursesbooks.org

American Nurses Association (ANA). (n.d.). *Leadership in nursing: Qualities & why it matters.* https://www.nursingworld.org/practice-policy/nursing-excellence/leadership-in-nursing/

Association of Public Health Nurses. (2021). *APHN public health policy advocacy guide book and tool kit.* https://www.phnurse.org/advocacy-toolkit

Ballard, M., Bancroft, E., Nesbit, J., Johnson, A., Holeman, I., Foth, J., Rogers, D., Yang, J., Nardella, J., Olsen, H., Raghavan, M., Panjabi, R., Alban, R., Maladba, S., Christiansen, M., Rapp, S., Schechter, J., Aylward, P., Rogers, A., … Palazuelos, D. (2020). Prioritising the role of community health workers in the COVD-19 response. *BMJ Global Health*, *5*, 1–7.

Bayot, M. L., & Varacallo, M. (2022). *Management skills.* In *StatPearls.* StatPearls Publishing. https://www.ncbi.nlm.nih.gov/books/NBK544227/

Carlson, K. (2023). Nurse entrepreneurship: No longer on the fringes. *American Nurse* (on-line). https://www.myamericannurse.com/nurse-entrepreneurship-no-longer-on-the-fringes/

Centers for Disease Control & Prevention (CDC). (2023). *10 essential public health services (revised).* Retrieved from https://www.cdc.gov/publichealthgateway/publichealthservices/essentialhealthservices.html

Centers for Disease Control and Prevention (CDC). (2019). *CDC research on SDOH: Neighborhood and the built environment.* Retrieved from https://www.cdc.gov/socialdeterminants/neighborhood/

Cherry, B., & Jacob, S. R. (2020). *Contemporary nursing: Issues, trends, and management* (8th ed.). Mosby.

Dahlin, C. (2021). *Palliative nursing: Scope and standards of practice* (6th ed.). Hospice & Palliative Nurses Association.

Fowler, M. (2016). *Nursing's social policy statement: Understanding the profession from social contract to social covenant.* American Nurses Association.

Giardino, A. P., & De Jesus, O. (2023). Case management. In *StatPearls* [Internet]. StatPearls Publishing. https://www.ncbi.nlm.nih.gov/books/NBK544227/

Institute of Medicine. (1988). *The future of public health.* National Academy Press.

Institute of Medicine. (2002). *The future of the public's health in the 21st century.* National Academy Press.

Ives Erickson, J., & Pappas, S. (2020). The value of nursing research. *The Journal of Nursing Administration*, *50*(5), 243–244.

Kalaitzidis, E., & Jewell, P. (2020). The concept of advocacy in nursing: A critical analysis. *Health Care Management*, *39*(2), 77–84.

Karimi, M., Lee, E. C., Couture, S. J., Gonzales, A., Grigorescu, V., Smith, S. R., DeLew, N., & Sommers, B. D. (2022). *National survey trends in telehealth use in 2021: Disparities in utilization and audio vs. video services.* [Issue Brief]. U.S. Department of health and Human Services. https://aspe.hhs.gov/sites/default/files/documents/4e1853c0b4885112b2994680a58af9ed/telehealth-hps-ib.pdf

Liou, Y. F., Lin, P. F., Chang, Y. C., & Liaw, J. J. (2021). Perceived importance of competencies by nurse managers at all levels: A cross-sectional study. *Journal of Nursing Management*, *30*(3), 633–642.

Management at Work. (2019). *Mintzberg's 10 managerial roles.* Retrieved from https://management.atwork-network.com/2008/04/15/mintzberg's-10-managerial-roles/

Maxell, A. (2022). *Home health agencies used multiple strategies to respond to the COVID-19 pandemic, although some challenges persist* (Report in Brief). U.S. Department of Health and Human Services. https://oig.hhs.gov/oei/reports/OEI-01-21-00110.pdf.

MindTools. (n.d.). *Mintzberg's management roles: Identifying the roles managers play.* Retrieved from https://www.mindtools.com/pages/videos/management-roles-transcript.htm

Mintzberg, H. (1973). *The nature of managerial work.* Harper & Row.

Murdaugh, C. L., Parsons, M. A., & Pender, N. J. (2019). *Health promotion in nursing practice* (8th ed.). Prentice Hall.

National Association of Clinical Nurse Specialists. (2023). *Definitions of transitional care.* https://nacns.org/resources/toolkits-and-reports/transitions-of-care/definitions-of-transitional-care/

Nsiah, C., Siakwa, M., & Ninnoni, J. (2019). Registered nurses' description of patient advocacy in the clinical setting. *Nursing Open*, *6*(3), 1124–1132. Retrieved from https://www.ncbi.nlm.nih.gov/pmc/articles/PMC6650676/

Ortiz, M. R. (2019). Transitional care: Nursing knowledge and policy implications. *Nursing Science Quarterly*, *32*(1), 73–77.

Orukwowu, U. (2022). Nursing leadership in healthcare: The impact of effective nurse leadership on quality healthcare outcomes. *IPS Interdisciplinary Journal of Social Sciences*, *1*(1), 1–6.

Public Health National Center for Innovations. (2020). Defining public health practice: 25 years of the 10 essential public health services. Retrieved from https://phnci.org/uploads/resource-files/EPHS-English.pdf

Quad Council Coalition Competency Review Task Force. (2018). *Community/public health nursing competencies.* Retrieved from http://www.quadcouncilphn.org/documents-3/2018-qcc-competencies/

Schneider, M. J. (2021). *Introduction to public health* (6th ed.). Jones & Bartlett Learning.

Stabler, H. (2023). Public health and multisectoral collaboration: Where's the evidence? *Journal of Public Health Management and Practice Direct.* https://jphmpdirect.com/2023/04/04/public-health-multisectoral-collaboration-wheres-the-evidence/

The Council on Linkages Between Academia and Public Health Practice. (2021). *Core competencies for public health professionals.* https://www.phf.org/resourcestools/Documents/Core_Competencies_for_Public_Health_Professionals_2021October.pdf

Thorton, L. (2019). A brief history and overview of holistic nursing. *Integrative Medicine: A Clinician's Journal*, *18*(4), 32–33.

U.S. Department of Health and Human Services (USDHHS). (2020). *Healthy people 2030: Public health infrastructure.* https://health.gov/healthypeople/objectives-and-data/browse-objectives/public-health-infrastructure

U.S. Department of Health and Human Services (USDHHS). (2023). *What is telehealth?* https://telehealth.hhs.gov/patients/understanding-telehealth

U.S. Department of Health and Human Services (USDHHS). (n.d.). *Types of evidence-based resources.* Retrieved from https://health.gov/healthypeople/tools-action/browse-evidence-based-resources/types-evidence-based-resources

Vázquez-Calatayud, M., Regaira-Martínez, E., Rumeu-Casares, C., Paloma-Mora, B., Esain, A., & Oroviogoicoechea, C. (2022). Experiences of frontline nurse managers during the COVID-19: A qualitative study. *Journal of Nursing Management*, *30*(1), 79–89.

Yakusheva, O., Czerwinski, M. A., & Buerhaus, P. (2022). Value-informed nursing practice is needed to make our healthcare systems more environmentally sustainable. *Nursing Outlook*, *70*(3), 377–380.

CHAPTER 3

Abrams, S. E. (2004). from function to competency in public health nursing, 1931 to 2003. *Public Health Nursing*, *21*(5), 507–510.

American Association for the History of Nursing (AAHN). (2018). *Isabel Adams Hampton Robb, 1860–1910.* Retrieved from https://www.aahn.org/robb

American Nurses Association. (n.d.). *Health system transformation.* https://www.nursingworld.org/practice-policy/health-policy/health-system-reform/

American Nurses Association, Community Health Nursing Division. (1980). *A conceptual model of community health nursing* (Publication No. CH-10 2M 5/80).

American Red Cross. (2020). *Red cross timeline.* Retrieved from https://www.redcross.org/about-us/who-we-are/history/significant-dates.html

Baker, J. H. (2011). *Margaret Sanger: A life of passion.* Hill and Wang.

Baker, J. P. (2019). When women and children made the policy agenda-The Sheppard-Towner Act, 100 years later. *The New England Journal of Medicine*, *385*(20), 1827–1829.

Beck, A. J., & Boulton, M. L. (2016). The public health nurse workforce in U.S. state and local health departments, 2012. *Public Health Reports*, *131*, 145–152.

Beck, A. J., Boulton, M. L., & Coronado, F. (2014). Public health workforce enumeration. *American Journal of Preventive Medicine*, 47(5 Suppl. 3), s306–s313.

Bowery Boys. (2018). Henry Street Settlement and the legacy of Lillian Wald. Retrieved from http://www.boweryboyshistory.com/2017/03/henry-street-settlement-legacy-lillian-wald.html

Brainard, A. M. (2012). *The many-sided opportunity of field nursing. Public Health Nursing*, 29(3), 283–285.

Buck, J. (2011). Policy and the re-formation of hospice: Lessons from the past for the future of palliative care. *Journal of Hospice and Palliative Nursing*, *13*(6), 35–43. 10.1097/NJH.0b013e3182331160

Buhler-Wilkerson, K. (2001). *No place like home: A history of nursing and home care in the United States.* The Johns Hopkins University Press.

Buhler-Wilkerson, K., Reverby, S. M., Fairman, J. A., & Lewenson, S. B. (2021). *False dawn: The rise and decline of public health nursing.* Rutgers University Press.

Bullough, V., & Bullough, B. (1978). *The care of the sick: The emergence of modern nursing.* Neale, Watson.

Cantelon, P. (2010). *NINR: Bringing science to life NIH Publication No. 10-7502.* https://www.ninr.nih.gov/sites/files/docs/NINR_History_Book_508.pdf

Carter, K. F. (2001). Trumpets of attack: Collaborative efforts between nursing and philanthropies to care for the child crippled with polio 1930 to 1959. *Public Health Nursing*, *18*(4), 253–261.

Carter, E. (September 20, 2018). The forgotten frontier: Nursing done in wild places. *Circulating Now: from the Historical Collection of the National Library of Medicine.* Retrieved from https://circulatingnow.nlm.nih.gov/2018/09/20/the-forgotten-frontier-nursing-done-in-wild-places/

Christy, T. W. (1970). Portrait of a leader: Lillian D. Wald. *Nursing Outlook*, *18*(3), 50–54.

Cueto, M., & Palmer, S. (2015). *Medicine and public health in Latin America: A history.* Cambridge University Press.

Curtis, M. (2008). Stricken village. *Public Health Nursing*, 25(4), 383–386.

D'Antonio, P. (2010). *American nursing: A history of knowledge, authority, and the meaning of work.* Johns Hopkins University Press.

D'Antonio, P. (2013). Cultivating constituencies: The story of the East Harlem Nursing and Health Service, 1928–1941. *American Journal of Public Health*, *103*(6), 988–996.

D'Antonio, P. (2017). *Nursing with a message: Public health demonstrations projects in New York City.* Rutgers University Press.

Dawley, K. (2003). Origins of nurse-midwifery in the United States and its expansion in the 1940s. *Journal of Midwifery and Women's Health*, *48*(2), 86–95.

Dickens, C. (1907). *Martin chuzzlewit.* Alfred A. Knopf Publishing.

Dix, D. (2006). "I tell what I have seen"—The reports of asylum reformer Dorothea Dix. 1843. *American Journal of Public Health*, 96(4), 622–625. https://doi:10.2105/ajph.96.4.622

Dolan, J. A. (1978). *Nursing in society: A historical perspective.* W. B. Saunders.

Donahue, M. P. (2011). *Nursing, the finest art: An illustrated history* (3rd ed.). Mosby Elsevier.

Duffy, J. (1992). *The sanitarians: A history of American public health.* University of Illinois Press.

Edmonds, J. K., Campbell, L. A., & Gilder, R. E. (2017). Public health nursing practice in the Affordable Care Act era: A national survey. *Public Health Nursing*, *34*(1), 50–58. https://doi:10.1111/phn.12286

Ellis, J. R., & Hartley, C. L. (2012). *Nursing in today's world: Trends, issues, and management* (10th ed.). Wolters Kluwer Health/Lippincott Williams & Wilkins.

Erwin, P. C., & Brownson, R. C. (2017). *Scutchfield & Keck's principles of public health practice* (4th ed.). Cengage.

Fee, E., & Bu, L. (2010). The origins of public health nursing: The Henry Street Visiting Nurse Service. *American Journal of Public Health*, *100*(7), 1206–1207.

Feld, M. N. (2008). *Lillian Wald: A biography.* University of North Carolina Press.

Florence Nightingale Museum Trust. (1997). *The Florence Nightingale Museum's school visit pack.*

Gardner, M. S. (1936). *Public health nursing* (3rd ed.). Macmillan.

Geister, J. (1957). The flu epidemic of 1918. *Nursing Outlook, 5*, 582–584.

Goodnow, M. (1930). *Outlines of nursing history* (4th ed.). W.B. Saunders Company.

Hamilton, D. (2007). The cost of caring: The Metropolitan Life Insurance Company's visiting nurse service, 1909–1953. In P. D'Antonio, E. D. Baer, S. D. Rinker & J. E. Lynaugh (Eds.), *Nurses' work: Issues across time and place* (pp. 141–164). Springer.

Hanes, P. (2016). Wildfire disasters and nursing. *Nursing Outlook, 51*(4), 625–645.

Hawkins, J. W., & Watson, J. C. (2010). School nursing on the Iron Range in a public health nursing model. *Public Health Nursing, 27*(6), 571–578.

Hogan, D. (2015). Public health nursing: A rich history. *The Florida Nurse, 63*(3), 10.

Howse, C. (2008). *Rural district nursing in Gloucestershire, 1880-1925*. Reardon Publishing.

Huaiquián-Silva, J. C., Siles-González, J., & Velandia-Mora, A. L. (2013). La enfermería de la Orden de San Juan de Dios en el Chile colonia. *Aquichan, 13*(2), 290–300.

Hughes, A. (1902). The origin, growth, and present status of district nursing in England. *American Journal of Nursing, 2*(5), 337–345.

Jamme, A. C. (1918). The Army School of Nursing. *The American Journal of Nursing, 19*(3), 179–184.

January, A. M. (2009). Friday at the Frontier Nursing Service. *Public Health Nursing*, 26(2), 202–203.

Kalisch, P. A., & Kalisch, B. J. (2004). *American nursing: A history* (4th ed.). Lippincott Williams & Wilkins.

Keeling, A. W. (2009). "When the city is a great field hospital": The influenza pandemic of 1918 and the New York City nursing response. *Journal of Clinical Nursing, 18*, 2732–2738.

Keeling, A. W., Hehman, J. C., & Kirchgessner, J. C. (2018). *History of professional nursing in the United States: Toward a culture of health*. Springer.

Keeling, A. W., & Wall, B. M. (2015). *Nurses and disasters*. Springer Publishing Company.

King, M. G. (2011). Four responsibilities of the tuberculosis nurse, circa 1919. *Public Health Nursing, 28*(5), 469–472.

Kulbok, P. A., & Glick, D. F. (2014). "Something must be done!" Public health nursing education in the United States from 1900 to 1950. *Family & Community Health, 37*(3), 170–178.

Kulbok, P. A., Thatcher, E., Park, E., & Meszaros, P. S. (2012). Evolving public health nursing roles: Focus on community participatory health promotion and prevention. *Online Journal of Issues in Nursing, 17*(2) Manuscript 1. https://doi:10.3912/OJIN.Vol17No02Man01

Lee, G., Clark, A. M., & Thompson, D. R. (2013). Florence Nightingale—Never more relevant than today. *Journal of Advanced Nursing, 69*(2), 234–246.

Lewinson, S. B., McAllister, A., & Smith, K. M. (Eds.). (2017). *Nursing history for contemporary role development*. Springer.

Liehr, P., Sopcheck, J., & Milbrath, G. (2016). Remembering Pearl Harbor at 75 years: Stories of Army and Navy nurses who were there. *The American Journal of Nursing, 116*(12), 54–57.

Lindenmeyer, K. (n.d.). *Children's bureau*. Retrieved from https://socialwelfare.library.vcu.edu/programs/child-welfarechild-labor/children's-bureau/

Lineberry, C. (May 7, 2013). *A brief history of female nurses in the military, from the American Revolution to World War II*. Retrieved from http://www.huffingtonpost.com/cate

Lippincott Williams & Wilkins. (1952). The 1952 Biennial. *The American Journal of Nursing, 52*(8), 960–977.

Mason, J. O., & McGinnis, J. M. (1990). "Healthy People 2000": An overview of the national health promotion and disease prevention objectives. *Public Health Reports, 105*(5), 441–446.

McIsaac, I. (1912). The Army Nurse Corps. *The American Journal of Nursing, 13*(3), 172–176.

Milbrath, G. R., & DeGuzman, P. B. (2015). Neighborhood: A conceptual analysis. *Public Health Nursing, 32*(4), 349–358.

Morman, E. T. (1984). Guarding against alien impurities: The Philadelphia Lazaretto 1854-1893. *The Pennsylvania Magazine of History and Biography, 108*(2), 131–151.

Mowbray, P. (1997). *Florence Nightingale museum guidebook*. The Florence Nightingale Museum Trust.

National Geographic Resource Library. (2008). *Mary Seacole*. Retrieved July 16, 2024 from https://education.nationalgeographic.org/resource/mary-seacole/

National Organization for Public Health Nursing (NOPHN). (1939). *Manual of public health nursing* (3rd ed.). Macmillan.

Nightingale, F. (1876). [*Letter to the editor*]. *The Times (London)*. Retrieved from https://www.ucl.ac.uk/bloomsbury-project/articles/archives/nightingale.pdf

Nightingale, F. (1969). *Notes on nursing: What it is, and what it is not*. Harrison. (Original work published 1859.).

Nursingtheory.org (2016). *Mary Ann Bickerdyke, Mother Bickerdyke*. Retrieved from http://www.nursing-theory.org/famous-nurses/Mary-Ann-Bickerdyke.php

Nutting, M. A., & Dock, L. L. (1907). *A history of nursing: The evolution of nursing systems from the earliest times to the foundation of the first English and American training schools for nurses* (2 volumes). G. P. Putnam's Sons.

Petry, L. (1945). The U.S. Cadet Nurse Corps: A summing up. *The American Journal of Nursing, 45*(12), 1027–1028.

Pugh, A. (2001). Men, monasteries, wars, and wards. *Nursing Times, 97*(44), 24–25.

Ramsay, A. G. (2012). The end of an era. *Public Health Nursing, 29*(4), 380–383.

Reddi, V. (2005). *Dorothea Lynde Dix (1802–1887)*. Retrieved from http://www.truthaboutnursing.org/press/pioneers/dix.html

Richardson, R. (2010). *Florence Nightingale and hospital design* Retrieved from http://www.kingscollections.org/exhibitions/specialcollections/nightingale-and-hospital-design/florence-nightingale-and-hospital-design

Robinson, T. M. (2009). *Your country needs you*. Xilbris.

Rooney, D. (2016). *Florence Nightingale: Pioneer statistician* Retrieved from https://beta.sciencemuseum.org.uk/stories/2016/11/4/florence-nightingalethe-pioneer-statistician

Rosenberg, C. E. (2008). Siting epidemic disease: 3 centuries of American history. *Journal of Infectious Diseases, 197*(Supplement 1), S4–S6. 10.1086/524985. Retrieved from https://academic.oup.com/jid/article/197/Supplement_1/S4/842514

Ruel, S. R. (2014). Lillian Wald. *Home Healthcare Nurse, 32*(10), 597–600.

Ruffing-Rahal, M. (1986). Margaret Sanger: Nurse and feminist. *Nursing Outlook, 34*, 246–249.

Sarnecky, M. T. (2018). *Miss Jane A* Delano, 2nd Superintendent, Army Nurse Corps. Retrieved from https://e-anca.org/History/Superintendents-Chiefs-of-the-ANC/Miss-Jane-A-Delano

Schwartz, C. C., Ajjarapu, A. S., Stamy, C. D., & Schwinn, D. A. (2018). Comprehensive history of 3-year and accelerated US medical school programs: A century in review. *Medical Education Online, 23*, 1530557. Retrieved from https://www.ncbi.nlm.nih.gov/pmc/articles/PMC6211283/pdf/zmeo-23-1530557.pdf

Spring, K. (2017). *Mary nutting*. National Women's History Museum. Retrieved from www.womenshistory.org/education-resources/biographies/mary-nutting

Staring-Derks, C., Staring, J., & Anionwu, E. N. (2014). Mary Seacole: Global nurse extraordinaire. *Journal of Advanced Nursing, 71*(3), 514–525. 10.1111/jan.12559

Staupers, M. K. (1961). *No time for prejudice: A story of the integration of Negroes in nursing in the United States*. The MacMillan Company.

Stegen, A. J., & Sowerby, H. (2019). *Nursing in today's world: Trends, issues, and management* (11th ed.). Wolters Kluwer.

The College of Physicians of Philadelphia. (2020). *The history of vaccines: Polio*. Retrieved from https://www.historyofvaccines.org/timeline/polio

Theofanidis, D., & Sapountzi-Krepia, D. (2015). Nursing and caring: An historical overview from ancient Greek tradition to modern times. *International Journal of Caring Sciences, 8*(3), 791–800.

Toering, J. (1919). Nursing work in the telephone company. *The Public Health Nurse, IX*(10), 793–796. Retrieved from https://archive.org/stream/publichealthnurs1110nati/publichealthnurs1110nati#page/n34/mode/1up

U.S. Bureau of Labor Statistics. (2020). *Occupational outlook handbook: Registered nurses*. Retrieved from https://www.bls.gov/ooh/healthcare/registered-nurses.htm

U.S. Department of Health and Human Services (USDHHS), Division of Nursing. (1984). *Consensus conference on the essentials of public health nursing practice and education: Report of the conference*.

U.S. Department of Health and Human Services, Office of Health Promotion and Disease Prevention. (n.d.). *Healthy people 2020*. Retrieved from www.healthypeople.gov/sites/default/files/HP2020Framework.pdf

Uribe, J. (2008). *Nurses, philanthropies, and governments: The public mission of Chilean nursing, 1900-1945*. Publication No. 3309517 [Doctoral dissertation, University of Pennsylvania]. ProQuest Dissertations and Theses database.

Vessey, J. A., & McGowen, K. A. (2006). A successful public health experiment: School nursing. *Pediatric Nursing, 32*(213), 255–258.

Wald, L. D. (1915). *The house on Henry Street*. Holt.

Wald, L. D. (1934). *Windows of Henry Street*. Little Brown.

Webb, B. (2011). Roaming through Virginia with the public health nurse. *Public Health Nursing, 28*(3), 291–293.

Woodham-Smith, C. (1951). *Florence Nightingale*. McGraw- Hill.

Ye, J., Stanford, S., Gousse, T., & Tosatto, R. J. (2014). Developing strong response capacity: Training volunteers in the Medical Reserve Corps. *Disaster Medicine and Public Health Preparedness, 8*(6), 528–532.

CHAPTER 4

Agency for Healthcare Research and Quality. (2015). *Quality improvement tip sheet for primary care*. qi-tip-sheet-primary-care-practices.pdf (ahrq.gov)

Altmiller, G. (2019). Care bundles, QSEN, and student learning. *Nurse Educator, 44*(1), 7–8.

American Association of Colleges of Nursing. (2021). *The essentials: Core competencies for professional nursing education*. https://www.aacnnursing.org/Portals/0/PDFs/Publications/Essentials-2021.pdf

American Nurses Association. (2015). *Code of ethics with interpretative statements*. http://www.nursingworld.org/MainMenuCategories/EthicsStandards/CodeofEthicsfor-Nurses/Code-ofEthics-For-Nurses.html

American Nurses Association. (n.d.). *What is evidence-based practice in nursing?* https://www.nursingworld.org/practice-policy/nursing-excellence/evidence-based-practice-in-nursing/#:~:text=Evidence%2Dbased%20practice%20in%20nursing%20involves%20providing%20holistic%2C%20quality%20care,from%20colleagues%2C%20or%20personal%20beliefs

Area Health Education Center (AHEC). (n.d.). https://www.nationalahec.org/

Bacon, F. (2013). Insatauratio magna. In *The words of Francis Bacon*. Cambridge University Press (Original work published 1621). https://www.cambridge.org/core/books/abs/works-of-francis-bacon/instauratio-magna/0E3C2D1D425ADCE1F9C625E98DD8A55C

Brucker, M. C. (2016). Applying evidence to health care with Archie Cochrane's legacy. *Nursing for Women's Health, 20*(5), 441–442.

Carper, B. A. (1978). Fundamental patterns of knowing in nursing. *Advances in Nursing Science, 1*(1), 13–23.

Centers for Disease Control and Prevention. (2021). *The US Public Health Service Untreated Syphilis Study at Tuskegee research implications*. https://www.cdc.gov/tuskegee/after.htm

Centers for Disease Control and Prevention. (2023). *Behavioral risk factor surveillance system ACE data*. https://www.cdc.gov/violenceprevention/aces/ace-brfss.html

Chickasaw Nation. (2024). *Hofanti chokma*. https://www.chickasaw.net/Services/Family/Hofanti-Chokma

Connor, L., Dean, J., McNett, M., Tydings, D. M., Shrout, A., Gorsuch, P. F., Hole, A., Moore, L., Brown, R., Melnyk, B. M., & Gallagher-Ford, L. (2023). Evidence-based practice improves patient outcomes and healthcare system return on investment: Findings from a scoping review. *Worldviews on Evidence-Based Nursing, 20*, 6–15. https://doi.org/10.1111/wvn.12621

Downstate Health Sciences University. (2023). *Evidence-based nursing practice guide*. https://guides.downstate.edu/c.php?g=868154&p=6230297

Duva, I. M., Murphy, J. R., & Grabbe, L. (2022). A nurse-led, well-being promotion using the community resiliency model, Atlanta, 2020-2021. *American Journal of Public Health, 112*(S3), S271–S274.

Eckenrode, J., Campa, M., Luckey, D., Henderson, C., Cole, R., Kitzman, H., Anson, E., Sidora-Arcoleo, K., Powers, J., & Olds, D. L. (2010). Long-term effects of prenatal and infancy nurse home visitation on the life course of youths. *Archives of Pediatrics and Adolescent Medicine, 164*(1), 9–15.

Fain, J. A. (2021). *Reading, understanding, and applying nursing research* (6th ed.). F. A. Davis.

Felitti, V. J., Anda, R. F., Nordenberg, D., Williamson, D. F., Spitz, A. M., Edwards, V., Koss, M. P., & Marks, J. S. (1998). Relationship of childhood abuse and household dysfunction to many of the leading causes of death in adults: The Adverse Childhood Experiences (ACE) study.

American Journal of Preventive Medicine, *14*(4), 245–258. https://doi.org/10.1016/S0749-3797(98)00017-8

Gamble, V. N. (2014). *It's not just about Tuskegee: The history of African Americans and Medicine*. https://youtu.be/6_l0w0AfGh0

Guevarra, J. P., Peden, A., & Franklin, R. C. (2021). Application of the PRECEDE-PROCEED model in the development of evidence-informed interventions for drowning prevention: A mixed-methods study protocol. *BMJ Open*, *11*(7), e050688. https://doi.org/. 10.1136/bmjopen-2021-050688

Heller, J. (2017). *Black men untreated in Tuskegee Syphilis Study*. https://apnews.com/article/business-science-health-race-and-ethnicity-syphilis-e9dd07eaa4e74052878a68132c-d3803a

Hockenberry, M. (2014). Quality improvement and evidence-based practice change projects and the Institutional Review Board: Is approval necessary? *Worldviews on Evidence-Based Nursing*, *11*(4), 217–218.

Indian Health Service. (n.d.). *Adverse childhood experiences*. https://www.ihs.gov/womenshealth/maternalchildhealth/ace/

Institute for Healthcare Improvement. (2023). *How to improve: Model for improvement*. https://www.ihi.org/resources/how-to-improve

Johns Hopkins University. (2024). *Evidence-based practice model*. https://www.hopkinsmedicine.org/evidence-based-practice/model-tools

Johns Hopkins University Welch Medical Library. (2020). *Expert methodologies & review types*. https://browse.welch.jhmi.edu/searching/other-review-types

Karoly, L. A. (2017). *Investing in the early years: The costs and benefits of investing in early childhood in New Hampshire*. RAND Corporation. https://www.rand.org/pubs/research-reports/RR1890.html

Kitzman, H., Olds, D., Henderson, C., Hanks, C., Cole, R., Tatelbaum, R., McConnochie, K. M., Sidora, K., Luckey, D. W., Shaver, D., Engelhardt, K., James, D., & Barnard, K. (1997). Effect or prenatal and infancy home visitation by nurses on pregnancy outcomes, childhood injuries, and repeated childbearing: A randomized controlled trial. *Journal of the American Medical Association*, *278*(8), 644–652.

Kitzman, H. J., Olds, D. L., Cole, R. E., Hanks, C. A., Anson, E. A., Arcoleo, K. J., Luckey, D. W., Knudtson, M. D., Henderson Jr., C. R., & Holmberg, J. R. (2010b). Enduring effects of prenatal and infancy home visiting by nurses on children: Follow up of a randomized trial among children at age 12 years. *Archives of Pediatrics & Adolescent Medicine*, *164*(5), 412–418.

Kroshus, E. (2015). *Weighing the evidence: One university takes a hard look at disordered eating among athletes*. https://www.hsph.harvard.edu/wp-content/uploads/sites/1267/2015/02/RevFINAL-Advanced-Teach-Note-Athletes-Case-Feb-20-15.pdf

Leslie, H., Hirschhorn, L., Marchant, T., Doubova, S., Gueje, O., & Kruk, M. (2018). Health systems thinking: A new generation of research to improve healthcare quality. *PLoS Medicine*, *15*(10), 1–4.

Li, S., Liu, S., Zhang, X., Chen, Y., & Ren, X. (2022). Effectiveness of the PRECEDE-PROCEED model for improving the care knowledge, skill, and sense of competence in mothers of preterm infants. *Journal of International Medical Research*, *50*(7), 1–14. https://doi.org/10.1177/03000605221110699

March of Dimes. (2024). *What is neonatal abstinence syndrome?* https://www.marchofdimes.org/find-support/topics/planning-baby/neonatal-abstinence-syndrome-nas#:~:text=What%20is%20Neonatal%20Abstinence%20Syndrome,drugs%20called%20opioids%20during%20pregnancy

Massi, L., Hickey, S., Maidment, S., Roe, Y., Kildea, S., & Kruske, S. (2023, June 9). "This has changed me to be a better mum": A qualitative study exploring how the Australian nurse-family partnership program contributes to the development of first nations women's self-efficacy. *Women Birth*, *36*(6), e613–e622. https://doi.org/10.1016/j.wombi.2023.05.010

McMaster University. (2024). *Evidence-based practice*. McMaster University Health Sciences Library. https://hslmcmaster.libguides.com/ebm/ebp

Melnyk, B., & Fineout-Overholt, E. (2023). *Evidence-based practice in nursing and healthcare: A guide to best practice* (5th ed.). Wolters Kluwer.

National Institute for Nursing Research. (n.d.). *What we do*. https://www.ninr.nih.gov/aboutninr/what-we-do

National Institutes of Health. (n.d.). *Ten landmark nursing research studies*. https://www.ninr.nih.gov/sites/www.ninr.nih.gov/files/10-landmark-nursing-research-studies.pdf

Nicholson, S., Aksana, W., Moon, D., & Haris-Haman, P. (2023). Abstinence syndrome with the eat, sleep, console method. *Advances in Neonatal Care*, *23*(6), 509–515.

Nicole, C., MacMillan, H., Cullen, A., Zheng, Y., Xie, H., Boyle, M., Sheehan, D., Lever, R., Jack, S. M., Gonzalez, A., Gafni, A., Tommyr, L., Barr, R., Marcellus, L., Varcoe, C., & Waddell, C. (2023). Effectiveness of nurse-home visiting in improving child and maternal outcomes prenatally to age two years: A randomized controlled trial (British Columbia Healthy Connections Project). *The Journal of Child Psychology and Psychiatry*, *65*(5), 644–655. https://doi.org/10.1111/jcpp.13846

Nightingale, F. (1898). *Notes on nursing: What it is, and what it not*. https://www.fulltextarchive.com/book/Notes-on-Nursing/

Nurse-Family Partnership. (2024). *Research and the nurse-family partnership program*. https://www.nursefamilypartnership.org/about/proven-results/research-inquiries/

Olds, D., Eckenrode, J., Henderson, C., Kitzman, H., Powers, J., Cole, R., Sidora, K., Morris, P., Pettitt, L. M., & Luckey, D. (1997). Long-term effects of home visitation on maternal life course and child abuse and neglect: Fifteen-year follow-up of a randomized trial. *Journal of the American Medical Association*, *278*(8), 637–643.

Olds, D. L., Holmberg, J. R., Donelan-McCall, N., Luckey, D. W., Knudtson, M. D., & Robinson, J. (2014a). Effects of home visits by paraprofessionals and by nurses on children: Follow-up of a randomized trial at ages 6 and 9 years. *JAMA Pediatrics*, *168*(2), 114–121.

Olds, D. L., Kitzman, H., Knudtson, M. D., Anson, E., Smith, J. A., & Cole, R. (2014b). Effect of home visiting by nurses on maternal and child mortality: Results of a 2-decade follow-up of a randomized clinical trial. *JAMA Pediatrics*, *168*(9), 800–806.

Oyesanya, T., Loflin, C., Byom, L., Harris, K. D., Rink, L., & Bettger, J. P. (2021). Transitions of care interventions to improve quality of life among patients hospitalized with acute conditions: A systematic literature review. *Health and Quality of Life Outcomes*, *19*(1), 36. https://doi.org/10.1186/s12955-021-01672-5

Pascua Yaqui Tribe. (2021). *2021 Health Needs Assessment*. https://www.pascuayaqui-nsn.gov/health-services/

Public Health Foundation. (n.d.). *Quality improvement in public health*. https://www.phf.org/focusareas/qualityimprovement/Pages/Quality_Improvement.aspx

Purdue Global. (2023). *What is the evidence-based practice pyramid of resources?* https://library.purdueglobal.edu/ecNU310/EBP

Roelcke, V. (2004). Nazi medicine and research on human beings. *The Lancet Online*, *364*, 6–7.

Rural Health Information Hub. (2024). *Precede-Proceed model*. https://www.ruralhealthinfo.org/toolkits/health-promotion/2/theories-and-models/precede-proceed

Sackett, D. (1981). How to read clinical journals: I. why to read them and how to start reading them critically. *Journal of the Canadian Medical Association*, *124*(5), 555–558.

Sackett, D. L., Richardson, S. W., Rosenberg, W. R., & Haynes, R. B. (1997). *Evidence-based medicine: How to practice and teach EBM*. Churchill-Livingstone.

Sadler, B. L., Joseph, A., Keller, A., & Rostenberg, B. (2009). *Using evidence-based environmental design to enhance safety and quality* [White paper]. IHI Innovation Series white paper. Institute for Healthcare Improvement. www.IHI.org

School Health Institute for Education and Leadership Development. (2024). *SBIRT in schools*. https://shield.bu.edu/content/sbirt-schools-0

Shuster, E. (2018). American doctors at the Nuremberg medical trial. *American Journal of Public Health*, *108*(1), 47–52. https://doi.org/10.2105/AJPH.2017.304104

Sierau, S., Dahne, V., Brand, T., Kurtz, V., von Klitzing, K., & Jungmann, T. (2016). Effects of home visitation on maternal competencies, family environment, and child development: A randomized controlled trial. *Prevention Science*, *17*(1), 40–51.

Thal, W., & Jimenez, R. (2019). Applying the plan-do-study-act (PDA) approach to community health worker job satisfaction: Local and global perspectives. *Journal of Refugee & Global Health*, *2*(2), 1–5. https://doi.org/10.18297/rgh/vol2/iss2/12

The Community Guide. (n.d.). *Your online guide to what works to promote healthy communities*. https://www.thecommunityguide.org

The Deming Institute. (2024). *Enriching society through the Deming philosophy*. https://deming.org/explore/pdsa/

The World Medical Association. (1964, amended last 2013). *Declaration of Helsinki: Medical research involving human subjects*. https://www.wma.net/what-we-do/medical-ethics/declaration-of-helsinki/

Tyson, P. (2000). *The experiments*. https://www.pbs.org/wgbh/nova/holocaust/experiside.html

U.S. Department of Health and Human Services (USDHHS). (1979). *The Belmont report: Ethical principles and guidelines for the protection of human subjects of research*. Read the Belmont Report | HHS.gov

U.S. Department of Health and Human Services (USDHHS). (2021). *Office for human research protections. Lesson 3: What are IRBs?* https://www.hhs.gov/ohrp/education-and-outreach/online-education/human-research-protection-training/lesson-3-what-are-irbs/index

WHO. (2023). *How health policy and systems research can advance universal health coverage*. file:///Users/joey-stanleyhotmail.com/Downloads/HPSR-and-UHC-web-final.pdf

CHAPTER 5

Abbaspoor, Z., Sharifipour, F., Siahposh, A., Nazaralivand, R., Mohaghegh, Z., & Siahkal, S. F. (2022). Effects of aromatherapy with citrus aurantium lavender on sexual function of postmenopausal women: A randomized controlled trial. *J Family Reprod Health*, *16*(2), 147–154. https://doi.org/10.18502/jfrh.v16i2.9485

Agency for Healthcare Research and Quality (AHRQ). (2019). *Cultural competence and patient safety*. https://psnet.ahrq.gov/perspective/cultural-competence-and-patient-safety

Agency for Healthcare Research and Quality (AHRQ). (2022). *Culturally and linguistically appropriate service*. https://www.ahrq.gov/sdoh/clas/index.html

Altman, M. R., Oseguera, T., McLemore, M. R., Kantrowits-Gordon, I., Franck, L. S., & Lyndon, A. (2019). Information and power: Women of color's experiences interacting with health care providers in pregnancy and birth. *Social Sciences and Medicine*, *238*, 112491. https://doi.org/10.1016/j.socscimed.2019.112491

American Nurses Association (ANA). (2021). *Nursing: Scope and standards of practice* (4th ed.). Nursesbooks.org

American Psychiatric Association. (2023). *Working with indigenous/native American patients*. https://www.psychiatry.org/psychiatrists/diversity/education/best-practice-highlights/working-with-native-american-patients

Andraska, E. A., Alabi, O., Dorsey, C., Erben, Y., Velazquez, G., Franco-Mesa, C., & Sachdev, U. (2021). Health care disparities during the COVID-19 pandemic. *Seminars in Vascular Surgery*, *34*(3), 82–88. https://doi.org/10.1053/j.semvascsurg.2021.08.002

Andrews, M., Boyle, J., & Collins, J. (2020). *Transcultural concepts in nursing care* (8th ed.). Wolters Kluwer.

Attum, B., Hafiz, S., Malik, A., & Shamoon, Z. (2023). Cultural competence in the care of muslin patients and their families. *StatPearls*. https://www.ncbi.nlm.nih.gov/books/NBK499933/

Batalova, J., Blizzard, J., & Bolter, B. (2023, March 14). *Frequently requested statistics on immigrants and immigration in the United States*. Migration Policy Institute. https://www.migrationpolicy.org/article/frequently-requested-statistics-immigrants-and-immigration-united-states?gclid=EAIaIQobChMIoeecsKDr6AIVHz2tBh37ogAIEAAYASAAEgI6Q_D_BwE

Bellagamba, A., Greene, S. E., & Klein, M. A. (2020). *African voices on slavery and the slave trade* (Vol. 2). Cambridge University Press.

Berger, J. T., & Miller, D. R. (2021). Health disparities, systemic racism, and failures of cultural competence. *The American Journal of Bioethics*, *21*(9), 4–10. https://doi.org/10.1080/15265161.2021.1915411

Blair, K. (2019). *Advanced practice nursing: Core concepts for professional role development* (6th ed.). Springer Publishing Company.

Bolter, J. (2022). *Immigration has been a defining, often contentious element throughout U.S. history*. https://www.migrationpolicy.org/article/immigration-shaped-united-states-history

Boyle, J., S., Collins, J. W., Ludwig-Beymer, P., & Andrews, M. M. (2025). *Transcultural concepts in nursing care* (9th ed.). Wolters Kluwer.

Brar-Josan, N., & Yohani, S. (2019). Cultural brokers' role in facilitating formal and informal mental health supports for refugee youth in school and community context: A Canadian case study. *British Journal of Guidance and Counseling, 47*(4), 512–523. https://doi.org/10.1080/03069885/2017.1403010

Center for Disease Control & Prevention (CDC). (2023). *Three overarching principles for global public health communication.* https://www.cdc.gov/globalhealth/equity/guide/overarching-principles.html

Centers for Disease Control & Prevention. (CDC). (2022a). *CDC's efforts to address racism as a fundamental drivers of health disparities.* https://www.cdc.gov/minorityhealth/racism-disparities/cdc-efforts.html

Centers for Disease Control & Prevention. (CDC). (2022b). *Lead in foods, cosmetics, and medicines.* https://www.cdc.gov/nceh/lead/tips/folkmedicine.htm

Cleveland Clinic. (2023). *Herbal supplements.* https://my.clevelandclinic.org/health/articles/17095-herbal-supplements-helpful-or-harmful

Condon, E. M., Tobon, A. L., Jackson, B., Holland, M. L., Slade, A., Mayes, L., & Lois, S. (2021). Maternal experiences of racial discrimination, child indicators of toxic stress, and the minding the baby early home visitation intervention. *Nursing Research, 70*(55), s43–s52. http://doi.org./10.1097/NNR.0000000000000529

Council of Public Health Nursing Organizations. (2018). *Community/public health nursing competencies.* https://www.cphno.org/wp-content/uploads/2020/08/QCC-C-PHN-COMPETENCIES-Approved_2018.05.04_Final-002.pdf

Coyle, D. (2022). *The cultural playbook: 60 highly effective actions to help your group succeed.* Bantam Books.

Dau, J. B., & Sweeney, M. S. (2008). *God grew tired of us: A memoir.* National Geographic.

Fadiman, A. (1998). *The spirit catches you and you fall down.* Farrar, Straus, & Giroux.

Fawzy, A., Wu, T. D., & Wang, K. (2022). Racial and ethnic disparities in pulse oximetry and delayed identification of treatment eligibility among patients with COVID-19. *JAMA Internal Medicine, 182*(7), 730–738. https://doi.org/10.1001/jamainternmed.2022.1906

Fitzgerald, E., & Campinha-Bacote, J. (2019, May). An intersectionality approach to the process of cultural competemility—part ll. *OJIN, 24*(2). https://doi.org/10.3912/OJIN.Vol24No02PPT202

Gamelin, R., Hebert, M., Tratt, E., & Brassard, P. (2022). Ethnographic study of the barriers and facilitators to implementing human papillomavirus (HPV) self-sampling as a primary screening strategy for cervical cancer among Intuit women of Nunavik, northern Quebec. *International Journal of Circumpolar Health, 81*(1). https://doi.org/10/1080/22423982.2022.2032930

Garcha, E., Qureshi, A., O'Driscoll, C., & Shaikh, M. (2023, May 2). The impact of cultural frame switching on well-being—Systematic review. https://doi.org/10.31219/osf.io/95gmr

Giger, J. N., & Haddad, L. G. (2021). *Transcultural nursing, assessment and intervention* (8th ed.). Elsevier.

Hall, E. T. (1959). *The silent language.* Doubleday.

Homeland Security. (2022). *2021 yearbook of immigration statistics.* https://www.dhs.gov/sites/default/files/2023-03/2022_1114_plcy_yearbook_immigration_statistics_fy2021_v2_1.pdf

Hong, Y.-Y., Morris, M. W., Chiu, C.-Y., & Benet-Martinez, V. (2000). Multicultural minds: A dynamic constructivist approach to culture and cognition. *American Psychologist, 55*, 709–720. https://doi.org/10.1037/0003-066X.55.7.709

Illamola, S. M., Amaeze, O. U., Krepkova, L. V., Birmbaum, A. K., Karanam, A., Job, K. M., Bortnikova, V. V., Sherwin, C., & Eniotina, E. Y. (2019). Use of herbal medicine by pregnant women: What physicians need to know. *Frontiers in Pharmacology, 10*, 1483. https://doi.org/10.3389/fphar.2019.01483

Johns Hopkins. (2023). *Herbal medicine.* https://www.hopkinsmedicine.org/health/wellness-and-prevention/herbal-medicine

Jones, N., Marks, R., Ramirez, R., & Rios-Vargas, M. (2021). *Improved race and ethnicity, measures reveals U.S population is much more multiracial.* https://www.census.gov/library/stories/2021/08/improved-race-ethnicity-measures-reveal-united-states-population-much-more-multiracial.html

Kark, S. L. (1974). *Epidemiology and community medicine.* Appleton-Century-Crofts.

Kaya, Y., Arslan, S., Erbas, A., Yasa, B. N., & Kucukkelepce, G. E. (2021). The effect of ethnocentrism on moral sensitivity on intercultural sensitivity in nursing students, descriptive cross-sectional research study. *Nurse Education Today, 20* https://doi.org/10.1016/j.nedt.2021.104867

Kiang, L., & Witkow, M. R. (2018). Identifying as American among adolescents from Asian backgrounds. *Journal of Youth and Adolescence, 47*(1), 64–76.

Kottack, C. (2022). *Cultural anthropology: Appreciating cultural diversity* (18th ed.). McGraw-Hill ebook.

Krosch, A. R., Park, S. J., Walker, J., & Lisner, A. R. (2022). The threat of majority–minority U.S. alters white Americans' perception of race. *Journal of Experiential Psychology, 99.* https://doi.org/10.1016/j.jesp.2021.104266

Lee, E. L., Richards, N., Harrison, J., & Barnes, J. (2022). Prevalence of use of traditional, complementary, and alternative medicine by the general population: A systematic review of National studies published from 2010-2019. *Drug Safe, 45*(7), 713–735. https://doi.org/10.1007/s40264-022-00189-w

Les Elfes International. (2021). *What are the benefits of understanding different cultures?* https://www.leselfes.com/understanding-different-cultures/

Lindquist, R., Tracy, M., & Snyder, M. (2022). *Complementary therapies in nursing: Promoting integrative care* (9th ed.). Springer Publishing Company.

Mantyselka, P., Kautiainen, H., & Miettola, J. (2019). Beliefs and attitudes towards lifestyle change and risk in primary care—A community-based study. *BMC Public Health, 19*(1049). https://doi.org/10.1186/s12889-01907377-x

McCluskey, L. (2020). *Culture shock stages: Everything you need to know.* https://www.now-health.com/en/blog/culture-shock-stages/

Meadows, V. (2023). *The ultimate holistic health guide: Achieving balance and harmony in every aspect of your life.* Q21 Media Group.

Merriam Webster Dictionary. (2020). Ethnicity. https://www.merriam-webster.com/dictionary/ethnicity

Merriam Webster Dictionary. (2023). Microculture. https://www.merriam-webster.com/dictionary/microculture

Miton, H., & Dedeo, S. (2022). The cultural transmission of tacit knowledge. *Journal of the Royal Society Interface, 19*(195). https://doi.org/10.1098/rsif.20220238

Mizrahi, I. (2020). *The minority-majority shift. Two decades that will change America. The surge of multi-racial families.* Forbes. https://www.forbes.com/sites/isaacmizrahi/2020/09/23/the-minority-majority-shift-two-decades-that-will-change-america-the-surge-of-multi-racial-families/?sh=203c244b6ba5

Murdock, G. (1972). The science of culture. In M. Freilich (Ed.), *The meaning of culture: A reader in cultural anthropology* (pp. 252–266). Xerox College Publishing.

Natarajan, A., Moslimani, M., & Lopez, M. H. (2022). *Key facts about recent trends in global migration* Pew Research Center. https://www.pewresearch.org/short-reads/2022/12/16/key-facts-about-recent-trends-in-global-migration/

Needy Meds. (2020). *Prescription assistance.* https://www.needymeds.org/pap?gclid=EAIaIQobChMI1Ifu2ffw_wIVQgV9Ch21uQahEAAYAiAAEgLeNPD_BwE

Nkwata, A. K., Song, X., Zhang, M., & Ezeamama, A. E. (2020). Change in quality of life over eight years in a nationally representative sample of US adults with heart disease and type 2 diabetes: Minority race and toxic stress as key social determinants. *BMC Public Health, 20*(684), 1–12. http://doi.org/10.1186/s12889-020-08842-y

Novosanis. (2022). *Urine—A preferred sample type for HPV detection for cervical cancer screening.* https://novosanis.com/blog/urine-preferred-sample-type-hpv-detection-cervical-cancer-screening

Ontology Search. (2023). *Ethnic group.* https://www.ebi.ac.uk/ols/ontologies/genepio/terms?iri=http%3A%2F%2Fwww.ebi.ac.uk%2Fefo%2FEFO_0001799

Pappas, S., & McKelvie, C. (2022). *What is culture?* https://www.livescience.com/21478-what-is-culture-definition-of-culture.html

Perez, A. D., & Hirschman, C. (2009). The changing racial and ethnic composition of the US population: Emerging American identities. *Population and Development Review, 35*(1), 1–15.

Pizzorno, J., & Murray, M. (2020). *Textbook of natural medicine—2 volume addition* (5th ed.). Elsevier.

Qu, Y., Lin, L. C., & Telzer, E. H. (2019). Culture modulates the neural correlates underlying risky exploration. *Frontiers in Human Neurosciences, 13*(171). https://doi.org/10.3389/fnhum.2019.00171

Roy, D. (2022). Ten graphics that explain the U.S. struggle with migrant flows in 2022. https://www.cfr.org/article/ten-graphics-explain-us-struggle-migrant-flows-2022?gclid=EAIaIQobChMIh6-gur_w_wIVLwGtBh3dYQ2kEAAYASAAEgK-G_D_BwE

Sabin, J. A. (2022). Tackling implicit bias in healthcare. *The New England Journal of Medicine, 387*(2), 105–107.

Santoro, H. (2023). *More states may soon require psychologists to be trained in equity, diversity, and inclusion.* https://www.apa.org/monitor/2023/06/states-equity-diversity-inclusion-training-psychologists

Schuerger, B. (2022). *When blood transfusion isn't an option.* https://www.myamericannurse.com/when-blood-transfusion-isnt-an-option-jehovahs-witnesses/

Searle, W., & Ward, C. (1990). The prediction of psychological and sociocultural adjustment during cross-cultural transitions. *International Journal of Intercultural Relations, 14*, 449–464. https://doi.org/Doi. 10.1016/0147-1767(90)90030-Z

Shahzad, S., Ali, N., Younas, A., & Tayaben, J. (2021). Challenges and approaches to transcultural care: An integrative review of nurses' and nursing students' experiences. *Journal of Professional Nursing, 37*(6), 1119–1131. https://doi.org/0.1016/j.profnurs.2021.10.001

Shonkoff, J. P., Slopen, N., & Williams, D. T. (2021). Early childhood adversity, toxic stress, and the impacts of racism on the foundations of health. *Annual Review of Public Health, 42*, 115–134. http://doi.org/10.1146/annurev-publhealth-0904190101940

Soyeon, S., Kang, B., Park, J., Kim, S., Park, E., Lee, S. H., & Kawachi, I. (2023). Racial/Ethnic disparity in association between fetal alcohol syndrome and alcohol intake during pregnancy: Multisite retrospective cohort study. *JMIR Public Health and Surveillance, 9*, e45358. https://doi.org/10.2196?45358

Stubbe, E. (2020). Practicing culturally competence and cultural humility in the care of diverse patients. *Focus, 18*(1), 49–51. https://doi.org/10.1176/appi.focus.20190041

Supreme Court of the United States. (2022). *19-1392 Dobbs v. Jackson Women's Health Organization.* https://www.supremecourt.gov/opinions/21pdf/19-1392_6j37.pdf

Tabatabaeichehr, M., & Mortazavi, H. (2020). The effectiveness of aromatherapy in the management of labor pain and anxiety: A systematic review. *Ethiopian Journal of Health Sciences, 30*(3), 449–459. https://doi.org/10.4314/ejhs.v30i3.16

Transcultural Nursing Society. (2023). *Standards.* https://tcns.org/standards/

U.S. Census Bureau. (2022). *2020 U.S. population more racially and ethnically diverse than measured in 2010.* https://www.census.gov/library/stories/2021/08/2020-united-states-population-more-racially-ethnically-diverse-than-2010.html

U.S. Department of Health and Human Services (USDHHS). (2020). *Browse 2030 objectives.* https://health.gov/healthypeople/objectives-and-data/browse-objectives

U.S. Department of Health and Human Services (USDHHS)—National Institute of Health (NIH). (2023). *Complementary, Alternative or Integrative Health: What's in a name?* https://www.nccih.nih.gov/health/complementary-alternative-or-integrative-health-whats-in-a-name#:~:text=Integrative%20health%20aims%20for%20well,care%20for%20the%20whole%20person

U.S. Equal Employment Opportunity Commission. (n.d.-a). *Laws enforced by EEOC.* https://www.eeoc.gov/statutes/laws-enforced-eeoc

U.S. Equal Employment Opportunity Commission. (n.d.-b). *Examples of court decisions supporting coverage of LGBT-related discrimination under title VII.* https://www.eeoc.gov/wysk/examples-court-decisions-supporting-coverage-lgbt-related-discrimination-under-title-vii

U.S. Food and Drug Administration (USFDA). (2022a). *Drug applications for nonprescription drugs.* https://www.fda.gov/drugs/types-applications/drug-applications-over-counter-otc-drugs

U.S. Food and Drug Administration (USFDA). (2022b). *Is it really 'FDA approved'?* https://www.fda.gov/consumers/consumer-updates/it-really-fda-approved

Vela, M. B., Erondu, A. I., & Smith, N. A. (2022). Eliminating explicit and implicit biases in healthcare: Evidence and research needs. *Annual Review of Public Health, 43*(1), 477–501.

Ward, N., & Batalova, J. (2023, March 14). *Frequently requested statistics on immigrants and immigration in the United States.* Migration Policy Institute. https://www.migrationpolicy.org/article/frequently-requested-statistics-immigrants-and-immigration-united-states

Warren, C. M., Turner, P. J., Chinthrajah, R. S., & Gupta, R. S. (2021). Advancing food allergy through epidemiology: understanding and addressing disparities in food allergy management and outcomes. *Journal of Allergy and Clinical Immunology: In Practice*, *9*(1), 110–118. https://doi.org/10.1016/j.jaip.2020.09.064

West, A. L., Zhang, R., Yampolsky, M. A., & Sasaki, J. Y. (2018). The potential cost of cultural fit: Frame switching undermines perceptions of authenticity in western contexts. *Frontiers in Psychology*, *9*, 2622. https://doi.org/10.3389/fpsyg.2018.02622

CHAPTER 6

Administration for Community Living. (2022a, November). *2021 profile of older Americans*. https://acl.gov/sites/default/files/Profile%20of%20OA/2021%20Profile%20of%20OA/2021ProfileOlderAmericans_508.pdf

Administration for Community Living. (2022b, May 4). *Projected future growth of older population*. https://acl.gov/aging-and-disability-in-america/data-and-research/projected-future-growth-older-population

Aetna. (n.d.). *HMO, POS, PPO, EPO and HDHP with HSA: What's the difference?* https://www.aetna.com/health-guide/hmo-pos-ppo-hdhp-whats-the-difference.html

Agency for Healthcare Research and Quality. (2019a, September). *Health care-associated infections*. https://psnet.ahrq.gov/primers/primer/7/health-care-associated-infections

Agency for Healthcare Research and Quality. (2019b, September 7). *Patient safety primer: Never events*. https://psnet.ahrq.gov/primers/primer/3/never-events

Alexander, D., Currie, J., & Schnell, M. (2019). Check up before you check out: Retail clinics and emergency room use. *Journal of Public Economics*, *178*, 104050. https://doi:10.1016/j.jpubeco.2019.104050

Ali, H. R., Valero-Elizondo, J., Wang, S. Y., Cainzos-Achirica, M., Bhimaraj, A., Khan, S. U., Khan, M. S., Mossialos, E., Khera, R., & Nasir, K. (2022). Subjective financial hardship due to medical bills among patients with heart failure in the United States: The 2014–2018 medical expenditure panel survey. *Journal of Cardiac Failure*, *28*(9), 1424–1433. https://doi:10.1016/j.cardfail.2022.06.009

Allan, T., & Lakey, D. (n.d.). *Exemplars of community health needs assessment collaboration Action Collaborative on Bridging Public Health, Health Care & Community*. https://www.nationalacademies.org/documents/embed/link/LF2255DA3DD1C41C0A42D3BEF0989ACAECE3053A6A9B/file/D1D9E442A128C44852498B243F3A90F90CEF9CDF7A3E?noSaveAs=1

American Association for Medicare Supplement Insurance (AAMSI). (2020). *Medicare Supplement Insurance Statistics Data—2023*. https://medicaresupp.org/information/medicare-advantage/medicare-advantage-2023-statistics/

American Hospital Association (AHA). (2022, February). *Fact sheet: Uncompensated hospital care cost*. https://www.aha.org/fact-sheets/2020-01-06-fact-sheet-uncompensated-hospital-care-cost

American Hospital Association (AHA). (2023, May). *Fast facts on US hospitals, 2023*. https://www.aha.org/statistics/fast-facts-us-hospitals

American Hospital Association (AHA). (n.d.). *Regulatory overload report: Assessing the regulatory burden on health systems, hospitals, and post-acute care providers*. https://www.aha.org/guidesreports/2017-11-03-regulatory-overload-report

American Medical Association (AMA). (2020). *Summary of research: Medicaid physician payment and access to care*. https://www.ama-assn.org/system/files/2020-10/research-summary-medicaid-physician-payment.pdf

American Nurses' Association (ANA). (2022). *Public health nursing: Scope and standards of practice* (3rd ed.).

American Public Health Association (APHA). (2019, March 11). *President's budget would hinder public health programs, says APHA*. https://www.apha.org/news-and-media/news-releases/apha-news-releases/2019/president-budget-proposal

American Public Health Association (APHA). (2023, July). *House FY 2024 labor-HHS-education spending bill would threaten public health and safety*. https://www.apha.org/News-and-Media/News-Releases/APHA-News-Releases/2023/House-FY-2024-Labor-HHS-Education-Spending-Bill

American Public Health Association (APHA). (n.d.-a). *Our History*. https://www.apha.org/about-apha/our-history

American Public Health Association (APHA). (n.d.-b). *Social justice and health*. https://apha.org/what-is-public-health/generation-public-health/our-work/social-justice

America's Health Rankings. (2022). *2022 annual report*. https://www.americashealthrankings.org/learn/reports/2022-annual-report

Anderson, G. F., Hussey, P., & Petrosyan, V. (2019). It's still the prices, stupid: Why the US spends so much on health care, and a tribute to Uwe Reinhardt. *Health Affairs*, *38*(1), 87–95.

Aron-Dine, A. (2019, November 6). *New research: Medicaid expansion saves lives*. Center on Budget and Policy Priorities. https://www.cbpp.org/blog/new-research-medicaid-expansion-saves-lives

Arrow, K. (2004). Uncertainty and the welfare economics of medical care. *Bulletin of the World Health Organization*, *82*(2), 141–149. http://www.who.int/bulletin/volume/82/2/PHCBP.pdf (Original work published 1964)

Association of American Medical Colleges. (2021, June 11). *AAMC report reinforces mounting physician shortage*. https://www.aamc.org/news/press-releases/aamc-report-reinforces-mounting-physician-shortage

Association of State and Territorial Health Officials (ASTHO). (2017). *ASTHO profile of state public health: Volume four*. Retrieved from https://www.astho.org/Profile/Volume-Four/2016-ASTHO-Profile-of-State-and-Territorial-Public-Health/

Association of State and Territorial Health Officials (ASTHO). (2020). *State health agency expenditures: 2010-2018*. https://www.astho.org/globalassets/pdf/state-health-agency-expenditures-2010-2018.pdf

Association of State and Territorial Health Officials (ASTHO). (n.d.-a). *About us*. https://www.astho.org/about/

Association of State and Territorial Health Officials (ASTHO). (n.d.-b). *ASTHO member directory*. https://www.astho.org/members/member-directory/

Association of State and Territorial Health Officials (ASTHO). (n.d.-c). *Profile of state and territorial public health*. https://www.astho.org/topic/public-health-infrastructure/profile/#finance

Bai, G., & Anderson, G. F. (2016). A more detailed understanding of factors associated with hospital profitability. *Health Affairs*, *35*, 889–897.

Balio, C., Yeager, V., & Beitsch, L. (2019). Perception of Public Health 3.0: Concordance between public health agency leaders and employees. *Journal of Public Health Management and Practice*, *25*, S103–S112. 10.1097/PHH.0000000000000903

Ballard, J., George, L., Zazueta-Lara, E., Turner, L., Aguado, J., Law, J., & Alger, R. (2019). Trauma informed public health nursing visits to parents and children. *Public Health Nursing*, *36*, 694–701.

Ballard, J., Turner, L., Cuca, Y. P., Lobo, B., & Dawson-Rose, C. S. (2022). Trauma-informed home visiting models in public health nursing: An evidence-based approach. *American Journal of Public Health*, *112*(S3), S298–S305. https://doi:10.2105/AJPH.2022.306737

Bartz, D., & Stempel, J. (2020, June 10). *U.S. States accuse 26 drugmakers of generic drug price fixing in sweeping lawsuit*. https://www.reuters.com/article/us-usa-drugs-antitrust-lawsuit-idINKBN23H2TR

Bekemeier, B., Singh, S. R., & Schoemann, A. W. (2018). A uniform chart of accounts for public health agencies: An "essential ingredient" for a strong public health system. *Journal of Public Health Management and Practice*, *24*, 289–291. https://doi:10.1097/PHH.0000000000000793

Benitez, J. A., Perez, V., & Seiber, E. (2020). Medicaid access during economic distress: Lessons learned from the great recession. *Medical Care Research and Review*, *78*, 490–501. https://doi:10.1177/1077558720909237

Berchik, E. R., Barnett, J. C., & Upton, R. D. (2019, November). *Health insurance coverage in the United States: 2018*. U.S. Census Bureau. https://www.census.gov/content/dam/Census/library/publications/2019/demo/p60-267.pdf

Bernard, D., Banthin, J., & Encinosa, W. (2009). Wealth, income, and the affordability of health insurance. *Health Affairs*, *28*, 887–896.

Bhatia, N. (2020). We need to talk about rationing: The need to normalize discussion about healthcare rationing in a post COVID-19 era. *Journal of Bioethical Inquiry*, *17*, 731–735. https://doi:10.1007/s11673-020-10051-6

Bihari, M. (2023). Prior authorization: Overview, purpose, process: Why some health insurers may deny a claim if you don't take this step. *Very Well Health*. https://www.verywellhealth.com/prior-authorization-1738770

Birkhead, G. S., Morrow, C. B., & Pirani, S. (2021). *Essentials of public health* (4th ed.). Jones & Bartlett.

Blavin, F., & Ramos, C. (2021). Medicaid expansion: Effects on hospital finances and implications for hospitals facing COVID-19 challenges. *Health Affairs*, *40*, 82–90. https://doi:10.1377/hlthaff.2020.00502

Bloom, D. E., Canning, D., Kotschy, R., Prettner, K., & Schunemann, J. (2022, November). *Health and economic growth: Reconciling the micro and macro evidence*. National Bureau of Economic Research. https://www.nber.org/papers/w26003

Blue Cross Blue Shield. (n.d.). *Leading the way in health insurance*. https://www.bcbs.com/about-us/industry-pioneer

Blumberg, A., & Davidson, A. (2009, October 22). *Accidents of history created U.S. health system*. NPR. https://www.npr.org/templates/story/story.php?storyId=114045132

Blumenthal, D., & Abrams, M. K. (2020, February 26). *The affordable care act at 10 years: What's changed in health care delivery and payment?* Commonwealth Fund. https://www.commonwealthfund.org/publications/journal-article/2020/feb/aca-at-10-years-changed-health-care-delivery-payment

Blumenthal, D., Collins, S. R., & Fowler, E. J. (2020). The affordable care act at 10 years—Its coverage and access provisions. *The New England Journal of Medicine*, *382*, 963–969. https://doi:10.1056/NEJMhpr1916091

Bowser, R. (2015). Race and rationing. *Health Matrix*, *25*(1), 87–107. https://scholarlycommons.law.case.edu/cgi/viewcontent.cgi?article=1019&context=healthmatrix

Brown, A. M., & Nanni, M. B. (2020, April). *Risky business: Recognizing the flaws of employer-based health insurance during COVID-19*. Lerner Center for Public Health Promotion and Population Health, Syracuse University. https://www.maxwell.syr.edu/research/lerner-center/population-health-research-brief-series/article/risky-business-recognizing-the-flaws-of-employer-based-health-insurance-during-covid-19

Buettgens, M., & Ramchandani, U. (2022, August). *3.7 Million people would gain health coverage in 2023 if the remaining 12 states were to expand Medicaid eligibility*. The Urban Institute. https://www.urban.org/research/publication/3-7-million-people-would-gain-health-coverage-2023-if-remaining-12-states-were

Bureau of Labor Statistics. (2022, September). *National compensation survey: Glossary of employee benefit terms*. https://www.bls.gov/ebs/

Button, P., Khan, M. R., & Penn, M. (2022). Do stronger employment discrimination protections decrease reliance on social security disability insurance? Evidence from the US. social security reforms. *The Journal of the Economics of Ageing*, *22*, 100370.

Cai, C., Runte, J., Ostrer, I., Berry, K., Ponce, N., Rodriguez, M., Bertozzi, S., White, J. S., & Kahn, J. G. (2020). Projected costs of single-payer healthcare financing in the United States: A systematic review of economic analysis. *PLoS Medicine*, *17*(1), e1003013. 10.1371/journal.pmed.1003013

California Department of Insurance. (n.d.). *Common health insurance terms*. http://www.insurance.ca.gov/01-consumers/110-health/10-basics/terms.cfm

California Department of Managed Care. (2020). *Your health care rights*. https://www.dmhc.ca.gov/HealthCareinCalifornia/YourHealthCareRights.aspx

Center on Budget and Policy Priorities (CBPP). (2020, February 7). *Sabotage watch: Tracking efforts to undermine the ACA*. https://www.cbpp.org/sabotage-watch-tracking-efforts-to-undermine-the-aca

Centers for Disease Control and Prevention (CDC). (2014). *United States public health 101*. https://www.cdc.gov/publichealthgateway/docs/usph101.pdf

Centers for Disease Control and Prevention (CDC). (2018, October). *CDC's 6|18 Initiative: Accelerating evidence into action*. https://www.cdc.gov/sixeighteen/index.html

Centers for Disease Control and Prevention (CDC). (2023b, June 26). *Health insurance coverage*. https://www.cdc.gov/nchs/hus/topics/health-insurance-coverage.htm#featured-charts

Centers for Disease Control and Prevention (CDC). (2024, May 16). *10 Essential Public Health Services*. https://www.cdc.gov/public-health-gateway/php/about/index.html

Centers for Disease Control and Prevention (CDC) (2024a). *Community planning for health assessment: Data & benchmarks*. https://www.cdc.gov/public-health-gateway/php/public-health-strategy/public-health-strategies-for-community-health-assessment-data-benchmarks.html

Centers for Disease Control and Prevention (CDC). (2024b). *Legal authorities for isolation and quarantine*. https://www.cdc.gov/port-health/legal-authorities/isolation-quarantine.html

Centers for Medicare & Medicaid Services (CMS). (n.d.-a). *Children's Health Insurance Program (CHIP)*. https://www.medicaid.gov/chip/index.html

Centers for Medicare & Medicaid Services (CMS). (n.d.-b). *National Health Expenditures 2017 highlights*. https://www.cms.gov/Research-Statistics-Data-and-Systems/Statistics-Trends-and-Reports/NationalHealthExpendData/downloads/highlights.pdf

Centers for Medicare & Medicaid Services (CMS) (n.d.-c). *Pre-existing conditions could affect 1 in 2 Americans*. The Center for Consumer Information & Insurance Oversight. https://www.cms.gov/CCIIO/Resources/FormMedicares-Reports-and-Other-Resources/preexisting

Centers for Medicare & Medicaid Services (CMS). (2018, June 5). *Declines in hospital-acquired conditions save 8,000 lives and $2.9 billion in costs*. https://www.cms.gov/newsroom/press-releases/declines-hospital-acquired-conditions-save-8000-lives-and-29-billion-costs

Centers for Medicare & Medicaid Services (CMS). (2021a, December 1). *History: CMS' program history*. https://www.cms.gov/about-cms/agency-information/history

Centers for Medicare & Medicaid Services (CMS). (2021c, December 1). *National health expenditure data*. https://www.cms.gov/Research-Statistics-Data-and-Systems/Statistics-Trends-and-Reports/NationalHealthExpendData

Centers for Medicare & Medicaid Services (CMS). (2022, December 15). *National health expenditure data: Historical*. https://www.cms.gov/Research-Statistics-Data-and-Systems/Statistics-Trends-and-Reports/NationalHealthExpendData/NationalHealthAccountsHistorical

Centers for Medicare & Medicaid Services (CMS). (2023a, April 18). *About the CMS innovation center*. https://innovation.cms.gov/about

Centers for Medicare & Medicaid Services (CMS). (2023b, March). *CMS fast facts*. https://www.cms.gov/research-statistics-data-and-systems/statistics-trends-and-reports/cms-fast-facts/index.html

Centers for Medicare & Medicaid Services (CMS). (2023c, July 31). *CMS releases 2024 projected Medicare part D premium and bid information*. https://www.cms.gov/newsroom/news-alert/cms-releases-2024-projected-medicare-part-d-premium-and-bid-information

Centers for Medicare & Medicaid Services (CMS). (2023d, April). *Monthly Medicare enrollment*. https://data.cms.gov/summary-statistics-on-beneficiary-enrollment/medicare-and-medicaid-reports/medicare-monthly-enrollment

Centers for Medicare & Medicaid Services (CMS). (2023e, July 21). *NHE fact sheet*. https://www.cms.gov/research-statistics-data-and-systems/statistics-trends-and-reports/nationalhealthexpenddata/nhe-fact-sheet

Chandra, A., Flack, E., & Obermeyer, Z. (2021). *The health costs of cost-sharing*. Working Paper 28439. National Bureau of Economic Research. http://www.nber.org/papers/w28439

Cheng, J., Kim, J., Bieber, S. D., & Lin, E. (2020). Four years into MACRA: What has changed? *Seminars in Dialysis*, *33*, 26–34. 10.1111/sdi.12852

Chernew, M. E., He, H., Mintz, H., & Beaulieu, N. (2021). The potential for consolidation-induced cost shifting. *Health Affairs*, *40*, 1277–1285. https://doi:10.1377/hlthaff.2021.00201

Chidambaram, P., & Burns, A. (2022, September 15). *10 Things about Long-Term Services and Supports (LTSS)* https://www.kff.org/medicaid/issue-brief/10-things-about-long-term-services-and-supports-ltss/

Clifton, G. L. (2009). *Flatlined: Resuscitating American Medicine*. Rutgers University Press.

Collins, S. R., Haynes, L. A., & Masitha, R. (2022). *The state of U.S. health insurance in 2022*. https://www.commonwealthfund.org/sites/default/files/2022-09/Collins_state_of_coverage_biennial_survey_2022_db.pdf

Colon-Morales, C. M., Giang, W. C. W., & Alvarado, M. (2021). Informed decision-making for health insurance enrollment: Survey study. *JMIR Formative Research*, *5*(8), e27477. https://doi:10.2196/27477

Commonwealth Fund. (2019, February 7). *Underinsured rate rose from 2014–2018, with greatest growth among people in employer health plans*. https://www.commonwealthfund.org/press-release/2019/underinsured-rate-rose-2014-2018-greatest-growth-among-people-employer-health

Commonwealth Fund. (n.d.). *International health care systems profiles*. https://international.commonwealthfund.org/countries/united_states/

Congress.gov (2010). HR 3590 (Public Law [PL] 111–148). *The Patient Protection and Affordable Care Act*, on March, 23, 2010. https://www.congress.gov/bill/111th-congress/house-bill/3590

Constantin, J., & Wehby, G. L. (2023). Effects of recent Medicaid expansions on infant mortality by race and ethnicity. *American Journal of Preventive Medicine*, *64*, 377–384. 10.1016/j.amepre.2022.09.026

Council of Public Health Nursing Organizations (CPHNO). (n.d.). *Council of Public Health Nursing Organizations*. https://www.cphno.org/

Crowley, R., Daniel, H., Cooney, T. G., & Engel, L. S. (2020). Envisioning a better U.S. health care system for all: Coverage and cost of care. *Annals of Internal Medicine*, *172*(2S), S7–S32. https://doi:10.7326/M19-2415

Cubanski, J., Koma, W., Damico, A., & Neuman, T. (2019, November 4). *How much do Medicare beneficiaries spend out of pocket on health care*. Kaiser Family Foundation. https://www.kff.org/medicare/issue-brief/how-much-do-medicare-beneficiaries-spend-out-of-pocket-on-health-care/

Cubanski, J., Neuman, T., & Freed, M. (2023, January 19). *What to know about Medicare spending and financing*. Kaiser Family Foundation. https://www.kff.org/medicare/issue-brief/the-facts-on-medicare-spending-and-financing/

Definitive Healthcare. (2023a, April 14). *How many retail clinics are in the U.S.?* https://www.definitivehc.com/resources/healthcare-insights/retail-clinics-us

Definitive Healthcare. (2023b, July 4). Top 50 Hospitals by Net Patient Revenue in the U.S. https://www.definitivehc.com/resources/healthcare-insights/top-50-hospitals-by-net-patient-revenue

DeSalvo, K., Parekh, A., Hoagland, G. W., Dilley, A., Kaiman, S., Hines, M., & Levi, J. (2019). Developing a financing system to support public health infrastructure. *American Journal of Public Health*, *109*, 1358–1361. https://doi:10.2105/AJPH.2019.305214

Dillon, D. M. (2021). A decade of the ACA: The progress, obstacles, and successes. *Health Care Finance*, *47*(3).

Disability Secrets. (n.d.). *SSDI overview*. https://www.disabilitysecrets.com/topics/ssdi-social-security-disability-overview

Donohue, J. M., Cole, E. S., & James, C. V. (2022). The US Medicaid program: Coverage, financing, reforms, and implications for health equity. *Journal of the American Medical Association*, *328*, 1085–1099. https://doi:10.1001/jama.2022.14791

Dowling, W. L. (1979). Prospective rate setting: Concept and practice. *Topics in Health Care Financing*, *3*(2), 35–42.

Edwards, C. (n.d.). *Department of health and human services timeline*. https://www.downsizinggovernment.org/hhs/timeline#:~:text=1878%3A%20Congress%20passes%20the%20National,today's%20National%20Institutes%20of%20Health

Edwards, E., & Dunn, L. (2019, June 30). Is Germany's health care system a model for the US? *NBC News*. https://www.nbcnews.com/health/health-news/germany-s-health-care-system-model-u-s-n1024491

Emerson, J. (2023, February 9). *Big Payers Ranked by 2022 Profit*. Becker's. https://www.beckerspayer.com/payer/big-payers-ranked-by-2022-profit.html

Erickson, S. (2022). Inequity in healthcare: Coverage denials for lifesaving and quality-of-life improving medications and treatments. *Journal of Health and Biomedical Law*, *19*, 52–79.

Erwin, P. C., & Brownson, R. C. (Eds.) (2017). *Scutchfield and Keck's Principles Of public health practice* (4th ed.). Cengage Learning.

Falkson, S. R., & Srinivasan, V. N. (2023). *Health Maintenance Organization*. https://www.ncbi.nlm.nih.gov/books/NBK554454/

Fan, W., Jiang, Y., Pei, J., & Qiu, L. (2023). The impact of medical insurance payment systems on patient choice, provider behavior, and out-of-pocket rate: Fee-for-service versus diagnosis-related groups. *Decision Sciences*, *00*, 1–17. https://doi:10.1111/deci.12593

Fehr, R., & Cox, C. (January 6, 2020). *Individual insurance market performance in late 2019*. Kaiser Family Foundation. https://www.kff.org/private-insurance/issue-brief/individual-insurance-market-performance-in-late-2019/

Fels, M. (2019). Why people buy insurance: A modern answer to an old question. *SSRN*. https://doi:10.2139/ssrn.3352604

Fitzgerald, M. P., & Yencha, C. (2019). A test of policy makers' formal and lay theories regarding health care prices. *Journal of Public Policy & Marketing*, *38*(1), 3–18. https://doi:10.1177/0743915618820573

Fox, K., Benes, L. L., & Harrington, E. (2022). Innovation and partnerships: Meeting the health care needs of a houseless population. *Public Health Nursing*, *39*, 1115–1118. https://doi:10.1111/phn.13068

Frieden, T. R. (2015). The future of public health. *New England Journal of Medicine*, *373*, 1748–1754. https://doi:10.1056/NEJMsa1511248

Gai, Y., & Jones, K. (2020). Insurance patterns and instability from 2006 to 2016. *BMC Health Services Research*, *20*, 334. https://doi:10.1186/s12913-020-05226-1

Gan, N., Xiong, Y., & Mackintosh, E. (2020, January 20). *China confirms new coronavirus can spread between humans*. CNN. https://www.cnn.com/2020/01/19/asia/china-coronavirus-spike-intl-hnk/index.html

Garfield, R., Orgera, K., & Damico, A. (2020, January 14). *The coverage gap: Uninsured poor adults in states that do not expand medicaid*. Kaiser Family Foundation. https://www.kff.org/medicaid/issue-brief/the-coverage-gap-uninsured-poor-adults-in-states-that-do-not-expand-medicaid/

Garfield, R., Rudowitz, R., & Musumeci, M. (2018, June 27). *Implications of a Medicaid work requirement: National estimates of potential coverage losses*. Kaiser Family Foundation. https://www.kff.org/medicaid/issue-brief/implications-of-a-medicaid-work-requirement-national-estimates-of-potential-coverage-losses/

Gast, A., & Mathes, T. (2019). Medication adherence influencing factors: An (updated) overview of systematic reviews. *Systematic Reviews*, *8*, 112. https://doi:10.1186/s13643-019-1014-8

Gee, E. (2019, June 26). *The high price of hospital care*. Center for American Progress. https://www.americanprogress.org/issues/healthcare/reports/2019/06/26/471464/high-price-hospital-care/

Giving USA. (n.d.). *2022 Giving overview*. https://givingusa.org/giving-usa-limited-data-tableau-visualization/

Gladwell, M. (2005, August 29). *The moral-hazard myth*. The New Yorker. http://www.newyorker.com/archive/2005/08/29/050829fa_fact

Globalnewswire. (2020, December 9). *United States urgent care centers markets, 2020-2025: What is the market for urgent care centers? What services are they selling? Who is selling testing and vaccine products to urgent care?* https://www.globenewswire.com/news-release/2020/12/09/2142221/28124/en/United-States-Urgent-Care-Centers-Markets-2020-2025-What-is-the-Market-for-Urgent-Care-Centers-What-Services-are-they-Selling-Who-is-Selling-Testing-and-Vaccine-Products-to-Urgent-.html

Goldsteen, R. L., Goldsteen, K., & Goldsteen, B. Z. (2020). Jonas'. *Introduction to the US health care system* (9th ed.). Springer Publishing.

Grimm, C. A. (2022). Adverse events in hospitals: A quarter of Medicare patients experienced harm in October 2018. *Office of the Inspector General*. OEI-06-18-00400.

Guinan, S. (2023, July 18). *Largest health insurance companies of 2023*. https://www.valuepenguin.com/largest-health-insurance-companies

Guindon, G. E., Fatima, T., Garasia, S., & Khoee, K. (2022). A systematic umbrella review of the association of prescription drug insurance and cost-sharing with drug use, health services use, and health. *BMC Health Services Research*, *22*, 297. https://doi:10.1186/s12913-022-07554-w

Haley, J. M., Long, J., & Kenney, G. M. (2022, January). *Parents with low incomes faced greater health challenges and problems accessing and affording needed health care in spring 2021*. Urban Institute. https://www.urban.org/sites/default/files/publication/105304/lowinc1_0.pdf

Hall, M. A., & McCue, M. J. (2019, July 2). *How the ACA's medical loss ratio rule protects consumers and insurers against ongoing uncertainty*. Commonwealth Fund. https://www.commonwealthfund.org/publications/issue-briefs/2019/jul/how-aca-medical-loss-ratio-rule-protects-consumers-insurers

Hamel, L., Munana, C., & Brodie, M. (2019, May). *Kaiser Family Foundation/L.A. times survey of adults with employer-sponsored health insurance*. Kaiser Family Foundation. http://files.kff.org/attachment/Report-KFF-LA-Times-Survey-of-Adults-with-Employer-Sponsored-Health-Insurance

Harmon, M., Joyce, B. L., Johnson, R. H., Hicks, V., Brown-Schott, N., Pilling, L., Collinge, R., & Brownrigg, V. (2020). An exploratory survey of public health nurses' knowledge, skills, attitudes, and application of the Quad Council Competencies. *Public Health Nursing*, *37*, 581–595. https://doi:10.1111/phn.12716

Hayes, S. L., Collins, S. R., & Radley, D. C. (2019, May 23). *How much US households with employer insurance spend on premiums and out-of-pocket costs: A state-by-state look*. Commonwealth Fund. https://www.commonwealthfund.org/publications/issue-briefs/2019/may/

how-much-us-households-employer-insurance-spend-premiums-out-of-pocket

Healthcare.gov. (2019, October 23). *About the affordable care act.* http://www.hhs.gov/healthcare/facts-and-features/key-features-of-aca/index.html

Healthcare.gov. (n.d.-a). *Glossary: Community rating.* https://www.healthcare.gov/glossary/community-rating/

Healthcare.gov. (n.d.-c). *Glossary: Recession.* https://www.healthcare.gov/glossary/rescission/

Healthcare.gov. (n.d.-d). *The Children's Health Insurance Program (CHIP).* https://www.healthcare.gov/medicaid-chip/childrens-health-insurance-program/

Henderson, J. W. (2022). *Health economics and policy* (8th ed.). Cengage Learning.

Hiltzik, M. (2019, September 4). *Medical bankruptcy is an American scandal that's not debatable.* Los Angeles Times. https://www.latimes.com/business/story/2019-09-04/hiltzik-medical-bankruptcy-american-scandal

Himmelstein, D. U., Dickman, S. L., McCormick, D., Bor, D. H., Gaffney, A., & Woolhandler, S. (2022). Prevalence and risk factors for medical debt and subsequent changes in social determinants of health in the US. *JAMA Network Open, 5*(9), e2231898. https://doi:10.1001/jamanetworkopen.2022.31898

Himmelstein, D. U., Lawless, R. M., Thorne, D., Foohey, P., & Woolhandler, S. (2019). Medical bankruptcy: Still common despite the Affordable Care Act. *American Journal of Public Health, 109,* 431–433. https://doi:10.2105/AJPH.2018.304901

Hinton, E., & Raphael, J. (2023, March 1). *10 Things to know about Medicaid managed care.* Kaiser Family Foundation. https://www.kff.org/medicaid/issue-brief/10-things-to-know-about-medicaid-managed-care/

Hoagland, G. W., & Parekh, A. (2019, November 18). *Patient-Centered Outcomes Research Institute: Healthcare's Savior?* MedPage Today. https://www.medpagetoday.com/publichealthpolicy/healthpolicy/83408

Hoffer, E. P. (2019a). America's health care system is broken: What went wrong and how we can fix it. Introduction to the series. *The American Journal of Medicine, 132,* 675–677. https://doi:10.1016/j.amjmed.2019.01.040

Hoffer, E. P. (2019b). America's health care system is broken: What went wrong and how we can fix it. Part 2: Health insurance. *The American Journal of Medicine, 132,* 791–794. https://doi:10.1016/j.amjmed.2019.02.039

Holgash, K., & Heberlein, M. (2019, April 10). *Physician acceptance of new Medicaid patients: What matters and what doesn't.* Health Affairs Blog. https://www.healthaffairs.org/do/10.1377/hblog20190401.678690/full/

InsureKidsNow.gov. (n.d.). *Frequently asked questions.* https://www.insurekidsnow.gov/find-coverage-your-family/frequently-asked-questions/index.html#haveJob

Jaggannathan, M. (2019, May 13). *Most of the profit in healthcare industry is going to drug companies: Here's why you should care.* MarketWatch. https://www.marketwatch.com/story/most-of-the-profit-in-the-health-care-industry-is-going-to-drug-companies-heres-why-you-should-care-2019-05-13

Jenkins, D., & Ho, V. (2023). Nonprofit hospitals: Profits and cash reserves grow, charity care does not. *Health Affairs, 42,* 866–869. https://doi:10.1377/hlthaff.2022.01542

Johns Hopkins. (n.d.). *What is health economics?* https://publichealth.jhu.edu/academics/academic-program-finder/masters-degrees/master-of-health-science-in-global-health-economics/what-is-health-economics#

Johnson, S. R. (2019, April 23). *Report: Public health funding falls despite increasing threats.* Modern Healthcare. https://www.modernhealthcare.com/government/report-public-health-funding-falls-despite-increasing-threats

Johnson, J. A., Davey, K. S., & Greenhill, R. G. (2022). *Sultz & Young's Health Care USA: Understanding its organization and delivery* (9th ed.). Jones & Bartlett Learning.

Johnson, A., Reising, V., Cruz, C., Franklin, C., & Martin, A. (2023). Implementation of nursing services in community corrections: A community-academic partnership. *Public Health Nursing, 40,* 511–516. https://doi:10.1111/phn.13195

Kaiser Family Foundation (KFF). (2012). *Focus on health reform.* https://www.kff.org/wp-content/uploads/2013/01/8347.pdf

Kaiser Family Foundation (KFF). (2019c, September 25). *Section 8: High-deductible health plan with savings option.* 2019 Employer Health Benefits Survey. https://www.kff.org/report-section/ehbs-2019-section-8-high-deductible-health-plans-with-savings-option/

Kaiser Family Foundation (KFF). (2019a, February 13). *An overview of Medicare.* https://www.kff.org/medicare/issue-brief/an-overview-of-medicare/

Kaiser Family Foundation (KFF). (2019b). *Employer health benefits annual survey, 2019.* http://files.kff.org/attachment/Report-Employer-Health-Benefits-Annual-Survey-2019

Kaiser Family Foundation (KFF). (2022a, October 27). *2022 Employer benefits survey.* https://www.kff.org/health-costs/report/2022-employer-health-benefits-survey/

Kaiser Family Foundation (KFF). (2022b, December 19). *Key facts about the uninsured population.* http://kff.org/uninsured/fact-sheet/key-facts-about-the-uninsured-population/

Kaiser Family Foundation (KFF). (2023a, August 9). *Medicare advantage in 2023: Enrollment update and key trends.* https://www.kff.org/medicare/issue-brief/medicare-advantage-in-2023-enrollment-update-and-key-trends/

Kaiser Family Foundation (KFF). (2023c, July 27). *Status of state Medicaid expansion decisions: Interactive map.* https://www.kff.org/medicaid/issue-brief/status-of-state-medicaid-expansion-decisions-interactive-map/

Kaiser Family Foundation (KFF). (n.d.-a). *Timeline: History of health reform in the US.* https://www.kff.org/wp-content/uploads/2011/03/5-02-13-history-of-health-reform.pdf

Kaiser Family Foundation (KFF). (n.d.-b). *Health coverage of the total population.* https://www.kff.org/other/state-indicator/total-population/?currentTimeframe

Kaiser Family Foundation (KFF). (n.d.-d). *Total Medicaid spending.* https://www.kff.org/medicaid/state-indicator/total-medicaid-spending/?currentTimeframe

Kaiser Health News. (August 13, 2019). *More patients are getting hit with surprise medical bills, and the price tags are going up, too.* https://khn.org/morning-breakout/more-patients-are-getting-hit-with-surprise-medical-bills-and-the-price-tags-are-going-up-too/

Kamal, R., Cox, C., McDermott, D., Ramirez, M., & Sawyer, B. (2019, March 29). *US health system is performing better, though still lagging behind other countries.* Health System Tracker. https://www.healthsystemtracker.org/brief/us-health-system-is-performing-better-though-still-lagging-behind-other-countries/

Kee, D., Wisnivesky, J., & Kale, M. S. (2021). Lung cancer screening uptake: Analysis of BRFSS 2018. *Journal of General Internal Medicine, 36,* 2897–2899. https://doi:10.1007/s11606-020-06236-9

Keehan, S. P., Fiore, J. A., Poisal, J. A., Cuckler, G. A., Sisko, A. M., Smith, S. D., Madison, A. J., & Rennie, K. E. (2023). National health expenditure projections, 2022–31: Growth to stabilize once the COVID-19 public health emergency ends. *Health Affairs, 42,* 886–898. https://doi:10.1377/hlthaff.2023.00403

Kinney, E. D. (2013). The Affordable Care Act and the Medicare program: The engines of true health reform. *Yale Journal of Health Policy, Law, and Ethics, 13,* 253–325.

Kirzinger, A., Muñana, C., Wu, B., & Brodie, M. (2019). *Data note: Americans' challenges with health care costs.* Kaiser Family Foundation. Retrieved from https://www.kff.org/health-costs/issue-brief/data-note-americans-challenges-health-care-costs/

Kisacky, J. (2019). An architectural history of US community hospitals. *AMA Journal of Ethics, 21,* e288–e296. https://doi:10.1001/amajethics.2019.288

Knickman, J. R., & Kovner, A. R. (Eds.). (2019). *Jonas & Kovner's health care delivery in the United States* (12th ed.). Springer.

Kramer, L. (2019, June 25). *How does the law of supply and demand affect prices?* https://www.investopedia.com/ask/answers/033115/how-does-law-supply-and-demand-affect-prices.asp

Kub, J. E., Kulbok, P. A., Miner, S., & Merrill, J. A. (2017). Increasing the capacity of public health nursing to strengthen the public health infrastructure and to promote and protect the health of communities and populations. *Nursing Outlook, 65,* 661–664. https://doi:10.1016/j.outlook.2017.08.009

Kumar, W., & Schulman, K. (2022). An intergenerational evaluation of Medicare. *The American Journal of Medicine, 136,* 132–133. https://doi:10.1016/j.amjmed.2022.09.032

Kurani, N., & Wager, E. (2021, September 30). *How does the quality of the US health system compare to other countries?* Health System Tracker. https://www.healthsystemtracker. org/chart-collection/quality-us-healthcare-system-compare-countries

Laurence, B. K. (2023, August 14). *How much in social security disability benefits can you get?* https://www.disabilitysecrets.com/how-much-in-ssd.html

Lee, A., Ruhter, J., Peters, C., De Lew, N., & Sommers, B. D. (2022, August). *National uninsured rate reaches all-time low in early 2022.* U.S. Department of Health and Human Services, Office of Health Policy. HP-2022-23. https://www.aspe.hhs.gov/sites/default/files/documents/15c1f989 9b3f203887deba90e3005f5a/Uninsured-Q1-2022-Data-Point-HP-2022-23-08.pdf

Leider, J. P., Resnick, B., McCullough, M., Alfonso, N., & Bishai, D. (2020). Inaccuracy of official estimates of public health spending in the United States, 2000-2018. *American Journal of Public Health, 110*(S2), S194–S196. https://doi:10.2105/AJPH.2020.305709

Lopez, L., Dhodapkar, M., & Gross, C. P. (2021). US nonprofit hospitals' community health needs assessments and implementation strategies in the era of the Patient Protection and Affordable Care Act. *JAMA Network Open, 4*(8), e2122237. https://doi:10.1001/jamanetworkopen.2021.22237

Lovelace, B. (2020, February 28). *WHO raises coronavirus threat assessment to its highest level: 'Wake up, get ready. This virus may be on its way'.* CNBC. https://www.cnbc.com/2020/02/28/who-raises-risk-assessment-of-coronavirus-to-very-high-at-global-level.html

Madden, J. M., Bayapureddy, S., Briesacher, B. A., Zhang, F., Ross-Degnan, D., Soumerai, S. B., Gurwitz, J. H., & Galbraith, A. A. (2021). Affordability of medical care among Medicare enrollees. *JAMA Health Forum, 2*(12), e214104. https://doi:10.1001/jamahealthforum.2021.4104

Manatt, P., & Phillips, L. L. P. (2019, February 1). *Medicaid's role in children's health.* Robert Wood Johnson Foundation. https://www.rwjf.org/en/library/research/2019/02/medicaid-s-role-in-children-s-health.html

Mathauer, I., Vinyals Torres, L., Kutzin, J., Jakab, M., & Hanson, K. (2020). Pooling financial resources for universal health coverage: Options for reform. *Bulletin of the World Health Organization, 98*(2), 132–139. https://doi:10.2471/BLT.19.234153

Mather, M., Scommegna, P., & Kilduff, L. (2019, July 15). *Fact sheet: Aging in the United States.* Population Reference Bureau. https://www.prb.org/aging-unitedstates-fact-sheet/

Mazurenko, O., Buntin, M. J. B., & Menachemi, N. (2019). High-deductible health plans and prevention. *Annual Review of Public Health, 40,* 411–421. https://doi:10.1146/annurev-publhealth-040218-044225

McNerney, W. J. (1980). Control of health care costs in the 1980s. *New England Journal of Medicine, 303,* 1088–1095. https://doi:10.1056/NEJM198011063031904

McPake, B., Normand, C., Smith, S., & Nolan, A. (2020). *Health economics: An international perspective* (4th ed.). Routledge.

Meachum, M. R. (2020). *Longest's Health policymaking in the United States* (7th ed.). Health Administration Press.

Medicaid and CHIP Payment and Access Commission (MACPAC). (n.d.). *CHIP eligibility.* https://www.macpac.gov/subtopic/eligibility-2/

Medicaid.gov. (2020, September). *Federal Fiscal Year (FFY) 2020 Statistical Enrollment Data System (SEDS) reporting.* https://www.medicaid.gov/sites/default/files/2019-12/fy-2018-childrens-enrollment-report.pdf

Medicaid.gov. (2023, April). *Medicaid.* https://www.medicaid.gov/medicaid/index.html

Medicaid.gov. (n.d.). *Mandatory & optional Medicaid benefits.* https://www.medicaid.gov/medicaid/benefits/mandatory-optional-medicaid-benefits/index.html

Medicare.gov. (n.d.-a). *About Medicare health plans.* https://www.medicare.gov/sign-up-change-plans/medicare-health-plans/medicare-health-plans.html

Medicare.gov. (n.d.-c). *Costs in the coverage gap.* https://www.medicare.gov/drug-coverage-part-d/costs-for-medicare-drug-coverage/costs-in-the-coverage-gap

Medicare.gov. (n.d.-d). *Medicare coverage of skilled nursing facility care.* https://www.medicare.gov/Pubs/pdf/10153-Medicare-Skilled-Nursing-Facility-Care.pdf

Medicare.gov. (n.d.-e). *Costs.* https://www.medicare.gov/basics/costs/medicare-costs

Medicare.gov. (n.d.-f). *Monthly premium for drug plans.* https://www.medicare.gov/drug-coverage-part-d/costs-for-medicare-drug-coverage/monthly-premium-for-drug-plans

Medicare.gov. (n.d.-g). *What's Medicare Supplement Insurance (Medigap)?* https://www.medicare.gov/health-drug-plans/medigap

Medicare.gov. (n.d.-h). *Yearly deductible for drug plans.* https://www.medicare.gov/drug-coverage-part-d/costs-for-medicare-drug-coverage/yearly-deductible-for-drug-plans

Mendelson, D. (2019, January 29). *Are health plans the future of public health?* Forbes. https://www.forbes.com/sites/

danielmendelson/2019/01/29/are-health-plans-the-future-of-public-health/#38178938318c

Mondesir, F. L., Kilgore, M. L., Shelley, J. P., Levitan, E. B., Huang, L., Riggs, K. R., Pisu, M., Li, Y., Bronstein, J. M., Agne, A., & Cherrington, A. L. (2019). Medicaid expansion and hospitalization for ambulatory care–sensitive conditions among nonelderly adults with diabetes. *The Journal of Ambulatory Care Management*, *42*, 312–320. https://doi:10.1097/JAC.0000000000000280

Moon, J., & Shugan, S. M. (2020). Nonprofit versus for-profit health care competition: How service mix makes nonprofit hospitals more profitable. *Journal of Marketing Research*, *57*, 193–210. https://doi:10.1177/0022243719901169

Moosa, M. R., & Luyckx, V. A. (2021). The realities of rationing in health care. *Nature Reviews Nephrology*, *17*, 435–436. https://doi:10.1038/s41581-021-00404-8

Morenz, A. M., Zhou, L., Wong, E. S., & Liao, J. M. (2023). Association between capitated payments and preventive care among U.S. adults. *AJPM Focus*, 2, https://doi:100116.10.1016/j.focus.2023.100116

Morton, F. S., Kandula, K., & Kang, K. (2022). Do we need a new Sherman Act? *Columbia Business Law Review*, *2022*, 42–71.

Muir, K. J. (2019). Historical perspectives informing modern day nursing innovation and economics. *Nursing Economics*, *37*, 284.

Muntner, P., Hardy, S. T., Fine, L. J., Jaeger, B. C., Wozniak, G., Levitan, E. B., & Colantonio, L. D. (2020). Trends in blood pressure control among US adults with hypertension, 1999-2000 to 2017-2018. *Journal of the American Medical Association*, *324*, 1190–1200. https://doi:10.1001/jama.2020.14545

Naik, Y., Baker, P., Ismail, S. A., Tillmann, T., Bash, K., Quantz, D., Hillier-Brown, F., Jayatunga, W., Kelly, G., Black, M., Gopfert, A., Roderick, P., Barr, B., & Bambra, C. (2019). Going upstream: An umbrella review of the macroeconomic determinants of health and health inequalities. *BMC Public Health*, *19*, 1678. https://doi:10.1186/s12889-019-7895-6

National Academies of Sciences, Engineering, and Medicine (NASEM). (2017). *Communities in action: Pathways to health equity in the United States*. National Academies Press.

National Academies of Sciences, Engineering, and Medicine (NASEM). (2019). *Integrating social care into the delivery of health care: Moving upstream to improve the nation's health*. The National Academies Press. https://doi:10.17226/25467

National Association of County and City Health Officials (NACCHO). (n.d.). *About*. https://www.naccho.org/about

National Association of County and City Health Officials (NACCHO). (2020). *NACCHO's 2019 profile study interactive report*. https://www.naccho.org/profile-report-dashboard

National Conference of State Legislatures (NCSL). (2020). *Health savings accounts*. https://www.ncsl.org/research/health/hsas-health-savings-accounts.aspx

National Council on Aging (NCA). (2022a, October). *Medicare advantage/Medicare part C costs*. https://www.ncoa.org/article/medicare-advantage-medicare-part-c-costs ?

National Council on Aging (NCA). (2022b, March 16). *SSI vs. SSDI: The differences, benefits, and how to apply*. https://www.ncoa.org/article/ssi-vs-ssdi-what-are-these-benefits-how-they-differ

National Council on Aging (NCA). (2023a, July 19). *A guide to social security disability insurance benefits*. https://www.ncoa.org/article/a-guide-to-social-security-disability-insurance-benefits

National Council on Aging (NCA). (2023b, January 19). *What is supplemental security income?* https://ncoa.org/article/what-is-supplemental-security-income-ssi

National Institutes of Health (NIH). (2019). *Who we are*. https://www.nih.gov/about-nih/who-we-are

Nickitas, D. M., Middaugh, D. J., & Feeg, V. D. (Eds.) (2020). *Policy and politics for nurses and other health professionals: Advocacy and action* (3rd ed.). Jones & Bartlett Publishers.

O'Day, S. (2021, June 28). *Is an EPO plan right for you?* https://healthcareinsider.com/what-is-an-epo-health-plan-216010

Organization for Economic Cooperation and Development (OECD). (2019). *Health for Everyone?: Social Inequalities in Health and Health Systems, OECD Health Policy Studies*. OECD Publishing. https://doi:10.1787/3c8385d0-en

Owen, L., Pennington, B., Fischer, A., & Jeong, K. (2019). The cost-effectiveness of public health interventions examined by NICE from 2011 to 2016. *Journal of Public Health*, *40*(3), 557–566. https://doi:10.1093/pubmed/fdx119

Park, E., Dwyer, A., Brooks, T., Clark, M., & Alker, J. (2023, January). *Consolidated appropriations act, 2023: Medicaid and CHIP provisions explained*. https://ccf.georgetown.edu/wp-content/uploads/2023/01/Consolidated-Approp-v3a-1.pdf

Parmar, D., & Banerjee, A. (2019). How do supply- and demand-side interventions influence equity in healthcare utilization? Evidence from maternal healthcare in Senegal. *Social Science and Medicine*, 241, 112582. https://doi:10.1016/j.socscimed.2019.112582

Patient Safety Network. (2019, September 7). *Never events*. https://psnet.ahrq.gov/primer/never-events

Patient-Centered Outcomes Research Institute (PCORI). (n.d.). *Our programs*. https://www.pcori.org/about-us/our-programs

Pena, M. T., Mohammed, M., Burns, A., Fuglesten Biniek, J., Ochieng, N., & Chidambaram, P. (2023, January 31). *A profile of Medicare-Medicaid enrollees (dual eligibles)*. Kaiser Family Foundation. https://www.kff.org/medicare/issue-brief/a-profile-of-medicare-medicaid-enrollees-dual-eligibles/

Perkins, B. B. (1998). Economic organization of medicine and the Committee on the Costs of Medical Care. *American Journal of Public Health*, *88*, 1721–1726. https://doi:10.2105/ajph.88.11.1721

Perry, M. J. (2022, May 14). *What economic lessons about health care costs can we learn from the competitive market for aesthetic plastic surgery?* American Enterprise Institute. https://www.aei.org/carpe-diem/what-economic-lessons-about-health-care-costs-can-we-learn-from-the-competitive-market-for-aesthetic-plastic-surgery-2/

Pestaina, K., Wallace, R., & Long, M. (2024). *The regulation of private health insurance*. https://www.kff.org/health-policy-101-the-regulation-of-private-health-insurance/?entry=table-of-contents-introduction

Physicians for a National Health Program. (n.d.). *Does the U.S. ration health care?* https://pnhp.org/2016/08/01/does-the-u-s-ration-health-care/

Pittman, P., & Park, J. (2021). Rebuilding community-based and public health nursing in the wake of COVID-19. *Online Journal of Issues in Nursing*, 26(2), 1–10. https://doi:10.3912/OJIN.Vol26No02Man07

Pollitz, K. (2021, December 10). *No surprises act implementation: What to expect in 2022*. Kaiser Family Foundation. https://www.kff.org/health-reform/issue-brief/no-surprises-act-implementation-what-to-expect-in-2022/

Pollitz, K., Lopes, L., Kearney, A., Rae, M., Cox, C., Fehr, R., & Rousseau, D. (2020). US statistics on surprise medical billing. *Journal of the American Medical Association*, *323*, 498. https://doi:10.1001/jama.2020.0065

Public Agenda. (2020, February 5). *America's Hidden common ground on improving health care*. https://publicagenda.org/resource/americas-hidden-common-ground-on-improving-health-care/

Public Health Accreditation Board (PHAB). (n.d.). *Accreditation activity*. https://phaboard.org/accreditation-recognition/accreditation-activity/?gclid=CjwKCAjw8ZKmBhArEiwAspcJ7gHE6kMnwNbDicAprCmKW79kTH2qpG6s-GHhx86w7sALn-6JpsGKeexoCQh8QAvD_BwE

Public Health Law Center. (2015, April). *State and local public health: An overview of regulatory authority*. https://www.publichealthlawcenter.org/sites/default/files/resources/phlc-fs-state-local-reg-authority-publichealth-2015_0.pdf

Rajkumar, S. V. (2020). The high cost of prescription drugs: Causes and solutions. *Blood Cancer Journal*, *10*, 71. https://doi:10.1038/s41408-020-0338-x

Rambur, B. (2022). *Health care finance, economics, and policy for nurses: A foundational guide* (2nd ed.). Springer Publishing.

Rao, P., Fischer, S. H., Vaiana, M. E., & Taylor, E. A. (2022). Barriers to price and quality transparency in health care markets. *Rand Health Quarterly*, *9*(3), 1.

Resnick, B., Morlock, L., Diener-West, M., Stuart, E., Spencer, M., & Sharfstein, J. M. (2019). PH WINS and the future of public health education. *Journal of Public Health Management*, *25*, S10–S12. https://doi:10.1097/PHH.0000000000000955

Rhodes, J. H., Buchmueller, T. C., Levy, H. G., & Nikpay, S. S. (2020). Heterogeneous effects of the ACA Medicaid expansion on hospital financial outcomes. *Contemporary Economic Policy*, *38*, 81–93. https://doi:10.1111/coep.12428

Rodrigo, G. C. (n.d.). *Micro and macro: The economic divide*. International Monetary Fund. https://www.imf.org/en/Publications/fandd/issues/Series/Back-to-Basics/Micro-and-Macro

Rodziewicz, T. L., & Hipskind, J. E. (2019, January). *Medical Error Prevention. StatPearls*. StatPearls Publishing. http://www.saludinfantil.org/Postgrado_Pediatria/Pediatria_Integral/papers/Medical%20Error%20Prevention%20-%20StatPearls%20-%20NCBI%20Bookshelf.pdf

Rook, D. (2020, August 27). *A brief history of employer-sponsored healthcare: from the 1930s to now*. http://www.griffinbenefits.com/employeebenefitsblog/history-of-employer-sponsored-healthcare

Rose-Jacobs, R., Ettinger de Cuba, S., Bovell-Ammon, A., Black, M. M., Coleman, S. M., Cutts, D., ... Sandel, M. (2019). Housing instability among families with young children with special health care needs. *Pediatrics*, *144*(2), e20181704. https://doi:10.542/peds.2018-1704

Rosen, G. (2015). *A history of public health* (rev. expanded ed.). Johns Hopkins University Press.

Rothbaum, J., & Edwards, A. (2019, September 10). *U.S. median household income was $63,179 in 2018, not significantly different from 2017*. U.S. Census Bureau. https://www.census.gov/library/stories/2019/09/us-median-household-income-not-significantly-different-from-2017.html

Roughley, T. G. (2023, August 21). *Indemnity insurance*. U.S. News and World Report. https://www.usnews.com/insurance/glossary/indemnity-insurance

Rudowitz, R., Burns, A., Hinton, E., & Mohamed, M. (2023, June 30). *10 things to know about Medicaid*. Kaiser Family Foundation. https://www.kff.org/medicaid/issue-brief/10-things-to-know-about-medicaid/

Rudowitz, R., Drake, P., Tolbert, J., & Damico, A. (2023, March 31). *How many uninsured are in the coverage gap and how many could be eligible if all states adopted the Medicaid expansion?* Kaiser Family Foundation. https://www.kff.org/medicaid/issue-brief/how-many-uninsured-are-in-the-coverage-gap-and-how-many-could-be-eligible-if-all-states-adopted-the-medicaid-expansion/

Saltzman, E. (2019). Demand for health insurance: Evidence from the California and Washington ACA exchanges. *Journal of Health Economics*, *63*, 197–222. https://doi:10.1016/j.jhealeco.2018.11.004

Saltzman, E. (2021). Managing adverse selection: Underinsurance versus underenrollment. *The RAND Journal of Economics*, *52*, 359–381. https://doi:10.1111/1756-2171.12372

Schneider, A. (2019, February 28). *Medicaid and state budgets: Checking the facts (yet again)*. Georgetown University Health Policy Institute. https://ccf.georgetown.edu/2019/02/28/medicaid-and-state-budgets-checking-the-facts-yet-again/

Schneider, E. C., Sarnak, D. O., Squires, D., Shah, A., & Doty, M. M. (2017, July). *Mirror, mirror 2017: International comparison reflects flaws and opportunities for better U.S. Health Care*. Commonwealth Fund. https://interactives.commonwealthfund.org/2017/july/mirror-mirror/assets/Schneider_mirror_mirror_2017.pdf

Schneider, E. C., Shah, A., Doty, M. M., Tikkanen, R., Fields, K., & Williams, R. D. (2021, August 4). *Mirror, mirror 2021: reflecting poorly: Health care in the U.S. compared to other high-income countries*. Commonwealth Fund. https://www.commonwealthfund.org/publications/fund-reports/2021/aug/mirror-mirror-2021-reflecting-poorly

Schpero, W., Wiener, T., & Carter, S. (2022). Lobbying expenditures in the US health care sector, 2000–2020. *JAMA Health Forum*, *3*(10), e223801. https://doi:10.1001/jamahealthforum.2022.3801

Schuchat, A. (2020). Public health response to the initiation and spread of pandemic COVID-19 in the United States, February 24–April 21, 2020. *Morbidity and Mortality Weekly Report*, *69*, 551–556. http://dx.doi.org/10.15585/mmwr.mm6918e2

Shi, L., & Singh, D. (2019). *Essentials of the U.S. Health Care System* (5th ed.). Jones & Bartlett.

Smith, L., Atherly, A., Campbell, J., Flattery, N., Coronel, S., & Krantz, S. (2019). Cost-effectiveness of a statewide public health intervention to reduce cardiovascular disease risk. *BMC Public Health*, *19*, 1234. https://doi:10.1186/s12889-019-7573-8

Sneed, R. S., Stubblefield, A., Gardner, G., Jordan, T., & Mezuk, B. (2022). Chronic disease, functional limitations, and workforce participation among Medicaid enrollees over 50: The potential impact of Medicaid work requirements post-COVID-19. *Journal of Aging & Social Policy*. https://doi:10.1080/08959420.2023.2226291

Social Security Administration (SSA). (2023a). *Medicare*. Publication No. 095-10043. https://www.ssa.gov/pubs/EN-05-10043.pdf

Social Security Administration (SSA). (2023b). *A guide to Supplemental Security Income (SSI) for groups and organizations*. https://www.ssa.gov/pubs/EN-05-11015.pdf

Social Security Administration (SSA). (n.d.-a). *Historical background and development of Social Security*. http://www.ssa.gov/history/briefhistory3.html

Social Security Administration (SSA). (n.d.-b). *SSI Federal payment amounts for 2023*. https://www.ssa.gov/oact/cola/SSI.html

Sommers, B. D. (2020). Health insurance coverage: What comes after the ACA? An examination of the major gaps in health insurance coverage and access to care that remain ten years after the Affordable Care Act. *Health Affairs*, *39*, 502–508. https://doi:10.1377/hlthaff.2019.01416

Sonfield, A., Frost, J. J., Dawson, R., & Lindberg, L. D. (2020, August 3). *COVID-19 job losses threaten insurance coverage and access to reproductive health care for millions*. Health Affairs Blog. https://www.healthaffairs.org/do/10.1377/hblog20200728.779022/full/

Speer, M., McCullough, J. M., Fielding, J. E., Faustino, E., & Teutsch, S. M. (2020). Excess medical care spending: The categories, magnitude, and opportunity costs of wasteful spending in the United States. *American Journal of Public Health*, *110*, 1743–1748. https://doi:10.2105/AJPH.2020.305865

Sullivan, T. (2022, October 23). *Teva reaches settlement with two more states over price-fixing allegations*. https://www.policymed.com/2022/11/teva-reaches-settlement-with-two-more-states-over-price-fixing-allegations.html

Tikkanen, R., & Osborn, R. (2019, July 11). *Does the United States ration health care?* Commonwealth Fund. https://www.commonwealthfund.org/blog/2019/does-united-states-ration-health-care

Tolbert, J., & Ammula, M. (2023, June 9). *10 things to know about the unwinding of the Medicaid continuous enrollment provision*. Kaiser Family Foundation. https://www.kff.org/medicaid/issue-brief/10-things-to-know-about-the-unwinding-of-the-medicaid-continuous-enrollment-provision/

Tolbert, J., Orgera, K., Singer, N., & Damico, A. (December, 2019). *Key facts about the uninsured population*. Kaiser Family Foundation. http://files.kff.org/attachment/Issue-Brief-Key-Facts-about-the-Uninsured-Population

Torrey, T. (2020, February 27). *Understanding Healthcare Reimbursement*. Verywellhealth. https://www.verywellhealth.com/reimbursement-2615205

Trust for America's Health (TFAH). (2022). *The impact of chronic underfunding on America's public health system: Trends, risks, and recommendations, 2019*.

Trust for America's Health (TFAH). (n.d.). *Ten top priorities for prevention*. https://www.tfah.org/report-details/ten-top-priorities-for-prevention/

U.S. Census Bureau. (2023). *2020 ACS 5-year estimates subject tables*. data.census.gov

U.S. Department of Health & Human Services (USDHHS). (2023, August 17). *HHS organizational chart: HHS agencies & offices*. Retrieved from http://www.hhs.gov/about/agencies/hhs-agencies-and-offices/index.html

U.S. Department of Health & Human Services (USDHHS). (n.d.-b). *Commissioned corps of the U.S. Public Health Service: HHS offices and agencies*. https://www.usphs.gov/

U.S. Department of Health & Human Services (USDHHS). (n.d.-d). *HHS organizational charts office of secretary and divisions*. https://www.hhs.gov/about/agencies/orgchart/index.html

U.S. Department of Health & Human Services (USDHHS). (n.d.-e). *Non-HHS agencies and programs*. https://www.usphs.gov/aboutus/agencies/non-hhs.aspx

U.S. Department of Health & Human Services (USDHHS). (2022). *New reports show record 35 million people enrolled in coverage related to the affordable care act, with historic 21 million people enrolled in Medicaid expansion coverage*. https://www.hhs.gov/about/news/2022/04/29/new-reports-show-record-35-million-people-enrolled-in-coverage-related-to-the-affordable-care-act.html

U.S. Department of State. (2021, January 20). *Non-Governmental Organizations (NGOs) in the United States*. https://www.state.gov/non-governmental-organizations-ngos-in-the-united-states/

U.S. Office of Personal Management. (n.d.-a). *Fast facts: High Deductible Health Plans (HDHP)*. https://www.opm.gov/healthcare-insurance/fastfacts/high-deductible-health-plans.pdf

U.S. Office of Personal Management. (n.d.-b). *Health savings accounts*. https://www.opm.gov/healthcare-insurance/healthcare/health-savings-accounts/

United States Courts (2023, May 5). *Bankruptcies rise, but stay lower than pre-COVID*. Administrative Office of the U.S. Courts. https://www.uscourts.gov/news/2018/03/07/just-facts-consumer-bankruptcy-filings-2006-2017

Voran, D. (2023). Effect of retail and urgent care clinics on primary care in Missouri. *Missouri Medicine*, *120*(2), 96–101.

Weber, L., Ungar, L., Smith, M. R., Recht, H., & Barry-Jester, A. M. (2020, August 24). *Hollowed-out public health system faces more cuts amid virus*. Kaiser Health News. https://khn.org/news/us-public-health-system-underfunded-under-threat-faces-more-cuts-amid-covid-pandemic/

White, C., & Whaley, C. M. (2019). *Prices paid to hospitals by private health plans are high relative to Medicare and vary widely: Findings from an employer-led transparency initiative*. RAND Corporation. https://doi:10.7249/RR3033

Whitehouse.gov. (2023, February 28). *Fact sheet: The congressional republican agenda: Repealing the affordable care act and slashing Medicaid*. https://www.whitehouse.gov/briefing-room/statements-releases/2023/02/28/fact-sheet-the-congressional-republican-agenda-repealing-the-affordable-care-act-and-slashing-medicaid/

Whitman, A., De Lew, N., Chappel, A., Aysola, V., Zuckerman, R., & Sommers, B. D. (2022). *Addressing social determinants of health: Examples of successful evidence-based strategies and current federal efforts*. United States Department of Health and Human Services, Office of Health Policy. HP-2022-12. https://www.aspe.hhs.gov/sites/default/files/documents/e2b650cd64cf84aae8ff0fae7474af82/SDOH-Evidence-Review.pdf

Witters, D. (2019, January 23). *US uninsured rate rises to four-year high*. Gallup. https://news.gallup.com/poll/246134/uninsured-rate-rises-four-year-high.aspx

Wolfe, I. D., & Pope, T. M. (2020). Hospital mergers and conscience-based objections—Growing threats to access and quality of care. *New England Journal of Medicine*, *382*, 1388–1389. https://doi:10.1056/NEJMp1917047

World Health Organization (WHO). (n.d.). *About WHO*. https://www.who.int/about

World Travel & Tourism Council. (n.d.). *Economic impact reports*. https://wttc.org/Research/Economic-Impact

Yabroff, K. R., Zhao, J., Han, X., & Zheng, Z. (2019). Prevalence and correlates of medical financial hardship in the USA. *Journal of General Internal Medicine*, *34*, 1494–1502. https://doi:10.1007/s11606-019-05002-w

Yakusheva, O., Rambur, B., O'Reilly-Jacob, M., & Buerhaus, P. I. (2022). Value-based payment promotes better patient care, incentivizes health care delivery organizations to improve outcomes and lower costs, and can empower nurses. *Nursing Outlook*, *70*, 215–218. https://doi:10.1016/j.outlook.2021.12.012

Yale School of Public Health. (2019). *NGOs and nonprofits*. https://publichealth.yale.edu/career/toolkit/resources/ngos/

Yeager, V. A., Wharton, M. K., & Beitsch, L. M. (2020). Maintaining a competent public health workforce: Lessons learned from experiences with public health accreditation domain 8 standards and measures. *Journal of Public Health Management and Practice*, *26*(1), 57–66. https://doi:10.1097/PHH.0000000000000750

Zewde, N., & Wimer, C. (2019). Antipoverty impact of Medicaid growing with state expansions over time. *Health Affairs*, *38*, 132–138. https://doi:10.1377/hlthaff.2018.05155

Zhang, A., Prang, K. H., Devlin, N., Scott, A., & Kelaher, M. (2020). The impact of price transparency on consumers and providers: A scoping review. *Health Policy*, *124*, 819–825. https://doi:10.1016/j.healthpol.2020.06.001

Zhang, P., & Zhu, L. (2021). Does the ACA Medicaid expansion affect hospitals' financial performance? *Public Finance Review*, *49*, 779–814. https://doi:10.1177/10911421211064676

CHAPTER 7

Abubakar, I., Stagg, H. R., Cohen, T., & Rodrigues, L. C. (Eds.) (2016). *Infectious disease epidemiology*. Oxford University Press.

Administration for Strategic Preparedness & Response (ASPR). (2022, April 4). *Renewal of determination that a public health emergency exists*. https://aspr.hhs.gov/legal/PHE/Pages/Opioid-4Apr22.aspx

Agency for Toxic Substances and Disease Registry (ATSDR). (2019, February 20). *Exposure and health registries*. https://www.atsdr.cdc.gov/publications_health_registries.html

Aiyer, S. M., Zimmerman, M. A., Morrel-Samuels, S., & Reischl, T. M. (2015). from broken windows to busy streets: A community empowerment perspective. *Health Education & Behavior*, *42*(2), 137–147.

American Academy of Pediatrics. (2021). *Red book®*.

American Diabetes Association. (2023). *Genetics of diabetes*. https://diabetes.org/diabetes/genetics-diabetes

Bain, L. E., & Awah, P. K. (2014). Eco-epidemiology: Challenges and opportunities for tomorrow's epidemiologists. *The Pan African Medical Journal*, *17*, 317. https://doi.org/10.11604/pamj.2014.17.317.4080

Bryant, J. H., & Rhodes, P. (2023, May 11). *Public health: Beginnings in antiquity*. https://www.britannica.com/topic/public-health#ref412417

Butelman, E. R., Huang, Y., Epstein, D. H., Shaham, Y., Goldstein, R. Z., Volkow, N. D., & Alia-Klein, N. (2023, June 15). *Overdose mortality rates for opioids and stimulant drugs are substantially higher in men than in women: State-level analysis. Neuropsychopharmacology*, *48*, 1639–1647. https://doi.org/10.1038/s41386-023-01601-8. https://www.nature.com/articles/s41386-023-01601-8

Celentano, D. D., & Szklo, M. (2019). *Gordis epidemiology* (6th ed.). Saunders/Elsevier.Fret.

Centers for Disease Control and Prevention (CDC). (1999). Adult lead poisoning from an Asian remedy for menstrual cramps—Connecticut, 1997. *Morbidity and Mortality Weekly Report*, *48*(20), 27–29. https://www.cdc.gov/mmwr/preview/mmwrhtml/00056277.htm

Centers for Disease Control and Prevention (CDC). (2006). *Principles of epidemiology in public health practice: An introduction to applied epidemiology and biostatistics* (3rd ed.). https://stacks.cdc.gov/view/cdc/6914/cdc_6914_DS1.pdf

Centers for Disease Control and Prevention (CDC). (2019a, April 10). *Frequently asked questions about the Laboratory Response Network (LRN)*. https://emergency.cdc.gov/lrn/faq.asp

Centers for Disease Control and Prevention (CDC). (2021a, August 6). *Plague: History*. https://www.cdc.gov/plague/index.html

Centers for Disease Control and Prevention (CDC) (2022a, June 10). Characteristics of adults aged ≥18 years evaluated for substance use and treatment planning—United States, 2019. *Morbidity and Mortality Weekly Report (MMWR)*, *71*(23), 749–756. https://www.cdc.gov/mmwr/volumes/71/wr/mm7123a1.htm

Centers for Disease Control and Prevention (CDC). (2022b, April 14). *U.S. Zika pregnancy & infant registry*. https://www.cdc.gov/pregnancy/zika/research/registry.html

Centers for Disease Control and Prevention (CDC). (2023a, April 20). *CDC's disease detectives give first-hand accounts from the front lines of public health*. https://www.cdc.gov/media/releases/2023/p0419-eis.html

Centers for Disease Control and Prevention (CDC). (2023b, March 6). *10 essential public health services*. https://www.cdc.gov/publichealthgateway/publichealthservices/essentialhealthservices.html

Centers for Disease Control and Prevention (CDC). (2023c, April 28). *Current avian influenza (bird flu) situation in humans in the United States*. https://www.cdc.gov/flu/avianflu/inhumans.htm

Centers for Disease Control and Prevention (CDC). (2023d, June 13). *West Nile virus*. https://www.cdc.gov/westnile/index.html

Centers for Disease Control and Prevention (CDC). (2023e, March 10). *National wastewater surveillance system*. https://www.cdc.gov/nwss/index.html

Centers for Disease Control and Prevention (CDC). (2023f, March 28). *Pregnancy risk assessment monitoring system (PRAMS)*. https://www.cdc.gov/prams/index.htm

Centers for Disease Control and Prevention (CDC). (2023g, February 8). *Traveler-based genomic surveillance for early detection of new SARS-CoV-2 variants. (TGS)*. https://wwwnc.cdc.gov/travel/page/travel-genomic-surveillance

Centers for Disease Control and Prevention (CDC). (n.d.). *Principles of epidemiology in public health practice* (3rd ed.). https://stacks.cdc.gov/view/cdc/6914/cdc_6914_DS1.pdf

Centers for Disease Control and Prevention (CDC)/National Center for Health Statistics (NCHS). (2022, December). *Drug overdose deaths in the United States, 2001–2021*. NCHS Data Brief No. 457. https://www.cdc.gov/nchs/products/databriefs/db457.htm

Ciccarone, D. (2021, July). The rise of illicit fentanyls, stimulants and the fourth wave of the opioid overdose crisis. *Current Opinion in Psychiatry, 34*(4), 344–350. https://journals.lww.com/co-psychiatry/Fulltext/2021/07000/The_rise_of_illicit_fentanyls,_stimulants_and_the.4.aspx

Clayton, A. (2023, June 15). *California seizes enough fentanyl in San Francisco to kill city's population three times over. The Guardian.* https://www.theguardian.com/us-news/2023/jun/15/california-fentanyl-overdose-newsom-supervised-drug-use-san-francisco

Community Preventive Services Task Force (CPSTF). (2023, May 31). *About the community guide.* https://www.thecommunityguide.org/pages/about-community-guide.html

Dutta, S. S. (2023, June 28). Public health concerns as highly pathogenic avian influenza A (H5N1) virus found in cat in France. *Medical & Life Sciences News.* https://www.news-medical.net/news/20230628/Public-health-concerns-as-highly-pathogenic-avian-influenza-A(H5N1)-virus-found-in-cat-in-France.aspx

Egger, G. (2012). *In search of a germ theory equivalent for chronic disease.* https://www.cdc.gov/pcd/issues/2012/11_0301.htm

Environmental Protection Agency. (2022, September 12). *Air pollution and cardiovascular disease basics.* https://www.epa.gov/air-research/air-pollution-and-cardiovascular-disease-basics

Facher, L. (2023, June 21). *Xylazine, or 'tranq,' is making opioid overdoses harder to reverse.* STAT. https://www.statnews.com/2023/06/21/xylazine-tranq-opioid-overdose-naloxone/

Frieden, J. (2023, July 11). *White House drug czar releases plan to combat xylazine-laced fentanyl. Medpage Today.* https://www.medpagetoday.com/publichealthpolicy/washington-watch/105414

Friis, R. H. (2018). *Epidemiology 101* (2nd ed.). Jones and Bartlett Learning.

Friis, R. H., & Sellers, T. (2021). *Epidemiology for public health practice* (6th ed.). Hones and Bartlett.

Hackett, K. M. (2023, July 1). *20 cats confirmed with bird flu in Poland.* https://www.precisionvaccinations.com/2023/07/01/20-cats-confirmed-bird-flu-poland

Haley, D. F., Wingood, G. M., Kramer, M. R., Haardoirfer, R., Adimora, A. A., Rubtsova, A., Edmonds, A., Goswamy, N. D., Ludema, C., Hichson, D. A., Ramirez, C., Ross, Z., Bolivar, H., & Cooper, H. L. F. (2018). Associations between neighborhood characteristics, social cohesion, and perceived sex partner risk and non-monogamy among HIV-seropositive and HIV-seronegative women in the southern U.S. *Archives of Sexual Behavior, 47*(5), 1451–1463.

Harvard Health Publishing (HHP). (2018). *How to boost your immune system.* https://www.health.harvard.edu/staying-healthy/how-to-boost-your-immune-system

Harvard Medical School & Brigham and Women's Hospital. (n.d.). *Women's health study.* http://whs.bwh.harvard.edu

Heymann, D. L. (Ed.). (2022). *Control of communicable diseases manual* (21st ed.). American Public Health Association.

History of Vaccines. (2022). *The human immune system and infectious disease.* https://historyofvaccines.org/vaccines-101/what-do-vaccines-do/human-immune-system-and-infectious-disease

HIV.gov. (2022). *Global statistics: The global HIV/AIDS epidemic.* https://www.hiv.gov/hiv-basics/overview/data-and-trends/global-statistics/

Jung, B. C. (2023a). *COVID-19 Internet resources.* https://www.bettycjung.net/COVID-19.htm

Jung, B. C. (2023b). *Koo Sar pills epidemiological investigation.* https://www.bettycjung.net/Koosarnet.htm

Kacha-Ochana, A., Jones, C. M., Green, J. L., Dunphy, C., Govoni, T. D., Robbins, R. S., & Guy Jr., G. P. (2022). Characteristics of adults aged ≥18 years evaluated for substance use and treatment planning—United States, 2019. *Morbidity and Mortality Weekly Report, 71*(23), 749–756. https://www.cdc.gov/mmwr/volumes/71/wr/mm7123a1.htm

Karlawish, J. (2020, May 17). *A pandemic plan was in place. Trump abandoned it—and science—in the face of Covid-19.* STAT. https://www.statnews.com/2020/05/17/the-art-of-the-pandemic-how-donald-trump-walked-the-u-s-into-the-covid-19-era/

King, L. S. (1952). Dr. Koch's postulates. *Journal of Historical Medicine,* 350–361. As cited in Friis, R. H., & Sellers, T. A. (2021). *Epidemiology for public health practice* (6th ed.). Jones and Bartlett Learning.

LaMorte, W. W. (2021, October 19). *PH717-module 3–Measuring frequency and association.* https://sphweb.bumc.bu.edu/otlt/MPH-Modules/PH717-QuantCore/PH717-Module3-Frequency-Association/PH717-Module3-Frequency-Association2.html

Madigan Library at Penn College. (2023, July 3). *Epidemiology: Experimental studies.* https://pct.libguides.com/epidemiology/clinical-research/experimental-studies

Marks, H. (2022). *What is holistic medicine?* https://www.webmd.com/balance/guide/what-is-holistic-medicine#1

McGlone, P. (2023, July 6). *These animal interactions are risks for future pandemics.* Futurity. https://www.futurity.org/zoonotic-disease-future-pandemics-2940062-2/

MedlinePlus. (2021). *Reportable diseases.* https://medlineplus.gov/ency/article/001929.htm

Merrill, R. M. (2021). *Introduction to epidemiology* (8th ed.). Jones & Bartlett Learning.

National Cancer Institute (NCI). (2020). *BRCA1 and BRCA2: Cancer risk and genetic testing.* https://www.cancer.gov/about-cancer/causes-prevention/genetics/brca-fact-sheet

National Cancer Institute (NCI). (n.d.). *About the SEER registries.* https://seer.cancer.gov/registries/index.html

National Center for Health Statistics (NCHS). (2023a, August 9). *National health interview survey. About NHIS.* https://www.cdc.gov/nchs/nhis/index.htm

National Center for Health Statistics (NCHS). (2023b). *National center for health statistics.* https://www.cdc.gov/nchs/

National Institute on Drug Abuse (NIDA). (2022, May 12). *What is fentanyl?* https://nida.nih.gov/research-topics/trends-statistics/infographics/what-fentanyl

National Institute on Drug Abuse (NIDA). (2023, June 30). *Drug overdose death rates.* https://nida.nih.gov/research-topics/trends-statistics/overdose-death-rates

National Institutes of Health (NIH). (2023, June 14). *Men died of overdose at 2-3 times greater a rate than women in the U.S. in 2020–2021.* News Releases. https://www.nih.gov/news-events/news-releases/men-died-overdose-2-3-times-greater-rate-women-us-2020-2021

Nickson, C. (2020, November 3). *Retrospective studies and chart reviews.* https://litfl.com/retrospective-studies-and-chart-reviews/

Nurses' Health Study (NHS). (2021). *Selected publications.* http://www.nurseshealthstudy.org/selected-publications

Perez, L. G., Conway, T. L., Bauman, A., Kerr, J., Elder, J., Arredondo, E. M., & Sallis, J. (2018). Sociodemographic moderators of environment-physical activity associations: Results from the International Prevalence Study. *Journal of Physical Activity and Health, 15*(1), 22–29.

Poison Control. (2023). *Unusual sources of lead poisoning.* https://www.poison.org/articles/2011-dec/unusual-sources-of-lead-poisoning

Resnick, B. (2020, May 5). *Covid-19 is way, way worse than the flu.* Vox. https://www.vox.com/science-and-health/2020/5/5/21246567/coronavirus-flu-comparisons-fatality-rate-contagiousness

Seabert, D. M., McKenzie, J. F., & Pinger, R. (2021). *McKenzie's an introduction to community & public health* (10th ed.). Jones & Bartlett Learning.

Smith, D., & Moore, L. (2020). *The SIR model for the spread of disease: The differential equation model.* Mathematical Association of America. https://www.maa.org/press/periodicals/loci/joma/the-sir-model-for-spread-of-disease-the-differential-equation-model

Straub, R. H., & Schradin, C. (2016). Chronic inflammatory systemic diseases: An evolutionary trade-off between acutely beneficial but chronically harmful programs. *Evolution, Medicine, & Public Health, 1*(1), 37–51.

Substance Abuse and Mental Health Services Administration (SAMHSA). (2023, June). *Drug abuse warning network: Findings from drug-related emergency department visits, 2022.* https://store.samhsa.gov/product/drug-abuse-warning-network-findings-drug-related-emergency-department-visits-2022/pep23-07-03-001

Suryawanshi, R., & Ott, M. (2022, August 9). SARS-CoV-2 hybrid immunity: Silver bullet or silver lining? *Nature Reviews Immunology, 22,* 591–592. https://www.nature.com/articles/s41577-022-00771-8

Susser, M., & Stein, Z. (2009). *Eras in epidemiology: The evolution of ideas.* Oxford University Press.

Susser, M., & Susser, E. (1996a). Choosing a future for epidemiology: I. Eras and paradigms. *American Journal of Public Health, 86*(5), 668–673.

Susser, M., & Susser, E. (1996b). Choosing a future for epidemiology: II. From black box to Chinese boxes and eco-epidemiology. *American Journal of Public Health, 86*(5), 674–677.

Szklo, M., & Nieto, J. (2019). *Epidemiology: Beyond the basics* (4th ed.). Bartlett & Jones Learning.

The National Archives. (n.d.). *Florence Nightingale. Why do we remember her?* https://www.nationalarchives.gov.uk/education/resources/florence-nightingale/

Tulchinsky, T. H. (2018). *John snow, cholera, the broad street pump; waterborne diseases then and now* (pp. 77–99). Case Studies in Public Health. http://doi.org/10.1016/B978-0-12-804571-8.00017-2

U.S. Department of Health and Human Services (USDHHS). (2022, December 16). *Opioid facts and statistics.* https://www.hhs.gov/opioids/statistics/index.html

U.S. Department of Health and Human Services (USDHHS). (2023a). *Healthy People 2030—Framework.* https://health.gov/healthypeople/about/healthy-people-2030-framework

U.S. Department of Health and Human Services (USDHHS). (2023b). *Healthy People 2030—Community.* https://health.gov/healthypeople/objectives-and-data/browse-objectives/community

U.S. Department of Health and Human Services (USDHHS). (2023c). *Healthy People 2030—Public health infrastructure.* https://health.gov/healthypeople/objectives-and-data/browse-objectives/public-health-infrastructure

U.S. Department of Justice/Drug Enforcement Administration. (2022). *The growing threat of xylazine and its mixture with illicit drugs.* https://www.dea.gov/sites/default/files/2022-12/The%20Growing%20Threat%20of%20Xylazine%20and%20its%20Mixture%20with%20Illicit%20Drugs.pdf

U.S. Drug Enforcement Administration (USDEA). (n.d.). *DEA reports widespread threat of fentanyl mixed with xylazine.* https://www.dea.gov/alert/dea-reports-widespread-threat-fentanyl-mixed-xylazine

U.S. Environmental Protection Agency (USEPA). (2023). *Federal agencies and organizations addressing environmental asthma.* https://www.epa.gov/asthma/federal-agencies-and-organizations-addressing-environmental-asthma

U.S. Food and Drug Administration (USFDA). (2022). *FDA alerts health care professionals of risks to patients exposed to xylazine in illicit drugs.* https://www.fda.gov/drugs/drug-safety-and-availability/fda-alerts-health-care-professionals-risks-patients-exposed-xylazine-illicit-drugs

U.S. Government Accountability Office (USGAO). (2018, October 23). *Opioid crisis: Status of public health emergency authorities.* https://www.gao.gov/products/gao-18-685r

White House. (2023, July). *Fentanyl adulterated with or associated with xylazine response plan.* https://www.whitehouse.gov/wp-content/uploads/2023/07/FENTANYL-ADULTERATED-OR-ASSOCIATED-WITH-XYLAZINE-EMERGING-THREAT-RESPONSE-PLAN-Report-July-2023.pdf

Wiley Online Library. (2023). *Cochrane database of systematic reviews.* https://www.cochranelibrary.com/cdsr/about-cdsr

Wilkin, J. A., Sondermeyer, G., Shusterman, D., McNary, J., Vugia, D., McDowell, A., Borenstein, P., Gilliss, D., Ancock, B., Prudhomme, J., Gold, D., Windham, G. C., Lee, L., & Materna, B. L. (2015). Coccidioidomycosis among workers constructing solar power farms, California, USA, 2011–2014. *Emerging Infectious Diseases, 21*(11), 1997–2005. https://doi.org/10.3201/eid2111.150129. https://pubmed.ncbi.nlm.nih.gov/26484688/

Wilson, C. (2023, June 28). *Bird flu viruses have mutations that might help with them spread to humans.* New Scientist. https://www.newscientist.com/article/2380281-bird-flu-viruses-have-mutations-that-might-help-them-spread-to-humans/

Wodi, A. P., & Morelli, V. (2021). *Chapter 1: Principles of vaccination.* https://www.cdc.gov/vaccines/pubs/pinkbook/prinvac.html

World Health Organization (WHO). (2020, December 9). *WHO reveals leading causes of death and disability worldwide: 2000–2019.* https://www.who.int/news/item/09-12-2020-who-reveals-leading-causes-of-death-and-disability-worldwide-2000-2019

Xiang, L., & Diamond, S. (2022, January/February). *Developing and using computer models to understand epidemics.* https://www.nsta.org/science-teacher/science-teacher-januaryfebruary-2022/developing-and-using-computer-models

Yates, C. (2020, April 1). *How to model a pandemic.* EarthSky. https://earthsky.org/human-world/how-to-model-a-pandemic

Zhao, X., Wang, Y., & Liang, C. (2022). *Cigarette smoking and risk of bladder cancer: A dose-response meta-analysis.* https://pubmed.ncbi.nlm.nih.gov/35332429/

CHAPTER 8

Ahasan, R., Alam, M. S., Chakraborty, T., & Hossain, M. M. (2022). Applications of GIS and geospatial analyses in

COVID-19 research: A systematic review. *F1000Research*, *9*, 1379. https://doi.org/10.12688/f1000research.27544.2

Anderson, E., Daugherty, M., Pickering, L., Orenstein, W. A., & Yogev, R. (2018). Protecting the community through child vaccination. *Clinical Infectious Diseases*, *67*(3), 464–471. https://doi.org/10.1093/cid/ciy142

Baines, A., Ittefaq, M., & Abwao, M. (2021). #Scamdemic, #plandemic, or #scaredemic: What parler social media platform tells us about COVID-19 vaccine. *Vaccines*, *9*(5), 421. http://doi.org/10.3390/vaccines9050421

Bloom, D. E., & Cadarette, D. (2019). Infectious disease threats in the twenty-first century: Strengthening the global response. *Frontiers in Immunology*, *10*, 549. https://doi.org/10.3389/fimmu.2019.00549

Boyce, M. R., Katz, R., & Standley, C. J. (2019). Risk factors for infectious diseases in urban environments of Sub-Saharan Africa: A systematic review and critical appraisal of evidence. *Tropical Medicine and Infectious Disease*, *4*(4), 123.

Brock, E. (2022). 2001 Anthrax attacks revealed the need to develop countermeasures against biological threats. *National Institutes of Health Record (NIH Record)*, *LXXIV*(10), 8. https://nihrecord.nih.gov/2022/05/13/2001-anthrax-attacks-revealed-need-develop--19 countermeasures-against-biological-threats

Brownson, R., Burke, T., Colditz, G., & Samet, J. M. (2020). Reimagining public health in the aftermath of a pandemic. *American Journal of Public Health*, *110*, 1605–1610. https://doi.org/10.2105/AJPH.2020.305861

Califf, R. M. (2023). *Preparing for and responding to future public health risks*. https://www.fda.gov/news-events/congressional-testimony/preparing-and-responding-future-public-health-risks-05112023

California Department of Public Health (CDPH). (2020). *Health officer resources*. https://www.cdph.ca.gov/Programs/CCLHO/Pages/HealthOfficerResources.aspx

Cason, D., & Williams, P. (2021). Vaccinating the unvaccinated adult. *Cleveland Clinic Journal of Medicine*, *88*(5), 279–285. https://doi.org/https://doi.org/10.3949/ccjm.88a.20046

Carrico, R. M., Garrett, H., Balcom, D., & Glowicz, J. B. (2018). Infection prevention and control core practices: A roadmap for nursing practice. *Nursing*, *48*(8), 28–29. https://doi.org/10.1097/01.NURSE.0000544318.36012.b2

Coccia, M. (2021). Pandemic prevention: Lessons from COVID-19. *Encyclopedia*, *1*(2), 433–444. https://doi.org/10.3390/encyclopedia1020036

Centers for Disease Control and Prevention (CDC). (2019a, November 19). *HIV risk factors*. https://www.cdc.gov/hiv/risk/estimates/riskbehaviors.html

Centers for Disease Control and Prevention (CDC). (2019b, August 2). *Middle East respiratory syndrome (MERS): About MERS*. https://www.cdc.gov/coronavirus/mers/about/index.html

Centers for Disease Control and Prevention (CDC). (2020a, August 1). *About the division of vector-borne diseases*. https://www.cdc.gov/ncezid/dvbd/index.html

Centers for Disease Control and Prevention (CDC). (2020b, May 13). *Advisory Committee on Immunization Practices (ACIP)*. https://www.cdc.gov/vaccines/acip/index.html

Centers for Disease Control and Prevention (CDC). (2020c, November 12). *Emergency preparedness and response: Bioterrorism*. https://emergency.cdc.gov/bioterrorism/

Centers for Disease Control and Prevention (CDC). (2020d, July 14). *Foodborne germs and illnesses*. https://www.cdc.gov/foodsafety/foodborne-germs.html

Centers for Disease Control and Prevention (CDC). (2020e, April 11). *Global health: CDC and the global health security agenda*. https://www.cdc.gov/globalhealth/security/index.htm

Centers for Disease Control and Prevention (CDC). (2020f, January 9). *Health communication basics*. https://www.cdc.gov/healthcommunication/healthbasics/WhatIsHC.html

Centers for Disease Control and Prevention (CDC). (2020g, July 28). *Hepatitis A questions and answers for health professionals*. https://www.cdc.gov/hepatitis/hav/havfaq.htm#A2

Centers for Disease Control and Prevention (CDC). (2020h, August 7). *Hepatitis B: For health professionals*. https://www.cdc.gov/hepatitis/hbv/index.htm

Centers for Disease Control and Prevention (CDC). (2020i, August 7). *Hepatitis C information: Hepatitis C questions and answers for health professionals*. https://www.cdc.gov/hepatitis/hcv/hcvfaq.htm#accordion-1-collapse-4

Centers for Disease Control and Prevention (CDC). (2020j, March 18). *Nationally notifiable infectious conditions, United States 2020*. http://www.cdc.gov/nndss/conditions/notifiable/2020/

Centers for Disease Control and Prevention (CDC). (2020k, July 20). *Quarantine and isolation: History of quarantine*. https://www.cdc.gov/quarantine/historyquarantine.html#:~:text=The%20practice%20of%20quarantine%2C%20as,for%2040%20days%20before%20landing

Centers for Disease Control and Prevention (CDC). (2020l, December 11). *Tuberculosis (TB): Latent TB infection and TB disease*. https://www.cdc.gov/tb/topic/basics/tbinfectiondisease.html

Centers for Disease Control and Prevention (CDC). (2020m, November 2). *Tuberculosis (TB): Tuberculin skin testing fact sheet*. https://www.cdc.gov/tb/publications/factsheets/testing/skintesting.htm

Centers for Disease Control and Prevention (CDC). (2021a, April 8). *CDC global health strategy*. https://www.cdc.gov/globalhealth/strategy/

Centers for Disease Control and Prevention (CDC). (2021b, June 1). *HIV: HIV prevention*. https://www.cdc.gov/hiv/basics/prevention.html

Centers for Disease Control and Prevention (CDC). (2021c, September 24). *Immunity types*. https://www.cdc.gov/vaccines/vac-gen/immunity-types.htm

Centers for Disease Control and Prevention (CDC). (2021d, April 6). *Plague*. https://www.cdc.gov/plague/index.html

Centers for Disease Control and Prevention (CDC). (2021e, July 22). *Sexually transmitted diseases (STDs): Herpes*. https://www.cdc.gov/std/herpes/stdfact-herpes-detailed.htm

Centers for Disease Control and Prevention (CDC). (2021f, July 22). *Sexually transmitted diseases (STDs): Human papillomavirus (HPV) infection*. https://www.cdc.gov/std/treatment-guidelines/hpv.htm

Centers for Disease Control and Prevention (CDC). (2021g, August 4). *Sexually transmitted diseases (STDs): State statutory and regulatory language regarding prenatal syphilis screenings in the United States*. https://www.cdc.gov/std/treatment/syphilis-screenings.htm?CDC_AA_refVal=https%3A%2F%2Fwwwdev.cdc.gov%2Fstd%2Ftreatment%2Fsyphilis-screenings-2018.htm

Centers for Disease Control and Prevention (CDC). (2021h, July 22). *Sexually transmitted infections treatment guidelines, 2021: Expedited partner therapy*. https://www.cdc.gov/std/treatment-guidelines/clinical-EPT.htm

Centers for Disease Control and Prevention (CDC). (2021i, October 18) *Smallpox: Research*. https://www.cdc.gov/smallpox/research/index.html

Centers for Disease Control and Prevention (CDC). (2021j, February 16). *Vaccines & immunizations*. https://www.cdc.gov/vaccines/index.html

Centers for Disease Control and Prevention (CDC). (2022a, September 20). *About flu*. https://www.cdc.gov/flu/about/index.html

Centers for Disease Control and Prevention (CDC). (2022c, September 20). *Campaign approach to reaching Latino audiences*. https://wecandothis.hhs.gov/resource/campaign-approach-to-reaching-latino-audiences

Centers for Disease Control and Prevention (CDC). (2022d, October 26). *COVID-19: Symptoms of COVID-19*. https://www.cdc.gov/coronavirus/2019-ncov/symptoms-testing/symptoms.html

Centers for Disease Control and Prevention (CDC). (2022e, July 12). *HIV basics: What is PEP?* https://www.cdc.gov/hiv/basics/pep/about-pep.html

Centers for Disease Control and Prevention (CDC). (2022f, September 15). *Diseases you almost forgot about (thanks to vaccines)*. https://www.cdc.gov/vaccines/parents/diseases/forgot-14-diseases.html

Centers for Disease Control and Prevention (CDC). (2022g, June 1). *Division of vector-borne diseases. Prevent mosquito bites*. https://www.cdc.gov/ncezid/dvbd/media/stop-mosquitoes.html

Centers for Disease Control and Prevention (CDC). (2022h, October 13). *Drug-resistant TB*. https://www.cdc.gov/tb/topic/drtb/default.htm

Centers for Disease Control and Prevention (CDC). (2022i, October 21). *Foodborne outbreaks: Investigating outbreaks*. https://www.cdc.gov/foodsafety/outbreaks/investigating-outbreaks/index.html

Centers for Disease Control and Prevention (CDC). (2022j, December 28). *Gonorrhea: Antimicrobial-resistant gonorrhea basic information*. https://www.cdc.gov/std/gonorrhea/drug-resistant/basic.htm

Centers for Disease Control and Prevention (CDC). (2022k, September 21) *Gonococcal infections*. https://www.cdc.gov/std/treatment-guidelines/gonorrhea-adults.htm

Centers for Disease Control and Prevention (CDC). (2022l, August 25). *Influenza: Flu & people 65 years and older*. https://www.cdc.gov/flu/highrisk/65over.htm

Centers for Disease Control and Prevention (CDC). (2022m, August 5). *Influenza (flu): Live attenuated influenza vaccine [laiv] (the nasal spray flu vaccine)*. https://www.cdc.gov/flu/prevent/nasalspray.htm

Centers for Disease Control and Prevention (CDC). (2022n, July 27). *National Notifiable Diseases Surveillance System: What is case surveillance?* https://www.cdc.gov/nndss/about/conduct.html

Centers for Disease Control and Prevention (CDC). (2022o, August 15). *PulseNet: Whole genome sequencing*. https://www.cdc.gov/pulsenet/pathogens/wgs.html

Centers for Disease Control and Prevention (CDC). (2022p, August 8). *Smallpox: Prevention and treatment*. https://www.cdc.gov/smallpox/prevention-treatment/index.html

Centers for Disease Control and Prevention (CDC). (2022q, October 13). *Tuberculosis: Drug resistant TB*. https://www.cdc.gov/tb/topic/drtb/default.htm#:~:text=Drug%2Dresistant%20TB%20is%20caused,)%20and%20rifampin%20(RIF).

Centers for Disease Control and Prevention (CDC). (2022r, November 29). *Tuberculosis (TB): Reported Tuberculosis in the United States, 2021*. https://www.cdc.gov/tb/statistics/reports/2021/risk_factors.htm

Centers for Disease Control and Prevention (CDC). (2023a, July 10). *About COVID-19*. https://www.cdc.gov/coronavirus/2019-ncov/your-health/about-covid-19.html

Centers for Disease Control and Prevention (CDC). (2023b, May 11). *About COVID-19: Understanding your risk: People with certain medical conditions*. https://www.cdc.gov/coronavirus/2019-ncov/need-extra-precautions/people-with-medical-conditions.html

Centers for Disease Control and Prevention (CDC). (2023c, March 15). *CDC museum COVID-19 timeline*. https://www.cdc.gov/museum/timeline/covid19.html

Centers for Disease Control and Prevention (CDC). (2023d, April 11). *Chlamydia*. https://www.cdc.gov/std/chlamydia/stdfact-chlamydia-detailed.htm

Centers for Disease Control and Prevention (CDC). (2023e, March 2). *Childhood immunization resources*. https://www.cdc.gov/vaccines/partners/childhood/stayingontrack.html

Centers for Disease Control and Prevention (CDC). (2023f, August 7). *Common questions about vaccines*. https://www.cdc.gov/vaccines/parents/FAQs.html

Centers for Disease Control and Prevention (CDC). (2023g, March 23). *Ebola disease*. https://www.cdc.gov/vhf/ebola/index.html

Centers for Disease Control and Prevention (CDC). (2023h, April 20). *Fast facts on global immunization*. https://www.cdc.gov/globalhealth/immunization/data/fast-facts.html#:~:text=4%20million%20deaths%20worldwide%20are,immunization%20between%202021%20and%202030

Centers for Disease Control and Prevention (CDC). (2023i, August 22). *FoodCORE: Foodborne diseases*. https://www.cdc.gov/foodcore/index.html

Centers for Disease Control and Prevention (CDC). (2023j, March 14). *Foodborne diseases centers for outbreak response enhancement: Colorado stops a multistate salmonella outbreak linked to seafood*. https://www.cdc.gov/foodcore/successes/colorado-stops-outbreak.html

Centers for Disease Control and Prevention (CDC). (2023k, May 3). *Gateway to health communication*. https://www.cdc.gov/healthcommunication/index.html

Centers for Disease Control and Prevention (CDC). (2023l, April 11). *Gonorrhea*. https://www.cdc.gov/std/gonorrhea/default.htm

Centers for Disease Control and Prevention (CDC). (2023m, March 9). *Hepatitis B*. https://www.cdc.gov/hepatitis/hbv/index.htm

Centers for Disease Control and Prevention (CDC). (2023n, August 8). *High-impact prevention (HIP: A promising hip intervention-electronic directly observed therapy for active TB disease)*. https://www.cdc.gov/nchhstp/highimpactprevention/promising-hip-intervention.html

Centers for Disease Control and Prevention (CDC). (2023o, March 21). *HIV: HIV pre-exposure prophylaxis (PrEP) care system*. https://www.cdc.gov/hiv/effective-interventions/prevent/prep/

Centers for Disease Control and Prevention (CDC). (2023p, February 10). *HPV infection*. https://www.cdc.gov/hpv/parents/about-hpv.html

Centers for Disease Control and Prevention (CDC). (2023q, February 10). *Immunization schedules.* https://www.cdc.gov/vaccines/schedules/

Centers for Disease Control and Prevention (CDC). (2023r, August 9). *Influenza (Flu): Interim guidance for the use of masks to control seasonal influenza virus transmission.* https://www.cdc.gov/flu/professionals/infectioncontrol/maskguidance.htm

Centers for Disease Control and Prevention (CDC). (2023s, April 29). *Mission, role, and pledge.* http://www.cdc.gov/about/organization/mission.htm

Centers for Disease Control and Prevention (CDC). (2023t, August 8). *Mpox.* https://www.cdc.gov/poxvirus/mpox/clinicians/index.html

Centers for Disease Control and Prevention (CDC). (2023u, March 27). *National Notifiable Diseases Surveillance System (NNDSS).* https://www.cdc.gov/nndss/about/index.html

Centers for Disease Control and Prevention (CDC). (2023v, April 18). *PulseNet.* https://www.cdc.gov/pulsenet/index.html

Centers for Disease Control and Prevention (CDC). (2023w, April 11). *Sexually transmitted disease surveillance 2021.* https://www.cdc.gov/std/statistics/2021/figures.htm

Centers for Disease Control and Prevention (CDC). (2023x, April 11). *Sexually transmitted diseases (STDs): Syphilis.* https://www.cdc.gov/std/syphilis/default.htm

Centers for Disease Control and Prevention (CDC). (2023y, April 11). *STDs & infertility.* https://www.cdc.gov/std/infertility/default.htm#:~:text=STDs%20%26%20Infertility,-STDs%20%26%20Infertility&text=Chlamydia%20and%20gonorrhea%20are%20important,tube%20infection%20without%20any%20symptoms

Centers for Disease Control and Prevention (CDC). (2023z, May 12). *Traveler advice.* https://wwwnc.cdc.gov/travel/page/traveler-information-center

Centers for Disease Control and Prevention (CDC). (2023aa, March 30). *Types of influenza viruses.* https://www.cdc.gov/flu/about/viruses/types.htm

Centers for Disease Control and Prevention (CDC). (2023bb, March 22). *Tuberculosis (TB).* https://www.cdc.gov/tb/

Centers for Disease Control and Prevention (CDC). (2023cc, March 22). *Tuberculosis (TB): Supplemental information for video directly observed therapy (vDOT).* https://www.cdc.gov/tb/topic/treatment/vDOT.htm#:~:text=vDOT%20is%20reported%20under%20electronic,patients%20and%20health%20care%20workers

Centers for Disease Control and Prevention (CDC). (2023dd, January 20). *Vaccines and preventable diseases: Pneumococcal vaccination: What everyone should know.* https://www.cdc.gov/vaccines/vpd/pneumo/public/index.html

Centers for Disease Control and Prevention (CDC). (2023ee, July 5). *Vaccine recommendations and guidelines of the ACIP: COVID-19 ACIP vaccine recommendations.* https://www.cdc.gov/vaccines/hcp/acip-recs/vacc-specific/covid-19.html

Centers for Disease Control and Prevention (CDC). (2023ff, May 1). *Yellow book.* https://wwwnc.cdc.gov/travel/yellowbook/2018/introduction/introduction-to-travel-health-the-yellow-book#4924

Chan, J., Gidding, H., Blyth, C., Fathima, P., Jayasinghe, S., McIntyre, P. B., Moore, H. C., Mulholland, K., Nguyen, C. D., Andrews, R., & Russell, F. M. (2021). Levels of pneumococcal conjugate vaccine coverage and indirect protection against invasive pneumococcal disease and pneumonia hospitalisations in Australia: An observational study. *PLOS Medicine, 18*(8), e1003733. https://doi.org/10.1371/journal.pmed.1003733

County of Los Angeles Department of Public Health. (n.d.). *Communicable disease reporting system.* http://publichealth.lacounty.gov/acd/procs/ReportPage.htm

Dadonaite, B., & Roser, M. (2019). *Pneumonia. Our world in data.* https://ourworldindata.org/pneumonia#citation

Decker, M. D., & Edwards, K. M. (2021). Pertussis (whooping cough). *The Journal of Infectious Diseases, 224*(12 Suppl 2), S310–S320. https://doi.org/10.1093/infdis/jiaa469

Desai, A., & Majumder, M. (2020). What is herd immunity? *JAMA, 324*(20), 2113. https://doi.org/10.1001/jama.2020.20895

Di Mattia, G., Nicolai, A., Frassanito, A., Petrarca, L., Nenna, R., & Midulla, F. (2018). Pertussis: New preventive strategies for an old disease. *Paediatric Respiratory Reviews, 29*, 68–73. https://www.clinicalkey.com/#!/content/playContent/2-s2.0-29914744?returnurl=null&referrer=null

Dominquez, B. C., Hernandez, A., Fernandez-Pacheco, A., Taylor, L., Kahar, P., & Khanna, D. (2022). A survey of public health failures during COVID-19. *Cureus, 14*(12), e32437. https://doi.org/10.7759/cureus.32437

Donovan, D. (2023). *Johns Hopkins COVID-19 data hub ends after three years.* https://hub.jhu.edu/2023/03/10/coronavirus-resource-center-data-hub-ends/

Emrick, P., Gentry, C., & Morowit, L. (2016). Ebola virus disease: International perspective on enhanced health surveillance, disposition of the dead, and their effect on isolation and quarantine practices. *Disaster and Military Medicine, 2*, 13. https://doi.org/10.1186/s40696-016-0023-6

Fauci, A. S., & Folkers, G. K. (2023). Pandemic preparedness and responses: Lessons from COVID-19. *Journal of Infectious Disease, 228*(4), 422–425. http://doi.org/10.1093/infdis/jiad095

Fernandes, E., Rodrigues, C., Sartori, A., De Soárez, P. C., & Novaes, H. M. D. (2019). Economic evaluation of adolescents and adults' pertussis vaccination: A systematic review of current strategies. *Human Vaccines & Immunotherapeutics, 15*(1), 14–27. https://doi.org/10.1080/21645515.2018.1509646

Filip, R., Gheorghita Puscaselu, R., Anchidin-Norocel, L., Dimian, M., & Savage, W. K. (2022). Global challenges to public health care systems during the COVID-19 pandemic: A review of pandemic measures and problems. *Journal of Personalized Medicine, 12*(8), 1295. https://doi.org/10.3390/jpm12081295

Fouque, F., & Reeder, J. C. (2019). Impact of past and on-going changes on climate and weather on vector-borne diseases transmission: A look at the evidence. *Infectious Diseases of Poverty, 8*, 51. https://doi.org/10.1186/s40249-019-0565-1

Frith, J. (2012). The history of plague—Part 1. The three great pandemics. *Journal of Military and Veterans' Health, 20*(2), 11–16. https://jmvh.org/article/the-history-of-plague-part-1-the-three-great-pandemics/

Gholizadeh, O. A. (2023). Hepatitis A: Viral structure, classification, life cycle, clinical symptoms, diagnosis error and vaccination. *Canadian Journal of Infectious Diseases and Medical Microbiology, 2023*, 17. https://doi.org/10.1155/2023/4263309

Granade, C., Lindley, M. C., Jatlaoui, T., Asif, A. F., & Jones-Jack, N. (2022). Racial and ethnic disparities in adult vaccination: A review of the state of evidence. *Health Equity, 6*(1), 206–223. https://doi.org/10.1089/heq.2021.0177

Hall, E., & Wodi, A. (2021). *Epidemiology and prevention of vaccine-preventable diseases* (14th ed.). Public Health Foundation. https://www.cdc.gov/vaccines/pubs/pinkbook/index.html

Hamson, E., Forbes, C., Wittkopf, P., Pandey, A., Mendes, D., Kowalik, J., Czudek, C., & Mugwagwa, T. (2023). Impact of pandemics and disruptions to vaccination on infectious diseases epidemiology past and present. *Human Vaccines & Immunotherapeutic, 19*(2), 2219577. https://doi.org/10.1080/21645515.2023.2219577

Han, S., Zhang, T., Lyu, Y., Lai, S., Dai, P., Zheng, J., Yang, W., Zhou, X.-H., & Feng, L. (2023). Influenza plummeting during the COVID-19 pandemic: The roles of mask-wearing, mobility change, and SARS-CoV-2 interference. *Engineering, 21*, 195–202. https://doi.org/10.1016/j.eng.2021.12.011

Immunization Action Coalition. (2023). *State laws and mandates by vaccine.* https://www.immunize.org/laws/exemptions.asphttp://www.immunize.org/laws/

Iwasaki, A., & Omer, S. B. (2020). Why and how vaccines work. *Cell, 183*(2), 290–295. https://doi.org/10.1016/j.cell.2020.09.040

Jennings, W., Stoker, G., Bunting, H., Valgarðsson, V. O., Gaskell, J., Devine, D., McKay, L., & Mills, M. C. (2021). Lack of trust, conspiracy beliefs, and social media use predict covid-19 vaccine hesitancy. *Vaccines, 9*(6), 593. https://doi.org/10.3390/vaccines9060593

Jernigan, D. (2018). *100 years since 1918: Are we ready for the next pandemic?* [PowerPoint] Centers for Disease Control and Prevention. https://www.cdc.gov/flu/pandemic-resources/1918-commemoration/pdfs/1918-pandemic-webinar.pdf

Johns Hopkins University & School of Medicine. (2020). *Coronavirus resource center.* Retrieved from https://coronavirus.jhu.edu

John Hopkins University & School of Medicine. (2023). *Coronavirus resource center.* https://coronavirus.jhu.edu/

Jones, D. S. (2020, March 12). History in a crisis: Lessons for COVID-19. *New England Journal of Medicine, 382*(18), 1681–1683. https://www.nejm.org/doi/pdf/10.1056/NEJMp2004361?articleTools=true

Kanchan, S., & Gaidhane, A. (2023). Social media role and its impact on public health: A narrative review. *Cureus, 15*(1), e33737. https://doi.org/10.7759/cureus.33737

Kisling, L., & Das, J. (2023 Jan). Prevention strategies. [Updated 2023 Aug 1. In *StatPearls [Internet]*. StatPearls Publishing. https://www.ncbi.nlm.nih.gov/books/NBK537222/

Kombe, A. J., Li, B., Zahid, A., Mengist, H. M., Bounda, G.-A., Zhou, Y., & Jin, T. (2021). Epidemiology and burden of human papillomavirus and related diseases, molecular pathogenesis, and vaccine evaluation. *Frontiers in Public Health, 8*, 552028. https://doi.org/10.3389/fpubh.2020.552028

Kuehn, B. M. (2020). Emerging drug-resistant meningitis detected in the US. *JAMA, 324*(6), 540. https://doi.org/10.1001/jama.2020.13761

Kulkarni, A., Desai, R., Alcalá, H., & Balkrishnan, R. (2021). Persistent disparities in immunization rates for the seven-vaccine series among infants 19-35 months in the United States. *Health Equity, 5*(1), 135–139. https://doi.org/10.1089/heq.2020.0127

Lederberg, J. (2000). Summary and assessment. In Institute of Medicine (US) Forum on Emerging Infections, J. R. Davis & J. Lederberg (Eds.), *Public health systems and emerging infections: Assessing the capabilities of the public and private sectors: Workshop summary.* National Academies Press (US). https://www.ncbi.nlm.nih.gov/books/NBK100244/

Liao, C., Francoeur, A., Kapp, D., Caesar, M. A. P., Huh, W. K., & Chan, J. K. (2022). Trends in human papillomavirus–associated cancers, demographic characteristics, and vaccinations in the US, 2001–2017. *JAMA Network Open, 5*(3), e222530. https://doi.org/10.1001/jamanetworkopen.2022.2530

Manns, M., & Maasoumy, B. (2022). Breakthroughs in hepatitis C research: from discovery to cure. *Nature Reviews Gastroenterology & Hepatology, 19*, 533–550. https://doi.org/10.1038/s41575-022-00608-8

MacDonald, N. (2015). *Anti-vaccine movement: Strategies to address vaccine hesitancy presentation.* Canadian Centre for Vaccinology. https://www.ammi.ca/Annual-Conference/2015/Presentations/2015-04-18.START%20-%20Noni%20MacDonald.pdf

Martin, B. (2018). Evidence-based campaigning. *Archives of Public Health, 76*(54) https://doi.org/10.1186/s13690-018-0302-4

Mayo Clinic. (2020). *Hepatitis A.* https://www.mayoclinic.org/diseases-conditions/hepatitis-a/symptoms-causes/syc-20367007

McArthur, D. B. (2019). Emerging infectious diseases. *The Nursing Clinics of North America, 54*(2), 297–311. https://doi.org/10.1016/j.cnur.2019.02.006

MedlinePlus. (2020). *Pneumonia.* https://medlineplus.gov/pneumonia.html

Meier, B., Evans, D., & Phelan, A. (2020). Rights-based approaches to preventing, detecting, and responding to infectious disease. In M. Eccleston-Turner & I. Brassington (Eds.), *Infectious diseases in the new millennium. International Library of Ethics, Law, and the New Medicine* (Vol. 82). Springer. https://doi.org/10.1007/978-3-030-39819-4_10

Meites, E., Szilagyi, P., Chesson, H., Unger, E. R., Romero, J. R., & Markowitz, L. E. (2019). Human papillomavirus vaccination for adults: Updated recommendations of the advisory committee on immunization practices. *MMWR Morbidity Mortality Weekly Report, 68*, 698–702. https://doi.org/10.1111/ajt.15633

Merrill, R. M. (2021). *Introduction to epidemiology* (8th ed.). Jones & Bartlett Learning.

Migliori, G. B., Wu, S. J., Matteelli, A., Zenner, D., Goletti, D., Ahmedov, S., Al-Abri, S., Allen, D. M., Balcells, M. E., Garcia-Basteiro, A. L., Cambau, E., Chaisson, R. E., Chee, C. B. E., Dalcolmo, M. P., Denholm, J. T., Erkens, C., Esposito, S., Farnia, P., Friedland, J. S., ... Ong, C. W. M. (2022). Clinical standards for the diagnosis, treatment and prevention of TB infection. *The International Journal of Tuberculosis and Lung Disease, 26*(3), 190–205. https://doi.org/10.5588/ijtld.21.0753

Minnesota Department of Health. (2019). *Public health interventions: Applications for public health nursing practice* (2nd ed.). Minnesota Department of Health Community Health Division. https://www.health.state.mn.us/communities/practice/research/phncouncil/docs/PHInterventions.pdf

Mizock, L., Kenner, C., DiStefano, A., Harway, M., Kaya, K., & Gurse, C. (2021). LGBTQ community needs and assets assessment of a sexual health clinic: A brief report. *Sexuality & Culture*, *25*, 1673–1689. https://doi.org/10.1007/s12119-021-09842-9

Msemburi, W., Karlinsky, A., Knutson, V., Aleshin-Guendel, S., Chatterji, S., & Wakefield, J. (2023). The WHO estimates of excess mortality associated with the COVID-19 pandemic. *Nature*, *613*, 130–137. https://doi.org/10.1038/s41586-022-05522-2

National Cancer Institute (NCI). (2019). *Human papillomavirus (HPV) vaccines*. https://www.cancer.gov/about-cancer/causes-prevention/risk/infectious-agents/hpv-accine-fact-sheet

National Conference of State Legislatures (NCSL). (2024, August 3). *State non-medical exemptions from school immunization requirements*. https://www.ncsl.org/health/state-non-medical-exemptions-from-school-immunization-requirements

National Heart, Lung, and Blood Institute (NHLBI). (2022, March 4). *Pneumonia*. https://www.nhlbi.nih.gov/health/pneumonia/causes

National LGBT Health Education Center. (2019, May 7). *Addressing HIV and sexually transmitted infections among LGBTQ people: A primer for health centers, 2019*. https://www.lgbtqiahealtheducation.org/publication/addressing-hiv-and-sexually-transmitted-infections-among-lgbtq-people-a-primer-for-health-centers/

National Tuberculosis Controllers Association (NTCA). (n.d.). *TB law*. https://www.tbcontrollers.org/resources/archives/tb-law/

Nelson, K., Skinner, A., Stout, C., Raderman, W., Unger, E., Raifman, J., Agénor, M., Ybarra, M. L., Dunsiger, S. I., Bryn Austin, S., & Underhill, K. (2023). Minor consent laws for sexually transmitted infection and human immunodeficiency virus services in the United States: A comprehensive, longitudinal survey of US state laws. *American Journal of Public Health*, *113*(4), 397–407. https://doi.org/10.2105/AJPH.2022.307199

New York City Department of Health & the NYC STD Prevention Training Center. (2019, March). *The diagnosis, management, and prevention of syphilis: An update and review*. https://www.nycptc.org/x/Syphilis_Monograph_2019_NYC_PTC_NYC_DOHMH.pdf

Night, S. S. (2007). Public health emergencies and HIPAA: When is the disclosure of individual health information lawful? *Houston Journal of Health Law & Policy*. https://www.law.uh.edu/healthlaw/perspectives/2007/(SN)SpeakerHIPAA.pdf

Nuwarda, R., Ramzan, I., Weekes, L., & Kayser, V. (2022). Vaccine hesitancy: Contemporary issues and historical background. *Vaccines*, *10*(10), 1595. https://doi.org/10.3390/vaccines10101595

Occupational Safety & Health Administration (OSHA). (n.d.). *Workers' protections against occupational exposure to infectious diseases*. https://www.osha.gov/SLTC/bloodbornepathogens/worker_protections.html

Occupational Safety & Health Administration (OSHA). (2011). *OSHA's bloodborne pathogens standard. OSHA Factsheet*. https://www.osha.gov/OshDoc/data_BloodborneFacts/bbfact01.pdf

Office of Disease Prevention and Health Promotion (ODPHP). (2018). *Proposed objectives for inclusion in Healthy People 2030*. https://www.healthypeople.gov/sites/default/files/ObjectivesPublicComment508_1.17.19.pdf

Office of Disease Prevention and Health Promotion (ODPHP). (2020). *Healthy People 2030 framework*. https://www.healthypeople.gov/2020/About-Healthy-People/Development-Healthy-People-2030/Framework

Oliveira, C., Feemster, K., & Ulloa, E. (2022). Pediatric COVID-19 health disparities and vaccine equity. *Journal of the Pediatric Infectious Diseases Society*, *11*(4), 141–147. https://doi.org/10.1093/jpids/piac091

Opel, D. J., Brewer, N. T., Buttenheim, A. M., Callaghan, T., Carpiano, R. M., Clinton, C., Elharake, J. A., Flowers, L. C., Galvani, A. P., Hotez, P. J., Schwartz, J. L., Benjamin, R. M., Caplan, A., DiResta, R., Lakshmanan, R., Maldonado, Y. A., Mello, M. M., Parmet, W. E., Salmon, D. A., ... Omer, S. B. (2022). The legacy of the COVID-19 pandemic for childhood vaccination in the USA. *The Lancet*, *401*(10370), 75–78. https://doi.org/10.1016/S0140-6736(22)01693-2

Open Stax. (2019). 12.3 Modes of disease transmission. *Allied health microbiology* (1st ed.). Oregon State University. https://open.oregonstate.education/microbiology/chapter/16-3modes-of-disease-transmission/

Pan American Health Organization (PAHO). (2023, May 11). *WHO declares end of Mpox emergency, calls for sustained efforts for long-term management of the disease*. https://www.paho.org/en/news/11-5-2023-who-declares-end-mpox-emergency-calls-sustained-efforts-long-term-management-disease

Puri, N., Coomes, E., Haghbayan, H., & Gunaratne, K. (2020). Social Media and vaccine hesitancy: New updates for the era of covid-19 and globalized infectious diseases. *Human Vaccines & Immunotherapeutic*, *16*(11), 2586–2593. https://doi.org/10.1080/21645515.2020.1780846

Reichler, M. R., Awal, K., Yuan, Y., Chen, B., McAuley, J., Mangura, B., Sterling, T. R., & Tuberculosis Epidemiologic Studies Consortium Task Order 2 Team. (2020). Duration of exposure among close contacts of patients with infectious tuberculosis and risk of latent tuberculosis infection. *Clinical Infectious Diseases*, *71*(7), 1627–1634. https://doi.org/10.1093/cid/ciz1044

Rosner, D. (2010). Public health in the early 20th century. *Public Health Reports*, *125*(Suppl 3), 37–47.

Sakai, T., & Morimoto, Y. (2022). The history of infectious diseases and medicine. *Pathogens (Basel, Switzerland)*, *11*(10), 1147. https://doi.org/10.3390/pathogens11101147

Schuchat, A. (2020). *Public health response to the initiation and spread of pandemic COVID-19 in the United States, February 24–April 21, 2020*. https://www.cdc.gov/mmwr/volumes/69/wr/mm6918e2.htm

Stop TB Partnership. (2022). *The global plan to end TB 2023-2030*. https://www.stoptb.org/global-plan-to-end-tb/global-plan-to-end-tb-2023-2030

Swire-Thompson, B., & Lazer, D. (2020). Public health and online misinformation: Challenges and recommendations. *Annual Review of Public Health*, *41*(1), 433–451. https://doi.org/10.1146/annurev-publhealth-040119-094127

The College of Physicians of Philadelphia. (2019). *Typhoid Mary. The history of vaccines*. https://www.historyofvaccines.org/content/typhoid-mary

Toebes, B. (2020). Mediating tensions between public health and individual rights. *European Journal of Public Health*, *30*(5). https://doi.org/10.1093/eurpub/ckaa165.044

Troeger, C. (2023, February 15). *Just how do deaths due to COVID-19 stack-up?* Think Global Health. https://www.thinkglobalhealth.org/article/just-how-do-deaths-due-covid-19-stack

Tuckerman, J., Kaufman, J., & Danchin, M. (2022). Effective approaches to combat vaccine hesitancy. *The Pediatric Infectious Disease Journal*, *41*(5), e243–e245. https://doi.org/10.1097/INF.0000000000003499

U.S. Department of Agriculture (USDA). (2015, March). *Kitchen companion: Your food safe handbook*. https://www.fsis.usda.gov/wps/wcm/connect/6c55c954-20a8-46fd-b617-ecffb4449062/Kitchen_Companion_Single.pdf?MOD=AJPERES

U.S. Equal Employment Opportunity Commission (EEOC). (n.d.). *Questions and answers about the association provision of the Americans with Disabilities Act*. http://www.eeoc.gov/facts/association_ada.html

U.S. Food and Drug Administration (FDA). (2023, July 21). *Anthrax*. https://www.fda.gov/vaccines-blood-biologics/vaccines/anthrax

U.S. Food and Drug Administration (FDA). (2020, September 21). *Countering bioterrorism and emerging infectious diseases*. https://www.fda.gov/vaccines-blood-biologics/safety-availability-biologics/countering-bioterrorism-and-emerging-infectious-diseases

United States Geological Survey (USGS). (2021, July 14). *USGS-led study helps in the fight against the coronavirus pandemic*. https://www.usgs.gov/news/national-news-release/usgs-led-study-helps-fight-against-coronavirus-pandemic

U.S. Preventive Services Task Force (USPSTF). (2018, August 21). *Final recommendation statement: Cervical cancer screening*. https://www.uspreventiveservicestaskforce.org/Page/Document/RecommendationStatementFinal/cervical-cancer-screening2

Wang, X., Du, Z., Huang, G., Pasco, R. F., Fox, S. J., Galvani, A. P., Pignone, M., Claiborne Johnston, S., & Meyers, L. A. (2020). Effects of cocooning on coronavirus disease rates after relaxing social distancing. *Emerging Infectious Diseases*, *26*(12), 3066–3068. https://doi.org/10.3201/eid2612.201930

Wodi, A., Murthy, N., Bernstein, H., McNally, V., Cineas, S., & Ault, K. (2022). Advisory committee on immunization practices recommended immunization schedule for children and adolescents aged 18 years or younger—United States, 2022. *MMWR. Morbidity and Mortality Weekly Report*, *71*(7), 234–237. https://doi.org/10.15585/mmwr.mm7107a2

Woodfield, M., Pergam, S., & Shah, P. (2021). Cocooning against COVID-19: The argument for vaccinating caregivers of patients with cancer. *Cancer*, *127*(16), 2861–2863. https://doi.org/10.1002/cncr.33598

World Health Organization (WHO). (n.d.-a). *About WHO: What we do*. http://www.who.int/about/what-we-do/en/

World Health Organization (WHO). (n.d.-c). *Global influenza surveillance and response system (GISRS)*. Retrieved September 1, 2023, from https://www.who.int/influenza/gisrs_laboratory/updates/GISRS_one_pager_2018_EN.pdf?ua=1

World Health Organization (WHO). (n.d.-e). *Ten threats to global health in 2019*. Retrieved September 4, 2023, from https://www.who.int/news-room/spotlight/ten-threats-to-global-health-in-2019

World Health Organization (WHO). (n.d.-f). *Smallpox*. https://www.who.int/health-topics/smallpox#tab=tab_3

World Health Organization (WHO). (2019). *Global tuberculosis report 2019*. https://apps.who.int/iris/bitstream/handle/10665/329368/9789241565714-eng.pdf?ua=1

World Health Organization (WHO). (2020). *Immunization*. Retrieved from http://www.who.int/topics/immunization/en/

World Health Organization (WHO). (2022b, October 27). *Global tuberculosis report 2022*. https://www.who.int/teams/global-tuberculosis-programme/tb-reports/global-tuberculosis-report-2022

World Health Organization (WHO). (2023a, April 7). *75 Years of improving public health: World health day 2023*. https://www.who.int/campaigns/75-years-of-improving-public-health

World Health Organization (WHO). (2023b, August 16). *Coronavirus (COVID-19) dashboard*. https://covid19.who.int/

World Health Organization (WHO). (2023c, August 9). *Coronavirus disease (COVID-19): Key facts*. https://www.who.int/news-room/fact-sheets/detail/coronavirus-disease-(covid-19)

World Health Organization (WHO). (2023d, July 8). *Fact sheets: Hepatitis C*. http://www.who.int/news-room/fact-sheets/detail/hepatitis-c

World Health Organization (WHO). (2023e, April 21). *Fact sheet: Tuberculosis*. http://www.who.int/en/news-room/fact-sheets/detail/tuberculosis

World Health Organization (WHO). (2023f, July 20). *Hepatitis A: Key facts*. https://www.who.int/news-room/fact-sheets/detail/hepatitis-a

World Health Organization (WHO). (2023g, July 18). *Hepatitis B: Key facts*. https://www.who.int/news-room/fact-sheets/detail/hepatitis-b

World Health Organization (WHO). (2023h, July 13). *HIV and AIDS*. https://www.who.int/news-room/fact-sheets/detail/hiv-aids

World Health Organization (WHO). (2023i, April 18). *Mpox (monkeypox)*. https://www.who.int/news-room/fact-sheets/detail/monkeypox

World Health Organization (WHO). (2023j, August 13). *Tracking SARS-CoV-2 variants*. https://www.who.int/activities/tracking-SARS-CoV-2-variants

WHO. (2024a). *2022–2024 Mpox (MonkeyPox) outbreak: Global trends*. https://www.cdc.gov/mpox/situation-summary/index.html#anchor_79452

WHO. (2024b). *WHO Covid-19 dashboard*. https://data.who.int/dashboards/covid19/deaths?n=o

CHAPTER 9

Abouk, R., & Adams, S. (2018). Birth outcomes in Flint in the early stages of the water crisis. *Journal of Public Health Policy*, *38*(1), 68–85.

Adamiec, E., Jarosz-Krzemińska, E., & Bilkiewicz-Kubarek, A. (2022). Adverse health and environmental outcomes of cycling in heavily polluted urban environments. *Scientific Reports*, *12*(1), 148. https://doi.org/10.1038/s41598-021-03111-3

Agency for Toxic Substances and Disease Registry (ATSDR). (2023a). *Asbestos and your health*. https://www.atsdr.cdc.gov/asbestos/

Agency for Toxic Substances and Disease Registry (ATSDR). (2023b). *ATSDR petition process*. https://www.atsdr.cdc.gov/hac/petitionatsdrdchi.html

Agency for Toxic Substances and Disease Registry (ATSDR). (2023c). *Partners and other environmental medicine resources*. https://www.atsdr.cdc.gov/emes/partners.html#:~:text=The%20Pediatric%20Environmental%20

Health%20Specialty,United%20States%2C%20Canada%20and%20Mexico.

Agency for Toxic Substances and Disease Registry (ATSDR). (2023d). *Social vulnerability index*. https://www.atsdr.cdc.gov/placeandhealth/svi/index.html

Agency for Toxic Substances and Disease Registry (ATSDR). (2023e). *What are the health effects of PFAS?* https://www.epa.gov/pfas/pfas-explained

Alliance of Nurses for Healthy Environments (ANHE). (2019). *History of AHNE*. https://envirn.org/about/

American Hospital Association. (2023). *Sustainability road map for health care*. https://www.aha.org/sustainability

American Nurses Association (ANA). (2021). *Nursing: Scope and standards of practice* (4th ed.).

American Nurses Association (ANA). (2022). *Public Health Nursing: Scope and standards of practice* (3rd ed.).

American Public Health Association (APHA). (2023). *Environmental health*. https://www.apha.org/topics-and-issues/environmental-health

American Public Health Association (APHA). (2005). *Environmental health principles for public health nursing*.

American Association of Occupational Health Nurses. (2020). *What is occupational & environmental health nursing?* http://aaohn.org/page/profession-of-occupational-and-environmental-health-nursing

American Lung Association. (2023). *State of the air*. https://www.lung.org/research/sota

Amiri, A. (2023). Contamination pathways. In R. McDermott-Levy, K. P. Jackman-Murphy, J. Leffers & A. G. Cantu (Eds.), *Environmental health in nursing* (3rd ed., pp. 46–51). Alliance of Nurses for a Healthy Environment.

Anderko, L., & Pennea, E. (2023). Perfluoroalkyl and polyfluoroalkyl substances (PFAS): Forever chemicals and health effects. In R. McDermott-Levy, K. P. Jackman-Murphy, J. Leffers & A. G. Cantu (Eds.), *Environmental health in nursing* (3rd ed., pp. 95–101). Alliance of Nurses for a Healthy Environment.

Bender, M., Grace, P. J., Green, C., Hopkins-Walsh, J., Kirkevold, M., Petrovskaya, O., Paljevic, E. D., & Sellman, D. (2021). The role of philosophy in the development and practice of nursing: Past, present and future. *Nursing Philosophy: an international journal for healthcare professionals*, *22*(4), e12363. https://doi.org/10.1111/nup.12363

Blackburn, K., & Green, D. (2022). The potential effects of microplastics on human health: What is known and what is unknown. *Ambio*, *51*(3), 518–530. https://doi.org/10.1007/s13280-021-01589-9

Bloom, M. (2020). Environmental epidemiology. In J. O. Nriagu (Ed.), *Encyclopedia of environmental health* (2nd ed., pp. 419–427). Elsevier. https://doi.org/10.1016/B978-0-444-63951-6.01002-0

Bullard, R. (2023). *About environmental justice*. https://drrobertbullard.com/

Butterfield, P. G. (2017). Thinking upstream: A 25-year retrospective and conceptual model aimed at reducing health inequities. *Advances in Nursing Science*, *40*(1), 2–11.

Butterfield, P. G., Hill, W., Postma, J., Butterfield, P. W., & Odom-Maryon, T. (2011). Effectiveness of a household environmental health intervention delivered by rural public health nurses. *American Journal of Public Health*, *101*(S1), S262–S270.

Butterfield, P., Leffers, J., & Vásquez, M. D. (2021). Nursing's pivotal role in global climate action. *British Medical Journal*, *373*(1049). https://doi.org/10.1136/bmj.n1049

Caba-Flores, M. D., Martínez-Valenzuela, C., Cárdenas-Tueme, M., & Camacho-Morales, A. (2023). Micro problems with macro consequences: Accumulation of persistent organic pollutants and microplastics in human breast milk and in human milk substitutes. *Environmental Science and Pollution Research International*, *30*(42), 95139–95154. https://doi.org/10.1007/s11356-023-29182-5

Cardarelli, K. M., Ickes, M., Huntington-Moskos, L., Wilmhoff, C., Larck, A., Pinney, S. M., & Hahn, E. J. (2021). Authentic youth engagement in environmental health research and advocacy. *International Journal of Environmental Research and Public Health*, *18*(4), 2154. https://doi.org/10.3390/ijerph18042154

Centers for Disease Control and Prevention (CDC). (2017). *National biomonitoring program*. https://www.cdc.gov/biomonitoring/index.html

Centers for Disease Control and Prevention (CDC). (2020). *Foodborne germs and illnesses*. http://www.cdc.gov/foodsafety/foodborne-germs.html

Centers for Disease Control and Prevention (CDC). (2023a). *10 essential environmental public health services*. https://www.cdc.gov/publichealthgateway/publichealthservices/essentialhealthservices.html

Centers for Disease Control and Prevention (CDC). (2023b). *Health disparities*. https://www.cdc.gov/healthyyouth/disparities/index.htm

Centers for Disease Control and Prevention (CDC). (2023c). *List of multistate foodborne outbreak notices*. https://www.cdc.gov/foodsafety/outbreaks/lists/outbreaks-list.html

Centers for Disease Control and Prevention (CDC). (2023d). *One health basics*. https://www.cdc.gov/onehealth/basics/index.html

Centers for Disease Control and Prevention (CDC). (2023e). *Sources of lead exposure*. https://www.cdc.gov/nceh/lead/prevention/sources.htm

Chesney, M. L., & Duderstadt, K. (2022). Children's rights, environmental justice, and environmental health policy in the United States. *Journal of Pediatric Health Care: official publication of National Association of Pediatric Nurse Associates & Practitioners*, *36*(1), 3–11. https://doi.org/10.1016/j.pedhc.2021.08.006

Chigwada, A. D., & Tekere, M. (2023). The plastic and microplastic waste menace and bacterial biodegradation for sustainable environmental clean-up a review. *Environmental Research*, *231*(Pt 1), 116110. https://doi.org/10.1016/j.envres.2023.116110

Costello, A., Abbas, M., Allen, A., Ball, S., Bell, S., Bellamy, R., Friel, S., Groce, N., Johnson, A., Kett, M., Lee, M., Levy, C., Maslin, M., McCoy, D., McGuire, B., Montgomery, H., Napier, D., Pagel, C., Patel, J., … Patterson, C. (2009). Managing the health effects of climate change: Lancet and University College London Institute for Global Health Commission. *Lancet*, *33*, 1693–1733.

Costello, A., Montgomery, H., & Watts, N. (2013). Climate change: The challenge for healthcare professionals. *British Medical Journal*, *347*, f6060. https://doi.org/10.1126/bmj.f6060

Crear-Perry, J., Correa-de-Araujo, R., Lewis Johnson, T., McLemore, M. R., Neilson, E., & Wallace, M. (2021). Social and structural determinants of health inequities in maternal health. *Journal of Women's Health*, *30*(2), 230–235. https://doi.org/10.1089/jwh.2020.8882

Dennis, B. (2019, October 10). For the first time in decades, EPA is overhauling how communities must test for lead in water. *The Washington Post*. https://www.washingtonpost.com/climate-environment/2019/10/10/first-time-decades-epa-is-overhauling-how-communities-must-test-lead-water/

De Pinto, A., Cenacchi, N., Kwon, H. Y., Koo, J., & Dunston, S. (2020). Climate smart agriculture and global food-crop production. *PLoS One*, *15*(4), e0231764. https://doi.org/10.1371/journal.pone.0231764

Desmond, S. (2016). Implementing climate change mitigation in health services: The importance of context. *Journal of Health Services Research & Policy*, *21*(4), 257–262.

Dórea, J. G. (2021). Exposure to environmental neurotoxic substances and neurodevelopment in children from Latin America and the Caribbean. *Environmental Research*, *192*, 110199. https://doi.org/10.1016/j.envres.2020.110199

Dovjak, M., & Kukec, A. (2019). Health outcomes related to built environments. In *Creating healthy and sustainable buildings*. Springer. https://doi.org/10.1007/978-3-030-19412-3_2

Duchenne-Moutien, R. A., & Neetoo, H. (2021). Climate change and emerging food safety issues: A review. *Journal of Food Protection*, *84*(11), 1884–1897. https://doi.org/10.4315/JFP-21-141

Dzau, V. J., Levine, R., Barrett, G., & Witty, A. (2021). Decarbonizing the U.S. health sector—A call to action. *The New England Journal of Medicine*, *385*(23), 2117–2119. https://doi.org/10.1056/NEJMp2115675

Edwards, M. (2015, September 8). *Our sampling of 252 homes demonstrates a high lead in water risk: Flint should be failing to meet the EPA Lead and Copper Rule*. http://flintwaterstudy.org/2015/09/our-sampling-of-252-homes-demonstrates-a-high-lead-in-water-risk-flint-should-be-failing-to-meet-the-epa-lead-and-copper-rule/

Elton, C. (2023). World Refugee Day: How will climate change force us to rethink attitudes to mass migration? *Euronews*. https://www.euronews.com/green/2023/06/20/climate-change-will-displace-millions-of-people

Environmental Working Group. (2019). *Nurses' health: A survey on health and chemical exposures*. https://www.ewg.org/research/nurses-health

Federal Emergency Management Agency (FEMA). (2023). *PrepToolkit and National Preparedness System*. https://preptoolkit.fema.gov/web/guest

Fitzsimmons, E. G. (2019, August 12). In echo of Flint lead crisis, Newark offers bottled water after long denial. *The New York Times (Late Edition; East Coast)*, A17.

Friis, R. H. (2019). *Essentials of environmental health* (3rd ed.). Jones & Bartlett Learning.

Frumkin, H. (2016). *Environmental health: from global to local* (3rd ed.). John Wiley.

Gilbert, H. A. (2020). Florence nightingale's environmental theory and its influence on contemporary infection control. *Collegian*, *27*(6), 626–633.

Gómez-Roig, M. D., Pascal, R., Cahuana, M. J., García-Algar, O., Sebastiani, G., Andreu-Fernández, V., Martínez, L., Rodríguez, G., Iglesia, I., Ortiz-Arrabal, O., Mesa, M. D., Cabero, M. J., Guerra, L., Llurba, E., Domínguez, C., Zanini, M. J., Foraster, M., Larqué, E., Cabañas, F., … Vento, M. (2021). Environmental exposure during pregnancy: Influence on prenatal development and early life: A comprehensive review. *Fetal Diagnosis and Therapy*, *48*(4), 245–257. https://doi.org/10.1159/000514884

Haines, A. (2016). Addressing challenges to human health in the Anthropocene epoch—an overview of the findings of the Rockefeller/Lancet Commission on Planetary Health. *Public Health Reviews*, *37*, 14. https://www.ncbi.nlm.nih.gov/pmc/articles/PMC5810099/pdf/40985_2016_Article_29.pdf

Hanna-Attisha, M. (2019). *What the eyes don't see: A story of crisis, resistance, and hope in an American City*. One World Trade Paperback Edition.

Hanna-Attisha, M., LaChance, J., Sadler, R. C., & Schnepp, A. C. (2016). Elevated blood lead levels in children associated with the Flint drinking water crisis: A spatial analysis of risk and public health response. *American Journal of Public Health*, *106*(2), 283–290.

Health Care Without Harm. (2018). *Leading the global movement for environmentally responsible healthcare*. https://noharm.org/

Health Care Without Harm. (2023). *Waste management*. https://noharm-uscanada.org/issues/us-canada/waste-management

Heard-Garris, N. J., Roche, J., Carter, P., Abir, M., Walton, M., Zimmerman, M., & Cunningham, R. (2017). Voices from Flint: Community perceptions of the Flint water crisis. *Journal of Urban Health*, *94*(6), 776–779.

Hill, E. L., & Ma, L. (2022). Drinking water, fracking, and infant health. *Journal of Health Economics*, *82*, 102595. https://doi.org/10.1016/j.jhealeco.2022.102595

Hopkins, E. E., & Zangrilli, N. (2023). Epigenetics. In R. McDermott-Levy, K. P. Jackman-Murphy, J. Leffers & A. G. Cantu (Eds.), *Environmental health in nursing* (3rd ed., pp. 65–69). Alliance of Nurses for a Healthy Environment.

Intergovernmental Panel on Climate Change (IPCC). (2018). *Special report: Global warming of 1.5° Celsius*. https://www.ipcc.ch/sr15/

Intergovernmental Panel on Climate Change (IPCC). (2021). *6th Assessment report: Physical science basis*. https://www.ipcc.ch/report/sixth-assessment-report-working-group-i/

Intergovernmental Panel on Climate Change (IPCC). (2023). *Climate change 2023 synthesis report*. https://www.ipcc.ch/report/ar6/syr/downloads/report/IPCC_AR6_SYR_SPM.pdf

Jackman-Murphy, K. (2023). Community survey for population health. In R. McDermott-Levy, K. P. Jackman-Murphy, J. Leffers & A. G. Cantu (Eds.), *Environmental Health in Nursing* (3rd ed., pp. 246–250). Alliance of Nurses for a Healthy Environment.

Jarvie, J. (2019, April 23). On a sinking Louisiana island, many aren't ready to leave. *Los Angeles Times*. https://www.latimes.com/nation/la-na-jean-charles-sinking-louisiana-island-20190423-htmlstory.html

Jenkins, D., Grossman, D., Slusky, D., & Danagoulian, S. (2022). Blood lead testing in flint before and after water contamination. *Pediatrics*, *150*(6), e2022056541. https://doi.org/10.1542/peds.2022-056541

Kampman, H., Whitlock, A., & Hosler, H. (2022). Health impact assessment: The impacts of increasing tree canopy coverage in Marion County, Indiana. *Chronicles of Health Impact Assessment*, 7(1). https://journals.iupui.edu/index.php/chia/article/view/26368

Kennedy, M. (2016, April 20). *Lead-laced water in Flint: A step-by-step look at the makings of a crisis*. https://www.npr.org/sections/I-way/2016/04/20/465545378/lead-laced-water-in-flint-a-step-by-step-look-at-the-makings-of-a-crisis

Keuhn, B. M. (2016). Pediatrician sees long road ahead for Flint after lead poisoning crisis. *JAMA*, *315*(10), 967–969.

Kurth, A. E. (2017). Planetary health and the role of nursing: A call to action. *Journal of Nursing Scholarship*, *49*(6), 598–605. https://doi.org/10.1111/jnu.12343

LeClair, J., & Potter, T. (2022). Planetary health nursing. *The American Journal of Nursing*, *122*(4), 47–52. https://doi.org/10.1097/01.NAJ.0000827336.29891.9b

Leffers, J. (2023). Harmful environmental exposures and vulnerable populations. In R. McDermott-Levy, K.P. Jackman-Murphy, J. Leffers, & A.G. Cantu (Eds.), *Environmental health in nursing* (3rd ed., pp. 19–29). Alliance of Nurses for a Healthy Environment.

Leffers, J., McDermott-Levy, R., Nicholas, P., & Sweeney, C. (2017). Mandate for the nursing profession to address climate change through nursing education. *Journal of Nursing Scholarship*, *49*(6), 679–687.

Leffers, J., McDermott-Levy, R., Smith, C. M., & Sattler, B. (2014). Nursing education's response to the 1995 Institute of Medicine report: Nursing, health, and the environment. *Nursing Forum*, *49*(44), 214–224. https://doi.org/10.1111/nuf.12072

Lynch, A., & Sachs, J. (2021). *The United States Sustainable Development Report 2021*. SDSN. https://s3.amazonaws.com/sustainabledevelopment.report/2021/United+States+Sustainable+Development+Report+2021.pdf

Macheka, L. R., Abafe, O. A., Mugivhisa, L. L., & Olowoyo, J. O. (2022). Occurrence and infant exposure assessment of per and polyfluoroalkyl substances in breast milk from South Africa. *Chemosphere*, *288*(Pt 2), 132601. https://doi.org/10.1016/j.chemosphere.2021.132601

McDermott-Levy, R., Murphy, K., Leffers, J., & Cantu, A. (2023). *Environmental health in nursing* (3rd ed.). ANHE e-book. https://envirn.org/e-textbook/

McDermott-Levy, R., Scolio, M., Shakya, K. M., & Moore, C. H. (2021). Factors that influence climate change-related mortality in the United States: An integrative review. *International Journal of Environmental Research and Public Health*, *18*(15), 8220. https://doi.org/10.3390/ijerph18158220

McDermott-Levy, R. (2023). Introduction to toxicology in environmental health nursing. In R. McDermott-Levy, K. P. Jackman-Murphy, J. Leffers & A. G. Cantu (Eds.), *Environmental health in nursing* (3rd ed., pp. 50–54). Alliance of Nurses for a Healthy Environment.

McKinley, J. (1979, June). A case for focusing upstream: The political economy of illness. *Proceedings of the American Heart Association Conference: Applying Behavioral Science to Cardiovascular Risk, Seattle, WA*.

Merriam Webster On-Line Dictionary. (2023). *Risk*. https://www.merriam-webster.com/dictionary/risk

Mooney, C., Muyskens, J., Dennis, B., & Freedman, A. (2020). Pollution is plummeting in Italy in the wake of coronavirus, emissions data show. *New York Times*. https://www.washingtonpost.com/climate-environment/2020/illa/italy-emissions-coronavirus/?arc404=true

Moyer, A. (2023). Using nursing process to guide advocacy for environmental health. In R. McDermott-Levy, K. P. Jackman-Murphy, J. Leffers & A. G. Cantu (Eds.), *Environmental health in nursing* (3rd ed., pp. 50–54). Alliance of Nurses for a Healthy Environment.

National Association of School Nurses (NASN). (2018). *The role of the 21st century school nurse*. https://www.nasn.org/advocacy/professional-practice-documents/position-statements/ps-role

National Geographic. (2023). *Ecosystem*. https://education.nationalgeographic.org/resource/ecosystem/

National Institute of Environmental Health Sciences. (2023). *Toxicology*. https://www.niehs.nih.gov/health/topics/science/toxicology/index.cfm

National Institute for Occupational Safety and Health (NIOSH). (2017). *Health and safety practices*. Survey of Healthcare Workers. https://www.cdc.gov/niosh/topics/healthcarehsps/default.html

National Institute for Occupational Safety and Health (NIOSH). (2023). *Chemical hazards for health care workers*. https://www.cdc.gov/niosh/topics/healthcare/chemical.html

National Oceanic and Atmospheric Administration. (2023). *What are microplastics?* https://oceanservice.noaa.gov/facts/microplastics.html

Occupational Safety and Health Administration. (2012). *Hazard communication standard: Safety data sheets*. OSHA Brief. https://www.osha.gov/sites/default/files/publications/OSHA3514.pdf

Office of Disease Prevention and Health Promotion. (2019). *Healthy people*. https://health.gov/our-work/healthy-people/

Office of Disease Prevention and Health Promotion. (2020). *Healthy people 2030 framework*. https://www.healthypeople.gov/2020/About-Healthy-People/Development-Healthy-People-2030/Framework

Partnership for Food Safety Education. (2023). *Food safety*. http://www.fightbac.org/

Pesticide Action Network. (2023). *What's on my food?* http://whatsinmyfood.org/index.jsp

Podesta, J. (2019, July 25). *The climate crisis, migration, and refugees* Brookings. https://www.brookings.edu/research/the-climate-crisis-migration-and-refugees/

Pope, A. M., Snyder, M. A., & Mood, L. H. (1995). *Nursing, health and the environment: Strengthening the relationship to improve the public's health*. National Academy Press.

Practice Green Health. (2023). *Waste*. https://practicegreenhealth.org/topics/waste/waste-0

Ramsay, J. M., Fendereski, K., Horns, J. J., VanDerslice, J. A., Hanson, H. A., Emery, B. R., Halpern, J. A., Aston, K. I., Ferlic, E., & Hotaling, J. M. (2023). Environmental exposure to industrial air pollution is associated with decreased male fertility. *Fertility & Sterility*, *120*(3), 637–647. https://doi-org.ezp1.villanova.edu/10.1016/j.fertnstert.2023.05.143

RAND Health. (2015). *Understanding the upstream social determinants of health*. https://www.rand.org/content/dam/rand/pubs/working_papers/WR1000/WR1096/RAND_WR1096.pdf

Rosner, D. (2016). Flint, Michigan: A century of environmental injustice. *American Journal of Public Health*, *106*(2), 200–201.

Saberi, P., & Becker, J. (2023). *Physicians for Social Responsibility PA; OCAREER* A practitioner's tool for evaluating climate and health.

Santiago, E. (2018, November 14). *Allyn Pierce, Camp Fire hero: 5 fast facts you need to know*. https://heavy.com/news/2018/11/allyn-pierce-camp-fire-hero-toyota/

Science and Environmental Health Network (SEHN). (2023). *Precautionary principle*. https://www.sehn.org/precautionary-principle-understanding-science-in-regulation

Sen, A., Heredia, N., Senut, M. C., Land, S., Hollocher, K., Lu, X., Dereski, M. O., & Ruden, D. M. (2015). Multigenerational epigenetic inheritance in humans: DNA methylation changes associated with maternal exposure to lead can be transmitted to the grandchildren. *Scientific Reports*, *5*, 14466.

Smith, K. R., Corvalán, C. F., & Kjellström, T. (1999). How much global ill health is attributable to environmental factors? *Epidemiology (Cambridge, Mass.)*, *10*(5), 573–584.

Stein, Y., & Udasin, I. G. (2020). Electromagnetic hypersensitivity (EHS, microwave syndrome)—Review of mechanisms. *Environmental Research*, *186*, 109445. https://doi.org/10.1016/j.envres.2020.109445

Su, Z., McDonnell, D., Ahmad, J., & Cheshmehzangi, A. (2023). Disaster preparedness in healthcare professionals amid COVID-19 and beyond: A systematic review of randomized controlled trials. *Nurse Education in Practice*, *69*, 103583. https://doi.org/10.1016/j.nepr.2023.103583

Taiwo, K. T., Lein, P., & Yaghoobi, B. (2023). *COVID-19, environmental justice & institutionalized racism*. https://environmentalhealth.ucdavis.edu/research/covid-19-environmental-injustice-racism

The Weather Chanel. (2023). *2023 Shattered record number of US billion-dollar disasters, with four months to go*. https://weather.com/news/climate/news/2023-09-11-billion-dollar-disasters-record-2023-august

Titus, L. (2021). Evidence of intergenerational transmission of diethylstilbestrol health effects: Hindsight and insight. *Biology of Reproduction*, *105*(3), 681–686. https://doi.org/10.1093/biolre/ioab153

Tomkins, C. M., Anderko, L., & Patten, M. (2016). *Air quality flag program influences behavioral change on poor air quality days* Mid Atlantic Center for Children's Health and the Environment. http://www.enviro.center/epas-air-quality-flag-program-influences-behavioral-change-poor-outdoor-air-quality-days-d-c-elementary-school-2/

Troisi, R., Hatch, E., Titus, L., Strohsnitter, W., Gail, M. H., Huo, D., Adam, E., Robboy, S. J., Hyer, M., Hoover, R. N., & Palmer, J. R. (2019). Prenatal diethylstilbestrol exposure and cancer risk in women. *Environmental and Molecular Mutagenesis*, *60*(5), 395–403. https://doi.org/10.1002/em.22155

UC Davis. (n.d.). *Science & climate: Climate change terms & definitions*. https://climatechange.ucdavis.edu/science/climate-change-definitions/

United Nations (UN). (2020). *About the sustainable development goals*. https://www.un.org/sustainabledevelopment/sustainable-development-goals/

United Nations. (2023). *Water*. https://www.un.org/en/global-issues/water

United Nations Environmental Programme. (2023). *Our planet is choking on plastic*. https://www.unep.org/interactives/beat-plastic-polluti

U.S. Department of Housing and Urban Development (USHUD). (2023). *Healthy homes program*. https://www.hud.gov/program_offices/healthy_homes/hhi

U.S. Environmental Protection Agency (EPA). (2017). *News releases from headquarters: EPA awards $100 million to Michigan for Flint water infrastructure upgrades*. https://archive.epa.gov/epa/newsreleases/epa-awards-100-million-michigan-flint-water-infrastructure-upgrades.html

U.S. Environmental Protection Agency (EPA). (2018a). *Management weaknesses delayed response to Flint water crisis, Report 18-P0221*. https://www.epa.gov/sites/production/files/2018-07/documents/_epaoig_20180719-18-p-0221.pdf

U.S. Environmental Protection Agency (EPA). (2018b). *What is superfund?* https://www.epa.gov/superfund/what-superfund

U.S. Environmental Protection Agency (EPA). (2019). *Advisories and technical resources for fish and shellfish consumption*. http://www2.epa.gov/fish-tech

U.S. Environmental Protection Agency (EPA). (2020a). *Environmental justice*. http://www.epa.gov/environmental-justice/

U.S. Environmental Protection Agency (EPA). (2020b). *Environmental justice equals healthy, sustainable, and equitable communities*. http://www3.epa.gov/environmentaljustice/sustainability/index.html

U.S. Environmental Protection Agency (EPA). (2020c). *Indoor air quality*. http://www2.epa.gov/indoor-air-quality-iaq

U.S. Environmental Protection Agency (EPA). (2020d). *Natural disasters and weather emergencies*. http://www2.epa.gov/natural-disasters

U.S. Environmental Protection Agency (EPA). (2020e). *Overview of the Clean Air Act and air pollution*. https://www.epa.gov/clean-air-act-overview

U.S. Environmental Protection Agency (EPA). (2021). *EPA report shows disproportionate impacts of climate change on socially vulnerable populations in the United States*. https://www.epa.gov/newsreleases/epa-report-shows-disproportionate-impacts-climate-change-socially-vulnerable

U.S. Environmental Protection Agency (EPA). (2023a). *Air topics*. https://www.epa.gov/environmental-topics/air-topics

U.S. Environmental Protection Agency (EPA). (2023b). *Air quality flag program*. https://cfpub.epa.gov/airnow/index.cfm?action=flag_program.index

U.S. Environmental Protection Agency (EPA). (2023c). *Creating healthy indoor air quality in schools*. https://www.epa.gov/iaq-schools

U.S. Environmental Protection Agency (EPA). (2023d). *Facts and figures about materials, waste, and recycling*. https://www.epa.gov/facts-and-figures-about-materials-waste-and-recycling/advancing-sustainable-materials-management-0

U.S. Environmental Protection Agency (EPA). (2023e). *Framework for cumulative risk assessment*. https://www.epa.gov/risk/framework-cumulative-risk-assessment#:~:text=Cumulative%20risk%20assessment%20is%20an,from%20multiple%20agents%20or%20stressors

U.S. Environmental Protection Agency (EPA). (2023f). *Ground water and drinking water*. https://www.epa.gov/ground-water-and-drinking-water

U.S. Environmental Protection Agency (EPA). (2023g). *Health impact assessments*. https://www.epa.gov/healthresearch/health-impact-assessments

U.S. Environmental Protection Agency (EPA). (2023h). *Human health risk assessment*. https://www.epa.gov/risk/human-health-risk-assessment

U.S. Environmental Protection Agency (EPA). (2023i). *Indoor air quality*. https://www.epa.gov/report-environment/indoor-air-quality

U.S. Environmental Protection Agency (EPA). (2023j). *Indoor air quality: What are the trends in indoor air quality and their effects on human health?* https://www.epa.gov/report-environment/indoor-air-quality#health

U.S. Environmental Protection Agency (EPA). (2023k). *Integrated pest management (IPM) principles.* https://www.epa.gov/ipm

U.S. Environmental Protection Agency (EPA). (2023l). *Our nation's air: Trends through 2022.* https://gispub.epa.gov/air/trendsreport/2022/#sources

U.S. Environmental Protection Agency (EPA). (2023m). *Overview of EPA's Brownfields Program.* https://www.epa.gov/brownfields/overview-epas-brownfields-program

U.S. Environmental Protection Agency (EPA). (2023n). *Radiation basics.* https://www.epa.gov/radiation/radiation-basics

U.S. Environmental Protection Agency (EPA). (2023o). *Radon frequently asked questions.* https://www.epa.gov/radon/radon-frequently-asked-questions

U.S. Environmental Protection Agency (EPA). (2023p). *Sources of electric and magnetic radiation.* https://www.epa.gov/radtown/sources-electric-and-magnetic-radiation

U.S. Environmental Protection Agency (EPA). (2023q). *Using the air quality index.* https://www.airnow.gov/aqi/aqi-basics/using-air-quality-index/

U.S. Food and Drug Administration (FDA). (2022). *FDA shares results on PFAS testing in seafood.* https://www.fda.gov/food/cfsan-constituent-updates/fda-shares-results-pfas-testing-seafood

U.S. Food and Drug Administration (FDA). (2023a). *Food.* https://www.fda.gov/food

U.S. Food and Drug Administration (FDA). (2023b). *How GMOs are regulated in the United States.* https://www.fda.gov/food/agricultural-biotechnology/how-gmos-are-regulated-united-states

U.S. Geological Survey (USGS). (2023a). *The water in you.* https://water.usgs.gov/edu/propertyyou.html

U.S. Geological Survey (USGS). (2023b). *Water quality data for pharmaceuticals, hormones and other organic wastewater contaminants in streams, 1999–2000.* http://toxics.usgs.gov/pubs/OFR-02-94/index.html

U.S. Global Change Research Program. (2023). *Fifth national climate assessment.* https://www.globalchange.gov/nca5

Wani, N. R., Rather, R. A., Farooq, A., Padder, S. A., Baba, T. R., Sharma, S., Mubarak, N. M., Khan, A. H., Singh, P., & Ara, S. (2023). New insights in food security and environmental sustainability through waste food management. *Environmental Science and Pollution Research International, 31*(12), 17835–17857. https://doi.org/10.1007/s11356-023-26462-y

Whitmee, S., Haines, A., Beyrer, C., Boltz, F., Capon, A. G., de Souza Dias, B. H., Ezeh, A., Frumkin, H., Gong, P., Head, P., Horton, R., Mace, G. M., Marten, R., Myers, S. S., Nishtar, S., Osofsky, S. A., Pattanayak, S. K., Pongsiri, M. J., Romanelli, C., ... Yach, D. (2015). Safeguarding human health in the Anthropocene epoch: Report of The Rockefeller Foundation-Lancet Commission on planetary health. *The Lancet, 386*(10007), 1973–2028. https://www.thelancet.com/journals/lancet/article/PIIS0140-6736(15)60901-1/fulltext

Wood, M. R. (2019, July 2). How the Flint water crisis set students back: Lead-poisoned children struggle to keep up with their peers academically and socially. *Pittsburgh Post-Gazette*, A-9.

World Bank. (2021). *Millions on the move in their own countries: The human face of climate change.* https://www.worldbank.org/en/news/feature/2021/09/13/millions-on-the-move-in-their-own-countries-the-human-face-of-climate-change

World Health Organization (WHO). (2023). *Drinking water.* https://www.who.int/news-room/fact-sheets/detail/drinking-water

Zhu, C., Kobayashi, K., Loladze, I., Zhu, J., Jiang, Q., Xy, X., Liu, G., Seneweera, S., Ebi, K. L., Drewnowski, A., Fukagawa, N. K., & Ziska, L. (2018). Carbon dioxide (CO_2) levels this century will alter the protein, micronutrients, and vitamin content of rice grains with potential health consequences for the poorest rice-dependent countries. *Science Advances, 4*(5), eaaq 1012.

CHAPTER 10

Ackley, B. J., Ladwig, G. B., Makic, M. B., Martinez-Kratz, M., & Zanotti, M. (2020). *Nursing diagnosis handbook: An evidence-based guide to planning care* (12th ed.). Elsevier.

Addicks, S. H., & McNeil, D. W. (2019). Randomized controlled trial of motivational interviewing to support breastfeeding among Appalachian women. *Journal of Obstetric, Gynecologic, and Neonatal Nursing, 48*(4), 418–432.

Agency for Healthcare Research and Quality (AHRQ). (2019). *Cultural competence and patient safety.* https://psnet.ahrq.gov/perspective/cultural-competence-and-patient-safety

Agency for Healthcare Research and Quality (AHRQ). (2021). *Approach to improving patient safety: Communication.* https://psnet.ahrq.gov/perspective/approach-improving-patient-safety-communication

American Society for Quality. (2023). *What is nominal group technique?* https://asq.org/quality-resources/nominal-group-technique

American Telemedicine Association. (2019). *Telehealth nursing: A position statement from the Telehealth Special Interest Group of the American Telemedicine Association.* https://www.americantelemed.org/?s=Telehealth+Nursing%3A+A+position+statement

Analytics Insight. (2021). *The 4 V's of big data- what is big data?* https://www.analyticsinsight.net/the-four-vs-of-big-data-what-is-big-data/

Apperson, A., Stellefson, M., Paige, S. R., Chaney, B., Chaney, J. D., Wang, M. Q., & Mohan, A. (2019). Facebook groups on chronic obstructive pulmonary disease: Social media content analysis. *International Journal of Environmental Research and Public Health, 16*(20), 3789. https://doi:10.3390/ijerph16203789

Arais, A. (2021). *NCG medical- a healthcare practice's guide to texting patients.* https://education.ncgmedical.com/blog/texting-patients-how-to-handle-communication-preferences-in-a-digital-world#hipaa-texting-rules

ArcUser Online. (n.d.). *GIS for healthcare: Using GIS for public health.* https://www.esri.com/news/arcuser/0499/umbrella.html

Arnold, E. C., & Boggs, K. U. (2020). *Interpersonal relationships: Professional communication skills for nurses* (8th ed.). Elsevier.

Association of State and Territorial Health Officials (ASTHO). (2023). *Telehealth.* https://www.astho.org/topic/population-health-prevention/healthcare-access/telehealth/

Bevilacqua, R., Strano, S., Rosa, M. D., Giammarchi, C., Cerna, K. K., Mueller, C., & Maranesi, E. (2021). E-health literacy: from theory to clinical application for digital health improvement. Results from the ACCESS training experience. *International Journal of Environmental Research and Public Health, 18*(22), 11800. https://doi:10.3390/ijerph182211800

Bilkey, G., Burns, B., Coles, E., Mahede, T., Baynam, G., & Nowak, K. (2019). Optimizing precision medicine for public health. *Frontiers in Public Health*, 7(42) 10.3389/fpubh.2019.00042

Bryne, A., Baldwin, A., & Harvey, C. (2020). Whose centre is it anyway? Defining person-centered in nursing: An integrative review. *PLoS One, 15*(3), e0229923. https://doi:10.1371/journal.pone.0229923

Cain, C. L., Surbone, A., Elk, R., & Kagawa-Singer, M. (2018). Culture and palliative care: Preferences, communication, meaning, and mutual decision making. *Journal of Pain and Symptom Management, 55*(5), 1408–1491. https://doi:10.1016/j.jpainsymman.2018.01.007

Call, G. (2022). *Medical Economics- telehealth post-COVID: Going digital to reduce costs.* from https://www.medicaleconomics.com/view/telehealth-post-covid-going-digital-to-reduce-costs-

Center for Creative Leadership. (2022). *6 steps for more effective active listening.* https://www.ccl.org/articles/leading-effectively-articles/coaching-others-use-active-listening-skills/

Centers for Disease Control and Prevention (CDC). (2020). *GIS at CDC.* https://www.cdc.gov/gis/gis-at-cdc.htm

Centers for Disease Control and Prevention (CDC). (2021). *Cultural Competence in Health and Human Service.* https://npin.cdc.gov/pages/cultural-competence#what

Centers for Disease Control and Prevention (CDC). (2022a). *Health effects of lead exposure.* https://www.cdc.gov/nceh/lead/prevention/health-effects.htm

Centers for Disease Control and Prevention (CDC). (2022b). *eHealth literacy.* https://www.cdc.gov/healthliteracy/researchevaluate/eHealth.html

Centers for Disease Control and Prevention (CDC). (2023a). *The CDC clear communication index.* https://www.cdc.gov/ccindex/

Centers for Disease Control and Prevention (CDC). (2023b). *What is health literacy?* https://www.cdc.gov/healthliteracy/learn/index.html

Central Intelligence Agency (CIA). (2021). *The world factbook: Mobile cellular telephone subscribers.* https://www.cia.gov/the-world-factbook/field/telephones-mobile-cellular/

Cole, J. (1990). *Filtering people: Understanding and confronting our prejudice.* New Society Publishers.

Colorado Department of Health and Environment. (2023). *Exposure notifications.* https://covid19.colorado.gov/Exposure-notifications

Community Toolbox. (2023). *Training for conflict resolution.* https://ctb.ku.edu/en/table-of-contents/implement/provide-information-enhance-skills/conflict-resolution/main

Coughlin, S., Vernon, M., Hatzigeorgiou, C., & George, V. (2020). Health literacy, social determinants of health, and disease prevention and control. *Journal of Environmental Health Science*, 6(1), 3061. from https://www.ncbi.nlm.nih.gov/pmc/articles/PMC7889072/

Council of Public Health Nurse Organizations (CPHNO). (2018). *Community/public health nursing competencies.* https://www.cphno.org/wp-content/uploads/2020/08/QCC-C-PHN-COMPETENCIES-Approved_2018.05.04_Final-002.pdf

Davidson, A., Kelly, J., Ball, L., Morgan, M., & Reidlinger, D. (2022). What do patients experience? Interprofessional collaborative practice for chronic conditions in primary care: An integrative review. *BMC Primary Care, 23*(8). https://bmcprimcare.biomedcentral.com/articles/10.1186/s12875-021-01595-6

Decker, M. J., Harrison, S., Price, M., Gutmann-Gonzalez, A., Yarger, J., & Tenney, R. (2022). Educator's perspectives on integrating technology into sexual health education: Implementation study. *JMIR Human Factors, 9*(1), e31381. https://doi:10.2196/31381

DePriest, K., Shields, T. M., & Curriero, F. C. (2019). Returning to our roots: The use of geospatial data for nurse-led community research. *Research in Nursing & Health, 42*(6), 467–475. https://doi:10.1002/nurs.21984

Dobber, J., Latoour, C., Snaterse, M., van Meijel, B., Ter Riet, G., Reimer, W. S., & Peters, R. (2019). Developing nurses' skills in motivational interviewing to promote a healthy lifestyle in patients with coronary artery disease. *European Journal of Cardiovascular Nursing, 18*(1), 38–37. https://doi:10.1177/1474515118784102

Donelan, K., Barreto, E. A., Sossong, S., Michael, C., Estrada, J. J., Cohen, A. B., ... Schwamm, L. H. (2019). Patient and clinician experiences with telehealth for patient follow-up care. *American Journal of Managed Care, 25*(1), 40–44.

Environmental Factor. (2024). *Responding to the East Palestine, Ohio, train derailment.* https://factor.niehs.nih.gov/2024/3/feature/1-feature-train-derailment-research

Erunal, M., Ozkaya, B., Mert, H., & Kucukguclu, O. (2019). Investigation of health literacy levels of nursing students and affecting factors. *International Journal of Caring Sciences, 12*(1), 270–277.

FAIR Health. (2019). *FH healthcare indicators and FH medical price index 2019: An annual review of place of service trends and medical pricing.* FAIR Health White Paper. https://s3.amazonaws.com/media2.fairhealth.org/whitepaper/asset/FH%20Healthcare%20Indicators%20and%20FH%20Medical%20Price%20Index%202019%20-%20A%20FAIR%20Health%20White%20Paper.pdf

Fernandez-Gonzalez, M., Monge-Pereira, E., Collado-Vazquez, S., Baeza, P., Cuesta-Gomez, A., Ona-Simbana, E. D., ... Cano-dela Cuerda, R. (2019). Leap motional controlled video game-based therapy for upper limb rehabilitation in patients with Parkinson's disease: A feasibility study. *Journal of NeuroEngineering and Rehabilitation, 16*(1), 133.

Gaines, K. (2023). *Updated map: Enhanced Nursing Licensure Compact (eNLC).* April 2023 Retrieved from https://nurse.org/articles/enhanced-compact-multi-state-license-eNLC/

Gallagher, E., Alvarez, E., Jin, L., Guenter, D., Hatcher, L., & Furlan, A. (2022). Patient contracts for chronic medical conditions: A scoping review. *Canadian Family Physician*, 68(5), e169–e177. https://doi:10.46747/cfp.6805e169

Gomez, H., Borgialli, D., Sharman, M., Shah, K., Scolpino, A., Oleske, J., & Bogden, J. (2019). Analysis of blood lead levels in Flint, Michigan before and during the 18-month switch to Flint River water. *Clinical Toxicology, 57*(9), 790–797. https://doi:10.1080/15563650.2018.1552003

Graetz, I., Huang, J., Brand, R., Hsu, J., & Reed, M. (2019). Mobile-accessible personal health records increase the frequency and timeliness of PHR use for patients with diabetes. *Journal of the American Medical Informatics Association*, 26(1), 50–54. https://doi:10.1093/jamia/ocy129

Gulanik, M., & Myers, J. (2022). *Nursing care plans: Diagnosis, interventions and outcomes* (10th ed.). Elsevier.

Haque, S. F., & D'Souza, A. (2019). Motivational interviewing: The RULES, ACE, and OARS. *Current Psychiatry*, *18*(1), 27–28. https://cdn.mdedge.com/files/s3fs-public/issues/articles/cp01801027.pdf

Harmon, M., Joyce, B., Johnson, R., & Hicks, V. (2020). An exploratory survey of public health nurses' knowledge, skills, attitudes, and application of the Quad Council Competencies. *Public Health Nursing*, *37*(4). https://doi:10.111/phn.12716

Harolds, J., & Miller, L. (2022). Quality and safety in health care, part LXXX: The national database for nursing quality indicators and the practice environment scale of the nursing work index. *Clinical Nuclear Medicine*, *47*(6), e472–e474. https://doi:10.1097/RLU0000000000003275

Health Information and Management Systems Society. (2019). *Connected health: It's personal*. https://www.himss.org/resources/connected-health-its-personal

Health Resources and Services Administration (HRSA) (2022). *Health literacy*. https://www.hrsa.gov/about/organization/bureaus/ohe/health-literacy#:~:text=Personal%20health%20literacy%20is%20the,actions%20for%20themselves%20and%20others.

Hersh, E. (2019). *Improving patient experience and reducing cost by measuring outcomes*. Harvard T. H. Chan School of Public Health. https://www.hsph.harvard.edu/ecpe/improving-patient-experience-and-reducing-cost-by-measuring-outcomes/

Hu, Y. (2019). Helping is healing: Examining relationships between social support, intended audiences, and perceived benefits of mental health blogging. *Journal of Communication in Healthcare*, *12*(2), 112–120. https://doi:10.1080/17538068.2019.1588491

Interexy. (2023). *9 hottest healthcare mobile app trends to watch for in 2023*. https://interexy.com/8-hottest-healthcare-mobile-app-trends-to-watch-for-in-2023/

Jen, M., Mechanic, O., & Teoli, D. (2022). *Informatics*. StatPearls. https://www.ncbi.nlm.nih.gov/books/NBK470564/

Johansson, B., & Martensson, L. B. (2019). Ways of strategies to knowing the patient described by nursing students. *Nurse Education in Practice*, *38*, 120–125.

Kearly, A., & Oputa, J. (November 5, 2019). *Telehealth state capacity survey*. Association of State and Territorial Health Officials (ASTHO). http://www.astho.org/Programs/Clinical-to-Community-Connections/Documents/ASTHO-Telehealth-Capacity-Survey_2019-APHA-Presentation/

Kernebeck, S., Busse, T. S., Bottcher, M. D., Weitz, J., Ehlers, J., & Bork, U. (2022). Impact of mobile health and medical applications on clinical practice in gastroenterology. *World Journal of Gastroenterology*, *26*(29), 4182–4197. https://doi:10.3748/wjg.v26.i29.4182

Knowles, M., Krasniansky, A., & Nagappan, A. (2023). *Consumer adoption of digital health in 2022: Moving at the speed of trust*. https://rockhealth.com/insights/consumer-adoption-of-digital-health-in-2022-moving-at-the-speed-of-trust/#:~:text=In%20our%202022%20Survey%2C%2080,long%20been%20underserved%20within%20healthcare

Kossenniemi, J., Leino-Kilpi, H., Puukka, P., & Suhonen, R. (2019). Respect and its associated factors as perceived by older patients. *Journal of Clinical Nursing*, *28*(21-22), 3848–3857. https://doi:10.1111/jocn.15013

Kumar, R., Sahu, M., & Rodney, T. (2022). Efficacy of motivational interviewing and brief interventions on tobacco use among healthy adults: A systematic review of randomized controlled trials. *Nursing Research and Education*, *40*(3), e03. https://doi:10.17533/udea.iee.v40n3e03

Lee, J. E., Zeng, N., Oh, Y., Lee, D., & Gao, Z. (2021). Effects of Pokémon GO on physical activity and psychological and social outcomes: A systematic review. *Journal of Clinical Medicine*, *10*(9), 1860. https://doi:10.3390/jcm10091860

Lopes, J. B., Duarte, N., Lazzari, L. D., & Oliveria, C. S. (2020). Virtual reality in the rehabilitation process for individuals with cerebral palsy and downs syndrome: A systematic review. *Journal of Bodywork and Movement Therapies*, *24*(4), 479–483. https://doi:10.1016/j.jbmt.2018.06.006

Lyamu, I., Tu, A., Gomez-Ramirez, O., Ablona, A., Chang, H., McKee, G., & Gilbert, M. (2021). Defining digital public health and the role of digitization, digitalization, and digital transformation: Scoping review. *JMIR public health and surveillance*, 7(11), e30399. https://doi:10.2196/30399

Mansouri, F., & Darvishpour, A. (2023). Mobile health applications in the COVID-19 pandemic: A scoping review of the reviews. *Medical Journal of the Islamic Republic of Iran*, *37*, 8. https://doi:10.47176/mjiri.37.8

Masri, S., Jia, J., Li, C., Zhou, G., Lee, M. C., Yan, G., & Wu, J. (2019). The use of twitter data to improve Zika surveillance in the United Stated during the 2016 epidemic. *BMC Public Health*, *19*(1), 761. https://doi: 10.1186/s12889-019-7103-8

Mataxen, P. A. (2019). Licensure barriers to telehealth nursing practice. *Nursing2020*, *49*(11), 67–68.

McCool, J., Dobson, R., Whittaker, R., & Paton, C. (2022). Mobile Health (mHealth) in low-and middle-income countries. *Annual Review of Public Health*, *43*, 525–539. https://doi:10.1146/annurev-publhealth-052620-093850

McGreevy, S., Murray, M., Montero, L., Gibson, C., Comfort, B., Barry, M., Kirmer-Voss, K., Coy, A., Zufer, T., Rampon, K., & Woodward, J. (2023). Assessing the immunization information system and electronic health records interface accuracy for COVID-19 vaccination. *JAMIA*, *6*(2), ooad026. https://doi:10.1093/jamiaopen/ooad026

Mesters, I., van Keulen, H. M., de Vries, H., & Brug, J. (2022). Intervention fidelity of telephone motivational interviewing on physical activity fruit intake and vegetable consumption in Dutch outpatients with and without hypertension. *International Journal of Behavioral Medicine*, *30*, 108–121.

mHealth Intelligence. (2022). *Key features of mHealth apps and trends in use*. From https://mhealthintelligence.com/features/key-features-of-mhealth-apps-trends-in-use

Miller, W. R., & Rollnick, S. (2013). *Motivational interviewing: Helping people change*. The Guilford Press.

Mills, J., Fox, J., Damarell, R., Tieman, J., & Yates, P. (2021). Palliative care providers use of digital health and perspectives on technological innovation: A national study. *BMC Palliative Care*, *20*(124). https://doi:10.1186/s12904-021-00822-2

Minnesota Department of Health. (2022a). *Multivoting*. https://www.health.state.mn.us/communities/practice/resources/phqitoolbox/nominalgroup.html#:~:text=Sources-,What%20is%20multivoting%3F,equal%20participation%20in%20the%20process

Minnesota Department of Health. (2022b). *Public Health Interventions: Applications for public health nursing practice* (2nd ed.). https://www.health.state.mn.us/communities/practice/research/phncouncil/docs/PHInterventions.pdf

Mobile Health Technologies and Global Markets. (2022). *Mobile health technologies and global markets report*. from https://www.researchandmarkets.com/reports/4556072/mobile-health-mhealth-technologies-and-global?utm_source=GNOM&utm_medium=PressRelease&utm_code=3l6lvj&utm_campaign=1707150+-+Key+Trends+and+Opportunities+in+the+Global+mHealth+Market+to+2026%3a+Focus+on+Medical+Devices+and+Mobile+Health+Apps+&utm_exec=cari18prd

Molina-Mula, J., & Gallo-Estrada, J. (2020). Impact of nurse-patient relationship on quality of care and patient autonomy in decision-making. *International Journal of Environmental Research and Public Health*, *17*(3), 835. https://doi:10.3390/ijerph17030835

National Institute of Health (NIH). (2018). *Community-based participatory research*. https://www.nimhd.nih.gov/programs/extramural/community-based-participatory.html

National Patient-Centered Clinical Research Network (PCORnet). (n.d.). *Home*. https://pcornet.org/

Ngiam, K. Y., & Khor, I. W. (2019). Big data and machine learning algorithms for health-care delivery. *Lancet Oncology*, *20*(6), 293. https://doi:10.1016/s1470-2045(19)30149-4

Norman, C. D., & Skinner, H. A. (2006). eHealth literacy: Essential skills for consumer health in a networked world. *Journal of Medical Internet Research*, *8*(2), e9.

Office of the National Coordinator for Health Information Technology (ONC). (2023). *What is an electronic health record (EHR)?* Retrieved from https://www.healthit.gov/faq/what-electronic-health-record-ehr

Oz, H. S., & Buyuksoy, G. D. (2022). The effects of motivational interview on healthy behaviors and quality of life in the uncontrolled type 2 diabetes patient. I*nternational Journal of Caring Sciences*, *15*(2), 1194–1201.

Perrin, A. (2021). *Some digital divides exist between rural, urban and suburban America*. Pew Research Center. https://www.pewresearch.org/fact-tank/2019/05/31/digital-gap-between-rural-and-nonrural-america-persists/

Pew Research Center. (April 7, 2021). *Mobile fact sheet*. https://www.pewresearch.org/internet/fact-sheet/mobile/

Pratt, H., Moroney, T., & Middleton, R. (2020). The influence of engaging authentically on nurse-patient relationships: A scoping review. *Nursing Inquiry*, *29*(2), e12388. https://doi:10.1111/nin.12388

Psychology today. (2023). *Motivational interviewing*. https://www.psychologytoday.com/us/therapy-types/motivational-interviewing

Public Health Leadership Forum. (2020). *Partnering to catalyze comprehensive community wellness: An actionable framework for health care and public health collaboration*. Retrieved from https://hcttf.org/wp-content/uploads/2018/06/Comprehensive-Community-Wellness-Report.pdf

Pyron, L., & Carter-Templeton, H. (2019). Improved patient flow and provider efficiency after the implementation of an electronic health record. *Computers, Informatics, Nursing*, *17*(10), 513–521.

Reddy, G., & Barbalat, G. (2021). Bottom-up and top-down development: Nexus between asset-based community development and unconditional cash transfers. *Development in Practice*, *32*(1), 82–91. https://doi:10.1080/09614524.2021.1937544

Richwine, C., Johnson, C., & Patel, V. (2023). Disparities in patient portal access and the role of providers in encouraging access and use. *Journal of the American Medical Informatics Association*, *30*(2), 308–317. https://doi:10.1093/jamia/ocac227

Ruckart, P. Z., Ettinger, A. S., Hanna-Attisha, M., Jones, N., Davis, S., & Breysse, P. N. (2019). The Flint water crisis: A coordinated public health emergency response and recovery initiative. *Journal of Public Health Management and Practice*, *25*(1), s84–s90. https://doi:10.1097/PHH.0000000000000871

Salik, I., & Ashurst, J. V. (2023). *Closed loop communication training in medical simulation*. StatPearls Publishing. https://www.ncbi.nlm.nih.gov/books/NBK549899/

SAS. (2023). *Big data analytics: What it is and why it matters*. https://www.sas.com/en_us/insights/analytics/big-data-analytics.html

Serin, E. K., & Tuluce, D. (2021). Determining nursing students' attitudes and empathetic tendencies regarding age discrimination. *Perspectives in Psychiatric Care*, *57*(1), 380–389. https://doi:10.111/ppc.12652

Shahid, R., Shoker, M., Chu, L. M., Frelick, R., Ward, H., & Pahwa, P. (2022). Impact of low health literacy on patients' health outcomes: A multicenter cohort study. *BMC Health Services Research*, *22*(1), 1148. https://doi:10.1186/s12913-022-08527-9

Siwicki, B. (September 9, 2019). *How asynchronous telemedicine saved SSM Health 18 minutes per visit*. Healthcare IT News. https://www.healthcareitnews.com/news/how-asynchronous-telemedicine-saved-ssm-health-18-minutes-visit

Sormunen, Y., Westerbotn, M., Aanesen, A., Fossum, B., & Karlgren, K. (2021). Social media in the infertile community—Using a text analysis tool to identify the topics of discussion on the multitude of infertility blogs. *Women's Health*, *17*. https://doi:10.1177/17455065211063280

Suleiman-Martos, N., Garcia-Lara, R., Albendin-Garcia, L., Romero-Bejar, J., Canadas-Del la Fuente, G., Monsalve-Reyes, C., & Gomez-Urquiza, J. (2022). Effects of active video games on physical function in independent community-dwelling older adults: A systematic review and meta-analysis. *Journal of Advanced Nursing*, *78*(5), 1228–1244. https://doi:10.1111/jan.15138

Symanski, E., Han, H. A., McCurdy, S., Hopkins, L., Flores, J., Han, I., Smith, M. A., Caldwell, J., Frontenot, C., Wyatt, B., & Markham, C. (2023). Data to action: Community-based participatory research to address concerns about metal air pollution in overburdened neighborhoods near metal recycling facilities in Houston. *Environmental Health Perspectives*, *131*(6), 67006. https://doi:10.1289/EHP11405

Tao, G., Garrett, B., Taverner, T., Cordingley, E., & Sun, C. (2021). Immersion virtual reality health games: A narrative review of game design. *Journal of NeuroEngineering and Rehabilitation*, *18*(31). https://doi:10.1186/s12984-020-00801-3

TEConomy Partners. (2020). *Video games in the 21st century: A 2020 economic impact report*. https://www.theesa.com/wp-content/uploads/2019/02/Video-Games-in-the-21st-Century-2020-Economic-Impact-Report-Final.pdf

The Arts Development Company. (2023). *Working together for creative change*. https://theartsdevelopmentcompany.org.uk/resources/good-to-know-1/what-is-vlogging-2/

The HIPAA Journal. (2023). *Text messaging in healthcare*. https://www.hipaajournal.com/text-messaging-in-health-care/

Tornetta, T. (2021). *Physicians practice- texting patients is now an expectation*. https://www.physicianspractice.com/view/texting-patients-is-now-an-expectation

Tsai, C. H., Eghdam, A., Davoody, N., Wright, G., Flowerday, S., & Koch, S. (2020). Effects of electronic health records implementation and barriers to adoption and use: A scoping review and qualitative analysis of the content. *Life, 10*(12), 327. https://doi:10.3390/life10120327

U.S Government Accountability Office. (2021). *COVID-19 exposure notification apps are available. But are they working?* https://www.gao.gov/blog/covid-19-exposure-notification-apps-are-available.-are-they-working

U.S. Department of Health and Human Services (USDHHS). (2020a). *Browse 2030 objectives*. Retrieved from https://health.gov/healthypeople/objectives-and-data/browse-objectives

U.S. Department of Health and Human Services (USDHHS). (2020b). *2030 Health communication and health information technology*. https://health.gov/healthypeople/about/workgroups/health-communication-and-health-information-technology-workgroup

U.S. Department of Health and Human Services: Office of Disease Prevention & Promotion. (2021). *National action plan to improve health literacy*. Retrieved from https://health.gov/our-work/national-health-initiatives/health-literacy/national-action-plan-improve-health-literacy

U.S. Department of Health and Human Services: Office of Disease Prevention & Promotion. (2023). *The promise of precision medicine*. https://www.nih.gov/about-nih/what-we-do/nih-turning-discovery-into-health/promise-precision-medicine#:~:text=Precision%20medicine%20is%20an%20innovative,grown%20directly%20from%20biomedical%20research.

U.S. Food and Drug Administration. (2020). *What is digital health?* https://www.fda.gov/medical-devices/digital-health-center-excellence/what-digital-health

U.S. Food and Drug Administration. (2022). *Device software functions including mobile medical applications*. https://www.fda.gov/medical-devices/digital-health-center-excellence/device-software-functions-including-mobile-medical-applications#:~:text=exercise%20enforcement%20discretion.-,Does%20the%20FDA%20regulate%20mobile%20devices%2C%20such%20as%20smartphones%20or,use%20of%20smartphones%20or%20tablets.

United States Geological Service (SGS). (n.d.). *What is geographic information system (GIS)?* https://www.usgs.gov/faqs/what-geographic-information-system-gis

Valdez, R., & Rogers, C. (2022). Consumer health informatics for racial and ethnic minoritized communities: Minor progress, major opportunities. *Yearbook of Medical Informatics, 31*(1), 167–172. https://doi:10.1055/s-0042-1742520

Verwijs, M. H., Puijk-Hekman, S., van der Heijden, H., Vasse, E., de Groot, L., & de van der Schueren, M. (2020). Interdisciplinary communication and collaboration as key to improved nutritional care of malnourished older adults across health care settings: A qualitative study. *Health Expectations, 23*, 1096–1107. https://doi:10.1111/hex.13075

Vowell, C. (2020). *Motivational interviewing: 30+ tools, affirmations and more*. from https://positivepsychology.com/motivational-interviewing-exercises/

Wagner, B., Rosenberg, N., Hofmann, L., & Maass, U. (2020). Web-based bereavement care: A systematic review and meta-analysis. *Frontiers in Psychiatry, 11*, 525. https://doi:10.3389/fpsyt.2020.00525

Wang, G., Zhao, Y., & Xie, F. (2022). Study on nursing effects if diabetic health education nursing methods applied to diabetes patients in the endocrinology department. *Journal of Healthcare Engineering, 4* https://doi:10.1155/2022/3363096

West Chester University (WCU). (2022). *Tuckman's stages of group development*. https://www.wcupa.edu/coral/tuckmanStagesGroupDelvelopment.aspx

Whittington, K., Walker, J., & Hirsch, B. (2020). Promoting interdisciplinary education as a vital function of effective team work to positively impact patient outcomes, satisfaction, and employee engagement. *Journal of Medical Imaging and Radiation Sciences, 51*(4), s107–s111. https://doi:10.1016.j.jmir.2020.07.002

Wilson, J. (2022). 10 effective brainstorming techniques for teams. https://www.wework.com/ideas/professional-development/creativity-culture/effective-brainstorming-techniques

Winn, R. (2023). What is a podcast and how do they work? https://www.podcastinsights.com/what-is-a-podcast/

Yeung, A. W., Kletecka-Pulker, M., Eibensteiner, F., Plunger, P., Volkl-Kernstock, S., Willschke, H., & Atanasov, A. (2021). Implications of twitter in health-related research: A landscape analysis of the scientific literature. *Frontiers in Public Health, 9*, 654481. https://doi:10.3389/fpubh.2021.654481

Zeydeni, A., Atashzadeh-Shoorideh, F., Abdi, F., Hosseini, M., Zohari-Anboohi, S., & Skerrett, V. (2021). Effects of community-based education on undergraduate nursing students' skills: A systematic review. *BMC Nurse, 20*. https://doi:10.1186/s12912-021-00755-4

Zhu, R., Han, S., Su, Y., Zhang, C., & Duan, Z. (2019). The application of big data and the development of nursing science: A discussion paper. *International Journal of Nursing Science, 6*(2), 229–234. https://doi:10.1016/j.ijnss.2019.03.001

CHAPTER 11

Agency for Healthcare Research and Quality. (2020a). *Health literacy universal precautions toolkit* (2nd ed.). https://www.ahrq.gov/health-literacy/improve/precautions/tool5.html#:~:text=The%20teach%2Dback%20method%20is,a%20manner%20your%20patients%20understand

Agency for Healthcare Research and Quality. (2020b). *The SHARE approach-using the teach-back method: A reference guide for healthcare professionals*. https://www.ahrq.gov/health-literacy/professional-training/shared-decision/tool/resource-6.html

Association of American Medical Colleges (AAMC). (2023). *2022 Physician specialty data report*. https://www.aamc.org/media/63371/download?attachment

Bandura, A. (1977). *Social learning theory*. Prentice-Hall

Bandura, A. (1986). *Social foundations of thought and action: A social cognitive theory*. Prentice-Hall

Barrow, J. M., Annamaraju, P., & Toney-Butler, T. J. (2022). *Change management*. National Library of Medicine. https://www.ncbi.nlm.nih.gov/books/NBK459380/

Bartholomew, L. K., Markham, C., Mullen, P., & Fernandez, M. E. (2015). Planning models for theory-based health promotion interventions. In K. Glanz, B. K. Rimer & K. Viswanath (Eds.), *Health behavior: Theory, research, and practice* (5th ed., pp. 359–388). Jossey-Bass

Bastable, S. B., Gramet, P., Sopczyk, D. L., Jacobs, K., & Braungort, M. M. (2020). *Health professional as educator: Principles of teaching and learning* (2nd ed.). Jones & Bartlett Learning

Bechard, L. E., Bergelt, M., Neudorf, B., DeSouza, T. E., & Middleton, L. E. (2021). Using the Health Belief Model to understand age differences in perceptions and responses to the COVID-19 pandemic. *Frontiers in Psychology, 12*, 609893. https://doi.org/10.3389/fpsyg.2021.609893

Bloom, B. (Ed.). (1956). Taxonomy of educational objectives: The classification of educational goals. *Handbook I: Cognitive domain*. Longman

Centers for Disease Control and Prevention (CDC). (2019). *Health communication basics*. https://www.cdc.gov/healthcommunication/healthbasics/WhatIsHC.html

Centers for Disease Control and Prevention (CDC). (2022a). *Social determinants of health at CDC*. https://cdc.gov/about/sdoh/index.html

Centers for Disease Control and Prevention (CDC). (2022b). *Health communication strategies and resources*. https://npin.cdc.gov/pages/health-communication-strategies#planning

Centers for Disease Control and Prevention (CDC). (2022c). *Health equity guiding principles for inclusive communication*. https://www.cdc.gov/healthcommunication/Health_Equity.html

Centers for Disease Control and Prevention (CDC). (2023a). *Adolescent and school health*. https://www.cdc.gov/healthyyouth/disparities/index.htm

Centers for Disease Control and Prevention (CDC). (2023b). *Social determinants of health*. https://www.cdc.gov/publichealthgateway/sdoh/index.html

Comen, E. (2022). Greatest public health achievements of the 21st century. *24/7 Wallstreet: Special report*. https://247wallst.com/special-report/2022/06/23/greatest-public-health-achievements-of-the-21st-century/

Duran, D. G., & Pérez-Stable, E. J. (2019). Novel approaches to advance minority health and health disparities research. *American Journal of Public Health, 109*, S8–S10. https://doi.org/10.2105/AJPH.2018.304931

Glanz, K., Rimer, B. K., & Viswanath, K. (Eds.). (2015). *Health behavior: Theory, research, and practice*. Jossey-Bass

Green, J., Cross, R., Woodall, J., & Tones, K. (2019). *Health promotion: Planning and strategies* (4th ed.). Sage

Green, L. W., Gielen, A. C., Ottoson, J. M., Peterson, D. V., & Kreuter, M. W. (Eds.). (2022). *Health program planning, implementation, and evaluation: Creating behavioral, environmental, and policy change* (p. 17). Johns Hopkins University Press

Green, L. W., & Kreuter, M. W. (2005). *Health program planning: An educational and ecological approach* (4th ed.). McGraw Hill

Havelock, R. G., & Havelock, M. C. (1973). *Training for change agents: A guide to the design of training programs in education and other fields*. Inst for Social Research the Univ.

Health Resources & Service Administration (HRSA). (2019). *Health literacy*. https://www.hrsa.gov/about/organization/bureaus/ohe/health-literacy/index.html

Huerto, R., & Lindo, E. (2020). Minority patients benefit from having minority doctors, but that's a hard match to make. *The Conversation*. https://theconversation.com/minority-patients-benefit-from-having-minority-doctors-but-thats-a-hard-match-to-make-130504#:~:text=Mounting%20evidence%20suggests%20when%20physicians,patient%20perceptions%20of%20treatment%20decisions

Institute of Medicine. (2003). *Unequal treatment: Confronting racial and ethnic disparities in healthcare*. The National Academies Press. Iowa State University Center for Excellence in Learning and Theory. 2019. Revised Bloom's taxonomy. http://www.celt.iastate.edu/teaching/effective-teaching-practices/revised-blooms-taxonomy/

Kaiser Family Foundation. (2023a). *What is driving widening racial disparities in life expectancy?* https://www.kff.org/racial-equity-and-health-policy/issue-brief/what-is-driving-widening-racial-disparities-in-life-expectancy/

Kaiser Family Foundation. (2023b). *Health coverage by rage and ethnicity, 2010-2021*. https://www.kff.org/racial-equity-and-health-policy/issue-brief/health-coverage-by-race-and-ethnicity/#:~:text=Coverage%20by%20Race%20and%20Ethnicity%20as%20of%202021&text=Nonelderly%20AIAN%20and%20Hispanic%20people,their%20White%20counterparts%20(7.2%25)

Kitchie, S. (2019). Determinants of learning. In S. B. Bastable, P. Gramet, K. Jacobs & D. L. Sopczyk (Eds.), *Health professional as educator: Principles of teaching and learning* (5th ed., pp. 119–168). Jones & Bartlett Learning.

Knowles, M. (1980). *The modern practice of adult education: Andragogy versus pedagogy* (2nd ed.). Follett.

Knowles, M. (1984). *The adult learner: A neglected species* (3rd ed.). Gulf.

Knowles, M. (1989). *The making of an adult educator: An autobiographical journey*. Jossey-Bass.

Knowles, M. (1990). *The adult learner: A neglected species* (4th ed.). Gulf Publishing.

Knowles, M. S., Holton, E. F., & Swanson, R. A. (2015). *The adult learner: The definitive classic in adult education and human resource development* (8th ed.). Routledge.

Kotter, J. P. (2012). *Leading change*. Harvard Business Review Press.

Lewin, K. (1947). Frontiers in group dynamics: Concept, method, and reality in social science; social equilibria and social change. *Human Relations, 1*(1), 5–41.

Lewin, K. (1951). *Field theory in social science: Selected theoretical papers*. Harper & Row.

Li, X., Yang, S., Wang, Y., Yang, B., & Zhang, J. (2020). Effects of a transtheoretical model-based intervention and motivational interviewing on the management of depression in hospitalized patients with coronary heart disease: a randomized controlled trial. *BMC Public Health, 20*, 420.

Lippitt, G. L. (1973). *Visualizing change: Model building and the change process*. University Associates.

Lippitt, R., Watson, J., & Westley, B. (1958). *The dynamics of planned change*. Harcourt.

Maslow, A. H. (1970). *Motivation and personality* (2nd ed.). Harper and Row.

Mayer, K. (2023). *Employees are delaying health care. Here's how employers can help*. SHRM. https://www.shrm.org/resourcesandtools/hr-topics/benefits/pages/employees-delaying-medical-health-care-employer-strategies.aspx

Medline Plus. (2019). *How to write easy-to-read health materials*. https://medlineplus.gov/etr.html

Miller, D. M., Linn, R., & Gronlund, N. E. (2021). *Measurement and assessment in teaching* (11th ed.). Pearson.

Miller, M. A., & Stoeckel, P. R. (2019). *Client education: Theory and practice* (3rd ed.). Jones & Bartlett.

Murdaugh, C. L., Parsons, M. A., & Pender, N. J. (2019). *Health promotion in nursing practice* (8th ed.). Prentice Hall.

National Association of Secondary School Principals. (2023). *Adolescent numeracy*. https://www.nassp.org/top-issues-in-education/position-statements/adolescent-numeracy/

Ndugga, N., & Artiga, S. (2023). *Disparities in health and health care: 5 key questions and answers*. Kaiser Family Foundation. https://www.kff.org/racial-equity-and-health-policy/issue-brief/disparities-in-health-and-health-care-5-key-question-and-answers/

Network of the National Library of Medicine. (n.d.). *Health literacy*. https://www.nnlm.gov/guides/intro-health-literacy

Office of Disease Prevention and Health Promotion. (2022). *Take a page out of Move Your Way's playbook: Actionable strategies to promote physical activity in your community*. https://health.gov/news/202210/take-page-out-move-your-ways-playbook-actionable-strategies-promote-physical-activity-your-community

Office of Disease Prevention and Health Promotion. (n.d.-a). *Browse Healthy People 2030 objectives*. https://health.gov/healthypeople/objectives-and-data/browse-objectives

Office of Disease Prevention and Health Promotion. (n.d.-b). *Healthy People 2030 framework*. https://health.gov/healthypeople/about/healthy-people-2030-framework#:~:text=Healthy%20People%202030's%20overarching%20goals,and%20well%2Dbeing%20of%20all

Office of Disease Prevention and Health Promotion. (n.d.-c). *Healthy People 2030: Social determinants of health*. https://health.gov/healthypeople/priority-areas/social-determinants-health

Office of Disease Prevention and Health Promotion. (n.d.-d). *Educational and community-based programs workgroup*. https://health.gov/healthypeople/about/workgroups/educational-and-community-based-programs-workgroup

Office of Disease Prevention and Health Promotion. (n.d.-e). *Health equity in Healthy People 2030*. https://health.gov/healthypeople/priority-areas/health-equity-healthy-people-2030

Office of Disease Prevention and Health Promotion. (n.d.-f). *Increase the health literacy of the population-HC-HIT-RO1*. https://health.gov/healthypeople/objectives-and-data/browse-objectives/health-communication/increase-health-literacy-population-hchit-r01

Olscamp, K., Pompano, L., Piercy, K. L., Oh, A., Barnett, E. Y., Lee, M. S., Fisher, D. G., & Bevinton, F. (2022). Understanding the impact of Move Your Way® campaign exposure on key physical activity outcomes: Results form a multi-site pilot evaluation. *Journal of Healthy Eating and Active Living*, *2*(3), 12–23.

Pavlov, I. P. (1957). *Experimental psychology and other essays*. Philosophical Library.

Pender, N. L., Murdaugh, C. L., & Parsons, M. A. (2015). *Health promotion in nursing practice* (7th ed.). Prentice Hall.

Piaget, J. (1966). *The origin of intelligence in children*. Norton.

Piaget, J. (1970). *Child's conception of movement and speed*. Routledge.

Prochaska, J. O., Norcross, J. C., & DiClemente, C. C. (2007). *Changing for good: A revolutionary six-stage program for overcoming bad habits and moving your life positively forward* (reprint ed.). William Morrow Paperbacks.

Raihan, N., & Cogburn, M. (2023). *Stages of change theory*. StatPearls Internet. National Library of Medicine. https://www.ncbi.nlm.nih.gov/books/NBK556005/

Readability Formulas. (2020). *The SMOG readability formula, a simple measure of gobbledygook*. https://readabilityformulas.com/smog-readability-formula.php

Robert Wood Johnson Foundation. (2023). *Racial, ethnic, and language concordance between patients and their usual healthcare providers*. https://www.rwjf.org/en/insights/our-research/2022/03/racial-ethnic-and-language-concordance-between-patients-and-their-usual-healthcare-providers.html

Rodriguez, S. (2023). *Rural-urban disparities in SUD treatment marked by rising inpatient care*. Patient Engagement Hit. https://patientengagementhit.com/news/rural-urban-disparities-in-sud-treatment-marked-by-rising-inpatient-care

Rogers, C. (1969). *Freedom to learn*. Merrill.

Rogers, C. (1989). *Freedom to learn for the eighties*. Merrill.

Rogers, E. M. (2003). *Diffusion of innovations* (5th ed.). Simon & Schuster.

Rosenstock, I. M. (1966). Why people use health services. *Milbank Memorial Fund Quarterly*, *44*, 94–127.

Roussel, L. A., Harris, J. L., & Thomas, T. (2020). *Management and leadership for nurse administrators* (7th ed.). Jones & Bartlett.

Rural Health Information Hub. (2023a). *Defining health promotion and disease prevention*. https://www.ruralhealthinfo.org/toolkits/health-promotion/1/definition

Rural Health Information Hub. (2023b). *The health belief model*. https://www.ruralhealthinfo.org/toolkits/health-promotion/2/theories-and-models/health-belief

Schunk, D. H. (2020). *Learning theories: An educational perspective*. Pearson.

Skinner, B. F. (1974). *About behaviorism*. Knopf.

Skinner, B. F. (1987). *Upon further reflection*. Prentice-Hall.

Spradley, B. W. (1980). Managing change creatively. *Journal of Nursing Administration*, *10*(5), 32–37.

Stevanovic, M., Weiste, E., & Uusitalo, L. L. (2022). Challenges of client participation in the co-development of social and health care services: Imbalances of control over action and the management of the interactional agenda. *SSM-Qualitative Research in Health*, *2*, 1–14.

The National Social Marketing Centre. (n.d.). *What is social marketing*. https://www.thensmc.com/content/what-social-marketing-1

The Omaha System. (2023). *Omaha system overview*. Retrieved from https://www.omahasystem.org/overview

Thorndike, E. L. (1932). *The fundamentals of learning*. Teachers College Press.

Thorndike, E. L. (1969). *Educational psychology*. Arno Press.

Tolbert, J., Drake, P., & Damico, A. (2022). *Key facts about the uninsured population*. Kaiser Family Foundation. https://www.kff.org/uninsured/issue-brief/key-facts-about-the-uninsured-population/

Vanderbilt University Center for Teaching. (2019). *Bloom's taxonomy*. https://cft.vanderbilt.edu/guides-sub-pages/blooms-taxonomy/

VARK Learn Limited. (2023). *VARK modalities: What do visual, aural, read/write, and kinesthetic really mean?* https://vark-learn.com/introduction-to-vark/the-vark-modalities/#:~:text=The%20acronym%20VARK%20stands%20for,experiences%20of%20students%20and%20teachers

West Health. (2022, March 31). *112 million Americans struggle to afford healthcare*. [Press release]. https://www.westhealth.org/press-release/112-million-americans-struggle-to-afford-healthcare/#:~:text=31%2C%202022%20%E2%80%94%20An%20estimated%20112,is%20not%20worth%20the%20cost.

Wolters Kluwer. (2022). *Five key barriers to healthcare access the United States*. https://www.wolterskluwer.com/en/expert-insights/five-key-barriers-to-healthcare-access-in-the-united-states

World Health Organization. (n.d.-a). *Social determinants of health*. https://www.who.int/health-topics/social-determinants-of-health#tab=tab_1

World Health Organization. (n.d.-b). *Quality of care*. https://www.who.int/health-topics/quality-of-care#tab=tab_1

Zhang, L., Yuan, X., & Dong, B. (2022). Analysis effects of Pender Health Promotion Model education on health behaviors and maternal and infant of cardiac disease in pregnancy. *Biotechnology & genetic engineering reviews*, 1–13. Advance online publication. https://doi.org/10.1080/02648725.2022.2159325

CHAPTER 12

Agency for Healthcare Research and Quality. (2022). *Collecting health data with electronic and paper chart audits*. Retrieved from: https://www.ahrq.gov/evidencenow/tools/data-collection.html

American Association of Colleges of Nursing. (2021). *The essentials. Domain 3: Population health*. Retrieved from https://www.aacnnursing.org/essentials/tool-kit/domains-concepts/population-health

American Nurses Association. (2022). *Public health nursing: Scope and standards of practice* (3rd ed.). Nursesbooks.

Arnos, D., Kroll, E., Jaromin, E., Daly, H., & Falkenburger, E. (2021, October 19). *Tools and resources for project-based community advisory boards*. Urban Institute. Retrieved from https://www.urban.org/research/publication/tools-and-resources-project-based-community-advisory-boards

Boulos, M. N. K., & Wilson, J. P. (2023). Geospatial techniques for monitoring and mitigating climate change and its effects on human health. *International Journal of Health Geographics*, *22*(2023), Article 2. https://doi:10.1186/s12942-023-00324-9

Brooks, D. (2020). Finding the road to character. *Y Magazine*. Retrieved from https://magazine.byu.edu/article/seeing-each-other-deeply/

Calanan, R. M., Bonds, M. E., Bedrosian, S. R., Laird, S. K., Satter, D. S., & Penman-Aguilar, A. (2023). CDC's guiding principles to promote an equity-centered approach to public health communication. *Prevention of Chronic Disease*, 20, e1-11. doi:10.5888/pcd20.230061

Castrucci, B. C., & Lupi, M. V. (2020, May 19). *When we need them most, the number of public health workers continues to decline*. deBeaumont. Retrieved from https://debeaumont.org/news/2020/when-we-need-them-most-the-number-of-public-health-workers-continues-to-decline/#:~:text=Since%20the%20Great%20Recession%2C%20state,fifth%20of%20the%20total%20workforce.&text=The%20number%20of%20employees%20in,is%20also%2

Centers for Disease Control and Prevention. (2020, April 9). Where malaria occurs. *Global health, division of parasitic diseases and malaria*. Retrieved from https://www.cdc.gov/malaria/about/distribution.html

Centers for Disease Control and Prevention. (2022, December 30). *Centers for disease control and prevention*. Gestational diabetes. Retrieved from https://www.cdc.gov/diabetes/basics/gestational.html#:~:text=Gestational%20diabetes%20is%20a%20type,are%20affected%20by%20gestational%20diabetes.

Centers for Disease Control and Prevention (CDC). (2023a, January 6). *QuickStats: Percentage of mothers with gestational diabetes,* by maternal age, National Vital Statistics System, United States, 2016 and 2021*. Morbidity and Mortality Weekly Report. Retrieved from https://www.cdc.gov/mmwr/volumes/72/wr/mm7201a4.htm#:~:text=Increases%20in%20gestational%20diabetes%20were,%3C20%20years%20(2.7%25)

Centers for Disease Control and Prevention (CDC). (2023b, October 3). *NCHS provide timely and accurate health statistics for the United States*. National Center for Health Statistics. Retrieved from https://www.cdc.gov/nchs/index.htm

Centers for Disease Control and Prevention (CDC). (2023c, August 30). *Quick facts on the risks of e-cigarettes for kids, teens and young adults*. Office on Smoking and Health, National Center for Chronic Disease Prevention and Health Promotion. Retrieved from https://www.cdc.gov/tobacco/basic_information/e-cigarettes/Quick-Facts-on-the-Risks-of-E-cigarettes-for-Kids-Teens-and-Young-Adults.html

Centers for Disease Control and Prevention (CDC). (2023d, August 23). *Office of policy, performance, and evaluation*. https://www.cdc.gov/evaluation/

Centers for Disease Control and Prevention (CDC). (2023e, October 2). *Social marketing guidance*. https://www.cdc.gov/stophivtogether/partnerships/social-marketing-toolkit.htm

Centers for Disease Control and Prevention (CDC). (2023f, May 3). *Gateway to health communication*. Retrieved from https://www.cdc.gov/healthcommunication/index.html

Centers for Disease Control and Prevention (CDC). (2023g, July 3). Digital and social media. Office of Communications. Retrieved from https://www.cdc.gov/digital-social-media-tools/index.html

Centers for Disease Control and Prevention (CDC). (2023h, September 26). *CDC's social media channels*. Office of Communications. Retrieved from https://www.cdc.gov/digital-social-media-tools/Social-Media-Channels.html

Community Preventive Services Task Force (CPSTF). (2023). About the community guide. *The Guide to Community Preventive Sources*. Retrieved from https://www.thecommunityguide.org/pages/about-community-guide.html

Conduent Healthy Communities Institute. (2023). *Community action research: An effective practice*. Retrieved from https://cdc.thehcn.net/promisepractice/index/view?pid=30159

Cusack, C., Cohen, B., Mignone, J., Chartier, M. J., & Lutfiyya, Z. (2018). Participatory action as a research method with public health nurses. *Journal of Advanced Nursing*, *74*(7), 1544–1553. https://doi:10.1111/jan.13555

deChesnay, M. (Ed.). (2015). *Nursing research using participatory action research: Qualitative designs and methods in nursing*. Springer Publishing.

Donabedian, A. (2003). *An introduction to quality assurance in health care*. Oxford University Press.

Doran, G. T. (1981). There's a S.M.A.R.T. way to write management's goals and objectives. *Management Review (American Management Association Forum)*, *70*(11), 35–36.

Dunham-Taylor, J. (2015). Organizations: Surviving within a chaotic, complex, value-based environment. In J. Dunham-Taylor & J. Z. Pinczuk (Eds.), *Financial management for nurse managers: Merging the heart with the dollar* (3rd ed., pp. 81–165). Jones and Bartlett.

Fairchild, A. L., Bayer, R., & Lee, J. S. (2019). The e-cigarette debate: What counts as evidence? *American Journal of Public Health*, *109*(7), 1000–1006. https://doi:10.2105/AJPH.2019.305107

Gharamani, A., de Courten, M., & Prokofieva, M. (2022). The potential of social media in health promotion beyond creating awareness: An integrative review. *BMC Public Health*, *22*(2022), Article 2402. https://doi:10.1186/s12889-022-14885-0

Goan, M. B. (2015). *Mary Breckinridge: The frontier nursing service and rural health in Appalachia*. The University of North Carolina Press.

Grants.gov. (n.d.). *Grants 101: A short summary of federal grants*. Retrieved from http://www.grants.gov/web/grants/learn-grants/grants-101.html

Green, L. W., & Kreuter, M. W. (2005). *Health program planning: An educational and ecological approach* (4th ed.). McGraw-Hill.

Green, L. W., Ottoson, J. M., & Roditis, M. L. (2014). Public health education and health promotion. In L. Shi & J. A. Johnson (Eds.), *Novick & Morrow's public health administration: Principles for population-based management* (3rd ed., pp. 477–504). Jones & Bartlett Learning.

Health Resources & Services Administration. (2023, September). *Uniform data system (UDS) resources*. HRSA Health Center Program. Retrieved from https://bphc.hrsa.gov/datareporting/reporting/index.html

Herrington, C. R., & Hand, M. W. (2019). Impact of nurse peer review on a culture of safety. *Journal of Nursing Care Quality*, *34*(2), 158–162. https://doi:10.1097/ncq.0000000000000361

Hill, L., & Artiga, S. (2021, April 9). *COVID-19 vaccination among American Indian and Alaskan Native people. KFF*. Retrieved from https://www.kff.org/racial-equity-and-health-policy/issue-brief/covid-19-vaccination-american-indian-alaska-native-people/

Holroyd, T., Limaye, R. J., Gerber, J. E., Rimal, R. N., Musci, R. J., Brewer, J., Sutherland, A., Blunt, M., Geller, G., & Salmon, D. (2021). Development of a scale to measure trust in public health authorities: Prevalence of trust and association with vaccination. *Journal of Health Communication*, *26*(4), 272–280. https://doi:10.1080/10810730.2021.1927259

International Union for Health Promotion and Education. (n.d.). *Mission*. Retrieved from http://www.iuhpe.org/index.php/en/

Jaykus, L. A. (2017). Keys to successful grant writing. *Journal of Food Science*, *82*(7), 1511–1512. https://doi:10.1111/1750-3841.13457

Kanshan, S., & Gaidhane, A. (2023). Social media role and its impact on public health: A narrative review. *Cureus*, *15*(1), Article e33737. https://doi:10.7759/cureus.33737

Karsh, E., & Fox, A. S. (2019). *The only grant-writing book you will ever need* (5th ed.). Basic Books.

Martin, K. S. (2005). *The Omaha System: A key to practice, documentation, and information management* (2nd ed.). Health Connections Press.

National Association for Healthcare Quality. (2023). National healthcare quality competency framework. Retrieved from. https://nahq.org/nahq-intelligence/competency-framework/

National Association of County & City Health Officials. (2023b). *Social media toolkit: A primer for local health department PIOs and communications professionals*. Retrieved from https://www.naccho.org/uploads/downloadable-resources/Social-Media-Toolkit-for-LHDs-2019.pdf

National Association of County and City Health Officials. (2017). *Local health department – Community health center toolkit*.

National Institutes of Health. (2023, April 11). Grants & funding: Types of grant programs. Retrieved from https://grants.nih.gov/grants/funding/funding_program.htm

National Prevention Information Network. (2022, April 15). *Health communication strategies and resources*. Centers for Disease Control and Prevention. Retrieved from https://npin.cdc.gov/pages/health-communication-strategies

Nock, B. (2016, August 2). Auditing medical records in 8 easy steps. *Ease the Way Blog* Retrieved from https://www.gebauer.com/blog/auditing-medical-records

Office of Disease Prevention and Health Promotion. (2022). *Healthy people*. National Health Initiatives. Retrieved from https://health.gov/our-work/national-health-initiatives/healthy-people

Pelletier, L. C., & Beaudin, C. L. (2018). *HQ solutions: Resource for the healthcare quality professional* (4th ed.). Wolters Kluwer.

Pew Research Center. (2021, April 7). Social media fact sheet. *Fact Sheet*. Retrieved from https://www.pewinternet.org/fact-sheet/social-media/

Phillips, B., Baker, L., Faherty, L. J., Ringel, J. S., & Kranz, A. M. (2023). *Mapping changes in inequities in COVID-19 vaccinations relative to deaths in Chicago, Illinois*. Centers for Disease Control and Prevention: Preventing Chronic Disease. Retrieved from https://www.cdc.gov/pcd/issues/2023/22_0319.htm

Pittman, P., & Park, J. (2021). Rebuilding community-based and public health nursing in the wake of COVID-19. *The Online Journal of Issues in Nursing*, *26*(7). https://doi:10.3912/OJIN.Vol26No02Man07

Public Health Accreditation Board. (2023a). *Accreditation activity*. Retrieved from https://phaboard.org/who-is-accredited/

Public Health Accreditation Board. (2023b). *Accreditation and recognition*. Retrieved from https://phaboard.org/accreditation-recognition/

Quality and Safety Education for Nurses. (2022). *Quality and Safety Education for Nurses*. Retrieved from https://qsen.org/about-qsen/project-overview/

Read, S. H., Rosella, L. C., Berger, H., Feig, D. S., Fleming, K., Ray, J. G., Baiju, R. S., & Lipscombe, L. L. (2021). BMI and risk of gestational diabetes among women of South Asian and Chinese ethnicity: A population-based study. *Diabetalogia*, *64*(2021), 805–813. https://doi:10.1007/s00125-020-05356-5

Seneres, G. (2023). *Case study: Using social marketing to improve public health*. University of Michigan School of Public Health. *The Pursuit*. Retrieved from https://sph.umich.edu/pursuit/2023posts/using-social-marketing-to-improve-public-health.html

Shewalte, R. (2023). *Social media users – Global demographics (2023, September 12)*. Demand Sage. Retrieved from https://www.demandsage.com/social-media-users/

The Omaha System. (2023). *Omaha system overview*. Retrieved from https://www.omahasystem.org/overview

United South and Eastern Tribes, Inc. (n.d.). *Vax-a-nation vaccine campaign*. https://www.usetinc.org/vax-a-nation-vaccine-campaign/

United States Environmental Protection Agency. (2023). Climate change and human health. *Climate Change Impacts* Retrieved from https://www.epa.gov/climateimpacts/climate-change-and-human-health#:~:text=The%20health%20effects%20of%20climate,illnesses%2C%20and%20injuries%20and%20deaths

University of Kansas. (n.d.-a). *Section 16. Geographical Information Systems: Tools for community mapping*. Community Tool Box. Retrieved from https://ctb.ku.edu/en/table-of-contents/assessment/assessing-community-needs-and-resources/geographic-information-systems/main

University of Kansas. (n.d.-b). *About the tool box*. Community Tool Box. Retrieved from https://ctb.ku.edu/en/about-the-tool-box

University of Kansas. (n.d.-c). *Section 13. MAPP: Mobilizing for action through planning and partnerships*. Community Tool Box. Retrieved from https://ctb.ku.edu/en/table-of-contents/overview/models-for-community-health-and-development/mapp/main

University of Kansas. (n.d.-d). *Section 1. Developing a logic model or theory of change*. Community Tool Box. Retrieved from https://ctb.ku.edu/en/table-of-contents/overview/models-for-community-health-and-development/logic-model-development/main

Urban Indian Health Institute. (2021). *Results from a national COVID-19 vaccination survey: Strengthening vaccine efforts in Indian Country*. Urban Health Institute. Retrieved from file:///C:/Users/dc338/Downloads/UIHI-COVID-Survey-Report.pdf

Walsh, M. J., Baker, S. A., & Wade, M. (2022). Evaluating the elevation of authoritative health content online during the COVID-19 pandemic. *Online Information Review*, *47*(4), 782–800. https://doi:10.1108/OIR-12-2021-0655

Wang, J. W., Cap, S. S., & Hu, R. Y. (2019). Smoking by family members and friends and electronic-cigarette use in adolescence: A systematic review and meta-analysis. *Tobacco Induced Diseases*, *16*, 5. https://doi:10.18332/tid/84864

Zhan, F. B., Liu, Y., Yang, M., Kluz, N., Olmstad, T. A., Spencer, J., Shokar, N. K., Cruz, R. L., & Pignone, M. P. (2023, March 2). *Using GIS to identify priority sites for colorectal cancer screening programs in Texas health centers*. Centers for Disease Control and Prevention: Preventing Chronic Disease. Retrieved from https://www.cdc.gov/pcd/issues/2023/22_0205.htm

CHAPTER 13

American Association of Colleges of Nursing (AACN). (2017). *Diversity, inclusion, and equity in academic nursing*.

American Association of Colleges of Nursing. (2021). *The essentials: Core competencies for professional nursing education*. https://www.aacnnursing.org/Portals/0/PDFs/Publications/Essentials-2021.pdf

American Nurses Association. (1994). *Nursing's agenda for health care reform*. http://ojin.nursingworld.org/MainMenuCategories/ANAMarketplace/ANAPeriodicals/OJIN/TableofContents/Vol31998/No1June1998/References.html

American Nurses Association. (2022). *Public health nursing: Scope and standards of practice*. https://www.nursingworld.org/nurses-books/public-health-nursing-scope-and-standards-of-prac/

American Nurses Association (ANA). (2015). *Code of ethics for nurses with interpretive statements (revised)*.

American Nurses Association (ANA). (n.d.-a). *ANA historical review*. http://www.nursingworld.org/history

American Nurses Association (ANA). (n.d.-b). *Health system reform resources*. https://www.nursingworld.org/practice-policy/health-policy/health-system-reform/resources/

American Public Health Association (APHA). (2023). *Health in all policies*. https://www.apha.org/topics-and-issues/health-in-all-policies

American Public Health Association, PHN Section. (2013). *Definition of public health nursing*. https://www.nursingworld.org/practice-policy/workforce/public-health-nursing/

APHN. (2021). *Public health advocacy guidebook and toolkit*. https://efaidnbmnnnibpcajpcglclefindmkaj/https://www.phnurse.org/assets/docs/APHN%20Public%20Health%20Policy%20Advocacy%20Guidebook%20and%20Toolkit%20_May%202021.pdf

Arias, E., Tejada-Vera, B., Kochanek, K. D., & Ahmad, F. B. (2022, August). *Provisional life expectancy estimates for 2021*. Vital Statistics Rapid Release; no 23. National Center for Health Statistics. https://dx.doi.org/10.15620/cdc:118999

Association of Public Health Nurses (APHN). (2021). *Public health policy advocacy guide book and tool kit*. https://www.phnurse.org/assets/docs/APHN%20Public%20Health%20Policy%20Advocacy%20Guide%20Book%20and%20Tool%20Kit%202016.pdf

Birkland, T. (2019). *An introduction to the policy process* (5th ed.). Routledge.

Carthon, J. M. B., Barnes, H., & Sarik, D. A. (2015). Federal policies influence access to primary care and nurse practitioner workforce. *Journal for Nurse Practitioners*, *11*(5), 526–531.

Center for Civic Education. (2023). *What is public policy?* https://civiced.org/project-citizen/what-is-public-policy

Center for Medicare and Medicaid Services (CMS). (2022a). *Historical*. https://www.cms.gov/Research-Statistics-Data-and-Systems/Statistics-Trends-and-Reports/NationalHealthExpendData/NationalHealthAccountsHistorical

Center for Medicare and Medicaid Services (CMS). (2022b). *Hospital acquired condition (HAC) reduction program.* https://www.cms.gov/Medicare/Quality-Initiatives-Patient-Assessment-Instruments/Value-Based-Programs/HAC/Hospital-Acquired-Conditions.html

Center to Champion Nursing in America (CCNA). (n.d.). Retrieved August 15, 2023, from https://campaignforaction.org/about/our-team/a-nursing-center-at-aarp/

Centers for Disease Control and Prevention (CDC). (2016). *Health in all policies.* https://www.cdc.gov/policy/hiap/index.html

Centers for Disease Control and Prevention (CDC). (2023a). *Data overview.* https://www.cdc.gov/opioids/data/index.html

Centers for Disease Control and Prevention (CDC). (2023b). *Smoking and tobacco use.* https://www.cdc.gov/tobacco/basic_information/policy/legislation/index.htm

Centers for Disease Control and Prevention (CDC). (2024). *Drug overdose deaths in the United States 2002-2022.* https://www.cdc.gov/nchs/products/databriefs/db491.htm#:~:text=Data%20from%20the%20National%20Vital%20Statistics%20System&text=Between%202021%20and%202022%2C%20the,semisynthetic%20opioids%2C%20and%20methadone%20declined

Centers for Disease Control and Prevention (CDC). (n.d.). *Step by step—Evaluating violence and injury prevention policies.* https://www.cdc.gov/injury/pdfs/policy/brief%201-a.pdf

City of Chicago. (2023). *Tobacco.* https://www.chicago.gov/city/en/depts/bacp/provdrs/enforce/svcs/tobacco.html#:~:text=It%20is%20illegal%20to%20furnish,sign%20must%20be%20conspicuously%20posted

Civic Impulse. (2023). *Statistics and historical comparison: Bills by final status.* https://www.govtrack.us/congress/bills/statistics

Cohen, S. S., Mason, D. J., Kovner, C., Leavitt, J. K., Pulcine, J., & Sochalshi, J. (1996). Stages of nursing's political development: Where we've been and where we ought to go. *Nursing Outlook*, *44*(6), 259–266.

Collins, S., Bhupal, H., & Dhoty, M. (2019). *Health insurance coverage eight years after the ACA.* https://www.commonwealthfund.org/publications/issue-briefs/2019/feb/health-insurance-coverage-eight-years-after-aca

Corlette, S., & Alker, J. (2023). A midterm assessment of President Biden's promise to build on the ACA. *Health Affairs Forefront*, February, *3*, 2023. https://doi.org/10.1377/forefront.20230202.274348

deChesnay, M., & Anderson, B. A. (2016). *Caring for the vulnerable: Perspectives in nursing theory, practice, and research* (4th ed.). Jones & Bartlett Learning.

Dimock, M., & Wilke, R. (2020). *America is exceptional in the nature of its political divide.* Pew Research Center. https://pewrsr.ch/2JZY9fb

Environmental Protection Agency. (2023). *Climate change regulatory actions and initiatives.* https://www.epa.gov/climate-change/climate-change-regulatory-actions-and-initiatives

Federal Election Commission (FEC). (n.d.). *Policy and other guidance.* https://www.fec.gov/legal-resources/policy-other-guidance/

Furlong, S. R., & Kraft, M. E. (Eds.). (2020). *Public policy: Politics, analysis, and alternatives* (7th ed.). SAGECQ Press.

Gallup. (2022). *Military Brass, Judges Among Professions at New Image Lows.* https://news.gallup.com/poll/388649/military-brass-judges-among-professions-new-image-lows.aspx#:~:text=The%20least%20revered%20professions%20are,are%20clearly%20the%20worst%20rated

Gunja, M. Z., Guzman, E. D., & Williams, R. D. (2023). *U.S. health care from a global perspective, 2022: Accelerating spending, worsening outcomes.* https://www.commonwealthfund.org/publications/issue-briefs/2023/jan/us-health-care-global-perspective-2022

Halfon, N., Long, P., Chang, D., Hester, J., Inkelas, M., & Rodgers, A. (2014). Applying A 3.0 transformation framework to guide large-scale health system reform. *Health Affairs*, *33*(11), 2003–2011. https://doi.org/10.1377/hlthaff.2014.0485

Health equity solutions. (2023). *Transformational community engagement to advance health equity.* https://www.shvs.org/wp-content/uploads/2023/03/SHVS_Transformational-Community-Engagement-to-Advance-Health-Equity.pdf

Inouye, L. (2021). Lobbying policymakers: Individual and collective strategies. Chap. 40. In D. J. Mason, E. Dickson, M. R. McLemore & A. Perez (Eds.), *Policy and politics* (8th ed.). Elsevier.

Institute of Medicine (IOM). (2011). *The future of nursing: Leading change, advancing health.* National Academics Press.

Johnson, K., Barolin, N., Ogbue, C., & Verlander, K. (2022, August 8). Lessons from five years of the CMS accountable health communities model. *Health Affairs Forefront.* https://doi.org/10.1377/forefront.20220805.764159

Joint Commission. (2023). *CLABSI toolkit.* https://www.jointcommission.org/resources/patient-safety-topics/infection-prevention-and-control/central-line-associated-bloodstream-infections-toolkit-and-monograph/clabsi-toolkit---introduction/

Kacic, A., & Castellucci, M. (2018, December 18). ACA repeal wouldn't stop transition to value based payment, efforts to lower drug spending. *Modern HealthCare.* https://www.modernhealthcare.com/article/20181219/NEWS/181219885/aca-repeal-wouldn-t-stop-transition-to-value-based-payment-efforts-to-lower-drug-spending

Kaiser Family Foundation. (2023). *Status of state medicaid expansion decisions: An interactive map.* https://www.kff.org/medicaid/issue-brief/status-of-state-medicaid-expansion-decisions-interactive-map/

Kalaitzidis, E., & Jewell, P. (2020). *The concepts of advocacy in nursing: A critical analysis.* http://doi.org/10.1097/HCM.0000000000000292

Kingdon, J. W. (2010). *Agendas, alternatives and public policies.* http://marieljohn.blogspot.com/2010/02/agendas-alternatives-and-public.html

Kingdon, J. W. (2011). *Agendas, alternatives and public policies* (2nd ed.). Pearson/Longman.

Kleinpell, R., Myers, C. R., & Schorn, M. N. (2023). Addressing barriers to APRN practice: Policy and regulatory implications during COVID-19. *Journal of Nursing Regulation*, *14*(1), 13–20. https://doi.org/10.1016/S2155-8256(23)00064-9

LaPointe, J. (2019). *Social determinants of health key to value based purchasing success.* https://revcycleintelligence.com/news/social-determinants-of-health-key-to-value-based-purchasing-success

Lasswell, H. (19360). *Politics; who gets what, when, how.* McGraw-hill book Co.

Lewenson, S. B. (2015). Overview and summary: Cornerstone documents in healthcare: Our history, our future. *Online Journal of Issues in Nursing*, *20*(2). http://www.nursingworld.org/MainMenuCategories/ANAMarketplace/ANAPeriodicals/OJIN/TableofContents/Vol-20-2015/No2-May-2015/OS-Cornerstone-Documents.html

Longest, B. B. (2004). An international constant: The crucial role of policy competence in the effective strategic management of health services organizations. *Health Services Management Research*, *17*(2), 71–78. https://doi.org/10.1258/095148404323043109

Longest, B. B. (2016). *Health policymaking in the United States* (6th ed.). Health Administration Press.

Milio, N. (1981). *Promoting health through public policy.* F. A. Davis.

Minnesota Hospital Association. (2020). *Quality and patient safety.* https://www.mnhospitals.org/quality-patient-safety/quality-patient-safety-improvement-topics/infections/clabsi#/videos/list

Narayan, M. M. (2023). *Community engagement helps drive much-needed infrastructure investments.* https://www.pewtrusts.org/en/research-and-analysis/articles/2023/04/03/community-engagement-helps-drive-much-needed-infrastructure-investments

Nash, D., & Wohlforth, C. (2022). *How covid crashed the system.* Rowman and Littlefield, Lanham, MD.

National Academy for State Health Policy. (2023). *State laws passed to lower prescription drug costs: 2017–2023.* https://nashp.org/state-drug-pricing-laws-2017-2023/

National Institute of Environmental Health Sciences. (2023). *Climate change.* https://www.niehs.nih.gov/health/topics/agents/climate-change/index.cfm

National Institute on Drug Abuse. (2021). *Prescription opioids drug facts.* https://nida.nih.gov/publications/drugfacts/prescription-opioids

National League for Nursing. (2016). *Overview.* http://www.nln.org/about

National League of Cities. (2023). *Cities 101-delegation of power.* https://www.nlc.org/resource/cities-101-delegation-of-power

National Nurses United. (2018). *Your handy guide to CAN lobby day, 2018.* https://www.nationalnursesunited.org/blog/your-handy-guide-cna-lobby-day-201

Nickitas, D. M., Middaugh, D. J., & Aries, N. (2016). *Policy and politics for nurses and other health professionals* (2nd ed.). Jones & Bartlett Learning.

NINR. (n.d.). https://www.ninr.nih.gov/aboutninr/who-we-are

Office of the Federal Register. (n.d.). *A guide to the rulemaking process.* https://www.federalregister.gov/uploads/2011/01/the_rulemaking_process.pdf

Organization for Economic Cooperation & Development (OECD). (2023). *OECD Health Statistics 2023.* https://www.oecd.org/els/health-systems/health-data.htm

Pate, K., Brelewski, K., Rutledge, S., Rankin, V., & Layell, J. (2022). CLABSI Rounding Team. *Journal of Nursing Care Quality*, *37*(3), 275–281. https://doi.org/10.1097/NCQ.0000000000000625

Peterson-KFF. (2023). *Health system tracker.* https://www.healthsystemtracker.org/

Pew Research Center. (2023). *What the data says about gun deaths in the U.S.* https://www.pewresearch.org/short-reads/2023/04/26/what-the-data-says-about-gun-deaths-in-the-u-s/

Positive Behavioral Interventions and Support. (2024). *Opioid crisis and substantive misuse.* https://www.pbis.org/topics/opioid-crisis-and-substance-misuse#:~:text=In%20the%20late%201990s%2C%20pharmaceutical%20companies%20reassured%20the,became%20clear%20these%20medications%20could%20be%20highly%20addictive

Public Health Law Center. (2019). *U.S. E-cigarette regulations—50 state review.* https://www.publichealthlawcenter.org/resources/us-e-cigarette-regulations-50-state-review

Rasheed, S. P., Younas, A., & Medhi, F. (2020). Challenges, extent of involvement, and the impact of nurses' involvement in politics and policy making in in last two decades: An integrative review. *Journal of Nursing Scholarship*, *52*(4), 446–455. https://doi.org/10.1111/jnu.12567

Rhodes, D. (2016, January 17). Raising cigarette-buying age to 21 a new strategy in fighting addiction. *Chicago Tribune.* http://www.chicagotribune.com/news/ct-minimum-tobacco-age-emanuel-met-20160117-story.html

Robert Wood Johnson Foundation. (2010, November 30). *Robert Wood Johnson Foundation launches national campaign to advance health through nursing.* https://www.rwjf.org/en/library/articles-and-news/2010/11/robert-wood-johnson-foundation-launches-national-campaign-to-adv.html

Rutgers Center for American Women and Politics. (2023). *Current numbers.* https://cawp.rutgers.edu/facts/current-numbers

Swider, S. M. (2023). Community engagement for health and development: Perspective of community organization leaders. Manuscript in preparation.

Tolbert, J., Drake, P., & Damico, An. (2023). *Key facts about the uninsured population.* https://www.kff.org/uninsured/issue-brief/key-facts-about-the-uninsured-population/

Tomsich, E. A., Pear, V. A., Schleimer, J. P., & Wintemute, G. J. (2023). The origins of California's gun violence restraining order law: A case study using Kingdon's multiple streams framework. *BMC Public Health*, *23*(1), 1275. https://doi.org/10.1186/s12889-023-16043-6

U.S. Department of Transportation. (2022). *Rulemaking process.* https://www.transportation.gov/regulations/rulemaking-process#:~:text=prepare%20effective%20comments%3F-,What%20is%20rulemaking%3F,repeal%20of%20an%20existing%20rule

U.S. Federal Drug Administration (FDA). (2016). *The facts on the FDA's new tobacco rule.* https://www.fda.gov/consumers/consumer-updates/facts-fdas-new-tobacco-rule

U.S. House of Representatives. (n.d.). *The legislative process.* http://www.house.gov/content/learn/legislative_process/

USAgov. (2023a). *How laws are made.* https://www.usa.gov/how-laws-are-made

USAgov. (2023b). *Branches of government.* https://www.usa.gov/branches-of-government

Wakefield, M. K., Williams, D. R., Le Menestrel, S., & Flaubert, J. L. (2021). *The future of nursing 2020-2030: Charting a path to achieve health equity.* National Academies Press. https://www.nationalacademies.org/our-work/the-future-of-nursing-2020-2030

Williamson-Younce, H. (2023). Learning lessons from COVID-19: Upstream fishing to mend downstream implications. In S. B. Hasmiller & G. A. Daniel (Eds.), *Taking action: Top ten priorities to promote health equity and well being in nursing.* Sigma.

World health Organization (WHO). (2019). *Community empowerment*. https://www.who.int/healthpromotion/conferences/7gchp/track1/en/

World Health Organization (WHO). (2023). *Promoting health in all policies and intersectoral action capacities*. https://www.who.int/activities/promoting-health-in-all-policies-and-intersectoral-action-capacities

WHO. (2024). *Promoting health in all policies and intrasectoral action capacities*. https://www.who.int/activities/promoting-health-in-all-policies-and-intersectoral-action-capacities

Xue, Y., & Intrator, O. (2016). Cultivating the role of nurse practitioners in providing primary care to vulnerable populations in an era of health-care reform. *Policy, Politics & Nursing Practice*, *17*(1), 24–31.

CHAPTER 14

American Nurses Association. (n.d.). *The nursing process*. Retrieved from https://www.nursingworld.org/practice-policy/workforce/what-is-nursing/the-nursing-process/

Association of Public Health Nurses. (2022). *Mission and Vision*. Retrieved from https://www.phnurse.org/mission-and-vision

Centers for Disease Control and Prevention. (2021). *Reproductive health: Teen pregnancy*. Retrieved from https://www.cdc.gov/teenpregnancy/about/index.htm

Centers for Disease Control and Prevention (CDC). (2024b). *About family health history*. https://www.cdc.gov/family-health-history/about/index.html

Children's Defense Fund, The State of America's Children. (2023). Retrieved from https://www.childrensdefense.org/the-state-of-americas-children/soac-2023-child-welfare/

Childstats Forum on Child and Family Statistics. (2021). *Family structure and children's living arrangements*. https://www.childstats.gov/americaschildren21/family1.asp

Cohn, D., Horowitcz, J. M., Minkin, R., Fry, R., & Hurst, K. (2022). *Financial issues top the list of reasons U.S. adults live in multigenerational homes*. Pew Research Center. Retrieved from https://www.pewresearch.org/social-trends/2022/03/24/financial-issues-top-the-list-of-reasons-u-s-adults-live-in-multigenerational-homes/

Collier, C. E., & Villareal, P. (2022). Family unit functioning questionnaire: Development and initial validation. *Australian and New Zealand Journal of Family Therapy*, *43*, 223–242.

Duvall, E. M., & Miller, B. (1985). *Marriage and family development* (6th ed.). Lippincott Williams & Wilkins.

Edelman, C. L., & Kudzma, E. E. (Eds.). (2021). *Health promotion throughout the life span* (10th ed.). Mosby.

Fadeyi, D., & Horowitz, J. M. (2022). *Americans more likely to say it's a bad thing than a good thing that more young adults live with their parents*. Pew Research Center. Retrieved from https://www.pewresearch.org/short-reads/2022/08/24/americans-more-likely-to-say-its-a-bad-thing-than-a-good-thing-that-more-young-adults-live-with-their-parents/

Federal Interagency Forum on Aging-Related Statistics (Agingstats). (2020). *Older Americans 2020: Key indicators of well-being*. U.S. Government Printing Office.

Fry, R. (2023). *A record-high share of 40-year-olds in the US have never been married*. Pew Research Center. Retrieved from https://www.pewresearch.org/short-reads/2023/06/28/a-record-high-share-of-40-year-olds-in-the-us-have-never-been-married/

Gryn, T., Kreider, R. M., Washington, C., & Anderson, L. (2023). *Family households still the majority*. U.S. Census Bureau. Retrieved from https://www.census.gov/library/stories/2023/05/family-households-still-the-majority.html

Habitat for Humanity. (2023). *What does home mean to you?* Retrieved from https://www.habitat.org/stories/what-does-home-mean-to-you

Harpin, S. B., Artmann, A. L., Neal, M., Robertson, G., & Barton, A. J. (2022). Program implementation and outcomes from three cohorts of the nurse-family partnership nurse residency program. *Public Health Nursing Wiley Periodicals LLC*, *39*, 1000–1008.

Healthy Families America. (n.d.) *Our approach; home visiting*. Retrieved from https://www.healthyfamiliesamerica.org/our-approach/.

International Family Nursing Association (IFNA). (2015). *IFNA position statement on generalist competencies for family nursing practice*. Retrieved from https://internationalfamilynursing.org/2015/07/31/ifna-position-statement-on-generalist-competencies-for-family-nursing-practice/

International Family Nursing Association (IFNA). (2013). *IFNA position statement on pre-licensure family nursing education*. Retrieved from https://internationalfamilynursing.org/2015/07/25/ifna-position-statement-on-pre-licensure-family-nursing-education

National Alliance to End Homelessness (2023a). *State of homelessness: 2023 Edition*. Retrieved from https://endhomelessness.org/homelessness-in-america/homelessness-statistics/state-of-homelessness/

National Alliance to End Homelessness. (2023b). *Who experiences homelessness*. Retrieved from https://endhomelessness.org/homelessness-in-america/who-experiences-homelessness/children-and-families/

National Responsible Fatherhood Clearinghouse. (n.d.). *Young fathers*. U.S. Department of Health and Human Services. Retrieved from https://www.fatherhood.gov/for-programs/young-fathers

Nurse Family Partnership. (2023). *Dads need help, too: Your personal nurse can help him be a great dad*. Retrieved from https://www.nursefamilypartnership.org/first-time-moms/expectant-fathers/

Osterman, M. J. K., Hamilton, B. E., Martin, J. A. M., Driscoll, A. K., & Valenzuela, C. P. (2022). Births: Final data for 2021. *National Vital Statistics Report*, *70*(17).

Pino-Gavidia, L. A., Seens, H., Fraser, J., Sivagurathan, M., MacDermid, J. C., Brunton, L., & Doralp, S. (2023). COVID-19 attributed changes of home and family responsibilities among single mothers. *Journal of Family Issues*, *44*(9), 2492–2503.

Robinson, M., Padgett, D., & Smith, P. (2022). *Family health nursing care: Theory, practice, and research* (10th ed.). F.A. Davis.

Rodriguez-Gonzalez, M., Lampis, J., Murdock, N. L., Schweer-Collins, M. L., & Lyons, E. R. (2020). Couple adjustment and differentiation of self in the United States, Italy, and Spain: A Cross Cultural Study. *Family Process*, *59*(4), 1552–1568.

Scherer, Z. (2022). *Same sex couple households exceeded one million*. U.S. Census Bureau. Retrieved from https://www.census.gov/library/stories/2022/11/same-sex-couple-households-exceeded-one-million.html

SmithBattle, L., Phengnum, W., Shagavah, A. W., & Okawa, S. (2019). Fathering on tenuous ground: A meta-synthesis on teen fathering. *MCN: The American Journal of Maternal/Child Nursing*, *44*(4), 186–194.

U.S. Department of Health & Human Services (USDHHS). (2020). *Healthy People 2030: Browse objectives*. Retrieved from https://health.gov/healthypeople/objectives-and-data/browse-objectives

United States Census Bureau. (2021). *Subject Definitions*. U.S. Department of Commerce. Retrieved from https://www.census.gov/programs-surveys/cps/technical-documentation/subject-definitions.html

Washington, C., & Anderson, L. (2023). *Is your state in step with national marriage and divorce trends?* U.S. Census Bureau. Retrieved from https://www.census.gov/library/stories/2023/07/marriage-divorce-rates.html

CHAPTER 15

American Nurses Association (ANA). (2022). *Public health nursing: Scope and standards of practice* (3rd ed.). Nursesbooks.org

American Public Health Association, Public Health Nursing Section. (2013). *The definition and practice of public health nursing: A statement of the public health nursing section*. American Public Health Association.

Anderson, E. T., & McFarlane, J. (2019). *Community as partner: Theory and practice* (8th ed.). Lippincott Williams & Wilkins.

Carnegie, E., Inglis, G., Taylor, A., Bak-Klimek, A., & Okoye, O. (2022). Is population density associated with non-communicable disease in wester developed countries? A systematic review. *International Journal of Environmental Research and Public Health*, *19*(5), 2638. http://dx.doi.org/10.3390/ijerph19052638

Centers for Disease Control and Prevention (CDC). (2022a). *Assessment & planning models, frameworks & tools*. https://www.cdc.gov/public-health-gateway/php/public-health-strategy/public-health-strategies-for-community-health-assessment-health-improvement-planning.html?CDC_AAref_Val=https://www.cdc.gov/publichealthgateway/cha/plan.html

Centers for Disease Control and Prevention (CDC). (2022b). *Why is addressing social determinants of health important for CDC and public health?* https://www.cdc.gov/about/priorities/why-is-addressing-sdoh-important.html?CDC_AAref_Val=https://www.cdc.gov/about/sdoh/addressing-sdoh.html

Centers for Disease Control and Prevention (CDC). (2022c). *Data and statistics*. https://www.cdc.gov/datastatistics/index.html

Centers for Disease Control and Prevention (CDC). (2023). *Populations and vulnerabilities*. https://ephtracking.cdc.gov/showPcMain

Centers for Disease Control and Prevention (CDC). (2024). *Behavioral risk factor surveillance system*. https://www.cdc.gov/brfss/index.html

Community Toolbox. (n.d.). *Section 6: Participatory evaluation*. http://ctb.ku.edu/en/table-of-contents/evaluate/evaluation/participatory-evaluation/main

Dawes, D. E. (2020). *The political determinants of health*. Johns Hopkins University Press.

Donabedian, A. (2005). Evaluating the quality of medical care. *Milbank Quarterly*, *83*(4), 691–729.

Duran, B., Oetzel, J., Magarati, M., Parker, M., Zhou, C., Roubideaux, Y., Muhammad, M., Pearson, C., Belone, L., Kastelic, S., & Wallerstein, N. (2019). Toward health equity: A national study of promising practices in community-based participatory research. *Progress in Community Health Partnerships: Research, Education, and Action*, *13*(4), 337–352. https://doi:10.1353/cpr.2019.0067

Ervin, N. E., & Kulbok, P. A. (2018). *Advanced public and community health nursing practice: Population assessment, program planning, and evaluation* (2nd ed.). Springer Publishing Company.

Harvard University. (2023). *Center for geographic analysis*. https://gis.harvard.edu/gis-institute

Hertz, M., & Barrios, L. (2021). Adolescent mental health, COVID-19, and the value of school-community partnerships. *Injury Prevention*, *27*(1), 85–86.

Higgins, E., & Cooper, R. (2021). *State cross-agency collaboration during the COVID-19 pandemic response*. https://nashp.org/state-cross-agency-collaboration-during-the-covid-19-pandemic-response/#:~:text=Some%20states%20have%20used%20cross,Bureau%2C%20latest%20American%20Community%20Survey

Kavanagh, S., Shiell, A., Hawe, P., & Garvey, K. (2022). Resources, relationships, and systems thinking should inform the way community health promotion is funded. *Critical Public Health*, *32*(3), 273–282. https://doi:10.1080/09581596.2020.1813255

Kirst-Ashman, K., & Hull, G. H. (2018). *Empowerment series: Human behavior in the macro social environment* (5th ed.). Cengage Learning.

Kretzman, J., & McKnight, J. (1993). *Building communities from the inside out: A path toward finding and mobilizing a community's assets*. ACTA Publications.

Larijani, F., Fotokian, Z., Jahanshahi, M., Tabi, S. R. (2021). Application of Neuman's model on anxiety of older adults waiting for colonoscopy. *Nursing and Midwifery Studies*, *10*(4), 236–242. https://doi.org/10.4103/nms.nms_77_20

Live Healthy South Carolina. (2019). *Collaborative health improvement toolkit transforming the health of your community*. https://livehealthy.sc.gov/sites/livehealthy/files/Documents/Call%20to%20Action/chi_toolkit_2019.pdf

Martin, K. S. (2005). *The Omaha system: A key to practice, documentation, and information management* (2nd ed.). Health Connections Press.

Michener, L., Aguilar-Gaxiola, S., Alberti, P. M., Castañeda, M. J., Castrucci, B. C., Macon Harrison, L. M., Hughes, L. S., Richmond, A., & Wallerstein, N. (2020). Peer reviewed: engaging with communities—Lessons (re) learned from COVID-19. *Preventing Chronic Disease*, *17*.

Minnesota Department of Health. (2019). *Public health interventions: Applications for public health nursing practice* (2nd ed.). https://www.health.state.mn.us/communities/practice/research/phncouncil/wheel.html

Minnesota Department of Health. (n.d.-a). *Local public health assessment and planning*. https://www.health.state.mn.us/communities/practice/assessplan/index.html

Minnesota Department of Health. (n.d.-b). *SMART and meaningful objectives*. http://www.health.state.mn.us/divs/opi/qi/toolbox/objectives.html

National Academies of Sciences, Engineering, and Medicine; National Academy of Medicine; Committee on the Future of Nursing 2020–2030. (2021). *The future of nursing 2020-2030: Charting a path to achieve health equity*. National Academies Press (US). 5, The role of nurses in improving health equity. Available from: https://www.ncbi.nlm.nih.gov/books/NBK573898/

National Association of County & City Health Officials (NACCHO). (2023). *Developing a community health improvement plan.* http://www.naccho.org/topics/infrastructure/CHAIP/chip.cfm

National Association of County & City Health Officials (NACCHO). (n.d.). *Guide to prioritization techniques.* https://www.naccho.org/uploads/downloadable-resources/Gudie-to-Prioritization-Techniques.pdf

National Institutes of Health (NIH). (2023). *National institute of health.* https://www.nih.gov/

New Mexico Department of Health. (n.d.). *Community health, assessment, prioritization and planning phase of the community health improvement process.* https://www.nmhealth.org/publication/view/training/8108/

Nieves, C., Chan, J., Dannefer, R., De La Rosa, C., Diaz-Malvido, C., Realmuto, L., Libman, K., Brown-Dudley, L., & Manyindo, N. (2020). *Health in action: Evaluation of a participatory grant-making project in east Harlem.* Health Promotion Practice, March 7, Online. https://doi.org/10.1177/1524839919834271

Northwest Center for Public Health Practice. (n.d.). *Module one: An overview of public health data.* Retrieved from http://www.nwcphp.org/docs/bcda_series/data_analysis_mod1_transcript.pdf

Office of Disease Prevention and Health Promotion (ODPHP). (n.d.). *Healthy People 2030.* U.S. Department of Health and Human Services. https://health.gov/healthypeople

Office of the Assistant Secretary for Planning and Evaluation. (n.d.). *Strategic planning.* Retrieved from https://aspe.hhs.gov/strategic-planning

Polit, D. F., & Beck, C. T. (2021). *Essentials of nursing research: Appraising evidence for nursing practice* (8th ed.). Lippincott Williams & Wilkins. ISBN-13 978-1975141851.

Public Health Accreditation Board. (2022). *Standards & measures for initial accreditation, version 2022.* https://phaboard.org/wp-content/uploads/Standards-Measures-Initial-Accreditation-Version-2022.pdf

Public Health Foundation. (2020). *Programs.* http://www.phf.org/Pages/default.aspx

Public Health Professionals Gateway. (n.d.). *Community planning for health assessment: Frameworks & tools.* https://www.cdc.gov/public-health-gateway/php/public-health-strategy/public-health-strategies-for-community-health-assessment-models-frameworks-tools.html

Quad Council Coalition of Public Health Nursing. (2018). *Community/public health nursing competencies.* Retrieved from http://www.quadcouncilphn.org/wp-content/uploads/2018/05/QCC-C-PHN-COMPETENCIES-Approved_2018.05.04_Final-002.pdf

RAND Corporation. (n.d.). *Community health and well-being.* https://www.rand.org/topics/community-health-and-well-being.html

Ravaghi, H., Guisset, A. L., Elfeky, S., Nasir, N., Khani, S., Ahmadnezhad, E., & Abdi, Z. (2023). A scoping review of community health needs and assets assessment: Concepts, rationale, tools and uses. *BMC Health Services Research, 23*(1), 44. https://doi:10.1186/s12913-022-08983-3

Robert Wood Johnson Foundation. (2024). *County health rankings and roadmaps: 2024 National findings report.* https://www.countyhealthrankings.org/findings-and-insights/2024-national-findings-report

Rural Health Information Hub. (2024). *Conducting rural health research, needs assessments, and program evaluations.* https://www.ruralhealthinfo.org/topics/rural-health-research-assessment-evaluation

Salmon, M. E. (1982). Construct for public health: Where is it practiced, in whose behalf, and with what desired outcome. *Nursing Outlook, 30*(9), 527–530. (Originally published under the author name Marla Salmon White.).

Salmon, M. E. (1993). Public health nursing: The opportunity of a century. *American Journal of Public Health, 83*(12), 1674–1675.

Schaffer, M. A., Strohschein, S., & Glavin, K. (2022). Twenty years with the public health intervention wheel: Evidence for practice. *Public Health Nurse, 39*(1), 195–201. https://doi:10.1111/phn.12941

Sherif, B., Awaisu, A., & Kheir, N. (2022). Refugee healthcare needs and barriers to accessing healthcare services in New Zealand: A qualitative phenomenological approach. *BMC Health Services Research, 22*(1), 1310. doi:10.1186/s12913-022-08560-8. PMID: 36329410; PMCID: PMC9632582

South Oaks Hospital Northwell Health. (2023). *School-based mental health services: Information for parents.* https://southoaks.northwell.edu/school-based-mental-health-services

U.S. Census Bureau. (2023). *Data.* Retrieved from http://www.census.gov/data.html

U.S. Drug Enforcement Administration (USDEA). (n.d.). *Coalitions 101: Getting started.* https://www.dea.gov/sites/default/files/DEA360/Coalition_101_Getting_Started%5B1%5D_0.pdf

World Health Organization. (2023). *Climate change and health.* https://www.who.int/news-room/fact-sheets/detail/climate-change-and-health

World Health Organization. (n.d.). *WHO GIS Centre for heath.* https://www.who.int/data/GIS

World Health Organization (WHO) GIS Center for Health. (2021). *Cutting Edge GIS Technologies for COVID-19 Vaccine Delivery: How do we equitably distribute vaccines across 90+ countries unless we have accurate, actionable spatial data and tools?* https://storymaps.arcgis.com/stories/7b3e36d2f4a04eaf9be1c3cb936e6681

Yasmin, S., Haque, R., Kadambaya, K., Maliha, M., & Sheikh, M. (2022). Exploring how public health partnerships with community-based organizations (CBOs) can be leveraged for health promotion and community health. *The Journal of Health Care Organization, Provision, and Financing., 2022,* 59. https://doi:10.1177/00469580221139372

Zeydani, A., Atashzadeh-Shoorideh, F., Hosseini, M., & Zohari-Annboohi, S. (2023). Community-based nursing: A concept analysis with Walker and Avant's approach. *BMC Medical Education, 23,* 762. https://doi.org/10.1186/s12909-023-04749-5

Zhu, R., Han, S., Su, Y., Zhang, C., Yu, Q., & Zhiguang, D. (2019). The application of big data and the development of nursing science: A discussion paper. *International Journal of Nursing Sciences, 3,* 229–234.

CHAPTER 16

Adovor, E., Czaika, M., Docquier, F., & Moullan, Y. (2021). Medical brain drain: How many, where and why? *Journal of Health Economics, 76.* https://doi:10.1016/j.jhealeco.2020.102409

Agarwal, P. (2022). *The demographic transition model.* https://www.intelligenteconomist.com/demographic-transition-model/

Agency for Toxic Substances and Disease Registry. (2023a). *Place and health.* US Department of Health and Human Services, Centers for Disease Control and Prevention. https://www.atsdr.cdc.gov/placeandhealth/index.html

Agency for Toxic Substances and Disease Registry. (2023b). *Environmental Justice Index (EJI).* US Department of Health and Human Services, Centers for Disease Control and Prevention. https://www.atsdr.cdc.gov/placeandhealth/eji/index.html

Agency for Toxic Substances and Disease Registry. (2023). *Environmental justice index.* https://www.atsdr.cdc.gov/placeandhealth/eji/index.html

American Nurses Association (ANA). (2019). Ethics Advisory Board. ANA position statement: Ethical considerations for local and global volunteerism. *The Online Journal of Issues in Nursing, 25*(1). https://ojin.nursingworld.org/table-of-contents/volume-25-2020/number-1-january-2020/ethical-considerations-for-volunteerism/

Association of Public Health Laboratories. (2022). *Influenza Virologic surveillance right size roadmap* (2nd ed.). https://www.aphl.org/aboutAPHL/publications/Documents/ID-Influenza-Right-Size-Roadmap-Edition2.pdf

Bill and Melinda Gates Foundation. (n.d.). *Our work.* https://www.gatesfoundation.org/our-work

Breslow, L. (2006). Health measurement in the third era of health. *American Journal of Public Health,* 96(1), 17–19.

Centers for Disease Control and Prevention (CDC). (2022a). *CDC 24/7.* US Department of Health and Human Services, CDC. https://www.cdc.gov/about/index.html

Centers for Disease Control and Prevention (CDC). (2022b). *About CDC: Advancing science & health equity.* US Department of Health and Human Services, CDC. https://www.cdc.gov/about/index.html

Centers for Disease Control and Prevention (CDC). (2022c). *International Health Regulations (IHR): Protecting people every day.* https://www.cdc.gov/globalhealth/healthprotection/ghs/ihr/index.html

Centers for Disease Control and Prevention (CDC). (2023a). *One Health basics.* https://www.cdc.gov/onehealth/basics/index.html

Centers for Disease Control and Prevention (CDC). (2023b). *CDC moving forward.* US Department of Health and Human Services, CDC. https://www.cdc.gov/about/organization/cdc-moving-forward

Centers for Disease Control and Prevention (CDC). (2023c). *Ebola disease.* https://www.cdc.gov/vhf/ebola/index.html

City-Data. (2023). *Montana languages.* http://www.city-data.com/states/Montana-Languages.html

Division of Global Health Protection. (2022). *CDC and WHO leverage partner resources to respond to humanitarian emergencies.* Centers for Disease Control and Prevention. https://www.cdc.gov/globalhealth/healthprotection/stories/CDC-and-WHO-Leverage-Partner-Resources-to-Respond-to-Humanitarian-Emergencies.html

Doctors Without Borders USA. (n.d.). *Commitment to our supporters.* https://www.doctorswithoutborders.org/who-we-are/accountability-reporting/commitment-our-supporters

Downey, E., Fokeladeh, H. S., & Catton, H. (2023). *What the COVID-19 pandemic has exposed: the findings of five global health workforce professions.* World Health Organization. (Human Resources for Health Observer Series No. 28). License: CC BY-NC-SA 3.0 IGO.

Food and Agriculture Organization of the United Nations. (2023). *Animal health.* http://www.fao.org/animal-health/en/

Global Health Security Agenda. (2023). *Home.* https://globalhealthsecurityagenda.org/

Global Outbreak Alert and Response Center (GOARN). (2023). *About us.* https://goarn.who.int/#aboutus

Institute for Health Metrics and Evaluation. (2020). *Global burden of disease.* https://www.healthdata.org/research-analysis/gbd

Institute for Health Metrics and Evaluation. (n.d.). *GBD concepts and terms defined.* https://www.healthdata.org/research-analysis/about-gbd

Institute for Health Metrics and Evaluation. (2024). *Global Burden of Disease 2021: Findings from the GBD 2021 Study.* https://www.healthdata.org/sites/default/files/2024-05/GBD_2021_Booklet_FINAL_2024.05.16.pdf

International Conference on Primary Health Care. (1978). *Declaration of Alma-Ata. Paper presented at the International Conference on Primary Health Care, Alma-Ata, USSR.* https://www.who.int/publications/almaata_declaration_en.pdf?ua=1

International Council of Nurses. (2020). *Who we are.* https://www.icn.ch/who-we-are/icn-mission-vision-and-strategic-plan

Johnson, S., & Sabo, S. (2022). *US Census Bureau: Deaths outnumbered births in half of all states b2020 and 2021.* https://www.census.gov/library/stories/2022/03/deaths-outnumbered-births-in-half-of-states-between-2020-and-2021.html

Kaiser Family Foundation. (January 24, 2019). *The US government and the World Health Organization.* https://www.kff.org/global-health-policy/fact-sheet/the-u-s-government-and-the-world-health-organization/

Lin, T. K., Kafri, R., Hammoudeh, W., Mitwalli, S., Jamaluddine, Z., Ghattas, H., Giacaman, R., & Leone, T. (2022). Pathways to food insecurity in the context of conflict: the case of the occupied Palestinian territory. *Conflict and Health, 16,* 38. https://doi:10.1186/s13031-022-00470-0

Los Angeles Almanac (2023). *Los Angeles Unified School District by the numbers.* Given Place Media. https://www.laalmanac.com/education/ed721.php

Office of Disease Prevention and Health Promotion (ODPHP). (n.d.). *Healthy People 2030.* U.S. Department of Health and Human Services. https://health.gov/healthypeople

Omran, A. R. (2005). The epidemiologic transition: A theory of the epidemiology of population change. *Milbank Quarterly, 83*(4), 731–757.

Pan American Health Organization (PAHO). (n.d.). *About the Pan American Health Organization (PAHO).* https://www.paho.org/hq/index.php?option=com_content&view=article&id=91:about-paho&Itemid=-220&lang=en

Partners in Health. (n.d.). *Our mission at PIH.* https://www.pih.org/pages/our-mission

Pereira, A., Biscaia, A., Calado, I., Freitas, A., Costa, A., & Coelho, A. (2022). Healthcare equity and commissioning: A four-year national analysis of Portuguese primary healthcare units. *International Journal of Environmental Research and Public Health, 19*(22), 14819. https://doi:10.3390/ijerph192214819

Prakash, A., Butani, D., Zayar, N. N., Eiamsakul, B., Dabak, S. V., & Isaranuwatchi, W. (2023). *Building a global*

framework for telehealth. Health Affairs Forefront. https://doi:10.1377/forefront.20230621.134595
RBM Partnership to End Malaria. (2020). *RBM Partnership Strategic Plan 2021–2025*. United Nations Office for Project Services. https://endmalaria.org/sites/default/files/RBM%20Partnership%20to%20End%20Malaria%20Strategic%20plan%20for%202021-2025_web_0.pdf
RBM Partnership to End Malaria. (2022). *RBM Partnership to end malaria overview*. United Nations Office for Project Services. https://endmalaria.org/about-us/overview1
Tracey, P., Rajaratnam, E., Varughese, J., Venegas, D., Gombachika, B., Pindani, M., Ashbourne, E., & Martiniuk, A. (2022). Guidelines for short-term medical missions: perspectives from host countries. *Globalization and Health, 18*(19). https://globalizationandhealth.biomedcentral.com/articles/10.1186/s12992-022-00815-7#citeas
UNICEF. (n.d.). *For every child*. https://www.unicef.org
United Nation (UN). (2023a). *With highest number of violent conflicts since second world war, United Nations must rethink efforts to achieve, sustain peace, speakers tell security council*. https://press.un.org/en/2023/sc15184.doc.htm
United Nation (UN). (2023b). Security council adopts presidential statement addressing Conflict-induced food insecurity in situations of armed conflict. https://press.un.org/en/2023/sc15377.doc.htm
United Nations (UN). (n.d.-a). *17 goals to transform our world*. https://www.un.org/sustainabledevelopment/
United Nations (UN). (n.d.-b). *United Nations Charter, Chapter 1: Purposes and principles*. https://www.un.org/en/about-us/un-charter/chapter-1
United Nations (UN). (n.d.-c). *Strategy*. https://www.un.org/en/genocideprevention/office-strategy.shtml
United Nations (UN). (n.d.-d). *International migration*. https://www.un.org/en/global-issues/migration#:~:text=Some%20people%20move%20in%20search,large%2Dscale%20human%20rights%20violations
United Nations AIDS (UNAIDS). (2024). *Let communities lead*. https://www.unaids.org/en/aboutunaids/unaidscosponsors
United Nations Development Programme. (2023). *What are the sustainable development goals?* https://www.undp.org/sustainable-development-goals
United Nations Global Market Place. (2024). *The Directory of the UN system organizations*. https://www.ungm.org/Shared/KnowledgeCenter/Pages/VBS_UNSystem
United States Department of Health and Human Services (USDHHS). (2022). *U.S. summary of the 75th World Health Assembly [Blog]*. https://www.hhs.gov/blog/2022/06/09/us-summary-of-the-75th-world-health-assembly.html
Wenham, C., & Stout, L. (2024). A legal mapping of 48 WHO member states' inclusion of public health emergency of international concern, pandemic, and health emergency terminology within national emergency legislation in responding to health emergencies. *The Lancet, 403*(10435). https://www.thelancet.com/journals/lancet/article/PIIS0140-6736(24)00156-9/fulltext
Woldie, M., & Yitbarek, K. (2021). Informal care and community volunteer work in global health. In I. Kickbusch, D. Ganten & M. Moeti (Eds.), *Handbook of global health*. Springer. 10.1007/978-3-030-45009-0_110
World Bank Group. (n.d.). *What we do*. http://www.worldbank.org/en/about/what-we-do
World Health Organization (WHO). (2010). *WHO global code of practice on the international recruitment of health personnel*. https://www.who.int/publications/i/item/wha68.32
World Health Organization (WHO) (2017). WHO country office for India. Brain Drain to brain gain migration of nursing and midwifery workforce in the State of Kerala .https://cdn.who.int/media/docs/default-source/health-workforce/migration-code/migration-of-nursing-midwifery-in-kerala.pdf?sfvrsn=fe2ca7ef_5&download=true
World Health Organization (WHO) (2020). Constitution of the World Health Organization. In *Basic documents: forty-ninth edition (including amendments adopted up to 31 May, 2019)* https://apps.who.int/gb/bd/pdf_files/BD_49th-en.pdf#page=6
World Health Organization (WHO). (2021). *Global strategy on digital health 2020-2025*. https://www.who.int/docs/default-source/documents/gs4dhdaa2a9f352b0445bafbc79ca799dce4d.pdf
World Health Organization (WHO). (2022a). *Consolidated telemedicine implementation guide*. https://www.who.int/publications/i/item/9789240059184
World Health Organization (WHO). (2022b). *70 years of GISRS: GISRS today: A public health resource for the world*. https://www.who.int/news-room/feature-stories/detail/seventy-years-of-gisrs---the-global-influenza-surveillance---response-system
World Health Organization (WHO). (2022c). *Implementing the end TB strategy: the essentials, 2022 update*. https://www.who.int/publications/i/item/9789240065093
World Health Organization (WHO). (2022d). *Vector alert: Anopheles stephensi invasion and spread in Africa and Sri Lanka*. https://iris.who.int/bitstream/handle/10665/365710/9789240067714-eng.pdf?sequence=1&isAllowed=y
World Health Organization (WHO). (2023a). *Primary health care policy and practice: Implementing for better results. International conference celebrating the 45th anniversary of Alma-Ata and 5th anniversary of Astana declarations*. https://www.who.int/europe/news-room/events/item/2023/10/23/default-calendar/international-conference-commemorating-alma-ata-45-and-astana-5---on-primary-health-care-policy-and-practice--implementing-for-better-results
World Health Organization (WHO). (2023b). *Primary health care*. https://www.who.int/health-topics/primary-health-care#tab=tab_1
World Health Organization (WHO) (2023c). Response tips and checklists. In *Managing epidemics: Key facts about major deadly diseases* (2nd ed., pp. 20–26) License: CC BY-NC-SA 3.0 IGO. https://iris.who.int/bitstream/handle/10665/374062/9789240083196-eng.pdf?sequence=1
World Health Organization (WHO). (2023d). *Social determinants of health: WHO called to return to the declaration of Alma-Ata*. https://www.who.int/social_determinants/tools/multimedia/alma_ata/en/
World Health Organization (WHO). (2023e). *WHO Coronavirus (COVID-19) dashboard*. Retrieved November 23, 2023 https://covid19.who.int/
World Health Organization (WHO). (2023f). *Tuberculosis* [Fact sheet]. https://www.who.int/news-room/fact-sheets/detail/tuberculosis
World Health Organization (WHO). (2023g). *World malaria report 2023*. https://www.who.int/teams/global-malaria-programme/reports/world-malaria-report-2023
World Health Organization (WHO). (2023h). *HIV and AIDS*. https://www.who.int/news-room/fact-sheets/detail/hiv-aids
World Health Organization (WHO). (2023i). *Rabat Declaration adopted to improve refugee and migrant health*. https://www.who.int/news/item/16-06-2023-rabat-declaration-adopted-to-improve-refugee-and-migrant-health
World Health Organization (WHO). (2024a). *Malaria*. https://www.who.int/news-room/questions-and-answers/item/malaria
World Health Organization (WHO). (2024b). *Promoting Health in All Policies and intersectoral action capacities*. https://www.who.int/activities/promoting-health-in-all-policies-and-intersectoral-action-capacities
World Health Organization (WHO). (n.d.) *WHO called to return to the Declaration of Alma-Ata*. https://www.who.int/teams/social-determinants-of-health/declaration-of-alma-ata
World Telehealth Initiative. (2023). *Stories of impact* [Blog]. https://www.worldtelehealthinitiative.org/blog
Ye, L., Liao, Z., & Yu, Y. (2023). *How Peace Corps volunteers influence the United States: an analysis based on pragmatism*. https://www.scielo.br/j/trans/a/FHTF6tRrDZ8tP5XGgSFNnSj/?lang=en

CHAPTER 17

Administration for Strategic Preparedness and Response. (2024). *The medical reserve corps*. https://aspr.hhs.gov/MRC/Pages/index.aspx
Administration for Strategic Preparedness and Response. (n.d.). *Emergency prescription assistance program*. https://aspr.hhs.gov/EPAP/Pages/default.aspx
Alghamdi, A. A. (2022). The psychological challenges of emergency medical service providers during disasters: A mini review. *Front Psychiatry, 13*, 773100. https://doi.org/10.3389/fpsyt.2022.773100. PMID: 35295786; PMCID: PMC8918654.
American Psychiatric Association (APA). (2023). *Resilience*. https://www.apa.org/topics/resilience
American Red Cross. (2023). *Survival kit supplies: I your emergency preparedness kit ready?* https://www.redcross.org/get-help/how-to-prepare-for-emergencies/survival-kit-supplies.html
American Red Cross. (2024). *Nursing and health*. https://www.redcross.org/about-us/who-we-are/nursing-health.html
American Red Cross. (n.d.). *American Red Cross guide to services*. http://www.redcross.org/images/MEDIA_CustomProductCatalog/m3140117_GuideToServices.pdf
Association of Public Health Nurses. (2014). *The role of the public health nurse in disaster preparedness, response, and recovery: A position paper*. Public Health Preparedness Committee. https://www.phnurse.org/assets/docs/Role%20of%20PHN%20in%20Disaster%20PRR_APHN%202014%20Ref%20updated%202015.pdf
Campinoti, M. S. (2023). *FDNY first responder deaths from 9/11-related diseases now equal FDNY deaths from attacks*. https://www.cnn.com/2023/09/24/us/9-11-firefighters-illnesses-deaths/index.html
Centers for Disease Control and Prevention (CDC). (2021). *Global health protection and security. Why it matters: The pandemic threat*. https://www.cdc.gov/globalhealth/healthprotection/fieldupdates/winter-2017/why-it-matters.html#:~:text=Investing%20in%20global%20health%20security,could%20avert%20these%20catastrophic%20costs
Centers for Disease Control and Prevention (CDC). (2024a). *Preparedness and planning*. https://emergency.cdc.gov/planning/index.asp#print
Centers for Disease Control and Prevention (CDC). (2024b). *Coronavirus disease 2019: Covid-19. How to protect yourself and others*. https://www.cdc.gov/coronavirus/2019-ncov/prevent-getting-sick/prevention.html
County of San Luis Obispo Emergency Medical Services Agency. (2023). *Multi-casualty incident response plan*. https://www.slocounty.ca.gov/Departments/Health-Agency/Public-Health/Emergency-Medical-Services/Emergency-Medical-Services-Agency/Forms-Documents/Policies,-Procedures,-and-Protocols-(includes-Form/200-299-OPERATIONS/210-Multi-Casualty-Incident-Response-Plan-7-01-202.pdf
Department of Homeland Security. (2019). *National response framework* (4th ed., pp. 39–42). https://www.fema.gov/sites/default/files/2020-04/NRF_FINALApproved_2011028.pdf
Department of Homeland Security. (2023). *Creation of the Department of Homeland Security*. https://www.dhs.gov/creation-department-homeland-security
Federal Bureau of Investigation (FBI). (n.d.). *Definitions of terrorism in the U.S. code*. https://www.fbi.gov/about-us/investigate/terrorism/terrorism-definition
Federal Bureau of Investigation and the Advanced Law Enforcement Rapid Response Training (ALERRT) Center at Texas State University. (2023). *Active Shooter Incidents in the United States in 2022*. https://www.fbi.gov/file-repository/active-shooter-incidents-in-the-us-2022-042623.pdf/view
Federal Emergency Management Agency (FEMA). (2021a). *History of FEMA*. https://www.fema.gov/about/history
Federal Emergency Management Agency (FEMA). (2021b). *National response framework* (4th ed.). https://www.fema.gov/emergency-managers/national-preparedness/frameworks/response#esf
Federal Emergency Management Agency (FEMA). (2021c). *Canines' role in urban search & rescue*. https://www.fema.gov/emergency-managers/national-preparedness/frameworks/urban-search-rescue/canines
Federal Emergency Management Agency (FEMA). (2023a). *How a disaster gets declared*. https://www.fema.gov/disaster/how-declared
Federal Emergency Management Agency (FEMA). (2023b). *National Incident Management System*. https://www.fema.gov/emergency-managers/nims
Federal Emergency Management Agency (FEMA). (2023c). *Are you "Petpared" for disasters?* https://www.fema.gov/fact-sheet/are-you-petpared-disasters
Federal Emergency Management Agency (FEMA). (2024a). *Social media*. https://www.fema.gov/social-media
Federal Emergency Management Agency (FEMA). (2024b). *Programs to support disaster survivors*. https://www.fema.gov/assistance/individual/disaster-survivors#case
Généreux, M., Schluter, P. J., Takahash, I. S., Usami, S., Mashino, S., Kayano, R., & Kim, Y. (2019). Psychosocial management before, during, and after emergencies and disasters-results from the Kobe Expert Meeting. *International Journal of Environmental Research and*

Public Health, *16*(8), 1309. https://doi.org/10.3390/ijerph16081309

Gross, I. T., Coughlin, R. F., Cone, D. C., Bogucki, S., Auerbach, M., & Cicero, M. X. (2019). GPS devices in a simulated mass casualty event, prehospital emergency care. *Prehospital Emergency Care*, *23*(2), 290–295. https://doi.org/10.1080/10903127.2018.1489018

International Charter. (n.d.). *Charter activations*. http://www.disasterscharter.org/

Joint Counterterrorism Assessment Team. (2020). *Chemical and biological threats to food retailers*. https://www.dni.gov/files/NCTC/documents/jcat/firstresponderstoolbox/First_Responders_Toolbox_Food_Attacks_8_MAY_Update.pdf

National Academies of Sciences, Engineering, and Medicine. (2021). *The future of nursing 2020-2030: Charting a path to achieve health equity*. The National Academies Press. https://doi.org/10.17226/25982

Office of Disease Prevention and Health Promotion (n.d.). *Browse objectives. Healthy People 2030*. U.S. Department of Health and Human Services. https://health.gov/healthypeople/objectives-and-data/browse-objectives

Office of the Assistant Secretary for Preparedness and Response. (2019). *ASPR TRACIE disaster behavioral health self care for healthcare workers modules*. https://files.asprtracie.hhs.gov/documents/aspr-tracie-dbh-self-care-for-healthcare-workers-modules-description-final-8-19-19.pdf

Office of the Assistant Secretary for Preparedness and Response. (n.d.). *Public health emergency: Strategic national stockpile*. https://www.phe.gov/about/sns/Pages/default.aspx

Organisation for the Prohibition of Chemical Weapons (OPCW). (2020). *What is a chemical weapon?* https://www.opcw.org/our-work/what-chemical-weapon

Pan American Health Organization (PAHO). Regional Office for the Americas of the World Health Organization (WHO). (n.d.) *Health in all policies*. https://www.paho.org/en/topics/health-all-policies

Prepare your pets for disasters. (2023). www.Ready.gov/pets

Ritter, M., Vance, M., & Iskander, J. (2023). *Moral injury among us public health service first responders during the COVID-19 pandemic*. Public Health Reports. https://doi.org/10.1177/00333549231176294

San Diego County Office of Emergency Services. (n.d.). *Family disaster plan and personal survival guide*. https://www.readysandiego.org/content/dam/oesready/en/Resources/Family-Disaster-Plan-English.pdf

Sen, H. E., Colucci, L., & Browne, D. T. (2022). Keeping the faith: Religion, positive coping, and mental health of caregivers during COVID-19. *Frontiers in Psychology*, *12*, 805019. https://doi.org/10.3389/fpsyg.2021.805019. PMID: 35126256; PMCID: PMC8811163.

Substance Abuse and Mental Health Services Administration (SAMHSA). (2019). *Supplemental research bulletin: Disasters and people with serious mental illness*. https://www.samhsa.gov/sites/default/files/disasters-people-with-serious-mental-illness.pdf

Substance Abuse and Mental Health Services Administration (SAMHSA). (2020). *Social media and disasters*. https://www.samhsa.gov/find-help/disaster-distress-helpline/social-media

Substance Abuse and Mental Health Services Administration (SAMHSA). (2024a). *Diversity, equity, and inclusion in disaster planning and response*. https://www.samhsa.gov/dtac/disaster-planners/diversity-equity-inclusion

Substance Abuse and Mental Health Services Administration (SAMHSA). (2024b). *Survivors of disasters resource portal*. Disaster Technical Assistance Center. https://www.samhsa.gov/dtac

U.S. Department of Health and Human Services (USDHHS). (2024). *Management of the deceased*. https://chemm.hhs.gov/deceased.htm

U.S. Department of Justice (2024a). *Critical Incident Review: Active Shooter at Robb Elementary School*. Office of Community Oriented Policing Services. https://cops.usdoj.gov/uvalde

U.S. Department of Justice. (2024b). *Domestic radicalization and violent extremism*. https://nij.ojp.gov/topics/articles/domestic-radicalization-and-violent-extremism

U.S. Public Health Service (USPHS). (n.d.). *U.S. Public Health Service Commissioned Corps*. https://www.usphs.gov/about-us

Wang, J. N., Lu, W. J., Hu, J. T., Xi, W., Xu, J. B., Wang, Z. N., & Zhang, Y. F. (2022). The usage of triage systems in mass casualty incident of developed countries. *Open Journal of Emergency Medicine*, *10*, 124–137. https://doi.org/10.4236/ojem.2022.102011

World Health Organization (WHO). (2024). *WHO coronavirus disease (COVID-10) dashboard*. https://covid19.who.int/?gclid=Cj0KCQjw6ar4BRDnARIsAITGzlC07PXVBWo7aExbhEy1eIi0wXAKyhy8Ju0Z6amxvLOKwozDj_suCJcaAieyEALw_wcB

CHAPTER 18

Abdurrachid, N., & Gama Marques, J. (2022). Munchausen syndrome by proxy (MSBP): A review regarding perpetrators of factitious disorder imposed on another (FDIA). *CNS Spectrums*, *27*(1), 16–26. https://doi.org/10.1017/S1092852920001741

American Association of Neurological Surgeons (AANS). (2023). *Shaken baby syndrome*. https://www.aans.org/en/Patients/Neurosurgical-Conditions-and-Treatments/Shaken-Baby-Syndrome

American College of Obstetricians and Gynecologist (ACOG). (reaffirmed in 2022). *Intimate partner violence*. https://www.acog.org/clinical/clinical-guidance/committee-opinion/articles/2012/02/intimate-partner-violence

American Psychiatric Association (APA). (2022a). *Bullying*. https://www.apa.org/topics/bullying

American Psychiatric Association (APA). (2022b). *Statement on the bipartisan safer communities act* 2022. https://www.psychiatry.org/news-room/news-releases/apa-statement-on-the-bipartisan-safer-communities

American Public Health Association (APHA). (2023). *Gun violence*. https://www.apha.org/topics-and-issues/gun-violence

Arizona Law. (n.d.). *Myths and realities of domestic abuse*. https://law.arizona.edu/sites/default/files/myths_and_realities_of_domestic_abuse.pdf

Banyard, V., Mitchell, K. J., & Ybarra, M. L. (2021). Exposure to self-directed violence: Understanding intention to help and helping behaviors among adolescents and emerging adults. *International Journal of Environmental Research and Public Health*, *18*(16), 8606. https://doi.org/10.3390/ijerph18168606. PMID: 34444354; PMCID: PMC8391527

Basile, K. C., De Gue, S., Jones, K., Freire, K., Dills, J., Smith, S. G., & Raiford, J. L. (2016). *Sexual violence prevention resource for action: A compilation of the best available evidence*. National Center for Injury Prevention and Control, Centers for Disease Control and Prevention.

Boone, R. (2023). *Attacks at US medical centers show why health care is one of the nation's most violent fields*. https://apnews.com/article/hospitals-workplace-violence-shootings-aa6918569ff8f76ff8a15b9813e31686

Burns, C. J., Borah, L., Terrell, S. M., James, L. N. Erkkinen, E., & Owens, L. (2023). Trauma-informed care curricula for the health professions: A scoping review of best practices for design, implementation, and evaluation. *Academic Medicine*, *98*(3), 401–409. https://doi.org/10.1097/ACM.0000000000005046

California Department of Education. (2020). *Child abuse and identification reporting guidelines*. https://www.cde.ca.gov/ls/ss/ap/childabusereportingguide.asp

Casanova-Perez, R., Apodaca, C., Bascom, E., Mohanraj, D., Lane, C., Vidyarthix, D., Beneteau, E., Sabin, J., Pratt, W., Weibel, N., & Hartzler, A. L. (2022). Broken down by bias: Healthcare biases experienced by BIPOC and LGBTQ+ patients. *AMIA Annual Symposium Proceeding*, 2021, 275–284.

Center for Strategic and International Studies. (2024). *Pushed to extremes: Domestic terrorism amid polarization and protest*. https://www.csis.org/analysis/pushed-extremes-domestic-terrorism-amid-polarization-and-protest

Centers for Disease Control and Prevention (CDC). (2024a). *About violence prevention*. https://www.cdc.gov/violence-prevention/about/?CDC_AAref_Val=https://www.cdc.gov/violenceprevention/about/social-ecologicalmodel.html

Centers for Disease Control and Prevention (CDC). (2024b). *Risk and protective factors*. https://www.cdc.gov/youth-violence/risk-factors/?CDC_AAref_Val=https://www.cdc.gov/violenceprevention/youthviolence/riskprotectivefactors.html

Centers for Disease Control and Prevention (CDC). (2024c). *About abusive head trauma*. https://www.cdc.gov/child-abuse-neglect/about/about-abusive-head-trauma.html?CDC_AAref_Val=https://www.cdc.gov/violenceprevention/childabuseandneglect/Abusive-Head-Trauma.html

Centers for Disease Control and Prevention (CDC). (2024d). *About school violence*. https://www.cdc.gov/youth-violence/about/about-school-violence.html?CDC_AAref_Val=https://www.cdc.gov/violenceprevention/youthviolence/schoolviolence/fastfact.html

Centers for Disease Control and Prevention (CDC). (2024e). *About bullying*. https://www.cdc.gov/youth-violence/about/about-bullying.html?CDC_AAref_Val=https://www.cdc.gov/violenceprevention/youthviolence/bullyingresearch/fastfact.html

Centers for Disease Control and Prevention (CDC). (2024f). *Intimate partner violence, sexual violence, and stalking among men*. https://www.cdc.gov/intimate-partner-violence/about/intimate-partner-violence-sexual-violence-and-stalking-among-men.html?CDC_AAref_Val=https://www.cdc.gov/violenceprevention/intimatepartnerviolence/men-ipvsvandstalking.html

Centers for Disease Control and Prevention (CDC). (2024g). *About teen dating violence*. https://www.cdc.gov/intimate-partner-violence/about/about-teen-dating-violence.html?CDC_AAref_Val=https://www.cdc.gov/violenceprevention/intimatepartnerviolence/teendatingviolence/fastfact.html

Centers for Disease Control and Prevention (CDC). (2024h). *About abuse of older persons*. https://www.cdc.gov/elder-abuse/about/?CDC_AAref_Val=https://www.cdc.gov/violenceprevention/elderabuse/fastfact.html

Centers for Disease Control and Prevention (CDC). (2024i). *Fast facts: Firearm injury and death*. https://www.cdc.gov/firearm-violence/data-research/facts-stats/?CDC_AAref_Val=https://www.cdc.gov/violenceprevention/firearms/fastfact.html

Centers for Disease Control and Prevention (CDC). (2024j). *Program: Rape prevention and education (RPE) program*. https://www.cdc.gov/sexual-violence/programs/?CDC_AAref_Val=https://www.cdc.gov/violenceprevention/sexualviolence/rpe/

Centers for Disease Control and Prevention (CDC). (n.d.-a). *Principles of prevention guide*. https://vetoviolence.cdc.gov/apps/pop/assets/pdfs/pop_notebook.pdf

Centers for Disease Control and Prevention (CDC). (n.d.-b). *Suicide prevention*. https://www.cdc.gov/suicide/?CDC_AAref_Val=https://www.cdc.gov/violenceprevention/suicide/fastfact.html

Cheung, S. P., & Huang, C. C. (2023). Childhood exposure to intimate partner violence and teen dating violence. *Journal of Family Violence*, *38*, 263–274. https://doi.org/10.1007/s10896-022-00377-7

Child Welfare Information Gateway. (2021). *Infant safe haven laws*. https://www.childwelfare.gov/resources/infant-safe-haven-laws/

Child Welfare Information Gateway. (2022). *Definitions of child abuse and neglect*. U.S. Department of Health and Human Services, Administration for Children and Families, Children's Bureau. https://www.childwelfare.gov/topics/systemwide/laws-policies/statutes/define/

Cox, J. W., Rich, S., Trevor, L., Muyskens, J., & Ulmanu, M. (2024). More than 370,000 students have experienced gun violence at school since columbine. *Washington Post*. https://www.washingtonpost.com/education/interactive/school-shootings-database/

Domestic Abuse Intervention Programs. (n.d.). *What is the Duluth Model?* https://www.theduluthmodel.org/

Doroudchi, A., Zarenezhad, M., Hosseininezhad, H., Malekpour, A., Ehsaei, Z., Kaboodkhani, R., & Valiei, M. (2023). Psychological complications of the children exposed to domestic violence: A systematic review. *Egyptian Journal of Forensic Science*, *13*, 26. https://doi.org/10.1186/s41935-023-00343-4

Ethier, K. (2023). *CDC releases the youth risk behavior survey data summary & trends report: 2011-2021 letter*. https://www.cdc.gov/nchhstp/dear_colleague/2023/DSRT-DCL.html

Federal Bureau of Investigation (FBI). (2022). *Elderly fraud report*. https://www.ic3.gov/Media/PDF/AnnualReport/2022_IC3ElderFraudReport.pdf

Federal Bureau of Investigation (FBI). (2023). *FBI releases 2022 crime in the nation statistics*. https://www.fbi.gov/news/press-releases/fbi-releases-2022-crime-in-the-nation-statistics

Federal Bureau of Investigation (FBI). (n.d.-a). *What we investigate: Gangs*. https://www.fbi.gov/investigate/violent-crime/gangs

Federal Bureau of Investigation (FBI). (n.d.-b). *Parents, caregivers, and teachers: Protecting your kids*. https://www.fbi.gov/how-we-can-help-you/parents-and-caregivers-protecting-your-kids

Felitti, V. J., Anda, R. F., Nordenberg, D., Williamson, D. F., Spitz, A. M., Edwards, V., Koss, M. P., & Marks J. S. (1998). Relationship of childhood abuse and household dysfunction to many of the leading causes of death in adults: The adverse childhood experiences (ACE) study. *American Journal of Preventive Medicine, 14*(4), 245–258. https://doi.org/10.1016/s0749-3797(98)00017-8

Fricke, J., Siddique, S. M., Douma, C., Ladak, A., Burchill, C. N., Greysen, R., & Mull, N. K. (2023). Workplace violence in healthcare settings: A scoping review of guidelines and systematic reviews. *Trauma, Violence, & Abuse, 24*(5), 3363–3383. https://doi.org/10.1177/15248380221126476

Government of Canada. (2022). *Statistics on sexual assault*. https://www.justice.gc.ca/eng/rp-pr/csj-sjc/ccs-ajc/rr06_vic2/p3_4.html

Gramlich, J. (2023). *What the data says about gun deaths in the U.S.* Pew Research Center. https://www.pewresearch.org/short-reads/2023/04/26/what-the-data-says-about-gun-deaths-in-the-u-s/

Hainaut, M., Thompson, K. J., Ha, C. J., Herzog, H. L., Roberts, T., & Ades, V. (2022). *Are screening tools for identifying human trafficking victims in health care settings validated? A scoping review*. Public Health Reports. https://doi.org/10.1177/00333549211061774

Health Resources and Services Administration (HRSA). (2022). *Women's preventive services guidelines. Affordable care act expands prevention coverage for women's health and well-being*. https://www.hrsa.gov/womens-guidelines

Holmes, M. R., Berg, K. A., Bender, A. E., Evans, K. E., O'Donnell, K., & Miller, E. K. (2022). Nearly 50 years of child exposure to intimate partner violence empirical research: Evidence mapping, overarching themes, and future directions. *Journal of Family Violence, 37*, 1207–1219. https://doi.org/10.1007/s10896-021-00349-3

Hunt, K. E., Robinson, L. E., Valido, A., Espelage, D. L., & Hong, J. S. (2022). Teen dating violence victimization: Associations among peer justification, attitudes toward gender inequality, sexual activity, and peer victimization. *Journal of Interpersonal Violence, 37*(9–10), 5914–5936. https://doi.org/10.1177/08862605221085015

International Association of Forensic Nurses. (n.d.). *What is forensic nursing?* https://www.forensicnurses.org/page/WhatisFN/

Joint Commission on Accreditation of Healthcare Organizations (JCAHO). (2021). *Quick safety issue 24: Bullying has no place in health care*. https://www.jointcommission.org/resources/news-and-multimedia/newsletters/newsletters/quick-safety/quick-safety-issue-24-bullying-has-no-place-in-health-care/bullying-has-no-place-in-health-care/

Kah, K., Dailey-Provost, J., Stanford, J. B., Rogers, C. R., & Schliep, K. (2022). Association between pre-pregnancy and pregnancy physical abuse, partner-related stress, and post-partum depression: Findings from the Utah pregnancy risk assessment and monitoring system (UT-PRAMS), 2016-2018. *Utah Womens Health Review, 6*(10). https://doi:10.26054/0d-0tbc-7vhj

Kidpower. (2021). *Stranger abduction & kidnapping prevention*. https://www.kidpower.org/library/article/safety-tips-kidnapping/

Legal Information Institute (n.d.). *U.S. code 5106g. Definitions*. Cornell Law School. https://www.law.cornell.edu/uscode/text/42/5106g

Lo Iacono, L., Trentini, C., & Carola, V. (2021). Psychobiological consequences of childhood sexual abuse: Current knowledge and clinical implications. *Frontiers in Neuroscience, 15*, 771511. https://doi.org/10.3389/fnins.2021.771511. PMID: 34924938; PMCID: PMC8678607.

Los Angeles Police Department (LAPD). (n.d.). *Domestic violence: Understanding the cycle of violence*. https://www.lapdonline.org/domestic-violence-understanding-the-cycle-of-violence/

Macassa, G., Cormac McGrath, C., & Soares, J. (2023). *Violence as an object of teaching, research, and prevention practices, at the nexus between public health, social work, criminology, and psychology*. https://www.diva-portal.org/smash/get/diva2:1813220/FULLTEXT01.pdf

Merriam-Webster. (2020). *Cyberstalking*. https://www.merriam-webster.com/legal/cyberstalking

Morgan, R. E., & Truman, J. L. (2022). *Stalking victimization, 2019*. Bureau of Justice Statistics. https://bjs.ojp.gov/library/publications/stalking-victimization-2019

Mueller, I., & Tronick, E. (2020). The long shadow of violence: The impact of exposure to intimate partner violence in infancy and early childhood. *International Journal of Applied Psychoanalytic Studies, 17*(3), 232–245. Special Issue: Interdisciplinary Perspectives on Domestic Violence and Coercive Control. https://doi.org/10.1002/aps.1668

National Center for Healthy Safe Children. (2020). *Safe schools/healthy students (SS/HS) framework*. https://healthysafechildren.org/sshs-framework

National Center for Missing and Exploited Children. (2023). *CyberTipline*. http://www.cybertipline.com

National Center of Education Statistics School Crime. (2023). *School crime*. https://nces.ed.gov/fastfacts/display.asp?id=49

National Center on Elder Abuse (NCEA). (n.d.-a). *What is elder abuse*. https://ncea.acl.gov/elder-abuse#gsc.tab=0

National Center on Elder Abuse (NCEA). (n.d.-b). *Mistreatment of lesbian, gay, bisexual and transgender (LGBT) elders: Research brief*. http://www.centeronelderabuse.org/docs/ResearchBrief_LGBT_Elders_508web.pdf

National Child Traumatic Stress Network. (n.d.). *What is child trauma?* https://www.nctsn.org/what-is-child-trauma

National Council on Aging. (n.d.). *Elder abuse facts*. https://www.ncoa.org/public-policy-action/elder-justice/elder-abuse-facts/

National Human Trafficking Hotline. (n.d.). *Human trafficking*. https://humantraffickinghotline.org/type-trafficking/human-trafficking

National Institute of Mental Health. (2024). *Coping with traumatic events*. https://www.nimh.nih.gov/health/topics/coping-with-traumatic-events

New York City Department for the Aging & Lifespan of Greater Rochester, Inc. & Weill Cornell Medical Centre of Cornell University. (2011). *Under the radar: New York state elder abuse prevalence study*. https://www.ojp.gov/ncjrs/virtual-library/abstracts/under-radar-new-york-state-elder-abuse-prevalence-study

NSPCC. (n.d.). *Emotional abuse*. https://www.nspcc.org.uk/what-is-child-abuse/types-of-abuse/emotional-abuse/

Occupational Safety and Health Administration (OSHA). (n.d.). *Workplace violence*. https://www.osha.gov/SLTC/workplaceviolence/

Office of Disease Prevention and Health Promotion (ODPHP) (n.d.). *Violence*. Healthy People 2030. https://health.gov/healthypeople/search?query=violence:

Office of Justice Programs (OJP). (n.d.). *National criminal justice reference service: Special feature—Gangs*. https://www.ncjrs.gov/gangs

Office of Juvenile Justice and Delinquency Prevention (OJJDP). (n.d.). *Commercial sexual exploitation of children*. https://www.ojjdp.gov/programs/csec_program.html

Office of the United Nations High Commissioner for Human Rights. (2020). *Committee on the rights of the child*. https://www.ohchr.org/EN/HRBodies/CRC/Pages/CRCIntro.aspx

Office of Victim Crime. (n.d.). *What is vicarious trauma?* https://ovc.ojp.gov/program/vtt/what-is-vicarious-trauma

Omaha System. (2019). *The Omaha system. Solving the clinical date-information puzzle*. http://www.omahasystem.org/overview.html

Paisner, S. R. (2018). *Five myths about domestic violence*. The Washington Post. https://www.washingtonpost.com/outlook/five-myths/five-myths-about-domestic-violence/2018/02/23/78969748-1819-11e8-b681-2d4d462a1921_story.html

Pereira, M. G., Pereira, D., & Pedras, S. (2020). PTSD, psychological morbidity and marital dissatisfaction in colonial war veterans. *Journal of Mental Health, 29*(1), 69–76. https://doi.org/10.1080/09638237.2018.1487532

RAINN. (2023). *Warning signs for young children*. https://www.rainn.org/articles/warning-signs-young-children

Saavedia, N. (2023). *28 arrested, 19 children rescued after months-long operation targeting child sex abuse on internet in Montgomery County*. https://www.click2houston.com/news/local/2023/07/24/28-arrested-19-children-rescued-after-month-long-operation-targeting-child-sex-abuse-on-internet-in-montgomery-county/

Salinas, M. E., Moll-Ramirez, V., Kipreos, C. B., & Su, A. (2022). Survivor of deadliest human smuggling case in US history speaks out. *ABC news*. https://abcnews.go.com/US/survivor-deadliest-human-smuggling-case-us-history-speaks/story?id=91394907

Sanchini, V., Sala, R., & Gastmans, C. (2022). The concept of vulnerability in aged care: A systematic review of argument-based ethics literature. *BMC Medical Ethics, 23*, 84. https://doi.org/10.1186/s12910-022-00819-3

Schaeffer, K. (2023). *9 facts about bullying in the U.S.* Pew Research Center. https://www.pewresearch.org/short-reads/2023/11/17/9-facts-about-bullying-in-the-us/

Schrubbe, L., García-Moreno, C., Sardinha, L., & Stöckl, H. (2023). Intimate partner violence against women during pregnancy: A systematic review and meta-analysis protocol for producing global and regional estimates. *Systemic Review, 12*, 107. https://link.springer.com/content/pdf/10.1186/s13643-023-02232-2.pdf

SexInfo Online. (2017). *The cycle of domestic violence*. https://sexinfo.soc.ucsb.edu/article/cycle-domestic-violence

Smithfield, B. (2016). *The case of Mary Ellen—The first documented case of child abuse in the US was reported to the animal welfare agency in 1874. The Vintage News*. https://www.thevintagenews.com/2016/11/09/the-case-of-mary-ellen-the-first-documented-case-of-child-abuse-in-the-us-was-reported-to-the-animal-welfare-agency-in-1874/

Stanford Medicine. (n.d.). *Child abuse: Signs and symptoms of abuse/neglect*. http://childabuse.stanford.edu/screening/signs.html

Stop It Now! (2022). *Tip sheet: Warning signs of possible sexual abuse in a child's behavior*. https://www.stopitnow.org/ohc-content/tip-sheet-7

Storey, J. E. (2020). Risk factors for elder abuse and neglect: A review of the literature. *Aggression and Violent Behavior, 50*, 101339. https://doi.org/10.1016/j.avb.2019.101339

Substance Abuse and Mental Health Service Administration (SAMHSA). (2023). *Compassion fatigue and self-care for crisis counselors*. https://www.samhsa.gov/dtac/ccp-toolkit/self-care-for-crisis-counselors#:~:text=Compassion%20fatigue%20signs%20and%20symptoms,Disorientation%20or%20confusion

The White House. (2023). *Executive summary: Initial blueprint for the White House task force to address online harassment and abuse*. https://www.whitehouse.gov/briefing-room/statements-releases/2023/03/03/executive-summary-initial-blueprint-for-the-white-house-task-force-to-address-online-harassment-and-abuse/

Turgoose, D., Glover, N., & Maddox, L. (2021). Chapter 4—Burnout and the psychological impact of policing: Trends and coping strategies. In P. B. Marques & M. Paulino (Eds.), *Police psychology new trends in forensic psychological science* (pp. 63–86). Elsevier. https://doi.org/10.1016/B978-0-12-816544-7.00004-8

Turner, R., & Hammersjö, A. (2023). Navigating survivorhood? Lived experiences of social support-seeking among LGBTQ survivors of intimate partner violence. *Qualitative Social Work, 23*(2). https://doi.org/10.1177/14733250221150208

U.S. Agency for International Development. (2023). *Implementation of the trafficking victims protection act*. Statement of Johnny Walsh, Deputy Assistant Administrator, Center for Democracy, Human Rights, and Governance (DRG), before the House Foreign Affairs Subcommittee on Global Health, Global Human Rights, and International Organizations. https://www.usaid.gov/news-information/congressional-testimony/may-12-2023-implementation-trafficking-victims-protection-act

U.S. Department of Health and Human Services (USDHHS). (2023). *What is child abuse or neglect? What is the definition of child abuse and neglect?* https://www.hhs.gov/answers/programs-for-families-and-children/what-is-child-abuse/index.html

U.S. Department of Health and Human Services (USDHHS). (n.d.). *The community guide*. https://www.thecommunityguide.org/

U.S. Department of Justice (USDOJ). (2023a). *Elder justice initiative: Research and data*. https://www.justice.gov/elder-justice/eappa

U.S. Department of Justice (USDOJ). (2023b). *What is human trafficking*. https://www.justice.gov/humantrafficking/what-is-human-trafficking

U.S. Department of Justice (USDOJ). (2023c). *Human trafficking: Key legislation*. https://www.justice.gov/humantrafficking/key-legislation#:~:text=Critically%2C%20the%20TVPA%20established%20the,protection%2C%20prevention%2C%20and%20prosecution

U.S. Department of Justice (USDOJ). (n.d.-a). Amber alert. America's missing: Broadcast emergency response. http://www.amberalert.gov/

U.S. Department of Justice (USDOJ). (n.d.-b). *Domestic violence*. http://www.justice.gov/ovw/domestic-violence

U.S. Department of Justice (USDOJ). (n.d.-c). *Sexual assault*. https://www.justice.gov/ovw/sexual-assault

U.S. Department of Justice (USDOJ). (n.d.-d). *Stalking*. http://www.justice.gov/ovw/stalking

U.S. Department of Justice (USDOJ). (n.d.-e). *Project safe childhood*. https://www.justice.gov/psc

United Nations. (n.d.). *World elder abuse awareness day: 15 June*. https://www.un.org/en/observances/elder-abuse-awareness-day/

United Nations Office on Drugs and Crime. (2023). *Global study on homicide 2023*. https://www.unodc.org/documents/data-and-analysis/gsh/2023/Global_study_on_homicide_2023_web.pdf

UNWomen. (2023). *Facts and figures: Ending violence against women*. https://www.unwomen.org/en/what-we-do/ending-violence-against-women/facts-and-figures

Vogels, E. A. (2022). *Teens and cyberbullying*. Pew Research Center. https://www.pewresearch.org/internet/2022/12/15/teens-and-cyberbullying-2022/

Whirry, R., & Holt, S. (2020). *Finding safety*. Los Angeles LGBT Center. https://stopviolence.lalgbtcenter.org/wp-content/uploads/2022/08/Finding_Safety.pdf

White Ribbon Australia. (2019). *Cycle of violence: What is the cycle of violence?* https://www.youtube.com/watch?v=cFa0l1Zlio8

Williams, S. G., Fruh, S., Barinas, J. L., & Graves, R. J. (2022). Self-care in nurses. *Journal of Radiology Nurse*, *41*(1), 22–27. https://doi.org/10.1016/j.jradnu.2021.11.001. PMID: 35431686; PMCID: PMC9007545.

World Health Organization (WHO). (2022a). *COVID-19 and violence against women. What the health sector/system can do*. https://iris.who.int/bitstream/handle/10665/331699/WHO-SRH-20.04-eng.pdf?sequence=1

World Health Organization (WHO). (2022b). *Child maltreatment*. https://www.who.int/news-room/fact-sheets/detail/child-maltreatment#:~:text=It%20includes%20all%20types%20of,of%20responsibility%2C%20trust%20or%20power

World Health Organization (WHO). (2024a). *Violence against women*. https://www.who.int/news-room/fact-sheets/detail/violence-against-women

World Health Organization (WHO). (2024b). *Elder abuse*. https://www.who.int/news-room/fact-sheets/detail/elder-abuse

World Health Organization (WHO). (n.d.). *Definition and typology of violence*. https://www.who.int/groups/violence-prevention-alliance/approach#:~:text=%22the%20intentional%20use%20of%20physical,%2C%20maldevelopment%2C%20or%20deprivation.%22

Yoon, S., Lee, J., Jun, Y. H., & Jeon, G. W. (2022). Neonatal abusive head trauma without external injuries: Suspicion improves diagnosis. *Children*, *9*(6), 808. https://doi.org/10.3390/children9060808. PMID: 35740745; PMCID: PMC9221573.

CHAPTER 19

Albers, A. N., Thaker, J., & Newcomer, S. R. (2022). Barriers to and facilitators of early childhood immunization in rural areas of the United States: A systematic review of the literature. *Preventive Medicine Report*, *27*, 1–12.

American Academy of Pediatrics. (2022). *American Academy of Pediatrics updates recommendations on maintaining, improving children's oral health*. https://www.aap.org/en/news-room/news-releases/aap/2022/american-academy-of-pediatrics-updates-recommendations-on-maintaining-improving-childrens-oral-health/

American Academy of Pediatrics. (2023a). from *bottle to cup: Helping your child make a healthy transition*. https://www.healthychildren.org/English/ages-stages/baby/feeding-nutrition/Pages/Discontinuing-the-Bottle.aspx

American Academy of Pediatrics. (2023b). *Ten common childhood illnesses and their treatments*. https://www.healthychildren.org/English/health-issues/conditions/treatments/Pages/10-Common-Childhood-Illnesses-and-Their-Treatments.asp

American Association of Neurological Surgeons. (2023). *Shaken baby syndrome*. https://www.aans.org/en/Patients/Neurosurgical-Conditions-and-Treatments/Shaken-Baby-Syndrome

American Association of Poison Control Centers (AAPCC). (n.d.-a). *In the home safety tips*. https://poisoncenters.org/prevention/in-the-home

American Association of Poison Control Centers (AAPCC). (n.d.-b). *Prevention*. http://www.aapcc.org/prevention/

American Cancer Society. (2022). *What do we know about e-cigarettes?* https://www.cancer.org/cancer/risk-prevention/tobacco/e-cigarettes-vaping/what-do-we-know-about-e-cigarettes.html

American Dental Association. (2023). *Pregnancy*. https://www.ada.org/en/resources/research/science-and-research-institute/oral-health-topics/pregnancy

Anbalagan, S., & Mendez, M. (2020). *Neonatal abstinence syndrome*. Statpearls publishing. https://www.ncbi.nlm.nih.gov/books/NBK551498/

Bell, L., Whelan, M., Thomas, L., Edwards, E., Lycett, D., Hayward, K., Wilson, K., Harrison, R., & Patel, R. (2023). Use of e-cigarettes in pregnancy: A systematic review of evidence. *J Public Health (Berl.)*. https://doi.org/10.1007/s10389-023-02026-9

Boston Children's Hospital. (n.d.). *Sudden infant death syndrome (SIDS)*. https://www.childrenshospital.org/conditions/sudden-infant-death-syndrome-sids

Bright Futures. (2022). *Developmental, behavioral, psychosocial, screening, and assessment forms*. https://brightfutures.aap.org/materials-and-tools/tool-and-resource-kit/Pages/Developmental-Behavioral-Psychosocial-Screening-and-Assessment-Forms.aspx

California Department of Public Health. (2019). *The congenital syphilis morbidity & mortality review toolkit*. https://www.cdph.ca.gov/Programs/CID/DCDC/CDPH%20Document%20Library/Congenital_Syphilis_Morbidity_and_Mortality_Review_Toolkit.pdf

Carson, M. P. (2022). *Hypertension and pregnancy*. https://emedicine.medscape.com/article/261435-overview?form=fpf

Casey Family Programs. (2021). *How do parent partner programs instill hope and support prevention and unification?* https://www.casey.org/parent-partner-program/

Catherine, N. L. A., Boyle, M., Zheng, Y., McCandeless, L., Xie, H., Lever, R., Sheehan, D., Gonzales, A., Jack, S. M., Gafni, A., Tonmyr, L., Marcellus, L., Varcoe, C., Cullen, A., Hjertaas, K., Riebe, C., Rikert, N., Sunthoram, A., Barr, R., MacMillan, H., & Waddel, C. (2021). Nurse home visiting and prenatal substance use in a socioeconomically disadvantaged population in British Columbia: analysis of prenatal secondary outcomes in an ongoing randomized controlled trial. *Canadian Medical Association Journal*, *9*(4), E1040. https://doi.org/10.9778/cmajo.20200063

Centers for Disease Control and Prevention (CDC). (2020a). *Sexually transmitted disease preventive services coverage*. https://www.cdc.gov/nchhstp/highqualitycare/preventiveservices/std.html

Centers for Disease Control and Prevention (CDC). (2020b). *Thimerosal and vaccines*. https://www.cdc.gov/vaccinesafety/concerns/thimerosal/index.html#:~:text=Scientific%20research%20does%20not%20show,to%20the%20development%20of%20autism

Centers for Disease Control and Prevention (CDC). (2020c). *Awardee immunization websites*. https://www.cdc.gov/vaccines/imz-managers/awardee-imz-websites.html

Centers for Disease Control and Prevention (CDC). (2020d). *Immunization information systems (IIS)*. https://www.cdc.gov/vaccines/programs/iis/index.html

Centers for Disease Control and Prevention (CDC). (2021a). *Mortality in the United States, 2020*. https://www.cdc.gov/nchs/products/databriefs/db427.htm#section_5

Centers for Disease Control and Prevention (CDC). (2021b). *Injuries among children and teens*. https://www.cdc.gov/injury/features/child-injury/index.html#:~:text=Leading%20causes%20of%20child%20unintentional,poisoning%2C%20fires%2C%20and%20falls

Centers for Disease Control and Prevention (CDC). (2021c). *Childhood lead poisoning prevention: Populations at higher risk*. https://www.cdc.gov/nceh/lead/prevention/populations.htm

Centers for Disease Control and Prevention (CDC). (2021d). *Cavities*. https://www.cdc.gov/oralhealth/fast-facts/cavities/index.html

Centers for Disease Control and Prevention (CDC). (2021e). *Autism and vaccines*. https://www.cdc.gov/vaccinesafety/concerns/autism.html

Centers for Disease Control and Prevention (CDC). (2022b). *Weight gain during pregnancy*. http://www.cdc.gov/reproductivehealth/maternalinfanthealth/pregnancy-weight-gain.htm

Centers for Disease Control and Prevention (CDC). (2022c). *Substance use during pregnancy*. https://www.cdc.gov/reproductivehealth/maternalinfanthealth/substance-abuse/substance-abuse-during-pregnancy.htm

Centers for Disease Control and Prevention (CDC). (2022d). *Fetal alcohol spectrum disorders alcohol use in pregnancy*. https://www.cdc.gov/ncbddd/fasd/alcohol-use.html

Centers for Disease Control and Prevention (CDC). (2022e). *Incidence, prevalence, and cost of sexually transmitted infections in the United States*. Retrieved from <https://www.cdc.gov/nchhstp/newsroom/fact-sheets/std/STI-Incidence-Prevalence-Cost-Factsheet.html>

Centers for Disease Control and Prevention (CDC). (2022f). *STDs & pregnancy: CDC fact sheet detailed*. https://www.cdc.gov/std/pregnancy/stdfact-pregnancy-detailed.htm

Centers for Disease Control and Prevention (CDC). (2022g). *Gestational diabetes*. https://www.cdc.gov/diabetes/basics/gestational.html

Centers for Disease Control and Prevention (CDC). (2022h). *Adult obesity facts*. https://www.cdc.gov/obesity/data/adult.html

Centers for Disease Control and Prevention (CDC). (2022i). *Hypertensive disorders in pregnancy and mortality at delivery hospitalization-United States, 2017-2019*. https://www.cdc.gov/mmwr/volumes/71/wr/mm7117a1.htm#:~:text=The%20prevalence%20of%20pregnancy%2Dassociated,from%202.0%25%20to%202.3%25

Centers for Disease Control and Prevention (CDC). (2022j). *Drowning prevention*. https://www.cdc.gov/drowning/prevention/index.html

Centers for Disease Control and Prevention (CDC). (2022k). *Car passenger safety: Get the facts*. https://www.cdc.gov/transportationsafety/child_passenger_safety/cps-fact-sheet.html

Centers for Disease Control and Prevention (CDC). (2022l). *Violence prevention: Risk and protective factors*. https://www.cdc.gov/violenceprevention/childabuseandneglect/riskprotectivefactors.html

Centers for Disease Control and Prevention (CDC). (2022m). *Violence prevention: Preventing abusive head trauma*. https://www.cdc.gov/violenceprevention/childabuseandneglect/Abusive-Head-Trauma.html

Centers for Disease Control and Prevention (CDC). (2022n). *What is autism spectrum disorder (ASD)?* https://www.cdc.gov/ncbddd/autism/facts.html

Centers for Disease Control and Prevention (CDC). (2022o). *Food allergies*. https://www.cdc.gov/healthyschools/foodallergies/index.htm

Centers for Disease Control and Prevention (CDC). (2022p). *Cystic fibrosis*. https://www.cdc.gov/genomics/disease/cystic_fibrosis.htm

Centers for Disease Control and Prevention (CDC). (2022q). *Vaccines for children program (VFC)*. https://www.cdc.gov/vaccines/programs/vfc/index.html

Centers for Disease Control and Prevention (CDC). (2022r). *Violence prevention: Prevention strategies*. https://www.cdc.gov/violenceprevention/childabuseandneglect/prevention.html

Centers for Disease Control and Prevention (CDC). (2022s). *Fast facts: Preventing child abuse & neglect*. https://www.cdc.gov/violenceprevention/childabuseandneglect/fastfact.html

Centers for Disease Control and Prevention (CDC). (2022t). *Individuals with Disabilities Education Act (IDEA) services*. https://www.cdc.gov/ncbddd/cp/treatment.html

Centers for Disease Control and Prevention (CDC). (2023a). *National Center for Health Statistics: Birth weight and gestation*. http://www.cdc.gov/nchs/fastats/birthweight.htm

Centers for Disease Control and Prevention (CDC). (2023b). *Pregnancy mortality surveillance system*. https://www.cdc.gov/reproductivehealth/maternal-mortality/pregnancy-mortality-surveillance-system.htm

Centers for Disease Control and Prevention (CDC). (2023c). *Maternal mortality rates in the United States, 2021*. https://www.cdc.gov/nchs/data/hestat/maternal-mortality/2021/maternal-mortality-rates-2021.htm#:~:text=In%202021%2C%201%2C205%20women%20died,20.1%20in%202019%20(Table)

Centers for Disease Control and Prevention (CDC). (2023d). *Enhancing reviews and surveillance to eliminate maternal mortality (ERASE MM)*. https://www.cdc.gov/reproductivehealth/maternal-mortality/erase-mm/index.html

Centers for Disease Control and Prevention (CDC). (2023e). *National Center for Health Statistics: Health, United*

States, 2020-2021. https://www.cdc.gov/nchs/hus/topics/births.htm

Centers for Disease Control and Prevention (CDC). (2023f). *Fetal Alcohol Spectrum Disorders (FASDs).* https://www.cdc.gov/ncbddd/fasd/

Centers for Disease Control and Prevention (CDC). (2023g). *Polysubstance use during pregnancy.* https://www.cdc.gov/pregnancy/polysubstance-use-in-pregnancy.html

Centers for Disease Control and Prevention (CDC). (2023h). *Human Immunodeficiency Virus (HIV).* https://www.cdc.gov/breastfeeding/breastfeeding-special-circumstances/maternal-or-infant-illnesses/hiv.html

Centers for Disease Control and Prevention (CDC). (2023i). *Depression among women.* https://www.cdc.gov/reproductivehealth/depression/index.htm

Centers for Disease Control and Prevention (CDC). (2023j). *Sudden unexpected infant death and sudden infant death syndrome: Data and statistics.* https://www.cdc.gov/sids/data.htm

Centers for Disease Control and Prevention (CDC). (2023k). *Fast facts: Preventing adverse childhood experiences.* https://www.cdc.gov/violenceprevention/aces/fastfact.html

Centers for Disease Control and Prevention (CDC). (2023l). *Fast facts: Adolescent health.* https://www.cdc.gov/nchs/fastats/adolescent-health.htm

Centers for Disease Control and Prevention (CDC). (2023m). *Fast facts: Child health.* https://www.cdc.gov/nchs/fastats/child-health.htm

Centers for Disease Control and Prevention (CDC). (2023n). *Testing children for lead poisoning.* https://www.cdc.gov/nceh/lead/prevention/testing-children-for-lead-poisoning.htm

Centers for Disease Control and Prevention (CDC). (2023o). *Preventing RSV.* https://www.cdc.gov/rsv/about/prevention.html

Centers for Disease Control and Prevention (CDC). (2023q). *Autism Spectrum Disorder (ASD).* https://www.cdc.gov/ncbddd/autism/index.html

Centers for Disease Control and Prevention (CDC). (2023r). *Data and statistics on ASD.* https://www.cdc.gov/ncbddd/autism/data.html

Centers for Disease Control and Prevention (CDC). (2023s). *What is sickle cell disease?* https://www.cdc.gov/ncbddd/sicklecell/facts.html

Centers for Disease Control and Prevention (CDC). (2023u). *Prevention strategies.* https://www.cdc.gov/violenceprevention/aces/prevention.html

Centers for Disease Control and Prevention (CDC). (2023v). *Child development basics.* https://www.cdc.gov/ncbddd/childdevelopment/facts.html

Centers for Disease Control and Prevention (CDC). (2023w). *CDC's milestone tracker app.* https://www.cdc.gov/ncbddd/actearly/milestones-app.html

Centers for Disease Control and Prevention (CDC). (2023x). *Early brain development and health.* https://www.cdc.gov/ncbddd/childdevelopment/early-brain-development.html

Centers for Disease Control and Prevention (CDC). (2023y). *Developmental monitoring and screening.* https://www.cdc.gov/ncbddd/childdevelopment/screening.html

Centers for Disease Control and Prevention (CDC). (2023z). *Birth defects.* https://www.cdc.gov/ncbddd/birthdefects/index.html

Child Welfare Information Gateway. (n.d.-a.). *Parent education programs.* https://www.childwelfare.gov/topics/preventing/prevention-programs/parented

Child Welfare Information Gateway. (n.d.-b.). *How to report suspected child maltreatment.* https://www.childwelfare.gov/topics/responding/reporting/how/

Child Welfare Information Gateway. (n.d.-c). *Home visiting programs.* https://www.childwelfare.gov/topics/preventing/prevention-programs/homevisit/homevisitprog/

Child Welfare Information Gateway. (2019). *Mandatory reporters of child abuse and neglect.* https://www.childwelfare.gov/pubPDFs/manda.pdf

Connections for Families. (2023). *Helping parents who have learning challenges.* https://connectionsforfamilies.ca/learn-more/how-to-help-parents-with-developmental-disabilities/

Cornelius, M. E., Loretan, C. G., Jamal, A., Davis Lynn, B. C., Mayer, M., Alcantara, I. C., & Neff, L. (2023). Tobacco product use among adults—United States, 2021. *MMWR Morbidity and Mortality Week Report, 72*(18), 475–483. https://doi.org/10.15585/mmwr.mm7218a1

Crane, K. (2020). *Prevention programs and strategies: State legislative experiences.* https://preventchildabuse.org/resources/prevention-programs-and-strategies-state-legislative-experiences-kelly-crane/

Davidson, L. (2023). *Car seat statistics in 2023.* https://parentingmode.com/car-seats/

Dejong, K., Olyaei, A., & Lo, J. O. (2019, March). Alcohol use in pregnancy. *Clinical Obstetrics and Gynecology, 62*(1), 142–155. https://doi.org/10.1097/GRF.0000000000000414

Felitti, V., Anda, R., Nordenberg, D., Williamson, D., Spits, A., Edwards, V., Koss, M. P., & Marks, J. (1998). Relationship of childhood abuse and household dysfunction to many leading causes of death in adults. The Adverse Childhood Experiences (ACE) Study. *American Journal of Preventive Medicine, 14*(4), 245–258. https://doi.org/10.1016/s0749-3797(98)00017-8

First Things First. (2023). *Brain development.* https://www.firstthingsfirst.org/early-childhood-matters/brain-development/#:~:text=At%20birth%2C%20the%20average%20baby's,center%20of%20the%20human%20body

Galiatsatos, P., Brigham, E., Krasnoff, R., Rice, J., Van Wyck, L., Sherry, M., Rand, C. S., Hansel, N. N., & McCormack, M. (2020). Association between neighborhood socioeconomic status, tobacco store density and smoking status in pregnant women in an urban area. *Preventive Medicine, 136,* 106107. https://doi.org/10.1016/j.ypmed.2020.106107

Health and Human Services (HHS). (n.d.). *Trends in teen pregnancy and childbearing.* https://opa.hhs.gov/adolescent-health/reproductive-health-and-teen-pregnancy/trends-teen-pregnancy-and-childbearing#:~:text=In%202020%2C%20the%20teen%20birth,the%201991%20peak%20of%2061.8.&text=There%20were%20158%2C043%20births%20to,of%20all%20births%20in%202020

Health Resources and Services Administration (HRSA). (June 2023). *Maternal, infant, and early childhood home visiting (MIECHV) program.* https://mchb.hrsa.gov/programs-impact/programs/home-visiting/maternal-infant-early-childhood-home-visiting-miechv-program

Health Resources and Services Administration (HRSA). (2024). *How we improve maternal health.* https://www.hrsa.gov/maternal-health

Hill, L., Artiga, S., & Ranji, U. (2022). *Racial disparities in maternal and infant health: Current status and efforts to address them.* https://www.kff.org/racial-equity-and-health-policy/issue-brief/racial-disparities-in-maternal-and-infant-health-current-status-and-efforts-to-address-them/

HIV.gov. (2023). *Global Statistics: The global HIV/AIDS epidemic.* https://www.hiv.gov/hiv-basics/overview/data-and-trends/global-statistics

HIVinfo.gov. (2023). *HIV prevention: Preventing perinatal transmission of HIV.* https://hivinfo.nih.gov/understanding-hiv/fact-sheets/preventing-perinatal-transmission-hiv

Hoyert, D. L. (2023). *Maternal mortality rates in the United States, 2021.* NCHS Health E-Stats. https://doi.org/https://dx.doi.org/10.15620/cdc:124678

Hyman, S. L., Levy, S. E., Myers, S. M., & AAP Council on Children with Disabilities (2020). Identification, evaluation, and management of children with autism spectrum disorder. *Pediatrics, 145*(1), e20193447.

Illinois.gov. (2022). *Test, inspect, and replace broken or expired smoke alarms as you change the clock this weekend.* https://www.illinois.gov/news/press-release.25653.html

MacMillan, C., & Flom, J. (2023). *How to prevent food allergies in kids.* https://www.yalemedicine.org/news/how-to-prevent-food-allergies-in-kids

Le, K., & Nguyen, M. (2022). Son preference and health disparities in developing countries. *SSM: Population Health, 17,* 1–9.

Loudoun County, Virginia. Combined Fire and Safety System. (n.d.). *Smoke alarm program.* https://www.loudoun.gov/819/Smoke-Alarms

March of Dimes. (2020a). *Health insurance/income.* https://www.marchofdimes.org/peristats/data?reg=99&top=11&stop=154&lev=1&slev=1&obj=18

March of Dimes. (2020b). *Loss and grief: Stillbirth.* https://www.marchofdimes.org/complications/stillbirth.aspx

Martin J. A., Hamilton B. E., Osterman M. J. K., & Driscoll, A. K. (2019). Births: Final data for 2018. *National Vital Statistics Reports, 68*(3). National Center for Health Statistics. https://www.cdc.gov/nchs/data/nvsr/nvsr68/nvsr68_13-508.pdf

Martin J. A., & Osterman M. J. K. (2023). *Statistics reports: Changes in prenatal care utilizations: United States. 2019-2021.* https://www.cdc.gov/nchs/data/nvsr/nvsr72/nvsr72-04.pdf

Maternal and Child Health Bureau (MCHB). (n.d.-a). *Healthy start.* http://mchb.hrsa.gov/programs/healthystart/

Maternal and Child Health Bureau (MCHB). (n.d.-b). *Overview of funded projects.* http://mchb.hrsa.gov/research/about-projects.asp

Maternal and Child Health Bureau (MCHB). (n.d.-c). *The maternal, infant, and early childhood home visiting program: Partnering with parents to help children succeed.* https://mchb.hrsa.gov/sites/default/files/mchb/MaternalChildHealthInitiatives/HomeVisiting/pdf/programbrief.pdf

Maternal and Child Health Bureau (MCHB). (n.d.-d). *Funding by service level.* https://mchb.tvisdata.hrsa.gov/Financial/FundingByServiceLevel

Maternal and Child Health Bureau (MCHB). (n.d.-e). *Historical timeline.* http://www.mchb.hrsa.gov/timeline/

Melillo, G. (2020). *US ranks worst in maternal care, mortality compared with 10 other developed nations.* https://www.ajmc.com/view/us-ranks-worst-in-maternal-care-mortality-compared-with-10-other-developed-nations

National Alliance to End Homelessness. (2023). *Children and families.* https://endhomelessness.org/homelessness-in-america/who-experiences-homelessness/children-and-families/

National Center for Education Statistics. (2021). *Fast facts: Child care.* https://nces.ed.gov/fastfacts/display.asp?id=4

National Conference of State Legislatures. (2021). *State approaches to ensuring healthy pregnancies through prenatal care.* https://www.ncsl.org/health/state-approaches-to-ensuring-healthy-pregnancies-through-prenatal-care

National Fire Protection Association. (n.d.). *Know when to stop, drop, and roll.* http://www.nfpa.org/public-education/resources/education-programs/learn-not-to-burn/learn-not-to-burn-grade-1/know-when-to-stop-drop-and-roll

National Head Start Association. (2023). *Head Start facts and impacts.* https://www.nhsa.org/facts-and-impacts

National Highway Traffic Safety Administration. (n.d.). *Car seats and booster seats.* https://www.nhtsa.gov/equipment/car-seats-and-booster-seats

Nurse-Family Partnership. (n.d.-a). *The David Olds story: from a desire to help people, to a plan that truly does.* https://www.nursefamilypartnership.org/about/program-history/

Nurse-Family Partnership. (n.d.-b). *Guiding theories: Three theories that guide the nurse-family partnership.* https://www.nursefamilypartnership.org/nurses/guiding-theories/

Office of Disease Prevention and Health Promotion (ODPHP). (n.d.-a.). Pregnancy and childbirth. *Healthy People 2030.* U.S. Department of Health and Human Services. https://health.gov/healthypeople/pregnancy-and-childbirth

Office of Disease Prevention and Health Promotion (ODPHP). (n.d.-b.). National action plan for child injury prevention. *Healthy People 2030.* U.S. Department of Health and Human Services. https://health.gov/healthypeople/tools-action/browse-evidence-based-resources/national-action-plan-child-injury-prevention

Office of Disease Prevention and Health Promotion (ODPHP). (n.d.-c.). Reduce the rate of deaths in children and adolescents age 1-19 years. *Healthy People 2023.* U.S. Department of Health and Human Services. https://health.gov/healthypeople/objectives-and-data/browse-objectives/children/reduce-rate-deaths-children-and-adolescents-aged-1-19-years-mich-03

Orr, C., Ben-Davies, M., Ravanbakht, S., Yin, H., Sanders, L., Rothman, R., Delamater, A., Wood, C., & Perrin, E. (2019). Parental feeding beliefs and practices and household food insecurity in infancy. *Academic Pediatrics, 19*(1), 80–89.

Patel, J., & Rouster, A. S. (2022). Infant nutrition requirements and options. In *StatPearls.* StatPearls Publishing. https://www.ncbi.nlm.nih.gov/books/NBK560758/

Prince George's County, Maryland. (2023). *Fire safety education.* https://www.princegeorgescountymd.gov/departments-offices/fire-emergency-medical-services/resourceslinks/fire-safety-education

Román-Gálvez, R. M., Sandra Martín-Peláez Roman-Galves, R. M., Martin-Palaez, S., Martinez-Galiano, J. M., Khan, K. S., Bueno-Cavanillas, A. (2021). Prevalence of intimate partner violence in pregnancy: An umbrella review. *International Journal of Environmental Research and Public Health, 18*(2), 707. https://doi.org/10.3390/ijerph18020707

Rudderown, L. C. (2019). *STD and STI—What's the difference?* Nursing Center Blog. Lippincott Nursing Center. https://www.nursingcenter.com/ncblog/january-2019/std-and-sti

Quesada, J. A., Mendez, I., & Martin-Gil (2020). The economic benefits of increasing breastfeeding rates in Spain. *International Breastfeed Journal, 15*(34). https://doi.org/10.1186/s13006-020-00277-w

Safe to Sleep. (n.d.). *Fast facts about SIDS.* https://www.nichd.nih.gov/sts/about/SIDS/Pages/fastfacts.aspx

Schmidt, R., Carson, P. J., & Jansen, R. J. (2019). Resurgence of Syphilis in the United States: An assessment of contributing factors. *Infectious Diseases*, 12. https://doi.org/10.1177/1178633719883282

Smith, E., & Badireddy, M. (2022). Failure to thrive. In *StatPearls*. StatPearls Publishing. https://www.ncbi.nlm.nih.gov/books/NBK459287/#:~:text=Introduction-,Failure%20to%20thrive%20(FTT)%20is%20a%20common%20term%20used%20to,gain%20in%20pediatric%2Daged%20patients

Stierman, B., Afful, J. A., Carroll, M. D., Chen, T. C., Davy, O., Fink, S., Fryar, C. D., Qiuping, G., Hales, C. M., Hughes, J. P., Yechiam, O., Storandt, M. T., & Akinbami, L. J. (2021). National health and nutrition examination survey 2017-2020 prepandemic data files—Development of files and prevalence estimates for selected health outcomes. *National Health Statistics Reports, 158, 4.* https://stacks.cdc.gov/view/cdc/106273

The Children's Cabinet. (2020). *Finding childcare.* https://www.childrenscabinet.org/who-we-serve/i-am-a-parent/finding-child-care/

The Urban Child Institute. (2023). *Child care.* http://www.urbanchildinstitute.org/why-0-3/child-care

The White House. (2022). *White House blueprint for addressing the maternal health crisis.* https://www.whitehouse.gov/wp-content/uploads/2022/06/Maternal-Health-Blueprint.pdf

U.S. Agency for Healthcare Research and Quality. (2019). *HCUP Fast Stats—Map of Neonatal Abstinence Syndrome (NAS) among newborn hospitalizations.* https://www.hcup-us.ahrq.gov/faststats/NASMap

U.S. Breastfeeding Committee (USBC). (2022). *A closer look at the 2022 CDC breastfeeding report card.* https://www.usbreastfeeding.org/usbc-news--blogs/a-closer-look-at-the-2022-cdc-breastfeeding-report-card

U.S. Department of Agriculture. (n.d.). *Women, Infants, and Children (WIC).* https://www.fns.usda.gov/wic/women-infants-and-children-wic

Verduci, E., DiProfio, E., Corsello, A., Scatigno, L., Fiore, G., Bosetti, A., & Zuccotti, G. V. (2021). Which milk during the second year of life: A personalized choice for a healthy future? *Nutrients, 13*(10), 2–16.

U.S. Food & Drug Administration. (n.d.). *Frequently asked questions on children's cold and cough medications.* https://www.fda.gov/drugs/information-drug-class/frequently-asked-question-childrens-cough-and-cold-medicines

UNICEF. (2023). *Maternal Mortality: Maternal mortality declined by 34 percent between 2000 and 2020.* https://data.unicef.org/topic/maternal-health/maternal-mortality/

Whitman, A., De Lew, N., Chappel, A., Aysola, V., Zuckerman, R., Sommers, B. D. (2022). *Addressing social determinants of health: Examples of successful evidence-based strategies and current federal efforts.* https://aspe.hhs.gov/sites/default/files/documents/e2b650cd64cf84aae8ff0fae7474af82/SDOH-Evidence-Review.pdf

World Health Organization (WHO). (2022). *Fact Sheets: Child mortality (under 5 years).* https://www.who.int/news-room/fact-sheets/detail/levels-and-trends-in-child-under-5-mortality-in-2020

World Health Organization (WHO). (2023a). *Maternal mortality.* https://www.who.int/news-room/fact-sheets/detail/maternal-mortality

World Health Organization (WHO). (2023b). *Fact Sheets: Preterm birth.* https://www.who.int/news-room/fact-sheets/detail/preterm-birth#:~:text=Preterm%20is%20defined%20as%20babies,preterm%20(less%20than%2028%20weeks)

World Health Organization (WHO). (2023c). *Fact Sheets: HIV/AIDS.* https://www.who.int/en/news-room/fact-sheets/detail/hiv-aids

World Health Organization (WHO). (2024a). *Every newborn action plan.* https://www.who.int/initiatives/every-newborn-action-plan

World Health Organization (WHO). (2024b). *Ending preventable maternal mortality.* https://www.who.int/initiatives/ending-preventable-maternal-mortality

CHAPTER 20

Adeghe, E. P. (2024). Integrating pediatric oral health into primary care: A public health strategy to combat oral diseases in children across the United States. *International Journal of Multidisciplinary Research Updates, 7*(1), 27–36. https://doi.org/10.53430/ijmru.2024.7.1.0026

Administration on Children and Families. (2024). *Child abuse & neglect.* http://www.acf.hhs.gov/programs/cb/focus-areas/child-abuse-neglect

Agency for Healthcare Research and Quality. (2022). *National healthcare quality and disparities report: Child and adolescent mental health.* https://www.ncbi.nlm.nih.gov/books/NBK587174/

America, SPSS. (2024). *Child maltreatment statistics.* https://americanspcc.org/child-maltreatment-statistics/#:~:text=4.276%20million%20child%20maltreatment%20referral,prevention%20%26%20post%2Dresponse%20services

American Academy of Child and Adolescent Psychiatry. (2019). *Self injury in adolescents.* https://www.aacap.org/AACAP/Families_and_Youth/Facts_for_Families/FFF-Guide/Self-Injury-In-Adolescents-073.aspx

American Academy of Child and Adolescent Psychiatry. (2024). *Suicide in children and teens.* https://www.aacap.org/AACAP/Families_and_Youth/Facts_for_Families/FFF-Guide/Teen-Suicide-010.aspx

American Academy of Pediatrics. (2023). *Study: Teens not meeting nutritional, physical active guidelines.* https://publications.aap.org/aapnews/news/24273/Study-Teens-not-meeting-nutrition-physical

American Cancer Society. (2024a). *Key statistics for childhood cancer.* https://www.cancer.org/cancer/types/cancer-in-children/key-statistics.html

American Cancer Society. (2024b). *Risk factors and causes of childhood cancer.* https://www.cancer.org/cancer/types/cancer-in-children/risk-factors-and-causes.html#:~:text=A%20few%20environmental%20factors%2C%20such,to%20explore%20these%20possible%20links

American College and Obstetrics and Gynecology (ACOG). (2024). *Mental health disorders in adolescents.* https://www.acog.org/clinical/clinical-guidance/committee-opinion/articles/2017/07/mental-health-disorders-in-adolescents

American Diabetes Association. (n.d.). *Devices and technology.* https://diabetes.org/about-diabetes/devices-technology

American Family Physician. (2020). *Prevention of unintentional childhood injury.* https://www.aafp.org/pubs/afp/issues/2020/1001/p411.html#:~:text=Unintentional%20injury%20accounts%20for%20one,least%20two%20years%20of%20age.

American Lung Association. (2024). *Cigarette and tobacco taxes.* https://www.lung.org/policy-advocacy/tobacco/tobacco-taxes#:~:text=Increasing%20taxes%20on%20tobacco%20products,well%20as%20tobacco%20prevention%20programs.

Annie E. Casey Foundation. (2024a). *Leading causes of death in teens.* https://www.aecf.org/blog/teen-death-rates

Annie E. Casey Foundation. (2024b). *Social media and teen mental health.* https://www.aecf.org/blog/social-medias-concerning-effect-on-teen-mental-health?gad_source=1&gclid=EAIaIQobChMIzpCSleGLhwMVLNMWBR2Q5QCqEAAYASAAEgLUy_D_BwE

Anxiety and Depression Association of America (ADAA). (n.d.). *School refusal.* https://adaa.org/living-with-anxiety/children/school-refusal

Asthma and Allergy Foundation of America (AAFA). (2024). *Asthma facts.* https://aafa.org/asthma/asthma-facts/?gad_source=1&gclid=EAIaIQobChMI6KGp7sCGhwMVLiutBh3gxwfuEAAYASAAEgK7LvD_BwE

Attention Deficit Disorder Association. (2024). *Understanding ADHD.* https://add.org/untreated-adhd-in-adults/

Bagley. (2024). *Crime, violence, discipline, and safety in the U.S. public schools.* https://youthtoday.org/2024/01/crime-violence-discipline-and-safety-in-u-s-public-schools-2/#:~:text=Sixty%2Done%20percent%20of%20schools,the%202021%E2%80%9322%20school%20year

Ballard Brief. (2020). *Chronic poverty among youth in the United States.* https://ballardbrief.byu.edu/issue-briefs/effects-of-chronic-poverty-on-youth-in-the-united-states#:~:text=Areas%20with%20high%20levels%20of,ages%20of%2014%20and%2017.&text=Youth%20who%20are%20economically%20disadvantaged,of%20violence%20in%20their%20communities

Blair, C. (2012). Treating a toxin to learning. *Scientific American Mind, 23*, 64–67.

Bransteter, I., McVoy, M., Miller, D. W., Gubitosi-Klug, R. A., Segall, T. L., Divan, M. K., Surdam, J., Sajatovic, M., & Dusek, J. A. (2024). Barriers and facilitators to incorporating an integrative mind–body intervention in youth With Type 2 Diabetes. *JAACAP Open, 2*(3), 208–216. https://doi.org/10.1016/j.jaacop.2024.01.005

Carlson, S. (2022). *SNAP is linked with improved health outcomes and lower health care costs.* https://www.cbpp.org/research/food-assistance/snap-is-linked-with-improved-health-outcomes-and-lower-health-care-costs

Center on Budget and Policy Priorities (CBPP). (2022). *TANF cash assistance should reach millions more families to lessen hardship.* https://www.cbpp.org/research/family-income-support/cash-assistance-should-reach-millions-more-families

Centers for Disease Control and Prevention (CDC). (2019). *Funding opportunity announcement (FOA) PS115-1502: Comprehensive high-impact HIV prevention projects for community-based organizations.* https://www.cdc.gov/hiv/funding/announcements/ps15-1502/index.html

Centers for Disease Control and Prevention (CDC). (2021a). *Managing chronic health conditions.* https://www.cdc.gov/healthyschools/chronicconditions.htm

Centers for Disease Control and Prevention (CDC). (2021b). *Adverse childhood experiences (ACE).* https://www.cdc.gov/policy/polaris/healthtopics/ace/index.html#:~:text=ACEs%20have%20a%20tremendous%20impact,attempt%20or%20die%20by%20suicide

Centers for Disease Control and Prevention (CDC). (2021c). Emergency department visits for suspected suicide attempts among persons aged 12-25 years before and during the Covid-19 pandemic- United States, January 2019-May 2021. *Morbidity and Mortality Weekly Report, 70*(24), 888–894. https://www.cdc.gov/mmwr/volumes/70/wr/mm7024e1.htm

Centers for Disease Control and Prevention (CDC). (2022a). *Health and academics.* https://www.cdc.gov/healthyschools/health_and_academics/index.htm

Centers for Disease Control and Prevention (CDC). (2022b). *Care coordination.* https://www.cdc.gov/healthyschools/shs/care_coordination.htm

Centers for Disease Control and Prevention (CDC). (2022c). Mental health, suicidality, and connectedness among high school students during the COVID-19 pandemic- adolescent behaviors and experiences survey, United States January-June, 2021. *Morbidity and Mortality Weekly Report, 71*(3), 16–21. https://www.cdc.gov/mmwr/volumes/71/su/su7103a3.htm

Centers for Disease Control and Prevention (CDC). (2022d). National vaccine coverage among adolescents aged 13-17 years—national immunization survey-teen, United States, 2021. *Morbidity and Mortality Weekly Report, 71*(35), 1101–1108. https://www.cdc.gov/mmwr/volumes/71/wr/mm7135a1.htm

Centers for Disease Control and Prevention (CDC). (2022e). *School meals.* https://www.cdc.gov/healthyschools/nutrition/schoolmeals.htm

Centers for Disease Control and Prevention (CDC). (2022f). *Childhood nutrition facts.* https://www.cdc.gov/healthyschools/nutrition/facts.htm

Centers for Disease Control and Prevention (CDC). (2022g). *Body mass index (BMI) measurement in school.* https://www.cdc.gov/healthyschools/obesity/bmi/bmi_measurement_schools.htm

Centers for Disease Control and Prevention (CDC). (2022h). *Physical activity guidelines for school-aged children and adolescents.* https://www.cdc.gov/healthyschools/physicalactivity/guidelines.htm

Centers for Disease Control and Prevention (CDC). (2022i). *High risk substance use among youth.* https://www.cdc.gov/healthyyouth/substance-use/index.htm

Centers for Disease Control and Prevention (CDC). (2022j). *More than 3 million youth reported using a tobacco product in 2022.* https://www.cdc.gov/media/releases/2022/p1110-youth-tobaco.html

Centers for Disease Control and Prevention (CDC). (2023a). *Whole school, whole community, whole child (WSCC).* https://www.cdc.gov/healthyschools/wscc/index.htm

Centers for Disease Control and Prevention (CDC). (2023b). *Spotlight on new patterns in racial and ethnic differences emerges in autism spectrum disorder (ASD) identification among 8-year-old children.* https://www.cdc.gov/ncbddd/autism/addm-community-report/spotlight-on-racial-ethnic-differences.html

Centers for Disease Control and Prevention (CDC). (2023c). *Preventing type 2 diabetes in kids*. https://www.cdc.gov/diabetes/prevention-type-2/type-2-diabetes-in-kids.html

Centers for Disease Control and Prevention (CDC). (2023d). *Epilepsy*. https://www.cdc.gov/healthyschools/npao/epilepsy.htm

Centers for Disease Control and Prevention (CDC). (2023e). *Adolescents are experiencing violence, sadness, and suicide risk*. https://www.cdc.gov/healthyyouth/data/yrbs/feature/dstr-feature.htm

Centers for Disease Control and Prevention (CDC). (2023f). *Data and statistics on children's mental health*. https://www.cdc.gov/childrensmentalhealth/data.html

Centers for Disease Control and Prevention (CDC). (2023g). *Youth risk behavior survey*. https://www.cdc.gov/healthyyouth/data/yrbs/pdf/YRBS_Data-Summary-Trends_Report2023_508.pdf

Centers for Disease Control and Prevention (CDC). (2023h). *Unintentional firearm injury deaths among children and adolescents aged 0-17 years- national violent death reporting system, United States, 2003-2021*. https://www.cdc.gov/mmwr/volumes/72/wr/mm7250a1.htm#:~:text=NVDRS%20identified%201%2C262%20unintentional%20firearm,persons%20aged%206%E2%80%9310%20years.

Centers for Disease Control and Prevention (CDC). (2023i). *Suicide*. https://www.cdc.gov/nchs/hus/topics/suicide.htm

Centers for Disease Control and Prevention (CDC). (2023j). *Vaccine coverage by age 24 months among children born during 2018-2019- national immunization survey- child, United States, 2019-2021*. https://www.cdc.gov/mmwr/volumes/72/wr/mm7202a3.htm

Centers for Disease Control and Prevention (CDC). (2023k). *Oral health*. https://www.cdc.gov/healthyschools/npao/oralhealth.htm#:~:text=Cavities%20(tooth%20decay)%20are%20the,childhood%20in%20the%20United%20States.&text=By%20age%208%2C%20over%20half,their%20primary%20(baby)%20teeth.&text=Children%20from%20low%2Dincome%20families,children%20from%20higher%2Dincome%20families

Centers for Disease Control and Prevention (CDC). (2023l). *Table 4: Number and percentage of students, by sexual identity- United States and selected U.S. sites, Youth Risk Behavioral Surveys, 2021*. https://www.cdc.gov/healthyyouth/data/yrbs/supplemental-mmwr/students_by_sexual_identity.htm

Centers for Disease Control and Prevention (CDC). (2023m). *Youth and tobacco use*. https://www.cdc.gov/tobacco/data_statistics/fact_sheets/youth_data/tobacco_use/index.htm

Centers for Disease Control and Prevention (CDC). (2024a). *Exhale: Strategies to help people with asthma breathe easier*. https://www.cdc.gov/national-asthma-control-program/php/exhale/index.html

Centers for Disease Control and Prevention (CDC). (2024b). *Autism spectrum disorder (ASD)*. https://www.cdc.gov/autism/index.html

Centers for Disease Control and Prevention (CDC). (2024c). *Autism and vaccines*. https://www.cdc.gov/vaccinesafety/concerns/autism.html

Centers for Disease Control and Prevention (CDC). (2024d). *Diabetes in young people is on the rise*. https://www.cdc.gov/diabetes/data-research/research/young-people-diabetes-on-rise.html

Centers for Disease Control and Prevention (CDC). (2024e). *Developmental disability basics*. https://www.cdc.gov/child-development/about/developmental-disability-basics.html

Centers for Disease Control and Prevention (CDC). (2024f). *Attention-deficit/hyperactivity disorder in children 5-17 years: United States 2020-2022*. https://www.cdc.gov/nchs/products/databriefs/db499.htm#:~:text=Key%20findings-,Data%20from%20the%20National%20Health%20Interview%20Survey,prevalence%20than%20girls%20(8.0%25)

Centers for Disease Control and Prevention (CDC). (2024g). *Treatment of ADHD*. https://www.cdc.gov/adhd/treatment/index.html

Centers for Disease Control and Prevention (CDC). (2024h). *Risk factors for teen drivers*. https://www.cdc.gov/teen-drivers/risk-factors/index.html

Centers for Disease Control and Prevention (CDC). (2024i). *Methicillin-resistant staphylococcus aureus (MRSA) basics*. https://www.cdc.gov/mrsa/about/index.html

Centers for Disease Control and Prevention (CDC). (2024j). *Risk factors for obesity*. https://www.cdc.gov/obesity/php/about/risk-factors.html

Centers for Disease Control and Prevention (CDC). (2024k). *HIOPS for screen time limits*. https://www.cdc.gov/early-care-education/php/obesity-prevention-standards/screen-time-limits.html#:~:text=Limit%20total%20media%20time%20for,during%20meal%20or%20snack%20time

Centers for Disease Control and Prevention (CDC). (2024l). *Oral and dental health*. https://www.cdc.gov/nchs/fastats/dental.htm

Centers for Disease Control and Prevention (CDC). (2024m). *Health disparities in oral health*. https://www.cdc.gov/oral-health/health-equity/index.html

Centers for Disease Control and Prevention (CDC). (2024n). *Risk factors for teen drivers*. https://www.cdc.gov/teen-drivers/risk-factors/index.html

Centers for Disease Control and Prevention (CDC). (2024o). *About youth violence*. https://www.cdc.gov/youth-violence/about/index.html

Centers for Disease Control and Prevention (CDC). (2024p). *Cannabis and teens*. https://www.cdc.gov/cannabis/health-effects/cannabis-and-teens.html

Centers for Disease Control and Prevention (CDC). (2024q). *Youth and tobacco use*. https://www.cdc.gov/tobacco/data_statistics/fact_sheets/youth_data/tobacco_use/index.htm

Centers for Disease Control and Prevention (CDC). (2024r). About teen pregnancy. https://www.cdc.gov/reproductive-health/teen-pregnancy/index.html

Centers for Disease Control and Prevention (CDC). (2024s). *National overview of STIs, 2022*. https://www.cdc.gov/std/statistics/2022/overview.htm#:~:text=As%20in%20past%20years%2C%20there,adults%20aged%2015%E2%80%9324%20years

Centers for Disease Control and Prevention (CDC). (2024t). *Tuberculosis in children*. https://www.cdc.gov/tb/about/children.html

Centers for Disease Control and Prevention (CDC). (2024u). *Parents are the key*. https://www.cdc.gov/teen-drivers/parents-are-the-key/index.html#:~:text=Overview&text=Many%20parents%20don't%20realize,about%20eight%20teens%20a%20day

Centers for Disease Control and Prevention (CDC). (2024v). *Child passenger safety*. https://www.cdc.gov/child-passenger-safety/resources/index.html#:~:text=Make%20sure%20your%20child%20is%20always%20buckled.&text=Rear%2Dfacing%20car%20seat%3A%20Birth,offers%20the%20best%20possible%20protection

Chaves, E., Jeffrey, D. T., & Williams, D. R. (2023). Disordered eating and eating disorders in pediatric obesity: Assessment and next steps. International *Journal of Environmental Research and Public Health*, *20*(17). http://doi.org/10.3390/ijerph210176638

Chelak, K., & Chakole, S. (2023). The role of social determinants of health in promoting health equality: A narrative review. *Cureus*, *15*(1), e33425. https://doi.org/10.7759/cureus.33425

Child Stats. (2023). *Family structure and children's living arrangements*. https://www.childstats.gov/americaschildren/family1.asp

Child Trends. (2022). *State level data for understanding child poverty*. https://www.childtrends.org/publications/state-level-data-for-understanding-child-poverty?gad_source=1&gclid=EAIaIQobChMIoZm1paSGhwMV7tXCBB15aADTEAAYASAAEgKxsfD_BwE

Child Trends. (2024). *5 important things to know about children and supplemental nutritional assistance program (SNAP)*. https://www.childtrends.org/publications/5-important-things-to-know-about-children-and-the-supplemental-nutrition-assistance-program-snap?_gl=1*qvmrq4*_up*MQ..&gclid=EAIaIQobChMI4_eQ7qqGhwMVgy-tBh2bWQC9EAAYASAAEgIHbfD_BwE

Children's Bureau. (2019). *Children in poverty—Poverty and its effects on children*. https://www.all4kids.org/news/blog/poverty-and-its-effects-on-children/#:~:text=The%20Health%20Risks%20of%20Childhood%20Poverty&text=Children%20who%20directly%20or%20indirectly,even%20a%20shorter%20life%20expectancy

D'Souza, N. J., Kuswara, K., Zheng, M., Leech, R., Downing, K. L., Lioret, S., Campbell, K. J., & Hesketh, K. D. (2020). A systematic review of lifestyle patterns and their association with adiposity in children aged 5-12 years. *Obesity Reviews*, *21*(8). https://doi.org/10.1111/obr.13029

Desilver, D. (2023). *What the data says about food stamps in the U.S.* https://www.pewresearch.org/short-reads/2023/07/19/what-the-data-says-about-food-stamps-in-the-u-s/

Eating Disorder Hope. (2024). *Eating disorder in teens*. https://www.eatingdisorderhope.com/risk-groups/eating-disorders-teens#:~:text=Teenage%20Eating%20Disorder%20Statistics&text=Studies%20have%20determined%20that%3A,age%20of%2020%20%5B2%5D

Feeding America. (2024). *Facts about child hunger*. https://www.feedingamerica.org/hunger-in-america/child-hunger-facts

Felitti, V. J., Anda, R. F., Nordenberg, D., Williamson, D. F., Spitz, A. M., Edwards, V., Koss, M. P., & Marks, J. S. (1998). Relationship of childhood abuse and household dysfunction to many of the leading causes of death in adults: The adverse childhood experiences (ACE) study. *American Journal of Preventive Medicine*, *14*(4), 245–258.

Fleming, M. A., Kane, W. J., Meneveau, M. O., Ballantyne, C. C., & Levin, D. E. (2021). Food insecurity and obesity in U.S. adolescents: A population-based analysis. *Childhood Obesity*, *17*(2). https://doi.org/10.1089/chi.2020.0158

Food Allergy, Research, and Education (FARE). (n.d.). *Children with food allergies*. https://www.foodallergy.org/living-food-allergies/information-you/children-food-allergies

Geria, K., & Beitz, J. M. (2018). Application of a modified diabetes prevention program with adolescents. *Public Health Nursing*, *35*, 337–343.

Get Smart About Drugs. (2024). *What you should know about steroids and young people*. https://www.getsmartaboutdrugs.gov/family/what-you-should-know-about-steroids-and-young-people

Guttmacher Institute. (2023). *Sex and HIV education*. https://www.guttmacher.org/state-policy/explore/sex-and-hiv-education

Hadland, S. E., Xuan, Z., Sarda, V., Blanchette, J., Swahn, M. H., Heeren, T. C., Voas, R. B., & Naimi, T. S. (2017). Alcohol policies and alcohol-related motor vehicle crash fatalities among young people in the US. *Pediatrics*, *139*(3). pii: e20163037. https://doi.org/10.1542/peds.2016-3037

HIVinfo. (n.d.). *HIV overview*. National Institute of Health. https://hivinfo.nih.gov/understanding-hiv/fact-sheets/stages-hiv-infection

Hockenberry, M. J., Wilson, D., & Rodgers, C. C. (2019). *Wong's nursing care of infants and children* (11th ed.). Elsevier.

ISM. (2023). *Five ways school nurses can work to prevent substance abuse*. https://isminc.com/advisory/publications/the-source/five-ways-school-nurses-can-work-prevent-substance-abuse

Jacobson Vann, J. C., Jacobson, R. M., Coyne-Beasley, T., Asafu-Adjei, J. K., & Szilagyi, P. G. (2018). Patient reminder and recall interventions to improve immunization rates. *Cochrane Database of Systematic Reviews*, *1*, CD003941. https://doi.org/10.1002/14651858.CD003941.pub3

Kids Health Alliance. (2020). *How divorce affects your child*. https://kidshealthalliance.com/how-divorce-affects-your-child/

Koob, G. F. (2023). *Understanding how alcohol policies impact public health*. National Institute on Alcohol Abuse and Alcoholism. https://www.niaaa.nih.gov/about-niaaa/directors-page/niaaa-directors-blog/understanding-how-alcohol-policies-impact-public-health

Learning Disabilities Association of America. (n.d.). *New to LD*. https://ldaamerica.org/support/new-to-ld/

Lee, J., Su, Z., & Chen, Y. (2023). Mobile apps for children's health and wellbeing: Design features and future opportunities. *AMIA Annual Symposium Proceedings*, 2023, 1027–1036. PMID: 38222362; PMCID: PMC10785842.

Lee, L. K., Fleeger, E. W., Gayol, M. K., Doh, K. F., Laraque-Arena, D., & Hoffman, B. D. (2022). Firearm related injuries and deaths in children and youth: Injury prevention and harm reduction. *Pediatrics*, *150*(6). https://doi.org/10.1542/peds.2022-060070

Lowe, A. A., Gerald, J. K., & Gerald, L. B. (2021). Medication administration practices in United States Schools: A systematic review and meta-synthesis. *Journal of School Nursing*, *38*(1), 21–34. http://doi.org/10.1177/10598405211026300

Marcus, B. (2020). A nursing approach to the largest measles outbreak in recent U.S. history: Lessons learned battling homegrown vaccine hesitancy. *The Online Journal of Issue in Nursing*, *25*(1). http://doi.org/OJIN.Vol25No01Man03

Mark, N. D., & Wu, L. (2022). More comprehensive sex education reduced teen births: Quasi experimental evidence. *Proceedings of the National Academy of Sciences*, *119*(8). http://doi.org/10.1073/pnas.2113144119

Mateo, K., Greenberg, B., & Valenzuela, J. (2024). *Disordered eating behaviors and eating disorders in youth with type 2 diabetes: A systematic review*. American Diabetes Association. https://doi.org/10.2337/ds23-0064

Matin, B. K., Byford, S., Soltani, S., Kazemi-Karyani, A., Atafar, Z., Zereshki, E., Soofi, M., Rezaei, S., Rakhshan, S. T., & Jahangiri, P. (2022). Contributing factors to healthcare costs in individuals with autism spectrum disorder: A systematic review. *BMC Health Services Research*, *22*(1), 604. http://doi.org/10.1186/s12913-022-07932-4

Mayer, M. J., Nickerson, A. B., & Jimerson, S. R. (2021). Preventing school violence and promoting school safety: Contemporary scholarship advancing science, practice, and policy. *School Psychology Review*, *50*(2–3), 131–142. https://doi.org/10.1080/2372966X.2021.1949933

Mayo Clinic. (2022). *Pediatric epilepsy: Defining syndromes and applying innovative therapies*. https://www.mayoclinic.org/medical-professionals/neurology-neurosurgery/news/pediatric-epilepsy-defining-syndromes-and-applying-innovative-therapies/mac-20529922

McEvoy, D., Brannigan, R., Cooke, L., Butler, E., Walsh, C., Arensman, E., & Clarke, M. (2023). Risk and protective factors for self-harm in adolescents and young adults: An umbrella review of systematic reviews. *Journal of Psychiatric Research*, *168*, 353–380. https://doi.org/10.1016/j.jpsychires.2023.10.017

Micha, R., Karageorgou, D., Bakogianni, I., Trichia, E., Whitsel, L. P., Story, M., Peñalvo, J. L., & Mozaffarian, D. (2018). Effectiveness of school food environment policies on children's dietary behaviors: A systematic review and meta-analysis. *PLoS One*, *13*(3), e0194555. https://doi.org/10.1371/journal.pone.0194555

Nassar, Y., & Brizuela, M. (2023). *The role of fluoride on caries prevention*. STATPEARLS Publishing. https://www.ncbi.nlm.nih.gov/books/NBK587342/

National Academies of Sciences, Engineering, and Medicine; Health and Medicine Division; Board on Population Health and Public Health Practice; Committee on the Impact of Social Media on Adolescent Health. (2024, March 25). In A. Wojtowicz, G. J. Buckley & S. Galea (Eds.), *Social media and adolescent health*. National Academies Press (US). 1, Introduction. https://www.ncbi.nlm.nih.gov/books/NBK603432/

National Academies of Sciences, Engineering, and Medicine; Health and Medicine Division; Division of Behavioral and Social Sciences and Education; Board on Children, Youth, and Families; Committee on the Neurobiological and Socio-behavioral Science of Adolescent Development and Its Applications. (2019, May 16). In E. P. Backes & R. J. Bonnie (Eds.), *The promise of adolescence: Realizing opportunity for all youth*. National Academies Press (US). 2, Adolescent Development. https://www.ncbi.nlm.nih.gov/books/NBK545476/

National Association of School Nurses (NASN). (2021a). *Chronic health condition management*. https://www.nasn.org/nasn-resources/resources-by-topic/chronic-health-condition-management

National Association of School Nurses (NASN). (2021b). *School nurses play key role in treating and supporting students with cancer*. https://schoolnursenet.nasn.org/nasn/blogs/nasn-profile/2021/02/01/school-nurses-play-key-role-in-treating-and-suppor

National Association of School Nurses (NASN). (2022). *Diabetes in children*. https://www.nasn.org/nasn-resources/resources-by-topic/diabetes

National Association of School Nurses (NASN). (2023). *Prevention and intervention of bullying and cyberbullying in schools*. https://www.nasn.org/nasn-resources/professional-practice-documents/position-statements/ps-bullying

National Cancer Institute (NCI). (2021). *Care for childhood cancer survivors*. https://www.cancer.gov/about-cancer/coping/survivorship/child-care#2

National Cancer Institute (NCI). (2024). *Childhood cancers*. https://www.cancer.gov/types/childhood-cancers

National Center for Children in Poverty (NCCP). (2024). *Who are America's poor children: The official story*. https://www.nccp.org/publication/americas-poor-children/

National Center for Education Statistics (NCES). (2024a). *Racial/Ethnic Enrollment in Public Schools. Condition of Education*. U.S. Department of Education, Institute of Education Sciences. Retrieved May 30, 2024, from https://nces.ed.gov/programs/coe/indicator/cge

National Center for Education Statistics (NCES). (2024b). *Students with disabilities*. https://nces.ed.gov/programs/coe/indicator/cgg/students-with-disabilities

National Center for Health Statistics. (2024). *Percentage of ever having asthma for children under age 18 years, United States, 2019—2022*. National Health Interview Survey. Generated interactively: Jul 01 2024 from https://wwwn.cdc.gov/NHISDataQueryTool/SHS_child/index.html

National Gang Center. (2020). *Risk factors*. https://nationalgangcenter.ojp.gov/spt/Risk-Factors/FAQ#4-0

National Gang Center. (2021). *Gang resistance educate*. https://nationalgangcenter.ojp.gov/spt/Programs/68 ion and training

National Healthcare Quality and Disparities Report. (2022, October). *Child and adolescent mental health*. Agency for Healthcare Research and Quality (US). https://www.ncbi.nlm.nih.gov/books/NBK587174/

National Heart, Lung, and Blood Institute. (2024). *Asthma treatment and action plan*. https://www.nhlbi.nih.gov/health/asthma/treatment-action-plan

National Institute of Diabetes and Digestive and Kidney Diseases (NIDDK). (2023). *Helping your child who is overweight*. https://www.niddk.nih.gov/health-information/weight-management/helping-your-child-who-is-overweight

National Institute for Drug Abuse. (n.d.). *What are inhalants*. https://nida.nih.gov/publications/research-reports/inhalants/what-are-inhalants

National Institute of Environmental Health. (n.d.). *Autism*. https://www.niehs.nih.gov/health/topics/conditions/autism

National Institute of Health (NIH). (2024). *ADHD and complimentary health approaches*. https://www.nccih.nih.gov/health/providers/digest/adhd-and-complementary-health-approaches

National Institute on Drug Abuse. (2022). *Most reported substance use among adolescents held steady in 2022*. https://nida.nih.gov/news-events/news-releases/2022/12/most-reported-substance-use-among-adolescents-held-steady-in-2022

Nurse Family Partnership. (2024). *A lot's gonna change—You've got this*. https://www.nursefamilypartnership.org/first-time-moms/?gad_source=1&gclid=EAIaIQobChMImvrKx4eRhwMVjssWBR1aBAK5EAAYASAAEgImPfD_BwE

Office of Juvenile Justice and Delinquency. (n.d.). *Youth homicide victims by race*. https://ojjdp.ojp.gov/statistical-briefing-book/victims/faqs/qa02310

Office of Juvenile Justice and Delinquency Prevention. (2023). *Child homicide is a leading cause of death- and rates are rising*. https://ojjdp.ojp.gov/newsletter/ojjdp-news-glance-marchapril-2023/child-homicide-leading-cause-death-and-rates-are-rising#:~:text=a%20Second%20Chance-,Child%20Homicide%20Is%20a%20Leading%20Cause%20of%20Death%E2%80%94and%20Rates,violence%20to%20and%20by%20youth

Office of Juvenile Justice and Delinquency Prevention. (n.d.). *Statistical briefing book*. https://www.ojjdp.gov/ojstatbb//victims/qa02304.asp?qaDate=2020#:~:text=Between%201980%20and%202020%2C%20an,United%20States%20%E2%80%93%201%2C777%20in%202020.&text=Homicides%20of%20youth%20peaked%20in,all%20murder%20victims%20in%202020

Office of Population Affairs. (n.d.-a). *Healthy relationships in adolescents*. https://opa.hhs.gov/adolescent-health/healthy-relationships-adolescence

Office of Population Affairs. (n.d.-b). *Trends in teen pregnancy and childbearing*. https://opa.hhs.gov/adolescent-health/reproductive-health-and-teen-pregnancy/trends-teen-pregnancy-and-childbearing

Oranika, U. S., Adeola, O. L., Egbuchua, T. O., Okob, O. E., Alrowaili, D. G., Kajero, A., Koleowo, O. M., Okobi, E., David, A. B., & Ezeamii, J. C. (2023). The role of childhood obesity in early-onset type 2 diabetes mellitus: A scoping review. *Cureus*, *15*(10). http://doi.org/10.7759/cureus.48037

Ortiz-Morron, H., Ortiz-Pinto, M. A., Lanza, M. U., Pujadas, G. C., Del Pino, V. V., Cortes, S. B., Gascon, T. G., & Gavin, M. O. (2022). Household food insecurity and its association with overweight and obesity in children aged 2-14 years. *BMC Public Health*, *22*(1930). https://doi.org/10.1186/s12889-022-14308-0

Peterson, C., Xu, L., Leemis, R. W., & Stone, D. M. (2019). Repeated self-inflicted injury among U.S. youth in a large medical claims database. *American Journal of Preventative Medicine*, *56*(3), 411–419. http://doi.org/10.1016/j.amepre.2018.09.009

Pew Research Center. (2023). *Gun deaths among U.S. children and teens rose 50% in two years*. https://www.pewresearch.org/short-reads/2023/04/06/gun-deaths-among-us-kids-rose-50-percent-in-two-years/

Pignenburg, M. W., Frey, U., De Jongste, J. C., & Saglani, S. (2022). Childhood asthma: Pathogenesis and phenotypes. *European Respiratory Journal Series*, *59*, 2100731. http://doi.org/. https://doi:10.1183/13993003.00731-2021

Ravi, P., & Khan, S. (2020). Attention deficit hyperactivity disorder: Association with obesity and eating disorders. *Cureus*, *12*(12). http://doi.org/10.7759/cureus.12085

Rubenstein, E., Croen, L., Lee, L. C., Moody, E., Schieve, L. A., Soke, G. N., Thomas, K., Wiggins, L., & Daniels, J. (2019). Community-based service use in preschool children with autism spectrum disorder and associations with insurance status. *Research in Autism Spectrum Disorders*, *66*. http://doi.org/10.1016/j.rasd.2019.101410

Rudisill, T. M., Smith, G., Chu, H., & Zhu, M. (2018). Cellphone legislation and self-reported behaviors among subgroups of adolescent U.S. drivers. *Journal of Adolescent Health*, *62*, 618–625.

Salam, R. A., Padhani, Z. A., Das, J. K., Shaikh, A. Y., Zoodbhoy, Z., Jeelani, S. R., Lassi, Z. S., & Bhutta, A. Y. (2020). Effects of lifestyle modification interventions to prevent and manage childhood and adolescent obesity: A systematic review and meta-analysis. *Nutrients*, *12*. https://doi.org/10.3390/nu12082208

Sandy Hook Promise. (n.d.). *17 facts about gun violence and school shootings*. https://www.sandyhookpromise.org/blog/gun-violence/facts-about-gun-violence-and-school-shootings/

Schlack, R., Peerenboon, N., Neuperdt, L., Junker, S., & Beyer, A. K. (2021). The effects of mental health problems in children and adolescents in young adults: Results of the KiGGS cohort. *Journal of Health Monitoring*, *6*(4), 3–19. http://doi.org/10.25646/8863

Sliwa, S. A., Wheaton, A. G., Li, J., & Michael, S. L. (2023). Sleep duration, mental health, and increased difficulty doing schoolwork among high school students during the COVID-19 pandemic. *Preventing Chronic Disease*, *20*, 220344. http://dx.doi.org/10.5888/pcd20.220344

Stanford Medicine Children's Health. (2024). *Accident statistics*. https://www.stanfordchildrens.org/en/topic/default?-id=accident-statistics-90-P02853

Statista. (2024). *Annual prevalence of use of steroids for grades 8,10,12 combined from 1991 to 2023*. https://www.statista.com/statistics/696545/us-annual-prevalence-of-steroid-use-in-grades-8-10-12-since-1991/

Substance Abuse and Mental Health Services Administration Administration (SAMHSA). (2024). *Eating disorders*. https://www.samhsa.gov/mental-health/eating-disorders

Sumner, R., Ganz, M., Jacobs, M., Alessandro, C., Fuchs, D., Gamss, S., & Miller, D. (2022). Bullying victimization as a risk factor for gun carrying among U.S. adolescents. *Cureus*, *14*(11). http://doi.org/10.7759/cureus.31785

Taylor, N. L., & Blenner, J. A. (2021). Attitudes and behaviors associated with young drivers' texting and app use. *Transportation research part F: Traffic psychology and behaviour*, *78*, 326–339.

The Children's Partnership. (2022). *Racial justice in children's oral health*. https://childrenspartnership.org/news/racial-justice-in-childrens-oral-health/

Turanovic, J. J., & Siennick, S. E. (2022). *The causes and consequences of school violence: A review*. National Institute of Justice. https://www.ojp.gov/pdffiles1/nij/302346.pdf

U.S. Department of Education. (n.d.). *IDEA: Individuals with disabilities education act*. https://sites.ed.gov/idea/

U.S. Department of Health and Human Services (USDHHS). (2023). *Surgeon general issues new advisory about effects social media use has on youth mental health*. https://www.hhs.gov/about/news/2023/05/23/surgeon-general-issues-new-advisory-about-effects-social-media-use-has-youth-mental-health.html

U.S. Department of Justice. (2020). *Children exposed to violence*. https://ojp.gov/program/programs/cev#:~:text=The%20term%20poly%2Dvictimization%20describes,partner%20violence%20and%20physical%20abuse.

U.S. Food and Drug Administration. (n.d.). *Ingesting or inhaling nitrite "poppers" can cause severe injury or death*. https://

www.fda.gov/consumers/consumer-updates/ingesting-or-inhaling-nitrite-poppers-can-cause-severe-injury-or-death

United States Department of Health and Human Services (USDHHS). (n.d.). *Mental health for adolescents*. https://opa.hhs.gov/adolescent-health/mental-health-adolescents#:~:text=Visit%20NIMH's%20Help%20for%20Mental,some%20point%20in%20their%20lives

United Way. (2022). *Childhood poverty in the United States*. https://unitedwaynca.org/blog/child-poverty-in-america/#:~:text=Child%20poverty%20can%20have%20a,finding%20employment%20as%20an%20adult

Van Ryzin, M. J., Fishbein, D., & Biglan, A. (2018). The promise of prevention science for addressing intergenerational poverty. *Psychology, Public Policy, and Law*, *24*(1), 128–143.

Venditti, E. M., Tan, K., Chang, N., Laffel, L., McGinley, G., Miranda, N., Tryggestad, J. B., Walders-Abramson, N., Yasuda, P., & Delahanty, L. (2018). Barriers and strategies for oral medication adherence among children and adolescents with Type 2 diabetes. *Diabetes Research and Clinical Practice*, *139*, 24–31.

Wisconsin Office of Children's Mental Health. (2024). *School shootings and youth mental health*. https://children.wi.gov/Documents/ResearchData/OCMH%20Fact%20Sheet_April%202024_School%20Shootings.pdf

World Health Organization (WHO). (2022). *Older children and young adolescent mortality (5-14 years)*. https://www.who.int/news-room/fact-sheets/detail/older-children-and-young-adolescent-mortality-(5-to-14-years)

World Health Organization (WHO). (2024). *Sexually transmitted infections among adolescents. The need for adequate health services*. https://www.who.int/publications/i/item/9241562889#:~:text=Each%20year%20an%20estimated%20333,HIV%20and%20other%20viral%20infections

Youth.gov. (n.d.-a). *Adolescent health*. https://youth.gov/youth-topics/adolescent-health

Youth.gov. (n.d.-b). *Substance abuse prevention: Risk and protective factors*. https://youth.gov/youth-topics/youth-mental-health/risk-and-protective-factors-youth

Youth.gov. (n.d.-c). *Welcome to the teen pregnancy prevention evidence review*. https://youth.gov/evidence-innovation/tpper

CHAPTER 21

Abrahamowics, A. A., Ebinger, J., Whelton, S. P., Commodore-Mensah, Y., & Yang, E. (2023). Racial and ethnic disparities in hypertension: Barriers and opportunities to improve blood pressure control. *Hypertension*, *25*, 17–27. http://doi.org/10.1007/s11886-022-01826-x

Ahmad, F. B., & Anderson, R. N. (2021). The leading causes of death in the US for 2020. *JAMA*, *325*(18), 1829–1830.

Ahmad, F. B., Cisewski, J. A., Xu, J., & Anderson, R. N. (2023). Provisional mortality data—United States, 2022. *Morbidity and Mortality Weekly Report*, *72*(18), 488. http://dx.doi.org/10.15585/mmwr.mm7218a3

American Cancer Society (ACS). (2022). *American cancer society recommendations for early detection of breast cancer*. https://www.cancer.org/cancer/breast-cancer/screening-tests-and-early-detection/american-cancer-society-recommendations-for-the-early-detection-of-breast-cancer.html

American Cancer Society (ACS). (2023a). *Cancer treatment & survivorship facts & figures 2022-2024*. https://cancercontrol.cancer.gov/ocs/statistics#statistics

American Cancer Society (ACS). (2023b). *Guidelines for the early detection of cancer*. https://www.cancer.org/cancer/screening/american-cancer-society-guidelines-for-the-early-detection-of-cancer.html

American Cancer Society (ACS). (2023c). *Testicular cancer*. http://www.cancer.org/cancer/testicularcancer/detailedguide/testicular-cancer-detailed-guide-toc

American Cancer Society (ACS). (2023d). *Prostate cancer*. https://www.cancer.org/cancer/prostate-cancer.html

American Cancer Society (ACS). (2023e). *Screening tests for prostate cancer*. https://www.cancer.org/cancer/types/prostate-cancer/detection-diagnosis-staging/tests.html

American Cancer Society (ACS). (2023f). *Initial treatment of prostate cancer, by stage and risk group*. https://www.cancer.org/cancer/types/prostate-cancer/treating/by-stage.html

American Civil Liberties Union (ACLU). (2023). *Women's rights*. https://www.aclu.org/issues/womens-rights#:~:text=Today%2C%20gender%20bias%20continues%20to,end%20to%20gender%2Dbased%20violence.

American College of Cardiology. (2023). *Keto-like diet may be linked to higher risk of heart disease, cardiac events*. https://www.acc.org/About-ACC/Press-Releases/2023/03/05/15/07/Keto-Like-Diet-May-Be-Linked-to-Higher-Risk

American College of Obstetricians and Gynecologists (ACOG). (2020). *Committee opinion: Hormone therapy and heart disease*. https://www.acog.org/Clinical-Guidance-and-Publications/Committee_Opinions/Committee_on_Gynecologic_Practice/Hormone_Therapy-and-Heart-Disease

American College of Obstetricians and Gynecologists (ACOG). (2022). *ACOG recommendations: Management of postmenopausal osteoporosis*. https://www.obgproject.com/2022/07/17/acog-recommendations-management-of-postmenopausal-osteoporosis/#:~:text=Pharmacologic%20treatment%20is%20recommended%20for,pharmacotherapy%20until%20findings%20are%20stable

American Heart Association (AHA). (2023). *Go red for women*. https://www.goredforwomen.org/en/

American Lung Association (ALA). (2023). *Lung health and diseases: Asthma*. http://www.lung.org/lung-health-and-diseases/lung-disease-lookup/asthma/

American Psychological Association (APA). (2022a). *Sexual orientation and gender diversity*. https://www.apa.org/topics/lgbtq

American Psychological Association (APA). (2022b). *Proposed eating disorder and body image announces eating disorder awareness week*. Retrieved from https://www.apa.org/about/division/digest/share-members/eating-disorder-awareness-week

Asthma and Allergy Foundation of America. (2023). *Asthma facts*. https://aafa.org/asthma/asthma-facts/

Berberian, A. G., Gonzalez, D. J. X., & Cushing, L. J. (2022). Racial disparities in climate change-related health effects in the United States. *Curr Envir Health Rpt*, *9*, 451–464. https://doi:10.1007/s40572-022-00360-w

Berk, L. E. (2018). Emotional and social development in early adulthood. In *Development through the lifespan* (7th ed., pp. 468–506). Pearson Education.

Bone Health and Osteoporosis Foundation. (2022). *Evaluation of bone health/bone density testing*. https://www.bonehealthandosteoporosis.org/patients/diagnosis-information/bone-density-examtesting/

Bryant, K. B., Morna, A. E., Kazi, D. S., Zhang, Y., Penko, J., Ruiz-Negron, N., Coxson, P., ... Bellow, B. K. (2021). cost-effectiveness of hypertension treatment by pharmacists in black barbers. *Circulation*, *143*(24) https://doi.org/10.1161/CIRCULATIONAHA.120.051683

Cancer Statistic Center. (2023). *Estimated deaths, 2016–2020*. https://cancerstatisticscenter.cancer.org/#!/cancer-site/Breast

Case, A., & Deaton, A. (2021). Life expectancy in adulthood is falling for those without a BA degree, but as educational gaps have widened, racial gaps have narrowed. *Proceedings of the National Academy of Sciences*, *118*(11), e2024777118. https://www.pnas.org/doi/abs/10.1073/pnas.2024777118

Center for Men's Health. (2022). *Male menopause or andropause*. https://www.centreformenshealth.co.uk/mens-health-services/male-menopause

Centers for Disease Control and Prevention. (CDC). (n.d.). *Depression and aging*. https://www.cdc.gov/aging/olderadultsandhealthyaging/depression-and-aging.html#

Centers for Disease Control and Prevention (CDC). (2020a). *Men and heart disease fact sheet*. https://www.cdc.gov/dhdsp/data_statistics/fact_sheets/fs_men_heart.htm

Centers for Disease Control and Prevention (CDC). (2020b). *Human papillomavirus (HPV) vaccine*. https://www.cdc.gov/vaccinesafety/vaccines/hpv-vaccine.html

Centers for Disease Control and Prevention (CDC). (2021a). *National Center for Immunization and Respiratory Diseases (NCIRD)*. https://www.cdc.gov/flu/season/faq-flu-season-2020-2021.htm

Centers for Disease Control and Prevention (CDC). (2021b). *Which STD tests should I get?* https://www.cdc.gov/std/prevention/screeningreccs.htm

Centers for Disease Control and Prevention (CDC). (2021c). *Myalgic encephalomyelitis/chronic fatigue syndrome: Symptoms*. Retrieved from https://www.cdc.gov/me-cfs/symptoms-diagnosis/symptoms.htm

Centers for Disease Control and Prevention (CDC). (2021d). *Mortality in the United States, 2021*. https://www.cdc.gov/nchs/products/databriefs/db456.htm#:~:text=Statistics%20System%2C%20Mortality.-,Summary,2020%20to%20416%2C893%20in%202021

Centers for Disease Control and Prevention (CDC). (2022a). *Injuries and violence are leading causes of death*. National Center for Injury Prevention and Control. https://www.cdc.gov/injury/wisqars/animated-leading-causes.html

Centers for Disease Control and Prevention (CDC). (2022b). *NCHHSTP social determinants of health*. https://www.cdc.gov/nchhstp/socialdeterminants/index.html

Centers for Disease Control. (2022c). *Opioids/understanding the epidemic*. https://www.cdc.gov/opioids/basics/epidemic.html

Centers for Disease Control and Prevention (CDC). (2022e). *Overweight and obesity*. https://www.cdc.gov/obesity/data/prevalence-maps.html

Centers for Disease Control and Prevention (CDC). (2022f). *Overweight and obesity. Consequences of obesity*. https://www.cdc.gov/obesity/basics/consequences.html

Centers for Disease Control and Prevention (CDC). (2022f). *Collecting sexual orientation and Gender Identity Information*. https://www.cdc.gov/hiv/clinicians/transforming-health/health-care-providers/collecting-sexual-orientation.html

Centers for Disease Control and Prevention (CDC). (2022g). *HPV-associated cancer statistics*. https://www.cdc.gov/cancer/hpv/statistics/index.htm

Centers for Disease Control and Prevention (CDC). (2022h). *Breast cancer in men*. https://www.cdc.gov/cancer/breast/men/index.htm

Centers for Disease Control and Prevention (CDC). (2022i). *What are risk factors for breast cancer*. https://www.cdc.gov/cancer/breast/basic_info/risk_factors.htm

Centers for Disease Control and Prevention (CDC). (2022j). *Does osteoporosis run in your family?* https://www.cdc.gov/features/osteoporosis/index.html

Centers for Disease Control and Prevention (CDC). (2023a). *National Center for Health Statistics. National Health and Nutrition Survey (NHANES)*. https://www.cdc.gov/nchs/nhanes/index.htm

Centers for Disease Control and Prevention (CDC). (2023b). *Heart disease. Men and heart disease*. https://www.cdc.gov/heartdisease/men.htm

Centers for Disease Control and Prevention (CDC). (2023c). *Stroke facts*. https://www.cdc.gov/stroke/facts.htm

Centers for Disease Control and Prevention (CDC). (2023d). *Type 2 diabetes*. https://www.cdc.gov/diabetes/basics/type2.html#:~:text=More%20than%2037%20million%20Americans,them%20have%20type%202%20diabetes.

Centers for Disease Control and Prevention (CDC). (2023e). *Smoking and tobacco use: Health effects*. https://www.cdc.gov/tobacco/basic_information/health_effects/index.htm

Centers for Disease Control and Prevention (CDC). (2023f). *U.S. adult tobacco use decreased from 2019-2020*. https://www.cdc.gov/media/releases/2022/p0318-US-tobacco-use.html

Centers for Disease Control and Prevention (CDC). (2023g). *Smoking and tobacco: Adult data*. https://www.cdc.gov/tobacco/data_statistics/fact_sheets/adult_data/cig_smoking/index.htm

Centers for Disease Control and Prevention (CDC). (2023h). *Smoking and tobacco: Economics*. https://www.cdc.gov/tobacco/data_statistics/fact_sheets/economics/econ_facts/index.htm

Centers for Disease Control and Prevention (CDC). (2023i). *Smoking and tobacco use: Current data*. https://www.cdc.gov/tobacco/data_statistics/fact_sheets/adult_data/cig_smoking/index.htm

Centers for Disease Control and Prevention (CDC). (2023j). *Sexually transmitted disease surveillance, 2021*. https://www.cdc.gov/std/statistics/2021/overview.htm#Chlamydia

Centers for Disease Control and Prevention (CDC). (2023k). *Pregnancy complication*. https://www.cdc.gov/reproductivehealth/maternalinfanthealth/pregnancy-complications.html

Centers for Disease Control and Prevention (CDC). (2023l). *Preconception care*. https://www.cdc.gov/preconception/index.html

Centers for Disease Control and Prevention (CDC). (2023m). *Basic information about gynecological cancers*. https://www.cdc.gov/cancer/gynecologic/basic_info/index.htm

Centers for Disease Control and Prevention (CDC). (2023n). *Engaging young men in reproductive health*. https://www.cdc.gov/teenpregnancy/about/educating-engaging-young-men-reproductive-health.htm

Psychological Sciences and Social Sciences, *77*(9), 1710–1720. https://doi.org/10.1093/geronb/gbac057. PMID: 35385579; PMCID: PMC9434459.

Bureau of Labor Statistics, U.S. Department of Labor, The Economics Daily. (2021). *Number of people 75 and older in the labor force is expected to grow 96.5 percent by 2030*. https://www.bls.gov/opub/ted/2021/number-of-people-75-and-older-in-the-labor-force-is-expected-to-grow-96-5-percent-by-2030.htm

Caplan, Z. (2023). *U.S. older population grew from 2010 to 2020 at fastest rate since 1880 to 1890*. U.S Census Bureau. https://www.census.gov/library/stories/2023/05/2020-census-united-states-older-population-grew.html

Carlson, B., Kohon, J. N., Carder, P. C., Himes, D., Toda, E., & Tanaka, K. (2023). Climate change policies and older adults: An analysis of states' climate adaptation plans. *The Gerontologist*. gnad077. https://doi-org.libproxy.uccs.edu/10.1093/geront/gnad077

Centers for Disease Control and Prevention (CDC). (2023a). *About REACH*. https://www.cdc.gov/reach/php/about/

Centers for Disease Control and Prevention (CDC). (2023b). *Oral and dental health*. http://www.cdc.gov/nchs/fastats/dental.htm

Centers for Disease Control and Prevention (CDC). (2023c). *STEADI: Stopping elderly accidents, deaths & injuries*. https://www.cdc.gov/steadi/

Centers for Disease Control and Prevention (CDC). (2023d). *Important facts about falls*. https://www.cdc.gov/falls/facts.html

Centers for Disease Control and Prevention (CDC). (2023e). *Depression and aging*. https://www.cdc.gov/aging/olderadultsandhealthyaging/depression-and-aging.html#:~:text=Depression%20is%20a%20true%20and,to%20be%20diagnosed%20and%20treated

Center for Disease Control and Prevention. (2024a). *Recommended immunizations for adults aged 19 years and older, United States, 2024*. https://www.cdc.gov/vaccines/imz-schedules/adult-easyread.html

Centers for Disease Control and Prevention (CDC). (2024b). *Arthritis basics*. http://www.cdc.gov/arthritis/basics/index.html

Centers for Disease Control and Prevention Newsroom. (2024). *Media statement: CDC recommends updated 2024-2025 COVID-19 and flu vaccines for fall/winter virus season*. https://www.cdc.gov/media/releases/2024/s-t0627-vaccine-recommendations.html

Centers for Medicare and Medicaid Services. (CMS). (2023). *Medicare wellness visits*. https://www.cms.gov/Outreach-and-Education/Medicare-Learning-Network-MLN/MLN-Products/preventive-services/medicare-wellness-visits.html

Centers for Medicare and Medicaid Services. (CMS). (2024). *Medicare and Medicaid programs: Minimum staffing standards for long-term care facilities and Medicaid institutional payment transparency reporting final rule (CMS 3442-F)*. https://www.cms.gov/newsroom/fact-sheets/medicare-and-medicaid-programs-minimum-staffing-standards-long-term-care-facilities-and-medicaid-0

Central Intelligence Agency. (n.d.). *The world factbook: Dependency ratios*. https://www.cia.gov/the-world-factbook/field/dependency-ratios/

Chang, E., Kannoth, S., Levy, S., Wang, S., Lee, J. E., & Levy, B. R. (2020). Global reach of ageism on older persons' health: A systematic review. *PLOS ONE*. https://doi.org/10.1371/journal.pone.0220857

Chang, E. S., & Levy, B. R. (2021). High prevalence of elder abuse during the COVID-19 pandemic: Risk and resilience factors. *The American Journal of Geriatric Psychiatry: official journal of the American Association for Geriatric Psychiatry*, *29*(11), 1152–1159. https://doi.org/10.1016/j.jagp.2021.01.007

Cheng, C., Yu, H., & Wang, Q. (2023). Nurses' experiences concerning older adults with polypharmacy: A meta-synthesis of qualitative findings. *Healthcare (Basel)*. *11*(3), 334. https://doi.org/10.3390/healthcare11030334. PMID: 36766909; PMCID: PMC9914425.

Coalition for Compassionate Care of California. (2023). *FICA spiritual assessment tool*. https://coalitionccc.org/CCCC/CCCC/Resources/FICA-Spiritual-Assessment-Tool.aspx

Commonwealth Fund. (2021). *When costs are a barrier to getting health care: Reports from older adults in the United States and other high-income countries*. https://www.commonwealthfund.org/publications/surveys/2021/oct/when-costs-are-barrier-getting-health-care-older-adults-survey

Congress.gov. (2024). *H.R.7165—Credit for caring act of 2024*. https://www.congress.gov/bill/118th-congress/house-bill/7165

Cordell, C. B., Borson, S., Boustani, M., Chodosh, J., Reuben, D., Verghese, J., Thies, W., Fried, L. B., & Medicare Detection of Cognitive Impairment Workgroup. (2013). Alzheimer's Association recommendations for operationalizing the detection of cognitive impairment during the Medicare Annual Wellness Visit in a primary care setting. *Alzheimer's & Dementia*, *9*(2), 141–150.

Cottrill, A., Cubanski, J., Neuman, T., & Smith, K. (2024). *Income and assets of Medicare beneficiaries in 2023*. Kaiser Family Foundation (KFF). https://www.kff.org/medicare/issue-brief/income-and-assets-of-medicare-beneficiaries-in-2023/#:~:text=In%202023%2C%20half%20of%20all,incomes%20below%20%2421%2C000%20per%20person

Cubanski, J., & Neuman, T. (2023). *What to know about Medicare spending and financing*. Kaiser Family Foundation. https://www.kff.org/medicare/issue-brief/what-to-know-about-medicare-spending-and-financing/

Dai, F., Liu, Y., Ju, M., & Yang, Y. (2021). Nursing students' willingness to work in geriatric care: An integrative review. *NursingOpen*., *8*, 2061–2077. https://doi.org/10.1002/nop2.726

Doucet, G. E., Kruse, J. A., Hamlin, N., Oleson, J. J., & White, S. F. (2023). Changing role of the amygdala in affective and cognitive traits between early and late adulthood. *Frontiers in Psychiatry*, *14*, 1033543. https://doi.org/10.3389/fpsyt.2023.1033543

Duke Aging Center. (n.d.). *Older Americans resources and services (OARS)*. Duke University School of Medicine. https://agingcenter.duke.edu/oars

Epstein, L. H., Jimenez-Knight, T., Honan, A. M., Paluch, R. A., & Bickel, W. K. (2022). Imagine to remember: An episodic future thinking intervention to improve medication adherence in patients with type 2 diabetes. *Patient Preference and Adherence*, *16*, 95–104. https://doi.org/10.2147/PPA.S342118

Fantacone, M. L., Lowry, M. B., Uesugi, S. L., Michels, A. J., Choi, J., Leonard, S. W., Gombart, S. K., Gombart, J. S., Bobe, G., & Gombart, A. F. (2020). The effect of a multivitamin and mineral supplement on immune function in healthy older adults: A double-blind, randomized, controlled trial. *Nutrients*, *12*(8), 2447. https://doi.org/10.3390/nu12082447

Galvin, J. E. (2015). The Quick Dementia Rating System (QDRS): A rapid dementia staging tool. *Alzheimer's & Dementia: Diagnosis, Assessment & Disease Monitoring*, *1*(2), 249–259.

Genworth Financial. (2024). Monthly median costs: USA - National 2023. https://www.genworth.com/aging-and-you/finances/cost-of-care

Ghosh, A., Jagtap, T., & Issac, T. G. (2024). Cognitive benefits of physical activity in the elderly: A narrative review. *Journal of Psychiatry Spectrum*, *3*(1), 4–11. https://doi.org/10.4103/jopsys.jopsys_40_23

Goldy-Brown, S., & Clem, M. (2024). *Skilled Nursing Costs in 2024*. https://www.seniorliving.org/skilled-nursing/cost/

González-Bueno, J., Sevilla-Sánchez, D., Puigoriol-Juvanteny, E., Molist-Brunet, N., Codina-Jané, C., & Espaulella-Panicot, J. (2021). Factors associated with medication non-adherence among patients with multimorbidity and polypharmacy admitted to an intermediate care center. *International Journal of Environmental Research and Public Health*, *18*(18), 9606. https://doi.org/10.3390/ijerph18189606. PMID: 34574530; PMCID: PMC8464705.

Graf, C. (2008). The Lawton Instrumental Activities of Daily Living Scale. *American Journal of Nursing*, *108*(4), 53–62.

Hale, J. M., Schneider, D. C., Mehta, N. K., & Myrskylä, M. (2020). Cognitive impairment in the U.S.: Lifetime risk, age at onset, and years impaired. *SSM—Population Health*, *11*, 100577. https://doi.org/10.1016/j.ssmph.2020.100577

Halvorsen, C. J., Werner, K., McCullogh, E., & Yulikova, O. (2022). How the senior community service employment program influences participant well-being: A participatory research approach with program recommendations. *Research on Aging*, *45*(1), 77–91. https://doi.org/10.1177/016402752210986

Harris, E. (2023). Most COVID-19 deaths worldwide were among older people. *Journal of the American Medical Association*, *329*(9), 704. https://doi.org/10.1001/jama.2023.1554

Healthfinder.gov. (2023). *Lower your risk of falling*. https://health.gov/myhealthfinder/topics/everyday-healthy-living/safety/lower-your-risk-falling

Heisel, M. J., & Flett, G. L. (2022). Screening for suicide risk among older adults: Assessing preliminary psychometric properties of the Brief Geriatric Suicide Ideation Scale (BGSIS) and the GSIS-Screen. *Aging & Mental Health*, *26*(2), 392–406. https://doi.org/10.1080/13607863.2020.1857690

Help Starts Here. (211). (n.d.). https://www.211.org/

Hill, A. V., Dyer, H. P., Gianakas, J., Howze, R., King, A., Gary-Webb, T. L., & Méndez, D. D. (2023). Correlates of COVID-19 vaccine uptake in black adults residing in Allegheny County, PA. *Health Equity*, *7*(1), 419–429. https://doi.org/10.1089/heq.2022.0215

Hill, L., & Artiga, S. (2023). *What is driving widening racial disparities in life expectancy?* Kaiser Family Foundation. https://www.kff.org/racial-equity-and-health-policy/issue-brief/what-is-driving-widening-racial-disparities-in-life-expectancy/

Hung, M., Srivastav, A., Lu, P., Black, C. L., Lindley, M. C., & Singleton, J. A. (2022). *Vaccination coverage among adults in the United States, national health interview survey, 2022*. CDC. https://www.cdc.gov/vaccines/imz-managers/coverage/adultvaxview/pubs-resources/vaccination-coverage-adults-2022.html

Hwang, P. H., Longstreth, W. T., Jr., Thielke, S. M., Francis, C. E., Carone, M., Kuller, L. H., & Fitzpatrick, A. L. (2022). Longitudinal changes in hearing and visual impairments and risk of dementia in older adults in the United States. *JAMA Network Open*, *5*(5), e2210734. https://doi.org/10.1001/jamanetworkopen.2022.10734. PMID: 35511175; PMCID: PMC9073563.

International Osteoporosis Foundation. (n.d.). *Facts and statistics*. http://www.iofbonehealth.org/facts-statistics

Johnson, K. (2021). *Deaths exceeded births in a record number of states in 2020*. Carsey School of Public Policy. University of New Hampshire. https://carsey.unh.edu/publication/deaths-exceeded-births-record-number-states-2020#:~:text=As%20a%20result%2C%20more%20people,did%20so%20again%20in%202020

Johnson, S., & Sabo, S. (2022). *New Census Bureau population estimates show COVID-19 impact on fertility and mortality across the nation*. U.S. Census Bureau. https://www.census.gov/library/stories/2022/03/deaths-outnumbered-births-in-half-of-states-between-2020-and-2021.html

Katz, S. (1963). Studies of illness in the aged. The index of ADL: A standardized measure of biological and psychosocial function. *Journal of the American Medical Association*, *185*, 914–919.

Kiger, P. (2023). *What's it like to turn 65 in 2024?* AARP. https://www.aarp.org/retirement/planning-for-retirement/info-2023/silver-tsunami-late-boomers-turn-65.html

Killeen, O. J., De Lott, L. B., Zhou, Y., Hu, M., Rein, D., Reed, N., Swenor, B. K., & Ehrlich, J. R. (2023). Population prevalence of vision impairment in US adults 71 years and older: The National Health and Aging Trends Study. *JAMA Ophthalmology*, *141*(2), 197–204. https://doi/10.1001/jamaophthalmol.2022.5840.

Kim, J., & Parish, A. L. (2021). Nursing: Polypharmacy and medication management in older adults. *Clinics in Integrated Care*, *8*. https://doi.org/10.1016/j.intcar.2021.100070

Koffel, E., Ancoli-Israel, S., Zee, P., & Dzierzewski, J. M. (2023). Sleep health and aging: Recommendations for promoting healthy sleep among older adults: A National Sleep Foundation report. *Sleep Health: Journal of the National Sleep Foundation*, *9*(6). https://doi.org/10.1016/j.sleh.2023.08.018

Kotronia, E., Brown, H., Papacosta, A. O., Lennon, L. T., Weyant, R. J., Whincup, P. H., Wannamethee, S. G., & Ramsay, S. E. (2021). Oral health and all-cause, cardiovascular disease, and respiratory mortality in older people in the UK and USA. *Scientific Reports*, *11*(1), 16452. https://doi.org/10.1038/s41598-021-95865-z

Kritz, M., Thogersen-Ntoumani, C., Mullan, B., Stathi, A., & Ntoumanis, N. (2021). "It's better together": A nested longitudinal study examining the benefits of walking regularly with peers versus primarily alone in older adults. *Journal of Aging and Physical Activity*, *29*, 455–465. https://doi.org/10.1123/japa.2020-0091

Kübler-Ross, E. (1969). *On death and dying*. Scribner.

Lindeza, P., Rodrigues, M., Costa, J., Guerreiro, M., & Rosa, M. M. (2024). Impact of dementia on informal care: A systematic review of family caregivers' perceptions. *BMJ*

Supportive & Palliative Care, 14, e38–e49. https://spcare.bmj.com/content/bmjspcare/14/e1/e38.full.pdf

Lotas, L. J. (2021). Commentary: A study for the evaluation of a safety education program me for nursing students: Discussions using the QSEN safety competencies. *Journal of Research in Nursing: JRN, 26*(1–2), 116–117. https://doi.org/10.1177/1744987121999794

Lytle, A., Macdonald, J., Apriceno, M., & Levy, S. R. (2021). Reducing ageism with brief videos about aging education, ageism, and intergenerational contact. *The Gerontologist, 61*(7), 1164–1168. https://doi.org/10.1093/geront/gnaa167

Ma, C., Guerra-Smith, O., & Mohammadi, M. (2022). Smart home modification design strategies for aging in place: A systematic review. *Journal of Housing and Built Environment, 37*(2), 1–27. https://doi.org/10.1007/s10901-021-09888-z

Martínez-Angulo, P., Muñoz-Mora, M., Rich-Ruiz, M., Ventura-Puertos, P. E., Cantón-Habas, V., & López-Quero, S. (2023). "With your age, what do you expect?": Ageism and healthcare of older adults in Spain. *Geriatric Nursing, 51*, 84–94. https://doi.org/10.1016/j.gerinurse.2023.02.020

Medicaid.gov. (n.d.). Community First Choice (CFC) 1915 (k). https://www.medicaid.gov/medicaid/home-community-based-services/home-community-based-services-authorities/community-first-choice-cfc-1915-k/index.html

Miller, C. A. (2019). *Nursing for wellness in older adults* (8th ed.). Wolters Kluwer.

Murray, K.O., Mahoney, S.A., Venkatasubramanian, R., Seals, D.R., & Clayton, Z.S. (2023). Aging, aerobic exercise, and cardiovascular health: Barriers, alternative strategies and future directions. *Experimental Gerontology, 173*. https://doi.org/10.1016/j.exger.2023.112105. PMID: 36731386; PMCID: PMC10068966.

National Center for Assisted Living. (2023). *Assisted living state regulatory review*. https://www.ahcancal.org/Assisted-Living/Policy/Pages/state-regulations.aspx

National Council on Aging (NCOA). (2022). *Suicide and older adults: What you should know*. https://www.ncoa.org/article/suicide-and-older-adults-what-you-should-know

National Council on Aging (NCOA). (2023). *Healthy aging*. https://www.ncoa.org/article/get-the-facts-on-healthy-aging

National Foundation for Infectious Diseases. (2023). *Influenza*. http://www.nfid.org/influenza/

National Institute of Aging. (2024). *10 common misconceptions about aging*. https://www.nia.nih.gov/health/healthy-aging/10-common-misconceptions-about-aging

National Institute of Arthritis and Musculoskeletal and Skin Diseases (NIAMS). (2022a). *Arthritis*. http://www.niams.nih.gov/Health_Info/Arthritis/default.asp

National Institute of Arthritis and Musculoskeletal and Skin Diseases (NIAMS). (2022b). *Rheumatoid arthritis*. http://www.niams.nih.gov/Health_Info/Rheumatic_Disease/default.asp

National Institute on Aging. (2020). *Real-life benefits of exercise and physical activity*. https://www.nia.nih.gov/health/exercise-and-physical-activity/real-life-benefits-exercise-and-physical-activity

National Institute on Aging. (2023). *The caregiver's handbook*. https://order.nia.nih.gov/sites/default/files/2023-03/caregivers-handbook-nia_0.pdf

National Institution on Deafness and Other Communication Disorders. (2023). *Age-related hearing loss (Presbycusis)*. https://www.nidcd.nih.gov/health/age-related-hearing-loss

National Library of Medicine. (2023). *Mandatory reporting laws*. https://www.ncbi.nlm.nih.gov/books/NBK560690/

National PACE Association. (2023). *What is PACE care?* https://www.npaonline.org/what-is-pace-care

New World Encyclopedia. (n.d.). *Spirit*. http://www.newworldencyclopedia.org/entry/Spirit

Ndugga, N., Hill, L., & Artiga, S. (2022). *COVID-19 cases and deaths, vaccinations, and treatments by race/ethnicity as of Fall 2022*. Kaiser Family Foundation. https://www.kff.org/racial-equity-and-health-policy/issue-brief/covid-19-cases-and-deaths-vaccinations-and-treatments-by-race-ethnicity-as-of-fall-2022/

Norouzi, N. (2020). Architecture of a smart home for aging in place. *Innovation in Aging*, 4(Suppl 1), 39. https://doi.org/10.1093/geroni/igaa057.126

Office of Disease Prevention and Health Promotion. (n.d.-a). *Health equity in Healthy People 2030*. https://health.gov/healthypeople/priority-areas/health-equity-healthy-people-2030

Office of Disease Prevention and Health Promotion. (n.d.-b). *Dementias*. https://health.gov/healthypeople/objectives-and-data/browse-objectives/dementias

Office of Disease Prevention and Health Promotion. (n.d.-c). *Reduce the proportion of adults with obesity—NWS-03*. https://health.gov/healthypeople/search?query=adults+and+obesity

Office of Disease Prevention and Health Promotion. (n.d.-d). *Reduce the proportion of older adults with untreated root surface decay—OH-04*. https://health.gov/healthypeople/objectives-and-data/browse-objectives/oral-conditions/reduce-proportion-older-adults-untreated-root-surface-decay-oh-04

Office of Disease Prevention and Health Promotion. (n.d.-e). *Reduce the rate of motor vehicle crashes due to drowsy driving—SH-01*. https://health.gov/healthypeople/objectives-and-data/browse-objectives/sleep/reduce-rate-motor-vehicle-crashes-due-drowsy-driving-sh-01

Office of Disease Prevention and Health Promotion. (n.d.-f). *Pneumonia*. https://health.gov/healthypeople/search?query=pneumonia

Office of Disease Prevention and Health Promotion. (n.d.-g). *Health care*. https://health.gov/healthypeople/objectives-and-data/browse-objectives/health-care

Office of Inspector General. (2024). *Nursing homes*. https://oig.hhs.gov/reports-and-publications/featured-topics/nursing-homes/

Office of the Assistant Secretary for Planning and Evaluation. (2023). *Addressing homelessness among older adults*. https://aspe.hhs.gov/reports/older-adult-homelessness

Office of the Federal Register Publications. (2024). Part 483—Requirements for states and long term care. *Code of federal regulations: Title, 42* https://www.ecfr.gov/current/title-42/chapter-IV/subchapter-G/part-483

Omaha System. (n.d.). *Omaha system overview*. https://www.omahasystem.org/overview

Omnibus Budget Reconciliation Act. (1987). *Federal nursing home reform act from the Omnibus Budget Reconciliation Act of 1987*. www.ncmust.com/doclib/OBRA87summary.pdf

Pew Research Center. (2022). *How U.S. religious composition has changed in recent decades*. https://www.pewresearch.org/religion/2022/09/13/how-u-s-religious-composition-has-changed-in-recent-decades/

Phillips, A. Z., Carnethon, M. R., Bonham, M., Lovett, R. M., & Wolf, M. S. (2023). Hazardous drinking by older adults with chronic conditions during the COVID-19 pandemic: Evidence from a Chicago-based cohort. *Journal of the American Geriatrics Society, 71*(11), 3508–3519. https://doi.org/10.1111/jgs.18497

Rijal, S. (2022). Polypharmacy in elderly people: A simple review. *Journal of Pharmaceutical Research International, 34*(64), 40–49. https://doi.org/10.9734/jpri/2022/v34i647293

Scott, J., & Mayo, A. M. (2018). Instruments for detection and screening of cognitive impairment for older adults in primary care settings: A review. *Geriatric Nursing, 39*(3), 323–329. https://doi.org/10.1016/j.gerinurse.2017.11.001

Sears, B. (2023). *Timed up and go (TUG) test: An overview*. https://www.verywellhealth.com/the-timed-up-and-go-test-2696072

Sol Price School of Public Policy. (2023). *The baby boomer effect and controlling health care costs*. University of Southern California. https://healthadministrationdegree.usc.edu/blog/the-baby-boomer-effect-and-controlling-health-care-costs

Song, D., Yu, D., Liu, T., & Wang, J. (2024). Effect of an aerobic dancing program on sleep quality for older adults with mild cognitive impairment and poor sleep: A randomized controlled trial. *Journal of the American Medical Directors Association, 25*(3), 494–499. https://doi.org/10.1016/j.jamda.2023.09.020

Supporting Grandparents Raising Grandchildren Act of 2018, S. 1091, 115th Cong., Second Sess. (2018). https://acl.gov/sites/default/files/about-acl/2018-10/BILLS-115s1091enr%20-%20SGRG.pdf

The White House.gov. (2023). *Fact sheet: Biden-Harris administration takes steps to crack down on nursing homes that endanger resident safety*. https://www.whitehouse.gov/briefing-room/statements-releases/2023/09/01/fact-sheet-biden-harris-administration-takes-steps-to-crack-down-on-nursing-homes-that-endanger-resident-safety/

U.S. Bureau of Statics. (2023). *Celebrating national family caregivers month with BLS data*. https://www.bls.gov/blog/2023/celebrating-national-family-caregivers-month-with-bls-data.htm

U.S. Department of Agriculture (USDA). (n.d.-a). *Choose my plate*. https://www.choosemyplate.gov/

U.S. Department of Agriculture (USDA). (n.d.-b). *Older adults*. https://www.myplate.gov/life-stages/older-adults

U.S. Department of Justice (USDOJ). (n.d.). *State elder abuse statutes*. https://www.justice.gov/elderjustice/elder-justice-statutes-0

U.S. Food and Drug Administration (FDA). (2023). *OTC hearing aids: What you should know*. https://www.fda.gov/medical-devices/hearing-aids/otc-hearing-aids-what-you-should-know

U.S. Preventive Services Task Force. (n.d.-a). *USPSTF A and B recommendations*. https://www.uspreventiveservicestaskforce.org/Page/Name/uspstf-a-and-b-recommendations/

U.S. Preventive Services Task Force. (n.d.-b). *Information for health professionals*. https://www.uspreventiveservicestaskforce.org/uspstf/search_results?searchterm=information+health+professionals

United Nations Department of Economic and Social Affairs, Population Division. (2023). *World population ageing 2023: Challenges and opportunities of population ageing in the least developed countries*. UN DESA/POP/2023/TR/NO.5. https://www.un.org/development/desa/pd/sites/www.un.org.development.desa.pd/files/undesa_pd_2024_wpa2023-report.pdf

Vera-Toscano, E., & Meroni, E. C. (2021). An age–period–cohort approach to disentangling generational differences in family values and religious beliefs: Understanding the modern Australian family today. *Demographic Research, 45*, 653–692. https://www.jstor.org/stable/48640791

Vespa, J., Medina, L., & Armstrong, D. M. (2020). *Demographic turning points for the United States: Population projections for 2020 to 2060, Current population reports, P25-1144*. U.S. Census Bureau, Washington, DC. https://www.census.gov/content/dam/Census/library/publications/2020/demo/p25-1144.pdf

Village to Village Network. (2023). *The village movement*. https://www.vtvnetwork.org/content.aspx?page_id=0&club_id=691012

Willcoxon, N. (2022). *Older adults sacrificing basic needs due to healthcare costs*. https://news.gallup.com/poll/393494/older-adults-sacrificing-basic-needs-due-healthcare-costs.aspx

World Health Organization. (2021). *Global report on ageism*. Geneva. Licence: CC BY-NC-SA 3.0 IGO. https://iris.who.int/bitstream/handle/10665/340208/9789240016866-eng.pdf?sequence=1

CHAPTER 23

Abdalla, S. M., Yu, S., & Galea, S. (2020). Trends in cardiovascular disease prevalence by income level in the United States. *JAMA Network Open*, 3(9), e2018150. https://doi:10.1001/jamanetworkopen.2020.18150

Aday, L. (2001). *At risk in America: The health and health care needs of vulnerable populations in the United States* (2nd ed.). Jossey-Bass, San Francis-co.

Agency for Healthcare Research and Quality (AHRQ). (2010). *2009 National healthcare disparities report*. U.S. Department of Health & Human Services. Publication No. 10-0004. Retrieved from http://www.ahrq.gov/qual/nhdr09/nhdr09.pdf

Agency for Healthcare Research and Quality (AHRQ). (2023). *2022 National healthcare quality and disparities report*. U.S. Department of Health & Human Services. https://www.ahrq.gov/research/findings/nhqrdr/nhqdr22/index.html

American Association of Colleges of Nursing (AACN). (2023). *Enhancing diversity fact sheet*. https://www.aacnnursing.org/Portals/0/PDFs/Fact-Sheets/Enhancing-Diversity-Fact-sheet.pdf

American Cancer Society. (2022). *The costs of cancer for people with limited incomes*. https://www.fightcancer.org/policy-resources/costs-cancer-people-limited-incomes-0#:~:text=U.S.%20counties%20that%20experience%20persistent,duct%20(27.6%25%20higher)

American Lung Association. (2023). *Disparities in the impact of air pollution*. https://www.lung.org/clean-air/outdoors/who-is-at-risk/disparities

Australian Institute of Health and Welfare. (2022). *Health across socioeconomic groups*. https://www.aihw.gov.au/reports/australias-health/health-across-socioeconomic-groups systematic review.

Bates, B. (2023). *Learning theories simplified and how to apply them to teaching*. Sage.

Burg, M. A., & Oyama, O. (Eds.) (2016). *The behavioral health specialist in primary care: Skills for integrated practice*. Springer Publishing Company.

Bustamante, A. V., Chen, J., Félix Beltrán, L., & Ortega, A. N. (2021). Health policy challenges posed by shifting demographics and health trends among immigrants to the United States. *Health Affairs(Millwood)*, *40*(7), 1028–1037. https://doi:10.1377/hlthaff.2021.00037

Campbell, K., Van Borek, N., Marcellus, L., Landy, C., Jack, S. M., & British Columbia Healthy connections Project Process Evaluation Research Team. (2020). "The hardest job you will ever love": Nurse recruitment, retention, and turnover in the nurse-family partnership program in British Columbia, Canada. *PLoS One*, *15*(9). https://doi:10.1371/journal.pone.0237028

Cardoso Barbosa, H., de Queiroz Oliveira, J. A., Moreira da Costa, J., de Melo Santos, R. P., Gonçalves Miranda, L., de Carvalho Torres, H., Pagano, A. S., & Martins, M. A. P. (2021). Empowerment-oriented strategies to identify behavior change in patients with chronic diseases: An integrative review of the literature. *Patient Education and Counseling*, *104*(4). https://doi:10.1016/j.pec.2021.01.011

Center for Poverty Research, University of California, Davis. (2021). *What is deep poverty?* Center for Poverty and Inequality Research (ucdavis.edu). Retrieved from https://poverty.ucdavis.edu/faq/what-deep-poverty

Centers for Disease Control and Prevention (CDC). (2020). *Defining health disparities. Health Disparities in HIV, Viral Hepatitis, STDs, and TB*. https://www.cdc.gov/nchhstp/healthdisparities/default.htm

Centers for Disease Control and Prevention (CDC). (2021). *CDC healthy schools: School health guidelines*. https://www.cdc.gov/healthyschools/npao/strategies.htm

Centers for Disease Control and Prevention (CDC). (2022a). *Preterm birth*. https://www.cdc.gov/chronicdisease/index.htm

Centers for Disease Control and Prevention (CDC). (2022b). *Social determinants of health at CDC*. https://www.cdc.gov/about/sdoh/index.html

Centers for Disease Control and Prevention (CDC). (2023a). *Socioeconomic factors: Indictor profile. Division of heart disease and stroke prevention*. https://www.cdc.gov/dhdsp/health_equity/socioeconomic.htm

Centers for Disease Control and Prevention (CDC). (2023b). *Current cigarette smoking among adults in the United States*. https://www.cdc.gov/tobacco/data_statistics/fact_sheets/adult_data/cig_smoking/index.htm

Clay, S. L. (2021). Black/White disparities in low birth weight pregnancy outcomes: An exploration of differences in health factors within a vulnerable population. *International Journal of Health Promotion and Education*, *61*(3), 115–126. https://doi:10.1080/14635240.2021.1931934

Collins, S., Hayes, L. A., & Masitha, R. (2022). *The State of U.S. health insurance in 2022: Findings from the Commonwealth Fund Biennial Health Insurance Survey*. The Commonwealth Fund. https://www.commonwealthfund.org/publications/issue-briefs/2022/sep/state-us-health-insurance-2022-biennial-survey

Committee on the Future of Nursing. (2021). *The Future of Nursing 2020-2030: Charting a path to achieve health equity. The role of nurses in improving healthcare access and quality, 99-128*. Retrieved from https://www.ncbi.nlm.nih.gov/books/NBK573910/

Commodore-Mensah, Y., Shaw, B., & Ford, M. (2021). A nursing call to action to support the health of migrants and refugees. *Advanced Nursing*, *77*(12), e41–e43. https://doi.org/10.111/jan.14970

Connolly, C., & Cotter, P. (2023). Effectiveness of nurse-led clinics on healthcare delivery: An umbrella review. *Journal of Clinical Nursing*, *32*(9-10), 1760–1767. https://doi:10.1111/jocn.16186. https://pubmed.ncbi.nlm.nih.gov/34970816/

Curtin, S. C., Tejada-Vera, B., & Bastian, B. A. (2024). Deaths: Leading causes for 2021. *National Vital Statistics Reports*, *73*(4). https://www.cdc.gov/nchs/data/nvsr/nvsr73/nvsr73-04.pdf

Davis, A., Kim, R., & Crifasi, C. K. (2023). *A year in review: 2021 gun deaths in the U.S. Johns Hopkins Center for gun violence solutions*. Johns Hopkins Bloomberg School of Public Health. https://publichealth.jhu.edu/sites/default/files/2024-01/2023-june-cgvs-u-s-gun-violence-in-2021-v3.pdf

Falk-Rafael, A. R. (2001). Empowerment as a process of evolving consciousness: A model of empowered caring. *Advances in Nursing Science*, *24*(1), 1–16.

Fernandez, M. (2018). *A year after Hurricane Harvey, Houston's Poorest neighborhoods are slowest to recover*. New York Times. Retrieved from https://www.nytimes.com/2018/09/03/us/hurricane-harvey-houston.html

Flaskerud, J. H., & Winslow, B. J. (1998). Conceptualizing vulnerable populations health-related research. *Nursing Research*, *47*(2), 69–78.

Galvani-Townsend, S., Isabel Martinez, I., & Pandey, A. (2022). Is life expectancy higher in countries and territories with publicly funded health care? Global analysis of health care access and the social determinants of health. *Journal of Global Health*, *12*. https://doi:10.7189/jogh.12.04091

Gelberg, L., Andersen, R., & Leake, B. (2000). The behavioral model for vulnerable populations: Application to medical care use and outcomes for homeless people. *Health Services Research*, *34*(6), 1273–1302.

Griffith, D. M., Bergner, E. M., Fair, A. S., & Wilkins, C. H. (2021). Using mistrust, distrust, and low trust precisely in medical care and medical research advances health equity. *American Journal of Preventive Medicine*, *60*(3), 442–445. https://doi:10.1016/j.amepre.2020.08.019

Hajizadeh, M., Mitnitski, A., & Rockwood, K. (2016). Socioeconomic gradient in health in Canada: Is the gap widening or narrowing? *Health Policy*, *120*(9), 1040–1050. https://doi:10.1016/j.healthpol.2016.07.019

Hamed, S., Bradby, H., Ahlberg, B. M., & Thapar-Björkert, S. (2022). Racism in healthcare: A scoping review. *BMC Public Health*, *22*, 988. https://doi:10.1186/s12889-022-13122-y

Health Resources & Services Administration. (2023). *Health center program: Impact and growth*. https://bphc.hrsa.gov/about-health-centers/health-center-program-impact-growth

Healthcare.gov. (2024). *Federal poverty level (FPL)*. https://www.healthcare.gov/glossary/federal-poverty-level-fpl/

Hu, X., Wang, T., Huang, D., Wang, Y., & Li, Q. (2021). Impact of social class on health: The mediating role of health self-management. *PLoS One*, *16*(7). https://doi:10.1371/journal.pone.0254692

Hutchison, L. M., & Cox, R. L. (2020). Addressing the health needs of the uninsured: One community's solution. *The Permanente Journal*, *24*(19), 022. https://doi:10.7812/TPP/19.022

Indian Health Services. (n.d.). *IHS innovation projects address social factors in health*. U.S. Department of Health and Human Services. https://www.ihs.gov/office-of-quality/ipc/impacts-and-outcomes/innovation-projects/

Indian Health Services. (2019). *Disparities*. U.S. Department of Health and Human Services. https://www.ihs.gov/newsroom/factsheets/disparities/

Institute for Functional Medicine. (2023). *Food insecurity and chronic disease*. Retrieved from Food Insecurity and Chronic Disease | The Institute for Functional Medicine (ifm.org)

Institute of Medicine (IOM). (2001). *Crossing the quality chasm: A new health system for the 21st Century*. National Academy Press.

Institute of Medicine (IOM). (2003). *Unequal treatment: Confronting racial and ethnic disparities in healthcare*. The National Academies Press.

Institute of Medicine (IOM). (2012). *For the Public's Health: The Role of Measurement in Action and Accountability*. The National Academies Press.

Iorhen, P. (2021). Vulnerability: Types, causes and coping mechanisms. *International Journal of Science and Management Studies*, *4*(3), 187–194. https://doi.org/10.51386/25815946/ijsms-v4i3p116

Kaiser Family Foundation (KFF). (2023). *Key facts on health coverage of immigrants*. https://www.kff.org/racial-equity-and-health-policy/fact-sheet/key-facts-on-health-coverage-of-immigrants/

Kamarck, E., & Stenglein, C. (2019). *How many undocumented immigrants are in the United States and who are they?* Brookings Institute. https://www.brookings.edu/articles/how-many-undocumented-immigrants-are-in-the-united-states-and-who-are-they/

Kessler, R. (1979). Psychological consequences of stress. *Journal of Health and Social Behavior*, *20*, 100–108.

Kjolhede, C., & Lee, A. C. (2021). School-based health centers and pediatric practice. *Pediatrics*, *148*(4). https://doi:10.1542/peds.2021-053758. https://pubmed.ncbi.nlm.nih.gov/34544844/

Kodsup, P., & Godebo, T. R. (2023). Disparities in underlying health conditions and COVID-19 infection and mortality in louisiana, USA. *Journal of Racial and Ethnic Health Disparities*, *10*, 805–816. https://doi:10.1007/s40615-022-01268-9

Lewis, K. N., Tilford, J. M., Goudie, A., Beavers, J., Casey, P. H., & McKelvey, L. M. (2023). Cost-benefit analysis of home visiting to reduce infant mortality among preterm infants. *Journal of Pediatric Nursing*, *71*. https://doi:10.1016/j.pedn.2023.05.003

Lopez Vera, A., Thomas, K., Trinh, C., & Nausheen, F. (2023). A case study of the impact of language concordance on patient care, satisfaction, and comfort with sharing sensitive information during medical care. *Journal of Immigrant and Minority Health*, *25*, 1261–1269. https://doi:10.1007/s10903-023-01463-8

Lowrey, A. (2019). *What the camp fire revealed*. The Atlantic. Retrieved from httpps://www.theatlantic.com/ideas/archive/2019/01/why-natural-disasters-are-worse-poor/580846/

Marmot, M., Ryff, C. D., Bumpass, L. L., Shipley, M., & Marks, N. F. (1997). Social inequalities in health: Next questions and converging evidence. *Social Science and Medicine*, *44*(6), 901–910.

Maslow, A. (1987). *Motivation and personality* (3rd ed.). Addison-Wesley.

Matwick, A., & Woodgate, R. (2017). Social justice: A concept analysis. *Public Health Nursing*, *34*(2), 176–184.

Mullachery, P. H., Vela, E., Montse, C., Comin-Colet, J., Nasir, K., Diez Rouxc, A. V., Cainzos-Achirica, M., Mauri, J., & Bilal, U. (2022). inequalities by income in the prevalence of cardiovascular disease and its risk factors in the adult population of Catalonia. *Journal of the American Heart Association*, *11*(17). https://doi:10.1161/JAHA.122.026587

Nadeem, R. (2023). *A brief statistical portrait of U.S. Hispanics*. Pew Research Center Science & Society. https://www.pewresearch.org/science/2022/06/14/a-brief-statistical-portrait-of-u-s-hispanics/

National Academies of Sciences, Engineering, and Medicine; National Academy of Medicine; Committee on the Future of Nursing 2020-2030. (2021) https://www.ncbi.nlm.nih.gov/books/NBK573925/?report=printable

National Academy of Sciences. (2019). *Accessing progress on the institute of medicine report the future of nursing*. Retrieved from https://www.nap.edu/read/21838/chapter/1

National Center for Safe and Supportive Learning Environments. (2023). *Human trafficking in America's schools*. Retrieved from: Human Trafficking in America's Schools | National Center on Safe Supportive Learning Environments (NCSSLE) (ed.gov)

National Conference of State Legislators. (2021). *Health disparities overview*. https://www.ncsl.org/health/health-disparities-overview

Ndugga, N., & Artiga, S. (2023). *Disparities in health and health care: 5 key questions and answers*. Kaiser Family Foundation. https://www.kff.org/racial-equity-and-health-policy/issue-brief/disparities-in-health-and-health-care-5-key-question-and-answers/

Needham, B. L., Ali, T., Allgood, K. L., Ro, A., Hirschtick, J. L., & Fleischer, N. L. (2023). Institutional racism and health: A framework for conceptualization, measurement, and analysis. *Journal of Racial and Ethnic Health Disparities*, *10*, 1997–2019. https://doi:10.1007/s40615-022-01381-9

New Jersey Department of Human Services Office of Research & Evaluation. (2023). *Social isolation study*. https://www.nj.gov/humanservices/news/reports/DHS%20Social%20Isolation%20Report.pdf

Office of Disease Prevention and Health Promotion. (2020). *Social determinants of health*. Retrieved from https://www.healthypeople.gov/2020/topics-objectives/topic/social-determinants-of-health

Office of Disease Prevention and Health Promotion. (n.d.). *Health equity. Healthy people 2030*. https://health.gov/healthypeople/priority-areas/health-equity-healthy-people-2030

Olds, D. L., Eckenrode, J., Henderson Jr., C. R., Kitzman, H., Powers, L., Cole, R., Sidora, K., Morris, P., Pettitt, L. M., & Luckey, D. (1997). Long-term effects of home visitation on maternal life course and child abuse and neglect. Fifteen-year follow-up on a randomized trial. *Journal of the American Medical Association*, *278*(8), 637–643.

Petrosky, E., Mercer Kollar, L. M., Kearns, M. C., Smith, S. G., Carter, J. B., Fowler, K. A., & Satteret, D. E. (2021). Homicides of American Indians/Alaska Natives — National violent death reporting system, United States, 2003–2018.

MMWR Surveillance Summaries, 70(No. SS-8),1–19. http://dx.doi.org/10.15585/mmwr.ss7008a1

Ponce-Chazarri, L. P., once-Blandón, J. A., Immordino, P., Giordano, A., & Morales, F. (2023). Barriers to breast cancer-screening adherence in vulnerable populations. *Cancers, 15*, 604. https://doi:10.3390/cancers15030604

Powers, M., & Takagishi, J. (2021). Care of adolescent parents and their children. *Pediatrics, 147*(5). https://doi:10.1542/peds.2021-050919

Public Health Accreditation Board. (2022). *Foundational public health services factsheet*. https://phaboard.org/wp-content/uploads/FPHS-Factsheet-2022.pdf

Salerno, J., Williams, N., & Gattamorta, K. (2020). LGBTQ populations: Psychologically vulnerable communities in the COVID-19 pandemic. Psychological trauma: Theory, research, practice and policy. *Trauma Psychology, 12*, 239–242.

Schake, M., Sommers, B., Subramanian, S., Waters, M., & Arcava, M. (2019). Effects of gentrification on health status after Hurricane Katrina. *Health & Place, 15*, 102237.

Schwandt, H., Curriec, J., von Wachter, T., Kowarski, J., Chapman, D., & Woolf, S. H. (2022). Changes in the relationship between income and life expectancy before and during the COVID-19 pandemic, California, 2015-2021. *Journal of the American Medical Association, 328*(4), 360–366. https://doi:10.1001/jama.2022.10952

Sells, M. L., Blum, E., Perry, G. S., Eke, P., & Presley-Cantrell, L. (2023). Excess burden of poverty and hypertension, by race and ethnicity, on the prevalence of cardiovascular disease. *Preventing Chronic Disease, 20*, 230065. https://doi:10.5888/pcd20.230065

Shanahan, K. H., Subramanian, S. V., Burdick, K. J., Monuteaux, M. C., Lee, L. K., & Fleegler, E. W. (2022). Association of neighborhood conditions and resources for children with life expectancy at birth in the US. *JAMA Network Open, 5*(10), e2235912. https://doi:10.1001/jamanetworkopen.2022.35912

Shi, L., Stevens, G., Lebrun, L., Faed, P., & Tsai, J. (2008). Enhancing the measurement of health disparities for vulnerable populations. *Journal of Public Health Management and Practice, 14*(Suppl), s45–s52.

Shin, S. H., & Choi, C. (2023). Improving birth outcomes among low-income families: The effect of a home visiting intervention. *Clinical Pediatrics, 62*, 11. 10.1177/00099228231158367

Shortreed, S. M., Gray, R., Akosile, M. A., Walker, R. L., Fuller, S., Temposky, L., Fortmann, S. P., Albertson-Junkans, L., Floyd, J. S., Bayliss, E. A., Harrington, L. B., Lee, M. H., & Dublin, S. (2023). Increased COVID-19 infection risk drives racial and ethnic disparities in severe COVID-19 outcomes. *Journal of Racial and Ethnic Health Disparities, 10*(1), 149–159.

Small-Rodriguez, D., & Akee, R. (2021). Identifying disparities in health outcomes and mortality for American Indian and Alaska Native Populations using tribally disaggregated vital statistics and health survey data. *American Journal of Public Health, 111*, S126–S132. 10.2105/AJPH.2021.306427

States. (n.d.) https://datacenter.aecf.org/data/tables/44-children-in-poverty-by-race-and-ethnicity#detailed/1/any/false/2048,1729,37,871,870,573,869,36,868/187,11,9,12,1,185,13/324,323

Takian, A., Kiani, M. M., & Khanjankhani, K. (2020). COVID-19 and the need to prioritize health equity and social determinants of health. *International Journal of Public Health, 65*, 521–523. https://doi:10.1007/s00038-020-01398-z

The Annie E. Casey Foundation. (2023). *Children in poverty by race and ethnicity in United*. https://datacenter.aecf.org/data/tables/44-children-in-poverty-by-race-and-ethnicity

The White House. (2021). *Fact sheet: The national action plan to combat human trafficking (NAP)*. https://www.whitehouse.gov/briefing-room/statements-releases/2021/12/03/fact-sheet-the-national-action-plan-to-combat-human-trafficking-nap/

Tolbert, J., Drake, P., & Damico, A. (2022). *Key facts about the uninsured population. KFF the independent source for health policy and news*. Retrieved from Key Facts about the Uninsured Population – Supplemental Tables – 8488-08 | KFF

U.S. Census data. (2023). https://www.usa.gov/census-data

U.S. Department of Agriculture (USDA). (2023). *Food access research atlas*. https://www.ers.usda.gov/data-products/food-access-research-atlas

U.S. Department of Health and Human Services (USDHHS). (n.d.). *Social determinants of health*. Retrieved from https://health.gov/healthypeople/objectives-and-data/social-determinants-health

United Nations Human Rights. (2023). *Migrants in vulnerable situations. Migrants in vulnerable situations | OHCHR*

Velasco, R. A. F., Blakeley, A., Rostovsky, J., Skeete, K. J., & Copeland, D. (2023). Conceptualizing transgender and gender-diverse older adults as a vulnerable population: A systematic review. *Geriatric Nursing, 49*, 139–147. https://doi:10.1016/j.gerinurse.2022.11.018

Voice of a Witness. (2019). *Voices of the storm: the people of New Orleans on Hurricane Katrina and its aftermath*. Retrieved from https://voiceofwitness.org/oral-history-book-series/voices-from-the-storm/

Wasserman, J., Palmer, R. C., Gomez, M. M., Berzon, R., Ibrahim, S. A., & Ayanian, J. Z. (2019). Advancing health services research to eliminate health care disparities. *American Journal of Public Health, 109*(S1), S64–S69. https://doi:10.2105/AJPH.2018.304922

Whitman, A., De Lew, N., Chappel, A., Aysola, V., Zuckerman, R., & Sommers, B. D. (2022). *Addressing social determinants of health: Examples of successful evidence-based strategies and current federal efforts*. Office of Health Policy: Assistant Secretary for Planning and Evaluation. https://aspe.hhs.gov/sites/default/files/documents/e2b650cd64cf84aae8ff0fae7474af82/SDOH-Evidence-Review.pdf

Wiltz, J. L., Feehan, A. K., Molinari, N. M., Ladva, C. N., Truman, B. I., Hall, J., Block, J. P., Rasmussen, S. A., Denson, J. L., Trick, W. E., Weiner, M. G., Koumans, E., Gundlapalli, A., Carton, T. W., & Boehmer, T. K. (2022). Racial and ethnic disparities in receipt of medications for treatment of COVID-19—United States, March 2020–August 2021. *Morbidity and Mortality Weekly Report, 71*(3), 96.

Woolf, S. H. (2023). Falling behind: The growing gap in life expectancy between the United States and other countries, 1933–2021. *American Journal of Public Health, 113*, 970_980. https://doi:10.2105/AJPH.2023.307310

World Bank. (2020). *Poverty and shared prosperity 2020: Reversals of fortune – Frequently asked questions* (worldbank.org)

World Health Organization (WHO). (2017). *Human rights and health*. Retrieved from https://www.who.int/news-room/fact-sheets/detail/human-rights-and-health

World Health Organization (WHO). (2020a). *Health Impact Assessment (HIA): The determinants of health*. Retrieved from http://www.who.int/hia/evidence/doh/en/

World Health Organization (WHO). (2020b). *Social determinants of health?* Retrieved from http://www.who.int/social_determinants/sdh_definition/en/

World Health Organization (WHO). (2022). *New WHO report highlights scale of childhood cancer inequalities in the European Region*. https://www.who.int/europe/news/item/15-02-2022-new-who-report-highlights-scale-of-childhood-cancer-inequalities-in-the-european-region

World Health Organization (WHO). (2023). *Fact sheet: Asthma*. https://www.who.int/news-room/fact-sheets/detail/asthma

Zeidan, A. J., Smith, M., Leff, R., Cordone, A., Moran, T. P., Brackett, A., & Agraval, P. (2023). Limited english proficiency as a barrier to inclusion in emergency medicine-based clinical stroke research. *Journal of Immigrant and Minority Health, 25*, 181–189. https://doi:10.1007/s10903-022-01368-y

Zeller, J., Fruin, B., Newkirk, M. B., & Travers, E. (2024). The effect of simulation on attitudes and empathy related to persons experiencing homelessness among nursing students. *Teaching and Learning in Nursing, 19*(2). https://doi:10.1016/j.teln.2023.12.007

CHAPTER 24

Alzheimer's Association. (2023). *2023 Alzheimer's disease facts and figures*. Alzheimer's Dementia. https://doi:10.1002/alz.13016; https://www.alz.org/media/documents/alzheimers-facts-and-figures.pdf

American Academy of pediatrics. (2024). *What is medical home?* https://www.aap.org/en/practice-management/medical-home/medical-home-overview/what-is-medical-home/

American Psychological Association (APA). (2019). *Disability and socioeconomic status*. https://www.apa.org/pi/ses/resources/publications/disability

American Sign Language (ASL) University. (n.d.). *International sign language (Gestuno)*. http://www.lifeprint.com/asl101/pages-layout/gestuno.htm

Baruch, L., Bilitzky-Kopit, A., Rosen, K., & Adler, L. (2022). Cervical cancer screening among patients with physical disability. *Journal of Women's Health, 31*(8), 1173–1178. https://doi:10.1089/jwh.2021.0447

Bedewy, D. (2021). Examining and measuring sources of stress in a sample of caregivers of children with special needs in Egypt: The Perception of Caregivers Stress Scale. *Cogent Psychology, 8*, 1. https://doi:10.1080/23311908.2021.1911094

Bureau of Labor Statistics. (2023). *Persons with a disability: Labor force characteristics —2022*. https://www.bls.gov/news.release/pdf/disabl.pdf

Cacchione, P. Z. (2020). Innovative care models across settings: Providing nursing care to older adults. *Geriatric Nursing, 41*(1). https://pubmed.ncbi.nlm.nih.gov/32033809/

Center for Universal Design. (2016). *About the center: Ronald L. Mace*. Retrieved from https://www.ncsu.edu/ncsu/design/cud/about_us/usronmace.htm

Centers for Disease Control and Prevention (CDC). (2020a). *Disability and health related conditions*. https://www.cdc.gov/ncbddd/disabilityandhealth/relatedconditions.html

Centers for Disease Control and Prevention (CDC). (2020b). *Disability and health stories from people living with a disability*. https://www.cdc.gov/ncbddd/disabilityandhealth/stories.html

Centers for Disease Control and Prevention (CDC). (2020c). *Common barriers to participation experienced by people with disabilities*. https://www.cdc.gov/ncbddd/disabilityandhealth/disability-barriers.html

Centers for Disease Control and Prevention (CDC). (2020d). *Disability and health promotion*. Retrieved from https://www.cdc.gov/ncbddd/disabilityandhealth/index.html

Centers for Disease Control and Prevention (CDC). (2020e). *Disability & health information for family caregivers*. https://www.cdc.gov/ncbddd/disabilityandhealth/family.html

Centers for Disease Control and Prevention (CDC). (2023a). *Disability impacts all of us*. https://www.cdc.gov/ncbddd/disabilityandhealth/infographic-disability-impacts-all.html

Centers for Disease Control and Prevention (CDC). (2023b). *Caregiving for a person with Alzheimer's disease or a related dementia*. https://www.cdc.gov/aging/caregiving/alzheimer.htm

Centers for Disease Control and Prevention (CDC). (2023c). *Data and statistics about hearing loss in children*. https://www.cdc.gov/ncbddd/hearingloss/data.html

Centers for Medicare & Medicaid Services (CMS). (2023). *Improving access to care for people with disabilities*. https://www.cms.gov/priorities/health-equity/minority-health/resource-center/health-care-professionals-researchers/improving-access-care-people-disabilities

Chen, A. (2022). *11 global health issues to watch in 2023, according to IHME experts*. The Institute for Health Metrics and Evaluation. https://www.healthdata.org/news-events/insights-blog/acting-data/11-global-health-issues-watch-2023-according-ihme-experts

Chen, C., Bailey, C., Baikie, G., Dalziel, K., & Hua, X. (2023). Parents of children with disability: Mental health outcomes and utilization of mental health services. *Disability and Health Journal, 16*(4). https://doi:10.1016/j.dhjo.2023.101506

Coulter, D., Lynch, C., & Joosten, A. V. (2023). Exploring the perspectives of young adults with developmental disabilities about sexuality and sexual health education. *Australian Occupational Therapy Journal, 70*(3), 380–391. https://doi:10.1111/1440-1630.12862

Erickson, W., Lee, C., & von Schrader, S. (2024). *2022 Disability Status Report: United States*. Cornell University Yang Tan Institute on Employment and Disability (YTI). https://www.disabilitystatistics.org/report/pdf

Everett, C. (2023). Hearing loss is more common than diabetes. *Why aren't we addressing it? National Council on Aging*. https://www.ncoa.org/adviser/hearing-aids/hearing-loss-america/#:~:text=The%20state%20of%20hearing%20loss,Control%20and%20Prevention%20(CDC)

Fair Housing Accessibility First. (n.d.) *Frequently asked questions*. USDHUD. https://www.hud.gov/program_offices/fair_housing_equal_opp/faq_accessibility_first

Fang, Z., Cerna-Turoff, I., Zhang, C., Lu, M., Lachman, J. M., & Barlow, J. (2022). Global estimates of violence against children with disabilities: An updated systematic review and meta-analysis. *The Lancet Child & Adolescent Health*, *6*, 313–323. https://doi:10.1016/S2352-4642(22)00033-5

Federal Emergency Management Agency (FEMA). (2023). *People with disabilities. https://www.ready.gov/disability#informed*

Friedman, C. (2022). Financial hardship experienced by people with disabilities during the COVID-19 pandemic. *Disability and Health Journal*, *15*(4) https://doi:10.1016/j.dhjo.2022.101359

Goodman, N., Morris, Z., Morris, M., & McGarity, S. (2020). *The extra costs of living with a disability in the U.S. — Resetting the policy table.* https://www.nationaldisabilityinstitute.org/wp-content/uploads/2020/10/extra-costs-living-with-disability-brief.pdf

Harrell, E. (2021). *Crime against persons with disabilities, 2009–2019 – Statistical tables.* U.S. Department of Justice Office of Justice Programs Bureau of Justice Statistics. https://bjs.ojp.gov/library/publications/crime-against-persons-disabilities-2009-2019-statistical-tables

Iezzoni, L. I., Roa, S. R., Ressalam, J., Bolcic-Jankovic, D., Agaronnik, N. D., Lagu, T., Pendo, E., & Campbell, E. G. (2022). US physicians' knowledge about the Americans with disabilities act and accommodation of patients with disability. *Health Affairs*, *41*(1). https://DOI.ORG/10.1377/HLTHAFF.2021.01136

Ishbia, L. (2024). *25 Life-changing apps for people With disabilities.* The Mighty. https://themighty.com/topic/disability/apps-for-people-with-disabilities/

Keck Medicine of USC. (2023). *Top 10 apps for visually impaired people.* https://www.keckmedicine.org/blog/top-10-apps-visually-impaired-people/

Lagu, T., Haywood, C., Reimold, K., Dejong, C., Sterling, R. W., & Iezzoni, L. I. (2022). 'I am not the doctor for you': Physicians' attitudes about caring for people with disabilities. *Health Affairs*, *41*(10). https://DOI.ORG/10.1377/HLTHAFF.2022.00475

Medicaid.gov. (n.d.). *Medicaid provides health coverage for people with disabilities.* https://www.medicaid.gov/about-us/program-history/medicaid-50th-anniversary/entry/47691

Morris, Z. A., McGarity, S. V., Goodman, N., & Zaidi, A. (2022). The extra costs associated with living with a disability in the United States. *Journal of Disability Policy Studies*, *33*(3), 158–167.

Nageswaran, S., & Golden, S. L. (2018). Establishing relationships and navigating boundaries when caring for children with medical complexity at home. *Home Healthcare Now*, *36*(2), 93–102. https://doi:10.1097/NHH.0000000000000636

National Centers of Environmental Information (NCEI). (2024). *U.S. billion-dollar weather & climate disasters 1980-2024.* National Oceanic and Atmospheric Administration. https://www.ncei.noaa.gov/access/billions/events.pdf

National Council on Disability (NCD). (2022). *Medicaid oral health coverage for adults with intellectual & developmental disabilities – A fiscal analysis.* https://ncd.gov/sites/default/files/NCD_Medicaid:Report_508.pdf

National Council on Disability (NCD). (n.d.). *About us.* https://www.ncd.gov/about

National Federation of the Blind. (n.d.). *Braille–What is it? What does it mean to the blind?* http://www.nfb.org/images/nfb/Publications/fr/fr15/Issue1/f150113.html

National Institute on Deafness and Other Communication Disorders. (2021). *American sign language.* https://www.nidcd.nih.gov/health/american-sign-language

Office of Disability Employment Policy. (n.d.). *Universal design resources.* U.S. Department of Labor. https://www.dol.gov/agencies/odep/program-areas/employment-supports/universal-design/resources

Office of Disease Prevention and Health Promotion (ODPHP). (n.d.). *Healthy people 2030: People with disabilities.* https://health.gov/healthypeople/objectives-and-data/browse-objectives/people-disabilities

Pan American Health Organization (PAHO). (2019). *Mental health problems are the leading cause of disability worldwide, say experts at PAHO Directing Council event.* https://www3.paho.org/hq/index.php?option=com_content&view=article&id=15481:mental-health-problems-are-the-leading-cause-of-disability-worldwide-say-experts-at-paho-directing-council-side-event&Itemid=0&lang=en#gsc.tab=0

Perrin, A., & Atske, S. (2021). *Americans with disabilities less likely than those without to own some digital devices.* Pew Research Center. https://www.pewresearch.org/short-reads/2021/09/10/americans-with-disabilities-less-likely-than-those-without-to-own-some-digital-devices/

Perry, M., Cotes, L., Horton, B., Kunac, R., Snell, I., Taylor, B., Wright, A., & Devan, H. (2021). "Enticing" but not necessarily a "space designed for me": Experiences of urban park use by older adults with disability. *International Journal of Environmental Research and Public Health*, *18*(2), 552. https://doi:10.3390/ijerph18020552

Sisson, P. (2023). *What people with disabilities know about surviving climate disasters. Bloomberg.* https://www.bloomberg.com/news/features/2023-06-22/in-climate-disasters-people-with-disabilities-are-getting-left-behind

Social Security Administration. (n.d.). *Benefits for people with disabilities.* https://www.ssa.gov/disability/

U.S. Census Bureau. (2023). *Disability rates higher in rural areas than urban areas.* https://www.census.gov/library/stories/2-23/06/disability-rates-higher-in-rural-areas-than-urban-areas.html

U.S. Department of Health & Human Services (USDHHS). (2024). *HHS finalizes rule strengthening protections against disability discrimination.* https://www.hhs.gov/about/news/2024/05/01/hhs-finalizes-rule-strengthening-protections-against-disability-discrimination.html#:~:text=HHS%20Finalizes%20Rule%20Strengthening%20Protections%20Against%20Disability%20Discrimination,-Final%20Rule%20advances&text=Today%2C%20the%20U.S.%20Department%20of,on%20the%20basis%20of%20disability.

U.S. Department of Health and Human Services (USDHHS). (n.d.). *Category: Programs for families and children.* https://www.hhs.gov/answers/programs-for-families-and-children/index.html

U.S. Department of Health and Human Services (USDHHS), Office for Civil Rights. (2006, September). *Delivering on the promise: OCR's compliance activities promote community integration.* http://www.hhs.gov/civil-rights/for-individuals/special-topics/community-living-and-olmstead/compliance-activities-promote-integration/index.html

U.S. Department of Housing and Urban Development. (USDHUD). (n.d.). *Fair housing accessibility guidelines.* http://portal.hud.gov/hudportal/HUD?src=/program_offices/fair_housing_equal_opp/disabilities/fhefhag

U.S. Department of Justice (USDOJ) Civil Rights Division. (n.d.-a). *The Americans with Disabilities Act (ADA) protects people with disabilities from discrimination.* https://www.ada.gov/

U.S. Department of Justice (USDOJ) Civil Rights Division. (n.d.-b). *Disability Rights Cases.* https://www.justice.gov/crt/disability-rights-cases?page=9

U.S. Department of Justice Civil Rights Division. (USDOJ). (n.d.-a). *Information and technical assistance on the Americans with disabilities act.* Retrieved from https://archive.ada.gov/regs2016/movie_captioning_rule_page.html

U.S. Department of Justice (USDOJ) Civil Rights Division. (n.d.-c). *File a complaint.* https://www.ada.gov/file-a-complaint/

U.S. Department of Justice (USDOJ) Civil Rights Division. (2020). *Disability rights section. A guide to disability rights law.* https://www.ada.gov/cguide.htm

U.S. Department of Labor (USDOL). (n.d.). The family and medical leave act. https://www.dol.gov/agencies/whd/fmla

U.S. Department of Labor Office of Disability Employment Policy. (2023). *National Disability Employment Awareness Month (NDEAM).* https://www.dol.gov/agencies/odep/initiatives/ndeam

United Nations (U.N.). (2016, May 30). *Treaty collection: Chapter IV: Human rights—Convention on the rights of persons with disabilities.* https://treaties.un.org/Pages/ViewDetails.aspx?src=IND&mtdsg_no=IV-15&chapter=4&lang=en

United Nations (U.N.). (2021). *Leveraging digital technologies for social inclusion.* https://www.un.org/development/desa/dspd/2021/02/digital-technologies-for-social-inclusion/

United Nations (U.N.). (2022). *Convention on the rights of persons with disabilities: Conference of states parties to the convention on the rights of persons with disabilities.* https://documents-dds-ny.un.org/doc/UNDOC/GEN/N22/448/18/PDF/N2244818.pdf?OpenElement

University of Rhode Island. (2023). *URI team develops app for and with people with intellectual and developmental disabilities.* https://www.uri.edu/news/2023/07/uri-team-develops-app-for-and-with-people-with-intellectual-and-developmental-disabilities/

Utz, R. L. (2022). Caregiver respite: An essential component of home- and community-based long-term care. *Journal of the American Medical Directors Association*, *23*(2), 320–321. https://doi:10.1016/j.jamda.2021.12.020

Veitch, J., Ball, K., Rivera, E., Loh, V., Deforche, B., Best, K., & Timperio, A. (2022). What entices older adults to parks? Identification of park features that encourage park visitation, physical activity, and social interaction. Landscape and Urban Planning, *217*. https://www.sciencedirect.com/science/article/abs/pii/S0169204621002176

Wondemu, M. Y., Joranger, P., Hermansen, Å., & Brekke, I. (2022). Impact of child disability on parental employment and labour income: A quasi-experimental study of parents of children with disabilities in Norway. *BMC Public Health*, *22*. https://doi:10.1186/s12889-022-14195-5

World Health Organization. (2011). World report on disability. https://apps.who.int/iris/bitstream/handle/10665/70670/WHO_NMH_VIP_11.01_eng.pdf;jsessionid=E07AF4E7D44C47A86B7289C214FB404B?sequence=1

World Health Organization. (2022). *Global report on health equity for persons with disabilities.* https://www.who.int/publications/i/item/9789240063600

World Health Organization (WHO). (2019). *International classification of functioning, disability and health.* https://www.who.int/classifications/icf/en/

World Health Organization (WHO). (2023). *Disability.* https://www.who.int/news-room/fact-sheets/detail/disability-and-health

CHAPTER 25

Agency for Healthcare Research and Quality. (2012). *Five major steps to intervention (the "5 A's").* https://www.ahrq.gov/prevention/guidelines/tobacco/5steps.html

Agency for Healthcare Research and Quality. (n.d.). *The academy integrating behavioral health & primary care.* https://integrationacademy.ahrq.gov/

American Academy of Physician Assistants (AAPA). (2018). *President signs SUPPORT for patients and communities act.* https://www.aapa.org/news-central/2018/10/president-signs-support-patients-communities-act/

American Nurses Association (ANA). (2018). *The opioid epidemic: The evolving role of nursing.* Issue brief. https://www.nursingworld.org/~4a4da5/globalassets/practiceandpolicy/work-environment/health--safety/opioid-epidemic/2018-ana-opioid-issue-brief-vfinal-pdf-2018-08-29.pdf

American Psychiatric Association. (2013). *Diagnostic and statistical manual of mental disorders* (5th ed.).

American Psychiatric Association. (2018). *APA dictionary of psychology: Mental disorder.* https://dictionary.apa.org/mental-disorder

American Psychiatric Association (APA). (2020). *Patient health questionnaire (PHQ-9 & PHQ-2) construct: Depressive symptoms.* https://www.apa.org/pi/about/publications/caregivers/practice-settings/assessment/tools/patient-health

American Psychiatric Association (APA). (2022). *Stress in America 2022: Concerned for the future, beset by inflation.* https://www.apa.org/news/press/releases/stress/2022/concerned-future-inflation

Birdsey, J., Cornelius, M., Jamal, A., Park-Lee, E., Cooper, M. R., Wang, J., Sawdey, M. D., Cullen, K. A., & Neff, L. (2023). Tobacco product use among U.S. middle and high school students — National youth tobacco survey, 2023. *MMWR Morbidity and Mortality Weekly Report*, 72, 1173–1182. http://dx.doi.org/10.15585/mmwr.mm7244a1

Brown, R. L., Batty, E., Lofwall, M., Kiviniemi, M., & Kizewski, A. (2023). Opioid use-related stigma and health care decision-making. *Psychology of Addictive Behaviors*, *37*(2), 222–227. https://doi.org/10.1037/adb0000830

Carlini, B. H., & Garrett, S. B. (2018). Drug helplines and adult marijuana users: An assessment in Washington, Colorado, Oregon, and Alaska. *Substance Abuse*, *39*(1), 3–5. https://doi.org/. 10.1080/08897077.2017.1355872

Centers for Disease Control and Prevention (CDC). (2022). *Prevention strategies.* https://www.cdc.gov/suicide/pdf/preventionresource.pdf

Centers for Disease Control and Prevention (CDC). (2024a). *U.S. overdose deaths decrease in 2023, first time since 2018*. National Center for Health Statistics. https://www.cdc.gov/nchs/pressroom/nchs_press_releases/2024/20240515.htm

Centers for Disease Control and Prevention (CDC). (2024b). *Deaths occurring through May 25, 2024 as of June 02, 2024*. https://wonder.cdc.gov/controller/datarequest/D176;jsessionid=74C7926CFF751439C6C4547EC784

Centers for Disease Control and Prevention (CDC). (2024c). *Suicide data and statistics*. https://www.cdc.gov/suicide/facts/data.html?CDC_AAref_Val=https://www.cdc.gov/suicide/suicide-data-statistics.html

Centers for Disease Control and Prevention (CDC). (2024d). *About alcohol use during pregnancy*. https://www.cdc.gov/alcohol-pregnancy/about/index.html#:~:text=Alcohol%20use%20during%20pregnancy%20is,alcohol%20spectrum%20disorders%20(FASDs)

Chan, M., Jiang, Y., Lee, C. Y. C., Ramachandran, H. J., Teo, J. Y. C., Seah, C. W. A., Lin, Y., & Wang, W. (2022). Effectiveness of eHealth-based cognitive behavioural therapy on depression: A systematic review and meta-analysis. *Journal of Clinical Nursing, 31*(21–22), 3021–3031. https://doi.org/10.1111/jocn.16212

Congress.gov. (2018). *H.R.6—SUPPORT for patients and communities act 115th congress (2017–2018)*. https://www.congress.gov/bill/115th-congress/house-bill/6

Consult QD. (2017, October 16). *Nurses step up to fight opioid crisis*. Cleveland Clinic. https://consultqd.clevelandclinic.org/nurses-step-up-to-fight-opioid-crisis/

Consumer Notice.org. (2023). *Juul lawsuits & settlements*. https://www.consumernotice.org/legal/juul-lawsuits/

Corrigan, P. W., & Nieweglowski, K. (2018). Stigma and the public health agenda for the opioid crisis in America. *International Journal of Drug Policy, 59*, 44–49. https://doi.org/10.1016/j.drugpo.2018.06.015

Dane, W., Fahel, D., & Tiffany Epley, T. (2018). *The solution to opioids is treatment*. Brain Injury Association of America. https://www.biausa.org/public-affairs/media/the-solution-to-opioids-is-treatment

Dion, K., & Griggs, S. (2020). Teaching those who care how to care for a person with substance use disorder. *Nurse Educator, 45*(6), 321–325. https://doi.org/10.1097/NNE.0000000000000808

Dowdell, E. B. (2023). *Overview and summary: Gun violence from a public health perspective*. https://ojin.nursingworld.org/table-of-contents/volume-28-2023/number-3-september-2023/overview-and-summary/

Ebersole, J., Samburova, V., Son, Y., Cappelli, D., Demopoulos, C., Capurro, A., Pinto, A., Chrzan, B., Kingsley, K., Howard, K., Clark, N., & Khlystov, A. (2020). Harmful chemicals emitted from electronic cigarettes and potential deleterious effects in the oral cavity. *Tobacco Induced Diseases, 18*, 41. https://doi.org/10.18332/tid/116988. PMID: 32435175; PMCID: PMC7233525.

Elansary, M., Kistin, C. J., Antonio, J., Fernández-Pastrana, I., Lee-Parritz, A., Cabral, H., Miller, E. S., & Silverstein, M. (2023). Effect of immediate referral vs a brief problem-solving intervention for screen-detected peripartum depression: A randomized clinical trial. *JAMA Network Open, 6*(5), e2313151. https://doi:10.1001/jamanetworkopen.2023.13151

European Monitoring Centre for Drugs and Drug Addiction (EMCDDA). (2024). *European drug report 2024: Trends and developments*. https://www.emcdda.europa.eu/publications/european-drug-report/2024_en

Fuller-Tyszkiewicz, M., Richardson, B., Klein, B., Skouteris, H., Christensen, H., Austin, D., Castle, D., Mihalopoulos, C., O'Donnell, R., Arulkadacham, L., Shatte, A., & Ware, A. (2018). A mobile app–based intervention for depression: End-user and expert usability testing study. *JMIR Mental Health, 5*(3), e54. https://www.ncbi.nlm.nih.gov/pmc/articles/PMC6127496/

Gaylor, E. M., Krause, K. H., Welder, L. E., Cooper, A. C., Ashley, C., Mack, K. A., Crosby, A. E., Trinh, E., Ivey-Stephenson, A. Z., & Whittle, L. (2023). Suicidal thoughts and behaviors among high school students—Youth Risk Behavior Survey, United States, 2021. *Morbidity and Mortality Weekly Report Supplements, 72*(1), 45–54. https://doi.org/10.15585/mmwr.su7201a6. PMID: 37104546; PMCID: PMC10156155.

Gordon Jr., R. S. (1983). An operational classification of disease prevention. *Public Health Reports, 98*(2), 107. https://www.ncbi.nlm.nih.gov/pmc/articles/PMC1424415/

Hansen, C., Horus, A., & Davis Jr., E. (2023). *Where is marijuana legal? US news: A guide to marijuana legalization*. https://www.usnews.com/news/best-states/articles/where-is-marijuana-legal-a-guide-to-marijuana-legalization

Insel, T. (2023). *America's mental health crisis*. https://www.pewtrusts.org/en/trend/archive/fall-2023/americas-mental-health-crisis

Institute of Health Metrics and Evaluation. (2023). *Smoking and tobacco 2023*. https://www.healthdata.org/research-analysis/health-risks-issues/smoking-and-tobacco#:~:text=155%20million%20global%20smokers%20in,to%20smoked%20tobacco%20use%20globally

Jeste, D. V., & Pender, V. B. (2022). Social determinants of mental health: Recommendations for research, training, practice, and policy. *JAMA Psychiatry, 79*(4), 283–284. https://doi.org/10.1001/jamapsychiatry.2021.4385

Levengood, T. W., Yoon, G. H., Davoust, M. J., Ogden, S. N., Marshall, B. D. L., Cahill, S. R., & Bazzi, A. R. (2021). Supervised injection facilities as harm reduction: A systematic review. *American Journal of Preventive Medicine, 61*(5), 738–749. https://doi.org/10.1016/j.amepre.2021.04.017

Lindley, B., Cox, N., & Cochran, G. (2019). Screening tools for detecting problematic opioid use and potential application to community pharmacy practice: A review. *Integrated Pharmacy Research and Practice, 8*, 85–96. https://www.tandfonline.com/doi/pdf/10.2147/IPRP.S185663

National Center for Drug Abuse Statistics. (n.d.). *Marijuana addiction: Rates & usage statistics*. https://drugabusestatistics.org/marijuana-addiction/

National Center for Drug Abuse Statistics. (NCDAS). (2023). *Drug abuse statistics*. https://drugabusestatistics.org/

National Council for Community Behavioral Healthcare. (2009). *Behavioral health/primary care integration and the person-centered healthcare home*. https://www.thenationalcouncil.org/wp-content/uploads/2020/01/Behavioral-HealthandPrimaryCareIntegrationandthePCMH-2009.pdf?daf=375ateTbd56

National Institute on Drug Abuse (NIDA). (2024). *Drug overdose death rates*. https://nida.nih.gov/research-topics/trends-statistics/overdose-death-rates

National Institute on Drug Abuse (NIDA). (n.d.). *Marijuana research report series*. https://www.drugabuse.gov/drugs-abuse/marijuana

Office of Disease Prevention and Health Promotion (ODPHP). (n.d.-a). *Mental health and mental disorders*. https://health.gov/healthypeople/objectives-and-data/browse-objectives/mental-health-and-mental-disorders

Office of Disease Prevention and Health Promotion (ODPHP). (n.d.-b). *Healthy People 2023: Browse objectives*. https://health.gov/healthypeople/objectives-and-data/browse-objectives

Office of Disease Prevention and Health Promotion. (ODPHP). (n.d.-c.). *Suicide*. https://health.gov/healthypeople/search?query=suicide&f%5B0%5D=content_type%3Ahealthy_people_objective

Pallin, R., & Barnhorst, A. (2021). Clinical strategies for reducing firearm suicide. *Injury Epidemiology, 8*(1), 57. https://doi.org/10.1186/s40621-021-00352-8. PMID: 34607607; PMCID: PMC8489372.

Petzold, J., Pochon, J. B. F., Ghahremani, D. G., & London, E. D. (2024). Structural indices of brain aging in methamphetamine use disorder. *Drug and Alcohol Dependence, 256*, 111107. https://doi.org/10.1016/j.drugalcdep.2024.111107

Rajesh, A. M., & Pierson, B. (2023). Altria agrees to $235 million settlement to resolve Juul related cases. *Reuters*. https://www.reuters.com/legal/altria-reaches-agreement-resolve-juul-related-cases-2023-05-10/#:~:text=As%20of%20December%2C%20its%20share,and%20flashy%20social%20media%20campaigns

Ruch, D. A., Heck, K. M., Sheftall, A. H., Fontanella, C. A., Stevens, J., Zhu, M., Horowitz, L. M., Campo, J. V., & Bridge, J. A. (2021). Characteristics and precipitating circumstances of suicide among children aged 5 to 11 years in the United States, 2013-2017. *JAMA Network Open, 4*(7), e2115683. https://doi.org/10.1001/jamanetworkopen.2021.15683. PMID: 34313741; PMCID: PMC8317003.

Schauer, G. L., Dilley, J. A., Roehler, D. R., Sheehy, T. J., Filley, J. R., Broschart, S. C., Holland, K. M., Baldwin, G. T., Holmes-Chavez, A. K., & Hoots, B. E. (2021). Cannabis sales increases during COVID-19: Findings from Alaska, Colorado, Oregon, and Washington. *The International Journal on Drug Policy, 98*, 103384. https://doi.org/10.1016/j.drugpo.2021.103384

Siddiqui, H., & Rutherford, M. D. (2023). Belief that addiction is a discrete category is a stronger correlate with stigma than the belief that addiction is biologically based. *Substance Abuse Treatment, Prevention, Policy, 18*(3). https://doi.org/10.1186/s13011-022-00512-z

Strategic Prevention Technical Assistance Center. (n.d.). *The Institute of Medicine's continuum of care*. Substance Abuse and Mental Health Services Administration. https://www.samhsa.gov/sites/default/files/resourcefiles/sptac-continuum-of-care.pdf

Substance Abuse and Mental Health Services Administration (SAMHSA). (2023a). *Harm reduction*. https://www.samhsa.gov/find-help/harm-reduction

Substance Abuse and Mental Health Services Administration (SAMHSA). (2023b). *Key substance use and mental health indicators in the United States: Results from the 2022 National Survey on drug use and health* (HHS publication no PEP23-07-01-006, NSDUH series H-58). Center for Behavioral Health Statistics and Quality, Substance Abuse and Mental Health Services Administration. https://www.samhsa.gov/data/report/2022-nsduh-annual-national-report

Substance Abuse and Mental Health Services Administration (SAMHSA). (2023c). *Screening, brief intervention, and referral for treatment*. https://www.samhsa.gov/sbirt

Substance Abuse and Mental Health Services Administration (SAMHSA). (2023d). *Learn about marijuana risks*. https://www.samhsa.gov/marijuana

Substance Abuse and Mental Health Services Administration (SAMHSA). (2023e). *A guide to SAMHSA's strategic prevention framework*. https://www.samhsa.gov/sptac/strategic-prevention-framework

Swedo, E. A., D'Angelo, D. V., Fasula, A. M., Clayton, H. B., & Ports, K. A. (2023). Associations of adverse childhood experiences with pregnancy and infant health. *American Journal of Preventive Medicine, 64*(4), 512–524. https://doi:10.1016/j.amepre.2022.10.017

Thabrew, H., Stasiak, K., Hetrick, S. E., Wong, S., Huss, J. H., & Merry, S. N. (2018). E-health interventions for anxiety and depression in children and adolescents with long-term physical conditions. *Cochrane Database Systematic Reviews, 8*(8), CD012489. https://doi.org/10.1002/14651858.CD012489.pub2

U.S. Department of Agriculture (2020). *Dietary guidelines for Americans 2020–2025: Make every bite count with the dietary guidelines* (9th ed.). https://www.dietaryguidelines.gov/sites/default/files/2021-03/Dietary_Guidelines_for_Americans-2020-2025.pdf

U.S. Department of Health and Human Services (USDHHS). (2018). *Surgeon General's advisory on naloxone and opioid overdose*. https://www.surgeongeneral.gov/priorities/opioid-overdose-prevention/naloxone-advisory.html

U.S. Drug Enforcement Agency. (n.d.). *DEA reports widespread threat of fentanyl mixed with xylazine*. https://www.dea.gov/alert/dea-reports-widespread-threat-fentanyl-mixed-xylazine

U.S. Food & Drug Administration (FDA). (2023). *Results from the annual national youth tobacco survey*. https://www.fda.gov/tobacco-products/youth-and-tobacco/results-annual-national-youth-tobacco-survey

U.S. Forest Service. (n.d.). *Hallucinogens*. https://www.fs.usda.gov/wildflowers/ethnobotany/Mind_and_Spirit/hallucinogens.shtml

U.S. Preventive Services Task Force. (2021). *Tobacco smoking cessation in adults, including pregnant persons: Interventions*. https://www.uspreventiveservicestaskforce.org/uspstf/recommendation/tobacco-use-in-adults-and-pregnant-women-counseling-and-interventions

U.S. Surgeon General. (2023). *Know the risks*. https://e-cigarettes.surgeongeneral.gov/

United Nations of Drugs and Crime (UNODC). (2023). *Global report on cocaine 2023—Local dynamics, global challenges*. https://www.unodc.org/documents/data-and-analysis/cocaine/Global_cocaine_report_2023.pdf

Weiner, S. G., Lo, Y., Carroll, A., Zhou, L., Ngo, A., Hathaway, D., Rodriguez, C. P., & Wakeman, S. E. (2023). Then incidence and disparities in use of stigmatizing language in clinical notes for patients with substance use disorder. *Journal of Addiction Medicine, 17*(4), 424–430. https://doi.org/10.1097/ADM.0000000000001145

World Health Organization (WHO). (2018). *WHO launches SAFER alcohol control initiative to prevent and reduce alcohol-related death and disability*. https://www.who.int/substance_abuse/safer/launch/en/

World Health Organization (WHO). (2022b). *WHO digital mental health intervention effective in reducing depression among Syrian refugees in Lebanon*. https://www.who.int/news-room/feature-stories/detail/who-digital-mental-health-intervention-effective-in-reducing-depression-among-syrian-refugees-in-lebanon

World Health Organization (WHO). (2023). *Alcohol action plan 2022-2030*. https://cdn.who.int/media/docs/default-source/alcohol/final-text-of-aap-for-layout-and-design-april-2023.pdf?sfvrsn=6c5adb25_2

CHAPTER 26

American Association of Colleges of Nursing. (2021). *The Essentials: Core competencies for professional nursing education*. https://www.aacnnursing.org/Portals/42/AcademicNursing/pdf/Essentials-2021.pdf

Andrade, F. M. R., Simões Figueiredo, A., Capelas, M. L., Charepe, Z., & Deodato, S. (2020). Experiences of homeless families in parenthood: A systematic review and synthesis of qualitative evidence. *International Journal of Environmental Research and Public Health*, *17*(8), 2712.

Bekasi, S., Girasek, E., & Gyorffy, Z. (2022). Telemedicine in community shelters: Possibilities to improve chronic care among people experiencing homelessness in Hungary. *International Journal for Equity in Health*, *21*(181), 1–17. https://doi:10.1186/s12939-022-01803-4

Centers for Disease Control and Prevention. (2022). *Issue brief: The role of housing in ending the HIV epidemic*. https://www.cdc.gov/hiv/pdf/policies/data/cdc-hiv-issue-brief-housing.pdf

Children's Bureau: An Office of the Administration for Children & Families. (2023). *Highlights from the NYTD Survey: Outcomes reported by young people at ages 17, 19, and 21 (Cohort 3)*. https://www.acf.hhs.gov/cb/research-data-technology/reporting-systems/nytd

Creamer, J., Shrider, E., Burns, K., & Chen, F. (2022). *Poverty in the United States: 2021*. United States Census Bureau. Report Number P60-277. https://www.census.gov/library/publications/2022/demo/p60-277.html

Davis, J. C., Cromartie, J., Farrigan, T., Genetin, B., Sanders, A., & Winikoff, J. B. (2023). *Rural America at a Glance 2023 Edition*. (Report No. EIB-261). U.S. Department of Agriculture, Economic Research Service. https://www.ers.usda.gov/webdocs/publications/107838/eib-261.pdf?v=5081.9

Farrell, D. C., Kuerbis, A., Parulkar, A., Preda, M., Toledo-Liz, M., & Fuller, R. (2023). Reassessing measures of risk for homelessness among families with children in New York City. *Cities*, *137*, 104319. https://doi:10.1016/j.cities.2023.104319

GovInfo.gov. (n.d.). *McKinney-Vento homeless assistance act: Titles I–V, VII*. https://www.govinfo.gov/content/pkg/COMPS-10570/pdf/COMPS-10570.pdf

Green Doors. (n.d.). *Veteran homelessness facts*. https://www.greendoors.org/facts/veteran-homelessness.php

Gultekin, L., Brush, B., Ginier, E., Cordom, A., & Dowdell, E. (2020). Health risks and outcomes in school-age children and youth: A scoping review of the literature. *The Journal of School Nursing*, *36*(1), 10–18. https://doi:10.1177/1059840519875182

Gupta, P., Mohareb, A., Valdes, C., Price, C., Jollif, M., Regis, C., Munchi, N., Taborda, E., Lautenschlager, M., Fox, A., Hanscom, D., Kruse, G., LaRocque, R., Betancourt, J., & Taveras, E. (2022). Counseling, testing, and vaccination for medically underserved populations. *American Journal of Public Health*, *112*(11), 1556–1559. https://doi:10.2105/AJPH.2022.307021

Henderson, K., Manian, N., Rog, D. J., Robison, E., Jorge, E., & Al-Abdulmunem, M. (2023). *Addressing homeless among older adults: Final report*. Office of the Assistant Secretary for Planning and Evaluation (ASPE): U.S. Department of Health & Human Services. https://aspe.hhs.gov/sites/default/files/documents/9ac2d2a7e8c360b4e75932b96f59a20b/addressing-older-adult-homelessness.pdf

Herring, C. (2015). *Tent City, America*. https://placesjournal.org/article/tent-city-america/?gclid=EAIaIQobChMIzqmD9YOi_AIViv_ICh2_cAsuEAAYASAAEgIjDPD_BwE#0

Housing Assistance Council (HAC). (2022). *HAC's 2023 Rural housing policy priorities*. https://ruralhome.org/hacs-2023-rural-housing-policy-priorities/

Institute for Children, Poverty & Homelessness. (2024). *The McKinney-Vento Homeless Assistance Act*. https://www.icphusa.org/mkv/

Kesselman, L. (2021). Lock it or list it: Limiting landlord risk through the adoption of a uniform lock change law for domestic violence victims. *William & Mary Business Law Review*, *12*, 763. https://scholarship.law.wm.edu/wmblr/vol12/iss3/5

Kushel, M., Moore, T., Birkmeyer, J., Dhatt, Z., Duke, M., Knight, K. R., & Ponder, K. Y. (2023). *Toward a New Understanding: The California statewide study of people experiencing homelessness* UCSF Benioff homelessness and housing initiative. https://homelessness.ucsf.edu/sites/default/files/2023-06/CASPEH_Report_62023.pdf

Lashley, M. (2020). Economic impact of faith-based addiction recovery for the homeless. *Public Health Nursing*, *37*(5), 722–728.

Lassiter, K. (2021). *Bring America home act & economic justice in the 2021*. National Coalition for the Homeless. https://nationalhomeless.org/economic-justice-2021/

Leopold, J. (2019). *Five ways the HEARTH Act changed homelessness assistance*. Urban Institute. https://www.urban.org/urban-wire/five-ways-hearth-act-changed-homelessness

Liu, M., Luong, L., Lachaud, J., Edalati, H., Reeves, A., & Hwang, S. W. (2021). Adverse childhood experiences and related outcomes among adults experiencing homelessness: a systematic review and meta-analysis. *Lancet Public Health*., *6*(11), e836–e847. https://doi:10.1016/S2468-2667(21)00189-4. Epub 2021 Sep 30 PMID:-34599894.

McKinney-Vento Homeless Assistance Act. (1987). *U. S. Congress, Public Law 100-77*. http://www.gpo.gov/fdsys/pkg/STATUTE-101/pdf/STATUTE-101-Pg482.pdf

Mermin, J. (2023). *HIV outbreak among people experiencing homelessness*. National Center for HIV, Viral Hepatitis, STD, and TB Prevention. Centers for Disease Control Prevention. https://www.hud.gov/sites/dfiles/CPD/documents/HOPWA-Listserv-Joint-CDC-HUD-HRSA-HIV-Outbreak-Letter.pdf

Mosites, E., Harrison, B., Montgomery, M., Meehan, A., Leopold, J., Barranco, L., Schwerz, L., Carmichael, A., Clarke, K., & Butler, J. (2022). Public health lessons learned in responding to COVID-19 among people experiencing homelessness in the United States. *Public Health Reports*, *137*(4), 625–629. https://doi:10.1177/00333549221083643

Murran, S., & Brady, E. (2022). How does family homelessness impact on children's development? A critical review of the literature. Child & family. *Social Work*, *28*(2). https://doi:10.1111/cfs.12968

Myrick, D. (2016). *Why are there more homeless men than women?* https://www.culturalweekly.com/homeless-men-women/

National Alliance to End Homelessness. (2022a). *Domestic violence*. https://endhomelessness.org/homelessness-in-america/what-causes-homelessness/domestic-violence

National Alliance to End Homelessness. (2022b). *Health*. https://endhomelessness.org/homelessness-in-america/what-causes-homelessness/health

National Alliance to End Homelessness. (2022c). *Older adults*. https://endhomelessness.org/homelessness-in-america/who-experiences-homelessness/older-adults/?gclid=EAIaIQobChMIwMPNzbSa_AIVEJXICh2LKw61EAAYAiAAEgL-zAfD_BwE

National Alliance to End Homelessness. (2022d). *Housing first*. https://endhomelessness.org/resource/housing-first/

National Alliance to End Homelessness. (2022e). *Policy priorities*. https:endhomelessness.org/ending-homelessness/policy/priorities

National Alliance to End Homelessness. (2023). *Children and families*. https://endhomelessness.org/homelessness-in-america/who-experiences-homelessness/children-and-families/

National Center for Homeless Education. (n.d.) *The McKinney-Vento definition of homeless*. https://www.cde.ca.gov/sp/hs/homelessdef.asp#:~:text=The%20McKinney%2DVento%20Act%20defines,hardship%2C%20or%20a%20similar%20reason

National Coalition for the Homeless. (2022a). *Understanding LGBT homelessness*. http://www.nationalhomeless.org/issues/lgbt

National Coalition for the Homeless. (2022b). *Healthcare and homelessness*. https://nationalhomeless.org/issues/health-care/

National Coalition for the Homeless. (n.d.). *Homelessness in the US*. https://nationalhomeless.org/about-homelessness/

National Conference of State Legislators. (2022). *Child support and incarceration*. http://www.ncsl.org/research/human-services/child-support-and-incarceration.aspx

National Conference of State Legislators. (2023). *Youth homelessness overview*. https://www.ncsl.org/human-services/youth-homelessness-overview

National Healthcare for the Homeless Council. (2022). *FAQ*. https://nhchc.org/faq

National Housing Law Project. (n.d.). *Know your rights: Protect your safety by having your locks changed*. California Civil Code Sections 1941.5 and 1941.6. https://nhlp.org/files/CA-Lock-Changes-Packet-Advocates-and-Survivors.pdf

National Institute for Mental Health. (2021). *Substance use and co-occurring mental disorders*. https://www.nimh.nih.gov/health/topics/substance-use-and-mental-health

National Institute for Mental Health. (n.d.). *What is prevalence*. https://www.nimh.nih.gov/health/statistics/what-is-prevalence#:~:text=Prevalence%20is%20the%20proportion%20of,in%20a%20given%20time%20period

National Law Center on Homelessness and Poverty. (2017). *Tent City USA: The growth of America's homeless encampments and how communities are responding*. https://homelesslaw.org/wp-content/uploads/2018/10/Tent_City_USA_2017.pdf

National Low Income Housing Coalition. (2022a). *A shortage of affordable homes*. nlihc.org/gap

National Low Income Housing Coalition. (2022b). *Out of reach: The high cost of housing*. https://nlihc.org/oor

Office of Disease Prevention and Health Promotion (ODPHP). (n.d.). *Healthy People 2030: Objectives and data*. https://health.gov/healthypeople/objectives-and-data

Orsi-Hunt, R., Clemens, E. V., Thibodeau, H., & Belcher, C. (2024). Young adults with lived foster care experience who later experience houselessness: An exploratory latent class analysis. *International Journal on Child Maltreatment*, *7*, 35–59. https://doi:10.1007/s42448-023-00160-1

Padgett D. (2020). Homelessness, housing instability and mental health: Making the connections. *British Journal Psychiatric Bulletin*, *44*(5), 197–201. doi:10.1192/bjb.2020.49. PMID:32538335; PMCID:PMC7525583.

Ramirez, J., Petruzzi, L., Mercer, T., Gulbas, L., Sebastian, K., & Jacobs, E. (2022). Understanding the primary health care experiences of individuals who are homeless in non-traditional clinic settings. *BMC Primary Care*, *2*(338), 1–8. https://doi:10.1186/s12875-022-01932-3

Rizzo, D., Mu, T., Cotroneo, S., & Aronogiri, S. (2022). Barriers to accessing addiction treatment for women at risk of homelessness. *Frontiers in Global Women's Health*, *3*(795532), 1–10. https://doi:10.3389/fgwh2022.795532

Saldua, M. (2023). *Addressing social determinants of health among individuals experiencing homelessness*. Center for Behavioral Health Statistics and Quality. Substance Abuse and Mental Health Services Administration.

Saude, J., Baker, L., Axman, L., & Swider, S. (2020). Applying the chronic care model to improve patient activation at a nurse-managed student-run free clinic for medically underserved people. *SAGE Open Nursing*, 6, 1–6. https://doi.org/10.1177.2377960820902612

Savransky, B. (2021, May 21). *A lot of homeless people referred to shelters in Seattle don't go. These are some reasons why*. SeattlePI. https://www.seattlepi.com/homeless_in_seattle/article/A-lot-of-homeless-people-the-city-refers-to-14504490.php

Social Security Administration. (2024). *Spotlight on homelessness: 2024 edition*. https://www.ssa.gov/ssi/spotlights/spot-homeless.htm

Soucy, D., Janes, M., & Hall, A. (2024). *State of homelessness: 2024 edition* NAEH. https://endhomelessness.org/homelessness-in-america/homelessness-statistics/state-of-homelessness/

Substance Abuse and Mental Health Services Administration. (2022b). Center for Mental Health Services. https://www.samhsa.gov/about-us/who-we-are/offices-centers/cmhs

Substance Abuse and Mental Health Services Administration. (2022c). *Homeless and Housing Resource Center*. https://www.samhsa.gov/homeless-housing-resource-center

Substance Abuse and Mental Health Services Administration. (2022d). *Projects for Assistance in Transition from Homelessness (PATH)*. https://www.samhsa.gov/homelessness-programs-resources/grant-programs-services/path

Substance Abuse and Mental Health Services Administration (SAMHSA). (2014). *SAMHSA's concept of trauma and guidance for a trauma-informed approach*. HHS Publication

No. (SMA) 14-4884. https://store.samhsa.gov/sites/default/files/d7/priv/sma14-4884.pdf

Thompson, R., Aivadyan, C., Stohl, M., Aharonovich, E., & Hasin, D. (2020). Smartphone application plus brief motivational intervention reduces substance use and sexual risk behaviors among homeless young adults: Results from a randomized control trial. *Psychology of Addictive Behaviors, 34*(6), 641–649. https://doi:10.1037/adb0000570

Thorndike, A. L., Yetman, H. E., Thorndike, A. N., Jeffreys, M., & Rowe, M. (2022). Unmet health needs and barriers to health care among people experiencing homelessness in San Francisco's Mission District: a qualitative study. *BMC Public Health, 22*, 1071. https://doi:10.1186/s12889-022-13499-w

Tolbert, J., Drake, P., & Damico, A. (2022). *Key facts about the uninsured population.* Kaiser Foundation. https://www.kff.org/uninsured/issue-brief/key-facts-about-the-uninsured-population/

U.S. Department of Housing and Urban Development (USDHUD). (2024). *Community development block grant program.* https://www.hud.gov/program_offices/comm_planning/cdbg

United States 117th Congress. (2021–2022). *H.R. 603 – Raise the Wage Act of 2021.* https://www.congress.gov/bill/117th-congress/house-bill/603/text

United States Department of Education. (2018). *Education for homeless children and youth program: Non-regulatory guidance.* https://oese.ed.gov/files/2020/07/160240ehcyguidanceupdated082718.pdf

United States Department of Health and Human Services. (2024). *Head Start. -children-families-experiencing-homelessness*

United States Department of Health and Human Services. (n.d.). About the affordable care act. https://www.hhs.gov/healthcare/about-the-aca/index.html

United States Department of Housing and Urban Development. (2020). *Exploring homelessness among people living in encampments and associated cost: City approaches to encampments and what they cost.* https://www.huduser.gov/portal/sites/default/files/pdf/Exploring-Homelessness-Among-People.pdf

United States Department of Housing and Urban Development. (2022a). *The 2022 annual homelessness assessment report (AHAR) to Congress. Part 1: Point in time estimates of homelessness.* https://www.huduser.gov/portal/sites/default/files/pdf/2022-AHAR-Part-1.pdf

United States Department of Housing and Urban Development. (2022b). *The 2019-2020 annual homelessness assessment report (AHAR) to Congress. Part II: Estimates of homelessness in the United States.* https://www.huduser.gov/portal/sites/default/files/pdf/2020-AHAR-Part-2.pdf

United States Department of Housing and Urban Development. (2022c). *Homeless assistance programs.* HUD Exchange. https://www.hudexchange.info/homelessness-assistance/

United States Department of Housing and Urban Development. (2022d). *House America.* https://www.hud.gov/house_america

United States Department of Housing and Urban Development. (n.d.). *Housing choice vouchers fact sheet.* https://www.hud.gov/topics/housing_choice_voucher_program_section_8

United States Department of Veteran Affairs. (n.d.). *Strategic plan 2021-2025, Winter 2022 update.* https://www.va.gov/HOMELESS/VHA-Strategic-Plan-External-April-2022-Final.pdf

United States Interagency Council on Homelessness. (2015). *Opening doors: Federal strategic plan to prevent and end homelessness.* https://www.usich.gov/resources/uploads/asset_library/USICH_OpeningDoors_Amendment2015_FINAL.pdf

United States Interagency Council on Homelessness. (2021). *Making the most of the American Rescue Plan: A guide to the funding that impacts people experiencing homelessness.* https://www.usich.gov/resources/uploads/asset_library/USICH_American_Rescue_Plan_Guide.pdf

United States Interagency Council on Homelessness. (2022). *All in: The federal strategic plan to prevent and end homelessness.* https://www.usich.gov/All_In_The_Federal_Strategic_Plan_to_Prevent_and_End_Homelessness.pdf

Winiarski, D., Rufa, A., Bounds, D., Glover, A., Hill, K., & Karnik, N. (2020). Assessing and treating complex mental health needs among homeless youth in a shelter-based clinic. *BMC Health Services Research, 20*(109), 1–10. https://doi:10.1186/s12913-020-4953-9

Yakubovich, A., Bartsch, A., Metheny, N., Gesink, D., & O'Campo, P. (2022). Housing interventions for women experiencing intimate partner violence: A systematic review. *Lancet Public Health, 7*, e23–e35. https://doi:10.1016/52468-2667(21)00234-6

Youth.gov. (n.d.). *Homelessness and housing instability.* https://youth.gov/youth-topics/homelessness-and-housing-instability#:~:text=The%20number%20of%20youth%20who,experience%20homelessness%20within%20the%20United

Yusuf, H., Golkari, A., & Kaddour, S. (2023). Oral health of people experiencing homelessness in London: A mixed methods study. *BMC Public Health, 23*, 1701. https://link.springer.com/content/pdf/10.1186/s12889-023-16648-x.pdf

Zhao, E. (2022). The key factors contributing to the persistence of homelessness. *International Journal of Sustainable Development & World Ecology, 30*(1), 1–5. https://doi:10.1080/13504509.2022.2120109

CHAPTER 27

Adekug, A. P., & Ibeh, C. V. (2024). Optimizing dental health equity: Integrating business analytics and program management for underserved populations in the U.S. *International Journal of Frontiers in Life Science. Research, 6*(02), 11–20. https://doi.org/10.53294/ijflsr.2024.6.2.0031

Ahmad, M.F., Ahmad, F.A., Alsayegh, A.A., Zeyaullah, M., AlShahrani, A.M., Muzammil, K., Saati, A.A., Wahab, S., Elbendary, E.Y., Kambal, N., Abdelrahman, M.H., & Hussain, S. (2024). Pesticides impacts on human health and the environment with their mechanisms of action and possible countermeasures. *Heliyon, 10*(7), e29128. https://doi.org/10.1016/j.heliyon.2024.e29128

American Association for the History of Nursing. (2018). *Mary Breckenridge.* https://www.aahn.org/breckinridge

Association for American Medical Colleges (AAMC). (2023). *How academic medicine serves rural communities across the country.* https://www.aamc.org/media/69371/download?attachment

American Immigration Council. (n.d.). *Violence Against Women Act (VAWA) provides protections for noncitizen women and victims of crime.* https://www.americanimmigrationcouncil.org/sites/default/files/research/violence_against_women_act_provides_protections_for_noncitizen_women_and_victims_of_crime.pdf

American Public Health Association (APHA). (2020). *Creating the healthiest nation: Health and housing equity.* https://www.apha.org/-/media/Files/PDF/topics/equity/Health_and_Housing_Equity.pdf

American Public Health Association (APHA). (n.d.). *What is public health?* https://www.apha.org/what-is-public-health

Anderson, J. H. (2020). *Classification of urban, suburban, and rural areas in the national crime victimization survey.* Bureau of Statistics. https://bjs.ojp.gov/content/pub/pdf/cusrancvs.pdf

Arellano, G. (2018). *When the U.S. government tried to replace migrant farmworkers with high schoolers.* National Public Radio. https://www.npr.org/sections/thesalt/2018/07/31/634442195/when-the-u-s-government-tried-to-replace-migrant-farmworkers-with-high-schoolers

Biography. (2019). *Cesar Chavez.* https://www.biography.com/people/cesar-chavez-9245781

Briscoe, K. (2024). *Detroit is back: The rise, fall, and rise of Motor City.* Lynnwood Times. https://lynnwoodtimes.com/2024/04/03/detroit-240403/

Businessinsider.com. (2023). *Business insider.* http://www.businessinsider.com/jackson-mississippi-new-orleans-shrinking -cities-population-decline-2023-8

Caldwell, D. R. (2007). Bloodroot: Life stories of nurse practitioners in rural Appalachia. *Journal of Holistic Nursing, 25*(2), 73–79. https://doi:10.1177/0898010106293610

California Department of Pesticide Regulation. (n.d.). *Pesticide illness surveillance program.* http://www.cdpr.ca.gov/docs/whs/pisp.htm

Carnevale, A. P., Kam, L., & Van Der Werf, M. (2024). *Small towns, big opportunities: Many workers in rural areas have good jobs, but these areas need greater investment in education, training, and career counseling.* Georgetown University Center on Education and the Workforce. https://cew.georgetown.edu/wp-content/uploads/cew-small_towns_big_opportunity-full_report.pdf

Castillo, F., Mora, A. M., Kayser, G. L., Vanos, J., Hyland, C., Yang, A. R., & Eskenazi, B. (2021). Environmental health threats to Latino migrant farmworkers. *Annual Review of Public Health, 42*, 257–276.

CDC/National Institute for Occupational Safety & Health. (2024). *Pesticide illness and injury surveillance.* https://www.cdc.gov/niosh/surveillance/pesticide/?CDC_AAref_Val=https://www.cdc.gov/niosh/topics/pesticides/

Center for Disease Control and Prevention (CDC). (2024a). *Leading causes of death in rural America as a public health issue.* https://www.cdc.gov/rural-health/php/public-health-strategy/public-health-considerations-for-leading-causes-of-death-in-rural-america.html

Center for Disease Control and Prevention (CDC). (2024b). *Heart disease facts.* https://www.cdc.gov/heart-disease/data-research/facts-stats/index.html

Center for Disease Control and Prevention (CDC). (2024c). *Extreme heat and your health.* https://www.cdc.gov/extreme-heat/about/index.html

Center for Disease Control and Prevention/National Center for Health Statistics. (2022). *Heart disease mortality by state.* https://www.cdc.gov/nchs/pressroom/sosmap/heart_disease_mortality/heart_disease.htm

Center for Migration Studies (CMS). (2022). *A profile of undocumented agricultural workers in the United States.* https://cmsny.org/agricultural-workers-rosenbloom-083022/

Center for Sustainable Systems, University of Michigan. (2023). *U.S. cities factsheet. Pub. No. CSS09-06.* https://css.umich.edu/publications/factsheets/built-environment/us-cities-factsheet

Chadde, C., & Hettinger, J. (2022). *Spotty regulations leave migrant farmworkers living in poor conditions across the Midwest.* USA Today. https://www.usatoday.com/story/news/investigations/2022/12/28/migrant-farm-workers-face-poor-housing-conditions-lack-regulations/10955474002/

Chapman, M. (2023). *Housing for: Renters. National League of Cities. NLC 100 years.* https://www.nlc.org/article/2023/09/12/housing-for-renters/

Cheney, A. M., Barrera, T., Rodriguez, K., & Jaramillo López, A. M. (2022). The intersection of workplace and environmental exposure on health in Latinx farm working communities in rural inland southern California. *International Journal of Environmental Research and Public Health, 19*(19), 12940. https://doi.org/10.3390/ijerph191912940. PMID: 36232240; PMCID: PMC9566176.

Curl, C. L., Spival, M., Phinney, R., & Montrose, L. (2020). *Synthetic pesticides and health in vulnerable populations: Agricultural workers. Current Environmental Health Reports*, 7(1), 13–29. https://doi.org/10.1007./s40572-020-00266-5

Daly, C. S. (2023). *Days before new Florida law takes effect, undocumented workers fear for their future.* https://www.miamiherald.com/news/local/immigration/article275925506.html#storylink=cpy

Davis, J. C., Cromartie, J., Farrigan, T., Genetin, B., Sanders, A., & Winikoff, J. B. (2023). *Rural America at a glance 2023 edition.* U.S. Department of Agriculture, Economic Research Service (Report No. EIB-261). https://www.ers.usda.gov/webdocs/publications/107838/eib-261.pdf?v=3349.1

de-Assis, M. P., Barcella, R. C., Padilha, J. C., Pohl, H. H., & Krug, S. B. F. (2021). Health problems in agricultural workers occupationally exposed to pesticides. *Revista Brasileira de Medicina do Trabalho, 18*(3), 352–363. https://doi.org/10.47626/1679-4435-2020-532

Dobis, E. A., Krumel, T. P., Cromartie, J., Conley, K. L., Sanders, A., & Ortiz, R. (2021). *Rural America at a glance.* Economic Research Service. https://www.ers.usda.gov/webdocs/publications/102576/eib-230.pdf

Egan, L., Gardner, L. A., Newton, N., & Champion, K. (2024). A systematic review of eHealth interventions among adolescents of low socioeconomic and geographically remote backgrounds in preventing poor diet, alcohol use, tobacco smoking and vaping. *Adolescent Research Review, 9*, 1–32. https://doi.org/10.1007/s40894-023-00210-2

Federal Emergency Management Agency. (FEMA). (n.d.). *The national risk index.* https://hazards.fema.gov/nri/

Florida Department of Health. (2023). *Migrant farmworker housing: Basic guidelines.* https://www.floridahealth.gov/environmental-health/migrant-farmworker-housing/migrant-farm-workers-guidelines.html

Fried, C. (2024). *Historical case for immigrants sending home more than money.* UCLA Anderson Review. https://

anderson-review.ucla.edu/historical-case-for-immigrants-sending-home-more-than-money/

Governors Highway Safety Association. (2022). *America's rural roads: Beautiful and deadly*. https://www.ghsa.org/sites/default/files/2022-09/America%E2%80%99s%20Rural%20Roads%20-%20Beautiful%20and%20Deadly%20FNL.pdf

Head Start. (2022). *Migrant and seasonal head start collaboration office*. https://eclkc.ohs.acf.hhs.gov/state-collaboration/article/migrant-seasonal-head-start-collaboration-office

Indiana Department of Health. (2024). *Drug overdose deaths in rural and urban Indiana counties (2019-2022)*. https://www.in.gov/health/overdose-prevention/files/72_SUDORS-in-Rural-and-Urban-Counties-2024.pdf

JBS International. (2022). *Findings from the National Agricultural Workers Survey (NAWS) 2019-2020: A demographic and employment profile of United States Farmworkers. Research Report 16*. https://www.dol.gov/sites/dolgov/files/ETA/publications/ETAOP2022-16_NAWS_Research_Report_16_508c.pdf

Johns Hopkins Urban Health Institute. (n.d.). *"About Us"*. https://urbanhealth.jhu.edu/about-us

Johnson, K., & Lichter, D. (2022). *Growing racial diversity in rural America: Results from the 2020 census*. University of New Hampshire. https://carsey.unh.edu/publication/growing-racial-diversity-rural-america-results-2020-census

Joint Center for Housing Studies of Harvard University. (2024). *The state of the nation's housing*. https://www.jchs.harvard.edu/sites/default/files/reports/files/Harvard_JCHS_The_State_of_the_Nations_Housing_2024.pdf

Katz, K. D. (2023). Organophosphate toxicity clinical presentation. *Medscape*. https://emedicine.medscape.com/article/167726-clinical?form=fp.

Keisler-Starkey, K., Bunch, L. N., & Lindstrom, R. A. (2023). *Health insurance coverage in the United States: 2022*. Census Bureau. https://www.census.gov/library/publications/2023/demo/p60-281.html#:~:text=More%20people%20were%20insured%20in,91.7%20percent%20or%20300.9%20million

Keizer, K., Lindenberg, S., & Steg, L. (2008). The spreading of disorder. *Science*, *322*(5908), 1681–1685.

Knudsen, A., & Meit, M. (n.d.). *Public health nursing: Strengthening the core of rural public health (Policy Brief)*. National Rural Health Association.

Kruse-Diehr, A. J., Lee, M. J., Shackelford, J., & Hangadoumbo, F. S. (2021). The State of Research on faith community nursing in public health interventions: Results from a systematic review. *Journal of Religion and Health*, *60*, 1339–1374. https://doi.org/10.1007/s10943-020-01168-4

Leys, T. (2023). *Millions of rural Americans rely on private wells. Few regularly test the water*. Health News Florida. https://health.wusf.usf.edu/health-news-florida/2023-10-24/millions-of-rural-americans-rely-on-private-wells-few-regularly-test-the-water

Li, Y., & Whitacre, B. E. (2022). Economic growth and adult obesity rates in rural America. *Review of Regional Studies*, *52*(3), 387–410. https://doi.org/10.52324/001c.66201

Los Angeles Unified School District. (n.d.). *Migrant education program*. https://www.lausd.org/domain/1454

Matias, S. L., French, C. D., Gomez-Lara, A., & Schenker, M. B. (2022). Chronic disease burden among Latino farmworkers in California. *Front Public Health*, *10*, 1024083. https://doi:10.3389/fpubh.2022.1024083.

Migrant Clinicians Network (MCN). (n.d.). *Migrant health issues: Health care access*. https://www.migrantclinician.org/explore-migration/migrant-health-issues.html#:~:text=Migrants%20struggle%20with%20similar%20challenges,privately%20funded%20health%20care%20programs

Migrant Clinicians Network (MCN). (2024a). *Tuberculosis*. https://www.migrantclinician.org/explore-issues-migrant-health/tuberculosis.html

Migrant Clinicians Network (MCN). (2024b). *Children's health*. https://www.migrantclinician.org/explore-issues-migrant-health/childrens-health.html

Migrant Clinicians Network (MCN). (2024c). *Intimate partner violence*. https://www.migrantclinician.org/explore-issues-migrant-health/intimate-partner-violence.html

Migrant Policy Institute. (2020). *Agricultural workers and COVID-19: Unique vulnerabilities and unprecedented partnerships to address them*. https://www.migrantclinician.org/streamline/agricultural-workers-and-covid-19-unique-vulnerabilities-and-unprecedented-partnerships

Murphy, D. (2022). *Rollover protection for farm tractor operators*. PennState Extension. https://extension.psu.edu/rollover-protection-for-farm-tractor-operators

Nardocci, A. C., Thiago Nogueira, T., de Almeida Piai, K., Araújo Cavendish, T., & Kumar, P. (2023). Indoor environment exposure and children's health. *Current Opinion in Environmental Science & Health*, *32*, 100449. https://doi.org/10.1016/j.coesh.100449

National Cancer Institute (NCI). (n.d.). *Rural-urban disparities in cancer*. GIS portal for cancer research. https://gis.cancer.gov/mapstory/rural-urban/index.html

National Center for Farmworker Health (NCFH). (n.d.). *A guide for safe and adequate housing for agricultural workers*. https://www.ncfh.org/uploads/3/8/6/8/38685499/a_guide_for_safe_and_adequate_housing_for_ag_workers-final.pdf

National Center for Farmworker Health (NCFH). (2022a). *Facts about agricultural workers*. https://www.ncfh.org/facts-about-agricultural-workers-fact-sheet.html

National Center for Farmworker Health (NCFH). (2022b). *A profile of migrant health 2020*. Analysis of HRSA Health Center Data. https://www.ncfh.org/uploads/3/8/6/8/38685499/uds_report_2022.pdf

National Center for Farmworker Health (NCFH). (2023a). *Agricultural workers factsheet*. http://www.ncfh.org/fact-sheets--research.html

National Center for Farmworker Health (NCFH). (2023b). *Tuberculosis factsheet*. http://www.ncfh.org/tuberculosis-fact-sheet.html

National Center for Farmworker Health (NCFH). (2023c). *HIV/AIDS & U.S. agricultural workers*. https://www.ncfh.org/hiv-fact-sheet.html

National Center for Frontier Communities. (2020). *2000 Update: Frontier counties in the United States*. https://frontierus.org/wp-content/uploads/2019/10/Frontier-Counties-2000update.pdf

National Center for Health Statistics. (n.d.). *NCHS urban-rural classification scheme for counties*. https://www.cdc.gov/nchs/data_access/urban_rural.htm

National Institute on Minority Health and Health Disparities (NIMHHD). (2024). *Community-based participatory research program (CBPR)*. https://www.nimhd.nih.gov/programs/extramural/community-based-participatory.html

New York Academy of Medicine. (2020). *Institute for urban health*. https://www.nyam.org/journal-urban-health/

Nguyen, Q. C., Khanna, S., Dwivedi, P., Huang, D., Huang, Y., Tasdizen, T., Brunisholz, K. D., Li, F., Gorman, W., Nguyen, T., & Jiang, C. (2019). Using Google Street View to examine associations between built environment characteristics and US health outcomes. *Preventive medicine reports*, *14*, 100859.

Novoselov, A. (2022). *These pesticides may increase cancer risk in children*. University of California Los Angeles (UCLA). https://www.universityofcalifornia.edu/news/these-pesticides-may-increase-cancer-risk-children

Occupational Safety and Health Administration (OSHA). (n.d.). *Occupational safety and health standards for agriculture*. https://www.osha.gov/laws-regs/regulations/standardnumber/1928/1928.110

Odahowski, C. L., Crouch, E. L., Zahnd, W. E., Probst, J. C., McKinney, S. H., & Abshire, D. A. (2021). Rural-urban differences in educational attainment among registered nurses: Implications for achieving an 80% BSN workforce. *Journal of Professional Nursing*, *37*(2), 404–410. https://doi.org/10.1016/j.profnurs.2020.04.008. PMID: 33867098; PMCID: PMC8056089.

Office of Disease Prevention and Health Promotion (ODPHP). (n.d.-a). *Health care access and quality*. Health People 2030. https://health.gov/healthypeople/objectives-and-data/browse-objectives/health-care-access-and-quality

Office of Disease Prevention and Health Promotion (ODPHP). (n.d.-b). *Healthy People 2030 framework*. https://health.gov/healthypeople/about/healthy-people-2030-framework

Office of Disease Prevention and Health Promotion (ODPHP). (n.d.-c). *Healthy People 2023. Browse objectives*. https://health.gov/healthypeople/objectives-and-data/browse-objectives

Okobi, O. E., Ajayi, O. O., Okobi, T. J., Anaya, I. C., Fasehun, O. O., Diala, C. S., Evbayekha, E. O., Ajibowo, A. O, Olateju, I. V., Ekabua, J. J., Nkongho, M. B., Amanze, I. O., Taiwo, A., Okorare, O., Ojinnaka, U. S., Ogbeifun, O. E., Chukwuma, N., Nebuwa, E. J., Omole, J. A., Udoete, I. O., & Okobi, R. K. (2021) *The burden of obesity in the rural adult population of America*. *Cureus*, *13*(6), e15770. https://doi.org/10.7759/cureus.15770. PMID: 34295580; PMCID: PMC8290986.

Open Anesthesia. (2020). *Organophosphate poisoning: Diagnosis and treatment*. https://www.openanesthesia.org/organophosphate_poisoning_diagnosis_and_treatment/

Ornelas, I. J., Yamanis, T. J., & Ruiz, R. A. (2020). The health of undocumented Latinx immigrants: What we know and future directions. *Annual Review of Public Health*, *41*, 289–308. https://doi.org/10.1146/annurev-publhealth-040119-094211. PMID: 32237989; PMCID: PMC9246400.

Pacific Northwest Agricultural Safety and Health Center. (n.d.). *Sexual harassment prevention*. https://deohs.washington.edu/pnash/sexual-harassment#:~:text=Recent%20studies%20estimate%20female%20farmworkers,workers%20and%20are%20seeking%20assistance

Patterson, D. G., Shipman, S. A., Pollack, S. W., Andrilla, C. H. A., Schmitz, D., Evans, D. V., Peterson, L. E., & Longenecker, R. (2024). Growing a rural family physician workforce: The contributions of rural background and rural place of residency training. *Health Services Research*, *59*(1), e14168. https://doi.org/10.1111/1475-6773.14168. PMID: 37161614; PMCID: PMC10771894.

Pender, J., Kuhns, M., Yu, C., Larson, J., & Huck, S. (2023). *Linkages between rural community capitals and health-care provision: A survey of small rural towns in three U.S. regions*. EIB-251, U.S. Department of Agriculture, Economic Research Service. https://ers.usda.gov/webdocs/publications/106139/eib-251.pdf?v=7960.3

Porru, S., & Baldo, M. (2022). Occupational health and safety and migrant workers: Has something changed in the last few years? *International Journal of Environment Research and Public Health*, *19*(15), 9535. https://doi.org/10.3390/ijerph19159535. PMID: 35954890; PMCID: PMC9367908.

Rahal, S. (2024). *Packard Plant to be fully torn down by year's end as city seeks new auto plant: Duggan*. The Detroit News. https://www.detroitnews.com/story/news/local/detroit-city/2024/03/04/demo-update-detroits-packard-plant-to-be-torn-down-by-end-of-year-mayor-duggan-new-auto-suppliers-mi/72834989007/

Realestate.usnews. (2023). *U.S. news*. http://www.realestate.usnews.com

Rivera, S. (2024). *$63 billion in remittances sent to Mexico, mostly from US in 2023*. Fox 5. https://fox5sandiego.com/news/border-report/63-billion-in-remittances-sent-to-mexico-mostly-from-us-in-2023/#:~:text=SAN%20DIEGO%20(Border%20Report)%20%E2%80%94,hike%20from%20the%20previous%20year

Rodríguez-Carrillo, A., D'Cruz, S. C., Mustieles, V., Beatriz Suárez, B., Smagulova, F., David, A., Peinado, F., Artacho-Cordón, F., López, L. C., Arrebola, J. P., Olea, N., Fernández, M. F., & Freire, C. (2022). Exposure to non-persistent pesticides, BDNF, and behavioral function in adolescent males: Exploring a novel effect biomarker approach. *Environmental Research*, *211*, 113115. https://doi.org/10.1016/j.envres.2022.113115

Rojas, P., Ramírez-Ortiz, D., Wang, W., Daniel, E.V., Sánchez, M., Cano, M.Á., Ravelo, G.J., Braithwaite, R., Montano, N.P., & De La Rosa, M. (2020). Testing the efficacy of an HIV prevention intervention among Latina immigrants living in farmworker communities in South Florida. *Journal of Immigrant and Minority Health*, 22(4), 661–667. https://doi.org/10.1007/s10903-019-00923-4. PMID: 31493119; PMCID: PMC7058487.

Rural Health Information Hub. (2024a). *Recruitment and retention for rural health facilities*. https://www.ruralhealthinfo.org/topics/rural-health-recruitment-retention

Rural Health Information Hub. (2024b). *Critical access hospitals*. https://www.ruralhealthinfo.org/topics/critical-access-hospitals

Rural Health Information Hub. (n.d.-a). *Chronic obstructive pulmonary disease in rural areas*. https://www.ruralhealthinfo.org/toolkits/copd/1/rural-area

Rural Health Information Hub. (n.d.-b). *Promotora de salud/lay health worker model*. https://www.ruralhealthinfo.org/toolkits/community-health-workers/2/layhealth

Rural Health Information Hub (RHIH). (2022a). *What is rural?* https://www.ruralhealthinfo.org/topics/what-is-rural

Rural Health Information Hub (RHIH). (2022b). *Rural healthcare access*. http://ruralhealthinfo.org/topics/healthcare-access

Rural Health Information Hub (RHIH). (2023a). *Health and healthcare in frontier areas*. https://www.ruralhealthinfo.org/topics/frontier

Rural Health Information Hub (RHIH). (2023b). *Rural data explorer*. http://ruralhealthinfo.org/data-explorer

Rural Health Information Hub (RHIH). (2023c). *Rural agricultural health and safety*. https://www.ruralhealthinfo.org/topics/agricultural-health-and-safety

Rural Health Information Hub (RHIH). (2023d). *Rural health clinics (RHCs)*. https://www.ruralhealthinfo.org/topics/rural-health-clinics

Rural Health Information Hub (RHIH). (2024c). *Federally qualified health centers (FQHCs) and the health center program*. https://www.ruralhealthinfo.org/topics/federally-qualified-health-centers

Rural Health Information Hub (RHIH). (2024d). *Telehealth and health information technology in rural healthcare*. https://www.ruralhealthinfo.org/topics/telehealth-health-it#:~:text=Telehealth%20services%20allow%20rural%20healthcare,healthcare%20without%20traveling%20long%20distances

Rural Health Information Hub (RHIH). (2024e). *Factors that affect mental health in rural communities*. https://www.ruralhealthinfo.org/toolkits/mental-health/1/outside-factors

Rural Health Information Hub (RHIH). (2024f). *Migrant and seasonal farmworker health*. https://www.ruralhealthinfo.org/topics/migrant-health#msaw

Scott, A. (2023). *The average U.S. renter now spends 30% of their income on rent, a new all-time high*. Market Place. https://www.marketplace.org/2023/01/20/the-average-u-s-renter-now-spends-30-of-their-income-on-rent-a-new-all-time-high/

Stoklosa, H., Kunzler, N., Ma, Z.B., Luna Jimenez, J.C., de Vedia Martinez, G., & Erickson, T.B. (2020). Pesticide exposure and heat exhaustion in a migrant agricultural worker: A case of labor trafficking. *Annals of Emergency Medicine*, *76*(2), 215–218https://doi.org/10.1016/j.annemergmed.2020.03.007

Stopka, T. J., Estadt, A. T., Leichtling, G., Schleicher, J. C., Mixson, L. S., Bresett, J., Romo, E., Dowd, P., Walters, S. M., Young, A. M., Zule, W., Friedmann, P. D., Go, V. F., Baker, R., & Fredericksen, R. J. (2024). Barriers to opioid use disorder treatment among people who use drugs in the rural United States: A qualitative, multi-site study. *Social Science and Medicine*, *346*, 1–11. https://doi.org/10.1016/j.socscimed.2024.116660

Taylor, D. E., Bell, A., & Saherwala, A. (2024). Understanding food access in flint: An analysis of racial and socioeconomic disparities. *American Behavioral Scientist*, *68*(4), 503–549. https://doi.org/10.1177/00027642221142201

Touchton, M., & Wampler, B. (2023). Democratizing public health: Participatory policymaking institutions, mosquito control, and Zika in the Americas. *Tropical Medicine and Infectious Disease*, *8*(1), 38. https://doi.org/10.3390/tropicalmed8010038

Tulimiero, M., Garcia, M., Rodriguez, M., & Cheney, A. M. (2021). Overcoming barriers to health care access in rural Latino communities: An innovative model in the Eastern Coachella Valley. *Journal of Rural Health*, *37*(3). https://doi.org/10.1111/jrh.12483

U.S. Bureau of Labor Statistics. (2023). *The Economics Daily: Fatal injuries to agricultural workers in 2021 were the second lowest in a decade*. https://www.bls.gov/opub/ted/2023/fatal-injuries-to-agricultural-workers-in-2021-were-the-second-lowest-in-a-decade.htm

U.S. Census Bureau. (2022). *Nation's urban and rural populations shift following 2020 census*. https://www.census.gov/newsroom/press-releases/2022/urban-rural-populations.html#:~:text=Despite%20the%20increase%20in%20the,down%20from%2080.7%25%20in%202010

U.S. Census Bureau. (2023). *Poverty in states and metropolitan areas: 2022*. https://www.census.gov/content/dam/Census/library/publications/2023/acs/acsbr-016.pdf

U.S. Citizenship and Immigration Services. (n.d.). *Immigration and Nationality Act*. https://www.uscis.gov/laws-and-policy/legislation/immigration-and-nationality-act

U.S. Department of Agriculture (USDA). (2021). *Rural education*. https://www.ers.usda.gov/topics/rural-economy-population/employment-education/rural-education

U.S. Department of Agriculture (USDA). (2023a). *Economic research service*. https://www.ers.usda.gov/topics/rural-economy-population/rural-poverty-well-being/

U.S. Department of Agriculture (USDA). (2023b). *Farm labor*. https://www.ers.usda.gov/topics/farm-economy/farm-labor/#:~:text=In%20recent%20years%2C%20farmworkers%20have,the%20farm%20workforce%20is%20aging

U.S. Department of Agriculture (USDA). (2024a). *Frontier and remote area codes*. http://www.ers.usda.gov/data-products/frontier-and-remote-area-codes.aspx

U.S. Department of Agriculture (USDA). (2024b). *Overview*. https://www.ers.usda.gov/topics/crops/fruit-and-tree-nuts/

U.S. Department of Agriculture (USDA). (n.d.-a). *What is rural?* https://www.nal.usda.gov/ric/what-is-rural

U.S. Department of Agriculture (USDA). (n.d.-b). *e-Connectivity for all rural Americans is a modern-day necessity*. https://www.usda.gov/broadband#:~:text=Unfortunately%2C%2022.3%20percent%20of%20Americans,by%20the%20Federal%20Communications%20Commission

U.S. Department of Education. (n.d.). *Migrant student records exchange initiative (MSIX)*. https://www2.ed.gov/admins/lead/account/msixbrochure.pdf

U.S. Department of Health and Human Services (USDHHS). (2023). *HHS invests $11 million to expand medical residencies in rural communities*. https://www.hhs.gov/about/news/2023/07/26/hhs-invests-11-million-expand-medical-residencies-rural-communities.html

U.S. Department of Health and Human Services National Advisory Council on Migrant Health (NACMH). (2023). *Meeting minute*. https://www.hrsa.gov/sites/default/files/hrsa/advisory-committees/migrant-health/nacmh-may-2023-meeting-minutes.pdf

U.S. Department of Housing & Urban Development (USDHUD). (n.d.). *Common questions about migrant/farmworkers*. https://www.hud.gov/states/florida/working/farmworker/commonquestions

U.S. Department of Labor. (n.d.-a). *U.S. Department of Labor urges greater focus on safety by employers, workers as deaths, injuries in agricultural transportation incidents rises sharply*. https://www.dol.gov/newsroom/releases/whd/whd20220920-0

U.S. Department of Labor. (n.d.-b). *Migrant and Seasonal Agricultural Worker Protection Act (MSPA)*. https://www.dol.gov/agencies/whd/agriculture/mspa

U.S. Department of Labor (DOL). (2024). *H-2A temporary agricultural program*. https://www.dol.gov/agencies/eta/foreign-labor/programs/h-2a

U.S. Environmental Protection Agency (EPA). (2023a). *Reducing pesticide drift*. https://www.epa.gov/reducing-pesticide-drift/introduction-pesticide-drift

U.S. Environmental Protection Agency (EPA). (2023b). *Indoor air quality in multifamily housing*. https://www.epa.gov/indoor-air-quality-iaq/indoor-air-quality-multifamily-housing

U.S. Environmental Protection Agency (EPA). (2024). *Pesticides*. https://www.epa.gov/pesticides

U.S. Environmental Protection Agency (EPA). (n.d.). *Agricultural worker protection standard (WPS)*. https://www.epa.gov/pesticide-worker-safety/agricultural-worker-protection-standard-wps#:~:text=EPA's%20Agricultural%20Worker%20Protection%20Standard,at%20over%20600%2C000%20agricultural%20establishments

U.S. Equal Employment Opportunity Commission. (n.d.). *Title VII of the Civil Rights Act of 1964*. https://www.eeoc.gov/statutes/title-vii-civil-rights-act-1964

U.S. Federal Register. (2023). *The daily journal of the U.S. Government*. http://www.federalregister.gov/documents/2021/10/25/2021/rural-econnectivity-program

U.S. Health Resources and Services Administration (HRSA). (2023). *What is shortage designation?* https://bhw.hrsa.gov/workforce-shortage-areas/shortage-designation

United Nations (UN). (2023). *The sustainable development goals report special edition*. https://unstats.un.org/sdgs/report/2023/The-Sustainable-Development-Goals-Report-2023.pdf

United Nations (UN) Nasyonzini. (n.d.). *Majority of the world's cities highly exposed to disasters, UN DESA warns on World Cities Day*. Department of Economic and Social Affairs. https://www.un.org/ht/desa/majority-world%E2%80%99s-cities-highly-exposed-disasters-un-desa-warns-world-cities-day

USAFacts. (2023). *Where are crime victimization rates higher: Urban or rural areas?* https://usafacts.org/articles/where-are-crime-victimization-rates-higher-urban-rural-areas/

World Health Organization (WHO). (2022). *Ambient (outdoor) air pollution*. https://www.who.int/news-room/fact-sheets/detail/ambient-(outdoor)-air-quality-and-health#:~:text=The%20combined%20effects%20of%20ambient,premature%20deaths%20worldwide%20in%202019

World Health Organization (WHO). (2024). *Operational framework for monitoring social determinants of health equity. License: CC BY-NC-SA 3.0 IGO*. https://iris.who.int/bitstream/handle/10665/375732/9789240088320-eng.pdf?sequence=1

World Health Organization (WHO). (n.d.-a). *Providing cross-cutting solutions to improve health in urban areas*. https://www.who.int/activities/providing-cross-cutting-solutions-to-improve-health-in-urban-areas

World Health Organization (WHO). (n.d.-b). *Creating healthy cities*. https://www.who.int/activities/creating-healthy-cities

Xu, J., Liu, N., Polemiti, E., Garcia-Mondragon, L., Tang, J., Liu, X., Lett, T., Yu, L., Nöthen, M. M., Feng, J., Yu, C., Marquand, A., & Schumann, G. (2023). Effects of urban living environments on mental health in adults. *Nature Medicine*, 29, 1456–1467. https://doi.org/10.1038/s41591-023-02365-w

Yeo, A. J., Cohenuram, A., Dunsiger, S., Boergers, J., Kopel, S. J., & Koinis-Mitchell, D. (2023). The sleep environment, napping, and sleep outcomes among urban children with and without asthma. *Behavioral Sleep Medicine*, *22*(1), 76–86. https://doi.org/10.1080/15402002.2023.2184369

Zhang, H., & Li, J. (2024). Mapping the urban and rural planning response paths to pandemics of infectious diseases. *Humanity and Social Sciences Communications*, *11*, 408. https://doi.org/10.1057/s41599-024-02885-x

CHAPTER 28

American Academy of Nursing (AAN). (n.d.). *Have you ever served in the military?* https://www.haveyoueverserved.com/

American College of Preventive Medicine (ACPM). (2023). *Level I and level II military environmental exposures certifications*. https://www.acpm.org/Education-Events/Military-Environmental-Exposures-Certification

American Psychologist Association (APA). (n.d.). *Understanding military culture*. https://www.apaservices.org/practice/good-practice/military-culture.pdf

Cleveland-Stout, N. (2021). *The civilian-military divide and why you should care*. https://sites.coloradocollege.edu/blockfeatures/2021/03/13/the-civilian-military-divide-why-you-should-care/

Cohen, R. A., & Boersma, P. (2023). *Financial burden of medical care among veterans aged 25-64, by health insurance coverage: United States, 2019-2021*. National Health Statistics Reports. Number 182. https://www.cdc.gov/nchs/data/nhsr/nhsr182.pdf

Congress.gov. (2022). *H.R.3967—Honoring our PACT Act of 2022*. https://www.congress.gov/bill/117th-congress/house-bill/3967/text

Congressional Budget Office. (2021). *The veterans community care program: Background and early effects*. https://www.cbo.gov/publication/57583

Encyclopedia.com. (n.d.). *Veterans affairs hospital system*. https://www.encyclopedia.com/caregiving/encyclopedias-almanacs-transcripts-and-maps/veterans-affairs-hospital-system

Giefer, K. G., & Loveless, T. A. (2021). *Benefits received by veterans and their survivors: 2017*. U.S. Census Bureau. https://www.census.gov/content/dam/Census/library/publications/2021/demo/p70br-175.pdf

Hinojosa, R. (2019). Veteran's likelihood of reporting cardiovascular disease. *Journal of the American Board of Family Medicine*, *32*(1), 50–57. https://doi.org/10.3122/jabfm.2019.01.180148

Joint Service Committee on Military Justice. (2024). *The Manual for Courts-Martial (MCM), United States (2024 edition)*. https://jsc.defense.gov/Portals/99/2024%20MCM%20files/MCM%20(2024%20ed)%20(2024_01_02)%20(adjusted%20bookmarks).pdf?ver=WLZvJg--lbaFtAC5qOM1uA%3d%3d

Office of Health Equity. (2023). *National veteran health equity report*. https://www.va.gov/healthequity/nvher.asp

Office of Rural Health. (n.d.). *Rural promising practices*. U.S. Department of Veteran Affairs. https://www.ruralhealth.va.gov/providers/promising_practices.asp

Patzel, M., Barnes, C., Ramalingam, N., Gunn, R., Kenzie, E. S., Ono, S. S., & Davis, M. M. (2023). Jumping through hoops: Community care clinician and staff experiences providing primary care to rural veterans. *Journal of*

General Internal Medicine, *38*(Suppl 3), 821–828. https://doi.org/10.1007/s11606-023-08126-2

Reger, M. A., Brenner, L. A., & du Pont, A. (2022). Traumatic brain injury and veteran mortality after the war in Afghanistan. *JAMA Network Open*, *5*(2), e2148158. https://doi.org/10.1001/jamanetworkopen.2021.48158

Schaeffer, K. (2023). *The changing face of America's veteran population*. https://www.pewresearch.org/short-reads/2023/11/08/the-changing-face-of-americas-veteran-population/

Shane III, L. (2023). *Total number of VA claims lost in online systems tops 120,000*. https://www.federaltimes.com/veterans/2023/12/04/total-number-of-va-claims-lost-in-online-systems-tops-120000/

Substance Abuse and Mental Health Services Administration (SAMHSA). (2024). *2022 National survey on drug use and health: Among the veteran population aged 18 or older*. https://www.samhsa.gov/data/sites/default/files/reports/rpt44472/2022-nsduh-pop-slides-veterans.pdf

Thelan, A. (2022). *Studying stigma*. News—Central Michigan University. https://www.cmich.edu/news/details/studying-stigma#:~:text=Another%20factor%20impacting%20one's%20journey,trauma%20to%20health%20care%20providers

Thomas, M. (2023). *Military 101: Understanding the differences between active duty, national guard, and reserves*. The Council of State Governments. https://www.csg.org/2023/12/19/military-101-understanding-the-differences-between-active-duty-national-guard-and-reserves/

U.S. Department of Defense (DOD). (2022). *2022 Demographics profile of the military community*. https://www.militaryonesource.mil/data-research-and-statistics/military-community-demographics/2022-demographics-profile/

U.S. Department of Veterans Affairs (VA). (n.d.-a). *Polytrauma/TBI system of care*. https://www.polytrauma.va.gov/system-of-care/TBI_Screening

U.S. Department of Veterans Affairs (VA). (n.d.-b). *Traumatic brain injury*. https://www.publichealth.va.gov/exposures/traumatic-brain-injury.asp

U.S. Department of Veterans Affairs (VA). (n.d.-c). *Healthcare provider: Traumatic brain injury*. https://www.mentalhealth.va.gov/healthcare-providers/tbi.asp

U.S. Department of Veterans Affairs (VA). (n.d.-d). *PTSD: National center for PTSD*. https://www.ptsd.va.gov/index.asp

U.S. Department of Veterans Affairs (VA). (n.d.-e). *VA research on pain management*. https://www.research.va.gov/topics/pain.cfm

U.S. Department of Veterans Affairs (VA). (n.d.-f). *Substance use*. https://www.mentalhealth.va.gov/substance-use/

U.S. Department of Veterans Affairs (VA) Office of Academic Affiliation. (n.d.). *Military health history: Pocket card for health professional trainees and clinicians*. https://www.va.gov/oaa/docs/mhpcmobile.pdf

U.S. Department of Veteran Affairs (VA). (2019). *Determining-veteran-status*. https://www.va.gov/OSDBU/docs/Determining-Veteran-Status.pdf

U.S. Department of Veteran Affairs (VA). (2020). *Veteran population projections 2020-2040*. https://www.va.gov/vetdata/docs/Demographics/New_Vetpop_Model/Vetpop_Infographic2020.pdf

U.S. Department of Veterans Affairs (VA). (2022a). *National Veteran Health Equity Report, 2021*. https://www.va.gov/HEALTHEQUITY/docs/NVHER_2021_Report_508_Conformant.pdf

U.S. Department of Veterans Affairs (VA). (2022b). *Substance use treatment for veterans*. https://www.va.gov/health-care/health-needs-conditions/substance-use-problems/

U.S. Department of Veterans Affairs (VA). (2022c). *VA benefits for service members*. https://www.va.gov/service-member-benefits/

U.S. Department of Veterans Affairs (VA). (2023a). *America's wars*. https://www.va.gov/opa/publications/factsheets/fs_americas_wars.pdf

U.S. Department of Veterans Affairs (VA). (2023b). *Polytrauma/TBI system of Care (2023)*. https://www.polytrauma.va.gov/definitions.asp#:~:text=Polytrauma%3A%20Polytrauma

U.S. Department of Veterans Affairs (VA). (2023c). *2023 National veteran suicide prevention annual report*. https://www.mentalhealth.va.gov/docs/data-sheets/2023/2023-National-Veteran-Suicide-Prevention-Annual-Report-FINAL-508.pdf

U.S. Department of Veterans Affairs (VA). (2023d). *Military sexual trauma (MST)*. https://www.va.gov/health-care/health-needs-conditions/military-sexual-trauma/

U.S. Department of Veterans Affairs (VA). (2023e). *Spotlight on substance use disorders*. https://www.hsrd.research.va.gov/news/feature/sud2023.cfm

U.S. Department of Veterans Affairs (VA). (2023f). *VA homeless programs*. https://www.va.gov/homeless/nationalcallcenter.asp

U.S. Department of Veterans Affairs (VA). (2024a). *VA history*. https://department.va.gov/history/history-overview/

U.S. Department of Veterans Affairs (VA). (2024b). *Community care overview*. https://www.va.gov/COMMUNITYCARE/

U.S. Department of Veterans Affairs (VA) (2024c). *Applying for benefits and your character of discharge*. Veterans Benefits Administration. https://www.benefits.va.gov/benefits/character_of_discharge.asp

U.S. Department of Veterans Affairs (VA) (2024d). *2023 National veteran suicide prevention annual report*. VA Suicide Prevention. Office of Mental Health and Suicide Prevention. https://www.mentalhealth.va.gov/docs/data-sheets/2023/2023-National-Veteran-Suicide-Prevention-Annual-Report-FINAL-508.pdf

U.S. Department of Veterans Affairs (VA). (2024e). *Point-in-Time (PIT) count: Everyone counts in the effort to end veteran homelessness*. https://www.va.gov/homeless/pit_count.asp#:~:text=end%20of%202022.-,The%20January%202023%20PIT%20Count,declined%20by%2052.0%25%20since%202010

U.S. Department of Veterans Affairs (VA). (2024f). *Eligibility for VA health care*. https://www.va.gov/health-care/eligibility/#:~:text=You%20must%20have%20been%20called,qualify%20for%20VA%20health%20care

U.S. Department of Veterans Affairs (VA). (2024g). *VA priority groups*. https://www.va.gov/health-care/eligibility/priority-groups/

U.S. Department of Veterans Affairs (VA) (2024h). *Your VA transition assistance program (TAP)*. Outreach, Transition and Economic Development. https://www.benefits.va.gov/transition/tap.asp

U.S. Department of Veterans Affairs (VA). (2024i). *Eligibility for VA home loan programs*. https://www.va.gov/housing-assistance/home-loans/eligibility/

U.S. Department of Veterans Affairs (VA). (2024j). *Veterans benefits administration reports*. https://www.benefits.va.gov/reports/detailed_claims_data.asp

U.S. Senate (2024). *Sens. Ossoff, Collins, Thune introduce bipartisan bill to help veterans in rural areas access*. VA Health Care.

USAFacts.org. (2023). *Veterans data trends*. https://usafacts.org/topics/veterans/

Wounded Warrior Project. (2023). *Women Warriors Report*. https://filecache.mediaroom.com/mr5mr_woundedwarriorproject2/220405/WWP-23013_WWI_2023_Report_M-NoCrops-Spreads.pdf

INDEX

Note: Page numbers followed by "*f*" indicate figures, "*b*" indicate boxed material, and "*t*" indicate tables.

F

G

H

O

P

T